Your roadmap to...

DAVIS ESSENTIAL NURSING CONTENT + PRACTICE QUESTIONS | FUNDAMENTALS

STEP 1 | Not enough time to read your textbook?

- Succinct summaries focus on must-know information.
- "Alerts" highlight important information at a glance.
- "Key Terms" at the beginning of each chapter make reference quick and easy.

CASE STUDY: Putting It All Together

An 80-year-old man is admitted to the emergency department. He states that he has lived alone since his wife passed away a few years ago but that his son visits about once a month. He says, "I'm on a tight budget because my only income is Social Security. I hoped that I would get better and not have to pay for an emergency room visit. I finally came because I couldn't breathe, and my legs were very swollen." The client shares that, at times, he gets a little forgetful and does not remember his medication every day. The client brought all containers of the medications that he takes daily. The nurse identified the following medications that the client is taking at home and why and documented the medications on the medication reconciliation form.
- Furosemide (Lasix) 20 mg PO, daily (diuretic)
- Docusate sodium (Colace) 100 mg PO, bid (stool softener)
- Famotidine (Pepcid) 20 mg PO, bid (antiulcer agent for gastroesophageal reflux disease)
- 1 Tab Centrum Silver for Men daily (multivitamin for men)
- Metoprolol (Toprol XL) 50 mg PO, daily (beta-blocker for hypertension)

The client states that he has a history of hypertension. His blood pressure on admission is 180/90 mm Hg. He says that he does not always take the Lasix when he has to go out in the morning to do errands because he has to stop so often to urinate. He also has some urinary frequency, urinary urgency, and nocturia because of an enlarged prostate. When talking, the client stops frequently to catch his breath. Respirations are 30 breaths/min, the client is using accessory muscles to breathe, and capillary refill is longer than 3 seconds. Oxygen saturation is 90%.

The primary health-care provider writes and signs the following prescriptions:
- I&O
- 2-g sodium diet
- OOB to chair every shift with assistance
- VS (vital signs) every 8 hours
- IV lock—flush with 10 mL NS every 8 hours
- 2 L oxygen via nasal cannula
- Furosemide (Lasix) 40 mg IVPB
- Famotidine (Pepcid) 20 mg bid
- Docusate sodium (Colace) 1 tab PO, bid
- Metoprolol (Toprol XL) 50 mg PO, daily

STEP 3 | Struggling with your exams?

- 1,000 NCLEX®-style questions in the book and online at DavisPlus—including alternate-format questions—feature answers and rationales for both correct and incorrect responses to identify areas for additional study.
- 100-question final examination at the end of the text assesses your progress and prepares you for classroom tests.

Unlock your DavisPlus Resources Online

Follow the instructions on the inside front cover to use the access code to unlock the questions online at DavisPlus.com.

VI. Medication-Dispensing Systems

The introduction of individual packaging of medications (unit-dose) and the use of a medication cart with a drawer for each client provided [...] pare, and deliver medic[...] system of large bottles [...] ication errors. Automa[...] an additional level of sa[...]

KEY TERMS

Adverse effect—Unintended, usually unpredictable harmful response to a medication that is more severe than a side effect

Allergic reaction—Response of a client's immune system to the presence of a substance that produces a [...]

[...]—Conversion [...]n to a less active form

[...]s it takes for specific

[...]ncased in a substance

7. Implement emergency actions to support a client who has a serious nontherapeutic response until a primary health-care provider assumes responsibility for prescribing medical interventions; for example, activate the rapid response team, administer oxygen, elevate the head of the bed, and prepare for intubation and mechanical ventilation if a client is having difficulty breathing.

STEP 2 | Worried about clinical?

- "Putting It All Together," a case study at the end of most chapters, connects your knowledge to a common clinical scenario.
- Questions on the relevant objective and subjective data in the study ask you to identify a nursing diagnosis, interventions, and client evaluation.

REVIEW QUESTIONS

1. A nurse plans to administer an intramuscular injection to an obese client. What muscle should the nurse consider the least desirable site for an intramuscular injection in an obese adult?
   1. Vastus lateralis
   2. Rectus femoris
   3. Dorsoglute[...]
   4. Deltoid

REVIEW ANSWERS AND RATIONALES

1. **ANSWER: 3.**
   Rationales:
   1. The vastus lateralis site is appropriate for an intramuscular injection in an obese individual as long as the amount of fluid injected is 3 mL or less.
   2. The rectus femoris is an appropriate site for an intramuscular injection in an obese individual as long as the amount of fluid injected is 3 mL or less.
   3. **The dorsogluteal muscle has a thick fat layer, and an intramuscular injection will deposit the medication into subcutaneous tissue rather than a muscle.**
   4. The deltoid is an appropriate muscle for an intramuscular injection in an obese individual as long as the amount of fluid injected is 2 mL or less.

   TEST-TAKING TIP: Identify the word in the stem that indicates negative polarity. The word *least* in the stem indicates negative polarity.

SECOND EDITION

DAVIS ESSENTIAL NURSING CONTENT + PRACTICE QUESTIONS

Fundamentals

Patricia M. Nugent, RN, EdD
Professor Emeritus
Adjunct Professor
Nassau Community College
Garden City, New York
Private Practice—President of Nugent Books, Inc.

Barbara A. Vitale, RN, MA
Professor Emeritus
Nassau Community College
Garden City, New York
Private Practice—Professional Resources for Nursing

F.A. Davis Company · Philadelphia

F. A. Davis Company
1915 Arch Street
Philadelphia, PA 19103
www.fadavis.com

Printed in the United States of America

Last digit indicates print number: 10 9 8 7 6 5 4 3 2

Sponsoring Editor: Jacalyn C. Sharp
Content Project Manager II: Amy M. Romano
Illustration and Design Manager: Carolyn O'Brien

As new scientific information becomes available through basic and clinical research, recommended treatments and drug therapies undergo changes. The author(s) and publisher have done everything possible to make this book accurate, up-to-date, and in accord with accepted standards at the time of publication. The author(s), editors, and publisher are not responsible for errors or omissions or for consequences from application of the book, and make no warranty, expressed or implied, in regard to the contents of the book. Any practice described in this book should be applied by the reader in accordance with professional standards of care used in regard to the unique circumstances that may apply in each situation. The reader is advised always to check product information (package inserts) for changes and new information regarding dose and contraindications before administering any drug. Caution is especially urged when using new or infrequently ordered drugs.

Library of Congress Cataloging-in-Publication Data

Names: Nugent, Patricia Mary, 1944- author. | Vitale, Barbara Ann, 1944-
  author.
Title: Davis essential nursing content + practice questions. Fundamentals /
  Patricia M. Nugent, Barbara A. Vitale.
Other titles: Fundamentals of nursing | Davis essential nursing content plus
  practice questions. Fundamentals | Fundamentals
Description: Second. | Philadelphia, PA : F.A. Davis Company, [2017] |
  Preceded by Fundamentals of nursing : content review plus practice
  questions / Patricia M. Nugent, Barbara A. Vitale. [2014]. | Includes
  bibliographical references and index.
Identifiers: LCCN 2016055129| ISBN 9780803660694 (pbk.) | ISBN 0803660693
  (pbk.)
Subjects: | MESH: Nursing Care | Outlines | Examination Questions
Classification: LCC RT55 | NLM WY 18.2 | DDC 610.73076—dc23 LC record available at https://lccn.loc.gov/2016055129

*Dedicated to our
awesome grandchildren,
who inspire us,
who share their lives
and aspirations with us,
who communicate their energy to us,
and who give us their unconditional love!*

*Aidan, Alexander, Andie, Andrew,
Ava, Cade, Elle, James, Joseph, Nathan,
Ronan, Sean, William, and Carleigh,
our angel in heaven*

Why This Book Is Necessary

Most beginning nursing students have information over-load. In addition to nursing, they must possess knowledge about a variety of subjects such as anatomy and physiology, psychology, sociology, diagnostic and laboratory tests, and growth and development, to mention a few topics. Also, with the expanding roles and responsibilities of the nursing profession, the nursing information that beginning nursing students must learn is growing in depth and breadth exponentially. This is more information than any beginning nursing student can possibly explore, remember, and apply in a stressful clinical situation without additional educational support. The significant difference between the first edition and this, the second edition of *Davis Essential Nursing Content + Practice Questions: Fundamentals*, is that the content was reorganized within a conceptual framework. This textbook provides beginning nursing students with additional educational support by:

- Focusing on conceptual content!
- Including only need-to-know information!
- Addressing commonalities and differences!
- Eliminating content saturation!
- Minimizing repetition of content!
- Applying conceptual learning to examination items!
- Providing over 1,000 practice questions in the book and on the F. A. Davis website davisplus.fadavis.com; hundreds of the questions are NCLEX alternate-type questions!

Who Should Use This Book

Davis Essential Nursing Content + Practice Questions: Fundamentals provides beginning nursing students with need-to-know information as well as practice questions to use to apply that information in a simulated clinical situation. This textbook is designed to:

- Be required by a nursing program as the sole nursing textbook for a fundamentals of nursing course to be used in conjunction with reliable primary Internet sources for nursing information.
- Be required or recommended by a nursing program to be used in conjunction with a traditional fundamentals nursing textbook.
- Be used by beginning nursing students who want to focus on essential information contained in a fundamentals of nursing course.
- Be used by nursing students to learn how to be more successful when answering National Council Licensure

Examination (NCLEX)–type multiple-choice and alternate-item format nursing questions early in their nursing education.
- Be used by nursing students preparing for the NCLEX-RN or NCLEX-PN examination to review basic nursing theory and practice.

Students should use every resource available to facilitate the learning process. We believe that this text-book will meet the needs of beginning nursing students who experience information overload!

What Information Is Presented in This Textbook

Message to Test-Takers of Nursing Examinations

This textbook begins with "Message to Test-Takers of Nursing Examinations," which includes information to help students maximize their ability to study effectively and achieve success when taking nursing examinations. General study strategies, specific study strategies, test-taking tips for answering multiple-choice questions and alternate-format questions, and the test plan categories for the NCLEX examinations are discussed.

Conceptual Organization of the Textbook

The textbook is divided into five units. Each unit contains related concepts to provide a logical sequence for conceptual learning. The first four units contain chapters that reflect the common, nucleus concepts contained in a fundamentals of nursing course. The fifth unit contains an integrated fundamentals of nursing examination.

- Unit I: Essential Health-Care Concepts—This unit reviews concepts related to safety; communication, collaboration, and documentation; legal and ethical issues; the health-care system; and leadership and management.
- Unit II: Essential Nursing Care Concepts—This unit reviews concepts related to critical thinking and the nursing process; evidenced-based practice; teaching and learning; and medication.
- Unit III: Essential Psychosocial and Cultural Concepts—This unit reviews concepts related to development across the life span; diversity and spirituality/religion; psychosocial health; and grief and loss.
- Unit IV: Essential Physiological Concepts—This unit reviews concepts related to physical assessment; pain, comfort, rest, and sleep; inflammation, infection,

immunity, and wound care; mobility; tissue integrity and hygiene; oxygenation; nutrition; fluid, electrolyte, and acid-base balance; urinary elimination; bowel elimination; and perioperative care.

- Unit V: Comprehensive Final Exam—This unit contains a 100-item fundamentals of nursing examination that integrates questions spanning concepts and content throughout the textbook. Each question contains rationales for correct and incorrect answers. Metadata follow each test item and includes the chapter in the textbook where the content in the question is located, the concept that reflects the intent of the question, and the NCLEX test plan categories (e.g., Integrated Processes, Client Need, and Cognitive Level).

Each chapter presents need-to-know information in an outline format, eliminating nice-to-know, extraneous information. Just essential information is included, limiting the challenge of wading through excessive material. This approach assists students to focus on what is most important. In addition, each chapter includes concepts related to the content within the chapter, definitions of key words, a case study called "Putting It All Together," and practice questions specific to chapter content. Multiple-choice questions as well as all the alternate-type questions included on NCLEX examinations are incorporated. Every question has the rationales for correct and incorrect answers and the identical metadata presented in Unit 5 above. Studying rationales for the right and wrong answers to practice test items helps students learn new information or solidify previously learned information. The metadata reflect the classification of items used by NCLEX.

All questions in the textbook are included on line at davisplus.fadavis.com to provide the opportunity to practice taking NCLEX-type questions on a computer. In addition to these questions, two 75-item exams also are posted online at davisplus.fadavis.com. Like the practice questions in the book, each question includes rationales for correct and incorrect answers and metadata coding for the NCLEX test plan categories.

A variety of additional features are included to expand students' knowledge base or focus on evidenced-based practice, significant content, myths, or new information. "Did You Know" presents new or significant information nurses should know or additional content to clarify complex information. "Making the Connection" explores content in more depth to facilitate the connection between content presented and clinical practice.

Item Writers

JANE BRODY, PhD, RN
Professor Emeritus
Nassau Community College
Garden City, New York

MARY ANN HELLMER-SAUL, PhD, RN, CNE
Professor Emeritus, Adjunct Professor
Nassau Community College
Garden City, New York
Clinical Examiner
Excelsior College, New York

MICHAEL W. MANGINO, JR., RN, NP-PSYCHIATRY
Associate Professor
Suffolk Community College
Selden, New York

Medical Consultant

JOANNE M. VITALE, RPA-C
Physician Assistant
Plastic and Reconstructive Surgery
Huntington, New York

Reviewers

TINA K. ALLEN, BSN, MSN, EdD, RN
Associate Professor
School of Nursing/College of Health and Human
  Services
Troy University
Montgomery, Alabama

PAT FAHEY BACON, DNP, RN, FNP-BC
Coordinator Nursing Program and Nursing Faculty
Presentation College
Fairmont, Minnesota

CAROL BLAKEMAN, ARNP, MSN
Professor
College of Central Florida
Ocala, Florida

PEG BROADIE, MSN, CNE
Assistant Professor
Allen College
Waterloo, Iowa

REMYLIN BRUDER, DNP, RN
Associate Professor
Rochester College
Rochester Hills, Michigan

GLORIA BRUMMER, MS, RN, CNE, CEN
Assistant Professor
Department of Nursing
St. John's College
Springfield, Illinois

MARSHA CANNON, MSN, RN
Chairperson
University of West Alabama
Livingston, Alabama

EILEEN O. COSTELLO, MSN, RN
Dean, Health Sciences and Community Service Programs
Mount Wachusett Community College
Gardner, Massachusetts

MARNEE L. CRAWFORD, MSN, RN, CNE
Nursing Faculty
Northwest College
Powell, Wyoming

LEIGH ANN CREEL, RN, BSN, MSN
ADN Faculty/Nursing Instructor
Copiah Lincoln Community College
Wesson, Mississippi

CLAIRE CYRIAX, RN, MSN, LNC, CAPA
Nursing Faculty
Bergen Community College
Paramus, New Jersey

BONNIE DAVIS, PhD, RN
Director of Nursing
University of New England
Portland, Maine

KELLI DAVIS, RN, MSN
Nursing Instructor/Faculty
Gadsden State Community College
Gadsden, Alabama

DEBORAH K. DRUMMONDS, RN, MN, CCRN, CEN
Assistant Professor
Abraham Baldwin Agricultural College
Tifton, Georgia

VICTOR DUARTE, MSN, RN, CCRN
Nursing Instructor
Front Range Community College, Larimer Campus
Fort Collins, Colorado

JACQUELINE FROCK, MSN, RN
Professor of Nursing
Oklahoma City Community College
Oklahoma City, Oklahoma

BELINDA FULLER, RN, MSN
Level 1 Coordinator
Gadsden State Community College
Gadsden, Alabama

NORENE GACHIGNARD, RN, MSN
Professor
North Shore Community College
Danvers, Massachusetts

WENDY GREENSPAN, RN, MSN, CCRN, CNE
Assistant Professor of Nursing
Rockland Community College
Suffern, New York

RENEE HARRISON, RN, MS
Nursing Outreach Coordinator
Tulsa Community College
Tulsa, Oklahoma

MICHELLE HORNACK, RN, MSN
Assistant Professor of Nursing
Graceland University
Independence, Missouri

SUSAN A. HUMENIK-SCHMIDT, MSN, RN
Assistant Professor of Nursing
Joliet Junior College
Joliet, Illinois

SHIRLEY JEANDRON, MSN, MBA
Nursing Instructor
Charity School of Nursing
Delgado Community College
New Orleans, Louisiana

CAROL JELFO, MSN, APRN-BC
Instructor, Associate Degree Nursing Program
West Georgia Technical College
Waco, Georgia

MARY ANN JOHNSTON, RN, MSN
Lecturer/Clinical Instructor
California State University, Stanislaus
Turlock, California

ANNE-MARIE JONES, MSN, RN, CNE
Assistant Professor of Nursing
Western Carolina University
Cullowhee, North Carolina

ELIZABETH KEENE, MSN/ED, RN, CNE
Assistant Professor, Nursing Program
Montgomery County Community College
Blue Bell, Pennsylvania

ANGIE KOONTZ, MSN, RN
Nursing Instructor
Caldwell Community College and Technical Institute
Hudson, North Carolina

RAEANN G. LEBLANC, DNP, GNP-BC, ANP-BC
Assistant Clinical Professor
University of Massachusetts
Amherst, Massachusetts

DIANE LITTEN, ARNP, MSN
Instructor, Chair—Nursing Department
Lake Sumter Community College
Clermont, Florida

KAREN LOCASCIO, MS, RN-BC
Assistant Professor of Nursing
Southern Maine Community College
South Portland, Maine

KATRINA LUTHER, RN, MSN
Nursing Instructor
Miles Community College
Miles City, Montana

BUFFI BEASLEY MCCAMBRIDGE, RN, MSN, BSN, BS
Faculty—Instructor and PreNursing Advisor
College of Nursing
Valdosta State University
Valdosta, Georgia

MAGDA SANDRA MCCARTHY, MSN, RN, CNE
Professor
Houston Community College
Houston, Texas

CATHY MCCAUGHEY, MSN, RN
Nursing Faculty/Adjunct
Los Medanos College
Pittsburg, California

AMY HILBURN MILLS, RN, MSN, CRNP
Assistant Professor
Troy University
Troy, Alabama

HEATHER PAULSEN, RN, BSN
Level 2 Team Leader and ASN Coordinator
Salish Kootenai College
Pablo, Montana

GLENDA REEDY, MSN, RN
Nursing Faculty
Caldwell Community College
Boone, North Carolina

LAURA SAUCER, RN, MSN
Program Director of Nursing
South University
Montgomery, Alabama

BARBARA A. SPRACKLIN, RN, MSN
Associate Professor
Bunker Hill Community College
Boston, Massachusetts

GERALDINE M. TYRELL, MSN, RN
Assistant Professor of Nursing
Bethel College
North Newton, Kansas

GRACE WAY, MSN, RN-C
Professor of Nursing
Seminole State College
Altamonte Springs, Florida

JANNA WICKHAM, RN, MSN
Nursing Faculty—Simulation
Lake Sumter Community College
Clermont, Florida

LICIA W. WILLIAMSON, RN, MSN
Instructor/Level 1 Coordinator
Lawson State Community College
Birmingham, Alabama

Student Reviewers

SANDRA APRIL
Hillsborough Community College
Tampa, Florida

SABRINA COLTON
Northwest College
Powell, Wyoming

DELINDA HAWKINS
Delgado Charity School of Nursing
New Orleans, Louisiana

JAMIE MARDIS
County College of Morris
Randolph, New Jersey

ASHLEY MICKEL
County College of Morris
Randolph, New Jersey

PAMELA PARSONS
Ohio Valley Hospital School of Nursing
McKees Rocks, Pennsylvania

VICKY SEGHERS
Delgado Charity School of Nursing
New Orleans, Louisiana

BRANDY THIGPEN-JOHNSON
Columbus State University
Columbus, Georgia

DEBBIE URSIN
Delgado Charity School of Nursing
New Orleans, Louisiana

NICOLE WARD
Germanna Community College
Fredericksburg, Virginia

We met Terri Allen, Publisher Nursing, for the first time at the 2016 National Student Nurses Association Convention. What a wonderful occasion to establish a collaborative publishing relationship that produces textbooks for nursing students. From day one she worked with us to explore nursing students' perceived needs and preferences. She encouraged and supported our creative efforts to address content saturation by redesigning the first edition of this book to embrace a conceptual organization of the content in this, the second edition. We value her input and support and look forward to a continued innovative, productive relationship.

We would like to thank Jacalyn Sharp, our Sponsoring Editor at F. A. Davis Company, who was always available for consultation, supported us enthusiastically, which kept us motivated, and expertly kept the project on track.

We acknowledge the work of Amy Romano, Content Project Manager II, Nursing, for her invaluable efforts on our behalf. Her organizational skills and attention to detail were beyond excellent. In addition, she helped retrieve information after one of our hard drives failed and she had the patience of a saint answering a never-ending list of questions.

Thanks to Lynn Lusk, Project Manager at Progressive Publishing Services and her team of copyeditors and indexer for their detailed editing. Lynn was extremely patient and supportive throughout the copyediting process, and her efforts were greatly appreciated.

Cheers to Daniel Domzalski, Illustration Coordinator, for producing the fabulous art work that supports visual learning and managing all the art for this edition. A monumental task that was expertly accomplished.

Applause to Julia Gillespie, Marketing Manager, who creatively designed and implemented interest-provoking marketing strategies. Thank you Julia for your dedication to getting our text noticed.

Praise to the talented and dedicated production team at F. A. Davis Company. Dan Clipner, Production Manager, ensured excellence as the manuscript became a printed text. A special thanks to Dan.

We want to thank the reviewers for their constructive criticism and recommendations. Their feedback added to the quality of the product. We are especially thankful to students, who constantly said that, while their required fundamentals textbooks provided in-depth information, they felt overwhelmed by these textbooks. Students said that a textbook with just the need-to-know information would help them clearly focus on information essential to nursing theory and practice. In addition, the focus on the essential content and the testing of that content would help them prepare for their nursing examinations.

Finally, we want to thank our husbands, Neil Nugent and Joseph Vitale, for tolerating the time that we dedicated to writing, editing, and proofing the manuscript. This textbook would not have been accomplished without their love and support. Special thanks to our children and their spouses: Kelly Dall, Heather and James McCormack, Joseph and Nicole Vitale, John and JoAnne Vitale, and Christopher and Whitney Vitale ... we are proud of all of you. Love and kisses to our grandchildren: Joey, Andie, Andrew, Nathan, Alexander, William, and James Vitale; Sean, Ava, and Elle Dall; and Aidan, Cade, and Ronan McCormack, who all make our day with their smiles and accomplishments. A very special thanks to our grandsons Ronan McCormack and Joey Vitale for giving us permission to illustrate their surgical scars (badges of courage) in the physical assessment chapter.

Patricia M. Nugent
Barbara A. Vitale

Message to Test-Takers of Nursing Examinations

To progress in a nursing program, you must achieve passing grades on course examinations. To pass nursing examinations you must know not only theory and principles of nursing but also theory and principles associated with other disciplines upon which nursing is based, such as anatomy, physiology, microbiology, psychology, sociology, mathematics, growth and development, and so on. Many factors influence your ability to learn all this information, such as genetic endowment, maturation level, past experience, self-image, mental attitude, motivation, and readiness to learn. You might not be able to change some of these factors; however, implementing study and test-taking strategies can enhance personal internal control, purposeful learning, and success on nursing examinations. The most important element in test success is to be overprepared. This text presents various learning strategies that can help you maximize your learning so that you are overprepared for examinations. In addition, it presents test-taking tips that will help you to understand what a test question is asking, how to examine options in a multiple-choice question, and how to eliminate incorrect options (distractors). For additional information on the strategies presented in this introduction, refer to *Test Success: Test-Taking Techniques for Beginning Nursing Students* published by the F. A. Davis Company.

Use General Study Strategies to Maximize Learning

1. Set short- and long-term learning goals because doing so promotes planned learning with a purpose.
2. Control internal and external distractors.
   - Select a study environment that allows you to focus on your learning and is free from external interruptions.
   - Limit internally generated distractions by challenging negative thoughts. For example, rather than saying to yourself, "This is going to be a hard test," say, "I can pass this test if I study hard."
   - Establish a positive internal locus of control. For example, say, "I can get an A on my next test if I study hard and I am overprepared," rather than blaming the instructor for designing "hard" tests.
   - Use controlled breathing techniques, progressive muscle relaxation, and guided imagery to control anxious feelings.
3. Review content before class because doing so supports mental organization and purposeful learning.
4. Take class notes.
   - Review class notes within 48 hours after class because doing so ensures that the information is still fresh in your mind.
   - Use one side of your notebook for notes and use the opposite page to identify additional information from the textbook or other sources.
   - Identify questions that you still have, and ask the instructor for clarification.
5. Balance personal sacrifice and time for relaxation. A rigorous course of study requires sacrifices in terms of postponing vacations, having less time to spend with family members and friends, and having less time to engage in personal leisure activities. However, you should find a balance that supports your need to meet course requirements and yet allows you time to rest and reenergize.
6. Treat yourself to a reward when you meet a goal because doing so supports motivation. Your long-term reward is to graduate and become a nurse. However, that reward is in the distance so, to stimulate motivation now, build in rewards when short-term goals are achieved.
   - An external reward might be watching a television program that you enjoy, having a 10-minute break with a snack, or calling a friend on the phone.
   - An internal reward might be saying to yourself, "Wow, I finished outlining that whole chapter; I am terrific" or "I feel great because I now understand the principles presented in this chapter."
7. Manage time effectively.
   - Examine your daily and weekly routine to identify and eliminate barriers to your productivity, such as attempting to do too much, lacking organization, or being obsessive-compulsive.
   - Learn to delegate household tasks.
   - Learn to say "no" to avoid overcommitting yourself to activities that take you away from what you need to do to meet your learning needs.
   - Get organized. Identify realistic daily, weekly, and monthly "to do" calendars. Work to achieve deadlines with self-determination and self-discipline.

- Maintain a consistent study routine because doing so eliminates procrastination and establishes an internal readiness to learn.
- Recognize that you do not have to be perfect. If every waking moment is focused on achieving an "A," your relationship with family members and friends will suffer. The key is to find a balance and accept the fact that you do not have to have an "A" in every course to become a nurse.
- Capitalize on small moments of time to study by carrying flashcards, a vocabulary list, or a small study guide, such as one of the products in the *Notes* series by F. A. Davis Company.

8. Study in small groups. Sharing and listening increases understanding and allows for correction of misinformation.

Use Specific Study Strategies to Maximize Learning

1. Use acronyms, alphabet cues, acrostics, and mnemonics to help learn information that must be memorized for future recall.
2. When studying, continually ask yourself "how" and "why" because the nurse must comprehend the meaning of the "how" and "why" of information. For example, a nurse must know *how* much pressure compresses a capillary bed and *why* this level of compression will result in a pressure ulcer. Many questions on nursing examinations require the nurse to comprehend the how and why when identifying the correct option in a test question in terms of what the nurse should do first or next or what not to do.
3. Relate new information to something you already know to enhance learning. For example, if you are learning how to collect a sterile urine specimen from a urinary retention catheter, identify the principles that are common to those that you learned several weeks before about sterile technique when preparing a medication to be administered via a syringe.
4. Identify and study principles that are common among different nursing interventions because doing so maximizes the application of information in clinical situations. For example, the principle of gravity applies when elevating a client's legs on pillows to reduce edema, when holding an enema solution bag 12 inches above the level of the client's anus to increase the flow of enema solution, and when raising the head of a client's bed to lower abdominal pressure to facilitate ventilation.
5. Identify and study differences. For example, three clients may have an increase in blood pressure for three different reasons, such as obesity, acute pain stimulating the sympathetic nervous system, and decreased arterial compliance due to the aging process.

Use Test-Taking Tips to Maximize Success on Nursing Examinations

There is no substitute for being overprepared for a test. However, when you are uncertain of a correct answer, test-taking tips are strategies you can use to be test wise. By being test wise, you may be better able to identify what a question is asking and better able to eliminate one or more distractors. Your chances of selecting the correct answer increase when you are able to eliminate distractors from consideration. For example, when answering a traditional multiple-choice question that has four answer options, if you can eliminate one distractor from further consideration, you increase your chances of selecting the correct answer to 33%. If you are able to eliminate two distractors from further consideration, you increase your chances of selecting the correct answer to 50%.

Practice using the following test-taking tips to help you to understand what a question is asking and to eliminate distractors. Recognize that not all questions lend themselves to using test-taking tips. The practice questions in this textbook identify test-taking tips where applicable to help you learn how to apply them when answering a test question.

Test-Taking Tips for Multiple-Choice Items and Related Study Tips

A traditional multiple-choice item typically presents a statement (stem) that asks a question. Usually, four statements that are potential answers follow the stem (options); one of which is the correct answer and three of which are incorrect answers (distractors). The test-taker must select the option that is the correct answer to receive credit for answering a traditional multiple-choice item correctly.

Test-taking tips describe strategies that can be used to analyze a traditional multiple-choice item and improve a test-taker's chances of selecting the correct answer.

Test-Taking Tip #1: Identify Positive Polarity of a Stem

- A stem with positive polarity is asking, "What should the nurse do when … ?"
- The correct answer may be based on understanding what is accurate or comprehending the principle underlying the correct answer.
- For example, a stem with positive polarity might say, "Which nursing action should a nurse implement when a client who is being ambulated begins to fall?"
- **Study tip:** Change the stem so that it reflects a negative focus and then answer the question based on a stem with negative polarity. For example, "Which action should a nurse *not implement* when a client who is being ambulated begins to fall?"

Test-Taking Tip #2:
Identify Key Words in the Stem That Indicate Negative Polarity

- A stem with negative polarity asks such questions as what the nurse should not do; what is contraindicated, unacceptable, or false; or what is the exception.
- Words in a stem that indicate negative polarity include *not, except, never, contraindicated, unacceptable, avoid, unrelated, violate,* and *least.*
- For example, a negatively worded stem might say, "Which action violates the principles of sterile technique when collecting a specimen from a surgical wound?"
- **Study tip:** Change the word that indicates negative polarity to a positive word and then answer the question based on a stem with positive polarity. For example, if a stem says, "Which action implemented by the nurse *violates* a principle of surgical asepsis?" change the word *violates* to *reflects.* You have just changed a stem with negative polarity to a stem with positive polarity.

Test-Taking Tip #3:
Identify Words in the Stem That Set a Priority

- The correct answer is something that is significant.
- Words in the stem that set a priority include *first, best, main, greatest, most, initial, primary,* and *priority.*
- For example, a stem that sets a priority might say, "What should a nurse do first when administering a tube feeding to a client?"
- **Study tip:** After identifying the first step in the procedure for administering a tube feeding to a client, place the remaining three options in order of importance.

Test-Taking Tip #4:
Identify Options That Are Opposites

- Options that are opposites generally reflect extremes on a continuum.
- More often than not, *but not always,* an option that is an opposite is the correct answer.
- If you are unable to identify the correct answer, select one of the opposite options.
- Some opposites are easy to identify, such as hypervolemia and hypovolemia or bradycardia and tachycardia, whereas others are obscure, such as bradycardia and rapid pulse rate or flat neck veins (indicating deficient fluid volume) and bounding pulse (indicating excess fluid volume).
- **Study tip:** Make flashcards that reflect the clinical indicator on one side and identify all situations that can cause that sign or symptom on the other side.

Test-Taking Tip #5:
Identify Client-Centered Options

- Client-centered options focus on feelings, opportunities for clients to make choices, and actions that empower clients or support client preferences.
- More often than not, a client-centered option is the correct answer.
- For example, a client-centered option might say, "What spices would you like me to sprinkle on your food?" or "Do you want to walk after your bath or after your lunch?" These example options give a client an opportunity to make a choice, which supports independence. A nursing action that supports a client's independence is an example of a client-centered option.
- **Study tip:** Compose your own client-centered options that would be a correct answer for the scenario presented in the question. "I would be mad, too, if my food were cold, but what can I do for you right now to make it better?" or "Losing a leg can be difficult."

Test-Taking Tip #6:
Identify Options That Deny Clients' Feelings, Needs, or Concerns

- Options that avoid clients' feelings, change the subject, offer false reassurance, or encourage optimism cut off communication.
- Options that deny clients' feelings, needs, or concerns are always distractors unless the stem has negative polarity.
- For example, an option that says, "You will feel better tomorrow," fails to recognize the client's concerns about the pain that the client is feeling today.
- If a stem with negative polarity says, "What should the nurse **avoid** saying when clients express concerns about the pain they are experiencing?", then the option that says, "You will feel better tomorrow" is the correct answer. It is important to ensure that you identify the polarity of the stem.
- **Study tip:** Construct additional options that deny clients' feelings, needs, or concerns that relate to the scenario in the stem, such as, "Cheer up because things could be worse," "Don't worry; I promise that the pain will be less and less every passing day," or "The pain medication you are receiving should be adequate to relieve your pain."

Test-Taking Tip #7:
Identify Equally Plausible Options

- Equally plausible options are options that are so similar that one option is no better than the other.
- Both equally plausible options can be deleted from further consideration.

- For example, one option says "Dyspnea" and another option says "Difficulty breathing." These two options are saying the same thing. One option is no better than the other; therefore, you can eliminate both from further consideration. Another example is if one option states, "Encourage deep breathing exercises" and another option states, "Encourage the use of an incentive spirometer 10 times every hour." Both of these options present interventions that increase the depth of respirations. One option is no better than the other; therefore, you can eliminate both options from further consideration. By doing so, you increase your chances of selecting the correct answer to 50%.
- **Study tip:** Construct equally plausible options for the correct answer and identify equally plausible options for the options that are distractors.

Test-Taking Tip #8:
Identify Options With Specific Determiners (Absolutes)

- A specific determiner is a word or phrase that indicates no exceptions.
- Words that are specific determiners place a limit on a statement that generally is considered correct.
- Words in options that are specific determiners include *all, none, only, always,* and *never.*
- For example, options with a specific determiner might say, "Use only water when bathing the perineal area" or "Clients should always be expected to provide their own care."
- Most of the time, options with specific determiners are distractors. However, there are some exceptions that focus on universal truths in nursing, such as interventions that focus on clients as individuals and the use of standard precautions. For example, "Always believe what clients report about their pain experience" and "Never leave a client's room without implementing hand hygiene."
- **Study tip:** Construct examples of options with specific determiners so that you are able to recognize when an option has a specific determiner. Next, identify whether the option should be deleted or whether the option is an exception to the rule.

Test-Taking Tip #9:
Identify the Unique Option

- When one option is different from the other three options that are similar, examine the unique option carefully.
- More often than not, an option that is unique is the correct answer.
- For example, if a question is asking you to identify an expected client response to a problem and three of the options identify an increase in something

and one option identifies a decrease in something, examine the option that identifies the decrease in something because it is unique.
- **Study tip:** Construct options that are similar to the distractors and construct options that are similar to the unique option. Doing so can help you to distinguish among commonalities and differences.

Test-Taking Tip #10:
Identify the Global Option

- Global options are more broad and wide-ranging than specific options.
- One or more of the other options might be included under the umbrella of a global option.
- Examine global options carefully because they are often the correct answer.
- For example, a global option might say, "Keep clients clean and dry" versus a specific option, which might say, "Wash a client's perineal area after toileting."
- **Study tip:** Construct as many specific options as possible that could be included under the umbrella of a global option. Construct as many global options as possible in relation to the content presented in the stem. Doing so will increase your ability to identify a global option.

Test-Taking Tip #11:
Use Maslow's Hierarchy of Needs and the ABCs (Airway, Breathing, and Circulation) to Identify the Option That Is the Priority

- This tip is best used when answering a question that asks what the nurse should do first or which action is most important.
- Examine each option and identify which level of need according to Maslow is associated with each option. Identify whether any of the options are associated with maintaining a patent airway, and if not, examine each option from the perspective of maintaining breathing and so on.
- For example, in a question associated with postoperative care, an option that addresses the presence of an oral airway generally is the priority.
- **Study tip:** Start by identifying the action that is least important and work backward toward the option with the action that is most important. Then identify the reasoning behind the assigned order. This tip focuses on the how and why and helps you to clarify the reasoning underlying your critical thinking. This tip is best practiced when working in a small study group.

Test-Taking Tip #12:
Identify Duplicate Facts in Options

- Some options contain two or more facts. The more facts that are contained in an option, the greater your chances of selecting the correct answer.

- If you identify one correct fact, eliminate all options that do not contain this fact.
- If you identify one incorrect fact, eliminate all options that contain this fact.
- Focus on the options that contain at least one correct fact.
- By eliminating options, you increase your chances of selecting the correct answer, usually by 50%. By the process of elimination, you may even arrive at the correct answer even when unsure of all the facts in the correct answer.
- **Study tip:** Identify all the correct facts that you can that are associated with what the question is asking.

Test-Taking Tip #14:
Practice Test-Taking Using Test-Taking Tips

- Practicing test-taking is an effective way to achieve six outcomes.
  1. You will desensitize yourself to the discomfort or fear that you might feel in a testing situation.
  2. You will increase your stamina if you gradually increase the time that you spend practicing test-taking to 2 to 3 hours. This practice will enable you to concentrate more effectively for a longer period of time.
  3. You will learn how to better manage your time during a test so that you have adequate time to answer all the questions.
  4. You will increase your learning when studying the rationales for the right and wrong answers.
  5. You will become more astute in determining what a question is asking and better able to identify when a test-taking tip might help you eliminate a distractor and focus on an option that might be the correct answer. Remember the old adage—practice makes perfect!
  6. You will maximize your ability to apply test-taking tips when answering nursing test questions.

Test-Taking Tip #13:
Use Multiple Test-Taking Tips When Examining Test Questions and Options

- If using one test-taking tip to analyze a question is beneficial, think how much more beneficial it would be to use two or more test-taking tips to analyze a question.
- Examine the stem first for a test-taking tip. For example, ask yourself, "Does the stem have negative polarity?" or "Is the stem setting a priority?"
- Next, examine the options. For example, ask yourself, "Do any of the options contain a specific determiner?" or "Is there a global option?" or "Is there a client-centered option?"
- By using more than one test-taking tip, you can usually increase your success in selecting the correct answer.

Test-Taking Tips for Alternate-Format Items

Alternate-format items are purported by the National Council of State Boards of Nursing to evaluate some nursing knowledge more readily and authentically than possible with traditional multiple-choice items. To accomplish this, an alternate-format item does not construct a question with the same organization as a multiple-choice item. Each type of alternate-format item presents information along with a question using a distinctive format and requires the test-taker to answer the item in a unique manner. Some alternate-format items use multimedia approaches, such as charts, tables, graphics, sound, and video. Understanding the composition of alternate-format items and strategies to analyze these items can increase your chances of selecting the correct answer.

1. *Multiple-Response Item*
   - A multiple-response item presents a stem that asks a question.
   - It presents five or six options as potential answers.
   - The test-taker must identify all (two or more) correct answers to the question posed in the stem.
   - When answering a multiple-response item on a computer, each option is preceded by a square box. The test-taker must click the mouse in the box in front of an option being selected. After all options are selected, click *Next* to confirm your answers and move to the next item. When answering a multiple-response item in a textbook, place a mark in front of the options being selected.
   - **Test-taking tip:** Before looking at the options, quickly review information you know about the topic. Then compare what you know against the options presented. Another approach is to eliminate one or two options that you know are wrong; identify one option you know is correct; then eliminate another one or two options that you know are wrong. Finally, you should identify all the options you believe are correct. To do this, you can use some of the test-taking tips that apply to traditional multiple-choice questions, such as identifying options that are opposites; identifying client-centered options; identifying options that deny clients' feelings, needs, or concerns; and identifying options with specific determiners (absolutes) to either eliminate options or to focus on potential correct answers.

2. *Drag-and-Drop (Ordered Response) Item*
   - A drag-and-drop item makes a statement or presents a situation and then asks the test-taker to prioritize five or six options.
   - The item may ask the test-taker to indicate the order in which nursing interventions should be performed, the order of importance of concerns, or actual steps in a procedure.

- To be considered a correct answer, the test-taker must place all of the options in the correct order.
- When answering a drag-and-drop item on a computer, the test-taker may highlight and click on the option or actually drag the option from the left side of the screen to a box on the right side of the screen. Click *Next* to confirm your answer and move to the next test item. When practicing a drag-and-drop item in a textbook, the test-taker can only indicate the priority order by listing the options in order by number.
- **Test-taking tip:** Use the ABCs (Airway, Breathing, and Circulation), Maslow's hierarchy of needs, and the nursing process to help focus your ordering of options. Identify the option that you consider to be the priority option; identify the option that you consider to be the least important option; then, from the remaining options, select the next priority option and the least priority option. Keep progressing along this same line of thinking until all the options have received a placement on the priority list.

3. *Fill-in-the-Blank Calculation Item*
   - A fill-in-the-blank calculation item presents information and then asks the test-taker a question that requires the manipulation or interpretation of numbers.
   - Computing a medication dosage, intake and output, or the amount of IV fluid to be administered are examples of fill-in-the-blank calculation items.
   - The test-taker must answer the item with either a whole number or within a specified number of decimal points as requested by the item.
   - When answering a fill-in-the-blank item on a computer, type the number of your answer into the box following the word *Answer*. You do not have to type in the unit of measure. Click *Next* to confirm your answer and move to the next test item. When answering a fill-in-the-blank item in a textbook, write the number of your answer and the unit of measure.
   - **Test-taking tip:** Before answering a question, recall the memorized equivalents or formula that is required to answer the item, then perform a calculation to answer the item.

4. *Hot-Spot Item*
   - A hot-spot item presents an illustration or photograph and asks a question.
   - The test-taker must identify a location on the visual image presented to answer the question.
   - The answer must mirror the correct answer exactly to be considered a correct answer.
   - When answering a hot-spot item on a computer, the test-taker uses a mouse, places the cursor on the desired location, and left-clicks the mouse. These actions place an X on the desired location to answer the question. Click *Next* to confirm your answer and move to the next test item. When answering a hot-spot item in a textbook, the test-taker is asked to either place an X on the desired location or identify an option indicated by an a, b, c, or d label presented in the illustration or photograph.
   - **Test-taking tip:** Read and reread the item to ensure that you understand what the item is asking. When attempting to answer a question that involves anatomy and physiology, close your eyes and picture in your mind the significant structures and recall their functions before answering the item.

5. *Exhibit Item*
   - An exhibit item presents a scenario, usually a client situation.
   - The test-taker is then presented with a statement that asks a question.
   - The test-taker must access information from a variety of sources. The information must be analyzed to determine its significance in relation to the question being asked to arrive at an answer.
   - These items require the highest level of critical thinking (analysis and synthesis).
   - When answering an exhibit item on a computer, information is contained behind three tabs. The mouse is used to click each tab to access the information. Each option to answer the question is preceded by a circle. The test-taker must place the cursor in the circle and click the mouse to select the desired answer. Click *Next* to confirm your answer and move to the next test item. When answering an exhibit item in a textbook, the information in the tabs is visible and the answer must be selected from among the options offered.
   - **Test-taking tip:** Identify exactly what the item is asking. Access the collected data and dissect, analyze, and compare and contrast the data collected in relation to what you know and understand in relation to what the item is asking.

6. *Graphic Item*
   - A graphic item presents a question with several options that are illustrations, pictures, photographs, charts, or graphs rather than text.
   - The test-taker must select the option with the illustration that answers the question.
   - When answering a graphic item on a computer, each option is preceded by a circle. The test-taker must place the cursor in the circle and click the mouse to select the desired answer. Click *Next* to confirm your answer and move to the next test item. When answering a graphic item in a textbook, the test-taker is presented with an illustration and must select one answer from among several options, or the test-taker is asked a question and must select one answer from among several options, each having an illustration.

- **Test-taking tip:** When reading your textbook or other resource material visual images are presented to support written content. "A picture is worth a thousand words." Examine these images in relation to the content presented to reinforce your learning. Often similar illustrations may be used in either hot-spot or graphic alternate test items.

7. *Audio Item*
   - An audio item presents an audio clip that must be accessed through a head set. The test-taker must click the *Play* button to access the audio clip. After listening to the audio clip, the test-taker must select the answer from among the options presented.
   - When answering an audio item on a computer, each option is preceded by a circle. The test-taker must place the cursor in the circle and click the mouse to select the desired answer.
   - **Test-taking tip:** Listen to educational resources that provide audio clips of sounds that the nurse must be able to identify such as breath, heart, and bowel sounds. Engage in learning experiences using simulation manikins available in the on-campus nursing laboratory. When in the clinical area, use every opportunity to assess these sounds when completing a physical assessment of assigned clients. For additional resources, access audio clips at wwwDavisPlus.com.

NCLEX-RN Test Plan and Classification of Questions

The National Council Licensure Examinations for Registered Nurses (NCLEX-RN) and for Licensed Practical/Vocational Nurses (NCLEX-PN) Test Plans (2016) primarily were designed to facilitate the classification of examination items and guide candidates preparing for these examinations. These test plans were developed to ensure the formation of tests that measure the competencies required to perform safe, effective nursing care as newly licensed, entry-level registered nurses or licensed practical/vocational nurses. They are revised every 3 years after an analysis of the activities of practicing nurses, input from experts on the NCLEX Examination Committees, and National Council of State Board of Nursing's content staff and member boards of nursing to ensure that the test plans are relevant and consistent with state nurse practice acts. The detailed test plans for the NCLEX-RN and NCLEX-PN differ owing to differences in the scope of practice for these professions. Each of these test plans can be found on the National Council of State Board of Nursing's website at www.ncsbn.org/nclex.htm.

Davis Essential Nursing Content + Practice Questions: Fundamentals utilizes the NCLEX-RN Test Plan categories to analyze every question. This book contains more than 1,000 questions. The majority of the questions appear in the chapters that reflect the content in the question. In addition, there is a final examination in Unit 5 and two comprehensive examinations on davisplus.fadavis.com. All the questions presented in the book, including the 100-question Comprehensive Final Exam, can be found on davisplus.fadavis.com. In addition, two 75-item comprehensive examinations are on the website. Each question has the rationales for the correct and incorrect answers; offers a test-taking tip, if applicable; and is classified according to the following categories.

Integrated Processes Categories

Integrated processes are the basic factors essential to the practice of nursing, which are the nursing process, caring, communication and documentation, teaching/learning, and culture and spirituality. Because the nursing process provides a format for critical thinking, it is included for each question. Caring, communication and documentation, teaching/learning, and culture and spirituality are included when the intent of the question addresses one or more of these factors.

Nursing Process
- *Assessment:* Nursing care that collects objective and subjective data from primary and secondary sources.
- *Analysis:* Nursing care that groups significant data, interprets data, and comes to conclusions.
- *Planning:* Nursing care that sets goals, objectives, and outcomes; prioritizes interventions; and performs calculations.
- *Implementation:* Nursing care that follows a regimen of care prescribed by a primary health-care provider, such as administration of fluids, medications, and procedures, as well as performs nursing care within the legal scope of the nursing profession.
- *Evaluation:* Nursing care that identifies a client's responses to medical and nursing interventions.

Caring
Nursing care that provides support, encouragement, empathy, concern, hope, and compassion to clients and significant others.

Communication and Documentation
Nursing care that reflects verbal and nonverbal interactions between the nurse and the client, significant others, and members of the health team as well as documentation on a client's clinical record that adheres to legal and ethical standards.

Teaching/Learning
Nursing actions that facilitate the acquisition of knowledge, skills, or attitudes by clients, family members, significant others, or staff members. The outcome of these interventions should promote a change in behavior.

Culture and Spirituality
Nursing care that considers individual client preferences, adhering to applicable standards of care and legal parameters.

Client Need Categories

Client needs reflect activities most commonly performed by entry-level nurses.

Safe and Effective Care Environment

- *Management of Care:* Nursing care that provides or directs the delivery of nursing activities to clients, significant others, and other health-care personnel. Management of care items account for 17% to 23% of the items on the NCLEX-RN examination.
- *Safety and Infection Control:* Nursing care that protects clients, significant others, and health-care personnel from health and environmental hazards. Safety and infection control items account for 9% to 15% of the items on the NCLEX-RN examination.

Health Promotion and Maintenance

Nursing care to assist clients and significant others to prevent or detect health problems and achieve optimum health, particularly in relation to their developmental level. Health promotion and maintenance items account for 6% to 12% of the items on the NCLEX-RN examination.

Psychosocial Integrity

Nursing care that supports and promotes the emotional, mental, and social well-being of clients and significant others as well as those with acute or chronic mental health problems. Psychosocial integrity items account for 6% to 12% of the items on the NCLEX-RN examination.

Physiological Integrity

- *Basic Care and Comfort:* Nursing care that provides support during the performance of the activities of daily living, such as hygiene, rest, sleep, mobility, elimination, hydration, and nutrition. Basic care and comfort items account for 6% to 12% of the items on the NCLEX-RN examination.
- *Pharmacological and Parenteral Therapies:* Nursing care related to the administration of medication, intravenous fluids, and blood and blood products. Pharmacological and parenteral therapies items account for 12% to 18% of the items on the NCLEX-RN examination.
- *Reduction of Risk Potential:* Nursing care that limits the development of complications associated with health problems, treatments, or procedures. Reduction of risk potential items account for 9% to 15% of the items on the NCLEX-RN examination.
- *Physiological Adaptation:* Nursing care that meets the needs of clients with acute, chronic, or life-threatening physical health problems. Physiological adaptation items account for 11% to 17% of the items on the NCLEX-RN examination.

Cognitive Level Categories

This category reflects the thinking processes necessary to answer a question.

Knowledge

Information must be recalled from memory, such as facts, terminology, principles, and generalizations.

Comprehension

Information, as well as the implications and potential consequences of information identified, must be understood, interpreted, and paraphrased or summarized.

Application

Information must be identified, manipulated, or used in a situation, including mathematical calculations.

Analysis

A variety of information must be interpreted, requiring the identification of commonalities, differences, and interrelationship among the data.

Content Area Categories

Content area categories are not part of the NCLEX-RN Test Plan. These categories were added to indicate the name of the chapter in which the content being tested in the question can be found in this textbook.

Concept Categories

Concept categories are not part of the NCLEX-RN Test Plan. These categories are a collective list of concepts created by F. A. Davis for approaching nursing content from a conceptual pedagogy. This list can be found on the inside back cover of this textbook. The categories after the rationales for each test item include a concept category. Identifying the concept associated with the content in each test item supports conceptual understanding, reasoning, and learning across settings in which nurses' work, the life span, and the range of health and illness.

Essential Health-Care Concepts

Chapter 1

Safety

NURSING CONCEPTS

Cognition
Growth and Development
Health Promotion
Immunity
Mobility
Oxygenation

Perfusion
Safety
Sensory Perception
Tissue Integrity
Violence

KEY TERMS

Allergy—Hypersensitivity precipitated by exposure to an allergen that causes a harmful immunologic reaction with subsequent exposures

Anaphylaxis—Severe, sudden immune response that involves a decrease in blood pressure and can cause shock, unconsciousness, and death if untreated

Aspiration—Inhalation of a substance into the respiratory tract

Drowning—Filling of the lungs with fluid, which prevents gas exchange and results in suffocation

Orthostatic hypotension—Lack of adequate autonomic vasoconstriction of peripheral blood vessels when moving from a lying to a sitting or standing position, resulting in a temporary decrease in blood pressure and inadequate circulation to the brain

Restraint—Devices used to limit movement of a body limb or body activity

- **Level 1 restraint**—Restraint used to protect the client from injuring self or others while receiving acute medical or surgical care

- **Level 2 restraint**—Restraint used to manage violent behavior to protect a client from injuring self or others

Safety—Freedom from physical or emotional trauma or injury

Standard precautions—Actions recommended by the Centers for Disease Control and Prevention (CDC) for reducing the risk of transmission of pathogens via blood or body fluids

Suffocation (asphyxiation)—Failure of air to reach the lungs, causing lack of oxygen, excess carbon dioxide, loss of consciousness, cessation of breathing, and death

Syncope—Temporary loss of consciousness due to an inadequate level of oxygen in the brain

I. Client Safety and Nursing Care

To remain safe is a basic expectation and right of all clients. A health-care environment, whether it is in a health-care agency or created in the home, can be frightening, unfamiliar, and stressful for a client. Nurses must focus on the basic needs for safety and security so clients do not experience accidents or sustain injuries.

A. Introduction
   1. **Safety** is freedom from physical or emotional trauma or injury.
   2. Safety and security are second-level needs, after physiological needs, according to Maslow's hierarchy of needs.
   3. According to the CDC, unintentional injuries are the fourth leading cause of death in the United States.

4. Nursing interventions for promoting safety for all clients involve:
   a. Assessing for factors that can jeopardize safety.
   b. Maintaining a safe environment in a health-care facility.
   c. Providing client teaching about maintaining safety in the home.
5. The Joint Commission has identified goals and requirements to provide for client safety (National Patient Safety Goals [NPSG]); they include:
   a. Identify clients correctly.
   b. Improve communication among health-care workers.
   c. Administer pharmaceuticals safely.
   d. Identify clients at risk for injury.
   e. Prevent infection.
   f. Prevent falls.
   g. Prevent pressure ulcers.
   h. Reduce the risk of influenza and pneumococcal disease in older adults.
   i. Implement preprocedure verification processes.
   j. Improve responses to changes in a client's status.
   k. Encourage client involvement in own safety care.
6. Unfortunately, accidents do occur in health-care facilities, and they are documented in incident reports. **Incident reports** document details of situations that caused or have the potential to cause harm to clients, health-care providers, or visitors. These reports record the facts, provide data for overseeing agencies, and help identify trends and influence the development of measures to limit similar events in the future.

B. Nursing interventions to maintain client safety in health-care environments
1. Ensure personal knowledge of agency policies and procedures that relate to safety.
2. Be knowledgeable about the use of equipment; inspect all equipment before use.
3. Continuously assess for physical, biological, and chemical hazards in the environment.
4. Perform a risk-for-injury assessment, including developmental and individual factors, on each client.
5. Ensure that each client has an identity band on his or her wrist.
6. Ensure that the client has a separate alert wristband for each risk factor, such as one for an allergy, one for fall risk, and one alerting the health team to avoid trauma to an arm (e.g., arm on the side of a mastectomy, presence of fistula for dialysis).
7. Ensure safety within the client's bedside unit.
   a. Orient the client to the environment.
   b. Keep the bed in lowest position when not providing direct care.
   c. Keep wheels on bed and overbed table locked.
   d. Keep the call bell and personal items within the client's reach.
   e. Keep one to four side rails raised, as required by the client.
      (1) All side rails raised is considered a restraint and requires a prescription unless requested by the client.
      (2) Unnecessary use of side rails is considered false imprisonment.
   f. Maintain a clutter-free environment.
8. Ensure that tubing (e.g., IV catheters, chest tubes, urinary catheters, electrocardiogram lines, and portable wound drainage systems) is coiled on the bed with no dependent loops and is safeguarded during activities, particularly during transfers and when the client is ambulating.
9. Maintain adequate lighting in the environment for day, evening, and night.
10. Keep environmental noise to a minimum.
    a. Place handheld controllers that project sound near client's ear so as not to impose on roommates.
    b. Pull curtain or close door when appropriate.
11. Immediately answer call bells and check equipment that sets off alarms.
12. Explain to the client what is to be done before and/or during an activity.
13. Instruct the client to seek assistance when ambulating, as needed.
14. Employ the use of assistive devices, such as a mechanical lift, to transfer clients safely, as needed.
15. Protect oneself from harm, such as by using sharps containers; and following infection control guidelines, particularly hand hygiene.

II. Factors That Influence Client Safety and Related Nursing Care

A. Age
1. Significance.
   a. Each age-group has unique developmental factors (e.g., physical, emotional, and cognitive) that influence the ability to remain safe.
   b. Nurses must understand these age-related factors to anticipate safety precautions necessary for clients in each age group.
      (1) Infants.
         (a) Depend on others for care.
         (b) Initially cannot turn over.
         (c) Put things in mouths to explore the world.
         (d) Able to manipulate small objects.
         (e) Have immature body systems (e.g., neurological and musculoskeletal systems).

(f) Lack judgment due to limited experiences and immature cognition.

(g) Gain mobility, such as turning over, crawling, and walking.

(2) Toddlers.

(a) Increase in mobility, such as walking and climbing.

(b) Lack judgment due to limited experiences and immature cognition.

(c) Have increasing curiosity (e.g., intrigued by stairs).

(3) Preschoolers.

(a) Desire independence.

(b) Have continuing curiosity.

(c) Play in areas beyond the house, such as in pools, playgrounds, and front yards.

(d) Engage in magical thinking that overestimates their abilities.

(e) Still lack judgment but are a little more aware of physical dangers.

(f) Trust authority figures, which may increase the risk of being abducted.

(4) School-aged children.

(a) Are less fearful than toddlers and preschoolers, such as attempting new skills without instruction.

(b) Use tools and household items that can cause harm, such as knives and lawn mowers.

(c) Have increased involvement with the environment, such as traveling to school, staying at school for activities, and playing team sports on weekends.

(d) Are involved in more active and competitive play; often overestimate personal abilities.

(e) Begin learning to be wary of strangers but trusting authority figures still persists.

(5) Adolescents.

(a) Are at peak of physical, sensory, and psychomotor abilities.

(b) Believe they are invincible.

(c) Engage in risk-taking behaviors, such as smoking, drug and alcohol misuse, driving fast, and unprotected sex.

(d) Desire to be independent and in control.

(e) Are exposed to increased peer relationships and pressure and decreased parental influence.

(f) Begin driving; tend not to wear seatbelts.

(6) Adults.

(a) Have progressively declining physical, sensory, and psychomotor abilities.

(b) Engage in lifestyle habits that increase risk, such as smoking, alcohol and drug misuse, and unprotected sex.

(c) Have increased stress due to career, family responsibilities, and financial demands.

(d) May be at risk for injury at work (e.g., using heavy machinery, working at heights, or engaging in repetitive motions).

(7) Older adults.

(a) Have decreased musculoskeletal strength and mobility.

(b) Have declining voluntary and autonomic reflexes.

(c) Have declining sensory functions, such as impaired hearing, vision, and sensation.

(d) May have declining cognitive awareness or ability to manage multiple incoming stimuli simultaneously.

(e) May engage in polypharmacy, which can precipitate overdoses or drug interactions.

2. Nursing care: See safety-related nursing interventions under each age group in Chapter 10, Development Across the Life Span.

B. Impaired vision

1. Significance.

a. Impaired vision limits or eliminates visual cues regarding the environment that can result in client injury.

b. An inability to detect relevant visual stimuli and perceive spacial relationships can cause postural instability, increased sway, and impaired balance, resulting in a fall.

c. Impaired depth perception, judgment of distance, and contrast sensitivity contribute to an inability to identify hazards; therefore, avoid obstacles in the environment.

2. Nursing care.

a. Assess the client's visual acuity to determine the extent of the client's risk of injury and the level of assistance required by the client (see "Assessment of the Eyes" in Chapter 14, Physical Assessment).

b. Encourage the use of prescription eyeglasses, contact lenses, tinted eyeglasses, a magnifying glass, and other visual devices.

c. Provide adequate room lighting and a small light at night.

d. Use shades or blinds on windows during the day to reduce glare.

e. Describe and maintain the placement of furniture in the room.

f. Use a clock arrangement for placement of food on a plate or tray.

g. Ensure that food and liquids are warm, not hot.

h. Provide care standing on the side of the client's most effective vision; inform the client when entering or leaving the room.

i. When walking with the client, be next to and slightly in front of the client with the client holding your arm.

j. Provide or encourage the use of objects with large print, such as clocks, phones, and computers.

C. Impaired hearing

1. Significance.

a. Impaired hearing limits the reception of auditory stimuli, which can result in client injury.

b. Nurses must understand that impaired hearing also impacts a client's ability to communicate; therefore, nursing interventions must facilitate communication.

2. Nursing care.

a. Assess the client's hearing ability to determine the extent of the client's risk of injury and the level of assistance required by the client (see "Assessment of the Ears" in Chapter 14, Physical Assessment).

b. Encourage the use of a prescribed hearing aid.

c. Decrease background noise when communicating with the client, such as by turning off the TV and closing the door.

d. Face the client and speak clearly; do not overenunciate words.

e. Encourage the use of devices, such as a smoke detector, phone, and doorbell, that amplify sound or use motion or lights to communicate a message.

🛑 f. Ensure that the client hears and understands communication, especially instructions concerning activities.

D. Impaired mobility

1. Significance.

a. Mobility relates to body alignment, joint flexibility, gait, and balance, which includes center of gravity and base of support. Impairment in any one of these areas can result in a fall.

b. Falls are a major concern because they can cause injury, loss of function, and mortality.

c. Falls are the leading cause of injury resulting in death in older adults.

2. Nursing care.

a. Assess the client for factors that increase the risk of falls; preferably use a measurement tool (e.g., the Morse Fall Scale).

(1) History of falls.

(2) Secondary medical diagnosis (e.g., cardiopulmonary, musculoskeletal diseases).

(3) Use of ambulatory aids.

(4) Presence of one or more objects that hamper mobility (e.g., urinary catheter, IV, and venous compression device).

(5) Impaired gait, balance, or weight-bearing ability of lower extremities.

(6) Impaired cognition or judgment.

(7) Impaired vision.

(8) **Orthostatic hypotension** (significant decrease in blood pressure when moving from lying to sitting or standing positions), or dizziness.

(9) Medications that depress the central nervous system, such as sedatives and opioids, or promote hypotension, such as antihypertensives and diuretics.

(10) Age more than 65 years.

b. Perform the **"Get Up and Go Test."**

(1) Have the client move from a sitting to a standing position without using the arms for support.

(2) Instruct the client to walk several steps, turn, and return to the chair.

(3) Have the client sit down in the chair without using the arms for support.

(4) Perform a follow-up assessment if the test reveals that the client is unsteady.

(a) Have the client move from a sitting to a standing position without using the arms for support.

(b) Have the client stand in place with eyes closed for several seconds.

(c) Push gently on the sternum while the client has his or her eyes closed.

(d) Instruct the client to walk several steps, turn, return to the chair, and sit down without using the arms for support.

c. Use monitoring devices that alert others when the client attempts to get out of a bed or chair; use two, three, or four side rails, as indicated.

d. Have the client use an assistive device, such as a walker or cane, to maintain a wide base of support.

e. Implement hourly rounding on clients to reduce clients' anxiety and attend to their personal needs.

f. Ensure that the client has well-fitted footwear with nonskid soles.

g. Instruct the client to rise slowly to a standing position and allow time for blood pressure to adjust to change in position; encourage the client to sit down if dizzy.

h. Use assistive devices, such as a transfer belt (Fig. 1.1), mechanical lift (Fig. 1.2), or sit-to-stand lift (Fig. 1.3), when transferring clients.

i. Arrange physical therapy sessions in the morning before the client becomes fatigued.

Fig 1.1 Transfer belt. (From Wilkinson and Treas [2016]. *Fundamentals of nursing*, Vol. 1, 3rd ed. Philadelphia: F. A. Davis Company, with permission.)

Fig 1.3 Sit-to-stand lift. (From Burton and Ludwig [2015]. *Fundamentals of nursing care: Concepts, connections & skills*, 2nd ed. Philadelphia: F. A. Davis Company, with permission.)

Fig 1.2 Mechanical lift. (From Wilkinson and Treas [2016]. *Fundamentals of nursing*, Vol. 1, 3rd ed. Philadelphia: F. A. Davis Company, with permission.)

Fig 1.4 Guiding a falling client. (From Wilkinson and Treas [2016]. *Fundamentals of nursing*, Vol. 1, 3rd ed. Philadelphia: F. A. Davis Company, with permission.)

    j. Assist the client if the client begins to fall.
      (1) Place feet apart and project the hip and leg closest to the client, allowing the client to slide down the caregiver's leg to the floor (Fig. 1.4).
      (2) Protect the client's head.
      (3) Call for assistance.
      (4) Have the client examined by a primary health-care provider for injury.
      (5) Document the event and complete an incident report.
    k. Position commode near bed for toileting at night.
E. Impaired cognition (confusion, disorientation, impaired memory, lack of judgment)
    1. Significance.
      a. The ability to perceive external stimuli and react appropriately requires intact cognition,

which includes the thought processes of thinking, problem-solving, judgment, and insight; level of consciousness; memory; and orientation to time, place, and person.

b. Factors such as lack of sleep, impaired memory, an altered level of consciousness, disorientation, confusion, or taking medications such as narcotics, hypnotics, or sedatives that influence the central nervous system can impair thought processes.

c. When thought processes are impaired, a client is unable to perceive risk factors or use judgment to maintain safety, thereby increasing the risk of injury.

2. Nursing care.

a. Assess the client's cognitive functioning, including:

(1) Orientation to time, place, and person.

(2) Short-term and long-term memory.

(3) Ability to perceive danger and use judgment and problem-solving.

(4) Ability to understand and follow instructions.

(5) Mental health status (see "Mental Health Assessment" in Chapter 12, Psychosocial Health).

MAKING THE CONNECTION

Making Hourly Rounds and Reducing the Rate of Falls

Falls are the leading cause of injury and death among people who are 65 years of age and older. The CDC reported the following statistics for the year 2013:

- 2.5 million fall injuries requiring treatment in emergency departments occurred among people age 65 and older.
- 30% of these individuals required hospitalization.
- 250,000 hip fractures were reported, and 95% were caused by falls.
- 25,500 older adults died from falls.

Performing hourly rounds (intentional checking of clients at hourly intervals) can help reduce the risk of falls. Of nine studies that examined the implementation of hourly rounds, seven indicated that fall rates were reduced. In eight of the nine studies, improvements in overall client satisfaction with attention to personal needs and timeliness of nurses' response were identified. Hourly rounds helped to reduce clients' anxiety about getting needs met, and clients learned to trust the process. One study documented a 52% reduction in falls, 37% reduction in the use of call lights, and 14% reduction in the development of pressure ulcers.

b. Maintain consistency of staff members, activities, and the environment.

c. Use color as environmental clues.

🛑 d. Use position monitoring devices that alert others when the client attempts to get out of a bed or chair.

e. Use two, three, or four side rails as indicated.

f. Use restraints as prescribed and needed.

g. Assign one-to-one supervision if necessary.

F. Heat or cold applications

1. Significance.

a. Heat.

(1) Positive consequences.

(a) Causes vasodilation that increases circulation and capillary permeability.

(b) Brings oxygen and white blood cells to the area to promote healing and help remove waste products.

(c) Decreases muscle tension and joint stiffness and promotes relaxation.

(2) Negative consequences.

(a) Vasodilation and capillary permeability decrease the circulating blood volume, resulting in a decrease in blood to the brain and causing dizziness or fainting (**syncope**).

(b) Decreased muscle tension and relaxation may result in muscle weakness or lack of attention to personal abilities or factors in the environment, which may result in injury.

(c) The addition of moisture increases the intensity of heat.

(d) Excessive heat can cause tissue injury and cell death (thermal burn).

b. Cold.

(1) Positive consequences.

(a) Causes vasoconstriction that decreases circulation and capillary permeability.

(b) Reduces muscle tension and cell metabolism.

(c) Limits inflammation, pain, edema, oxygen requirements at the cellular level, and bleeding.

(2) Negative consequences.

(a) May limit transport of adequate oxygen and nutrients necessary for muscle contraction resulting in weakness due to vasoconstriction.

(b) Anesthetizes nerve endings, which diminishes the ability to perceive sensations, such as placement of feet on the floor.

(c) May result in tissue injury and cell death because excessive cold causes ischemia (cold burn).

2. Nursing care.
   a. Commonalities of care for clients exposed to interventions involving either heat or cold.
      (1) Identify clients at increased risk for non-therapeutic results, such as the very young and very old, those with sensory impairments, and those with injuries on highly vascular areas (e.g., hand, face, perineum), traumatized skin, or involvement of large surface areas.
      (2) Verify the primary health-care provider's prescription.
      (3) Assess the site before application.
      (4) Use a thermometer to measure water temperature.
      (5) Avoid direct contact with the skin; use a fitted sleeve or towel.
      (6) Apply intermittently for 15 minutes to prevent the opposite effect when the application reaches maximum therapeutic value (rebound phenomenon).
   b. Specific nursing care for clients exposed to interventions involving heat.
      (1) Apply heat, such as a heating pad or disposable hot packs, as prescribed and at a temperature of 105°F to 115°F; sitz bath should not exceed 110°F.
      (2) Assess for nontherapeutic responses, such as extreme redness, cyanosis, blanching, blistering, and decreased blood pressure.
   c. Specific nursing care for clients exposed to interventions involving cold.
      (1) Apply cold, such as a cool sponge bath, cold compresses, ice collar, or disposable ice packs, as prescribed and at the recommended temperature; cool sponge bath should be 65°F to 90°F.
      (2) Reduce the temperature extreme or discontinue treatment if the client begins to shiver because shivering increases body temperature.
      (3) Assess for nontherapeutic responses, such as blanching, mottled skin, numbness, pain, blisters, shivering, and increased blood pressure.

G. Allergies
   1. Significance.
      a. An **allergy** is a hypersensitivity precipitated by exposure to a stimulus (*allergen*) that can cause harmful immunologic reactions within the body.

MAKING THE CONNECTION

Heat and Cold Therapy and the Length of Application

Heat or cold can be applied to areas of the body for 20 to 30 minutes every 2 to 6 hours to achieve a local effect. When heat is applied, the blood vessels dilate, bringing more plasma, oxygen-carrying red blood cells, white blood cells, and nutrients to the treated area. When cold is applied, vasoconstriction occurs, which decreases blood flow to the area, resulting in reduced edema, discomfort and pain, muscle spasm, and a numbing sensation. However, when heat or cold is applied longer than 30 minutes, a rebound phenomenon occurs, causing an opposite effect. When heat therapy is applied too long, vasoconstriction occurs for unknown reasons, which then prevents the dissipation of the applied heat and in turn may cause a burn or worsen the condition. When cold therapy is applied too long, vasoconstriction initially persists, denying cells of oxygen and nutrients; when the local temperature decreases below 60°F, vasodilation occurs as a protective mechanism. These responses can worsen the condition and cause tissue injury and even tissue necrosis. To prevent tissue injury, nurses must understand, as well as teach clients about, the rebound phenomenon related to heat and cold therapy.

b. Mild and moderate reactions involve uncomfortable responses, such as sneezing, coughing, itching eyes, and conjunctivitis.
c. A rapid, severe reaction may include hives, swelling of respiratory passages that causes difficulty breathing, and wheezing and can progress to anaphylaxis.
d. **Anaphylaxis** is a sudden, severe allergic response that involves a decrease in blood pressure and can cause shock, unconsciousness, and death if untreated.

2. Nursing care.
   a. Assess for a history of allergies, such as to drugs (prescription and over the counter), foods (especially seafood), tape, skin care products, animals, and insects; obtain a description of the client's response to each.
   b. Identify the risk of a latex allergy. An increased risk is associated with asthma; allergies to bananas, kiwi, chestnuts, or avocados; and repeated exposure to latex in medical care settings. Use latex-free gloves and equipment.
   c. Assess for clinical indicators of mild to moderate allergic responses, such as a skin rash, urticaria, pruritus, nausea, vomiting, diarrhea, rhinitis, and lacrimal tearing.

d. Assess for clinical indicators of anaphylaxis, such as wheezing, dyspnea, angioedema, tachycardia, hypotension, and circulatory collapse.

🛑 e. **Apply an allergy alert wristband (usually red in color) that itemizes the offending agents.**

f. Communicate the allergy to other health team members, such as by documenting it in the medication administration record, history and physical, front of the clinical record, and the client's plan of care.

g. Ensure that the client is not exposed to any known offending agents.

h. Encourage the client to wear a medical alert band at all times.

i. Encourage the client to carry or have readily available an epinephrine auto-injector (EpiPen), if prescribed.

H. Increased risk for aspiration, drowning, or suffocation

1. Significance.

   a. **Aspiration** is the inhalation of a substance (e.g., foreign material, vomitus, blood, saliva) into the respiratory tract.

   b. **Drowning** occurs when the lungs fill with fluid, preventing gas exchange and resulting in suffocation.

   c. **Suffocation** (*asphyxiation*) occurs when no air reaches the lungs, causing lack of oxygen, excess carbon dioxide, loss of consciousness, cessation of breathing, and death. It can be caused by gas or smoke inhalation, strangulation, a foreign body in the trachea, drowning, and electric shock and also occurs when an infant's face is pressed against a sleeping caregiver, mattress, stuffed toy, or blanket.

   d. Nursing interventions for promoting safety in relation to these issues involve direct nursing interventions and health teaching for clients and parents.

2. Nursing care.

   a. Teach parents to:

      (1) Ensure that cribs meet regulations, such as having slats less than 2 3/8 inch apart and stationary side rails.

      (2) Keep cords out of reach, such as from mobiles, venetian blinds, neck ties, and sweatpants.

      (3) Ensure that toys are larger than a fist and have no small, removable parts.

      (4) Store plastic bags out of reach.

      (5) Cut food (e.g., grapes and hard cheese) into small pieces.

      (6) Do not give children chewing gum, hard candy, nuts, popcorn, marshmallows, soft cheese, or peanut butter.

      (7) Supervise play with balloons, and discard broken balloons immediately.

      (8) Ensure that pools have appropriate safety precautions, such as a high fence, pool cover, and splash sensor.

      (9) Supervise children around water such as tubs, pools, buckets, and toilets; provide Coast Guard–approved flotation devices.

   b. Provide specific nursing care for clients at risk for aspiration.

      (1) Assess for risk factors, such as dysphagia, dentures, and impaired cognition.

      (2) Position the client in a sitting position for meals, and ensure that the client swallows food before giving the next spoonful.

      (3) Teach the client to cut food into small pieces.

      (4) Teach the client to chew food thoroughly.

      (5) Use a thickening product to thicken liquids.

      (6) Identify whether a client with a neurological impairment has retained food in the buccal cavity (*cheeking*) to prevent aspiration.

   c. Teach the client to check the depth of water before jumping or diving.

   d. Teach older children and adults the universal choking sign. (See Fig. 19.17, in Chapter 19, Oxygenation.)

III. Safety of Health-Care Providers

Nursing is a profession that exposes its members to numerous work-related stressors that can impact their health. New devices have been developed, such as needleless syringes, passive guards on syringes, and sit-to-stand lifts, to address some workplace stressors. However, nurses increasingly are caring for more clients who are obese, acutely ill, and physically dependent and those receiving a variety of radiation and/or intravenous therapies that raise new concerns in relation to the safety of nurses. In addition, nurses must cope with clients who become verbally and physically aggressive because of delirium, cognitive impairment, mental illness, grief, caregiver role strain, and drug or alcohol misuse. The potential for musculoskeletal injuries, radiation exposure, puncture injuries, and violence toward nurses and other health-care providers still exists.

A. Introduction

1. The American Nurses Association (ANA), Occupational and Safety and Health Administration (OSHA), Joint Commission (JC), American Hospital Association (AHA), and Environmental

Protection Agency (EPA) all issue guidelines and regulations that address safety in health-care settings to protect health-care providers, clients, and visitors.

2. Agency policies and procedures must address such safety issues as infection control, handling of chemical and biological agents, disposal of sharps, equipment for moving clients, badges for measuring level of radiation exposure, and ways to manage violence in the workplace.

B. Hazards to health-care providers

1. Back injury.
   a. Most commonly results from activities that require bending and twisting the torso, such as lifting clients up in bed, transferring clients from a bed to a chair, and changing linens.
   b. Preventive measures.
      (1) Use appropriate body mechanics (see "Body Mechanics" in Chapter 17, Mobility)
      (2) Use client-handling devices when necessary, such as mechanical lifts (see Fig. 1.2), transfer boards, and sit-to-stand lifts (see Fig. 1.3).
2. Exposure to a client receiving radiation therapy.
   a. Types of radiation therapy.
      (1) Internal radiation therapy *(brachytherapy)*.
         (a) Interstitial implants (e.g., needle, seeds, wire).
         (b) Intracavitary implants (e.g., radioactive source contained within an applicator that is inserted into a body cavity).
      (2) External radiation therapy *(teletherapy)*: Radiation dose administered by a machine.
      (3) Radiopharmaceutical therapy: Radioactive medication administered orally or intravenously.
   b. Preventive measures to protect nurses caring for clients receiving internal radiation therapy.
      (1) Perform all care based on the concept of **"As Low As Reasonably Achievable" (ALARA).**
         (a) Understand that ALARA means making all reasonable efforts regarding controlling time, distance, and shielding to minimize exposure to ionizing radiation.
         (b) Monitor radiation dosimeter (badge) to ensure that it does not exceed the U.S. annual occupational dose limit of 5,000 millirem (5 rem); many agencies advocate exposure to less than 500 millirem yearly.
         🛑 (c) Ensure that pregnant women and women attempting to become pregnant do not

routinely care for clients receiving internal radiation.

(2) Control time.
   (a) Wear a radiation dosimeter (badge) when providing care if regularly exposed to radiation to measure the extent of radiation exposure.
   (b) Organize care to minimize the amount of time at the client's bedside, meeting only essential needs; keep time to less than 30 minutes in an 8-hour period per caregiver.
   (c) Rotate care among nurses.
(3) Control distance.
   (a) Place the client in a private room.
   (b) Stand as far away from the client as possible (at least 6 feet) unless giving direct care.
   (c) Provide care by standing at the head or foot of the bed as indicated, such as head and side of the client's bed for vaginal or prostate implants or seeds and foot of the bed if seeds are in the neck or tongue.
(4) Control shielding.
   (a) Wear a lead apron and protective shoe covers and gloves when in the room with the client.
   (b) Ensure that an internal radiation device is in place.
   (c) Inspect linens for displacement of radioactive seeds.
   (d) Maintain the client in the position prescribed to prevent displacement and promote comfort, such as supine for a vaginal implant and semi-Fowler's position for seed implants in the neck or tongue.
   (e) Notify the appropriate radiation team immediately if a radioactive device or seed is displaced; use a long-handled forceps to place a dislodged radioactive device in a lead container only if trained in this technique.
   🛑 (f) Never touch radioactive implant devices or seeds with the hands.

c. Preventive measures to protect nurses when caring for a client receiving external radiation therapy.
   (1) Wear a radiation dosimeter (badge) when providing care if regularly exposed to radiation to measure the extent of radiation exposure.

(2) Stand behind the designated shield/door or wear full body lead clothing during diagnostic tests that emit radiation.

d. Preventive measures to protect nurses and others when caring for a client receiving radiopharmaceutical therapy.

(1) Follow recommendations for time, distance, and shielding depending on the radioactive material used for diagnostic or therapeutic procedures. Recommendations depend on the half-life of the radioactive material.

(2) Teach clients and family members about precautions that should be followed when a client is discharged home after receiving radiopharmaceutical therapy (e.g., ^{131}I: oral and close contact with others should be avoided, urine and vomitus should be disposed of in a toilet and the toilet flushed twice, meticulous hand washing should be performed after urinating, and eating utensils should be washed thoroughly with soap and water).

3. Puncture injuries.

a. Can occur when handling anything sharp enough to pierce the skin; most occur as a result of the penetration of a needle of a syringe, hence the sometimes interrelated term *needlestick injury.*

b. Preventive measures.

(1) Encourage the adoption of needleless systems.

(2) Use devices that passively activate a safety guard over a needle rather than requiring the nurse to activate the guard.

(3) Use caution when working with sharp objects, such as scissors, clamps, scalpels, and syringes with needles.

(4) See also Box 9.3, "Preventing Needlestick Injuries," in Chapter 9, Medication.

4. Violence.

a. Can be precipitated by physical stressors (e.g., delirium, cognitive impairments, alcohol or drug use) and emotional stressors (e.g., manic episodes of bipolar disorder, grief, jealousy, and caregiver role strain).

b. Preventive measures.

(1) Stay with the client.

(2) Listen attentively and validate the client's feelings.

(3) Provide an atmosphere of caring and empathy.

(4) Remain calm and communicate in short, clear sentences.

(5) Give the client choices if possible and if the client is capable of decision making.

(6) Limit environmental stimuli, such as by reducing noise and people in the room.

(7) Identify whether the client's level of anxiety is escalating; be aware that behavior usually progresses to verbal and then physical aggression, such as agitation, pacing, pressured speech, gesturing wildly, sarcasm, swearing, verbal threats, pushing, and hitting.

🛑 **(8) Protect self and others when a client or visitor is angry.**

(a) Know how to access the help of agency safety control officers.

(b) Do not go into the room alone.

(c) Keep the door open and stand between the client and the door.

(d) Remain at least 3 feet away from and do not turn your back on an angry client.

(e) Do not wear anything that can be used to inflict harm, such as a stethoscope, dangling jewelry, and pointed objects.

(f) Avoid threatening, aggressive verbal or nonverbal communication; do not respond to anger with anger; avoid prolonged eye contact.

(g) Do not touch the client without permission.

(h) Offer first and then administer prescribed sedatives if necessary, using a calm, reassuring approach.

(i) Use mechanical restraints as prescribed and necessary to prevent injury to self and others.

🛑 **(9) Ensure safety in home-care settings.**

(a) Carry a cell phone and a minimal amount of money.

(b) Exit the car after determining the safety of the surroundings, such as adequate lighting and nonthreatening behavior of residents; drive away if you do not deem the area safe.

(c) Remain close to an exit after entering a home.

(d) Request that animals and visible weapons be kept in another room.

(e) Leave immediately if you suspect substance misuse, drug dealing, or intoxicated behavior.

(f) Leave immediately if a domestic argument occurs; do not attempt to intervene.

(g) Request a security escort if the area is considered potentially unsafe.

(h) Report to the appropriate authorities suspected child, domestic partner, or elder abuse or neglect (depends on state law and local agencies).

IV. Restraints

Restraints (e.g., physical, environmental, or chemical) are interventions used to limit movement of a body limb or body activity. They should be used only as a last resort to prevent injury to the client or others after other less-restrictive measures have failed.

A. Introduction

1. Two levels of restraints are used.

   a. **Level 1 restraints** are used to protect a client from injuring self and others while receiving acute medical or surgical care.

   b. **Level 2 restraints** are used to manage violent behavior to protect a client from injuring self and others.

2. Less-restrictive means to provide for client safety that should be attempted before restraint use include:

   a. Orienting the client to the environment.

   b. Planning nursing care with the client and explaining all procedures.

   c. Monitoring the client frequently.

   d. Keeping two side rails up and using additional rails cautiously because the client may attempt to climb over the rails if feeling confined.

DID YOU KNOW?

Raising all side rails is considered a restraint that requires a prescription from a primary health-care provider. If all side rails are raised at the request of a client, it is not considered a restraint and does not require a prescription. This request must be documented in the client's clinical record.

   e. Using verbal interventions.

   f. Using a weight- or position-sensitive device to alert caregivers of a client's attempt to ambulate.

   g. Using seclusion (e.g., locked, padded room) in a mental health setting.

   h. Providing one-to-one supervision.

3. Client rights include freedom from physical restraints or psychoactive medications for the purpose of discipline or convenience.

4. Restraints should be used only as a last resort because they can cause injury, actually do not reduce falls, and make client care more time consuming.

5. Prescriptions for as-needed restraints or seclusion are not acceptable.

B. Types of restraints

1. Physical restraints immobilize a limb or movement of a body part; examples include wrist restraint, ankle restraint, cloth vest, and material mitt (Table 1.1).

2. Environmental restraints confine a person to an area; examples include side rails, a wheelchair with an immovable tray, and a seclusion room.

3. Chemical restraints alter disruptive and aggressive behavior so that the client cannot cause harm to self or others; examples include sedatives and psychotropic medications.

C. Nursing care for clients who are restrained

1. Follow agency policies, state laws, and professional guidelines.

2. Use less-restrictive interventions first; document their use and the client's response.

3. Use restraints as a last resort to protect the client and others from harm.

4. Before application, obtain a primary health-care provider's prescription for the least restrictive restraint, except in an emergency.

5. Secure the restraint using a quick-release knot (Fig. 1.5), which should not constrict or slip with client movements but will untie rapidly in an emergency; tie the knot to the bed frame, not a movable object such as a bed rail, because tying to a movable object could injure a client when the object moves.

Fig 1.5 Quick release knot. (From Burton and Ludwig [2015]. *Fundamentals of nursing care: Concepts, connections & skill,* 2nd ed. Philadelphia: F. A. Davis Company, with permission.)

Table 1.1 Types of Physical Restraints

Type of Restraint	Nursing Care
Mitt Restraint • Limits use of fingers. • Prevents removal of tubes and scratching. 	• Apply to one or both hands, as prescribed. • Tie to an immobile object. • Ensure that the client can flex and extend the fingers. • Ensure that two fingers can be slid under the wrist strap to ensure that it is not too tight. • Remove the restraint every 2 hr to perform a neurovascular assessment and put the entire extremity through full range-of-motion (ROM) exercises.
Vest and Jacket Restraints • Prevent getting out of bed or chair. • Permit turning from side to side. 	• Place the device on with the V in the front and the closure at the back. • Ensure that the device does not impair breathing. • Ensure that the client can turn from side to side. • Encourage the client to cough and deep breathe every hour. • Remove the restraint every 2 hr and assess skin integrity.
Wrist and Ankle Restraints • Prevent removal of tubes. • Prevent hitting or kicking others. 	• Apply the restraints as prescribed, such as two-point (both arms) or four-point (all extremities) restraints. • Place padding around the wrists or ankles before applying the straps. • Make the straps tight enough to prevent removal without impairing circulation (but ensure that two fingers can be slid under the strap). • Remove the restraint every 2 hr to assess neurovascular status and tissue integrity, and put the extremity through full ROM exercises. • Follow guidelines for use of four-point restraints: limit use to 4 hr; continuously assess response, monitor for safety, and reevaluate need; ensure that the client is assessed by a primary health-care provider within 1 hr of institution of the restraint.

Photo credits: Wilkinson and Treas (2016). *Fundamentals of nursing,* Vol. 2, 3rd ed. Philadelphia: F. A. Davis Company, with permission.

6. Maintain supervision of a client in restraints or seclusion according to agency policy and procedures.
7. Release restraints every 2 hours or more frequently, especially if used for behavioral problems, to assess the site of application for impaired circulation, tissue injury, or nerve compression; perform range-of-motion (ROM) exercises to the limbs; and provide skin care.
8. Document all interventions and the client's response. Document continued need for restraints every few hours for a client in a mental health agency, according to state mental health laws, and at least every 24 hours in other health-care agencies; discontinue use as soon as possible.
9. Delegate application and reapplication of restraints only to assistive personnel who are educated to perform this skill; however, retain the responsibility to evaluate the client's response, which should be performed only by a registered professional nurse.
10. Meet hydration, nutrition, elimination, and emotional needs while the client is restrained or secluded.

V. Fire Safety

Fire is a risk in all health-care environments and in the home. Fires in health-care environments sometimes occur due to the presence of flammable gases and materials as well as electrical equipment. Oxygen supports combustion of flammable materials and intensifies the severity of a fire. Incapacitated or immobile individuals are particularly at risk for injury from a fire because they may be unable to evacuate themselves.

A. Fire prevention measures
1. Ensure that all electrical equipment has three-pronged grounded plugs.
2. Test electrical equipment before use.
3. Avoid overloading outlets.
4. Remove an electric plug by gripping the plug, not pulling on the cord.
5. Inspect electrical plugs and wires for signs of loss of integrity, such as visible damage and frayed wires.
6. Decommission damaged electrical equipment; discard, send home with family, or forward to appropriate maintenance department.
7. Keep rooms and halls free from clutter.
8. Participate in educational programs regarding fire prevention and safety measures.
9. Participate in routine fire drills, and know the protocol for evacuating a home or unit.
10. Know the location of fire alarms, chart of bell codes, exits, and fire extinguishers.
11. Know how to locate a fire using a bell code chart.
12. Know how to report a fire per agency protocol.
13. Ensure that caregivers are aware of where and when oxygen is in use and the location of oxygen shut-off valves in a facility.

B. Agency fires
1. Follow the **RACE mnemonic.**
   a. Rescue: Remove clients in the vicinity of a fire; evacuate clients beyond a fire safety door if necessary; evacuate horizontally and then vertically. Do not use elevators.
   b. Alarm: Activate the first alert, usually by pulling an alarm or via telephone; indicate the type and location of the fire and identify yourself; then, activate the agency-wide call-bell system and automatic notification of the fire department.
   c. Confine: Close all doors and windows on the unit; ensure that fire safety doors that close automatically have closed; shut off all oxygen valves after ensuring clients' oxygen needs.
   d. Extinguish: Extinguish the fire using the appropriate fire extinguisher.
2. Respond to a fire if you are on the response team (fire brigade); usually one person from each unit

of the agency in addition to maintenance personnel are members of the fire brigade.
   a. Bring your assigned equipment.
   b. Use the stairs, not an elevator.

C. Home fires
1. Be aware that home fires sometimes occur because of careless disposal of cigarettes and matches as well as kitchen grease, faulty electrical wiring, and defective heating equipment.
2. Teach individuals to:
   a. Install smoke alarms near the kitchen, stairs, and bedrooms, and change the batteries once a year.
   b. Keep the fire department's number on home phones.
   c. Have and practice a home fire escape plan.
   d. Keep a fire extinguisher readily available, especially in a kitchen or workshop.
   e. Avoid smoking inside or near the entrances and exits to the home.
   f. Attend to fireplace fires, barbeque fires, and burning candles at all times.
   g. Store flammable liquids in appropriate containers.
   h. Never pour water on a grease fire.
   i. Stop, Drop, and Roll when clothing is on fire.

D. Fire extinguishers
1. Types.
   a. A: Used for materials that burn, such as wood, cloth, and paper.
   b. B: Used for flammable materials, such as liquids, gases, grease, tar, solvents, and paint.
   c. C: Used for fires involving electrical equipment, such as toasters and electric stoves.
   d. ABC: Used for all types of fires.
2. Nursing interventions.
   a. Determine the type of fire and select the appropriate extinguisher; most agencies now use ABC fire extinguishers.
   b. Position yourself between the fire and an exit.
   c. Follow the **PASS** mnemonic when using a fire extinguisher.
      (1) **P**ull the pin on the fire extinguisher.
      (2) **A**im the nozzle at the base of the flames.
      (3) **S**queeze the handles of the fire extinguisher.
      (4) **S**weep the nozzle from side to side at the base of the flames.

VI. Standard Precautions

A. Introduction
1. **Standard precautions** are techniques used to limit the risk of transmission of microorganisms from all clients regardless of the absence of, suspicion of, or confirmed presence of infection.

2. Precautions are based on the concept that blood, body fluids, body secretions and excretions (except sweat), mucous membranes, and nonintact skin contain microorganisms.

B. Nursing care related to standard precautions

1. Perform hand hygiene after caring for a client or touching contaminated articles.
2. Wash hands in sinks with foot pedals, keep hands above the level of the sink; wash vigorously with friction for a minimum of 15 seconds and then rinse and dry hands; if faucet has handles, shut off faucets with a clean, dry paper towel.
3. Clean hands with an alcohol-based (minimum of 60%) antimicrobial gel; after application, briskly rub hands together until air dried; washing with soap and water is required when caring for a client with *Clostridium difficile (C. diff),* vancomycin-resistant enterococci (VRE), and other multidrug-resistant organisms because antimicrobial hand gels are ineffective.
4. Keep fingernails short and avoid wearing artificial nails, fingernail polish, and jewelry with stones.

DID YOU KNOW?

The CDC recommends that nurses "not wear artificial fingernails or extenders when having direct contact with clients at high risk" and that they "keep natural nail tips less than 1/4-inch long." The CDC documents that studies indicate that persons wearing artificial nails or long nails have been epidemiologically implicated in outbreaks of infection related to gram-negative bacilli and yeasts. In addition, studies indicate that chipped nail polish may support the growth of larger numbers of organisms on fingernails even after careful hand washing.

5. Wear clean gloves when potential exposure to blood or body fluids exists.
6. Use additional personal protective equipment (PPE) such as a mask, face shield, and fluid-impervious gown when there is potential for splashing of body fluids or if a client is receiving transmission-based precautions.
7. Routinely disinfect items that act as fomites, such as stethoscopes, clamps, eyeglasses, pens, and telephones.
8. Use respiratory hygiene and cough etiquette, such as covering the mouth and nose when coughing or sneezing, disposing of tissues in no-touch receptacles, and performing hand hygiene after hands come in contact with respiratory secretions; provide fluid-impervious bags at the bedside for disposal of used tissues by client.
9. Limit visitors with suspected respiratory infections or require them to wear masks.
10. Fold soiled linen into itself and place in a fluid-impervious hamper; carry linen without touching uniform.
11. Keep all items off the floor and off closet floors.
12. Dispose of urine and feces in appropriate receptacles, such as a client's toilet.
13. Place needles and needleless systems into puncture-proof containers (sharps containers).

CASE STUDY: Putting It All Together

A 72-year-old widow is admitted to the hospital to receive treatment for a fracture of the neck of the left femur. This is the second admission for the client, who was admitted 4 months ago for a right brain attack (cerebrovascular accident, stroke). She has residual left-sided hemiparesis, a sling on her left arm to prevent subluxation of the shoulder, and a below-the-knee foot brace on the lower left leg for foot drop and to facilitate ambulation. She has been receiving furosemide daily for hypertension. When interviewed, the client says that she heard the doorbell ring, got up quickly, stood at the side of the bed, slipped on the scatter rug next to the bed, and fell to the floor. She was able to activate her safety alert necklace to summon help. An x-ray confirms a fracture in the intertrochanteric area, below the neck of the left femur. The client is admitted to the surgical unit so that orthopedic surgery can be performed to stabilize the femur. When assessing the client after transfer from the postanesthesia care unit to her room after the surgery, the primary nurse on the surgical unit identifies that the client's dressing is dry and intact, vital signs are within expected limits, and urine output is more than 50 mL/hr (according to the hourly urine output via a urinary retention catheter). The client states that she has pain and rates it as a level 3 on a 0-to-10 pain scale. She is able to state her name but does not recognize that she is in the hospital or that she had surgery and that it is the afternoon. The client states, "Why is everyone trying to kill me?" In addition, the client is attempting to get out of bed.

Postoperative Prescriptions
- Position on back and left side.
- Vital signs every 4 hours.

CASE STUDY: Putting It All Together

- Neuro checks every 4 hours for 24 hours.
- Bed rest and range-of-motion exercises to all unaffected extremities BID.
- Full liquid diet; advance to regular diet as tolerated.
- Elevate left leg on two pillows.
- IV fluids: 0.9% normal saline solution 60 mL/hr.
- Heparin 5,000 units Sub-Q every 12 hours.
- Hydromorphone (Dilaudid) 2 mg Sub-Q every 4 hours prn for severe pain.

- Oxycodone and acetaminophen (Percocet) 5/325 mg, 1 tab for mild pain and 2 tabs for moderate pain, PO every 6 hours prn.
- Docusate sodium (Colace) 100 mg PO BID.
- Sennosides (Senokot) 8.6 mg per tab, 2 tabs PO at bedtime prn for constipation.

Case Study Questions

A. What factors increased the risk of the client falling at home?

1. _____
2. _____
3. _____
4. _____

B. Which of the following concerns is the priority, and what data support the nurse's conclusion: potential for hemorrhage, fluid balance, client safety, or pain management?

_____
_____
_____

C. Identify common nursing actions that should be implemented to ensure the safety of this client.

1. _____
2. _____
3. _____
4. _____
5. _____
6. _____
7. _____
8. _____
9. _____

D. Identify additional nursing interventions specific to this client that the nurse should implement before seeking a prescription for a restraint.

1. _____
2. _____
3. _____
4. _____
5. _____

continued.

CASE STUDY: Putting It All Together   *cont'd*

_____ **Case Study Questions** _____

E. Because nonrestrictive measures are ineffective in providing for the client's safety, the primary health-care provider writes a prescription for a vest restraint. What actions should the nurse implement when caring for this client while she is in the vest restraint?

1. _____

2. _____

3. _____

4. _____

5. _____

6. _____

7. _____

8. _____

9. _____

10. _____

REVIEW QUESTIONS

Be sure to read the Introduction for valuable test-taking tips.

1. A nurse has a prescription to apply wrist restraints to maintain a client's safety. What should the nurse do when applying this type of restraint? **Select all that apply.**
   1. Check the site of the restraint every 30 minutes.
   2. Remove the wrist restraints to provide skin care every 2 hours.
   3. Ensure that the wrists are well padded when applying wrist restraints.
   4. Permit 3 finger-widths to slide between the client's skin and the restraints.
   5. Tie the straps of the wrist restraints to the frame of the bed using a slip knot.

2. Which are important steps when transferring a client from a bed to a chair using a mechanical lift? **Select all that apply.**
   1. Position the chair as close as possible to the bed.
   2. Remove the sling after the transfer is completed.
   3. Position the sling from the middle of the client's back to the ankles.
   4. Spread the legs of the lift apart before lowering the client to the chair.
   5. Attach the longer straps to the lower grommets on each side of the sling.

3. A client who is legally blind says to the nurse, "I once was able to see a little bit, but now I can't see anything." What should the nurse encourage the client to do while hospitalized?
   1. Wear dark-tinted eyeglasses.
   2. Keep a light on in the room at all times.
   3. Close the window blinds during the day.
   4. Call for assistance when getting out of bed.

4. A nurse is caring for an older adult who is cognitively impaired and has a history of pulling out tubes and falling. List the following safety devices in the order of least restrictive to most restrictive that may be employed to ensure the safety of this client.
   1. Cloth vest
   2. Two wrist straps
   3. Four side rails up
   4. Bed exiting alarm device
   5. Four-point restraint tied to the bed frame
   Answer: _____

5. A client who is cognitively impaired is admitted to the hospital for pneumonia. The client has a history of wandering at night. What should the nurse do to meet the needs of this client? **Select all that apply.**
   1. Obtain a sedative to be administered to the client at bedtime.
   2. Apply a vest restraint when the client plans to go to sleep.
   3. Apply a radio frequency product to the client's wrist.
   4. Restrict fluids several hours before bedtime.
   5. Activate the bed alarm on the client's bed.
   6. Eliminate caffeine products from the diet.

6. An 87-year-old adult is admitted to the hospital for diagnostic tests and intravenous rehydration therapy after a fall in the home. The next day the client's prescription for "out of bed to chair" twice daily was changed to "out of bed ad lib." What should the nurse do before getting the client out of bed?
   1. Test the strength of the client's legs.
   2. Take the blood pressure while the client is supine.
   3. Give the client oxygen via a nasal cannula for several minutes.
   4. Disconnect the client's intravenous tubing from the venous access device.

Client's Clinical Record

Medical History

Diagnosed with hypothyroidism for 10 years and hypertension for 5 years. Taking levothyroxine 100 mcg PO once a day and hydrochlorothiazide 25 mg PO once a day. Came to the emergency department twice in the past year because of falls in the home. Both times blood work and x-rays were normal. Both times treated for cuts and bruises and discharged.

Serum Electrolyte Levels

Potassium: 3.4 mEq/L.
Sodium: 134 mEq/L.
Calcium: 9.6 mEq/L.

Progress Note

Out of bed to chair for 1 hour twice between 8:00 a.m. and 8:00 p.m. Required minimal assistance and did not experience lightheadedness or syncope. States, "I'm afraid to walk because I was admitted to the hospital when I fell walking from the living room to the bedroom." IVF 5% dextrose in water at 75 mL/hr.

7. A community-health nurse is providing a program about fire safety in the home. What recommendations should the nurse include in this program? **Select all that apply.**
   1. Practice a home fire escape plan.
   2. Smoke cigarettes in just 1 room of the home.
   3. Install smoke alarms near bedrooms and stairs.
   4. Install a Class A extinguisher close to the kitchen.
   5. Teach participants to stop, drop, and roll if clothing is on fire.

8. Which nursing interventions can give a client a sense of control regarding personal safety? **Select all that apply.**
   1. Inform the client why an identification band should be worn.
   2. Instruct the client how to lock the wheels on a wheelchair.
   3. Keep the client's bed in the lowest position.
   4. Teach the client how to use the call bell.
   5. Orient the client to the environment.

9. A nurse is caring for a client who has a vaginal radiation implant. What essential actions should the nurse implement when caring for the client? **Select all that apply.**
   1. Maintain the client in the semi-Fowler position.
   2. Have the client wear a detection badge while receiving care.
   3. Talk with the client while standing at the foot of the client's bed.
   4. Wear a lead apron when providing direct nursing care to the client.
   5. Instruct visitors that they can stay a half hour daily and to sit at the door.
   6. Keep soiled linens in the room until surveyed by a radiation safety staff member.

10. A nurse in the emergency department hears a client and a family member arguing with each other in a room at the end of the unit. What should the nurse do **first**?
   1. Get another staff member and go to the room together.
   2. Have a security guard handle the situation.
   3. Ask what is going on and then set limits.
   4. Go to the room and try to intervene.

11. Warm compresses are prescribed to be applied to the insertion site of an intravenous catheter that had become red and inflamed. What should the nurse explain to the client is the desired outcome of this therapy?
   1. "The area will feel less tense, which will decrease the risk of bleeding."
   2. "Circulation to the area will increase, which will promote healing."
   3. "Circulation to the area will decrease, which will limit edema."
   4. "The area will feel numb, which will decrease discomfort."

12. A nurse is caring for a client who has a prescription for a vest restraint. Which actions should the nurse implement? **Select all that apply.**
   1. Check the restraint every 2 hours.
   2. Release the restraint every 4 hours.
   3. Tie the restraint to the movable part of the bed frame.
   4. Provide skin care every 3 hours when a client has a restraint.
   5. Ensure that the cross-over of the vest restraint is in the front of the client.

13. Which intervention is effective in reducing the major cause of injury in the hospital setting for clients who are older adults?
   1. Assist all older adults with toileting activities.
   2. Elevate all bedside rails of older adults at night.
   3. Place a fall precaution sign on the door to a room with an older adult.
   4. Identify medications taken by an older adult that may increase the risk of falls.

14. A nurse just finished a complete bath for a client with limited mobility. Which action is **most** important for the nurse to perform before leaving the bedside of the client?
   1. Raise all of the bedside rails.
   2. Ensure that the water pitcher has fresh water.
   3. Lower the height of the bed to the lowest position.
   4. Position the bedpan in easy reach under the covers.

15. A nurse is caring for a client who is hearing impaired and legally blind. What should the nurse do to prevent a sensory deficit? **Select all that apply.**
   1. Encourage the client to wear prescribed hearing aids.
   2. Provide a telephone, radio, and talking books.
   3. Encourage purchase of a talking watch.
   4. Provide a foot bath and back massage.
   5. Speak in a high tone of voice.

16. A nurse is caring for a 60-year-old adult who is a resident in a rehabilitation center recovering from a right-sided brain attack (cerebrovascular accident, stroke). The client has a prescription for out-of-bed ambulating with assistance as tolerated. Which intervention is **most** important?
    1. Assessing balance
    2. Using a bed alarm
    3. Encouraging the use of a walker
    4. Teaching to rise slowly from a sitting to standing position

17. A nurse is caring for a client who is blind. What should the nurse do to facilitate client safety? **Select all that apply.**
    1. Encourage the client to have a bed bath rather than a shower.
    2. Walk about a foot ahead and have the client grasp your arm.
    3. Provide a small light in the room and bathroom at night.
    4. Remain nearby when the client is providing self-care.
    5. Orient the client to the physical environment.
    6. Provide cold rather than hot drinks.

18. A nurse is caring for a client who fell by the side of the bed when attempting to use a commode. What should the nurse do **first** when completing responsibilities associated with this situation?
    1. Initiate an incident report.
    2. Notify the nursing supervisor of the event.
    3. Document the incident in the client's clinical record.
    4. Have a primary health-care provider examine the client immediately.

19. Which nursing actions should the nurse implement when ambulating a client with a gait belt? **Select all that apply.**
    1. Position yourself slightly behind and next to the client when ambulating a client with a gait belt.
    2. Adjust the gait belt so that no fingers can be inserted between the belt and the client's waist.
    3. Stand on the client's weaker side when ambulating a client with a gait belt.
    4. Assess for activity intolerance while ambulating a client with a gait belt.
    5. Hold the gait belt in the middle of the client's back.

20. A nurse is caring for a client with wrist restraints. Which actions should the nurse implement when caring for this client? **Select all that apply.**
    1. Release the restraints every 3 hours and provide skin care.
    2. Provide additional padding when applying a wrist restraint.
    3. Offer fluids and assist the client to toilet every time the restraints are released.
    4. Check on the client every hour and ensure that circulation is not impaired by the restraints.
    5. Ensure that every 24 hours the primary health-care provider assesses the need for the restraints.

21. A nurse working on the night shift in a long-term care facility identifies a small fire in a magazine rack in the corner of a community lounge. Because all of the residents are in their rooms, the nurse activates the fire alarm and then instructs staff members to close all doors on the unit. The nurse then obtains a fire extinguisher to fight the fire. Place the following steps in the order in which they should be implemented.
    1. Pull the pin on the extinguisher.
    2. Drag the extinguisher on the floor to the area of the fire.
    3. Aim the nozzle of the extinguisher at the base of the flames.
    4. Squeeze the handles together to discharge water from the extinguisher.
    5. Sweep the nozzle of the extinguisher back and forth at the base of the flames.
    Answer: _____

22. A nurse is completing a client assessment for the purpose of determining factors that place the client at risk for falls. Which factor should cause the **most** concern when completing this assessment?
    1. Uses a walker
    2. Has a history of falls
    3. Takes a diuretic twice a day
    4. Has a urinary retention catheter

23. A nurse is teaching a class for a community group about how to prevent the **most** common cause of fatal accidents in the home. Which information is important to include that addresses this concern?
    1. Remove scatter rugs.
    2. Check for the presence of lead paint.
    3. Use gates at the bottom and top of stairs.
    4. Store cleaning products in a locked cabinet.

24. A hospitalized older adult who has left-sided weakness as the result of a brain attack (stroke, cerebrovascular accident) has the need to urinate several times during the night. What should the nurse do to ensure client safety?
    1. Encourage the use a bedpan at night.
    2. Keep the light on in the room at night.
    3. Assist the client to a commode at night.
    4. Encourage the client to use a walker at night.

25. An older adult is admitted to the hospital in heart failure. An IV of dextrose 5% water to infuse at 50 mL/hr is prescribed. The nurse uses a microdrip infusion set that has a drop factor of 60. At what rate should the nurse administer the intravenous solution? **Record your answer using a whole number.**
    Answer: _____ drops per minute

26. A home health-care nurse is visiting a client recently discharged from the hospital to the home. The client has a history of violence. What is important for the nurse to do when caring for this client?
    1. Apply restraints if the client engages in threatening behavior.
    2. Administer a prescribed sedative before providing client care.
    3. Identify when the level of anxiety is elevating.
    4. Use gentle touch communicating acceptance.

27. A nurse is transferring a weak, older adult from a bed to a toilet using the apparatus in the illustration. What is the **most** important reason why a nurse uses this device rather than a gait belt to transfer a client to a toilet?
    1. Encourage independence
    2. Protect the nurse from injury
    3. Promote muscle development
    4. Support psychological well-being

28. A client is confused and trying to pull out an indwelling urinary catheter. The nurse tried various interventions to protect the client from pulling out the catheter to no avail. The nurse notifies the primary health-care provider and asks for a prescription for a restraint. What type of restraint should the nurse anticipate will be prescribed?
    1. Belt
    2. Mitt
    3. Vest
    4. Wrist

29. Which actions are essential when maintaining standard precautions? **Select all that apply.**
    1. Putting on a gown when changing soiled linen
    2. Disposing of soiled tissues in a water-impervious bag
    3. Wearing gloves during contact with a client's body fluids
    4. Donning a mask with an eye shield when entering a client's room
    5. Washing hands with antimicrobial gel when hands are visibly soiled

30. A nurse is ambulating a client in the hall several rooms away from the client's room. During the walk, the client states, "I feel so dizzy and weak; I don't think that I will make it back to the room." What action should be implemented at this time?
    1. Return the client to bed quickly.
    2. Lower the client to the floor gently.
    3. Walk toward the client's room slowly.
    4. Call another nurse to assist with the client immediately.

REVIEW ANSWERS AND RATIONALES

1. ANSWER: 1, 2, 3, 5.
Rationales:
1. The site of the restraint should be checked every 30 minutes to ensure that circulation and/or breathing are not affected depending on the type of restraint as well as the client's response to the restraint.
2. Removing the wrist restraint should occur at least every 2 hours and more frequently if determined to be necessary. In addition, when restraints are released, skin care should be provided to promote tissue integrity.
3. Well-padded wrist restraints help to prevent injury to the wrists.
4. Three finger-widths between the client's wrist and the restraint will make the restraint too loose. Two finger-widths are sufficient to ensure that the client's circulation is not impaired and yet tight enough for the restraints to remain secured around the client's wrists.
5. A slip knot should be used to permit a quick release of the straps in the event of an emergency. Tying the straps of the wrist restraints to the immovable frame of the bed protects the client from injury when the bed position is altered or the side rails are raised or lowered.
TEST-TAKING TIP: Identify the clang association. The words *apply wrist restraints* in the stem and *applying wrist restraints* in option 3 is a clang association. Examine option 3 carefully. Also, the word *wrist* in the stem and in options 2, 3, and 5 are clang associations.
Content Area: Safety
Integrated Processes: Nursing Process: Implementation
Client Need: Safe and Effective Care Environment; Safety and Infection Control
Cognitive Level: Application
Concept: Safety

2. ANSWER: 4, 5.
Rationales:
1. It is not necessary to position the chair as close as possible to the client's bed. Mechanical lifts are designed to move a client completely across a room safely.
2. The sling remains under the client after the transfer. It would be difficult or even impossible to remove and then reposition the sling if the client were obese or immobile.
3. The sling should start at the shoulders and end at the knees. This completely supports the client for the transfer. If it is too high, the client could slide out from the bottom of the sling. If it is too low, the client could slide out from the top of the sling.
4. Spreading the legs of the lift apart widens the base of support increasing stability of the lift.
5. Attaching the longer straps to the lower grommets in each side of the sling is correct. When the longer straps are attached to the bottom of the sling and the shorter straps are attached to the top of the sling, the client will be raised to a sitting position when the lift raises the sling and the client up and off the bed.
TEST-TAKING TIP: Identify the clang associations. The word *chair* in the stem and options 1 and 4 as well as the word *lift* in the stem and in option 4 are clang

associations. Examine options 1 and 4 carefully. Option 4 has two clang associations.
Content Area: Safety
Integrated Processes: Nursing Process: Implementation
Client Need: Safe and Effective Care Environment; Safety and Infection Control
Cognitive Level: Analysis
Concept: Safety

3. ANSWER: 4.
Rationales:
1. Dark-tinted eyeglasses will not benefit a client who "can't see anything."
2. Keeping a light on in the room may help a client with partial vision, but it will be insignificant for a client who "can't see anything."
3. Closing window blinds will be beneficial for a client with partial vision who is affected by glare; this intervention will not benefit a client who "can't see anything."
4. A client who is in a strange environment and who has a visual impairment is at an increased risk for falls. The client should seek assistance with transfers and ambulating until the client feels comfortable engaging in these activities and the nurse determines that the client is safe to perform this activity unassisted.
TEST-TAKING TIP: Identify the option with a specific determiner. Option 2 contains the specific determiner *all*. Identify the unique option. Option 4 is unique because it is the only option that involves another person and it is the only option that does not engage in adjusting the light in the room. Identify options that are equally plausible. Options 1 and 3 are equally plausible. Both reduce light that meets the eye. Option 1 is no better than option 3. Eliminate both from further consideration.
Content Area: Safety
Integrated Processes: Teaching/Learning; Nursing Process: Implementation
Client Need: Safe and Effective Care Environment; Safety and Infection Control
Cognitive Level: Application
Concept: Safety

4. ANSWER: 4, 3, 1, 2, 5.
Rationales:
4. A bed-exiting alarm device will signal caregivers when the client attempts to exit the bed. These devices do not restrict the client's movement but will alert staff members that the client needs supervision. This is a safety device that does not require a prescription from a primary health-care provider.
3. Although four side rails will confine the client to the bed, the client is still able to turn and sit up with ease.
1. A cloth vest permits turning from side to side and sitting up but physically restricts the client to the bed by the use of straps tied to the bed frame.
2. Two wrist restraints restrict the movement of the upper extremities and prevent turning from side to side; also, they confine the client to the bed because the straps are tied to the bed frame.

5. A four-point restraint is the most restrictive physical restraint because the extremities are for all practical purposes immobilized; all four extremities are tied to the bed frame.

Content Area: Safety
Integrated Processes: Nursing Process: Analysis
Client Need: Safe and Effective Care Environment; Safety and Infection Control
Cognitive Level: Analysis
Concept: Safety

5. ANSWER: 3, 4, 5, 6.
Rationales:
1. A chemical restraint should be used as a last resort. Clients have a right to have the least restrictive restraint used to promote safety.
2. A vest restraint is too restrictive a device to use before a less restrictive method is proven unsuccessful.
3. A radio frequency product worn on the wrist or ankle or as a pendant alerts the caregiver when a client approaches an area of egress that is unsafe for the client.
4. Restricting fluids several hours before bedtime may reduce the need to void during the night. A cognitively impaired person may feel the need to void during the night and exit the bed to find a bathroom.
5. A bed-exiting device (e.g., position sensor on the leg, weight sensor under the mattress of a bed) should be used to alert caregivers when the client is attempting to exit the bed. A health team member should immediately assist the client and maintain safety when the alarm sounds.
6. Caffeine is a stimulant. Removing caffeine products from the diet may help reduce wandering at night.
Content Area: Safety
Integrated Processes: Nursing Process: Implementation
Client Need: Safe and Effective Care Environment; Safety and Infection Control
Cognitive Level: Application
Concept: Safety

6. ANSWER: 1.
Rationales:
1. The client's serum sodium (expected range 135 to 145 mEq/L) and potassium (expected range 3.5 to 5.0 mEq/L) are both low, which precipitates muscle weakness. The strength of the client's legs should be assessed to determine if the client can bear the body's weight. While the client is lying in bed, the client can be asked to exert pressure against the nurse's hands that are pressed against the soles of the client's feet. The nurse should assess the strength of the pressure exerted by the client. While the client is sitting on the side of the bed, the client can be instructed to extend the knee of one leg and hold it in extension for 15 seconds. Then the other leg should be assessed in the same manner. If the client can hold the legs in extension, then the client probably has the strength to bear the body's weight.
2. Taking the blood pressure while the client is supine is an incomplete assessment. When assessing the blood pressure to determine a client's risk of falls, the nurse should obtain orthostatic blood pressures. The client's blood pressure should be obtained while lying in bed, sitting up, and when standing. The client is experiencing orthostatic hypotension when the blood pressure drops to the level where it causes transient hypotension resulting in lightheadedness and dizziness (syncope).
3. The administration of oxygen is a dependent function of a nurse. Nurses may administer oxygen in an emergency situation, but this is not an emergency situation.
4. It is not necessary to interrupt the intravenous infusion. A client can be ambulated safely while receiving intravenous fluid therapy.
Content Area: Safety
Integrated Processes: Nursing Process: Implementation
Client Need: Safe and Effective Care Environment; Safety and Infection Control
Cognitive Level: Analysis
Concept: Patient-Centered Care; Safety

7. ANSWER: 1, 3, 5.
Rationales:
1. All residents in a home should develop a home fire escape plan. It includes the number of the local fire department on all phones, routes to take to exit each room of the home safely, and place to meet outside the home after exiting the home.
2. Residents should avoid smoking inside or near the entrances and exits to the home. This prevents accidently setting a fire in the home.
3. A smoke detector near the stairs will detect smoke from a fire as it rises. A smoke detector near bedrooms should alert people who are sleeping because of the close proximity of the alarm.
4. A Class ABC fire extinguisher, not a Class A fire extinguisher should be used in a kitchen. The water in a Class A fire extinguisher can cause a grease fire in the kitchen to spread. Also the water in a Class A fire extinguisher can conduct electricity and should avoid being used in a kitchen because many appliances are electric. A Class A fire extinguisher is appropriate for wood, paper, and cloth fires.
5. When a person's clothing is on fire the person should Stop, Drop, and Roll. Stopping limits movement that may fan the flames. Dropping positions the body on the ground in preparation for the next step in the firefighting technique. Rolling helps to deprive the fire of oxygen.
TEST-TAKING TIP: Identify the option with a specific determiner. Option 2 contains the word *just*, which is a specific determiner. Identify the clang associations. The word *fire* in the stem and in options 1 and 5 are clang associations.
Content Area: Safety
Integrated Processes: Teaching/Learning; Nursing Process: Planning
Client Need: Safe and Effective Care Environment; Safety and Infection Control
Cognitive Level: Analysis
Concept: Safety

8. ANSWER: 2, 4, 5.
Rationales:
1. Although wearing an identification band will provide for client safety, it does not give the client a sense of control.

2. Instructing the client how to lock the wheels on a wheelchair allows the client to provide safe self-care when in a wheelchair.

3. Keeping the client's bed in the lowest position will not give the client a sense of control.

4. The ability to call for help when needed gives the client a sense of control.

5. Having an understanding of the environment (e.g., how to use a call bell, how to raise and lower the bed, and how to use the side rails when turning or transferring) gives the client a sense of control.

Content Area: Safety
Integrated Processes: Teaching/Learning; Nursing Process: Implementation
Client Need: Safe and Effective Care Environment; Safety and Infection Control
Cognitive Level: Analysis
Concept: Safety

9. **ANSWER: 4, 5, 6.**
Rationales:

1. The semi-Fowler position may result in dislodgement of the implant, inappropriately exposing the nurse and client to the source of radiation. The supine position will help maintain the implant in the vaginal vault.

2. The nurse, not the client, should wear a radiation film badge.

3. When in the room, the nurse should stand across the room or at the head of the bed when giving care. When possible, the nurse should talk with the client through an intercom outside the room or from the doorway. These actions adhere to the principles of distance and shielding.

4. A lead apron provides a barrier between the nurse and the source of the radiation; it adheres to the principle of shielding.

5. Thirty-minute visits daily and sitting by the door protect a visitor from excessive exposure to radiation emanating from the client; these parameters follow the principles of time and distance.

6. All soiled linen should be held in the room until surveyed by radiation safety staff. This ensures that linen is safe for removal from the room.

Content Area: Safety
Integrated Processes: Nursing Process: Implementation
Client Need: Safe and Effective Care Environment; Safety and Infection Control
Cognitive Level: Application
Concept: Safety

10. **ANSWER: 1.**
Rationales:

1. The situation needs to be assessed, but a health team member should never enter a volatile situation alone. When entering the room, the health team members should stand between the client/visitor and the door.

2. Having a security guard handle the situation is premature and may cause the situation to escalate.

3. The nurse is in a vulnerable, unsafe position when going to a volatile situation alone. Setting limits may be unnecessary or may escalate an already volatile situation. Setting

limits should not be attempted without adequate staff members readily available.

4. The nurse is in a vulnerable, unsafe position when going to a volatile situation alone. Attempting to intervene may result in harm to the nurse.

TEST-TAKING TIP: Identify the word in the stem that sets a priority. The word *first* in the stem sets a priority. Identify options that are opposites. Options 1 and 4 are opposites. In option 1 the nurse gets another staff member to go to the room together. In option 4 the nurse goes to the room alone.

Content Area: Safety
Integrated Processes: Nursing Process: Implementation
Client Need: Safe and Effective Care Environment; Safety and Infection Control
Cognitive Level: Application
Concept: Violence

11. **ANSWER: 2.**
Rationales:

1. The application of heat causes vasodilation, which may increase the potential for bleeding. Cold applications cause vasoconstriction, which decreases the risk for bleeding.

2. Heat causes vasodilation, which increases circulation and capillary permeability in the area; this brings oxygen, nutrients, and WBCs to the area and removes toxic wastes.

3. Circulation to the area decreases with an application of cold, not heat.

4. The application of cold, not heat, influences nerve endings and precipitates an anesthetic effect, which decreases pain.

TEST-TAKING TIP: Identify options that are opposites. Options 2 and 3 are opposites.

Content Area: Safety
Integrated Processes: Communication and Documentation; Nursing Process: Evaluation
Client Need: Safe and Effective Care Environment; Safety and Infection Control
Cognitive Level: Application
Concept: Inflammation

12. **ANSWER: 3, 5.**
Rationales:

1. A client with a restraint should be checked every 30 minutes, not every 2 hours, to ensure client safety. The restraint should not be too tight or too loose. The nurse should check the client's circulation and ensure that there is room to insert two finger-widths between the restraint and the client.

2. Restraints should be released every 2, not 4, hours so that the client can receive exercise and skin care.

3. A vest restraint should be tied to the movable part of the bed frame. If the restraint is tied to the immovable part of the bedframe, the client may be injured or the restraint may become too tight and impair respirations when the head of the bed is raised. If the head of the bed is lowered, the restraint will become too loose.

4. Skin care should be provided every 2, not 3, hours when a restraint is removed and range-of-motion exercises provided.

5. The cross-over of a vest restraint should be in the front of the client, not the back. If the vest was applied with the cross-over in the back and the client should slide down in the bed, the collar edge could choke the client.

TEST-TAKING TIP: Identify options with specific determiners. Options 1, 2, and 4 contain the word *every*, which is a specific determiner. Rarely are options with specific determiners the correct answer. Identify the clang association. The word *vest* in the stem and in option 5 is a clang association. Examine option 5 carefully.

Content Area: Safety
Integrated Processes: Nursing Process: Implementation
Client Need: Safe and Effective Care Environment; Safety and Infection Control
Cognitive Level: Application
Concept: Safety

13. ANSWER: 4.
Rationales:
1. Assisting all older adults with toileting activities is not client centered. Not all older adults need to be assisted with toileting activities. This promotes dependence and violates the client's right to privacy if assistance is unnecessary.
2. Elevating all bedside rails of older adults at night is not client centered. Not all older adults need all side rails raised at night. Side rails are considered a restraint when all of them are raised. Unless it is requested by the client, the use of all side rails requires a prescription from a primary health-care provider for a specific reason that is documented.
3. Placing a fall precaution sign on the door to a room with an older adult is not client centered. Not all older adults require fall precautions beyond the average interventions implemented to maintain physical safety for all adult clients. In addition, a sign indicating fall precaution violates the client's right to privacy. Facilities generally use a sign such as a flower to indicate to staff that a client is at risk for falls.
4. Assessment is the first step in the nursing process. Assessments should be completed before planning and implementing care. Older adults often experience one or more chronic illness and receive a variety of medications. Polypharmacy is a risk factor for adverse reactions and drug interactions that may cause an older adult to fall.

TEST-TAKING TIP: Identify options with specific determiners. Options 1 and 2 contain the word *all*, which is a specific determiner. More often than not, options with specific determiners are distractors. Identify options that deny clients' feelings, concerns, and needs. Options 1 and 2 deny clients the right to be independent. Identify the option that is client centered. Option 4 is client centered because it involves an assessment specific to the client. Identify the unique option. Option 4 is unique. Options 1, 2, and 3 are interventions designed to reduce a fall. Option 4 is the only option that is an assessment. Assessment is the first step of the nursing process.

Content Area: Safety
Integrated Processes: Nursing Process: Assessment

Client Need: Safe and Effective Care Environment; Safety and Infection Control
Cognitive Level: Application
Concept: Medication; Safety

14. ANSWER: 3.
Rationales:
1. Raising all the side rails on a bed is considered a restraint. It can be requested by the client or prescribed by the primary health-care provider if necessary. This prescription must be rewritten every 24 hours. A progress note must address the reasons for the restraint and what other measures were tried that were ineffective.
2. Although it is important for a client to have fresh water and ice if preferred and permitted, it is not as important as another option.
3. All clients should have their beds maintained in the lowest position unless a member of the health-care team is providing direct care. This supports client safety. It enables mobile clients to more easily enter and exit the bed. Also, if a client should fall out of bed accidentally, the bed is closer to the floor, which may minimize client injury.
4. A client with limited mobility generally will not be able to use a bedpan unassisted.

TEST-TAKING TIP: Identify the word in the stem that sets a priority. The word *most* in the stem sets a priority. Identify the option with a specific determiner. Option 1 contains the word *all,* which is a specific determiner.

Content Area: Safety
Integrated Processes: Nursing Process: Implementation
Client Need: Safe and Effective Care Environment; Safety and Infection Control
Cognitive Level: Application
Concept: Safety

15. ANSWER: 1, 2, 3, 4.
Rationales:
1. Hearing aids will enhance hearing, which should help prevent the sense of isolation.
2. A telephone, radio, and talking books will help to stimulate the client (e.g., hearing, thinking, socialization).
3. When a button is pushed, a talking watch reports the time. This will help to keep the client oriented to time, which is stimulating.
4. A foot bath and back massage will provide for tactile interaction with the caregiver, increasing stimulation.
5. People with impaired hearing tend to have a reduced ability to hear high-pitched tones. The nurse should use a lower tone when speaking with a client who is hearing impaired.

TEST-TAKING TIP: Identify the clang association. The word *hearing* in the stem and in option 1 is a clang association. Examine option 1 carefully.

Content Area: Safety
Integrated Processes: Communication and Documentation; Nursing Process: Implementation
Client Need: Psychosocial Integrity
Cognitive Level: Application
Concept: Sensory Perception

16. ANSWER: 1.
Rationales:

1. Assessment is the first step of the nursing process. The nurse must first assess the client for the presence of problems with strength and balance before moving a client out of bed. People with problems with balance may not be able to maintain the sitting position while sitting on the side of the bed.

2. A bed alarm is unnecessary. There is no information in the stem that indicates that the client is confused or unwilling to call for assistance when getting out of bed.

3. Encouraging the use of a walker is implementing an intervention before the client's needs are assessed.

4. Although teaching a client to rise slowly from a sitting to standing position should be done, it is not as critical as another option.

TEST-TAKING TIP: Identify the word in the stem that sets a priority. The word *most* in the stem sets a priority. Identify the option that is unique. Option 1 is the only option that is an assessment. Options 2, 3, and 4 identify actions to prevent a fall.

Content Area: Safety
Integrated Processes: Nursing Process: Implementation
Client Need: Safe and Effective Care Environment; Safety and Infection Control
Cognitive Level: Application
Concept: Safety

17. ANSWER: 2, 4, 5.
Rationales:

1. With guidance or supervision, a client who is blind can shower safely.

2. Walking about a foot ahead and having the client grasp your arm is the proper way to assist a client who is blind with ambulation. By walking slightly ahead and with the client holding the nurse's arm, the nurse is able to guide the client around obstacles.

3. The client is blind. A nightlight will not help this client to see.

4. Remaining nearby enables the caregiver to intervene if the client's safety is jeopardized.

5. Orienting the client to where furniture and equipment are located in the room provides a frame of reference for the client.

6. Clients who are blind have a right to have hot drinks, such as coffee, tea, or soup. With guidance, they can be instructed regarding the location of hot drinks. In addition, suggesting the use of a commuter cup is a reasonable accommodation to help prevent spilling a hot drink, which may cause a burn.

Content Area: Safety
Integrated Processes: Nursing Process: Implementation
Client Need: Safe and Effective Care Environment; Safety and Infection Control
Cognitive Level: Application
Concept: Safety

18. ANSWER: 4.
Rationales:

1. Initiating an incident report is not the priority intervention when a client falls. However, this should be done eventually.

2. Although a nursing supervisor should be notified, it is not the first nursing responsibility associated with a client falling.

3. Documenting the incident in the client's clinical record is not the priority intervention when a client falls. However, eventually the incident should be documented in the client's clinical record.

4. Having a primary health-care provider examine the client immediately is the first action that the nurse should implement. The client needs to be examined by a primary health-care provider to ensure that the client has not sustained an injury.

TEST-TAKING TIP: Identify the clang association. The words *first* in the stem and *immediately* in option 4 is an obscure clang association. These words are closely related because they both are associated with the concept of a priority.

Content Area: Safety
Integrated Processes: Nursing Process: Implementation
Client Need: Safe and Effective Care Environment; Management of care
Cognitive Level: Application
Concept: Safety

19. ANSWER: 1, 3, 4, 5.
Rationales:

1. The caregiver should walk slightly behind and next to the client being ambulated with a gait belt. This enables the caregiver to hold the belt handle in the center of the back as well as grab the handle on the side if the client needs more assistance with balance.

2. A belt that does not allow fingers to be inserted between the belt and the client's body may cause discomfort and impair breathing. Three fingers should be able to be positioned between the belt and the client.

3. Walking on the client's weaker side provides better support of the client when the client shifts weight to the weaker side when ambulating.

4. Clients who need a gait belt when being ambulated generally have impaired balance or are weak and, therefore, must be assessed for clinical indicators of activity intolerance. It is not acceptable to just make this assessment after the completion of ambulation.

5. Holding a gait belt at the location of the client's back allows the caregiver to quickly control the client's balance.

TEST-TAKING TIP: Identify clang associations. The word *ambulating* in the stem and in options 1, 3 and 4 are clang associations.

Content Area: Safety
Integrated Processes: Nursing Process: Evaluation
Client Need: Safe and Effective Care Environment; Safety and Infection Control
Cognitive Level: Application
Concept: Safety

20. ANSWER: 2, 3, 5.
Rationales:

1. Restraints must be released every 2, not 3, hours.

2. Additional padding when applying a wrist restraint protects bony prominences from pressure and tissue abrasion.

3. When a restraint is removed, the nurse should assess for the presence of edema, capillary refill, sensation, function, skin integrity, and erythema. In addition, the client should be offered fluids and the opportunity to go to the bathroom. Finally, skin care and range-of-motion exercises should be provided and the client's position changed before restraints are reapplied.

4. Circulation should be checked every 30 minutes, not every hour.

5. A primary health-care provider must renew the prescription for restraints every 24 hours. In addition, a progress note should indicate why the restraint is still needed.

TEST-TAKING TIP: Identify the options with specific determiners. Options 1, 3, 4, and 5 contain the word *every*, which is a specific determiner; examine these options carefully because they are not all distractors. The word *wrist* in the stem and in option 2 is a clang association. Examine option 2 carefully.

Content Area: Safety
Integrated Processes: Nursing Process: Implementation
Client Need: Safe and Effective Care Environment; Safety and Infection Control
Cognitive Level: Application
Concept: Safety

21. ANSWER: 2, 1, 3, 4, 5.
Rationales:
2. An extinguisher can be heavy, and it is an acceptable practice to drag a fire extinguisher on the floor to the site of a fire.
1. Follow the acronym PASS. *Pulling* the pin between the handles is the first step when using an extinguisher and prepares the extinguisher for use.
3. Follow the acronym PASS. *Aiming* the nozzle of the extinguisher at the base of the flames is the second step when using an extinguisher. The base of a fire is the source of the flames.
4. Follow the acronym PASS. *Squeezing* the handles together to discharge the contents from the extinguisher is the third step when using an extinguisher.
5. Follow the acronym PASS. *Sweeping* the nozzle of the extinguisher back and forth across the base of the flames is the fourth step in using an extinguisher. This ensures that the discharge from the extinguisher makes contact with the entire source of the fire.

Content Area: Safety
Integrated Processes: Nursing Process: Planning
Client Need: Safe and Effective Care Environment; Safety and Infection Control
Cognitive Level: Analysis
Concept: Safety

22. ANSWER: 2.
Rationales:
1. Although a client using a walker is a concern in relation to safety, it is a less significant predictor of the potential for a fall than another option.
2. Most assessment tools indicate that a history of a recent fall is a significant factor regarding the risk for a future fall.

3. Although a client receiving a diuretic is at risk for hypotension, which is a concern, it is a less significant predictor of the potential for a fall than another option.
4. Although a urinary retention catheter is a concern in relation to safety, it is a less significant predictor of the potential for a fall than another option.

TEST-TAKING TIP: Identify the word in the stem that sets a priority. The word *most* in the stem sets a priority. Identify the clang association. The word *fall* in the stem and in option 2 is a clang association. Examine option 2 carefully.

Content Area: Safety
Integrated Processes: Nursing Process: Assessment
Client Need: Safe and Effective Care Environment; Safety and Infection Control
Cognitive Level: Application
Concept: Safety

23. ANSWER: 4.
Rationales:
1. Although it is important to remove scatter rugs from the home to prevent falls, falls are the third-leading cause of accidental deaths in the home.
2. Although it is important to check for the presence of lead paint in the home, it is not one of the top five leading causes of accidental death.
3. According to the National Safety Council, falls are the third leading cause of accidental death. It is important to teach the use of gates at the bottom and top of stairs until children can negotiate stairs safely.
4. Accidental poisoning and unintentional overdose are the *leading* causes of death in the *home* and are the *second* leading cause of death after motor vehicle accidents *overall*. Household cleaners are followed by medicine, houseplants, cosmetics, pesticides, kerosene, gasoline, furniture polish, lighter fluid, and other chemicals. The five leading causes of accidental death are motor vehicle accidents, accidental poisoning, falls, choking/suffocation, and drowning.

TEST-TAKING TIP: Identify the word in the stem that sets a priority. The word *most* in the stem sets a priority. Identify the key words in the stem that direct attention to content. The key words in the stem that direct attention to content are *fatal accidents in the home*.

Content Area: Safety
Integrated Processes: Teaching/Learning; Nursing Process: Implementation
Client Need: Health Promotion and Maintenance
Cognitive Level: Application
Concept: Health Promotion; Safety

24. ANSWER: 3.
Rationales:
1. Using a bedpan limits mobility, does not let the client assume the best position for voiding, and unnecessarily limits the client's independence.
2. Although having a night light on in the room at night helps with orientation, it does not provide as well for the client's safety needs as another option; the client has a problem with mobility, not vision.
3. The nurse should assist clients who are unstable or have impaired mobility. A commode at the bedside

limits the energy the client needs to expend at night when the risk for falls escalates.

4. Although a walker may help with client stability, the client should not be performing this activity independently, especially at night when the risk for falls escalates.

Content Area: Safety
Integrated Processes: Nursing Process: Implementation
Client Need: Safe and Effective Care Environment; Safety and Infection Control
Cognitive Level: Application
Concept: Safety

25. **ANSWER: 50.**
Rationale:

A microdrip infusion set is more accurate and safer to use than a macrodrip infusion set when administering small volumes of intravenous solutions. A microdrip infusion set delivers 60 drops per milliliter, whereas a macrodrip infusion set delivers 10 or 15 drops per milliliter, depending on the manufacturer.

$$\frac{\text{Volume to be infused} \times \text{drop factor}}{\text{Total time in minutes}}$$

$$\frac{50\ (\text{mL}) \times 60\ (\text{drop factor})}{60\ (\text{minutes in 1 hour})} = \frac{3{,}000}{60} = 50 \text{ drops per minute}$$

Content Area: Safety
Integrated Processes: Nursing Process: Planning
Client Need: Physiological Integrity; Pharmacological and Parenteral Therapies
Cognitive Level: Application
Concept: Medication; Safety

26. **ANSWER: 3.**
Rationales:

1. The nurse should not attempt to apply restraints in a client's home. The nurse should immediately leave the client's home and/or call 911 if the nurse feels in imminent danger.
2. This is not the first action of the nurse. Although the client has a history of violence, it does not mean that the client will be violent during this home visit.
3. **Identifying when the client's level of anxiety is increasing is the most important nursing action. Assessment is the first step of the nursing process. A client with a history of violence may resort to violence when coping with anxiety. As soon as a nurse identifies that the client's level of anxiety is elevating, the nurse should leave and return when the client is less anxious.**
4. The nurse should never touch a person with a history of violence without permission. Touch may be perceived as a threat and may precipitate a violent client reaction.

Content Area: Safety
Integrated Processes: Nursing Process: Assessment
Client Need: Safe and Effective Care Environment; Safety and Infection Control
Cognitive Level: Application
Concept: Violence

27. **ANSWER: 2.**
Rationales:

1. Although the client participates to some degree in a transfer with a sit-to-stand lift by partially bearing weight and holding onto the handles of the device, encouraging independence is not its primary purpose.
2. **Both the nurse and client are protected from injury when the nurse uses this device to transfer the client from a chair/bed to a commode/toilet. It is designed for individuals who can bear some weight in an upright position, but who are weak or recovering from surgery.**
3. Although weight bearing in the upright position and holding onto the handles of the sit-to-stand device may require muscle contraction promoting muscle strengthening, it is not its primary purpose.
4. Although the client participates to some degree in a transfer with a sit-to-stand lift by partially bearing weight and holding onto the handles of the device, encouraging independence and psychological well-being, it is not its primary purpose.

TEST-TAKING TIP: Identify the word in the stem that sets a priority. The word *most* in the stem sets a priority. Identify options that are equally plausible. Options 1 and 4 are equally plausible because they both address the psychosocial domain. Option 1 is no better than option 4. Eliminate both from further consideration. Identify the unique option. Option 2 is unique. It is the only option that addresses the nurse's need. Options 1, 3, and 4 address the client's needs.

Content Area: Safety
Integrated Processes: Nursing Process: Planning
Client Need: Safe and Effective Care Environment; Safety and Infection Control
Cognitive Level: Application
Concept: Safety

28. **ANSWER: 2.**
Rationales:

1. A belt restraint is applied around a client's abdomen and tied to the base of a bed or behind a chair to prevent a client from getting out of a bed or chair without assistance. The upper and lower extremities have free range of motion. It does not protect a client from pulling out a catheter.
2. **Mitt restraints are the least restrictive of the restraints presented in the options and are most appropriate for this client. A mitt restraint permits the client to move the upper extremities but will not permit the client to grasp a catheter.**
3. A vest restraint does not protect a client from pulling out a catheter. It protects the client from leaving a bed or chair without assistance. The upper arms and hands have free range of motion.
4. A wrist restraint is more restrictive than a restraint presented in another option. Although a wrist restraint may prevent pulling out a catheter, it unnecessarily prevents free range of motion of the upper extremities.

Content Area: Safety
Integrated Processes: Communication and Documentation; Nursing Process: Planning
Client Need: Safe and Effective Care Environment; Management of Care
Cognitive Level: Analysis
Concept: Safety

29. ANSWER: 2, 3.

Rationales:

1. A gown is not necessary to maintain standard precautions when changing soiled linen. However, the nurse should wear gloves and hold the linen away from the uniform to prevent contamination.

2. Soiled tissues are a reservoir (source) of microorganisms and need to be contained within an impervious bag.

3. A caregiver must always wear clean gloves when there is a likelihood of coming into contact with a client's body fluids, such as secretions, excretions, nonintact skin, mucous membranes, or contaminated items.

4. A mask with eye protection is only necessary if the caregiver is at risk for being splashed with the client's body fluids. A surgical mask is required within three feet of a client receiving droplet precautions, and an N95 respirator mask is required when entering a room with airborne precautions.

5. When hands are visibly soiled they must be vigorously washed with soap, water, and friction for a minimum of 15 seconds. Antimicrobial gel is sufficient for washing hands that are not visibly soiled.

Content Area: Safety
Integrated Processes: Nursing Process: Implementation
Client Need: Safe and Effective Care Environment; Safety and Infection Control
Cognitive Level: Application
Concept: Safety

30. ANSWER: 2.

Rationales:

1. Returning the client to bed quickly is inappropriate and unsafe. Rapid movements will exacerbate the client's feeling dizzy, and the client is feeling weak and will not be able to move quickly.

2. Lowering the client to the floor gently allows the nurse to prevent the client's head from hitting the floor. It controls the client's movement toward the floor, preventing injury to both the client and nurse.

3. Slowly walking back to the client's room when the client feels weak and dizzy may result in the client falling, injuring both the client and nurse.

4. Calling for another nurse to assist is an admirable intervention, but there may not be enough time for the nurse to arrive to be of assistance.

Content Area: Safety
Integrated Processes: Communication and Documentation; Nursing Process: Implementation
Client Need: Safe and Effective Care Environment; Safety and Infection Control
Cognitive Level: Application
Concept: Safety

Chapter 2

Communication, Collaboration, and Documentation

Collaboration
Communication
Informatics

Patient-Centered Care
Sensory Perception

KEY TERMS

Aphasia—Loss of or impairment in ability to communicate through speech, writing, or gestures

Channel of communication—Vehicle used to convey a message

Collaboration—Collegial working relationship among health-care professionals in the provision of client care

Communication—Dynamic, purposeful, reciprocal process of sending and/or receiving a message

Documentation—Act of creating a written record

Expressive aphasia—Inability to formulate and/or send a message

Feedback—Response from the receiver to the sender

Message—Information communicated

Nonverbal communication—Use of facial expression or other body language to convey a message

Plan of care—Written communication of strategies that should be implemented to meet client needs

Receiver—Person who acquires a message

Receptive aphasia—Inability to understand communicated information

Sender—Person who conveys a message

Therapeutic communication—Interaction between a nurse and a client in which the nurse focuses on the feelings, concerns, needs, and/or objectives of the client.

Verbal communication—Use of spoken or written words to communicate a message

I. Communication

Communication is a dynamic, purposeful, reciprocal process of sending and/or receiving a message. The need to communicate is universal because it is the way people convey and fulfill needs.

A. Concepts about communication
   1. All verbal communication and nonverbal communication transmits meaning.

   2. Communication is a learned process.
   3. Communication can occur within the self (intrapersonal); between two people (interpersonal); when sending a message (e.g., public speaking); or communicating within a group (e.g., self-help and social groups, and group therapy).
   4. Recurring ideas and thoughts (themes) communicated during an interaction provide insight to a client's feelings.

5. A trusting relationship is basic to effective communication.
6. A client's degree of expression (emotional affect) reflects the client's mood.
7. Humor is highly subjective; it can mean different things to different people.
8. Clients have a potential for growth as a result of verbal and nonverbal communication.
9. Previous patterns of communication can become inadequate when one is ill or under stress.
🛑 10. Communication is confidential information and should be shared only with health team members.

B. Elements of communication
   1. **Sender** (encoder/source): Person who conveys a message.
   2. **Message:** Information communicated; includes language, words, voice intonation, and gestures.
   3. **Channel of communication** (mode): Vehicle used to convey a message; includes written, oral, and touch.
   4. **Receiver** (decoder): Person who acquires a message.
   5. **Feedback** (response): Response from the receiver to the sender.

C. Factors affecting the communication process
   1. Attitudes, values, beliefs, and experiences.
   2. Culture, education, and language.
   3. Developmental level.
      a. The very young are concrete thinkers and have little or no experience.
      b. Adults are more abstract thinkers.
      c. Older adults may have vision and hearing loss that interferes with communication.
   4. Gender.
      a. Males and females generally communicate differently from an early age.
      b. Females seek intimacy and validation and reduce differences; boys use language to negotiate status and establish independence.
      c. Differences are changing as gender roles become less distinct.
   5. Authority one ascribes to a role (e.g., some see nurses as authority figures, whereas others see nurses as servants).
   6. Ineffective perception or selective inattention: May distort a message.

D. Barriers to communication
   1. Unwillingness to listen to another point of view.
   2. Physical factors, such as an uncomfortable environment (e.g., too hot or too cold), excessive noise, or distractions.
   3. Adaptation to disease, such as **aphasia,** an impaired ability to communicate through speech, writing, or signs because of brain dysfunction (e.g., receptive or expressive aphasia); impaired ability to say words

(dysarthria); impaired cognition (e.g., dementia or delirium); oral problems; fatigue; and pain.
   4. Treatment-related factors, such as laryngectomy, or artificial airways, such as tracheostomy or endotracheal tube.
   5. Psychological factors, such as lack of privacy, anxiety, and fear.

E. Phases of the communication process
   1. Preinteraction phase.
      a. This phase occurs before meeting the client.
      b. The nurse gathers information about the client.
   2. Orientation phase.
      a. Initially, the nurse is in the stranger role.
      b. The nurse meets a client and begins to establish a relationship of rapport and trust.
      c. Introductions and initial exchange of information occurs.
      d. The purpose of the visit is explained, roles are clarified, and an agreement or contract about the relationship may be formulated.
      e. The termination phase is initiated in this phase.
   3. Working phase.
      a. Most communication occurs during this phase.
      b. This phase is the active part of the relationship.
      c. The nurse and client work together to address client needs, feelings are shared, caring is demonstrated, and mutual respect is maintained.
      d. The nurse may function as caregiver, counselor, teacher, resource person, and so on.
      e. The nurse motivates a client by identifying progress and supporting movement toward independence.
      f. Anxiety may increase during this phase, as the client may need to learn new adaptive behaviors.
      g. Preparation for the termination phase continues.
   4. Termination phase.
      a. Actual termination occurs at the conclusion of a relationship.
      b. Termination occurs at discharge, at the end of a shift, or when the goals of the relationship are achieved.
      c. Goals and objectives are summarized, adaptive behavior is reinforced, and additional resources available are arranged for the client.
      d. Some clients become emotional during this phase because they feel angry, rejected, or fearful of leaving a safe environment; the nurse needs to address these feelings.

F. Modes of communication
   1. **Verbal communication:** Uses spoken or written words to communicate a message; characteristics include the:
      a. Clarity: Simple words and sentence structure are better understood.

b. Intonation: Reflects feeling behind words; loud or soft volume, cadence, and pitch can impart a message, such as anger, excitement, sarcasm, and fear.

c. Pacing: Speed, rhythm, and patterns of delivery can convey anxiety, indifference, and attention; pace must be fast enough to maintain interest but slow enough for receiver to decode the message.

d. Relevance: Message needs to be conveyed when the receiver is ready and able to receive the message; information has to be important to the client.

2. **Nonverbal communication:** Message that is sent and received without use of spoken or written words; involves use of body language; may be more accurate than verbal communication because it is less consciously controlled; characteristics include the following:

a. Facial expression: Can convey meaning or mask emotions; some expressions are universal, such as a smile (happiness) or a frown (displeasure); can be subtle, such as raising the eyebrows.

b. Gestures: Emphasize spoken word; some have same meaning regardless of culture, such as waving indicates hello or goodbye; different gestures may have similar meanings, such as shaking a fist versus cold, stillness when angry.

c. Eye contact: In Western cultures, indicates interest and attention, whereas downcast eyes may indicate low self-esteem, powerlessness, and sadness; however, in some cultures, downcast eyes show respect.

d. Posture and gait: Erect posture, head held up with a rapid gait indicates well-being and confidence; slumped, slow, shuffling gait with head held low indicates illness, depression, or impaired self-esteem; crossing legs and arms indicates a defensive posture.

e. Touch: Generally conveys caring, concern, encouragement; some clients do not like to be touched, and touching is unacceptable in some cultures (e.g., only relatives can touch an orthodox Jewish man).

f. Territoriality and space: People have a physical zone around the body that is culturally and individually defined.

(1) Intimate: 0 to 18 inches; used for providing nursing care or emotional support, such as hygiene and hand holding.

(2) Personal: 1.5 to 4 feet; used for therapeutic communication, such as nurse-client conversation, counseling, and teaching.

(3) Social and public: 4 feet and beyond; used when performing more formal interventions, such as making rounds, teaching a class, or facilitating a group.

II. Therapeutic Versus Nontherapeutic Communication

Therapeutic communication is interaction between a nurse and a client in which the nurse focuses on the feelings, concerns, needs, and/or objectives of the client. Nurses must develop a repertoire of verbal and nonverbal techniques that can be used to facilitate therapeutic communication as well as be aware of the various attitudes and approaches that can hinder communication. The therapeutic use of self is the most valuable tool that nurses have to facilitate therapeutic communication and ultimately develop an effective nurse-client relationship.

A. Therapeutic communication techniques and related nursing care: See Table 2.1

B. Nontherapeutic communication and preventive nursing care: See Table 2.2

III. Nursing Care Related to Communication

Effective communication is essential when developing a therapeutic relationship with clients. The nurse should communicate with all clients in a manner that supports respect and dignity using techniques that focus on the client and client needs. Basic principles that are common to communicating with all clients and principles related to nonverbal communication are presented.

A. Therapeutic use of self
1. Place oneself in the client's place mentally and emotionally (empathy).
2. Respect values and beliefs.
3. Maintain credibility and genuineness; be truthful, respond to needs promptly, and follow through on promises.
4. Use behaviors that exhibit active listening such as eye contact, caring facial expression, unhurried behavior, and open posture.
5. Ensure intonation and pace of words convey professional confidence, respect, interest, and acceptance of the client.

B. Environmental considerations that promote communication
1. Knock before entering a client's room, and ask permission before entering a client's closet or bedside drawer; these actions convey respect.
2. Provide privacy when communicating.
3. Reduce environmental noise and distractions.
4. Explain what is going to be done and why before entering a client's personal space; entering personal space may be perceived as a violation of a client's territory, and the client may feel uncomfortable, threatened, or anxious.

Table 2.1 Therapeutic Communication Techniques and Related Nursing Care

Therapeutic Communication Technique	Related Nursing Care
Silence • Provides time for the client to process what was said, reflect, and articulate a response. • Encourages the client to initiate or continue a conversation.	• Maintain an open posture. • Maintain an unhurried manner.
Offering Self • Indicates a nurse's attention and interest without expectations.	• Maintain an open posture. • Maintain an unhurried manner. • Example: Say, "I will sit with you for a while."
Open-Ended Questions • Allows the client to control the direction of the conversation to an area of concern.	• Ask questions that require more than one-word answers and invite a more detailed response. • Example: "Tell me about how you have been managing your illness."
Direct Questions • Facilitates collection of specific information. • May interfere with exploration of feelings because they may be too blunt and threatening.	• Keep questions short and simple. • Example: "Have you received the pneumococcal (PVC) vaccine?"
Paraphrasing • Encourages further discussion by repeating content in same or similar words. • Conveys that the message was understood. • Allows the client to hear what he or she said.	• Listen attentively. • Focus on content. • Example: The client says, "When I'm discharged, I might have a hard time because I live alone." The nurse responds, "You sound concerned about how you are going to manage."
Reflection • Encourages further discussion by focusing on emotional themes and feelings. • Indicates active listening. • Helps the client to identify emotional themes and feelings.	• Listen attentively. • Focus on feelings rather than content. • Example: The client says, "I don't understand how I had a heart attack. I don't smoke or eat fatty foods, and I exercise regularly." The nurse responds, "It must be frustrating to have a heart attack when you did everything right."
Clarifying • Encourages elaboration on unclear messages. • Ensures that the message is understood as intended; minimizes misunderstanding.	• Be nonjudgmental; do not place responsibility for lack of understanding on the client. • Example: "I don't understand what you mean when you say that your pain feels like melting lava."
Focusing • Directs conversation to areas of concern; targets discussion to key points. • Encourages the client to expand on an idea, thought, or feeling.	• Focus on the priority topic of concern. • Example: "Earlier you mentioned that you are having a problem with recurrent diarrhea."
Validating • Identifies and supports what the client feels or believes. • Demonstrates respect for the client. • Demonstrates empathy.	• Maintain a nonjudgmental, empathetic demeanor. • Example: "I can understand how difficult it must be to wait 5 days for a biopsy result."
Touch • Communicates caring, concern, and encouragement.	• Use touch cautiously because some clients prefer not to be touched, touch can be misunderstood, and touch invades a person's intimate space. • Examples: Hold a client's hand or place an arm around a client's shoulder.
Summarizing • Highlights important points in a conversation, such as progress made and tasks that may still need to be accomplished.	• Review just the most important points. • Provide a summary in writing when appropriate. • Example: "Let's review what we accomplished today."

Table 2.2 Nontherapeutic Communication and Preventive Nursing Care	
Nontherapeutic Communication	**Preventive Nursing Care**
Being Judgmental • *Imposes the nurse's opinions, values, beliefs, and standards on the client.* • *Demonstrates lack of respect for the client.*	• *Be aware of own values, beliefs, standards, and opinions and do not impose them on others.* • *Use words that demonstrate acceptance.* • *Maintain an empathetic demeanor.*
Using Medical Jargon • *Confuses clients.* • *Communicates that the nurse is not interested enough to make information understandable.* • *Demonstrates a demeanor of superiority and arrogance.*	• *Use words that can be understood; avoid use of medical jargon, such as medical terminology, acronyms, and slang.* • *Offer opportunities to ask questions; answer all questions to the client's satisfaction.* • *Seek feedback to ensure understanding.*
Using Ridicule or Sarcasm • *Conveys a hostile attitude through words, tone of voice, or actions.*	• *Avoid cutting, caustic, sarcastic, and hostile remarks.* • *Avoid gestures or actions that demean the client.*
Using Probing Questions • *Invades privacy because it attempts to obtain information to satisfy one's curiosity.* • *Pressures the client to discuss topics before he or she is ready.*	• *Ask questions based on the client's needs, not curiosity.* • *Use open-ended questions.*
Focusing on Self • *Demonstrates lack of interest in the client.* • *Demonstrates an attitude of self-importance and egocentricity.*	• *Remember that the client is the center of the health team.* • *Focus on the client's needs and not self-needs.*
Stereotyping • *Devalues client uniqueness and individuality.* • *Demonstrates opinions either blatantly or subtly, such as men who cry are not manly, and clients who are health-care professionals do not need health teaching.*	• *Assess own beliefs, such as stereotypes, biases, and prejudices, and ensure that they do not affect professional relationships.* • *Accept each client as unique.*
Changing the Subject • *Indicates lack of interest in the client's concerns or feelings.* • *Reflects that the nurse feels uncomfortable talking about the topic.* • *Cuts off communication when the client may be ready to discuss an emotionally charged topic.*	• *Identify health-care topics that cause anxiety within one's self and seek education or counseling to become therapeutic in the health-care role.* • *Listen attentively.* • *Focus on the client's concerns.*
Providing False Reassurance • *Minimizes the client's concerns.* • *Violates trust.*	• *Answer questions truthfully; base reassurance on facts.* • *Address underlying concerns.*
Minimizing Feelings • *Devalues the validity of the client's feelings.*	• *Use the communication technique of reflection.* • *Address feelings.*
Giving Advice • *Bases responses on one's own values and beliefs rather than on what is important to the client.* • *Limits the client's right to be a partner in problem-solving.* • *Supports dependence and is controlling.*	• *Assist the client to explore his or her own feelings, concerns, opinions, and options.* • *Assist the client to use critical thinking to arrive at a conclusion.*
Using Clichés, Colloquialisms, and Slang • *Trivializes the client's concerns.* • *Causes misunderstanding.*	• *Use words that the client can understand.* • *Avoid comments that may have ambiguous meanings or multiple interpretations.*
Using Terms of Endearment • *Demonstrates lack of respect.* • *Reflects an unprofessional demeanor.*	• *Call the client by his or her name.* • *Avoid use of intimate names (e.g., honey, dear, sweetie, mom, or pop).*
Responding Defensively by the Nurse • *Demonstrates the nurse's attempt to protect the self rather than focus on the client's concerns; defensive responses usually are precipitated by clients who are angry, demanding, or critical.* • *Minimizes the client's concerns.* • *Focuses on content rather than feelings.*	• *Identify the underlying cause of the client's behavior; clients' angry, demanding, or critical responses are attempts to protect the self; all behavior has meaning.* • *Focus on the client's feelings.* • *Involve the client in identifying a resolution, such as, "I am sorry that I did not meet your expectations. What can I do now to help you?"*

Continued

Table 2.2 Nontherapeutic Communication and Preventive Nursing Care—cont'd	
Nontherapeutic Communication	**Preventive Nursing Care**
Challenging the Client • *Requires the client to defend his or her feelings or point of view.* • *Ignores the client's feelings and rights.* • *Causes the client to abandon a coping mechanism that may be temporarily therapeutic.*	• *Accept the client's right to have his or her own feelings, beliefs, and point of view.* • *Support the client's coping mechanisms, unless they are destructive to self or others; abandoning a coping mechanism can leave a client defenseless.*
Asking "How" or "Why" • *Threatens or intimidates the client.* • *May leave the client unsure how to answer the question.*	• *Use open-ended questions.* • *Explore issues with the client so that he or she can develop insight and come to own conclusions about "how" or "why."*
Asking Too Many Questions • *Overwhelms the client emotionally and may invade the client's privacy or precipitate feelings of "being interrogated."* • *Overwhelms the client physically.*	• *Assess the client's physical and emotional stamina to engage in data collection.* • *Use several shorter sessions to collect data.*
Engaging in Nonprofessional Involvement • *Oversteps boundaries of the therapeutic nurse-client relationship.* • *Befriends the client, but actually abandons the client because the nurse is unable to fulfill professional role.*	• *Maintain a professional relationship with the client as the center of the health team; avoid personal and social relationships.* • *Minimize self-disclosure; use it judiciously.* • *Explain the nurse-client relationship, and set limits if necessary.*

C. Interventions that facilitate communication
  1. Address the client by name; avoid using terms of endearment, such as "grandma" and "honey."
  2. Acknowledge the client's individuality; be flexible when meeting needs.
  3. Let the client take the lead in the communication process.
  4. Ensure that message is relevant and a priority for the client.
  5. Stand in front of the client while making eye contact.
  6. Use simple words and sentence structures; keep messages brief.
  7. Repeat a message using different words if the message was not understood.
  8. Use humor carefully; although it may lighten the mood, it can be misunderstood and offend a client.
  9. Give the client adequate time to formulate a response to a message.
  10. Seek feedback to ensure that a message is received as intended.

D. Specific interventions related to nonverbal communication
  1. Be aware of a client's culture and its impact on nonverbal communication.
  2. Validate the meaning of body language to ensure messages are received as intended.
  3. Validate the meaning of a client's body language that is not congruent with the spoken word.
  4. Use touch cautiously so as not to offend the client; touching a client enters a client's personal space; religious beliefs may prohibit being touched by a person of another gender.

IV. Nursing Care for Clients With Special Communication Needs

A client's physical, emotional, or cultural status may result in a diminished or absent ability to receive, process, or send a message. When impaired communication occurs between a client and a nurse, it is the nurse's responsibility to identify what is interfering with the communication process. Once the cause has been identified, the nurse can formulate an individualized plan to promote communication.

A. Clients who are angry
  1. Assess for the cause of anger because all behavior has meaning.
  2. Assess for verbal and nonverbal signs of escalating aggression, such as a loud voice, clenched fist and jaw, narrowed eyes, and physical agitation.
  3. Model acceptable behaviors, such as keeping a calm voice with a normal volume, tone, and pace.
  4. Validate the client's feelings.
  5. Avoid touching the client because it may be perceived as a threat.
  6. Do not turn your back to an angry client; avoid prolonged eye contact but keep the client within your visual field; position yourself between the client and the door.

B. Clients who have aphasia
  1. Assess the client's ability to communicate through speech, writing, or alternative means of communication, such as gestures, a picture board, and computer programs.

2. Promote communication when the client has an inability to formulate and/or send a message (**expressive aphasia**).
   a. Use questions that require a one-word answer or a short response.
   b. Give the client ample time to formulate a message; do not complete sentences for the client.
   c. Use alternative means of communication, such as picture cards, blinking the eyes once for yes and twice for no, a computer, a puff-activated communication device, or a voice synthesizer.
3. Promote communication when the client has an inability to understand communicated information (**receptive aphasia**).
   a. Use simple words and sentences; vary words when repeating a message.
   b. Augment verbal messages with gestures and facial expressions.
   c. Augment verbal communication with picture cards or objects, such as holding up a cup of water to encourage fluid intake.

C. Clients who are confused
1. Use short sentences and convey concrete ideas.
2. Speak slowly.
3. Use questions that require a one-word answer or a short response.
4. Break down instructions into simple steps.
5. Augment verbal communication with picture cards or objects, such as holding up a comb to indicate the need for hair care.

D. Clients who are hearing impaired
1. Ensure that the client is wearing a hearing aid, if available; ensure that a hearing aid is functioning, is inserted properly, and is cleaned and stored with a label.
2. Stand on the side on which the client has more acute hearing; speak at a normal pace using a low tone because high-pitched sounds are harder to hear; use a slightly louder volume, but do not yell.
3. Face the client, enunciate words (without exaggeration), and to facilitate lip-reading avoid chewing gum or holding a hand in front of the mouth when speaking.
4. Use gestures and facial expression to augment verbal communication.
5. Determine whether the client knows sign language, and seek the assistance of sign-language specialists if applicable.
6. Provide writing materials to support communication if the client is able to write and is literate.

E. Clients who are unresponsive
🛑 1. Assume that the client's hearing is intact because hearing is believed to be the last sense lost before death. Never talk about a client or others in front of the client thinking that the client cannot hear.

2. Talk to the client using a normal volume, tone, and pace.
3. Explain what you are going to do and the reasons why before touching a client.

F. Clients who are visually impaired
1. Provide adequate lighting.
2. Verbally inform the client when you enter or are about to leave a room.
3. Speak in a normal volume because the client is not hearing impaired.
4. Explain what you are going to do if you have to touch the client, and seek permission first.
5. Orient the client to surroundings, such as furniture in room and food on a plate using a clock as a format (e.g., meat is at 12, green beans at 3, potatoes at 6).

G. Clients who do not speak English
🛑 1. Seek the help of a professional interpreter fluent in the client's language (e.g., use a telephone service that provides translation services); avoid the use of noneducated translators or family members because inaccuracies may occur (inadvertently or deliberately) and confidentiality may be jeopardized.

2. Use a translation book that presents common questions and answers in the nurse's and client's language.
3. Use pictures, body language, and environmental cues to communicate until an interpreter is available.

H. Clients with a physical barrier (e.g., endotracheal tube, laryngectomy)
1. Encourage the client to use eye blinks; hand squeezes; writing tools, such as a magic slate; flash cards or pictures; or a communication board to communicate.
2. Reinforce and praise efforts to communicate.

V. Types of Interactions Between the Nurse and Other Health-Care Team Members

Information about clients must be communicated between nurses and among nurses and other members of the health team, including clients and their families. Whether the interaction is verbal or written, a systematic approach is preferred so that the message is clearly, concisely, and accurately transmitted and received.

A. Systematic approach to communication
1. Framework to facilitate thorough communication among health-care professionals to provide a culture of safety for the client.
2. Current movement occurring in the health-care community toward setting standards related to interdisciplinary communication (e.g., The Joint Commission is requiring that a systematic approach be used during nursing change-of-shift

reports and when a nurse seeks a telephone prescription from a primary health-care provider).

3. Example: SBAR.
   a. Situation: Identify self, title, facility; identify client, date of birth, gender; reason for collaboration.
   b. Background: Client's present issue, relevant medical history, summary of background.
   c. Assessment: Vital signs and clinical indicators outside expected range, severity of client issue, nurse's clinical impression.
   d. Recommendation: Explain what is required and urgency of what is required; make suggestions.

B. Change of shift report
   1. Given by a nurse who is finishing a shift to a nurse who is responsible for continuing care of the client.
   2. May be verbal, written, or audiotaped; may include walking rounds where two or more nurses visit the client as part of the report.
   3. Includes basic data about the client, current assessment of the client's health status, recent interventions and client responses, dependent and independent nursing interventions to be implemented, report of clients who are off the unit temporarily (includes purpose, when they are expected to return, and nursing care that is anticipated), and clients who have been admitted, transferred, or discharged.

C. Telephone reports
   1. Method by which critical information, such as laboratory test results, may be communicated to the unit.
   2. Method by which nurses can report a change in a client's condition to a primary health-care provider.
   3. Require the nurse to identify self by name and title, state relationship with the client, and concisely and accurately report the client's condition, including vital signs, any clinical findings, and any intervention already performed for the client.

D. Transfer and discharge reports
   1. Concisely summarize all pertinent data about a client that are needed to implement immediate care.
   2. Include, but are not limited to, discharge from the postanesthesia care unit (PACU); discharge to another facility, such as a nursing home or rehabilitation center; discharge to another service within the facility; and discharge from the hospital to home.

E. Reports to family members
   1. Provide a progress report to designated family members; the client gives legal consent to disclose

---

MAKING THE CONNECTION

Systematic Approach to Communication and Clinical Practice

A client with no previous history of acute or chronic health problems is admitted to a hospital for surgical removal of a mass in the ascending colon. After an uneventful recovery in the postanesthesia care unit, the client is transferred to a surgical unit. The client is receiving a patient-controlled analgesia (PCA) intravenous infusion containing morphine. In addition to the basal dose of 1 mg/hr, the client is allowed a 0.2 mg on-demand dose with a lock-out interval of 10 minutes. The client can self-administer six 0.2 mg doses per hour, for a total of 1.2 mg/hr, with a maximum dose of 8.8 mg in 4 hours. As the postoperative period progresses, the nurse identifies that the client's personal pain rating scale has increased from a range of 2 to 3 to a range of 4 to 5, and the PCA pump history indicates that the client has been pressing the button every 5 minutes in the last hour. The nurse assesses the client. The client's vital signs are T—99.6°F; P—92 beats/minute and regular; R—22 breaths/minute, regular, and shallow; BP—134/88 mm Hg. The client states that the incisional pain is sharp and rates it as a 7 on a scale of 0 to 10. The client is lying in one position, has clenched fists, and is exhibiting a facial grimace. The client's oxygen saturation is 96%, the urinary catheter is draining an adequate amount of clear yellow urine, and the dressing is dry and intact. The nurse concludes that the client's analgesic prescription is inadequate to relieve the client's pain and places a phone call to the client's primary health-care provider. The nurse uses the SBAR format to provide a systematic approach when communicating with the primary health-care provider.

Situation: Hello, this is Ms. Jones. I am a registered nurse from Longview Medical Center. I am caring for Mr. Smith, who was born April 5, 1939, and I am calling about his patient-controlled analgesia.

Background: Mr. Smith had no acute or chronic health problems prior to this admission. He had surgery at 0800 this morning for resection of a tumor in his ascending colon. His PCA prescription is morphine basal dose of 1 mg/hr, and he is allowed a 0.2 mg on-demand dose with a lock-out interval of 10 minutes. The client can self-administer six 0.2 mg doses per hour, for a total of 1.2 mg/hr, with a maximum dose of 8.8 mg in 4 hours. In the last hour, Mr. Smith has pushed the trigger of the PCA pump every 5 minutes.

Assessment: Mr. Smith states that his pain is a 7 on a scale of 0 to 10. His vital signs are T—99.6°F; P—92 beats/minute and regular; R—22 breaths/minute, regular, and shallow; BP—134/88 mm Hg. He is lying in one position, has clenched fists, and is exhibiting a facial grimace. The client's oxygen saturation is 96%, the urinary catheter is draining an adequate amount of clear yellow urine, and the dressing is dry and intact. I think that Mr. Smith is in excessive pain and the prescribed dose of morphine is inadequate.

Recommendation: Mr. Smith has been in excessive pain for an hour and it is important to adjust the morphine prescription. Could you please increase the basal dose, increase the on-demand dose, or shorten the lock-out time?

confidential information to a designated person(s).
2. A code word, functioning as a PIN number, is required from a caller before a nurse can give information over the telephone.

DID YOU KNOW?

Nurses legally are not permitted to acknowledge that a person is admitted to a facility. Acknowledging a client's presence without the client's consent violates the client's right to confidentiality and Health Insurance Portability and Accountability Act (HIPAA) laws.

F. Nursing and interdisciplinary team conferences
  1. Nurses and other health team members discuss a client's needs and coordinate a client's care.
  2. Promote critical thinking from a multidisciplinary perspective.
G. Incident reports
  1. Are required in response to any occurrence that results in or is likely to result in harm to a client, employee, or visitor.
  2. Used for quality improvement activities, not for disciplinary actions against a staff member.
  3. Promote identification of high-risk trends, which promote the development of educational programs to address the prevention of the problem. (For more information, see "Incident Report" in Chapter 3, Legal and Ethical Issues.)

VI. Collaboration

Collaboration is the collegial working relationship among health-care professionals in the provision of client care. It involves joint planning, decision making, goal setting, and implementation of coordinated interdisciplinary care to facilitate a more positive outcome for the client. Communication is essential among health team members because it adds an additional dimension to the communication process.
A. Components of collaboration
  1. Mutual respect is essential to working collaboratively with members of an interdisciplinary team.

2. Each discipline must recognize and value the expertise that each professional brings to the partnership.
B. Personal skills essential to collaboration
  1. Ability to use effective interpersonal skills.
  2. Ability to keep communication open and ongoing.
  3. Willingness to work with others as a team.
  4. Ability to value and manage diversity.
  5. Willingness to use assertive communication or engage in conflict resolution to solve mutually satisfying solutions to a problem.

VII. Documentation

Documentation is the act of creating a written record. It involves the insertion of information about a client onto paper forms or electronically in a paperless charting system. Documentation should include information about client assessments, plans of care, interventions provided, and client responses. The written record is a legal document that also is used to promote quality assurance, reimbursement to third-party payers, education, and research.
A. Admission nursing assessment
  1. Initiates a database about the client.
  2. Provides information with which subsequent information can be compared.
B. Plan of care
  1. A **plan of care** documents client's problems and strategies to reduce or eliminate them. The plan individualizes care based on assessment, problem identification, expected outcomes, and planned interventions. The plan provides a base for evaluation.
  2. May be a nursing plan of care or an integrated health team plan.
  3. Is part of the client's permanent record.
C. Clinical pathways
  1. Collaborative, interdisciplinary case management plan for a client with a specific medical diagnosis or procedure.
  2. Includes expected outcomes, interventions to be implemented, and the sequence and timing of those interventions.
D. Flow sheets
  1. Document routine aspects of nursing care.
  2. Include forms, such as for vital signs, weight, I&O, skin assessment, and activities of daily living.
E. Medication administration record (MAR)
  1. Documents all the client's prescribed and administered or omitted medications.
  2. It contains a section to record why a drug was not administered or contains specific information relative to before or after administering a drug, such as blood pressure before an antihypertensive and

objective pain scale results before and after pain medication is administered.

F. Progress notes

1. Inform other members of the health-care team of the client's progress.
2. May use various formats.
   a. Charting by exception (PIE).
      (1) **PIE** includes:
          (a) Problem identification.
          (b) Interventions provided.
          (c) Evaluation of client outcomes.
      (2) Documents information other than routine care (routine care is documented on a separate flow sheet).
      (3) Assigns a number to each identified problem, providing easy reference.
      (4) Simplifies and streamlines documentation.
   b. Focus charting.
      (1) Uses format of data, action, and response.
      (2) Ensures a focus on planning (action) and evaluation (response).
   c. Case management—critical pathway.
      (1) Includes key elements used by all disciplines to monitor and document interventions performed on a daily schedule so that outcomes are achieved when expected.
      (2) When a goal is not met when expected because of a complication or unexpected event (variance), the event and actions in response to the event are documented.
      (3) Promotes collaboration, communication, and teamwork.
      (4) Attempts to ensure that interventions are implemented as expected, increasing quality of care and discharge in a timely manner.

G. Nursing responsibilities related to documentation

1. Documentation do's.
   a. Use only acceptable abbreviations.
   b. Use correct spelling and grammar.
   c. Document each entry with a signature/name and title.
   d. Indicate the date and time of each entry, using a 24-hour clock (military time); record events chronologically and as close as possible to the time they occur.
   e. Verify that client identification is on forms before charting.
   f. Record only pertinent information as concisely as possible; record facts, client statements, and nonjudgmental observations of the client's behavior.
   g. Record the client's response to visits by health-care providers, consultants, and other caregivers, such as speech, respiratory, and physical therapists.
   h. Record all telephone calls concerning the client.
   i. When inserting a late entry, identify that the note is a late entry.
   j. Record all care implemented and the client's response to care.

DID YOU KNOW?

If an intervention is not documented, it is considered not done. Charting should be thorough, clear, and concise. Entries in a clinical record document the care provided and the status and progress of a client.

2. Documentation don'ts.
   a. Never chart interventions before they are delivered.
   b. Avoid charting opinions or terms that label a client (e.g., "demanding," "uncooperative," and "unpleasant").
   c. Never chart for another nurse.
   d. Never alter a previous entry.
   e. Never backdate a note; instead, enter the current date and time with the word "addendum," and then add the note with the date and time it should have been documented; procedures vary by facilities.
   f. Avoid using the word "client" because it is unnecessary.
   g. Avoid judgmental words that mean different things to different people (e.g., "good," "poor," "sufficient," "decreased," "bad," "normal," "abnormal").
   h. Avoid terms of generalization (e.g., "seems to be" or "appears").
   i. Do not use abbreviations that are not included in the facility's policy and procedure manual or abbreviations disallowed by The Joint Commission (Table 2.3).

DID YOU KNOW?

In 2002, The Joint Commission identified a national client safety goal requiring accredited organizations to develop and implement a list of abbreviations not to use in their organization. In 2004, The Joint Commission identified a minimum list of dangerous abbreviations, acronyms, and symbols that must be included on an organization's do-not-use list of abbreviations as part of the requirement for meeting this goal.

Table 2.3 Abbreviations to Avoid in Documentation

Abbreviation	Meaning	Preferred Documentation
IU*	international unit	international unit
MS*	morphine sulfate	morphine sulfate
MSO_4, $MgSO_4$*	magnesium sulfate	magnesium sulfate
qd, q.d., QD, Q.D.*	every day	daily
qod, q.o.d., QOD, Q.O.D.*	every other day	every other day
u, U*	unit	unit
AS, AD, AU	left ear, right ear, both ears	left ear, right ear, each ear
cc	cubic centimeters	mL, milliliters
d/c, D/C, DC	discharge, discontinue	discharge, discontinue
hs, qhs	hour of sleep, bedtime	nightly, at bedtime
OS, OD, OU	left eye, right eye, each eye	left eye, right eye, each eye
sub q, SQ, SC	subcutaneous	subcutaneously, Sub-Q
TIW	three times a week	three times weekly, 3 times weekly
μg, mcg	microgram	microgram
@	at	at
&	and	and
°	hour	hour

Use of "0" in a Medication Dose

Eliminate trailing zero after a decimal point dose* 1.0 mg can be mistaken for 10 if decimal is not seen.	1 mg
Insert a leading zero before a decimal point dose* .5 mg can be mistaken for 5 mg if decimal is not seen.	0.5 mg

*Included on The Joint Commission's Official "Do Not Use" List of dangerous abbreviations, acronyms, and symbols. The Joint Commission. (2015). Facts about the official "Do Not Use" List. Retrieved May 10, 2016, from www.jointcommission.org/facts_do_not_use_list/.

CASE STUDY: Putting It All Together

On a Saturday evening, a tractor trailer loses control, crosses the median of a roadway, and causes a 10-car pileup in the oncoming lanes of a highway. The hospital disaster plan is activated, and many health team members respond to the emergency department of the local hospital. The emergency department is filled to capacity and has a lot of noise and commotion because of the presence of clients, family members, and health team members.

A client who reports severe pain in the hip as a result of the accident is placed on a stretcher in an alcove in the hallway until a room becomes available. The client is accompanied by her adult daughter and 5-year-old grandson. The daughter and grandson were passengers in the car, but they did not sustain any injuries and were not admitted to the emergency department. The nurse positions a curtain around the client's stretcher and stands near the head of the bed, facing the client. The nurse cannot sit because a chair would block the hallway, creating an unsafe situation. While making eye contact with the client, the nurse introduces himself by name and title and states that he is going to conduct an interview and perform a physical assessment. The nurse asks whether the client prefers that the daughter and grandson stay or step to the other end of the hall during the interview. The client says that it is all right for the daughter and grandson to stay during the interview.

The grandson appears anxious and is pulling on the linen at the foot of the grandmother's bed. The nurse observes the client grimacing and rubbing her right hip. Before the nurse can assess the client's pain, the client stated, "I am so angry. I was riding in the right lane, and I was on cruise control within the speed limit. Why did this have to happen?" The nurse responds, "It must be frustrating to know that you did everything right and still had something like this happen."

When beginning the pain assessment, the nurse asks, "What is the intensity of your pain on a scale of 0 to 10?" The nurse also says, "Tell me the location of the pain and

continued.

CASE STUDY: Putting It All Together   *cont'd*

what it feels like." The client is breathing in short, shallow breaths; shaking her head from side to side; and, with her eyes closed, states, "The pain in my right hip is crazy. It is unbearable." The nurse responds, "Can you explain in more detail what you mean by 'crazy'?"

After diagnostic tests have been completed, the primary health-care provider informs the client that surgery to repair the right hip will be performed in the morning. The nurse then transports the client to the orthopedic unit and reinforces the information about the client being scheduled for an open reduction internal fixation (ORIF) in the morning. After being transferred to a bed on the orthopedic unit, the client begins to cry and says, "I am sorry I'm crying. I am such a big baby." The nurse touches the client's arm and responds, "It's okay to cry. You had a lot happen to you today. Everything is going to be fine. Try to be strong and a good role model for your grandson."

Case Study Questions

A. Identify the nursing actions that facilitated communication and the rationales for why they are effective in promoting communication.

1. _____
2. _____
3. _____
4. _____
5. _____

B. Identify factors in this scenario that can be barriers to communication, and explain why.

1. _____
2. _____
3. _____
4. _____
5. _____

C. Identify the interviewing skills the nurse used when communicating with the client, and explain why these skills are effective in promoting communication.

1. _____
2. _____
3. _____
4. _____
5. _____
6. _____

D. Identify the nursing responses that were nontherapeutic.

1. _____
2. _____
3. _____

REVIEW QUESTIONS

Be sure to read the Introduction for valuable test-taking tips.

1. A nurse is caring for a client who is unconscious. Which is the sense that is **most** important to a person who appears to be unconscious?
   1. Taste
   2. Smell
   3. Touch
   4. Hearing

2. Which is **most** effective when the nurse is developing a therapeutic relationship with a client?
   1. Catharsis
   2. Confrontation
   3. Trustworthiness
   4. Recommendations

3. Which is **most** important for the nurse to do when assessing a client's nonverbal expressions?
   1. Increase the client's self-awareness.
   2. Validate their meaning.
   3. Remain observant.
   4. Explore feelings.

4. A nurse is caring for a client who is blind. What should the nurse do to facilitate communication? **Select all that apply.**
   1. Overarticulate when speaking.
   2. Speak slightly louder than usual.
   3. Indicate when you are going to leave the room.
   4. Announce your presence when entering the room.
   5. Explain your intentions before touching the client.

5. Which questions asked by the nurse will elicit the **most** specific information? **Select all that apply.**
   1. "How long ago did the pain in your left knee start?"
   2. "Please describe the characteristics of your last bowel movement."
   3. "I think I heard you say that you have concerns about going home."
   4. "Tell me more about yourself before you were admitted to the hospital."
   5. "Could you tell me more about the dark feeling that you say you have been having?"

6. Which fundamental concept about communication should the nurse include in a foundation for nursing practice?
   1. Communication is an instinctive process.
   2. Communication through humor is highly objective in nature.
   3. Previous patterns of communication may be ineffective when one is ill.
   4. Verbal communication is more meaningful than nonverbal communication.

7. A nurse is interacting with a client at a local mental health clinic. The nurse states, "So, you've come here today because you feel you cannot go on." Which phase of the nurse-client relationship does this interaction reflect?
   1. Working
   2. Termination
   3. Preinteraction
   4. Orientation phase

8. Which examples of documentation regarding the administration of medication are recorded accurately according to The Joint Commission? **Select all that apply.**
   1. Levothyroxine 100 mcg PO daily
   2. Heparin 5,000 units Sub-Q daily
   3. Warfarin 5 mg QOD for 7 days
   4. $MgSO_4$ 1.0 g for hypertension
   5. Calcium 600 mg PO qd

9. A nurse is working with a severely visually impaired client. Which approaches are effective when communicating with this client during a bed bath? **Select all that apply.**
   1. Speak in a louder volume.
   2. Enunciate every word slowly.
   3. Stand directly in front of the client.
   4. Tell the client exactly what will happen.
   5. Use touch to emphasize what is being done.

10. A nurse is attempting to identify a client's concerns. Which communication technique is **most** appropriate for the nurse to use?
    1. Silence
    2. Reflection
    3. Paraphrasing
    4. Open-ended question

11. A nurse is checking a client's graphic sheet (shown here) to verify when the client exhibited the lowest temperature. What time on May 6th was the client's temperature the lowest?
    1. 0800
    2. 1200
    3. 2000
    4. 2400

GRAPHICS

DATE	5/6/2011						
HOSPITAL DAY	2						
POSTOP DAY	2						
TIME	0400	0800	1200	1600	2000	2400	0400
C F							
40.0 104							
39.4 103							
38.8 102							
38.3 101							
37.7 100							
37.2 99							
36.6 98							
36.1 97							
35.5 96							
35.0 95							
PULSE		88	76	80	74		
RESPIRATIONS		16	14	18	16		
BLOOD PRESSURE		140/84	138/84	130/88	128/82		
HEIGHT 5'2"	WEIGHT 125						
TYPE OF DIET	Clear liquids						
%		B 80%	L 50%		S		

12. When talking with a client, a nurse states, "Since speaking with you for a while, it seems that you are very worried about your upcoming surgery." In which phase of the nurse-client relationship is this statement **most** appropriate?
    1. Working
    2. Orientation
    3. Termination
    4. Preinteraction

13. A client who is about to have a mastectomy is wringing her hands, and her eyes are darting around the preoperative unit. Which statements by the nurse are appropriate to explore the client's potential concerns? **Select all that apply.**
    1. "It is all right to be a little nervous before having surgery."
    2. "Do you have any concerns regarding your surgery?"
    3. "Tell me about the surgery you are about to have."
    4. "Have you thought about alternatives to surgery?"
    5. "You will feel better after the surgery is over."

14. Which interventions by the nurse are **least** appropriate during the orientation phase of the nurse-client relationship? **Select all that apply.**
    1. Discussing boundaries of the therapeutic alliance
    2. Explaining the time frame of their interaction
    3. Introducing themselves to each other
    4. Dealing with personal issues
    5. Exploring feelings

15. Which information is **most** informative when giving a change-of-shift report?
    1. A client with dementia is confused.
    2. A client reports that incisional pain is now tolerable.
    3. A client's blood pressure is within the expected range.
    4. A client walked down the hall with no activity intolerance.

16. A nurse is using the SBAR communication technique during a crisis. Which nursing intervention reflects the R step of this technique?
    1. Recording the reaction of the client to the event
    2. Reassessing the client after medical intervention
    3. Recommending a potential action to manage the event
    4. Reporting the situation to the primary health-care provider

17. An 86-year-old man is admitted to an intermediate care facility after discharge from the hospital for treatment of left-sided weakness and an inability to verbally express himself clearly. He is being assessed to identify his physical, occupational, and speech therapy needs. The nurse reviews the client's family history, performs a physical assessment, and interviews the client. Which nursing action addresses this client's **most** urgent need?
    1. Thicken all beverages and soups.
    2. Maintain the splint on the upper extremity.
    3. Explore interventions to facilitate communication.
    4. Encourage the children to participate in their father's rehabilitation.

Client's Clinical Record

Family History

An 86-year-old man had a brain attack, resulting in left hemiparesis and expressive aphasia. The client lives with his 78-year-old wife. The couple lives alone but are visited frequently by a daughter and a son, who both live approximately 30 minutes away.

Physical Assessment

The client has left hemiparesis and wears a hand and forearm splint on the left arm to prevent contractures. The client ambulates safely with the use of a tripod cane. The client needs assistance with activities of daily living. The client is continent of urine and feces. The ability to chew and swallow solid food safely is intact, but on infrequent occasions the client experiences dribbling from the corner of the mouth when drinking fluids.

Client Interview

The client was oriented to time, place, and person. He pointed to things for which he had difficulty finding the words, such as "pen" and "bathroom." He became frustrated and banged on the table when he could not communicate his thoughts clearly. He had an angry facial expression and turned away from his wife when she was unable to understand what he was saying.

---

18. A nurse asks a client, "How are you feeling?" The client responds, "I am doing fine," while looking toward the floor. The nurse identifies that the verbal and nonverbal communication are incongruent. What is the nurse's **most** appropriate response?
    1. "What is bothering you?"
    2. "Let's talk about your illness."
    3. "I am glad you are doing fine."
    4. "Are you sure nothing is bothering you?"

19. The nurse should anticipate that the client with what condition will **most** likely have difficulty conveying needs verbally?
    1. Hearing impairment
    2. Receptive aphasia
    3. Delirium
    4. Blind

20. Which nursing actions are common for clients who have impaired hearing or impaired vision? **Select all that apply.**
    1. Repeating the message using different words if the message was not understood
    2. Being alert for nonverbal cues and behavior
    3. Using gestures to augment verbal language
    4. Using a clock to orient food on a plate
    5. Providing for adequate lighting

21. A nurse is talking with a client about the client's concerns. Which nursing action reflects the **most** important component of verbal communication in this situation?
    1. Answering questions that the client is asking
    2. Taking the lead in the interaction
    3. Using simple sentence structure
    4. Speaking in a calm cadence

22. A nurse answers a client's question while standing by the side of the client's bed. The client responds saying, "Oh well, I just know that I am going to be fine," and then begins to cry, using a head-shaking gesture to indicate "no." What should the nurse do **first**?
    1. Pat the client's hand.
    2. Sit in a chair near the head of the client's bed.
    3. Get a tissue from the bedside drawer for the client.
    4. Use an open-ended question to explore the client's feelings.

23. A nurse is caring for an older adult who is hearing impaired but refuses to wear hearing aids. What are the appropriate ways to have a verbal interaction with this client? **Select all that apply.**
    1. Speak in a normal volume.
    2. Speak in a very loud volume.
    3. Use a soft, higher-pitched voice.
    4. Use a deep, slightly louder voice.
    5. Stand directly in front of the client.
    6. Ensure that the client knows that a conversation is to begin.

24. A client in the emergency department says to a nurse, "I have been so sick for a while with pain in my stomach and nothing seems to work." Which statement by the nurse demonstrates the use of an open-ended question?
    1. "Tell me what you have been doing to manage your illness."
    2. "Would you like for me to sit down with you for a little while?"
    3. "Can you tell me how long you have been experiencing this pain?"
    4. "It must be frustrating when nothing works to make you feel better."

25. A client says to a nurse, "I periodically get a weird feeling in my head. It is so frustrating not to have a specific diagnosis. I am not thrilled about having this test tomorrow, but maybe I will get some answers." Which statement by the nurse is an example of the interviewing technique of clarification?
    1. "You sound upset about the test that you are having tomorrow."
    2. "Can you describe what you mean by a strange feeling in your head?"
    3. "I can understand how frustrating it is not to have a definitive diagnosis."
    4. "Did your primary health-care provider say you would get the results of the test right away?"

26. An inservice educator is correcting a test taken by a newly hired nurse regarding the use of abbreviations. Which abbreviations disallowed by The Joint Commission did the nurse identify correctly? **Select all that apply.**
    1. qd
    2. IU
    3. mL
    4. Sub-Q
    5. $MgSO_4$

27. Which nursing action is considered acceptable nursing practice when documenting in a client's clinical record?
    1. Only chart for another nurse in the event of an emergency.
    2. Always initial an entry when adding a comment to a previously written progress note.
    3. When documenting an opinion, such as "The client is demanding," also include examples of the client's behavior.
    4. For an addendum to a note, enter the current date, the word "addendum," and the date and time it should have been documented.

28. A nurse working on the day shift receives a telephone call from the night nurse who just left the unit. While in the parking lot, the night nurse remembered the need to document nursing care given to a client. What is the **best** action by the day nurse?
    1. Leave room in the progress notes for the night nurse to enter the note on the nurse's return the next night.
    2. Enter the note dictated by the night nurse, note that it was dictated, and sign and date the note.
    3. Suggest that the night nurse enter an addendum note on the nurse's return the next night.
    4. Encourage the night nurse to return to the hospital to enter the progress note.

29. A nurse is providing preoperative teaching for a client who is scheduled for a pacemaker insertion in 3 days. The client tells the nurse, "I am so nervous. I never had surgery before." Which are therapeutic responses by the nurse? **Select all that apply.**
    1. "The unknown can be unsettling."
    2. "What is it that concerns you the most?"
    3. "Has anyone in your family had surgery before?"
    4. "Being anxious before surgery is a normal response."
    5. "Having a pacemaker inserted is a routine procedure."

30. A nurse is orienting a newly admitted client to the client's bedroom environment in a long-term care facility. The client tells the nurse, "I have difficulty hearing. I left my hearing aids at home." What is the nurse's **most** important intervention?
    1. Facing the client directly when speaking
    2. Speaking clearly when conversing with the client
    3. Ensuring that communicated information is understood
    4. Eliminating excess background noise when having a conversation

31. A nurse is documenting a variance associated with an interdisciplinary plan of care, describing the event and actions in response to the event. What type of documenting format is the nurse using?
    1. Clinical pathway
    2. Focused charting
    3. Charting by exception
    4. Problem-oriented charting

32. Which statements by a nurse are examples of non-therapeutic communication? **Select all that apply.**
    1. "I know you're angry about the cold coffee, but occasionally these things happen."
    2. "Take a deep breath. You are getting excited over very simple surgery."
    3. "Let's review what we accomplished today learning about insulin."
    4. "We are going to start an IV with a piggyback in a few minutes."
    5. "I can't believe that you didn't eat all of that beautiful dinner."

33. A nurse case manager is assessing an alert client who is a candidate for a nursing home. Which is the **best** source of information about this client?
    1. Primary health-care provider
    2. Family member
    3. Nurse
    4. Client

34. A nurse working in the emergency department of a hospital is interviewing an extremely agitated client who keeps standing up, pacing, and sitting down. Which statement by the nurse is **most** appropriate?
    1. "Please sit down so that we can discuss your concerns."
    2. "Your behavior is inappropriate and you have to try to control it."
    3. "Let's go to a quiet room because your anxiety may be contagious."
    4. "Come with me for a walk and you can describe what is bothering you."

35. A client who had a brain attack (stroke) has expressive aphasia. Which should the nurse do to facilitate communication? **Select all that apply.**
    1. Vary words when repeating a message that was previously communicated to the client.
    2. Ask questions that require a short response when communicating with the client.
    3. Give the client ample time to formulate a verbal response when communicating.
    4. Use simple words and sentences when communicating with the client.
    5. Assess the client's ability to communicate in ways other than words.

REVIEW ANSWERS AND RATIONALES

1. ANSWER: 4.
Rationales:
1. Although being able to taste is important, it is not the most important sense to an unconscious client. Food or fluid should not be placed in the mouth of an unconscious client because aspiration can occur.
2. Although being able to smell is important, it is not the most important sense to an unconscious client.
3. Although touch is important, it is not the most important sense to an unconscious client.
4. Hearing is the most important sense to an unconscious client because it is believed to be the last sense that is lost. The senses receive stimuli from the environment, and hearing keeps one in contact with others.
TEST-TAKING TIP: Identify the word in the stem that sets a priority. The word *most* in the stem sets a priority.
Content Area: Communication, Collaboration, and Documentation
Integrated Processes: Communication and Documentation; Nursing Process: Analysis
Client Need: Psychosocial Integrity
Cognitive Level: Knowledge
Concept: Sensory Perception

2. ANSWER: 3.
Rationales:
1. Catharsis should not occur before trust is developed because the client is vulnerable and must have faith that the nurse will be accepting and supportive.
2. Confrontation should not occur before trust is developed because the client is vulnerable and must have faith that the nurse will be accepting and supportive.
3. Trustworthiness results from being responsible and dependable. Trust is the foundation of a therapeutic relationship.
4. Recommendations and advice promote dependence; the client should be assisted to problem-solve.
TEST-TAKING TIP: Identify the word in the stem that sets a priority. The word *most* in the stem sets a priority.
Content Area: Communication, Collaboration, and Documentation
Integrated Processes: Caring; Communication and Documentation; Nursing Process: Implementation
Client Need: Psychosocial Integrity
Cognitive Level: Application
Concept: Communication

3. ANSWER: 2.
Rationales:
1. Self-awareness cannot be attained without first exploring the meaning of behavior.
2. The meaning and significance of behavior must be declared or clarified by the client; otherwise, they are just assumptions by the nurse.
3. Just remaining observant is inadequate; the nurse must explore the meaning of behavior.
4. Feelings may not be related to the nonverbal behavior.

TEST-TAKING TIP: Identify the word in the stem that sets a priority. The word *most* in the stem sets a priority.
Content Area: Communication, Collaboration, and Documentation
Integrated Processes: Communication and Documentation; Nursing Process: Assessment
Client Need: Psychosocial Integrity
Cognitive Level: Application
Concept: Communication

4. ANSWER: 3, 4, 5.
Rationales:
1. Overarticulation will not facilitate communication with a client who is blind. It may be perceived as condescending by the client who is blind.
2. Speaking slightly louder is unnecessary. The client is blind, not deaf.
3. This is common courtesy. A blind person may be unaware that you have left the room if not told.
4. This is common courtesy. Also, it supports a sense of security. The person who is blind has a right to know who is in the room and why the person is there.
5. Touching clients who are blind without first telling them what you are doing can be frightening for the client and should be avoided.
Content Area: Communication, Collaboration, and Documentation
Integrated Processes: Communication and Documentation; Nursing Process: Implementation
Client Need: Psychosocial Integrity
Cognitive Level: Application
Concept: Sensory Perception

5. ANSWER: 1, 2.
Rationales:
1. The question in option 1 is a direct question and is seeking specific information about when the pain started. It can be answered with a short answer.
2. This is a direct question that should elicit a short, direct answer. It is requesting specific information about the client's last bowel movement.
3. This question is used to validate whether what was heard was the message that was sent.
4. This question is an open-ended question that allows the client to determine the direction and extent of the information shared.
5. This question is clarifying previous information. It asks the client to expand on information already shared and invites the client to continue the discussion.
TEST-TAKING TIP: Identify the word in the stem that sets a priority. The word *most* in the stem sets a priority.
Content Area: Communication, Collaboration, and Documentation
Integrated Processes: Communication and Documentation; Nursing Process: Implementation
Client Need: Psychosocial Integrity
Cognitive Level: Analysis
Concept: Communication

6. **ANSWER: 3.**
Rationales:
1. Communication is learned; it is not instinctive.
2. Humor is subjective, not objective, in nature. Humor may be interpreted as having many different meanings. What is funny to one person may be insulting to another.
3. This is a true statement. The nurse should assess a client's communication pattern and determine if the client is able to express feelings and communicate needs effectively.
4. What people verbalize really may not be what they believe or feel. Nonverbal language (e.g., behavior, gestures) often is more meaningful and emotionally charged than what is spoken.
Content Area: *Communication, Collaboration, and Documentation*
Integrated Processes: *Communication and Documentation; Nursing Process: Analysis*
Client Need: *Psychosocial Integrity*
Cognitive Level: *Knowledge*
Concept: *Communication*

7. **ANSWER: 4.**
Rationales:
1. The working phase involves attempts at problem-solving with the client.
2. The termination phase involves summarization of goals and objectives.
3. The preinteraction phase occurs prior to the nurse meeting the client.
4. The orientation phase involves gathering information from the client and identifying client needs.
TEST-TAKING TIP: Identify the option with a clang association. The word *phase* in the stem and in option 4 is a clang association.
Content Area: *Communication, Collaboration, and Documentation*
Integrated Processes: *Communication and Documentation; Nursing Process: Implementation*
Client Need: *Psychosocial Integrity*
Cognitive Level: *Analysis*
Concept: *Communication*

8. **ANSWER: 1, 2.**
Rationales:
1. The use of mcg for micrograms and po for by mouth are allowed by The Joint Commission.
2. The use of Sub-Q for subcutaneously is allowed by The Joint Commission.
3. The Joint Commission requires that QOD be spelled out as *every other day*.
4. The Joint Commission requires that magnesium sulfate be spelled out. It disallows the use of a trailing 0 after a decimal. In addition, the route and frequency are not included in this prescription.
5. The Joint Commission requires that qd be spelled out as *daily*.
Content Area: *Communication, Collaboration, and Documentation*
Integrated Processes: *Communication and Documentation; Nursing Process: Implementation*

Client Need: *Safe and Effective Care Environment; Management of Care*
Cognitive Level: *Application*
Concept: *Communication*

9. **ANSWER: 4, 5.**
Rationales:
1. Speaking loudly to a visually impaired person will not facilitate communication with a client who is blind; it may be interpreted by the client as demeaning.
2. Enunciating more clearly will not facilitate communication for a client who is blind. This approach is appropriate for a client who is hearing impaired.
3. The nurse should be standing directly next to the client while giving a bed bath. It is the close proximity to the client rather than being in front of the client that is important.
4. Telling the client exactly what will happen before and during the bed bath provides both information and emotional support.
5. Using touch with a visually impaired person promotes communication because it engages another sense.
Content Area: *Communication, Collaboration, and Documentation*
Integrated Processes: *Caring; Communication and Documentation; Nursing Process: Implementation*
Client Need: *Psychosocial Integrity*
Cognitive Level: *Application*
Concept: *Sensory Perception*

10. **ANSWER: 4.**
Rationales:
1. Silence is not the most appropriate technique to identify concerns. It provides no direction to gather information.
2. Reflection is not the most appropriate technique to identify concerns. With this technique, a feeling that the nurse identified in the client's conversation is reflected back to the client. This may not be an accurate interpretation by the nurse, and it is more directive than another communication technique.
3. Paraphrasing is not the most appropriate technique to identify concerns. Paraphrasing restates the main idea of the client's message in similar but different words. This may be too directed in that the nurse decides what part of the client's message to rephrase.
4. Open-ended questions are the best way to identify a client's concerns because this technique allows a client to take the initiative and direct the conversation to any topic desired by the client.
TEST-TAKING TIP: Identify the word in the stem that sets a priority. The word *most* in the stem sets a priority. Identify the option that is unique. Option 4 is unique because it is the only option with 3 words and a hyphen.
Content Area: *Communication, Collaboration, and Documentation*
Integrated Processes: *Caring; Communication and Documentation; Nursing Process: Implementation*

Client Need: Psychosocial Integrity
Cognitive Level: Application
Concept: Communication

11. ANSWER: 4.

Rationales:

1. At 0800, the client's temperature was at its highest at 100.2°F.
2. The client's temperature at 1200 was not at its lowest. At 1200, the client's temperature was 99.2°F.
3. The client's temperature at 2000 was not at its lowest. At 2000, the client's temperature was 99.2°F.
4. The client's temperature at 2400 was at its lowest, at 98.4°F.

TEST-TAKING TIP: Identify the equally plausible options. Options 2 and 3 are equally plausible. They are both 99.2°F. One is no better than the other. Eliminate options 2 and 3 from further consideration.

Content Area: Communication, Collaboration, and Documentation
Integrated Processes: Communication and Documentation; Nursing Process: Evaluation
Client Need: Safe and Effective Care Environment; Management of Care
Cognitive Level: Analysis
Concept: Communication

12. ANSWER: 1.

Rationales:

1. This statement is most appropriate during the working phase because, by this phase, the client and nurse have talked for a while, which allows the nurse to verbalize the implied.
2. During the orientation phase, the nurse is just getting to know the client, and it is inappropriate to verbalize the implied.
3. This statement is inappropriate in the termination phase because, by the time the termination phase is reached, the client's issues and concerns should have been addressed.
4. This statement does not apply to the preinteraction phase; this phase involves gathering information before meeting with the client.

TEST-TAKING TIP: Identify the word in the stem that sets a priority. The word *most* in the stem sets a priority.

Content Area: Communication, Collaboration, and Documentation
Integrated Processes: Communication and Documentation; Nursing Process: Implementation
Client Need: Psychosocial Integrity
Cognitive Level: Application
Concept: Communication

13. ANSWER: 1, 2.

Rationales:

1. This statement lets the client know that it is all right to be nervous; it provides the client with an opportunity to express feelings if desired.
2. This statement invites the client to discuss her concerns about the surgery.
3. This statement assesses knowledge about the surgery but does not explore the client's anxiety or concerns.

4. This statement is inappropriate and may increase the client's anxiety.
5. This statement invalidates the client's anxiety. There is no way the nurse can predict that the client will feel better after the surgery.

TEST-TAKING TIP: Identify the option with a clang association. The word *concerns* in the stem and option 2 is a clang association. Identify the option that denies the client's concerns. Option 5 denies the client's concerns.

Content Area: Communication, Collaboration, and Documentation
Integrated Processes: Caring; Communication and Documentation; Nursing Process: Implementation
Client Need: Psychosocial Integrity
Cognitive Level: Analysis
Concept: Communication

14. ANSWER: 4, 5.

Rationales:

1. Defining limits and parameters is part of the orientation phase of a nurse-client relationship. It provides a guide for the future relationship.
2. Explaining the anticipated time frame of the relationship is part of the orientation phase of a nurse-client relationship.
3. Introducing oneself is part of the orientation phase of a nurse-client relationship. Clients have the right to know who is providing care.
4. Dealing with personal issues should take place during the working phase of the nurse-client relationship. Dealing with personal issues is inappropriate during the orientation phase of a nurse-client relationship. A therapeutic alliance must be established before addressing personal issues.
5. Exploring feelings should take place during the working phase of the nurse-client relationship. Exploring feelings is inappropriate during the orientation phase of the nurse-client relationship. The nurse must first develop a rapport and trust before transitioning into the working phase of the nurse-client relationship.

TEST-TAKING TIP: Identify the word in the stem that indicates negative polarity. The word *least* in the stem indicates negative polarity.

Content Area: Communication, Collaboration, and Documentation
Integrated Processes: Communication and Documentation; Nursing Process: Planning
Client Need: Psychosocial Integrity
Cognitive Level: Application
Concept: Communication

15. ANSWER: 2.

Rationales:

1. Although it is important to know that a client with dementia is confused and disoriented, these responses are commonly associated with a medical diagnosis of dementia.
2. Knowing that incisional pain is now tolerable is the evaluation step of the nursing process; ongoing evaluation of the effectiveness of the management of pain is the most important of the options presented.

3. Although a client's blood pressure being within the expected range is important to know, it is within a normal, not abnormal, range; this information is not as significant as information in another option.

4. Although knowing that a client walked down the hall with no activity intolerance is important to know, it is a normal, not abnormal, expectation; this is not as significant as information in another option.

TEST-TAKING TIP: Identify the word in the stem that sets a priority. The word *most* in the stem sets a priority.

Content Area: Communication, Collaboration, and Documentation

Integrated Processes: Communication and Documentation; Nursing Process: Evaluation

Client Need: Safe and Effective Care Environment; Management of Care

Cognitive Level: Application

Concept: Communication

16. **ANSWER: 3.**

Rationales:

1. The **A** step (**A**ssessment) in the SBAR communication framework includes the client's status in relation to the crisis.

2. There is no step in the SBAR communication framework that addresses a reassessment of the client.

3. The R in the SBAR communication framework stands for suggested Recommendations. Once the nurse explains the Situation (e.g., identify self, title, facility; identify the client's date of birth and gender; and reason for collaboration), provides Background information (e.g., client's present issue, relevant medical history, and summary of background), and provides an Assessment (e.g., vital signs and clinical indicators outside expected range, severity of client's issue, and nurse's clinical impression), then the nurse makes a Recommendation (e.g., explains what is required, urgency of what is required, and makes suggestions).

4. The **R** in the SBAR communication framework does not denote reporting the crisis. The entire SBAR technique is a reporting format; each step reports a specific piece of information regarding the crisis.

Content Area: Communication, Collaboration, and Documentation

Integrated Processes: Communication and Documentation; Nursing Process: Implementation

Client Need: Safe and Effective Care Environment; Management of Care

Cognitive Level: Analysis

Concept: Communication

17. **ANSWER: 3.**

Rationales:

1. Occasional difficulty with fluids is not the priority at this time. However, direct supervision should be provided to ensure that this occasional difficulty is not a serious problem. Clients should be encouraged to enjoy food and liquid until the difficulty progresses to a point where it presents a risk for aspiration.

2. Although use of the splint should be maintained, it is not the most serious concern at this time.

3. **This is the priority at this time. The client is exhibiting anger and frustration with his inability to express himself and communicate his feelings and needs.**

4. Although the nurse may explore the son's and daughter's interest in participating in their father's rehabilitation, this is not the priority.

TEST-TAKING TIP: Identify the word in the stem that sets a priority. The word *most* in the stem sets a priority. Identify the option with a specific determiner. Option 1 contains the word *all*, which is a specific determiner.

Content Area: Communication, Collaboration, and Documentation

Integrated Processes: Caring; Communication and Documentation; Nursing Process: Planning

Client Need: Psychosocial Integrity

Cognitive Level: Analysis

Concept: Patient-Centered Care; Communication

18. **ANSWER: 4.**

Rationales:

1. This statement is inappropriate because the nurse is making an assumption.

2. This response focuses on a topic that may not be the client's concern.

3. Since the verbal and nonverbal communications are incongruent, the nurse should not assume the client is doing fine.

4. This response seeks further information because the client's verbal and nonverbal communications are incongruent.

TEST-TAKING TIP: Identify the word in the stem that sets a priority. The word *most* in the stem sets a priority. Identify the options that deny the client's feelings. Options 2 and 3 ignore the client's behavior and therefore deny the client's feelings or concerns.

Content Area: Communication, Collaboration, and Documentation

Integrated Processes: Caring; Communication and Documentation; Nursing Process: Assessment

Client Need: Psychosocial Integrity

Cognitive Level: Application

Concept: Communication

19. **ANSWER: 3.**

Rationales:

1. People who are hearing impaired generally are able to verbalize a message; they may have difficulty receiving a message.

2. The client with expressive, not receptive, aphasia has an impaired ability to verbalize a message.

3. Of the four options presented, the client with delirium is the most likely person to have difficulty verbalizing needs effectively. Delirium is a temporary disturbance in cognition accompanied by incoherent speech and altered sensory perception. It may be caused by a variety of acute problems, such as hypoxia or a metabolic problem associated with such conditions as renal or liver impairment.

4. Most clients who are blind are able to encode and decode a verbal message.

TEST-TAKING TIP: Identify the word in the stem that sets a priority. The word *most* in the stem sets a priority.
Content Area: Communication, Collaboration, and Documentation
Integrated Processes: Communication and Documentation; Nursing Process: Analysis
Client Need: Psychosocial Integrity
Cognitive Level: Analysis
Concept: Cognition

20. **ANSWER: 1, 2, 5.**
   Rationales:
   1. Repeating the message using different words if the message was not understood is common nursing care for clients who are either hearing or visually impaired. Additional or different words help to clarify a message.
   2. Being alert to nonverbal cues and behavior is common nursing care for clients who are either hearing or visually impaired.
   3. Although many gestures have universal meanings that can augment verbal language, gestures are not helpful when a client is visually impaired. Using gestures in addition to the spoken word is most effective when communicating with clients who are hearing impaired.
   4. Using a clock to orient food on a plate is helpful to clients who are visually impaired. It is not necessary for clients who are hearing impaired.
   5. Providing for adequate lighting is common to caring for clients who are either hearing or visually impaired. Adequate lighting enables some clients who are considered legally blind, but who have some limited vision, to see shadows and outlines of people and objects in the environment. Clients who are hearing impaired may lip-read to facilitate reception of a message; adequate lighting promotes lip-reading.
   Content Area: Communication, Collaboration, and Documentation
   Integrated Processes: Communication and Documentation; Nursing Process: Analysis
   Client Need: Psychosocial Integrity
   Cognitive Level: Analysis
   Concept: Sensory Perception

21. **ANSWER: 1.**
   Rationales:
   1. Answering questions posed by a client is related to the concept of relevance. Although some of the other options are important to effective communication, providing answers to questions posed by the client is the priority.
   2. The nurse should not take the lead when discussing a client's concerns. The nurse should use open-ended and other nondirect interviewing techniques that encourage the client to lead the discussion to topics that concern the client.
   3. Although using simple words and sentence structure support clarity, another option is the priority.
   4. Although speaking in a calm cadence is important because it conveys professional competence and respect for the client, it is not the priority.

TEST-TAKING TIP: Identify the word in the stem that sets a priority. The word *most* in the stem sets a priority. Identify the clang association.
Content Area: Communication, Collaboration, and Documentation
Integrated Processes: Communication and Documentation; Nursing Process: Implementation
Client Need: Psychosocial Integrity
Cognitive Level: Application
Concept: Communication

22. **ANSWER: 2.**
   Rationales:
   1. This intervention is inappropriate at this time. Touch should be used carefully because some clients believe that it is an invasion of their personal space.
   2. The first step is to sit at the head of the bed. This indicates to the client that you are staying and interested.
   3. A nurse should not enter a client's bedside drawer without permission. The bedside cabinet and overbed table are the client's personal space.
   4. This is premature. Silence is more appropriate.
   TEST-TAKING TIP: Identify the word in the stem that sets a priority. The word *first* in the stem sets a priority.
   Content Area: Communication, Collaboration, and Documentation
   Integrated Processes: Caring; Communication and Documentation; Nursing Process: Implementation
   Client Need: Psychosocial Integrity
   Cognitive Level: Application
   Concept: Communication

23. **ANSWER: 4, 5, 6.**
   Rationales:
   1. If the nurse speaks at a normal volume, the client probably will not hear the message.
   2. A nurse should speak a little louder than usual, not very loud, to a client who is hearing impaired but does not wear a hearing aid. Speaking too loudly may be perceived by the client as aggression.
   3. This approach is inappropriate. As people age, they tend to lose the ability to hear higher-pitched sounds.
   4. Older adults hear lower-, rather than higher-, pitched voices as a result of the aging process. Speaking slightly louder and deeper will aid the client in hearing the message.
   5. Standing in front of the client will promote communication because the client will be able to see the nurse's lips, which may aid in the reception and comprehension of the message.
   6. Ensuring that the client knows when a conversation is going to begin allows the client to be prepared to listen.
   Content Area: Communication, Collaboration, and Documentation
   Integrated Processes: Communication and Documentation; Nursing Process: Implementation
   Client Need: Psychosocial Integrity
   Cognitive Level: Application
   Concept: Sensory Perception

24. ANSWER: 1.

Rationales:

1. This is an open-ended question. It requires more than just a yes-or-no answer. Open-ended questions permit the client to control the direction of the discussion.

2. This is an example of offering of the self. It indicates the nurse's attention and interest without expectations. It is not an open-ended question.

3. This is an example of a direct question. Direct questions generally are used to collect specific data.

4. This is an example of reflection. It lets the client know that the nurse has heard the message and is being empathetic.

Content Area: Communication, Collaboration, and Documentation
Integrated Processes: Communication and Documentation; Nursing Process: Implementation
Client Need: Psychosocial Integrity
Cognitive Level: Analysis
Concept: Communication

25. ANSWER: 2.

Rationales:

1. This statement does not seek clarification concerning the weird feeling in the client's head. This is an example of paraphrasing. It repeats content in the same or similar words (frustrating, upset) used by the client.

2. This is a clarifying question. It asks the client to elaborate on an unclear message, which helps to minimize misunderstanding.

3. This statement does not seek clarification concerning the weird feeling in the client's head. This is an example of reflection. It is a validating statement because it identifies and supports what the client feels and demonstrates empathy.

4. This statement does not seek clarification concerning the weird feeling in the client's head. This is a direct question that does not focus on the client's feelings.

TEST-TAKING TIP: Identify the equally plausible options. Options 1 and 3 are equally plausible. They both address the client's feelings—upset and frustrated.

Content Area: Communication, Collaboration, and Documentation
Integrated Processes: Communication and Documentation; Nursing Process: Implementation
Client Need: Psychosocial Integrity
Cognitive Level: Analysis
Concept: Communication

26. ANSWER: 1, 2, 5.

Rationales:

1. According to The Joint Commission, *every day* or *daily* must be written out. QD and qd are no longer acceptable abbreviations.

2. According to The Joint Commission the abbreviation IU must be written out as *international unit*.

3. According to The Joint Commission, milliliters or cubic centimeters (cc) may be abbreviated only as *mL* or written out as *milliliters*.

4. The Joint Commission does not specifically address the use of an abbreviation for subcutaneous. According to the Institute for Safe Medication Practices, Sub-Q must be written out as *subcutaneously*.

5. According to The Joint Commission, *magnesium sulfate* must be written out. MgSO$_4$ is no longer an acceptable abbreviation.

TEST-TAKING TIP: Identify the word in the stem that indicates negative polarity. The word *disallowed* indicates negative polarity. The question is asking, "What abbreviations cannot be used as directed by The Joint Commission?"

Content Area: Communication, Collaboration, and Documentation
Integrated Processes: Communication and Documentation; Nursing Process: Evaluation
Client Need: Safe and Effective Care Environment; Management of Care
Cognitive Level: Application
Concept: Communication

27. ANSWER: 4.

Rationales:

1. It is never acceptable to chart for another nurse. Nurses are responsible for only their own actions.

2. The nurse should never alter a previously written entry in the client's clinical record. When the correct procedure for adding an addendum to a note is followed, no one can claim that an attempt was made to alter the previous note surreptitiously.

3. A nurse should describe a client's behavior and avoid using judgmental words (e.g., demanding) to characterize behavior.

4. This is the correct procedure for entering an addendum to a progress note. This avoids a claim by another that a previous note was altered surreptitiously.

TEST-TAKING TIP: Identify options with specific determiners. The word *only* in option 1 and the word *always* in option 2 are specific determiners. Rarely are options with specific determiners the correct answer.

Content Area: Communication, Collaboration, and Documentation
Integrated Processes: Communication and Documentation; Nursing Process: Implementation
Client Need: Safe and Effective Care Environment; Management of Care
Cognitive Level: Knowledge
Concept: Communication

28. ANSWER: 4.

Rationales:

1. Blank spaces between entries and between the end of a note and one's signature should be avoided. This prevents anyone from entering a note later, which is an unacceptable practice.

2. A nurse should never enter a note for another person. A nurse should only enter notes for clients for whom the nurse is responsible.

3. This action should be suggested if the night nurse refuses to implement an action presented in another option.

4. This is the best advice the day nurse should give the night nurse. This avoids the need for the night nurse to add an "addendum" note the next night.

TEST-TAKING TIP: Identify the word in the stem that sets a priority. The word *best* in the stem sets a priority.

Content Area: Communication, Collaboration, and Documentation
Integrated Processes: Communication and Documentation; Nursing Process: Implementation
Client Need: Safe and Effective Care Environment; Management of Care
Cognitive Level: Application
Concept: Communication

29. **ANSWER: 1, 2.**

Rationales:

1. This statement uses reflective technique and provides the client with an opportunity to explore feelings. It focuses on the comment that the client is nervous and never had surgery before.

2. This response is open ended and allows the client to talk about whatever the client wants to discuss.

3. This response takes the focus away from the client.

4. This response minimizes the client's feelings and may cut off further communication.

5. This statement invalidates the client's concerns and may interfere with further communication.

TEST-TAKING TIP: Identify the options that deny the client's feelings. Options 4 and 5 minimize the client's feelings and concerns. Identify the equally plausible options. Options 4 and 5 are equally plausible.

Content Area: Communication, Collaboration, and Documentation
Integrated Processes: Caring; Communication and Documentation; Nursing Process: Assessment
Client Need: Psychosocial Integrity
Cognitive Level: Application
Concept: Communication

30. **ANSWER: 3.**

Rationales:

1. Although facing the client may facilitate lip-reading, it does not ensure that the client will receive the message accurately.

2. Although speaking clearly may be done, it will not ensure that the client will receive the message accurately.

3. Feedback from the client must be obtained to ensure that the instructions about the environment are understood. This is the primary outcome of any client teaching, regardless of the physical status of the client.

4. Although eliminating background noise helps to eliminate competing stimuli, it does not ensure that the message will be received accurately.

TEST-TAKING TIP: Identify the word in the stem that sets a priority. The word *most* in the stem sets a priority. Identify equally plausible options. Options 1, 2, and 4 are equally plausible because they all address how to improve the transmission of a verbal message to a person who has impaired hearing. Identify the unique option. Option 3 is unique because it is the only option that involves an intervention that obtains feedback from the client.

Content Area: Communication, Collaboration, and Documentation
Integrated Processes: Communication and Documentation; Nursing Process: Implementation
Client Need: Psychosocial Integrity
Cognitive Level: Application
Concept: Sensory Perception

31. **ANSWER: 1.**

Rationales:

1. A clinical pathway includes key elements used by all disciplines to monitor and document interventions performed on a daily schedule so that outcomes are achieved when expected. When an outcome is not achieved as expected, the health-care professional is required to document the variance, including the event and the action in response to the event. This approach is designed to ensure that interventions are implemented as expected, increasing quality of care and discharge in a timely manner.

2. This is not an example of focused charting. Focused charting uses the format of data, action, and response in a narrative note. It focuses on planning and evaluation.

3. This is not an example of charting by exception. Charting by exception documents information other than routine care. Routine care is documented on a separate flow sheet. It assigns a number to each identified problem, providing for easy reference. It streamlines documentation following the format of problem identification, interventions provided, and evaluation of client outcomes.

4. This is not an example of problem-oriented charting. Problem-oriented charting follows the SOAP format. **S**ubjective data, **O**bjective data, **A**ssessment, and **P**lan. This approach provides a structured, logical format to charting.

Content Area: Communication, Collaboration, and Documentation
Integrated Processes: Communication and Documentation; Nursing Process: Implementation
Client Need: Safe and Effective Care Environment; Management of Care
Cognitive Level: Comprehension
Concept: Communication

32. **ANSWER: 1, 2, 4, 5.**

Rationales:

1. This is a defensive nontherapeutic response to a client who is angry. The better response is, "I am sorry that your coffee was cold this morning. How about I get you a nice hot cup of coffee right now?"

2. This statement minimizes the client's concerns and violates trust. The better response is, "Let's talk about what concerns you have regarding the surgery so that you will feel more comfortable."

3. This is the therapeutic communication skill of summarization. It highlights important points in a conversation or teaching session and may identify what still needs to be accomplished.

4. The statement uses medical jargon that the client may not understand. Medical jargon may confuse a client and communicates that the nurse is not interested enough to

make information understandable. The nurse should use language that the client understands, offer opportunities for questions, and evaluate the client's understanding.
5. This is a judgmental statement and demonstrates a lack of respect for the client. The better response is, "I see that you did the best that you could with regard to eating your dinner." This is an empathetic response that demonstrates acceptance.

TEST-TAKING TIP: Identify the word in the stem that indicates negative polarity. The word *nontherapeutic* in the stem indicates negative polarity. The question is asking, "Which statements are inappropriate or do not promote communication?"

Content Area: Communication, Collaboration, and Documentation
Integrated Processes: Communication and Documentation; Nursing Process: Evaluation
Client Need: Psychosocial Integrity
Cognitive Level: Analysis
Concept: Communication

33. **ANSWER: 4.**
    Rationales:
    1. The primary health-care provider is a secondary source.
    2. The client's family member is a secondary source.
    3. The charge nurse is a secondary source.
    4. The client is the center of the health team and is the primary source for current objective and subjective data.
    TEST-TAKING TIP: Identify the word in the stem that sets a priority. The word *best* in the stem sets a priority. Identify the option that is unique. Option 4 is unique because the other options identify people other than the client.
    Content Area: Communication, Collaboration, and Documentation
    Integrated Processes: Communication and Documentation; Nursing Process: Assessment
    Client Need: Safe and Effective Care Environment; Management of Care
    Cognitive Level: Comprehension
    Concept: Communication

34. **ANSWER: 4.**
    Rationales:
    1. This statement by the nurse, although courteous, may make the client more agitated. This is an unrealistic request.
    2. Telling a client to control behavior may make the client more agitated. The client may not be able to control the behavior.
    3. Stating that the client's anxiety may be contagious is nontherapeutic and possibly may make the client feel worse.

4. Offering to walk with the client during the interview allows the client to expend energy while voicing concerns.

TEST-TAKING TIP: Identify the word in the stem that sets a priority. The word *most* in the stem sets a priority. Identify the option that denies the client's needs. Option 1 denies the client's need to move around. Identify the options that are not client centered. Option 2 is confrontational and not client centered. The client is unable to control the behavior. Option 3 is not client centered because by saying that the client's anxiety may be contagious implies that the client may harm others. Identify the client-centered option. Option 4 is client centered. It is the only option that allows the client to continue moving about while the nurse addresses the client's concerns.

Content Area: Communication, Collaboration, Documentation
Integrated Processes: Caring; Communication and Documentation; Nursing Process: Implementation
Client Need: Psychosocial Integrity
Cognitive Level: Application
Concept: Mood

35. **ANSWER: 2, 3, 5.**
    Rationales:
    1. Varying words when repeating a message is a technique used for clients with receptive, not expressive, aphasia.
    2. Questions that require short answers decrease the stress to formulate long responses.
    3. People with expressive aphasia require a longer period of time to choose words and formulate sentences. Rushing clients or finishing their sentences will emphasize their disability and may precipitate anxiety and frustration.
    4. Using simple words and sentences are techniques used for clients with receptive, not expressive, aphasia. Simple words and sentences with one noun and one verb are easier to decode.
    5. There are numerous channels of communication, such as gestures, facial expressions, and touch. In addition, aids such as picture boards and computer programs can facilitate communication.
    Content Area: Communication, Collaboration, and Documentation
    Integrated Processes: Communication and Documentation; Nursing Process: Implementation
    Client Need: Psychosocial Integrity
    Cognitive Level: Analysis
    Concept: Communication

Chapter 3

Legal and Ethical Issues

NURSING CONCEPTS

Collaboration
Ethics
Health-Care System
Legal
Patient-Centered Care

Professionalism
Safety
Violence

KEY TERMS

Abuse—When person is physically, emotionally, or sexually mistreated or exploited
  Emotional—Behavior by someone that results in an impairment of the social, emotional, or intellectual functioning of another
  Physical—Nonaccidental injury inflicted by one person on another
  Sexual—Actual or simulated sexual acts with a nonconsenting person; sexual exploitation for physical, psychological, or monetary gains
Assisted suicide—A competent person legally ends own life with prescribed medication
Autonomy—Right of people to have individual liberty and self-determination
Belief—Opinion about something that people accept as true
Beneficence—An ethical principle that addresses the concept that nursing actions should promote good
Common law—Laws based on judges' interpretation and application of constitutional and statutory laws to a set of facts presented in a court case
Ethical dilemma—When a decision must be made between two or more actions and the best action is unclear
Ethics—A structure of moral principles or standards that govern behavior
Euthanasia—Intentionally ending a life to relieve suffering from an incurable or terminal illness
Fidelity—Making only promises or commitments that can be kept

Incident report—Document that contains information related to an event that results in or is likely to result in harm to a client, employee, or visitor
Informed consent—Document that indicates that a client, or legal surrogate, understands what is to be done and why, including the risks and benefits of the procedure.
Justice—Fairness and equality
Malpractice—Professional negligence that occurs when a nurse fails to provide an expected level of care to a client consistent with professional standards of practice and/or fails to act how another nurse would in similar circumstances.
Morals—Personal or societal standards of what is right or wrong and good or bad
Neglect—When a person's physical and/or emotional needs are inadequately met.
Negligence—When a nurse fails to implement reasonable care as dictated by standards of care by omission or commission of an act and/or fails to act how a reasonable and prudent nurse would in similar circumstances.
Nonmaleficence—An ethical principle that refers to preventing harm, avoiding actions that cause harm to a client, or removing a client from harm
Nursing ethics—The study of ethical issues that occur in nursing and an attempt to provide standards or principles to guide professional behavior

Continued

KEY TERMS—cont'd

Personal values—Beliefs that are internalized into one's own life to help guide personal behavior

Professional values—Beliefs that help to guide professional behavior

Proxy—A person identified to make health-care decisions for another individual (health-care proxy) when the individual is no longer capable

Surrogate—Individual who legally is permitted to make health-care decisions for an incapacitated individual who does not have a health-care proxy

Tort—A civil wrong inflicted or imposed on another's person, property, or reputation

Value—Belief about the worth of something; a belief, ideal, or action respected by an individual, group, or society

Values clarification—Process by which individuals recognize, explore, and shape personal values

Veracity—Truthfulness

Vicarious liability—When accountability for a wrong is assigned to a person or entity that did not directly cause an injury but has a contractual relationship with the person who did cause the wrong

Whistle-blowing—Act of reporting workplace incompetence or unethical or illegal situations to someone who has the power to discontinue the wrongdoing

I. Sources of Law

Nursing practice is influenced by many legal concepts. Therefore, nurses must understand the sources of law established and enforced by the government.

A. Constitutional law
 1. **Constitutional law** is based on the U.S. Constitution, a group of laws that establish the powers and limits of each of the three branches of government (executive, legislative, and judicial).
 2. Grants broad individual rights and responsibilities.
 3. Is the foundation of the U.S. justice system.
 4. States can pass their own constitutions, but the laws and regulations contained within them must act in accordance with the principle precepts of the U.S. Constitution.

B. Statutory law (legislative)
 1. **Statutory law** is based on the laws enacted by federal and state legislative bodies, which are made up of elected individuals who represent the interests of voters.
 2. Federal laws supersede state laws, and state laws supersede local laws.
 3. Examples of federal and state laws are presented in this section "Specific Laws and Regulations That Guide Nursing Practice," page 63.

C. Administrative law (regulatory)
 1. **Administrative law** is based on rules and regulations designed to enforce the laws passed by legislative bodies.
 2. Developed by governmental administrative agencies.
 3. Example: Statutory law establishes nurse practice acts and authority for administrative functions of the state boards of nursing. The state board of nursing in each state is entrusted with the task of creating the rules and regulations detailing

how the profession of nursing is practiced in the state.

DID YOU KNOW?

Although none of the standards published by professional organizations are statutory laws, their guidelines factor into what is considered reasonable and prudent nursing care.

D. Common law
 1. **Common law** evolves from court decisions, not through legislation.
 2. Based on judges' interpretation and application of constitutional and statutory laws to a set of facts presented in a court case.
 3. Generally follow precedent, meaning that judges apply the same rules and principles relevant in previous similar cases (doctrine of *stare decisis*— "let the decision stand").

E. Criminal law
 1. **Criminal law** seeks to punish a person for an offense against society; usually involves actions that jeopardize public safety and welfare.
 2. Must have a verdict based on guilt beyond a reasonable doubt.
 3. Punishment for a minor crime (misdemeanor) generally is a fine or imprisonment for less than 1 year.
 4. Punishment for a major crime (felony) is imprisonment for more than 1 year or possibly even execution, depending on the severity of the crime.

II. Civil Law

Civil law seeks to resolve a disagreement between a private individual and another individual or group. Verdicts are based on a preponderance of the evidence, and punishment may include payment of money by the person being sued (defendant) to the person bringing the suit (plaintiff). Two types of civil law that influence standards for nursing practice are contract law and tort law.

A. Contract law
  1. **Contract law** is based on legally enforceable agreements (contracts) between individuals.
  2. Requires:
      a. An agreement between legally competent individuals that indicates the responsibilities of each party.
      b. Understanding of provisions and responsibilities by each party.
      c. Payment for contracted actions performed.
  3. Includes employment contracts, for example, in which:
      a. A nurse is expected to follow an employer's policies and standards consistent with federal and state law, satisfy the terms of agreed-upon tasks and responsibilities, and respect the tasks and responsibilities of other health team members.
      b. In return, the nurse can expect sufficient and competent support in the delivery of care, reasonable treatment by providers of care and clients, payment for services, a safe working environment, and adequate resources to complete the contracted service.
  4. Liability for a wrong may be assigned to a person or entity that did not directly cause an injury but has a contractual relationship with the person who did cause the wrong (vicarious liability). Examples include:
      a. *Respondeat superior* ("let the master answer"): When a hospital hires a nurse, the nurse functions as a representative of the institution and must perform within its policies and procedures; the hospital is responsible for the actions of the nurse.
      b. *Captain of the ship:* A health-care provider may be held liable for a nurse who is working under the direction of the health-care provider; however, the nurse is also still liable for his or her own actions.
      c. *Borrowed servant:* When an employer directs a nurse to work for a second employer, the second employer is held accountable for the nurse's actions (e.g., agency nurse); however, the nurse is also still liable for his or her own actions.

B. Tort law
  1. A **tort** is a civil wrong inflicted or imposed on another's person, property, or reputation.
  2. Types of torts (Table 3.1).
      a. *Intentional tort:* Commission of a deliberate improper act (actual or threatened) that is beyond the legal limits of what is considered acceptable. It must be executed on purpose and with intent; however, no harm has to occur for liability to exist.
      b. *Quasi-intentional tort:* Making false statements, verbally (slander) or in writing (libel), about another person that harms the person's reputation or causes the person to be avoided, ridiculed, or held in contempt.
      c. *Unintentional tort:* Commission or omission of an act that results in harm to another. However, there is no intent to do harm by the person committing or omitting the act. Negligence and malpractice are considered unintentional torts (see next section).

Table 3.1 **Types of Torts**	
Types and Definitions	**Examples**
Intentional Torts	
Assault Intentionally threatening to harm or touch a client in an insulting, unjustifiable, or offensive manner.	• *Stating, "Stop yelling, or I will move you to the end of the hall."* • *Stating, "If you don't behave, you can't have your pain medication."*
Battery Intentionally touching a client's body or clothing or anything held by or attached to a client in an angry, willful, negligent, or violent manner without consent.	• *Performing a procedure without informed consent.* • *Forcefully undressing a client.* • *Resuscitating a client who has a do-not-attempt-resuscitation order.* • *Administering a medication refused by a client.*
Fraud Engaging in purposeful misrepresentation or reckless disregard of the truth to produce unlawful gain.	• *Stating, "You should not feel any pain with this procedure," when it is commonly known that the procedure is painful.* • *Engaging in dishonesty when obtaining a nursing license.* • *Altering a medical record for the purpose of concealing the truth.*

Continued

Table 3.1 Types of Torts—cont'd

Types and Definitions	Examples
Intentional Torts	
False imprisonment Intentionally and unjustifiably preventing movement or retaining a client without consent or authority to do so.	• *Refusing to discharge a client from the hospital until he or she pays the bill.* • *Applying a restraint when doing so does not comply with the policies and procedures for restraint application.*
Invasion of privacy Disclosing confidential information about a client to an inappropriate person, sharing unnecessary information or gossip about a client, or not honoring a client's right to be left alone.	• *Discussing confidential information on an elevator used by visitors.* • *Releasing information about a client without consent.* • *Unnecessarily physically exposing a client.* • *Asking unnecessary probing questions.*
Quasi-Intentional Torts	
Defamation Communicating false, derogatory information that harms a person's reputation, holds the person up to ridicule or contempt, or causes the person to be avoided. *1. Slander* Occurs when false derogatory information is stated orally. *2. Libel* Occurs when false derogatory information is stated in writing.	1. Slander • *Maliciously stating that another nurse is incompetent without supportive data.* • *Commenting to another nurse that a client is a child molester after hearing gossip from another caregiver.* 2. Libel • *Documenting false information about the client's sexual orientation in the client's clinical record.* • *Documenting false, derogatory information about a client in an incident report.*
Unintentional Tort	
See section III, "Negligence and Malpractice," in this chapter.	

III. Negligence and Malpractice

The most common unintentional torts that affect nurses are negligence and malpractice. Both relate to failure to implement reasonable care according to standards that results in injury to another. The differentiating factor is that malpractice is considered "professional negligence."

A. Negligence
  1. **Negligence** occurs when a nurse fails to implement reasonable care as dictated by standards of care by omission or commission of an act and/or fails to act how a reasonable and prudent *nurse* would in similar circumstances.
  2. Must result in physical, emotional, or financial harm.

B. Malpractice
  1. **Malpractice** occurs when a nurse fails to provide an expected level of care to a client consistent with professional standards of practice and/or fails to act how another nurse would in similar circumstances.
  2. Malpractice is a professional form of negligence.
  3. Must result in physical, emotional, or financial harm.
  4. Litigation occurs when a client (the plaintiff) initiates a civil suit in court against a provider

of health care (the defendant). To prove malpractice, the plaintiff must establish by a preponderance of the evidence four elements of liability.
  a. *Duty:* The nurse-client relationship establishes that the nurse has a legal obligation to the client when the client seeks nursing care.
  b. *Breach of duty:* The nurse's actions by omission or commission of an act failed to meet standards of care established by a job description, agency policy or procedures, the state nurse practice act, standards established by professional organizations, and/or a text deemed to be authoritative.
  c. *Causation:* Involves two elements that must be proven by the plaintiff.
    (1) A nurse's action or inaction was the immediate cause of the plaintiff's injury (proximate cause).
    (2) A nurse should have known that the breach of the nursing standard could result in harm or injury (foreseeability).
  d. *Damages:* A plaintiff must prove that physical, emotional, or financial harm or injury, such as pain, suffering, disfigurement, disability, medical expenses, or lost wages, was the result of the breach of duty.

C. Common malpractice claims related to nursing practice
1. Failure to assess the client and identify client needs.
   a. Includes:
      (1) Failure to complete an admission assessment or assignment.
      (2) Failure to make ongoing assessments.
      (3) Failure to recognize a cluster of data that indicates a problem.
      (4) Failure to identify safety needs, such as a risk of falls or pressure ulcers.
      (5) Failure to listen to client concerns or requests.
   b. To minimize the risk of litigation, the nurse must:
      (1) Make a complete assessment.
      (2) Have a strong knowledge base of the science of nursing, anatomy and physiology, sociology, psychology, chemistry, and so forth; collect, analyze, and recognize the significance of data; and have the ability to identify a client's needs.
      (3) Make ongoing assessments until a client is stable.
      (4) Listen to a client's concerns or requests and respond appropriately.
2. Failure to plan appropriate nursing care.
   a. Includes:
      (1) Failure to design a plan of care according to facility policy and procedures.
      (2) Failure to include appropriate nursing interventions in the plan of care, such as failure to plan for assistance when a debilitated client moves from a bed to a chair and subsequently falls or failure to plan assistance with meals for a client who is at risk for aspiration and who subsequently aspirates.
   b. To minimize the risk of litigation, the nurse must:
      (1) Formulate a plan of care for every client, including problems/needs, goals/outcomes, and planned interventions.
      (2) Document the plan of care according to agency policy and procedures.
      (3) Include all appropriate nursing interventions in the plan of care to achieve the client's goals/outcomes based on professional standards of care.
3. Failure to implement a plan of care appropriately.
   a. Includes:
      (1) Failure to follow standards of practice and agency policy and procedures, such as unsafe use of equipment, improper application of restraints, medication error, or disregard for do-not-attempt-resuscitation (DNAR) orders.
      (2) Failure to follow state laws or regulations concerning the prescription of medications and performance of medical/surgical interventions.
      (3) Failure to function as an advocate, such as failure to protect a client's physical safety, report an impaired nurse, or report suspected abuse or neglect.
      (4) Failure to respond to a client's needs or requests in a timely manner, such as not providing pain medication or answering a call light.
      (5) Failure to document critical information about a client or a client response to care, such as drug allergies, falls, untoward reaction to treatment or nursing care, client status and progress, medication administration, response to interventions, and information provided by family members.
      (6) Failure to communicate with other members of the health-care team, such as failure to notify the primary health-care provider of a change in a client's condition or providing incomplete information at a change-of-shift report.
   b. To minimize the risk of litigation, the nurse must:
      (1) Know and understand acceptable legal limits of one's words or actions.
      (2) Know who has a prescriptive license in the state and accept and implement prescriptions only from these professionals.
      🛑 (3) Accept assignments only for which one is qualified to provide safe and appropriate nursing care.

DID YOU KNOW?

A nurse has the right to refuse to be temporarily reassigned (floated) to an area in which he or she is unqualified to work. Staff members on the unit accepting a reassigned nurse have a responsibility for orienting the nurse to the unit and supporting the nurse in the performance of nursing care.

      (4) Participate in continuing education to ensure competence in light of new technology and progress in nursing practice (e.g., know how to operate equipment before using it with a client).
      (5) Follow standards of care identified in the nurse practice act in the state in which the nurse works.

(6) Follow professional standards of care and agency policy and procedures (e.g., keep a bed in the lowest position, provide education and counseling, follow controlled-drug policies and procedures, maintain confidentiality and privacy, ensure that informed consent is obtained for procedures).

(7) Employ the nursing process when identifying client needs and providing client care:

(a) Assessment.

(b) Analysis.

(c) Planning.

(d) Implementation.

(e) Evaluation.

(8) Properly assign, delegate, and supervise subordinates, including assigning only tasks and responsibilities that are within the legal parameters of a person's role (e.g., only nurses are responsible for ongoing assessment, client education, and completion of tasks that require sterile technique; nurse aides can take vital signs and assist clients with uncomplicated activities of daily living).

(9) Treat a client with respect and dignity (e.g., address a client by name, pull a curtain, provide draping, support clients' rights, explain what you are going to do and why).

(10) Involve a client in the planning and implementation of care.

(11) Always function as a client advocate (e.g., help a client communicate wishes to other health-care providers and family members, question inappropriate medication and treatment prescriptions, follow an agency policy to report impaired coworkers, intervene on the behalf of clients when clients are unable to protect themselves).

(12) Always respond to client requests (e.g., assess the need for pain medication, answer call lights in a timely manner, arrange for an alternative meal if requested).

(13) Always follow the rights of medication administration and question incomplete or inappropriate prescriptions.

(14) Document all important information about a client, nursing care planned for and provided, client responses, and all events in the client's medical record (e.g., progress notes, medication administration record, flow sheets, admission assessment form, discharge form).

(15) Report to the primary health-care provider a change in a client's condition that requires immediate action.

(16) Notify the rapid response team (a group of professional health-care team members responsible for responding to emergency situations) when a client's condition deteriorates.

(17) Provide a thorough report at the end of a shift to the nurse responsible for the continued care of the client.

4. Failure to evaluate client responses to interventions.

a. Includes:

(1) Failure to observe for nontherapeutic and therapeutic responses.

(2) Failure to recognize significance of responses.

(3) Failure to respond appropriately to nontherapeutic responses.

(4) Failure to notify the primary health-care provider of a client's nontherapeutic responses.

(5) Failure to document the client's therapeutic or nontherapeutic responses.

b. To minimize the risk of litigation, the nurse must:

(1) Always assess for therapeutic and nontherapeutic responses to an intervention (e.g., chills, fever, low back pain, dyspnea, and facial flushing indicating a hemolytic reaction to a blood transfusion).

(2) Respond appropriately to a nontherapeutic response (e.g., immediately stop a blood transfusion and replace it with normal saline solution if a hemolytic reaction occurs).

(3) Notify the primary health-care provider of nontherapeutic responses to interventions (e.g., immediately notify the primary health-care provider if a client has a hemolytic reaction to a blood transfusion and then wait for treatment prescriptions).

(4) Document all therapeutic and nontherapeutic client responses to interventions (e.g., document medications given before a blood transfusion is initiated, client evaluation afterward, therapeutic and nontherapeutic responses, immediate notification of the primary health-care provider in the event of a negative reaction, and follow-up care provided along with ongoing assessments and client responses).

(5) Complete an incident report and follow facility policies and procedures when negative events occur (e.g., medication error, fall or injury involving a client, visitor, or staff member).

IV. Informed Consent

When a client agrees to be admitted to a hospital, the client gives approval for routine care. However, each specialized procedure requires the client to sign a special form called an informed consent. An **informed consent** indicates that the client, or the client's legal surrogate, has an understanding of what is to be done and why, including the risks and benefits of the procedure.

A. Elements that must be met for a client to give informed consent

1. *Disclosure:* The client must be provided with a thorough explanation of the risks, benefits, costs, and alternatives. It is the responsibility of the primary health-care provider to provide this information as well as answer all questions asked by the client.
2. *Comprehension:* The client must be able to repeat in his or her own words details about the procedure, including risks, benefits, costs, and alternatives.
3. *Voluntariness:* The client must give his or her consent willingly.
4. *Competence:* The client must be capable of understanding the information to make an informed decision.
   a. Understanding is dependent on the client being alert, having intact cognition, and being a minimum of 18 years of age.
   b. Minors younger than 18 years of age can sign a consent form if legally emancipated, a parent, or married.

B. Nursing care related to obtaining informed consent

1. Criteria that must be met to obtain an informed consent:
   a. *Disclosure:* Ensure that the primary health-care provider has discussed details about the procedure, including risks, benefits, costs, and alternatives in a language the client understands.
   b. *Comprehension:* Instruct the client, "State in your own words what you have been told about the procedure by your primary health-care provider." Determine if the information is consistent with details concerning the procedure.
   c. *Voluntariness:* Ask the client, "Are you signing this consent voluntarily without pressure from others?"
   d. *Competence:* Ensure that the client is at least 18 years of age or is an emancipated minor, a parent, or married and is alert with intact

cognition. When a client is incapable of participating in the decision-making process (e.g., intellectual disability, confusion, delirium, unconscious, sedated, emotionally incompetent), an alternative decision-maker must be identified. Most states specify the order of priority, such as durable power of attorney, court-appointed guardian, parents, spouse, and adult children.

2. Steps to obtain an informed consent:

🛑 a. Ensure that all the criteria related to an informed consent are met.

   b. Reinforce the primary health-care provider's information if necessary.
   c. Obtain the client's signature on the consent form.
   d. Sign the consent form as a witness. *Note:* The nurse's signature only indicates that the nurse was a witness to the client's signature.
   e. Ensure that the consent form is in the client's clinical record.

🛑 3. Notify the primary health-care provider if the criteria for consent are not met—for example, the client lacks understanding, is emotionally or mentally incompetent, or is not alert; a procedure is delayed until the primary health-care provider addresses concerns.

4. Document all nurse-client and nurse–primary health-care provider conversations and notifications in the clinical record.

DID YOU KNOW?

Clients have the right to sign a form that states that they do not want to be informed of the details of a procedure. In addition, if clients sign consent they have a right to withdraw the consent at any time before the procedure.

V. Specific Laws and Regulations That Guide Nursing Practice

Federal and state laws have been established to protect individual rights and public interests. Nurses must have knowledge and understanding of these laws because of their impact on the profession of nursing and nursing practice.

A. Examples of federal laws

1. Bill of Rights.
   a. First 10 amendments to the U.S. Constitution.
   b. Examples of rights especially relevant to nursing practice are the rights of privacy, freedom of speech, and due process.
2. Americans with Disabilities Act.
   a. Established a mandate for eliminating discrimination against people with disabilities.

b. Requires reasonable accommodation for individuals to perform their job and for clients (e.g., buildings must be wheelchair accessible, providers of care cannot discriminate against clients who have acquired immunodeficiency syndrome [AIDS]).

3. Comprehensive Drug Abuse Prevention and Control Act.
   a. Controls distribution and use of drugs that have a high potential for abuse or addiction, such as opioids, depressants, stimulants, and hallucinogens.
   b. Controlled drugs must be stored, handled, disposed of, and administered according to regulations established by the U.S. Drug Enforcement Administration (DEA).

4. Emergency Medical Treatment and Active Labor Act.
   a. Ensures access to emergency services despite an inability to pay for services.
   b. Forbids the transfer of indigent or uninsured individuals from a private to a public facility without adequate assessment and stabilization, except when:
      (1) The client requests a transfer.
      (2) The facility does not have the capacity to stabilize the client.
   c. Requires that, when transferred, a client must be attended to by competent personnel and with appropriate equipment.

5. Occupational Safety and Health Act (OSHA).
   a. Established the Occupational Safety and Health Administration (an agency of the U.S. Department of Labor), which identifies and enforces regulations that protect individuals from work-related injury.
   b. Protects nurses, who have the potential for injury because of exposure to such hazards as radiation, chemotherapeutic agents, blood-borne pathogens, electrical equipment, sharps, and moving and lifting clients.
   c. Sets specific standards and requires the availability of certain equipment (e.g., mechanical lifts, personal protective equipment) to maintain a safe and healthful workplace for nurses.

DID YOU KNOW?

Occupational nurses have an essential role in helping maintain the health and safety of workers within the work setting.

6. Health Care Quality Improvement Act.
   a. Provides public identification of primary health-care providers who are disciplined or penalized for failure to meet legal standards of care.
   b. Established the National Practitioner Data Bank, which tabulates data about medical malpractice payments, unfavorable actions taken against clinical privileges, and measures taken by professional organizations that negatively affect membership.

7. National Labor Relations Act.
   a. Gives individuals the legal right to bargain with an employer as a group to improve working conditions and salaries (collective bargaining).
   b. The American Nurses Association (ANA) in 1944 stated that each state's nurses association can perform collective bargaining for nurses.

8. Newborns' and Mothers' Health Protection Act.
   a. Increased the length of stay in a hospital or birthing center for a mother and infant to no less than 48 hours after a vaginal birth and no less than 96 hours after a cesarean birth.
   b. Attempts to limit maternal and neonatal morbidity and mortality.

9. Health Insurance Portability and Accountability Act (HIPAA).
   a. Provides regulations that protect the confidentiality of health information and medical records.
   b. Sets standards for organizational identifiers, electronic transfer of client information among organizations, uniform protection of all health information, and appropriate disclosure of protected health information.
   c. Requires nurses to:
      (1) Share client information (e.g., verbally, electronically, or in writing) with only those members of the health-care team responsible for the client. For example, nurses should:
         (a) Avoid posting signs that contain health-related information around clients' bed or on message boards in a nursing station.
         (b) Avoid talking about clients in areas where conversation can be overheard by others.
         (c) Avoid leaving client documents (i.e., electronic or paper) unsupervised.

DID YOU KNOW?

Information about a client's health-care status can be shared with people other than members of the health-care team when the client gives written permission. In addition, student nurses are held to the same rules and regulations as licensed health-care providers.

      (2) Inform clients verbally and in writing of their rights to privacy and confidentiality

regarding their health information. For example, a nurse should not disclose that a person is a client without expressed client permission.

    (3) Ensure that clients have the right to view and amend their own health records and obtain a copy of their clinical record upon written request. For example, a client may want a copy of his or her medical records sent to another health-care provider for a second opinion.

10. Patient Self-Determination Act.

    a. Requires health-care agencies to provide clients written information about their rights when making decisions regarding health care.

    b. Requires all health-care providers who receive Medicare funds to explain advance directives to staff and clients (e.g., client's wishes relative to health care should incapacitation or an inability to make decisions occur).

    c. Requires health-care providers to offer clients the opportunity to complete an advance directive.

B. Examples of state laws

1. Mandatory reporting laws.

    a. Require reporting of communicable diseases and suspected abuse (e.g., physical, sexual, emotional, or verbal abuse; financial exploitation; neglect) of children, elders, and mentally disabled people by health-care providers or family members to authorities (e.g., child protective services).

    b. Exist in most states.

    c. Vary by state, requiring nurses to know their own agency policy and state laws because, in some states, the employer is responsible for reporting suspected abuse or neglect.

    d. Provide for legal immunity from privacy laws if a nurse has made a report in good faith.

    e. Can charge nurses with a criminal or civil offense under the law if they do not report suspected abuse or neglect.

2. Good Samaritan laws.

🛑 a. Offer immunity from liability in malpractice litigation to health-care professionals who provide assistance at the scene of an accident or in an emergency when standards of practice are followed and the health-care professional acts in a prudent manner as would another professional in a similar circumstance.

    b. Nurses should:

      (1) Provide only first aid, if possible.

      (2) Employ only actions that they are educated to do.

      (3) Instruct someone to get additional help.

      (4) Stay until the injured person leaves or is transferred by ambulance or until another qualified person assumes responsibility for the injured person.

      (5) Not accept compensation.

    c. Gross divergence from normal standards of care or recklessly or intentionally injuring a person can lead to litigation.

    d. Do not require nurses to render care to people outside of their contractual responsibilities to an entity.

3. Nurse practice acts.

    a. Safeguard the public by legally defining the nature and scope of nursing practice, describing how the nursing profession is governed, and defining criteria for nursing education.

    b. Are specific to each state; therefore, nurses should know and understand the nurse practice act of the state or states in which they work; this is critical for travel nurses and other nurses who work in more than one state.

    c. Generally give state boards of nursing the authority to regulate nursing practice and education within the state, including licensing, credentialing, and disciplinary procedures.

    d. Licensing.

      (1) State boards of nursing have the authority to permit graduates of approved schools of nursing to take the National Council Licensure Examination (NCLEX-RN or NCLEX-PN).

      (2) After criteria for licensure are met (vary from state to state), the state board of nursing awards a nursing license that authorizes an individual the right to engage in the practice of nursing as a registered professional nurse or licensed practical nurse.

      (3) Certain states allow nurses to be licensed in one state and to practice in all states taking part in a multistate agreement (multistate compact).

    e. Credentialing: Voluntary self-regulation that attempts to ensure proficiency of its health-care providers and includes accreditation and certification.

      (1) Accreditation.

        (a) State boards of nursing examine and monitor a nursing program's ability to meet minimal expected standards for basic nursing education as well as evaluate ongoing efforts at continuous improvement of the program.

        (b) They generally require nursing programs to meet educational standards established by the National League for Nursing Accrediting Commission or the American Association of Colleges of Nursing.

    (c) Hospitals generally voluntarily seek accreditation by The Joint Commission, which ensures a minimum standard of quality of care is provided to clients.

  (2) Certification.

    (a) Professional organizations, such as the ANA, offer voluntary certification in specialty areas (e.g., oncology, geriatrics, pediatrics) when specific criteria are met, such as educational preparation, experience, evidence of continuing education, and a passing grade on an examination.

    (b) Some states permit a nurse to seek an advanced practice license only if first certified by an approved specialty organization.

  f. Disciplinary procedures.

    (1) State boards of nursing generally are responsible for enforcing requirements by establishing disciplinary procedures.

    (2) Unprofessional conduct is reported to the state board of nursing, which follows a set procedure to determine whether the nurse has violated the state's nurse practice act. Punitive action (e.g., suspension, revocation of a license, attendance at a drug rehabilitation program) may result if guilt is proven.

VI. Professional Guidelines for Nursing Practice

The role of the nurse has expanded dramatically because of the advent of new technology and changes in the delivery of health care within society. Client and nurse rights, standards of nursing care, and specific policies and procedures within an entity are designed to protect both clients and nurses.

A. ANA Nurse's Bill of Rights

1. Developed to "protect the dignity and autonomy of nurses in the workplace."
2. Identifies seven conditions nurses should expect from the workplace that address issues related to the provision of safe, competent, and ethical nursing care as well as personal nurse-related issues.

  a. Right to practice nursing in a way that fulfills their obligations to society.

  b. Right to practice nursing within the legal scope of nursing practice and professional standards.

  c. Right to practice nursing in accordance with the Code of Ethics for Nurses.

  d. Right to advocate for clients and themselves without fear of retribution.

  e. Right to have fair compensation for their work.

  f. Right to work in a safe environment.

  g. Right to individually or collectively negotiate the conditions of their employment.

B. The Patient Care Partnership

1. Asserts that clients have rights regarding their treatment when admitted to a health-care facility.
2. Originally published as the Patient's Bill of Rights by the American Hospital Association; has evolved and now addresses client expectations.
3. Briefly identifies that clients should expect:

  a. High-quality care.

  b. A clean, safe environment.

  c. Freedom from abuse and neglect.

  d. To be involved in decisions.

  e. To receive information about the right to refuse care and resources available to help make decisions.

  f. Protection of privacy and confidentiality.

  g. Help with billing and insurance claims.

  h. Preparation and information on discharge from the facility.

C. Standards of practice

1. Are specific stipulations that guide the practice of nursing by outlining the scope, function, and role of nurses and nursing practice.
2. May be general and relate to values within the profession or specific and relate to expectations of nursing care for an identified group of clients.
3. Published by various states (e.g., nurse practice acts), professional organizations (e.g., ANA, Emergency Nurses Association), and federal organizations (e.g., The Joint Commission, Centers for Medicare & Medicaid Services) to guide nursing practice.

D. Institutional policies and procedures

1. Are not law.
2. Are more specific than standards.
3. Include information specific to nursing practice that an employer expects a nurse to know and safely implement.

VII. Protection Against Litigation

By virtue of such factors as the complexity of nursing care, reengineering of health-care delivery, expanding role of the nurse, and expectations of clients and family members, as well as the litigiousness of society, nurses are at an increased risk for being accused of negligence or malpractice.

Various safeguards exist that protect nurses from legal actions.

A. Legal safeguards for nurses

1. Good Samaritan laws.
   a. Offer immunity from liability in malpractice litigation to health-care professionals who provide assistance at the scene of an accident or emergency if standards of practice are followed.
   b. Example: A nurse applies pressure with a shirt to a hemorrhaging wound that a person sustained in an automobile collision. Later, the person experiences a wound infection. The nurse is not libel for the person's infection because the nurse acted in a prudent manner consistent to what another nurse would have done in a similar situation.
2. "Safe harbor."
   a. Protects a nurse from suspension, termination, disciplinary action, and discrimination if the nurse refuses to do or not do something because he or she believes that it is inappropriate and could be harmful.
   b. Example: A nurse working on a medical-surgical unit who has no obstetrical nursing experience has a right to refuse to be floated to a birthing unit.
3. Professional liability insurance.
   a. Contract the nurse has with an insurance company, which pays for legal fees and for judgment or settlement costs to the extent of the policy in the event of litigation.
   b. Example: Provides a legal defense during litigation from claims that the nurse committed malpractice by an act of omission or commission; however, some liability contracts do not defend against claims of sexual abuse of a client, damages caused while a nurse is under the effect of drugs or alcohol, or unlawful actions by the nurse.
4. Incident report.
   a. An **incident report** clearly documents all the facts (e.g., date, time, location, and a brief description of the incident in factual terms) related to any occurrence out of the ordinary that results in or is likely to result in harm to a client, employee, or visitor.
   b. The nurse must document the event in the client's medical record, including how the injury occurred, the client's response, and any actions taken; the nurse does not need to reference in the client's clinical record that an incident report was completed.
   c. An incident report should include quoted statements by the client or individuals involved when possible; should not contain opinions, conclusions, or speculation; and should not place blame.
   d. Example: An incident report should be completed when a client climbs over a side rail or receives a medication intended for another; an incident report is required if a nurse sustains an injury while moving a client or a visitor falls on the floor.
   e. In the event of litigation, an incident report helps to remind individuals involved what the facts were and avoids blurring of the facts over time.
   f. Reports are used for quality improvement activities, not for disciplinary actions against a staff member; they facilitate identification of high-risk trends, which promotes the development of educational programs to address the prevention of the identified problem.
5. Informed consent.
   a. Protects a nurse from charges of battery if a client claims that permission was not given for an invasive procedure.
   b. In the event a client refuses to sign a consent form for a recommended intervention, the client should be informed of the consequences of inaction and then be asked to sign a form that releases the health-care team and agency from responsibility.
6. Nurse practice acts.
   a. Protect a nurse by clearly defining the nature and scope of nursing practice and conditions under which a person can practice the profession of nursing.
   b. Requires nurses to work within the legal definition of their role to be protected.
7. Controlled substance laws.
   a. Protects a nurse from involvement in a situation of missing or misused controlled drugs.
   b. Requires nurses to follow all the rules and regulations established by the DEA related to storage, handling, administration, and disposal of controlled drugs to be protected by these laws.
8. Laws to protect whistle-blowing.
   a. **Whistle-blowing** occurs when a person who unsuccessfully attempts to correct a quality-of-care issue within the normal channels of an organization and then resorts to going to an outside organization with the concern.
   b. Whistle-blowing should be a last resort when no action is taken in response to reported concerns, such as understaffing, reassignment, and excessive mandatory overtime.
   c. Some states have laws that protect whistle-blowers from reprisal.

B. Nursing actions to protect oneself from litigation

🛑 1. Know the legal parameters of the state nurse practice act in the state in which one works.

2. Follow laws that influence nursing practice.
3. Follow institutional policies and procedures.
4. Follow the ANA Standards of Nursing Practice.
5. Follow ethical parameters provided by the ANA Code of Ethics for Nurses.
6. Purchase professional liability insurance separate from what an employer provides to ensure that one's personal interests are protected.
7. Work only in a setting in which one is prepared to meet the challenges of delivering safe nursing care.
8. Keep current by attending educational and in-service programs.
9. Maintain competent nursing practice.
   a. Implement safe nursing care in the technical realm (e.g., perform skills safely and develop new skills in response to technological advances).
   b. Maintain cognitive competence (e.g., acquire new knowledge and apply it appropriately, especially in response to the results of evidence-based practice research).
   c. Ensure interpersonal competency (e.g., continue to develop communication skills to collaborate with clients and other members of the health-care team).
10. Be respectful of clients' rights, and deliver nursing care in a compassionate manner.
11. Use the nursing process to plan and implement comprehensive nursing care.
12. Document all nursing activities and client responses to interventions (see "Documentation" in Chapter 2, Communication, Collaboration, and Documentation for more information).

VIII. Abuse and Neglect

A. Individuals who are abused or neglected
1. **Abuse** occurs when a person is physically, emotionally, or sexually mistreated or exploited. **Neglect** occurs when a person's physical and emotional needs are inadequately met (e.g., insufficient food, health care, contact with others, environmental safety).
2. Most commonly are women, children, adults with an intellectual disability, or dependent older adults.
3. Have risk factors such as a relationship with another person who has a mental illness, an addiction (e.g., alcohol, drugs, gambling, sex), or a socioeconomic issue, such as excessive spending or lack of income.

B. Community resources that address the needs of abused or neglected individuals
1. The Victim Information Bureau that provides referrals to related services.
2. Rape crisis centers that provide counseling and comprehensive services 24 hours a day.
3. Emergency department companion programs that provide trained rape crisis counselors who meet children and adults in hospital emergency departments; the counselors provide nonjudgmental emotional support, information, referrals, and a change of clothes.
4. Sexual assault nurse examiner (SANE) programs that provide special education to nurses so that they can care for rape victims in a SANE center (designated hospitals) by providing victim-centered care, medical evaluations, preventive medication for pregnancy and sexually transmitted diseases, evidence collection and storage, and a change of clothes.
5. Referral to an agency that provides an emergency safe haven or shelter.
6. Access to counselors who provide support and advice as a victim and family members navigate the legal system.

C. Nursing care for individuals who are abused or neglected
1. Identify signs and symptoms of abuse or neglect (Box 3.1).
2. Provide privacy when interviewing clients; ensure that interviews take place out of sight and hearing of suspected abusers (abused people may fear retribution).

🛑 3. Encourage clients who are currently unwilling to leave their abusive environments to have an exit plan, including a packed bag of clothes and toiletries, in the event a quick escape is necessary.

4. Provide the telephone number of a domestic abuse hotline in the event immediate advice and emotional support is needed; instruct clients to memorize the phone number.
5. Encourage clients to call 911 if personal safety is in immediate jeopardy.
6. When sexual abuse of a child is suspected, ensure that a child protective services counselor and a sexual assault nurse examiner or a primary health-care provider are present.
7. For an adult who is sexually abused, ensure that a rape counselor and a primary health-care provider or sexual assault nurse examiner are present.
8. Arrange for clients to be sheltered in a safe environment.

Box 3.1	Signs of Abuse and Neglect

Child Sexual Abuse

- *Vaginal or penile discharge*
- *Pain, itching, or trauma in the genital area*
- *Sexually transmitted disease*
- *Recurrent urinary tract infections*
- *Regressed behavior*
- *Fear of certain people or places*
- *Play that re-creates sexual abuse*
- *Decreasing performance in school*

Older Adult Abuse and Neglect

- *Fractures or trauma inconsistent with stated cause*
- *Cigarette burns*
- *Scratches*
- *Injuries at different stages of recovery*
- *Chafing at ankles and wrists, indicating use of restraint*
- *Prolonged gap between injury and seeking of medical attention*
- *Dependence on caregiver*
- *Physical or cognitive impairment*
- *Combativeness*

Domestic Abuse

- *Fractures or trauma inconsistent with stated cause*
- *Multiple injuries involving face, head, breasts, and genitalia*
- *Ecchymotic areas around eyes, face, or neck*
- *Fractured nose or eye orbits*
- *Broken teeth*
- *Injuries at different stages of recovery*
- *X-ray evidence of old fractures*
- *Sense of helplessness, guilt, depression, or low self-esteem*
- *History of panic attacks, headaches, or anxiety*

9. Refer clients and family members to available community services.

🛑 10. Report abuse or neglect when appropriate.

DID YOU KNOW?

All states mandate that nurses report suspected abuse or neglect of children to appropriate authorities, and most states mandate that nurses report suspected abuse or neglect of older adults and developmentally or cognitively impaired individuals to appropriate officials. Laws concerning reporting spousal abuse (i.e., intimate partner violence) and rape vary widely because some people believe that reporting violates the autonomy of the person being abused. Also, an adult client who states that she or he is a victim of rape has to be the person who reports the rape to the authorities. However, a nurse should do everything possible to advocate for the client.

IX. Ethical Nursing Practice

Nurses must perform self-examination to identify personal beliefs and values because these foundations drive the formation of one's character, morals, and ethics, ultimately influencing one's behavior in society. Then nurses must develop a professional ethical platform that does not impose their personal beliefs and values about what is acceptable and unacceptable onto clients and their family members. Incorporating the concepts of autonomy, beneficence, nonmaleficence, justice, and fidelity in conjunction with adhering to the laws and standards associated with the profession of nursing promotes the delivery of ethically competent nursing care. Nursing care becomes a challenge when decision-making conflicts occur among clients and their family members and even among health-care providers.

A. Societal factors that contribute to ethical issues
1. Advances in technology, such as:
   a. In vitro fertilization.
   b. Genetic engineering.
   c. Organ transplantation.
   d. Life support interventions.
   e. Procedures that reveal fetal impairment.
2. Multicultural population issues, such as:
   a. Multifaith society.
   b. Increased ethnic diversity.
   c. Groups with vastly different values and beliefs.
3. Increased consumer awareness, such as:
   a. Increased client awareness of their rights.
   b. Internet availability of health information.
   c. Increased client self-advocacy.
   d. Internet chat rooms that facilitate discussion among people with the same disorder.
4. Cost-containment measures, such as:
   a. Nurses caring for increased numbers of more acutely ill clients, contributing to potentially unsafe situations.
   b. Decreased length of stay in health-care facilities, sending clients home while they still need skilled health-care services, which are not always readily available.

B. Principles related to ethical nursing practice
1. Autonomy.
   a. **Autonomy** refers to the right of people to have individual liberty and self-determination (i.e., clients have the right to make personal choices about treatment and care).
   b. Means that nurses should provide information so that clients can make personal choices regarding their care.
   c. Clients have a right to accept or refuse planned health care.
   d. Examples: Signing a consent form, continuing the intake of salt when a low-sodium diet is recommended, refusing blood products because of religious beliefs, signing one's self out of the hospital against medical advice.

2. Beneficence.
   a. **Beneficence** is an ethical principle that addresses a concept that nursing actions should promote good.
   b. Nursing actions should benefit others or support a positive outcome.
   c. Examples: Irrigating a wound, administering a medication, turning and positioning an immobile client.
3. Nonmaleficence.
   a. **Nonmaleficence** is a principle that refers to preventing harm, avoiding actions that can cause harm, and removing a client from harm.
   b. The positive outcome of an action must be measured against the risk of potential harm.
   c. Example: Medicating a postoperative client for pain and then ambulating the client using a two-person assist addresses the need to improve circulation and to prevent harm while minimizing the risk of pain or a fall.
4. Fidelity.
   a. **Fidelity** refers to making only promises or commitments that can be kept.
   b. Means that a client can expect that a nurse will honor agreements made verbally.
   c. Example: A nurse who promises to return immediately with pain medication is expected to honor that commitment.
5. Justice.
   a. **Justice** refers to fairness and equality.
   b. Means that all clients should be treated fairly and equally regardless of individual factors, such as age, gender, skin color, ethnic origin, religious beliefs, sexual orientation, and medical diagnosis.
   c. Example: All people should have access to health care whether they have medical insurance or are indigent; just and fair policies and procedures should guide the allocation of organs for transplantation.
6. Veracity.
   a. **Veracity** refers to being truthful, which is essential to a trusting nurse-client relationship.
   b. Demonstrates respect for the client.
   c. Necessary for a client's right to make informed decisions.
   d. Examples: Providing truthful answers to clients who are asking questions about their prognosis; informing a client when a procedure may be painful.

C. Guides to ethical decision making in nursing
1. Nursing codes of ethics.
   a. Officially state ideals and values of the profession, provide a framework for making ethical

decisions, and are a standard for professional actions.
   b. Examples: The ANA Code of Ethics for Nurses (see http:www.nursingworld.org/MainMenuCategories/EthicsStandards/CodeofEthicsforNurses.aspx); International Council of Nurses' (ICN) Code of Ethics for Nurses (see http://www.icn.ch/who-we-are/code-of-ethics-for-nurses/).
2. Institutional ethics committees.
   a. Generally consist of interdisciplinary health-care professionals, such as primary health-care providers, nurses, clergy, ethicists, and lay representatives.
   b. Establish guidelines, formulate policies and procedures, provide counseling and education, and conduct case reviews.
   c. Mediate in ethical dilemmas to facilitate resolution.
3. Nursing ethics forums.
   a. May be unit based or agency wide and are designed to provide opportunities for nurses to identify and discuss ethical issues associated with the provision of nursing care.
   b. Assist nurses in improving skills in ethical problem-solving and decision making.

D. Development of a personal ethical foundation
1. Nurses should identify and clarify their own values and beliefs.
2. Nurses should form a personal ethical foundation.
3. Nurses should integrate a personal ethical foundation with the ethics of the nursing profession (e.g., ANA Code of Ethics).
4. Nurses should be aware of sensitive ethical issues.
5. Nurses should continuously work at improving ethical decision-making abilities.

E. Nursing actions that support clients' ethical rights
1. Nurses should follow ethical codes provided by professional organizations.
2. **Nurses should support client autonomy, especially when a client's decision is not supported by family members. The nurse must remember that the client is the center of the health team and must be an advocate for the client above all others.**
3. Nurses should support clients and family members as they make decisions.
4. Nurses should accept clients' and family members' decisions, even if those decisions differ from the decisions a nurse would make personally; if unable to do so, nurses should remove themselves from responsibility for the care of the client and family members.

5. Nurses should use an ethical decision model for guidance to identify the best response to a dilemma.
6. Nurses should use and participate in an institutional ethics committee.

X. Legal Rights and Ethical Issues Related to End-of-Life Care

End-of-life issues have escalated dramatically due to advances in technology that prolong life, the increased number of older adults, and the desire of dying individuals to control their destinies with dignity. As a result, clients, family members, and health-care providers are faced with multiple ethical dilemmas, such as assisted suicide, euthanasia, withholding or termination of life-sustaining treatment, organ donation, and certification of death. Multiple legal instruments are available to address some of these issues, such as advanced health-care directives, health-care proxies, living wills, and DNAR orders.

A. Advance health-care directives
   1. **Advance health-care directives** are a set of instructions or directions stating a person's health-care requests if the person becomes incapacitated or unable to make decisions.
   2. Health-care providers are required to offer clients the opportunity to complete an advance health-care directive.
   3. Clients can cancel or make changes to advanced health-care directives at any time.
   4. People should complete an advanced health-care directive before they become ill so that personal wishes are carried out should they become ill.
   5. Health-care providers are protected from liability when they follow the instructions in an advance directive.
   6. Advance health-care directives include health-care proxy (durable power of attorney for health care), living will, and DNAR orders.
B. Health-care proxy (durable power of attorney for health care)
   1. A **health-care proxy** is a document that identifies a person to make health-care decisions for a client when the client is no longer able to make decisions.
   2. The contract may indicate certain conditions under which the proxy takes effect, such as irreversible coma or terminal illness.
   3. It may include specific instructions about issues, such as withholding hydration, medication, parenteral nutrition, and mechanical ventilation.
   4. It is a legal instrument signed by two witnesses.
C. Living will
   1. A **living will** is a document prepared by a competent person giving instructions associated with

medical care to be delivered or not delivered if the person becomes unable to make decisions in the future.
   2. A living will differs from a health-care proxy in that it does not identify a person as a proxy.
D. DNAR orders
   1. **DNAR orders** direct health-care providers not to attempt resuscitation in the event that a client suffers cardiac or respiratory failure in a health-care facility or the home.
   2. Health-care providers are not legally permitted to initiate DNAR orders without the consent of the client, surrogate, or proxy.
   3. Nurses and clients must know that a DNAR order does not mean "do not treat."
   4. DNAR orders may be suspended before surgery and reinstituted after surgery if the primary health-care provider has discussed this with and received consent from the client or proxy.
   5. Health-care professionals who initiate cardiopulmonary resuscitation in the presence of a DNAR order may be held accountable (i.e., sued by the family for pain and anguish; reported to the state board of nursing).
E. Assisted suicide
   1. **Assisted suicide** is the taking of one's own life after seeking and receiving a prescription from a primary health-care provider for a medication that will cause death.
   2. Various criteria are determined by state law; for example, the client must:
      a. State the intent to and be capable of self-administering medication that will end one's life.
      b. Be at least 18 years of age.
      c. Be terminally ill with fewer than 6 months to live, as determined by two physicians.
      d. Meet certain psychiatric criteria and be counseled regarding other options, including palliative and hospice care.
      e. Request a prescription from a physician for a medication that will cause death. Generally, there is a designated waiting period (e.g., 15 days) between the request for the prescription and the writing of the prescription by the physician.
   3. The states of Oregon, Washington, California, Montana, and Vermont have passed laws that permit physicians to prescribe medications that may be used by clients to cause their own death.
   4. Physicians, nurses, and pharmacists are not required to participate in assisted suicide.
   5. The ANA "prohibits nurses' participation in assisted suicide and euthanasia because these

acts are in direct violation of Code of Ethics for Nurses with Interpretive Statement. . . , the ethical traditions and goals of the profession, and its covenant with society. Nurses have an obligation to provide humane, comprehensive, and compassionate care that respects the rights of patients but upholds the standards of the profession in the presence of chronic, debilitating illness and at end-of-life." (ANA, 2013)

F. Euthanasia

1. **Euthanasia** is premeditated termination of the life of a person suffering from an incurable or terminal illness.
2. A person directly implements the cause of death.
3. The ANA prohibits nurses' participation in active euthanasia. (See "Assisted Suicide" section in this chapter.)

4. No state in the United States currently allows euthanasia.

G. Withholding or terminating life-sustaining treatment, food, and/or fluid

1. People have the right to refuse recommended treatment as well as interventions that are life sustaining.
2. When clients are incapable of speaking for themselves, legal surrogates can make the decision to refuse or withdraw treatments for clients; states have specific protocols to determine the order of surrogacy.

H. Certification of death, organ donation (upon death), and postmortem examination (autopsy) (For more information about these topics see "Certification of Death" and Box 13.1, "Legal Issues Related to Postmortem Care," in Chapter 13, Grief and Loss.)

CASE STUDY: Putting It All Together

A 17-year-old, accompanied by her mother, brings her 1-week-old infant to the emergency department. The infant's mother appears dazed, does not make eye contact, and rarely answers the nurse's questions. The grandmother tells the triage nurse that her daughter is a senior in high school, is unmarried, and lives at home. The nurse obtains the infant's vital signs, weighs the infant, and identifies that the infant is pale and lethargic. The grandmother, who is holding the infant, states, "The baby sleeps all the time and has difficulty sucking when given a bottle and stops a lot during a feeding." The triage nurse transports the infant and family members from the triage area to a room with a crib in the emergency department. When passing the main desk, the triage nurse says, loudly enough for other health team members to hear, "The baby's mother is on drugs. She had no business getting pregnant in the first place." Later, while the infant is waiting to be further assessed, the mother of the infant attempts to run out of the emergency department. A nurse grabs the mother's arm and pulls her back to the unit, saying firmly, "Where do you think you are going? Stay here. Your baby needs you!"

Case Study Questions

A. From whom should the informed consent be obtained to provide care to the infant? Why?

B. During the intake interview, the triage nurse asks the following questions. Which questions are appropriate or inappropriate, and why?

1. "Why didn't you get married?"

2. "Did you drink alcohol while you were pregnant?"

3. "Where is the father of the baby now?"

4. "Were you taking prescription or illegal drugs while you were pregnant?"

5. "Did you experience any health problems during your pregnancy?"

6. "Do you plan on going back to school or staying at home with your baby?"

C. Which nursing intervention is an example of an intentional tort, and why?

D. Which nursing intervention is an example of a quasi-intentional tort, and why?

REVIEW QUESTIONS

Be sure to read the Introduction for valuable test-taking tips.

1. A home care nurse is visiting an older adult who experienced a brain attack 2 years ago and now has a sacral pressure ulcer. The nurse identifies that the client and spouse both appear unkempt, and the spouse appears tired and irritated. The client is very quiet and avoids eye contact. Which nursing action is **most** appropriate?
   1. Explore with the client and spouse their concerns.
   2. Assess the client for signs of physical abuse and neglect.
   3. Discuss with the client and spouse additional resources to help with the client's care.
   4. Assess the client's pressure ulcer and report findings to the primary health-care provider.

2. A client is admitted to a home health-care program for palliative care. During the admission interview and nursing assessment, the client empathically states, "I want no intervention to extend my life other than keeping me comfortable." Family members, however, tell the nurse that they want the client to continue chemotherapy. What should the nurse do?
   1. Protect the client's right to self-determination.
   2. Initiate a referral to a psychiatric nurse practitioner.
   3. Ask the client to reconsider chemotherapy for the sake of the family.
   4. Refer family members to the primary health-care provider to resolve this issue.

3. A nurse is planning client care based on moral and ethical principles. Which nursing statement demonstrates an effort to implement the principle of fidelity?
   1. "Let's talk about foods that are healthy and that you should include in your daily diet."
   2. "I know that you are out of work, so I have arranged for you to get follow-up care at our outpatient clinic."
   3. "You said that your son wants you to have this surgery. What is important is what you believe is best for you."
   4. "It's been half an hour, and I am back as I promised to ensure that the pain medication I gave you is providing relief."

4. Which statements are associated with state nurse practice acts? **Select all that apply.**
   1. Nurse practice acts identify what a nurse can and cannot do.
   2. A purpose of state nurse practice acts is to regulate the practice of nursing.
   3. The federal government is the regulating agency responsible for state nurse practice acts.
   4. Student nurses are not obligated to meet the same standards of care as are licensed nurses.
   5. If a student nurse is involved in a disciplinary action by the state board of nursing, the student may be prohibited from taking the National Council Licensure Examination.

5. A nurse is caring for an adult client who is scheduled for surgery. Which actions are associated with the nurse ensuring a valid, legal consent? **Select all that apply.**
   1. Observe the client signing the consent form.
   2. Ensure that the client is signing the consent form voluntarily.
   3. Assess if the client has the capacity to make an informed consent.
   4. Review with the client the risks and benefits of the surgery before the consent is signed.
   5. Explore options other than surgery that may be beneficial in meeting the client's health needs.

6. Which situations should the nursing staff refer to the hospital ethics committee?
   1. The adult client with renal insufficiency who refuses dialysis
   2. The wife who wants her unconscious husband to have a drug that is available in a phase-three trial
   3. The parents of a developmentally disabled adult who disagree with the health-care decisions of the court-appointed guardian
   4. The adult client recently diagnosed with metastatic cancer who wants hospice care but whose family wants chemotherapy to be given immediately
   5. The members of a family who disagree on the medical course of action for a relative who is unconscious and did not identify a person to be a health-care proxy

7. A nurse is implementing care based on moral and ethical principles. What should the nurse do **first** to accomplish a personal professional code of ethics consistent with the American Nurses Association *Code of Ethics for Nurses?*
1. Deliver care that preserves and protects client autonomy and self-determination.
2. Explore personal values and beliefs because they affect nursing decisions.
3. Implement culturally competent and sensitive nursing care to clients.
4. Respect the inherent worth and uniqueness of each individual client.

8. Which actions meet obligations regarding the Health Insurance Portability and Accountability Act (HIPAA) of 1996? **Select all that apply.**
1. Allowing clients the right to review and copy their clinical record
2. Providing access to a client's clinical record to all members of the nursing team
3. Holding client rounds in a hallway out of the hearing range of the client being discussed
4. Explaining to a person inquiring about the condition of a client that information about the client is confidential
5. Giving medical information about an unconscious client to the client's daughter who is the person indicated in the client's proxy directive

9. An older adult is diagnosed with atrial flutter with a 4-to-1 block. The atrial rate is 280 beats/minute and the ventricular rate is 70 beats/minute. The client is admitted to the hospital and transferred to a medical unit. The client is being treated with diltiazem (Cardizem), an antidysrhythmic, as well as continuous electrocardiogram monitoring. Cardioversion is being considered if the client does not respond favorably to the antidysrhythmic. Later that evening, the client reports feeling strange, so the nurse obtains the client's vital signs and performs a physical assessment. The nurse concludes that the client is stable and continues to follow the primary health-care provider's prescription. During the night, the client dies. Eventually, the client's cause of death is determined to be a brain attack (cerebral vascular accident, stroke). The risk manager of the hospital reviews the client's clinical record, specifically the vital signs, progress notes, and electrocardiogram results. The risk manager concludes that the nurse can be accountable for which specific tort?
1. Assault
2. Battery
3. Negligence
4. Malpractice

Client's Clinical Record

Vital Signs

Temperature: 99.2°F
Pulse: 90 beats/minute, irregular rhythm
Respirations: 26 breaths/minute
Blood pressure: 98/60 mm Hg

Electrocardiogram

Atrial fibrillation

Progress Notes

Client reports feeling weak, tired, dizzy, and short of breath. States, "I feel very anxious and like my heart is pounding." Respirations are 26 breaths/minute but do not appear to be labored. Denies chest pain, nausea, and headache. Strength in both hands and feet are equal. Spoke with client to provide reassurance.

10. A client who has a history of schizophrenia and is hallucinating is brought to the emergency department of a community hospital. The primary health-care provider in charge refuses to admit the client. The nurse attempts to educate the primary health-care provider regarding the law involving clients who are grossly disabled. The primary health-care provider still refuses to admit the client. What is the nurse's **next** action?
1. Allow the client to stay against the primary health-care provider's wishes.
2. Refuse to discharge the client as per the primary health-care provider's decision.
3. Describe the primary health-care provider's behavior to the nursing supervisor and ask for guidance.
4. Call the primary health-care provider's supervisor and explain that the primary health-care provider is acting inappropriately.

11. Which statements associated with a client's clinical record are considered accurate? **Select all that apply.**
1. The clinical record belongs to the client.
2. The Joint Commission examines clients' clinical records to substantiate compliance with standards of care.
3. Clinical records are used by a quality assurance committee to monitor quality of care provided by the facility.
4. Clinical records serve as a legal document that can be used in a court of law to prove that a standard of care was met or not met.
5. Parts of a clinical record can be copied and used by student nurses only if the client's name and medical record number are removed.

12. A client with paralyzed lower extremities (paraplegia) as a result of a spinal cord injury states that the employer said, "You cannot come back to work because the office is not set up for employees using wheelchairs." Which nursing action is **most** supportive of this client?
    1. Instruct a social worker to intercede on behalf of the client.
    2. Report the client's situation to the hospital's legal department to negotiate a compromise.
    3. Suggest that the client seek employment where assistive devices are able to maneuver about the work environment.
    4. Explain to the client that employers must make reasonable accommodations to facilitate employment of disabled employees.

13. A nurse is caring for a client receiving hospice care for terminal cancer. The client has a transdermal opioid patch and a prescription for an oral opioid for breakthrough pain. The client reports that the pain is excruciating. The nurse assesses the client and identifies that the client's pulse is 85 beats/minute, respirations are 10 breaths/minute and shallow, and the blood pressure is 98/68 mm Hg. Which should the nurse do?
    1. Administer the prn opioid medication.
    2. Inform the primary health-care provider of the client's respiratory rate.
    3. Call the nursing supervisor to ask for guidance in dealing with this situation.
    4. Hold the pain medication until the respirations increase to an acceptable rate.

14. Which statements accurately pertain to nursing licensure? **Select all that apply.**
    1. A state board of nursing can never revoke a nursing license.
    2. A nursing license can be refused as a result of unlawful actions.
    3. A nursing license is not necessary when practicing nursing in the home setting.
    4. A nursing license allows a nurse to practice in the state in which the license was issued.
    5. A state board of nursing is responsible for ensuring that graduates of recognized schools of nursing take the NCLEX licensure examination.

15. A nurse is making every effort to implement nursing care based on moral concepts and principles of ethics. Which nursing statements demonstrate an effort to implement the principle of veracity?
    1. "Let's review the in-bed leg exercises that you need to perform after surgery."
    2. "Here is the pain medication that I promised I would get for you immediately."
    3. "After receiving this drug, you may feel bone pain, but it should subside in about a week."
    4. "I am going to move you to a room away from the nurses' station so that you sleep better at night."
    5. "With a permanent colostomy you will eliminate fecal material through an opening on your abdomen into a bag."

16. Which term describes the situation when a nurse says to a pediatric client, "If you don't be quiet, I will not let your parents visit you today"?
    1. Battery
    2. Assault
    3. Negligence
    4. Abandonment

17. Which actions are a violation of the Health Insurance Portability and Accountability Act of 1996 (HIPAA)? **Select all that apply.**
    1. Talking about a client to another health professional in an elevator
    2. Telling a neighbor about a famous person who currently is your client
    3. Documenting untrue information on purpose in a client's clinical record
    4. Leaving client data on a computer screen in a hallway while administering medication
    5. Completing an incident report about a client situation and asking the nurse manager to review it

18. Which must be reported to legal authorities in some states in North America?
    1. Release against medical advice
    2. Diagnosis of tuberculosis
    3. Suspected child neglect
    4. Abuse of older adults

19. A primary nurse is caring for a 70-year-old adult who suffered a brain attack 10 days ago and is unresponsive. The client did not sign a legal instrument identifying which adult child should make health-care decisions in the event of incapacitation. Two of the adult children are adamant about not wanting a feeding tube inserted for nutritional support, and two of the adult children are just as firm about wanting a feeding tube inserted. What should the nurse do to **best** help resolve this situation?
    1. Explain to the siblings all the advantages of inserting a feeding tube.
    2. Urge family members to discuss the matter of inserting a feeding tube with their spiritual advisor.
    3. Suggest that this issue about the feeding tube be presented to an ethics committee for consultation.
    4. Encourage the insertion of the feeding tube temporarily until the client's status can be determined.

20. Which of the following are designed to protect the nurse? **Select all that apply.**
    1. Occupational Safety and Health Act
    2. Americans with Disabilities Act
    3. Nurse practice acts
    4. Reporting of abuse
    5. Incident reports

21. A nurse accidentally administers a medication to the wrong client and the client experiences a serious untoward reaction. For which tort can the nurse be legally charged?
    1. Malpractice
    2. Assault
    3. Battery
    4. Fraud

22. Which are examples of violations of the Health Insurance Portability and Accountability Act (HIPAA)? **Select all that apply.**
    1. Failure to fill out an incident report after a client falls
    2. Discussing a plan of care with other student nurses in a debriefing conference
    3. Discussing test results with a client in a populated sitting area in the unit lounge
    4. Discussing a client's condition with a family member before checking if the person is a designated surrogate
    5. Temporarily misplacing a form with the names of clients and their scheduled surgeries that is returned by a visitor

23. Which statement is accurate regarding a nurse practice act?
    1. Educational criteria that must be met by schools of nursing are legislated exclusively by a state's nurse practice act.
    2. The National League for Nursing dictates the criteria for awarding licensure to state nurse practice acts.
    3. Rules and regulations regarding the practice of nursing are identified in each state's nurse practice act.
    4. A nurse practice act provides federal oversight of what a nurse can and cannot do.

24. A client who is staggering, slurring words, and is clearly incoherent is brought to the hospital via ambulance. A diagnostic evaluation reveals that the client is grossly intoxicated but is in no medical distress. When called, the wife says, "I've had it. I am done being an enabler. You handle it." The primary health-care provider refuses to admit the client because the client has no medical problem. What is the nurse's **most** appropriate action at this time?
    1. Request that the nursing supervisor talk with the primary health-care provider.
    2. Discharge the intoxicated client as per the primary health-care provider's decision.
    3. Have the primary health-care provider encourage the spouse to come to the emergency department.
    4. Inform the primary health-care provider that the client is gravely disabled and should not be released.

25. A nurse is a defendant in a lawsuit. The plaintiff must provide evidence in the four elements of liability. Place the statements presented in the options related to meeting the elements of liability in the order of duty, breach of duty, causation, and damages.
    1. The client experienced hypotension, fell, and fractured the head of the left femur as a result of receiving a diuretic that was not prescribed.
    2. The client required surgery to repair the fractured femur and experienced a delay of chemotherapy for lung cancer.
    3. The nurse administered a diuretic to the wrong client.
    4. The nurse is caring for a client in the hospital.
    Answer: _____

26. Which situation involving a nurse is reportable to the state board of nursing?
    1. Omission of documentation of a medication that was administered intravenously
    2. Discussion of confidential information at a grand rounds meeting without the client's consent
    3. Failure to monitor the blood glucose level of a client with diabetes who became comatose and died
    4. Not placing a mouth guard in the mouth of a client experiencing a tonic-clonic seizure who bites off the tip of the tongue

27. A nurse is caring for a client who was brought to the emergency department by her husband, who did not leave the wife's side and was overly solicitous. After a physical examination and an x-ray, the client was diagnosed with a fractured arm. The client stated that she is constantly clumsy. When the nurse assisted the client into a hospital gown, the nurse identified multiple old bruises. The nurse suspects physical abuse. What should the nurse do **first**?
    1. Suggest preparation of an exit plan if the client is reluctant to leave the abusive environment.
    2. Interview the client outside the vision and hearing of the suspected husband.
    3. Report the suspected physical abuse of the client to appropriate officials.
    4. Instruct the client to call the police if personal safety is in jeopardy.

28. A school nurse, when performing scoliosis screening on a 12-year-old female student, identifies that the girl has multiple bruises on the arms and thighs. The school nurse talks with the student, reviews the student's school file, and interviews the student's classroom teacher. What is the **best** nursing intervention based on the collected information?
    1. Arrange for the mother to come to the school for a parent-nurse conference.
    2. Telephone the boyfriend to confirm the student's accusations.
    3. Call the public health nurse to make a home visit.
    4. Notify the authorities of suspected child abuse.

Additional Information

Student Interview

"My mom and I moved in with my mom's new boyfriend a couple of months ago. He has an 8-year-old girl and a 17-year-old boy. I have to go home right after school to babysit the girl. I hate living with them. The boy gives me a hard time and has beaten me up a couple of times. My mom doesn't believe me and tells me to stop making trouble. I can hear my mom crying at night after her boyfriend hits her. A couple of weeks ago, he hit me too. I am afraid he is going to start hitting me again."

Student's School File

Has had three different home addresses in the last year
Grades have declined from a B average to a D+ average in the last 2 months
Has been absent from school for a total of 15 days in the last 3 months
Withdrew from participation in the marching band

Classroom Teacher Interview

"Over the past several months, I have noticed that she has become very quiet and has limited interaction with the boys in the class. Several times, I saw that she had some bruises. One time, she said she fell off her bike, and another time, she said she fell down the front steps at home. I know her grades have declined, but she is not doing her homework. I try to support her the best that I can in class."

29. A client is comatose and unable to make health-care decisions. Which decisions are permitted by a family member identified in a legally executed durable power of attorney to represent the client? **Select all that apply.**
    1. Withdraw ventilator support.
    2. Refuse the administration of a tube feeding.
    3. Administer medications that cause assisted suicide.
    4. Reject the insertion of an intravenous line for the administration of fluid.
    5. Do not attempt to resuscitate in the event that the client suffers cardiac or respiratory failure.

30. A mother brings her 7-year-old daughter to the emergency department. The child has a high fever, reports "It hurts when I pee," and is sucking her thumb. The mother states that her daughter clings to her when a man other than her father enters the room. The mother is concerned about possible sexual abuse because the daughter was cared for by an uncle while she and her husband were on vacation. What should the nurse do **first** before a physical examination of the child?
    1. Collect a urine specimen for a culture and sensitivity test.
    2. Interview the child to assess for clinical indicators of assault.
    3. Ask the mother to leave the bedside so that the child can be examined.
    4. Ensure that a sexual abuse health-care worker is present during the child's care.

31. The day before surgery, a male client signed the necessary forms giving permission for surgery. The next day at the ambulatory surgical center, the nurse administers the prescribed anxiolytic. Twenty minutes later, the client tells the nurse that he does not want to go through with the surgery. Which should the nurse do in this situation?
    1. Continue with the preoperative protocol because the client already signed the consent for surgery.
    2. Notify the surgeon about the client's preference not to have the surgery.
    3. Explore why the client has decided not to have the surgery.
    4. Encourage the client to go through with the surgery.

32. A nurse works in a state that permits assisted suicide. A 38-year-old woman who has had multiple sclerosis for 3 years states, "I can't stand my life anymore. I want a prescription for a drug so that I can commit suicide. What are the criteria for assisted suicide?" How should the nurse respond? **Select all that apply.**
    1. "You have to be over 21 years of age."
    2. "You have to meet certain psychiatric criteria."
    3. "You have to receive counseling regarding alternative options."
    4. "You have to have less than 6 months to live, as determined by 2 physicians."
    5. "You have to have a significant other who is willing to administer the medication."

33. Parents bring a 3-month-old infant to the pediatrician because the infant has been crying on and off for hours at a time for several weeks. One parent states that, after a bottle, the baby repeatedly draws up the legs, arches the back, and cries for 4 to 5 hours. Both parents convey being extremely frustrated and exhausted from lack of sleep. Which concern is **most** important that the nurse should include in a teaching program for these parents?
    1. Infant colic
    2. Failure to thrive
    3. Shaken baby syndrome
    4. Sudden infant death syndrome

34. Which of the following statements reflect ethical nursing practice when providing end-of-life care? **Select all that apply.**
    1. Clients in some states in the United States can legally take their own life.
    2. Euthanasia is acceptable if a client is suffering or has a terminal illness.
    3. Withholding food and fluid is acceptable practice near end-of-life care to allow a life to progress to its natural end.
    4. Titration of pain medication is acceptable as long as it does not cause respirations to fall below 10 breaths per minute.
    5. Discontinuing life support is acceptable if the client is dying and it is the decision of the client or the client's health proxy, or it is stated in the client's legal documents regarding end-of-life care.

35. A nurse working in the emergency department of a hospital is assessing a 3-year-old child with a burn injury. Which assessment should alert the nurse to collect additional information because of a concern regarding potential child abuse?
    1. Grease burn on the arm
    2. Evidence of a burned tongue
    3. Scalding burns on both hands
    4. Second degree sunburn on the back

1. ANSWER: 2.

Rationales:

1. If the client is being neglected or abused by the spouse, the client may not feel that this information can safely be conveyed to the nurse.

2. Protecting the client from neglect or abuse is the priority. The client should be assessed further for signs of neglect or abuse. The client's behavior may indicate fear. The spouse's appearance and behavior may indicate caregiver role strain. Inadequate turning and positioning, nutritional intake, and bathing and skin care can precipitate a pressure ulcer. Reporting suspected elder abuse or neglect to appropriate authorities is legally required by health-care professionals in most states.

3. This intervention is premature. Additional information is necessary for a comprehensive assessment. Respite care often is helpful in providing full-time caregivers an opportunity to experience a rest from providing 24/7 care to a family member.

4. Although assessing the pressure ulcer and reporting findings to the primary health-care provider should be done, it is not the priority.

TEST-TAKING TIP: Identify the word in the stem that sets a priority. The word *most* in the stem sets a priority. Identify the option that is most client centered. Although all of the options are client centered, option 2 is the only option that focuses on advocacy, which is an important role of the nurse.

Content Area: Legal and Ethical Issues
Integrated Processes: Caring; Nursing Process: Assessment
Client Need: Safe and Effective Care Environment; Management of Care
Cognitive Level: Application
Concept: Violence

2. ANSWER: 1.

Rationales:

1. The client has a right to refuse treatment and to be in charge of decisions regarding treatment and care. The nurse should support the decisions made by the client.

2. The client's behavior does not indicate a need for a referral for psychological counseling.

3. This action denies the client's feelings. Asking the client to reconsider chemotherapy for the sake of the family is not client centered.

4. This action defers interventions that are within the legal role of nursing practice to another health-care professional.

TEST-TAKING TIP: Identify the option that is client centered. Option 1 is the only option that focuses on the client; it is a client-centered intervention. Identify options that are opposites. Options 1 and 3 are opposites. Identify the option that denies the client's feelings. Option 3 denies the client's feelings.

Content Area: Legal and Ethical Issues
Integrated Processes: Caring; Communication and Documentation; Nursing Process: Implementation
Client Need: Safe and Effective Care Environment; Management of Care
Cognitive Level: Application
Concept: Ethics

3. ANSWER: 4.

Rationales:

1. This is an example of the ethics principle of beneficence, not fidelity. Beneficence refers to the performance of an action that benefits others or supports a positive outcome.

2. This is an example of the ethics principle of justice, not fidelity. Ensuring that clients are treated equally, regardless of such factors as economics, age, gender, skin color, ethnic origin, religious beliefs, and sexual orientation, is associated with the principle of justice.

3. This is an example of the ethics principle of autonomy, not fidelity. Autonomy refers to the right to have individual liberty and self-determination. Clients have a right to make personal choices about treatment and care.

4. This is an example of the ethics principle of fidelity. Fidelity is the duty to keep commitments. Clients need to know that nurses will honor verbal agreements.

TEST-TAKING TIP: Identify the clang associations. The words *nurse practice acts* in the stem and in options 1, 2, and 3 are clang associations. Examine options 1, 2, and 3 carefully.

Content Area: Legal and Ethical Issues
Integrated Processes: Caring; Communication and Documentation; Nursing Process: Implementation
Client Need: Safe and Effective Care Environment; Management of Care
Cognitive Level: Analysis
Concept: Ethics

4. ANSWER: 1, 2, 5.

Rationales:

1. Each state has its own nurse practice act, which identifies the scope of nursing practice within the state; they identify what a nurse can legally do or not do.

2. Although state nurse practice acts regulate the practice of nursing, the main purpose is to safeguard the health, safety, and well-being of people in the community from maltreatment or injury related to nursing care.

3. Each state, not the federal government, defines the nurse practice act in its own state.

4. Student nurses are held to the same standards of care as a licensed nurse.

5. Since student nurses are held accountable for ensuring that standards of care are met, they are subject to disciplinary actions by the state board of nursing. A student nurse may be prohibited from taking the National Council Licensure Examination if it is determined that the student nurse failed to meet standards of care identified in the state nurse practice act.

TEST-TAKING TIP: Identify the clang associations. The words *nurse practice acts* in the stem and in options 1, 2, and 3 are clang associations. Examine options 1, 2, and 3 carefully.

Content Area: Legal and Ethical Issues
Integrated Processes: Nursing Process: Analysis
Client Need: Safe and Effective Care Environment; Management of Care
Cognitive Level: Comprehension
Concept: Professionalism

5. ANSWER: 1, 2, 3.
Rationales:
1. It is the responsibility of the nurse to observe a client signing an informed consent form.
2. It is the nurse's responsibility to ensure that the client is agreeing freely and not being forced into having the surgery. Clients have the right to self-determination, which means they have the right to refuse treatment.
3. The client has to be cognitively intact (have capacity) to understand the risks, benefits, and ramifications associated with the surgery for a consent to be legally valid.
4. Explaining the risks and benefits of surgery is the responsibility of the surgeon, not the nurse.
5. Exploring options other than surgery is the responsibility of the primary health-care provider or surgeon, not the nurse.

TEST-TAKING TIP: Identify the clang associations. The word *consent* in the stem and in options 1, 2, 3, and 4 are clang associations. Examine options 1, 2, 3, and 4 carefully.

Content Area: *Legal and Ethical Issues*
Integrated Processes: *Communication and Documentation; Nursing Process: Implementation*
Client Need: *Safe and Effective Care Environment; Management of Care*
Cognitive Level: *Application*
Concept: *Legal*

6. ANSWER: 3, 5.
Rationales:
1. An adult client who is cognitively intact has the right to self-determination; this means that the client has a right to pursue or refuse medical treatment.
2. Requesting the use of an experimental drug by a person who has legal authority is not an ethical issue. However, to be accepted into a drug trial program, the client must meet the criteria established by the individuals responsible for the program.
3. Although the legal guardian has the right to make medical decisions for this developmentally disabled adult, the involvement of the hospital's ethics committee may help to resolve the dispute between the parents and the guardian.
4. An adult client who is cognitively intact has the right to self-determination; this means that the client has a right to pursue or refuse medical treatment regardless of what family members want.
5. An ethics committee can listen to and advise family members as well as negotiate a course of action for family members who do not agree on a course of action for a family member who is unable to make decisions.

Content Area: *Legal and Ethical Issues*
Integrated Processes: *Communication and Documentation; Nursing Process: Implementation*
Client Need: *Safe and Effective Care Environment; Management of Care*
Cognitive Level: *Application*
Concept: *Ethics*

7. ANSWER: 2.
Rationales:
1. Another step should be done before integrating ethical principles into one's nursing practice.

2. This is the first step in developing professional values. Professional values will develop and form as a student nurse expands knowledge and experience. First the nurse must identify personal values and beliefs before a conflict can be identified between personal values versus professional values. There may be times that personal values conflict with professional values, such as when a nurse who does not believe in abortion is asked to care for a client scheduled for an abortion. Issues arise, such as whether the nurse can care for the client in a nonjudgmental way.
3. Another step should be done before implementing culturally competent and sensitive nursing care to clients.
4. Another step should be done before integrating ethical principles, such as respecting the inherent worth and uniqueness of each individual client.

TEST-TAKING TIP: Identify the word in the stem that sets a priority. The word *first* in the stem sets a priority. Identify the option that is unique. Option 2 is unique. It is the only option that is associated just with the nurse; options 1, 3, and 4 include the client. Option 2 is the only option that presents a reason why the action is necessary, *because they affect nursing decisions.* For all these reasons, examine option 2 carefully.

Content Area: *Legal and Ethical Issues*
Integrated Processes: *Nursing Process: Analysis*
Client Need: *Safe and Effective Care Environment; Management of Care*
Cognitive Level: *Comprehension*
Concept: *Professionalism*

8. ANSWER: 1, 4, 5.
Rationales:
1. Clients have the right to examine, amend, and request a copy of their entire clinical record.
2. Only nursing team members directly responsible for caring for the client have a right to access the client's clinical record.
3. Rounds should be held in an area that is private so that only health team members can hear the conversation. If rounds are conducted in a hallway, visitors and other clients and nursing team members not responsible for the client's care may overhear confidential information about the client. Discussing clients in hallways, elevators, or dining areas violates HIPAA rules.
4. No information can be released to an inquiring individual without the permission of the client. Health-care workers are not permitted to share the fact that the person is currently admitted or not admitted to the hospital.
5. If a client is unable to participate in making personal health-care decisions, the client's designated health-care proxy is responsible for making these decisions. An individual who is a health-care proxy must know all the risks and benefits of health-care interventions before making informed decisions for the client.

TEST-TAKING TIP: Identify the option with a specific determiner. Option 2 contains the word *all*, which is a specific determiner. More often than not, an option with a specific determiner is a distractor.

Content Area: *Legal and Ethical Issues*
Integrated Processes: *Communication and Documentation; Nursing Process: Analysis*

Client Need: *Safe and Effective Care Environment;*
Management of Care
Cognitive Level: *Application*
Concept: *Legal*

9. **ANSWER: 4.**
Rationales:
1. This scenario does not reflect an assault. An assault occurs when a person unjustifiably threatens to touch or harm another.
2. This scenario does not reflect battery. Battery is the intentional touching of a client's body or clothing or anything held by or attached to a client in an angry, willful, negligent, or violent manner without consent.
3. Another option is more specific. Negligence does not require a nurse-client relationship.
4. The nurse had a professional relationship with and responsibility for the nursing care of the client. The nurse failed to provide an expected level of care consistent with professional standards of practice and failed to act how *another nurse* **would in similar circumstances. The client's vital signs and physical assessment revealed that the client was unstable, and the client's electrocardiogram results converted from atrial flutter to atrial fibrillation. Atrial fibrillation can be a precursor to a brain attack (stroke). The rapid response team and the primary health-care provider should have been notified so that appropriate medical intervention could be performed.**
Content Area: *Legal and Ethical Issues*
Integrated Processes: *Communication and Documentation; Nursing Process: Evaluation*
Client Need: *Safe and Effective Care Environment; Management of Care*
Cognitive Level: *Analysis*
Concept: *Patient-Centered Care; Legal*

10. **ANSWER: 3.**
Rationales:
1. The nurse cannot allow a client to stay in the emergency department or admit a client to the hospital.
2. Although this is something that the nurse should do, there is another option that should be implemented first. A nurse should refuse to be involved in a discharge or any other action if it is known to be against policy or is unethical.
3. If a nurse believes an action by another professional is inappropriate, the nurse should seek guidance from the nurse's immediate supervisor.
4. It is inappropriate for a nurse to contact the primary health-care provider's supervisor. This does not follow the nurse's chain of command within a facility.
TEST-TAKING TIP: Identify the word in the stem that sets a priority. The word *next* in the stem sets a priority.
Content Area: *Legal and Ethical Issues*
Integrated Processes: *Communication and Documentation; Nursing Process: Implementation*
Client Need: *Safe and Effective Care Environment; Management of Care*
Cognitive Level: *Application*
Concept: *Collaboration*

11. **ANSWER: 2, 3, 4.**
Rationales:
1. The clinical record belongs to a facility or to a primary health-care provider if it is in a primary health-care provider's office; it does not belong to the client. However, the information in the clinical record belongs to the client.
2. The Joint Commission, in the process of accrediting a health-care facility, will audit clients' clinical records to ensure compliance with standards by which quality of health care is measured.
3. Quality assurance committees examine clients' clinical records to determine if there are any undesirable trends that indicate where improvement can be made in the delivery of care, such as success rates of procedures, frequency of agency-acquired infections, occurrences of harmful events, and so on.
4. Comprehensive, detailed, and unambiguous documentation of the client's status, nursing care provided, and the client's response protect the nurse from false claims of negligence or malpractice.
5. A client's clinical record cannot be copied and removed from the unit, even after the client's name and medical record number are removed. This violates HIPAA regulations.
Content Area: *Legal and Ethical Issues*
Integrated Processes: *Communication and Documentation; Nursing Process: Analysis*
Client Need: *Safe and Effective Care Environment; Management of Care*
Cognitive Level: *Knowledge*
Concept: *Legal*

12. **ANSWER: 4.**
Rationales:
1. It is not the responsibility of a social worker to advocate for a client in this situation.
2. It is not the responsibility of the legal department of a hospital to advocate for a client in this situation.
3. It is not necessary for the client to seek new employment.
4. The Americans with Disabilities Act, passed in 1990, requires employers to make reasonable accommodations (e.g., ramps, bathrooms, parking, elevators) to facilitate employment of people with disabilities. The client should be made aware of one's rights indicated in the Americans with Disabilities Act and then be encouraged to seek compliance by the employer.
TEST-TAKING TIP: Identify the word in the stem that sets a priority. The word *most* in the stem sets a priority. Identify the options that are equally plausible. Options 1 and 2 are equally plausible. Identify opposite options. Options 3 and 4 are opposites.
Content Area: *Legal and Ethical Issues*
Integrated Processes: *Caring; Communication and Documentation; Nursing Process: Implementation*
Client Need: *Safe and Effective Care Environment; Management of Care*
Cognitive Level: *Application*
Concept: *Legal*

13. **ANSWER: 1.**

Rationales:

1. The American Nurses Association's *Code of Ethics* indicates that clients have the right to die in comfort. To be accepted into a hospice program, clients must complete a do-not-attempt-resuscitation form and understand that care is directed toward supporting comfort and dignity and is not curative. Medicating a client to achieve a comfortable and peaceful death is appropriate, even if by doing so it hastens death.

2. The primary health-care provider has already prescribed an intravenous opioid medication for the purpose of providing for a comfortable and peaceful death.

3. It is unnecessary to seek guidance from the nursing supervisor. In a situation where a client is receiving hospice care, pain medication may be administered, even though it may hasten death. The intention of providing opioid medication is relief of pain and support for a comfortable and peaceful death.

4. Withholding prescribed pain medication from a dying client who has agreed to hospice care is cruel, unethical, and unacceptable.

TEST-TAKING TIP: Identify opposite options. Options 1 and 4 are opposites. Identify equally plausible options. Options 2 and 3 are equally plausible. They both seek direction in what to do next. Identify the most client-centered option. Option 1 is the most client-centered option.

Content Area: Legal and Ethical Issues

Integrated Processes: Caring; Nursing Process: Implementation

Client Need: Safe and Effective Care Environment; Management of Care

Cognitive Level: Application

Concept: Patient-Centered Care; Professionalism

14. **ANSWER: 2, 4, 5.**

Rationales:

1. A nursing license can be revoked or suspended for professional misconduct.

2. This is an accurate statement. Candidates for licensure must self-report criminal convictions, chemical dependencies, and functional ability deficits.

3. A nursing license is required to practice the profession of nursing in all settings.

4. This is an accurate statement. Each state sets the criteria for the passing rate on the NCLEX examination. If a person meets the criteria to practice nursing in one state, another state may grant a license to practice nursing in that state upon the person's application for this privilege (reciprocity).

5. Each state's board of nursing is responsible for ensuring that only graduates of recognized schools of nursing take the NCLEX examination. Administrators of schools of nursing inform state boards of nursing of the names of individuals who have successfully completed a nursing program. The graduate then completes an application to take the NCLEX examination, which is submitted to the state board of nursing.

TEST-TAKING TIP: Identify options with a specific determiner. The word never in option 1 is a specific determiner.

Generally, an option with a specific determiner can be eliminated from consideration.

Content Area: Legal and Ethical Issues

Integrated Processes: Nursing Process: Analysis

Client Need: Safe and Effective Care Environment; Management of Care

Cognitive Level: Knowledge

Concept: Professionalism

15. **ANSWER: 3, 5.**

Rationales:

1. This statement is an example of the ethical principle of beneficence, not veracity. Performing an action that supports a positive outcome is an example of beneficence.

2. This statement is an example of the ethical principle of fidelity, not veracity. Fidelity refers to making only promises or commitments that can be kept. Promising to return immediately with pain medication and then immediately returning with the pain medication is an example of fidelity.

3. This statement is an example of the ethical principle of veracity. Veracity refers to being truthful, which is essential to a trusting nurse-client relationship. Informing a client when a procedure may be painful is an example of veracity.

4. This statement is an example of the ethical principle of nonmaleficence, not veracity. Removing a client from harm, preventing harm, and avoiding actions that may cause harm are associated with the principle of nonmaleficence. The positive outcome of an action must be measured against the risk of potential harm.

5. This statement is an example of the ethical principle of veracity. Veracity refers to being truthful, which is essential to a trusting nurse-client relationship. With a permanent colostomy, the client will always eliminate fecal material through a stoma on the abdomen rather than through the anus.

Content Area: Legal and Ethical Issues

Integrated Processes: Communication and Documentation; Nursing Process: Implementation

Client Need: Safe and Effective Care Environment; Management of Care

Cognitive Level: Analysis

Concept: Ethics

16. **ANSWER: 2.**

Rationales:

1. Battery occurs when a person unlawfully touches another person without consent.

2. Assault occurs when a person threatens harm to an individual. The client does not have to be touched for the nurse to be charged with assault.

3. Negligence occurs when a client suffers an injury when a nurse fails to meet a standard of care.

4. Abandonment occurs when a nurse leaves a client without an appropriate nursing replacement.

Content Area: Legal and Ethical Issues

Integrated Processes: Communication and Documentation; Nursing Process: Evaluation

Client Need: Safe and Effective Care Environment; Management of Care

Cognitive Level: Application

Concept: Legal

17. **ANSWER: 1, 2, 4.**
    Rationales:
    1. This action violates HIPAA. Confidential information should be discussed only in an area where privacy is provided.
    2. This action violates HIPAA. Information about a client should be discussed only with appropriate members of the health-care team and individuals for whom the client gives written consent.
    3. This action is fraud, not a violation of HIPAA.
    4. This action violates HIPAA. Information left on a computer screen that can be seen by people walking in a hallway violates confidentiality.
    5. Consulting with a nurse manager is an appropriate action and does not violate HIPAA.
    TEST-TAKING TIP: Identify the word in the stem that indicates negative polarity. The word *violation* in the stem indicates negative polarity.
    Content Area: Legal and Ethical Issues
    Integrated Processes: Communication and Documentation; Nursing Process: Evaluation
    Client Need: Safe and Effective Care Environment; Management of Care
    Cognitive Level: Application
    Concept: Legal

18. **ANSWER: 4.**
    Rationales:
    1. This event is not reportable to authorities in any state. A release against medical advice is a form that must be signed by a client who wants to leave a hospital when the client is advised not to do so by the primary health-care provider. It protects the health-care team members and the agency from legal liability in the event of negative consequences.
    2. Notifying an agency, such as the health department, about the presence of certain communicable diseases, such as tuberculosis and AIDS, is mandated in all states.
    3. All states have laws that mandate that suspected child abuse or neglect be reported to appropriate authorities; for example, child protective services.
    4. Not all states have mandatory reporting laws that protect adults over 60 years of age when abuse or neglect is suspected.
    Content Area: Legal and Ethical Issues
    Integrated Processes: Communication and Documentation; Nursing Process: Implementation
    Client Need: Safe and Effective Care Environment; Management of Care
    Cognitive Level: Knowledge
    Concept: Legal

19. **ANSWER: 3.**
    Rationales:
    1. The issue is beyond solving at the primary nurse level. The adult children on both sides of the issue have a determined position.
    2. Although this may be suggested to facilitate a different perspective of the issue that may help promote agreement, the spiritual advisor may have a limited focus that will not include the short- and long-term health-care issues.

3. This ensures that the two sides of this issue are explored in a nonconfrontational environment. The ethics committee will act as the client's advocate and protect the rights of the client, which is the focus of its activities.
    4. The nurse should not give advice.
    TEST-TAKING TIP: Identify the word in the stem that sets a priority. The word *best* in the stem sets a priority. Identify the option with a specific determiner. The word *all* in option 1 is a specific determiner. Rarely is an option with a specific determiner the correct answer.
    Content Area: Legal and Ethical Issues
    Integrated Processes: Communication and Documentation; Nursing Process: Implementation
    Client Need: Safe and Effective Care Environment; Management of Care
    Cognitive Level: Application
    Concept: Ethics

20. **ANSWER: 1, 2.**
    Rationales:
    1. The Occupational Safety and Health Act established the Occupational Safety and Health Administration (an agency of the U.S. Department of Labor), which identifies and enforces regulations that protect individuals from work-related injury.
    2. The Americans with Disabilities Act protects a person with a disability from discrimination by an employer. An employer is required by law to provide reasonable accommodation within the work setting to facilitate the job performance of a disabled person.
    3. Nurse practice acts protect clients and society. They establish the minimum standards of care to be delivered by working nurses.
    4. Mandatory reporting laws, such as the reporting of neglect or abuse of children, older adults, and people with mental illness or developmental impairments, are designed to protect those who are unable to protect themselves.
    5. Incident reports are designed to identify problems and areas for quality improvement, not protect the nurse.
    Content Area: Legal and Ethical Issues
    Integrated Processes: Nursing Process: Analysis
    Client Need: Safe and Effective Care Environment; Management of Care
    Cognitive Level: Comprehension
    Concept: Legal

21. **ANSWER: 1.**
    Rationales:
    1. The nurse can be charged with malpractice. Malpractice occurs when the nurse does not adhere to standards of nursing practice and it results in injury to the client. Nurses are expected to act in a way a reasonably prudent person with the same education and experience would act in a similar circumstance.
    2. Administering a medication to the wrong client is not an example of assault. Assault occurs when a nurse intentionally threatens to harm or touch a client in an insulting, unjustifiable, or offensive manner. An example is saying, "If you don't behave, you can't have your pain medication."
    3. Administering a medication to the wrong client is not an example of battery. Battery occurs when a nurse

intentionally touches a client's body or clothing or any-thing held by or attached to a client in an angry, willful, negligent, or violent manner without consent. Examples include forcefully undressing a client, resuscitating a client who has a do-not-attempt-resuscitation order, and admin-istering a medication refused by a client.

4. Administering a medication to the wrong client is not an example of fraud. Fraud occurs when there is purpose-ful misrepresentation intended to produce unlawful gain. Fraud is a reckless disregard of the truth. An example is stating, "You should not feel any pain with this proce-dure," when it is commonly known that the procedure is painful.

Content Area: Legal and Ethical Issues
Integrated Processes: Nursing Process: Analysis
Client Need: Safe and Effective Care Environment;
Management of Care
Cognitive Level: Application
Concept: Legal

22. **ANSWER: 3, 4, 5.**

Rationales:

1. Failure to complete an incident report after a client falls is not associated with HIPAA. This is related to failure to follow a policy or procedure of the agency.
2. Sharing clinical events and learning with other student nurses during a clinical postconference does not violate HIPAA as long as all members of the class maintain confi-dentiality of the client's protected health information.
3. Any health-care professional who discusses protected personal health information within the hearing of unauthorized individuals is in violation of maintaining protected personal health information.
4. Information can be shared only with those individuals who have legal authority to make health-care decisions for an incapacitated individual (legal surrogate). In addition, clients can identify individuals with whom information can be shared.
5. This is a violation of maintaining the confidentiality of protected health information. The information on the form was exposed to a visitor who is not a member of the health team.

TEST-TAKING TIP: Identify the word in the stem that reflects negative polarity. The word *violations* in the stem indicates negative polarity.
Content Area: Legal and Ethical Issues
Integrated Processes: Communication and Documentation;
Nursing Process: Evaluation
Client Need: Safe and Effective Care Environment;
Management of Care
Cognitive Level: Application
Concept: Legal

23. **ANSWER: 3.**

Rationales:

1. Educational criteria are established by the National League for Nursing Accrediting Commission (NLNAC) and the Commission on Collegiate Nursing Education (CCNE), which accredit schools of nursing.
2. The National League for Nursing is not involved with nurse licensure. Each state's board of nursing determines

the criteria for awarding licensure in their respective states based on satisfactory completion of a recognized school of nursing and achieving the passing rate determined by the state on the NCLEX-RN or NCLEX-PN examination.
3. This is an accurate statement. Each state has a nurse practice act that safeguards the public by legally defining the nature and scope of nursing practice, describing how the nursing profession is governed, and defining criteria for nursing education.
4. Nurse practice acts are legislated and enforced by each individual state, not the federal government.

TEST-TAKING TIP: Identify the option with a specific determiner. The word *exclusively* in option 1 is a specific determiner. Generally, options with specific determiners are distractors.
Content Area: Legal and Ethical Issues
Integrated Processes: Nursing Process: Analysis
Client Need: Safe and Effective Care Environment;
Management of Care
Cognitive Level: Knowledge
Concept: Professionalism

24. **ANSWER: 4.**

Rationales:

1. This is premature. The nurse should implement another option first.
2. This intervention may result in the client causing self-harm or harm to others. The nurse should refuse to be involved in this client's discharge.
3. The client's spouse clearly has indicated no desire to help the client at this time.
4. Clients who are visibly impaired are considered to be gravely disabled because they may cause self-harm or harm others; therefore, the person should not be released until sobriety is demonstrated. The nurse should explain this to the primary health-care provider.

TEST-TAKING TIP: Identify the word in the stem that sets a priority. The word *most* in the stem sets a priority.
Content Area: Legal and Ethical Issues
Integrated Processes: Caring; Communication and Documentation; Nursing Process: Implementation
Client Need: Safe and Effective Care Environment;
Management of Care
Cognitive Level: Application
Concept: Collaboration

25. **ANSWER: 4, 3, 1, 2.**

Rationales:

4. This meets the requirement of *duty* associated with litigation. A nurse working as a representative of an agency has an implied contract with clients receiving care provided by a staff member of the agency.
3. A nurse's actions by omission or commission that fails to meet standards of care meets the legal require-ment of *breach of duty* associated with litigation.
1. This statement indicates that the two elements of *causation* were met. The nurse administered a diuretic that was not prescribed by the primary health-care provider, and the diuretic caused dehydration and subsequent hypotension that resulted in a fall.

2. This statement addresses the *damages* suffered by the client as a result of receiving the diuretic that was not prescribed by the primary health-care provider. The surgery necessitated by the fall and the delay of the client's chemotherapy treatment resulted in pain, suffering, and additional medical expenses. The client experienced physical consequences of a longer hospitalization and recovery and the physical and psychological consequences associated with the delay of cancer treatment.

Content Area: Legal and Ethical Issues
Integrated Processes: Nursing Process: Analysis
Client Need: Safe and Effective Care Environment;
Management of Care
Cognitive Level: Analysis
Concept: Legal

26. **ANSWER: 3.**

Rationales:

1. This is not a reportable incident to a state board of nursing. However, the nurse may be counseled and be required to attend an in-service program on medication administration.

2. Confidential information may be shared among a group of health-care professionals for educational purposes without the consent of the client. In most cases, the initials, not names, of clients are used to help maintain confidentiality. Also, health-care professionals understand that maintaining confidentiality of information shared at professional meetings is a standard of care protected by the *Client Care Partnership: Understanding Expectations, Rights, and Responsibilities* and codes of ethics of various disciplines.

3. Monitoring a client and protecting a client from preventable complications are minimum standards of care and when violated can be reported to the state board of nursing. The nurse failed to meet these standards of care.

4. Placing a mouth guard in the mouth of a client experiencing a tonic/clonic seizure is contraindicated because it may cause broken teeth. It is unfortunate that the client bit off the tip of the tongue in this situation; however, the nurse's inaction was justified based on the nursing standard of care.

TEST-TAKING TIP: Identify the word in the stem that indicates negative polarity. The word *reportable* in the stem indicates negative polarity. The question is asking, "In what situation did a nurse *not* meet a nursing standard of care?"

Content Area: Legal and Ethical Issues
Integrated Processes: Communication and Documentation;
Nursing Process: Evaluation
Client Need: Safe and Effective Care Environment;
Management of Care
Cognitive Level: Application
Concept: Professionalism

27. **ANSWER: 2.**

Rationales:

1. Although this should be done if the nurse suspects physical abuse, it is not the priority.

2. This is the first thing the nurse should do if physical abuse is suspected. The client is more likely to discuss physical abuse when not threatened by the presence of the suspected abuser.

3. This is premature. The nurse should first assess the client in more detail. There is not enough evidence based on the data presented in the question to report suspected abuse to the appropriate officials. Most, not all, states require the reporting of domestic violence to law-enforcement authorities.

4. Although this should be done if a nurse suspects physical abuse, it is not the priority.

TEST-TAKING TIP: Identify the word in the stem that sets a priority. The word *first* in the stem sets a priority. Identify the clang associations. The word *husband* in the stem and in option 2 is a clang association. The word *abuse* in the stem and the word *abusive* in option 1 is a clang association. The words *suspected physical abuse* in the stem and in option 3 is a clang association. Examine options 1, 2, and 3 carefully because they all contain clang associations.

Content Area: Legal and Ethical Issues
Integrated Processes: Caring; Communication and Documentation; Nursing Process: Implementation
Client Need: Psychosocial Integrity
Cognitive Level: Application
Concept: Violence

28. **ANSWER: 4.**

Rationales:

1. The time it takes to arrange and conduct a parent-nurse conference may delay keeping the student safe. If confronted, the mother probably will deny the allegations. Also, this is not the role of a school nurse.

2. This is an unsafe intervention. Confronting the boyfriend to confirm the student's accusations will place the student in greater jeopardy. Also, this is not the role of a school nurse.

3. A school nurse does not have the authority to make a referral to a public health nurse. A person with a prescriptive license (e.g., primary health-care provider, nurse practitioner, physician's assistant) has the authority to make a referral to a public health nurse.

4. Nurses have the responsibility and authority to report suspected cases of child abuse to the authorities. The nurse must be an advocate for the student to protect her from further harm. A home assessment will be made by the authorities and appropriate actions taken if necessary.

Content Area: Legal and Ethical Issues
Integrated Processes: Caring; Communication and Documentation; Nursing Process: Implementation
Client Need: Safe and Effective Care Environment;
Management of Care
Cognitive Level: Analysis
Concept: Patient-Centered Care; Violence

29. **ANSWER: 1, 2, 4, 5.**

Rationales:

1. When clients are incapable of speaking for themselves, legal surrogates can make the decision to withdraw treatments, such as mechanical ventilation, especially if the client's desires are documented in a legally executed durable power of attorney for health care.

2. When clients are incapable of speaking for themselves, legal surrogates can make the decision to refuse

treatments, such as enteral feedings, especially if the client's desires are documented in a legally executed durable power of attorney for health care.

3. To meet the criteria for assisted suicide the client must be capable of self-administering the medication that would end one's life, meet certain psychiatric criteria, and engage in counseling regarding other options.

4. When clients are incapable of speaking for themselves, legal surrogates can make the decision to refuse treatments, such as intravenous fluids, especially if the client's desires are documented in a legally executed durable power of attorney for health care.

5. When clients are incapable of speaking for themselves, legal surrogates can make the decision to refuse treatments, such as resuscitation, especially if the client's desires are documented in a legally executed durable power of attorney for health care.

Content Area: *Legal and Ethical Issues*
Integrated Processes: *Nursing Process: Planning*
Client Need: *Safe and effective care environment; Management of care*
Cognitive Level: *Analysis*
Concept: *Legal*

30. **ANSWER: 4.**
Rationales:

1. This is not the priority at this time. However, this should be done before an antibiotic is initiated to treat an infection, such as a sexually transmitted infection or urinary tract infection.

2. An interview with the child should be conducted by a trained sexual abuse health-care worker after the sexual abuse health-care worker has established a relationship with the child.

3. The mother should remain with the daughter to provide emotional support at this time. If after further assessment there is a suspicion that the mother is the perpetrator of the sexual assault, the child should be interviewed out of the presence of the mother. This interview should be conducted by a sexual abuse health-care worker only after building a relationship with the child.

4. This is the first thing that the nurse should do. A sexual abuse health-care worker is trained to meet the emotional and physical needs of a client who has been sexually abused as well as meet the emotional needs of a nonabusive parent of a child who has been sexually abused.

TEST-TAKING TIP: Identify the word in the stem that sets a priority. The word *first* in the stem sets a priority. Identify the clang association. The words *sexual abuse* in the stem and in option 4 is a clang association. Examine option 4 carefully.

Content Area: *Legal and Ethical Issues*
Integrated Processes: *Caring; Nursing Process: Implementation*
Client Need: *Safe and Effective Care Environment; Management of Care*
Cognitive Level: *Application*
Concept: *Violence*

31. **ANSWER: 2.**
Rationales:

1. The members of the health-care team can be held libel for malpractice and battery if they proceed with the surgery against the client's wishes.

2. Clients have a right to cancel a signed consent. The client has already received the preoperative anxiolytic. The surgeon should be notified immediately.

3. The client has already received the preoperative anxiolytic. Having a discussion with the client at this time is inappropriate.

4. This action denies the client's feelings, concerns, and rights. The client has a right to cancel the surgery.

TEST-TAKING TIP: Identify the options that are equally plausible. Options 1 and 4 are equally plausible. Identify the options that deny the client's feelings, needs, and concerns. Options 1 and 4 deny the client's concerns and rights. Identify options that are opposites. Options 1 and 4 are opposite to option 2. Since options 1 and 4 are equally plausible and can be eliminated, examine option 2 carefully.

Content Area: *Legal and Ethical Issues*
Integrated Processes: *Communication and Documentation; Nursing Process: Implementation*
Client Need: *Safe and Effective Care Environment; Management of Care*
Cognitive Level: *Application*
Concept: *Legal*

32. **ANSWER: 2, 3, 4.**
Rationales:

1. A person who wants to receive a prescription for a medication to commit assisted suicide must be at least 18 years of age or older. Obviously, a minor cannot receive a prescription for a medication to commit assisted suicide.

2. Certain psychiatric criteria must be met before someone can receive a prescription for a medication to commit assisted suicide. Mental or emotional disorders that interfere with the ability to make an informed decision will prevent someone from receiving a prescription to commit assisted suicide. The client must be mentally competent.

3. A person who wants to commit assisted suicide must receive counseling regarding alternative options (e.g., hospice, palliative sedation) so that the final decision is an informed decision.

4. A person who wants to commit assisted suicide must be terminally ill and this status certified by two physicians.

5. The client must be capable of self-administering the prescribed medication. This prevents another person from performing involuntary or nonvoluntary euthanasia.

Content Area: *Legal and Ethical Issues*
Integrated Processes: *Communication and Documentation; Nursing Process: Implementation*
Client Need: *Safe and Effective Care Environment; Management of Care*
Cognitive Level: *Knowledge*
Concept: *Legal*

33. ANSWER: 3.
   Rationales:
   1. Although infant colic is a concern and should be addressed, it is not the priority in this situation.
   2. There is no evidence to support the conclusion that the infant is not thriving. Failure to thrive is suspected when an infant falls below the fifth percentile for height and weight.
   3. When exhausted, frustrated, and overwhelmed, a person, out of desperation, may resort to shaking a child who is constantly crying. The parents should be taught appropriate comforting techniques and told what can happen to an infant if shaken. It is also important for the parents to have a respite from the crying child to sleep, rest, or relax.
   4. Although implementing measures to prevent sudden infant death syndrome, such as avoiding the prone position when sleeping, is important, it is not the priority in this situation.
   TEST-TAKING TIP: Identify the word in the stem that sets a priority. The word *most* in the stem sets a priority. Identify the central person in the question. The parents are the central persons in the question.
   Content Area: Legal and Ethical Issues
   Integrated Processes: Teaching/Learning; Nursing Process: Implementation
   Client Need: Safe and Effective Care Environmental; Safety and Infection Control
   Cognitive Level: Application
   Concept: Family Dynamics

34. ANSWER: 1, 3, 5.
   Rationales:
   1. Assisted suicide is the taking of one's own life after seeking and receiving a prescription from a primary health-care provider for a medication that will cause death. Specific criteria must be met, such as having the ability to self-administer the medication that will end one's life, being at least 18 years of age, being terminally ill, and having received counseling regarding other options.
   2. A position statement on euthanasia by the American Nurses Association states that nurses are prohibited from participating in euthanasia. Euthanasia is the premeditated termination of the life of a person who is suffering from an incurable disease or terminal illness.
   3. Withholding food and fluid is acceptable practice near end-of-life care to allow a life to progress to its natural end. This is often a difficult decision for family members who equate providing food and fluid as nurturing and caring.

4. Titration of pain medication to achieve comfort is acceptable even if it hastens death. It is considered an ethical, justified intervention.
   5. Discontinuing life support is acceptable if the client is dying and it is the decision of the client or the client's designated health-care proxy, or it is stated in the client's legal documents regarding end-of-life care.
   TEST-TAKING TIP: Identify the clang associations. The words *end-of-life care* in the stem and in options 3 and 5 are clang associations. Examine options 3 and 5 carefully.
   Content Area: Legal and Ethical Issues
   Integrated Processes: Nursing Process: Analysis
   Client Need: Psychosocial Integrity
   Cognitive Level: Application
   Concept: Ethics

35. ANSWER: 3.
   Rationales:
   1. A grease burn generally is not a *red flag* indicating potential child abuse. Hot water and grease burns are the most common cause of burns in children younger than 3 years of age.
   2. A burned tongue indicates that the child most likely ingested food or fluid that was too hot. However, it could be considered child neglect if the caregiver provided the child with a nutrient that was hotter than intended and intentionally did not check its temperature first. This is often associated with heating food in a microwave, which should be avoided when heating food or liquids for infants and children. Intentional avoidance of providing physical or emotional care to another, such as a child or older adult, is considered neglect.
   3. Scalding burns on both hands or both feet and cigarette burns are most often associated with child and elder abuse than with an accident. Further assessments should be made to determine if abuse is the cause when these signs are identified. When a person causes harm or injury (e.g., physical, emotional, or sexual) to another person (usually a child, adult with an intellectual disability, woman, or older adult), it is called abuse.
   4. A sunburn is not a *red flag* indicating potential child abuse. However, it could be considered child neglect if the caregiver intentionally did not apply suntan protection on a sunny day.
   Content Area: Legal and Ethical Issues
   Integrated Processes: Nursing Process: Assessment
   Client Need: Psychosocial Integrity
   Cognitive Level: Application
   Concept: Violence

Chapter 4

Health-Care System

Addiction and Behaviors
Cognition
Collaboration
Culture
Evidenced-Based Practice
Health-Care System

Health Promotion
Leadership and Management
Patient-Centered Care
Professionalism
Safety

KEY TERMS

Community—Group of individuals who share some characteristics, engage in multifaceted relationships, and have the capacity to act collectively

Community-based health care—Provision of health care in settings near where individuals, families, or groups live, work, or play

Community-based nursing—Provision of health-care services to protect, promote, maintain, or improve the health and quality of life of individuals, families, and groups within the context of a population

Hospice—Interdisciplinary services that focus on maintaining comfort and quality of life of dying individuals and providing supportive care to grieving family members

Nursing care delivery model—Organizational system that provides a framework for how nursing care is implemented and which members of the nursing team deliver the care

Primary health care—Care that focuses on maintaining an optimum level of wellness

Public health nursing—Nursing interventions that focus on meeting the health needs of populations

Respite care—Total care for an individual is delegated to another for a specified time period to provide relief from the duty of providing care and to limit caregiver role strain

Role—Set of responsibilities and expected behaviors related to a position or status

Secondary health care—Care that focuses on early detection of and intervention to cure disease and minimize further impairment

Stigmatized population—Group of people who are unaccepted and discriminated against and lack status and power

Telehealth care—Health care provided via use of the Internet, telephone, or fax machine

Tertiary health care—Care that focuses on health restoration and palliation

Vulnerable population—A group of people who are at increased risk for health problems because of multiple stressors, unhealthy behaviors, and lack of economic, social, and/or health-related resources

I. Health-Care Delivery

The health-care delivery system provides a variety of services across various settings to meet the health-related needs of the members of society. It is complex and continually changing because of such factors as federal and state legislation, reengineering of organizations, cost-containment issues, emergence of new health-care professions, and expectations of clients and their family members. Recent changes in health care, such as the increased emphasis on the provision of care within the community rather than in hospitals and the focus on health rather than illness, have influenced the settings in which health care is provided.

A. Classification of health-care agencies
1. Are classified in a number of respects.
   a. By state license when criteria are met.
   b. By ownership.
      (1) Public/official: Federal, state, or local governmental control.
      (2) Voluntary: Nonprofit.
      (3) Proprietary: For profit.
   c. By focus of care or by mission, such as:
      (1) Orthopedic.
      (2) Pediatric.
      (3) Psychiatric.
      (4) General medicine and surgery.
      (5) Rehabilitation.
      (6) Hospice.
   d. Services offered generally are determined by the license, size, location, and mission of the agency.

B. Acute care hospitals
1. Generally are involved with the diagnosis and treatment of acute and chronic illnesses.
2. Services provided may include:
   a. Acute inpatient medical and surgical services.
   b. Outpatient care, such as ambulatory care services, diagnostic tests, day surgery, rehabilitative care, and emergency department administered care.
   c. Specialty services, such as a burn, spinal cord, or dialysis unit.

C. Outpatient settings
1. Include such settings as clinics, primary health-care provider's offices, ambulatory surgery centers, schools, occupational settings, and agencies that provide home-care services.
2. Provide such services as minor surgical procedures, physical examinations, physical therapy, medical screenings, counseling, teaching, day care, and primary care.
3. Examples of specific settings.
   a. Schools.
      (1) Provide health education, health promotion, and disease prevention interventions.
      (2) Coordinate with health-care professionals and implement assistance to ensure a meaningful learning experience within school settings for children with disabilities or health-care needs.
      (3) Engage in case-finding activities, such as head lice and scoliosis screening, and make referrals to other health agencies as needed.
   b. Occupational settings.
      (1) Provide programs to support safety in the work environment.
      (2) May provide annual employee health screenings.
      (3) May provide health education on topics such as weight reduction and hypertension.
      (4) May provide counseling services.
      (5) May provide follow-up care after an injury.

DID YOU KNOW?

Increasing numbers of employers are providing health-care services and related benefits, such as exercise facilities, to their employees. The underlying reason is the belief that productivity is related to the health of a worker.

D. Long-term care settings
1. Provide services on a continuum in a variety of inpatient and outpatient settings.
   a. Independent living setting.
      (1) Adults generally live in their own apartment, care for themselves, and may have meals and housekeeping services provided.
      (2) Some facilities provide for leisure activities, banking hours, hairdresser services, rehabilitation services, and access to primary health-care providers at one's own expense within the building.
   b. Assisted living setting.
      (1) Adults receive some assistance with activities such as dressing and bathing, in addition to the provision of meals and housekeeping services.
      (2) Some facilities provide for leisure activities, banking hours, hairdresser services, rehabilitation services, and access to primary health-care providers at one's own expense within the building.
   c. Subacute unit in a skilled nursing home.
      (1) Provides comprehensive care for a person with an acute illness, injury, or exacerbation of a disease process in lieu of hospitalization.
      (2) Provides treatment interventions to avoid unnecessary and recurrent hospitalizations.
   d. Intermediate care setting.
      (1) Provides care for people who are disabled, older adults, and people who are not

acutely ill but need less intensive care than
services provided by a hospital or skilled
nursing facility.

    (2) Care generally is provided by nonskilled
and unlicensed personnel.

    (3) Usually provides custodial care.

  e. Skilled nursing care provided in a nursing home.

    (1) Facilities that are certified to participate in
and receive remuneration from Medicare
or Medicaid.

    (2) Requires people to meet specific criteria
before admission, such as criteria regarding
insurance, prescribed treatment, nursing
services needed, and resources required.

    (3) Provides long-term care for people
who need ongoing medical and nursing
attention.

    (4) Provides short-term care for people
discharged from a hospital who still require
medical and nursing care to facilitate
recovery from an acute health event.

    (5) May specialize in services such as brain
injury care or orthopedic rehabilitation.

E. Hospice

  1. **Hospice** provides interdisciplinary services that
focus on maintaining comfort and quality of life
of dying individuals and providing supportive care
to grieving family members.

  2. Focuses on maintaining comfort and quality of
life, not curative treatment.

  3. Offers care in such settings as hospitals, skilled
nursing homes, intermediate care settings, freestanding hospice settings, and private homes;
locations vary depending on the client's condition
and the ability of family members to provide care
at home.

F. Community-based health care

  1. **Community-based health care** is associated with
agencies that provide care in the home as well as
outpatient services.

  2. Examples include urgent care centers, day-care
centers, use of hospital services and equipment on
an outpatient basis, and residential treatment
halfway houses where no treatment interventions
are provided.

G. Public health nursing

  1. **Public health nursing** focuses on meeting the
health needs of populations.

  2. Provides services such as prenatal care, immunizations for children, screening for illnesses
(e.g., tuberculosis, scoliosis) and helps to prevent
individual disability and disease (e.g., correct
use of automobile restraining devices for children, ways to reduce risk factors for cardiac
disease).

II. Community-Based Nursing

A **community** consists of a group of people living in the
same area or having a common characteristic or interest.
Community-based nursing focuses on caring for people
near where they live, work, and play. It is concerned with
protecting, promoting, maintaining, and improving the
health and quality of life of individuals, families, and
groups.

A. Community-based settings

  1. Mobile health clinics.

    a. Vans or buses with equipment and health-
care professionals who provide primary and
secondary health-care services at numerous
places within a geographic area.

    b. Bring health care to the people.

    c. Help to service migrant workers, who pose a
unique challenge to the provision of health-care
services because they move about the country
according to the timing of harvests.

  2. Faith-based organizations.

    a. Religious organizations that provide
health-care services to individuals.

    b. Address clients' physical, emotional, and
spiritual needs.

    c. Activities associated with faith-based
organizations.

      (1) Coordination and training of volunteers
who may provide such services as companionship visits and transportation to and
from appointments.

      (2) Development and facilitation of support
groups.

      (3) Referral services to community health-care
facilities and programs.

      (4) Presentation of programs involving health
education, illness prevention, and health
promotion.

      (5) Discussion and education about health
issues on an individual basis.

      (6) Facilitation of assimilation of faith and
health.

  3. Correctional and prison environments.

    a. Provide routine examinations and screenings as
well as acute care when needed.

    b. Generally require nurses to meet certain physi-
cal criteria and complete special training, such
as weapons training and security procedures,
to provide for their own safety.

  4. Telehealth care.

    a. **Telehealth care** provides services to geographic
areas where health care is not easily accessible.

    b. Allows data to be transmitted via the Internet,
telephone, or fax machine to primary health-
care providers and specialists for consultation.

c. Raises legal issues (e.g., who is responsible for the client, how confidentiality is protected, and whether the health-care provider must be licensed in the state in which the client lives).

DID YOU KNOW?

The National Council of State Boards of Nursing's position on telehealth is that regulations associated with the state in which the client lives are applicable.

B. Issues promoting the movement of health care into the community
   1. Federal legislation identified a prospective payment system for Medicare based on illnesses and diseases. The introduction of diagnosis-related groups (DRGs) into the U.S. health-care system, in an effort to control costs, has resulted in clients being discharged from the hospital to the community earlier than was the practice before DRGs were introduced and often when clients are still sick.
   2. The aging of the U.S. population has resulted in a larger percentage of individuals in the community having chronic illnesses and disabilities, requiring supportive care for the client and respite care for family members providing care.
   3. The number of people who do not seek or cannot afford health care is increasing. Examples include vulnerable populations, such as people who are immigrants, homeless, living below the poverty level, uninsured, cognitively impaired, or abused.
   4. The focus of health care is changing from treatment of diseases to health promotion and disease prevention, which emphasizes a nurse's teaching role and requires educating children before unhealthy habits become engrained.
   5. More people prefer to die at home rather than in a health-care facility, necessitating the provision of both physical and emotional care for clients and family members in the home.

C. *Healthy People 2020* (www.healthypeople.gov)
   1. A national initiative instituted in 1979, and updated every 10 years, that identifies health improvement goals and priorities and also includes new data on issues and progress achieved toward previous goals.
   2. *Healthy People 2020* contains 42 topic areas with more than 1,200 objectives; a subset of *Healthy People 2020* objectives, called *Leading Health Indicators*, communicates high-priority health issues and actions to address them.
   3. Provides objectives in a format that enables diverse groups to combine their efforts and work as a team.

   4. Has a major impact on all health-care programs but especially on activities and groups concerned with community health needs.

D. Characteristics of a healthy community
   1. Has an awareness of its members, populations, and subgroups as being part of the community.
   2. Provides opportunities for and encourages participation of individuals and groups in decision making related to issues affecting the community.
   3. Ensures that communication remains open and information flows among all members and groups in every direction within the community.
   4. Detects, investigates, and dissects problems and collaborates and coordinates a response among members and groups to meet their identified needs.
   5. Ensures that community resources are available to all members and groups within the community.
   6. Focuses on promoting a high level of wellness and health among all members and populations within the community.

MAKING THE CONNECTION

Healthy People 2020 and Improved Health and Quality of Life

Healthy People 2020 sets objectives to improve the health and quality of life of people and communities and to reduce health disparities associated with vulnerable populations. The Healthy People Consortium & Partners, instituted by the U.S. Department of Health and Human Services, is a rich resource for helping communities address health issues. In addition, the MAP-IT framework (Mobilize, Assess, Plan, Implement, Track) provides a foundation upon which to plan and evaluate community health initiatives. Nurses working in a community setting should have a thorough understanding of *Healthy People 2020* and the resources available to assist them in addressing the needs of their community. For example, a public health nurse completes a community assessment and identifies that the health-care needs of homeless people are not being met. The nurse uses data provided by *Healthy People 2020* to demonstrate the issues, networks with resources available through the Healthy People Consortium & Partners for advice and direction, and then uses the MAP-IT framework to design an initiative that addresses the needs of the homeless. Also, the nurse may use information from *Healthy People 2020* to identify funding sources to underwrite the cost of implementing the program for the homeless in the community. Once the initiative is implemented, the nurse can track the outcomes of the initiative using the track guidelines in the MAP-IT framework.

7. Has a well-organized base of community resources available to meet needs and to intervene in a crisis or natural disaster.

E. Components of a community assessment
1. Overview of a community assessment.
   a. Provision of care is based on the nursing process; assessment is the most significant step because it drives the rest of nursing interventions.
   b. Information is collected about the physical environment and infrastructure of the community, characteristics of its population, available resources and services, and the economic and social systems within the community.
   c. Conducted by a community health nurse or public health nurse in collaboration with others (e.g., various members of the health-care team, members of community organizations, and government officials).
2. Physical environment of the community.
   a. Natural boundaries and size of the community.
   b. Types of housing.
   c. Average household income.
   d. Location of agencies and resources.
3. Population of the community.
   a. Characteristics of community members, such as age, gender, and educational level.
   b. Growth trends.
   c. Predominant ethnic and religious groups represented.
   d. Population density.
4. Safety and transportation systems available to the population.
   a. Agencies and status of services provided regarding water and sanitation.
   b. Air quality.
   c. Telephone service.
   d. Numbers of police and emergency services available.
   e. Rail and bus systems.
5. Social services available to the community.
   a. Schools, health-care agencies, and recreational facilities and the programs they provide.
   b. Number of health-care providers and services available, such as sources of health-care information, extent of primary care, and home and long-term care services.
   c. Number and types of spiritual institutions.
   d. Recreational organizations and clubs, such as playgrounds, parks, beaches, and sports centers.
6. Status of the members of the community.
   a. Biological, emotional, and sociological nature of the community.

   b. Biological statistics, including data on illness (morbidity) and death (mortality) rates and life expectancy of members of the community.
   c. Emotional and sociological statistics, including data on indications of the general mental health of community members and satisfaction or dissatisfaction with characteristics or features of the community.
7. Economic status of the community.
   a. Industries, employers, and occupations within the community.
   b. Economic level of the community, such as average household income.
   c. Number of workplace health promotion and illness prevention programs.
   d. Number of population receiving public assistance.
8. Social system of the community.
   a. Statistics related to crime and drug misuse within the community.
   b. Percentage of population attending school.
   c. Ways communication flows.
   d. Extent of interaction among members and groups within the community.
   e. Kind of government that runs the community.
   f. Extent of participation of members in health-care decision making within the community.
   g. Availability of a welfare system to support the needy.
   h. Types and extent of volunteer programs.

F. Specific roles of community-based nurses
1. Nurse epidemiologist.
   a. Provides surveillance and monitoring activities to identify trends in health and risk factors that threaten the health of specific populations or the health of members of the general community.
   b. Performs such activities as examining sources of information, case findings, field studies, surveys, and investigations; tracking illnesses, diseases, and death rates; and providing information and reports to appropriate local, state, or national officials.
2. Case manager.
   a. Ensures that an appropriate plan of care is formulated and implemented to meet the needs of clients across a continuum of care in the community setting.
   b. Coordinates and promotes continuity of care among health-care disciplines.
3. Advocate.
   a. Assists clients to work their way through the health-care system and obtain appropriate services.

b. Engages in political action at the local, state, or national level to campaign on behalf of the community.
4. Change agent.
   a. Mediates within a family system or within the community, empowering people to effect change to better meet health-care needs.
   b. Utilizes information related to facilitating change and managing resistance to change to be a more effective change agent.
5. Teacher.
   a. Focuses on health promotion and disease prevention with individuals and groups through educational activities.
   b. Presents programs on such topics as prenatal classes, child safety, dental health, hypertension, and nutrition.
   c. Targets groups in schools, community organizations, and businesses.
G. Specific competencies of community-based nurses
   1. Collaborate with others.
      a. Recognize that partnerships, networks, and coalitions are essential to effectively address the heath-care needs of members and groups within a community.
      b. Maintain collegial working relationships with other health team members to ensure consultation and cooperation in management of the delivery of care.
      c. Collaborate with other health-care providers in identifying the need for change in social, political, economic, or health-care systems within the community.
      d. Offer suggestions for changes compatible with the norms and values of the community.
   2. Communicate with others.

      🛑 a. Have excellent communication skills when working in a collaborative relationship with other health team members and when communicating with members and groups within a community.

      b. Demonstrate respect verbally and nonverbally for the expertise that each professional brings to the team as well as for individual differences among members and groups within the community.
   3. Maintain continuity of care.
      a. Coordinate delivery of health-care services between settings (e.g., hospital to home, rehabilitation center to assisted-living facility, or nursing home to hospital) and between and among providers of health care within the community.

      🛑 b. Be involved in discharge planning as soon as a client is admitted to a hospital or extended-care facility when the person is expected to return to the community.

c. Know the resources, agencies, and services that are available in the community and make referrals on behalf of the client to support continuity of care.
      d. Ensure that, with the client's consent, family members and significant others are included in the planning process because family members often are the main caregivers.
   4. Provide care across the life span.
      a. Provide services to clients of all ages from the time they are born until they die.
      b. Provide health-care services to special needs populations within different age groups, such as adolescents (e.g., pregnant teens who give birth to low-birth-weight and premature infants), preschool and school-aged children (e.g., immunization programs, health screening, and nutrition services), and young adults (e.g., services for those who have sexually transmitted diseases or substance misuse problems).
      c. Coordinate hospice care to assist terminally ill members of the community to die a peaceful, dignified death.

DID YOU KNOW?

Hospice is a concept, not a place to go to die. Hospice care provides interdisciplinary services that focus on maintaining comfort and quality of life of dying individuals and providing supportive care to grieving family members. Hospice care can be provided in extended-care facilities, in freestanding hospices, or in the home. The location depends on the client's physical and emotional needs and the ability of family members to provide care in the home. Although clients of all ages receive hospice care, a large percentage of these clients are older adults.

III. Types of Health-Care Services

Numerous types of health-care services are available to meet the complex needs of clients. These services can be categorized into primary, secondary, and tertiary care, each with its own unique focus. The complexity of care in each depends on a client's individual needs, the primary health-care provider's knowledge and expertise, and the setting in which the health care is provided.
A. Primary: Health promotion and illness prevention
   1. **Primary health care** focuses on maintaining an optimum level of wellness.
   2. Interventions decrease the risk of disease and disability.
   3. Activities include sanitation, immunization, and lifestyle modifications, such as dietary counseling, smoking cessation, and exercise.

B. Secondary: Diagnosis and treatment
1. **Secondary health care** focuses on early detection and intervention to treat disease and minimize further impairment.
2. Involves acute medical care and surgical intervention.
3. Diagnostic activities include regular dental examinations, routine screenings (e.g., bone density testing and mammograms for women, HIV testing, blood pressure and cholesterol testing), and x-rays.
4. Treatment activities include prescribing and administering antibiotics and prescribing and administering wound irrigation.

C. Tertiary: Rehabilitation
1. **Tertiary health care** focuses on restoring function, maximizing results of treatment, and providing palliative care, such as supporting comfort and quality of life.
2. Aims to maximize abilities in light of chronic or irreversible conditions.
3. Activities include education and rehabilitation (e.g., learning how to use a wheelchair, learning to engage in activities of daily living to live independently, and making environmental modifications, such as installing grab bars and ramps and widening doorways in the home).

IV. Health Team Members

Client needs are multifaceted, complex, and require a multitude of people from a variety of health-care disciplines with specific expertise to assist clients to meet these needs. Because nurses have a unique relationship with clients, function as client advocates, and, depending on the setting, provide care 24/7, they are commonly responsible for coordinating client care. Nurses must know the members of the health team and the services they provide to perform the role of coordinator effectively. Although the nurse is the coordinator of the health team, the client is the center of the health team.

A. The client

🛑 1. The client is the center of the health team.

2. All members of the health team lend their expertise to assist the client in meeting health-care goals.

B. Nursing team members
1. Nurse administrators.
   a. Establish and manage achievement of organizational goals, particularly those of the department of nursing and other related agency departments.
   b. Examples include vice president for nursing, associate director of nursing, assistant director of nursing, nursing supervisor, nurse coordinator, and nurse manager.

2. Clinical nurse specialist (CNS).
   a. Functions as a resource to nurses caring for clients with complex nursing needs.
   b. Requires advanced education in a specific field.
   c. Examples include diabetic nurse educator, infection control nurse, and medical-surgical CNS.
3. Registered nurse (RN).
   a. Coordinates services provided by members of the health-care team.
   b. Provides direct nursing care.
   c. Supervises unlicensed nursing personnel.
4. Licensed vocational nurse (LVN) or licensed practical nurse (LPN).
   a. Provides uncomplicated bedside nursing care.
   b. Works in a structured setting under the supervision of an RN.
5. Unlicensed assistive personnel (UAP).
   a. Provides direct nursing care delegated by an RN or LPN.
   b. Performs activities generally related to assisting clients with activities of daily living and performing noncomplex tasks.
   c. Examples include nursing associate and nursing assistant.

C. Other professional team members
1. Primary health-care provider: Person who has a prescriptive license, such as medical doctor (MD), physician assistant (PA), and nurse practitioner (NP).
2. Pharmacist (RPh).
3. Dietitian (RD).
4. Respiratory therapist (RT).
5. Physical therapist (PT).
6. Occupational therapist (OT).
7. Social worker (SW).
8. Dentist (DDS).
9. Podiatrist (DPM).
10. Audiologist (Au.D).
11. Speech language pathologist (SLP).
12. Laboratory and radiology professionals (x-ray, ultrasound, and laboratory technicians).
13. Activity therapist (AT).
14. Certified child life specialist (CCLS).
15. Chaplain.

D. Supportive team members
1. Family members.
2. Unit secretary.
3. Transport staff.
4. Housekeeping personnel.
5. Security personnel.

V. Delivery of Nursing Care

Nurses comprise the largest number of health-care professionals in most health-care settings. Utilization of their professional expertise requires a clear delineation of their roles and responsibilities as well as the use of a system that delivers nursing care that is safe, competent, and cost effective.

A. Nursing care delivery models
   1. **Nursing care delivery models** are organizational systems that provide a framework for how nursing care is provided and which members of the nursing team deliver the care.
   2. Continuously evolving because of societal health-care initiatives, organizational reengineering, increasing acuity of clients, and the need to address cost containment.
   3. Types of nursing care delivery models.
      a. Primary nursing.
         (1) An RN is responsible for assigned clients throughout their hospitalization, 7 days a week, 24 hours a day (primary nurse).
         (2) The primary nurse does not deliver all care personally but is responsible for ensuring that comprehensive and individualized care is delivered.
         (3) Primary nursing requires more registered nurses; however, it might not cost more because it improves collaboration, avoids delays, and supports comprehensive care.
         (4) Communication is lateral; the primary nurse communicates directly with the nurses on the other shifts who are assigned to care for the client.
         (5) Variations of primary nursing.
            (a) Total client-care nursing: One nurse is responsible for the total care administered to a client, but the nurse changes from shift to shift.
            (b) Modular nursing: Nurses are assigned to clients within a small segment of a nursing unit to ensure that clients receive care from the same personnel on a regular basis.
      b. Team nursing.
         (1) An RN team leader is responsible for a group of clients' plans of care and nursing care delivered and makes assignments based on the abilities of each team member, such as RNs, LPNs, and unlicensed nursing personnel.
         (2) Team members share the work to be accomplished for a group of clients.
         (3) The team leader is responsible for coordinating the team, planning care, and collaborating with professionals in other disciplines and often does not provide direct client care.
         (4) Although the focus is on client assignments rather than tasks, tasks are assigned within the team.

      (5) Communication occurs in a matrix (i.e., between the team leader and members and among team members).
   c. Functional nursing.
      (1) Functional nursing is a task-oriented approach whereby tasks are assigned on the basis of a person's educational preparation.
      (2) It is based on clearly defined job descriptions, policies, and procedures.
      (3) The focus is efficiency and productivity, but can fragment care and fail to meet the emotional needs of clients.
      (4) Communication occurs in a hierarchy from the head nurse to subordinates.
   d. Case management (total care) model.
      (1) An RN is responsible for planning, implementing, and evaluating care for a specific client.
      (2) The case manager is responsible for client care across the continuum of practice settings to promote continuity of care and limit fragmentation and redundancy of care.
      (3) This model commonly relies on critical pathways to ensure appropriate delivery of care and facilitate evaluation of the achievement of expected outcomes.
B. Roles of the nurse (Table 4.1)
   1. A **role** is a set of responsibilities and expected behaviors related to a person's position or status.
   2. There are many common roles in the provision of nursing care regardless of the setting in which nurses work, and there are also differences in roles depending on the unique services provided by particular health-care settings.
   🛑 3. Nurses must have the knowledge and ability to assume appropriate roles when individualizing client care and ensure that the roles are within the legal definition of the state nurse practice act of the state in which they work.

VI. Caring for Vulnerable Populations

A **vulnerable population** is a group of people who are at an increased risk for health problems because of multiple stressors, unhealthy behaviors, or lack of economic, social, and/or health-related resources. Examples of vulnerable populations include those who are homeless or indigent; immigrants; those who are severely mentally ill, abused, or neglected; older adults; infants and children; substance misusers; and those within a stigmatized population. For traits of vulnerable populations, see Box 4.1.

Table 4.1 Roles of the Nurse

Role	Examples of Nursing Care
Direct Caregiver Implements activities that address a client's physical, psychosocial, developmental, sociocultural, and spiritual needs **Requires:** • Clinical proficiency • A supportive, empathetic, and caring bedside manner	• Assesses a client • Performs technical skills, such as dressing changes, mechanical ventilation, and inserting and managing tubes and catheters • Administers medications • Provides emotional support • Evaluates outcomes of care
Client Advocate Works with or on behalf of clients to meet their physical and emotional needs **Requires:** • Knowledge of human and legal rights • A nonjudgmental attitude • An assertive personality • Efficient communication skills	• Helps a client explore options • Supports a client's right to make decisions • Helps explain a client's position to a health-care provider or family member • Helps clients to stand up for themselves • Implements activities that protect the client's human and legal rights, including the development of policies and procedures • Teaches clients how to prepare for office visits and how to prepare a list of questions for the primary health-care provider • Illustrates how to communicate with providers in new situations
Teacher Communicates clearly and accurately (verbally and in writing) with clients and their family members and people in the community to help them learn about their health and health care **Requires:** • Effective communication skills • Knowledge of teaching and learning principles	• Presents information about health-care procedures to maintain or restore health • Teaches clients how to access credible and reliable health-care information • Teaches healthy lifestyle behaviors, such as weight-loss strategies, smoking cessation, and a heart-healthy diet • Teaches prenatal education classes • Provides preoperative teaching to prevent postoperative complications • Teaches self-administration of medications
Manager Influences others to achieve an identified goal **Requires:** • Knowledge of management theory • Knowledge of leadership theory • Effective communication skills • Ability to assume responsibility and accountability for the demands of the role	• Delegates and supervises nursing care activities of subordinate nursing team members • Evaluates outcomes of care delegated • Makes decisions regarding allocation of resources • Motivates staff members to achieve unit goals (See Chapter 5, Leadership and Management, for additional information.)
Case Manager Oversees a client's progress through the health-care system while ensuring that needs are identified and addressed **Requires:** • Organizational skills • Effective communication skills	• Oversees a client's plan of care and functions as an advocate throughout the client's hospitalization • Ensures that a client's needs are met within the facility • Ensures continuity of a client's health care within the community when preparing for discharge • Fulfills specific roles identified by the agency, such as discharge planning and managing referrals
Researcher Participates in planning and conducting evidence-based practice projects as well as implementing research results to the extent of one's educational preparation **Requires:** • Critical thinking ability • An inquisitive mind • Effective communication skills	• Participates as a member of a formal research committee • Assists in all phases of a research project • Incorporates findings into policy and procedure development • Facilitates the application of research results into practice (evidence-based practice) to improve client care
Expert An individual who has specialized education, training, or experience in a particular field or activity and functions as a resource or in an expanded role **Requires:** • An advanced educational degree or certification in a specialty • Extensive experiential background in a particular field or activity	• Collaborates with other health team members regarding a plan of care for a client with multiple or complex needs (e.g., clinical nurse specialist, diabetes nurse educator, enterostomal therapy nurse, infection control nurse, or dialysis nurse) • Provides primary care for a specific population, such as pregnant women, older adults, and children • Provides specialized services to clients (e.g., nurse anesthetist)

A. Commonalities of nursing care for vulnerable populations
   1. Provide emotional and culturally sensitive care.
   (!) 2. Provide dignified, respectful, and nonjudgmental care.
   3. Collaborate with other health-care professionals to ensure that comprehensive care is planned and implemented.
   4. Engage clients in the planning process to ensure that they have input and a vested interest in goal achievement.
   5. Involve family members in developing a plan of care to address client needs if the client gives consent or if the client is a minor.
   6. Establish priorities with the client's input because what the nurse believes is most important might not be what is most important to the client.
   7. Promote and acknowledge client abilities to foster independence and increase self-esteem.
   8. Make referrals to appropriate community resources and services.
   9. Arrange for transportation and child care to facilitate attendance at appointments.
   10. Coordinate home-based care if the client is unable to leave the home or if a vulnerable client is at risk for not attending health-care services.
   11. Arrange for participation in economic support programs, such as food stamps, Medicaid, and the Women, Infants, and Children (WIC) program.
   12. Provide assistance for vocational counseling if the client is able to maintain employment.
B. Individuals who are infants (birth to 1 year) or children
   1. Infants and children are dependent on others to meet their physiological and emotional needs.
   2. They have immature immune systems to protect themselves from infection.
   3. They lack depth and breadth of physiological responses to stress.
   4. They lack judgment, which may result in injury.
   5. They may be born into a hostile environment (e.g., inadequate nutrition, parents who misuse substances, poverty).
   6. Specific nursing care for infants and children.
      a. Ensure that infants and children receive immunizations.
      b. Ensure that they receive routine health care (e.g., initially monthly and then yearly) and dental care.
      c. Educate parents about positive health-care practices (e.g., nutrition, safety practices, and developmental expectations).
C. Individuals who are older adults
   1. Includes a rising percentage of adults over age 85 because of an increase in life span; older adults have multiple health problems, requiring comprehensive health care.
   2. Also includes a rising percentage of adults over age 65 because of the aging of the large number of people born between 1946 and 1960 (baby boomer generation); these people have health promotion and illness prevention needs to maintain health and independence.
   3. Demonstrate an increase in alcohol use in response to depression, lack of social support, and lack of companionship.
   4. Experience socioeconomic stressors, such as retirement, inadequate income, social isolation, downsizing of home and lifestyle, and relocation, which also can cause psychological and physiological stress.
   5. Generally live in their own homes but may have impaired mobility or lack of transportation, which may require services to be provided in the home.

DID YOU KNOW?

Home-care services support independence and help avoid institutionalization of older adults.

   6. Specific nursing care for older adults.
      a. Provide opportunities that support the developmental task associated with older adults (integrity versus despair).
      b. Assess clients for substance use (e.g., polypharmacy) and alcohol and prescription drug misuse.
      c. Encourage clients to engage in social activities available in the community.
      d. Arrange for home-care services so that older adults are able to remain in their own homes for as long as possible.

🛑 e. Arrange for respite care. **Respite care** temporarily relieves family members from the caregiving role; varies in duration, from as short as a few hours so a family member can go to a movie or shop to a week or more admission to a nursing home while a family attends an event or goes on vacation.

D. Individuals who are homeless or indigent
1. Generally live in substandard housing or in hazardous conditions, such as insect- or vermin-infested environments, or live outside in the elements.
2. Are less healthy because of such factors as inadequate nutrition, inaccessible facilities in which to bathe and wash clothes, inadequate rest, and absence of preventive health care, such as immunizations and health screenings.
3. Are at increased risk for accidental injury, assault, abuse, and infectious diseases, such as tuberculosis and skin and respiratory infections.
4. Have a higher incidence of severe mental illness, alcoholism, illegal drug use, and smoking than the general population.
5. Specific nursing care for homeless and indigent individuals and families.
   a. Help clients find mobile health clinics, soup kitchens, shelters, thrift shops, and housing.
   b. Teach the importance of and ways to maintain a clean, healthy environment.
   c. Teach homeless people ways to avoid violence.

E. Individuals who are immigrants
1. Generally do not speak English well enough to communicate needs or find resources that support health and wellness and treat illness.
2. If in the country illegally, often do not seek health care until acutely ill because of a fear of being deported.
3. Often cannot afford health insurance or health-care services because of low-paying jobs or dependence on day work.
4. Present with specific health problems, such as tuberculosis, intestinal parasites, dental decay, and hepatitis B.
5. May have experienced a traumatic event, such as war, natural disaster, lack of economic opportunity, or oppression, and are at risk for emotional distress.
6. Frequently engage in nontraditional healing practices that may or may not be helpful.
7. Specific nursing care for immigrant populations.
   a. Learn as much as possible about the client's culture and its impact on the client's health-care needs.

b. Be sensitive to cultural values and beliefs and demonstrate respect for nontraditional healing practices unless they are harmful to the client.
c. Assess the client for signs and symptoms of specific health problems unique to the client's history, culture, and environment.

🛑 d. Use a professional interpreter so that information can be correctly translated and confidentiality can be maintained; ensure that all questions are answered and understood to promote client participation in the planning process.

F. Individuals who engage in substance misuse
1. Includes individuals who misuse illegal or prescription drugs and alcohol.
2. Often have economic and legal issues as well as health problems related to substance misuse, such as the expense of supporting the habit, arrest and conviction related to illegal activities acquiring drugs, and infectious disease as a result of sharing drug supplies.
3. Often experience a breakdown of the family and loss of support systems as the substance misuse becomes the focus of activities or because of abusive behavior.
4. Often present with complex medical problems (e.g., cocaine use can cause nasal, sinus, and cardiac problems; alcohol misuse can cause liver cirrhosis).
5. Specific nursing care for clients who engage in substance misuse.
   a. Observe for signs and symptoms of substance misuse, such as multiple missed appointments, chief complaint of insomnia or "bad nerves," multiple health-care providers, medication bottles with different provider names, requests for frequent refills of sedatives or analgesics, history of frequent sexually transmitted infections, multiple abortions, gastrointestinal illnesses, chest pain or palpitations, and family history of addiction.
   b. Encourage client participation in a substance misuse program.
   c. Refer the client to appropriate legal services.

G. Individuals who are mentally ill
1. Are routinely cared for in the community rather than in psychiatric facilities.
2. Often refuse to take prescribed medications, which worsens their health status.
3. Often unable to self-perform activities of daily living.
4. Generally incapable of retaining a job, commonly resulting in their living below the poverty level and becoming homeless.
5. Often have many of the same needs as indigent and homeless people have.

6. Specific nursing care for severely mentally ill individuals.
   a. Arrange for the client to attend a day-care program for individuals with mental illness, if appropriate.
   ⓘ b. **Arrange for admission to a psychiatric facility if the client becomes a danger to self or others.**

H. Individuals who are within a stigmatized population
   1. A **stigmatized population** is a group of people who are unaccepted and discriminated against and lack status and power.
   2. Includes individuals who have communicable diseases (e.g., HIV, AIDS, tuberculosis, hepatitis C), are mentally ill, or engage in behaviors that are denounced (e.g., substance misuse).
   3. Specific nursing care for stigmatized populations.
   a. Teach individuals who engage in high-risk behaviors ways to protect themselves from infection, such as using condoms and avoiding needle sharing.
   b. Refer clients who have HIV or AIDS to an HIV coordinator because these professionals have expertise to meet the needs of this vulnerable population.
   c. Provide clients with choices and opportunities to participate in planning care in an effort to empower them.

CASE STUDY: Putting It All Together

A nurse in a primary-care clinic administered immunizations to all the members of a family. The children received immunizations that were appropriate for their ages, the parents asked to be immunized against hepatitis B, and the older adult parent (grandmother) received a vaccine for shingles and a flu vaccine. All of the members of the family received complete physical examinations with routine blood work. The two adult women received bone density tests and mammograms. Eight months later, the grandmother's physical mobility became impaired because of osteoarthritis and the aging process. The primary health-care provider prescribed physical therapy to help the grandmother learn how to use a walker. The family decided to make modifications to the house, adding grab bars in the bathroom and a ramp to the side door of the house so that the grandmother could walk out to the backyard independently. Two years later, the grandmother was diagnosed with stage IV ovarian cancer. The family was adamant about keeping her home to die.

Case Study Questions

A. Identify interventions associated with primary health care, and briefly discuss the focus of this type of health care.

_____

B. Identify interventions associated with secondary health care, and briefly discuss the focus of this type of health care.

_____

C. Identify interventions associated with tertiary health care, and briefly discuss the focus of this type of health care.

_____

D. What health-care service is available to assist the family with their goal of keeping the grandmother in the home to die, and how will this service meet the needs of the grandmother and family members?

_____

REVIEW QUESTIONS

Be sure to read the Introduction for valuable test-taking tips.

1. Under which category is the agency Alcoholics Anonymous (AA) classified?
   1. Proprietary
   2. Voluntary
   3. Official
   4. Private

2. A nurse is caring for a client who has shortness of breath because of chronic obstructive pulmonary disease and an upper respiratory infection. The client reveals having several cigarettes a day. Which nursing intervention is associated with a secondary health-care service?
   1. Talking about managing work responsibilities while convalescing
   2. Suggesting attending a smoking cessation program
   3. Administering the prescribed antibiotic regimen
   4. Implementing care that supports quality of life

3. Which interventions **most** likely are considered necessary by a company that provides health insurance? **Select all that apply.**
   1. Removal of an infected appendix.
   2. Off-label use of a chemotherapeutic medication.
   3. Bariatric surgery to promote weight loss of 100 lb.
   4. Laser therapy for facial brown pigmentation due to sun damage.
   5. Surgery to remove excess skin in the neck area after significant weight loss.

4. A client is recovering from a brain attack (cerebrovascular accident) and experiencing dysphasia and aspiration. For which professional should the nurse seek a consultation referral from the primary health-care provider?
   1. Clinical nurse specialist
   2. Respiratory therapist
   3. Nurse practitioner
   4. Speech therapist

5. A client experienced a brain attack (cerebrovascular accident) that resulted in a left hemiparesis. Which health-care professional is appropriate to teach this client how to recover and maintain abilities associated with activities of daily living?
   1. Occupational therapist
   2. Medical technician
   3. Physical therapist
   4. Primary nurse

6. An older adult who lives alone is recovering after surgery for a total hip replacement. Which is the **most** appropriate setting for this client after discharge from the hospital?
   1. Home
   2. Hospice
   3. Skilled nursing facility
   4. Assistive living apartment

7. Client needs are met in a variety of health-care settings. Place these settings in order, considering the progression from diagnosis to death.
   1. Hospice
   2. Outpatient clinic
   3. Acute care hospital
   4. Skilled nursing facility
   5. Intermediate care facility
   Answer: _____

8. Which setting has successfully reduced the overall cost of health care in the United States?
   1. Hospice
   2. Home care
   3. Rehabilitation facility
   4. Skilled nursing facility

9. An occupational nurse provides services related to primary prevention. Which actions by the occupational nurse are examples of this type of service?
   1. Administering yearly flu vaccines to employees
   2. Measuring employee cholesterol levels twice a year
   3. Providing an exercise program after work for employees
   4. Encouraging female employees to obtain routine mammograms
   5. Ensuring environmental accommodations for an employee who uses a wheelchair

10. Nurses working in acute care settings perform activities related to primary, secondary, and tertiary prevention. Which activities by a nurse in a hospital are related to secondary prevention?
    1. Teaching a client's spouse how to administer an opioid injection
    2. Counseling a client about a heart-healthy diet
    3. Obtaining a client's blood glucose level
    4. Instructing a client how to use a walker
    5. Assessing a client's vital signs

11. A public health nurse is performing a variety of activities within the community. Which activities are examples of tertiary prevention? **Select all that apply.**
    1. Assessing the home environment of a client with a spinal cord injury who is to be discharged
    2. Conducting a class at the local library about the importance of exercise
    3. Visiting a new mother who has a child with Down syndrome
    4. Teaching a client how to perform a colostomy irrigation
    5. Screening school-aged children for scoliosis

12. A nurse is caring for an older adult who was admitted to the hospital for treatment of a new acute cardiac problem and who has a history of chronic asthma, diabetes, and colitis. The client is having difficulty coping with the additional self-care responsibilities associated with the new health problem. With whom should the nurse consult to **best** explore strategies to assist this client to provide self-care?
    1. Nurse manager
    2. Clinical nurse specialist
    3. Licensed vocational nurse
    4. Primary health-care provider

13. A 76-year-old man is hospitalized for pneumonia. His daughter has a meeting with her father's case manager to explore what should be done when her father is discharged. The nurse manager speaks with the client's daughter, reviews the client's medical history and present physical status, and identifies the community resources in the client's community. What community resource should the nurse plan to explore with the client and his daughter?
    1. Independent living apartment in an older adult development
    2. Long-term care facility providing skilled nursing care
    3. Older adult day-care center
    4. Respite care center

Additional Information

Client's History

The client experienced a brain attack (cerebral vascular accident, stroke) 3 years ago. He has right-sided hemiplegia and must use a wheelchair for ambulation. He wears a brace on his right leg and a splint on his right hand and forearm and has periodic episodes of night time urine and fecal incontinence. He can perform some activities of daily living (ADLs) independently (e.g., brush teeth, shave face, feed self) but needs assistance completing other tasks (e.g., transfer from bed to wheelchair, toileting). He is mentally alert and is able to communicate effectively. The pneumonia is resolving, but he has activity intolerance.

Interview With the Client's Daughter

The client's daughter is 52 years old, single, and works full time as a teacher. She states, "I like my dad living with me and we have a wonderful home health aide who comes in from 8 a.m. to noon, Monday through Friday. My dad has a medical alert button in case anything happens when I am not there. The job of caring for my dad is getting more demanding. When I come home, I immediately take my dad to the bathroom, make our dinner, wash our clothes, and do all the chores around the house. The hardest part is cleaning him at night when he is incontinent. The 24/7 responsibility is tough, but I refuse to put him in a nursing home."

Community Resources

Independent living apartment in an older adult development
Long-term care facility with skilled nursing
Older adult day-care center
Respite care center

14. A public health nurse analyzes statistics about health issues in the community and identifies that domestic violence against women and their children is on the rise. Place the following interventions in the order in which they should be implemented to address this health-related problem.
    1. Design and implement outreach initiates to access the targeted population.
    2. Identify the social system of the community and the social services available.
    3. Make referrals to appropriate community resources and arrange for transportation if needed.
    4. Collaborate with health-care professionals and women who personally have successfully dealt with this issue.
    5. Engage each individual in developing a personal plan for safety and acknowledge client abilities to increase self-esteem.
    Answer: _____

15. A nurse is interviewing for a position as charge nurse for a medical-surgical unit. During the interview, the nurse manager mentions that primary nursing is the nursing care model used in the agency. Which statements are associated with this nursing care model? **Select all that apply.**
    1. The delivery of nursing care is task oriented.
    2. It minimizes the fragmentation of nursing care.
    3. Communication occurs in a hierarchy from head nurse to subordinate.
    4. One nurse is responsible for ensuring that comprehensive care is delivered.
    5. Responsibility for care is shared by nursing staff but directed by a team leader.

16. Which nursing action reflects the caregiver role? **Select all that apply.**
    1. Completes a dressing change ensuring that standards of care are met
    2. Assesses a client on return from the post-anesthesia care unit
    3. Participates in developing policies that protect human rights
    4. Supervises quality of care delegated to other team members
    5. Helps a client learn how to test a blood glucose level

17. A registered nurse graduated from an associate degree nursing program. The hospital in which the nurse works is requiring all registered nurses to attain a bachelor of science in nursing (BSN) degree within 5 years. Which educational program should the college counselor suggest is the **most** appropriate for this nurse to attend?
    1. Masters in science nursing program
    2. Continuing education program
    3. In-service education program
    4. General nursing program

18. A client who lives alone is scheduled to be discharged from the hospital with a large pressure ulcer that needs comprehensive nursing care. The service provided by which option is **most** appropriate for this client?
    1. Assisted living facility
    2. Hospice care program
    3. Skilled nursing home
    4. Day-care center

19. A Public Health Nurse is considering the needs of individual members of a community. Which stressor identified by the nurse possesses the greatest risk for precipitating illness?
    1. Change in marital status
    2. Teenage motherhood
    3. Single parent family
    4. Living on the street

20. With what is community health nursing mainly associated?
    1. Delivering home health-care services
    2. Assisting economically disadvantaged high-risk groups
    3. Addressing the nursing needs of individuals or groups within the community
    4. Providing interventions that help people on the health end of the health–illness continuum

21. In what way is a home health-care nursing practice different from the acute care setting?
    1. The family is encouraged to provide emotional support.
    2. The client is responsible for formulating outcomes.
    3. The nursing process is the framework for care.
    4. The nurse functions more autonomously.

22. The focus of the delivery of health care has changed from treatment to prevention. An increased emphasis on what aspect of nursing care will result?
    1. Intensive care services
    2. Community-based care
    3. Evidence-based practice
    4. Pathophysiology of illness

23. What focus is unique to community health practice when compared to acute health care?
    1. Family focused
    2. Individual focused
    3. Population focused
    4. Geographically focused

24. Which type of care is not designed to assist individuals and families with care in the home?
    1. Acute care
    2. Respite care
    3. Hospice care
    4. Restorative care

25. A nurse is preparing a health promotion class for individuals in the community. Which of the following topics should the nurse address because they are among the 10 indicators that are studied to determine if progress is made toward health goals identified in *Healthy People 2020*? **Select all that apply.**
    1. Obesity
    2. Tobacco use
    3. Heart disease
    4. Family planning
    5. Physical activity

26. Which is **most** important when providing services to homeless individuals?
    1. Being aware of cultural beliefs
    2. Helping to find a source of food
    3. Teaching how to bathe in a public restroom
    4. Arranging for attendance at a day-care program

27. A nurse working in the community is functioning as a nurse epidemiologist. Which actions implemented by the nurse are associated with this role? **Select all that apply.**
    1. Tracks illnesses, diseases, and death rates within a community.
    2. Monitors for risk factors that threaten the health of members of the community
    3. Engages in political action to represent health needs on behalf of members of the community
    4. Focuses on health promotion for groups of people as well as individuals within the community
    5. Ensures that plans of care meet clients' needs across the continuum of care within the community

28. A client is diagnosed with pulmonary tuberculosis and must attend a clinic every week for treatment and follow-up health care. Which is **most** important to ensure that the client is cured of tuberculosis when providing care in the community setting?
    1. Provide the client with assistance regarding vocational counseling.
    2. Seek economic support for the client, such as Medicaid, during recovery.
    3. Have the client set the outcome criteria for the plan of care independently.
    4. Arrange home-based care if the client is at risk for nonattendance at appointments.

29. A nurse is completing a community assessment. Which information is **most** significant when identifying the health needs of the community in relation to the status of its members?
    1. Natural boundaries and size of the community
    2. Employers and occupations within the community
    3. Morbidity and mortality rates related to the community
    4. Crime rates and drug abuse associated with the community

30. Which setting for the provision of health-care services in the community is at the highest risk for potential legal and ethical issues?
    1. Migrant services
    2. Telehealth services
    3. Faith-based services
    4. Prison-based services

REVIEW ANSWERS AND RATIONALES

1. ANSWER: 2.

Rationales:

1. Proprietary agencies are privately owned and operated to make a profit.

2. Alcoholics Anonymous (AA) is a voluntary organization. Voluntary agencies are nonprofits and rely on professional and lay volunteers in addition to a paid staff.

3. Official health agencies are supported by local, state, and/or national taxes.

4. Private agencies are privately owned and operated to make a profit.

TEST-TAKING TIP: Identify the equally plausible options. Options 1 and 4 are equally plausible. Agencies that make a profit are called *proprietary* or *private agencies.*

Content Area: *Health-Care System*
Integrated Processes: *Nursing Process: Analysis*
Client Need: *Safe and Effective Care Environment; Management of Care*
Cognitive Level: *Knowledge*
Concept: *Health-Care System*

2. ANSWER: 3.

Rationales:

1. Discussing concerns associated with responsibilities is related to facilitating health promotion, not restoring health.

2. Suggesting attending a smoking cessation program is related to preventing illness, not restoring health.

3. Antibiotics are curative and are given to restore health.

4. Tertiary (rehabilitation) health-care services includes interventions that focus on maximizing function and supporting comfort and quality of life, not restoring health.

Content Area: *Health-Care System*
Integrated Processes: *Nursing Process: Implementation*
Client Need: *Safe and Effective Care Environment; Management of Care*
Cognitive Level: *Application*
Concept: *Health-Care System*

3. ANSWER: 1, 3.

Rationales:

1. Surgery to remove an infected appendix is considered emergency surgery that is paid for by health insurance. Appendicitis can lead to perforation, peritonitis, and death if the appendix is not removed.

2. Off-label use of a medication generally is not covered by health insurance because efficacy has not been demonstrated.

3. Bariatric surgery to promote weight loss of 100 lb generally is covered by health insurance. Weight loss of less than 100 lb may be covered if the client has a concurrent medical condition, such as diabetes or hypertension. It is believed that successful weight loss after bariatric surgery improves functioning; helps prevent complications, such as diabetes and hypertension; and improves quality of life. Although costly to provide initially, the person probably will have fewer health issues in the future.

4. Laser therapy to remove brown pigmentation of facial skin is not considered medically necessary to diagnose, treat, or improve functioning; this generally is not covered by health insurance.

5. Surgery to remove excess skin around the neck after significant weight loss is considered cosmetic and not medically necessary; this generally is not covered by health insurance. An exception to coverage for cosmetic surgery includes removal of pendulous abdominal skin that causes constant excoriation of touching skin surfaces, even with meticulous skin care. Reconstructive cosmetic surgery after a burn injury is covered by health insurance.

TEST-TAKING TIP: Identify the word in the stem that sets a priority. The word *most* in the stem sets a priority.

Content Area: *Health-Care System*
Integrated Processes: *Nursing Process: Planning*
Client Need: *Safe and Effective Care Environment; Management of Care*
Cognitive Level: *Analysis*
Concept: *Health Care-System*

4. ANSWER: 4.

Rationales:

1. Although a clinical nurse specialist may provide care to a client with impairment in swallowing, a clinical nurse specialist is not the professional educated to diagnose the specific mechanism that is impaired.

2. Respiratory therapists assess and treat clients with impairments of heart and lung functioning, not swallowing and speech impairments.

3. A nurse practitioner is educationally prepared to diagnose illness and prescribe medications and treatments related to a client's problems. However, nurse practitioners should consult with another health-care professional who can best determine the mechanism that is impaired when a swallowing problem exists.

4. Swallowing involves a complex mechanism that speech therapists are educated to diagnosis and treat; speech therapists assess, diagnose, and treat problems associated with speaking, language, articulation, vocal sound, and swallowing.

Content Area: *Health-Care System*
Integrated Processes: *Communication and Documentation; Nursing Process: Implementation*
Client Need: *Safe and Effective Care Environment; Management of Care*
Cognitive Level: *Application*
Concept: *Collaboration*

5. ANSWER: 1.

Rationales:

1. An occupational therapist is the most appropriate professional to help this client regain, acquire, improve, and maintain abilities related to activities of daily living, such as eating, dressing, bathing, grooming, and cooking.

2. A medical technician works in a laboratory testing body fluid; activities may include evaluating blood levels of medication, cross-matching blood for blood transfusions, and examining tissues of the body.

3. A physical therapist is involved with preventing and limiting physical impairment and restoring function, strength,

and coordination associated with mobility, not helping a client cope with performing activities of daily living.

4. A primary nurse may be involved in coordinating the efforts of nursing team members with those of other health-care professionals involved in helping a client recover from an illness. A primary nurse provides nursing care and supports the plans of care established by professionals in other health-care disciplines.

Content Area: Health-Care System
Integrated Processes: Nursing Process: Planning
Client Need: Safe and Effective Care Environment; Management of Care
Cognitive Level: Application
Concept: Collaboration

6. **ANSWER: 3.**

Rationales:

1. This client lives alone and will not be capable of managing self-care.

2. There is no evidence in the stem that indicates that the client has a probability of only 6 months to live, which is the central criterion for admission to a hospice program.

3. **Several weeks of rehabilitation services generally are prescribed to promote strength, endurance, and mobility after a total hip replacement; the client will require skilled nursing care and physical therapy.**

4. An assistive living arrangement may be an appropriate setting in the future if it is determined after rehabilitation that the client can no longer live alone safely.

TEST-TAKING TIP: Identify the word in the stem that sets a priority. The word *most* in the stem sets a priority.

Content Area: Health-Care System
Integrated Processes: Nursing Process: Planning
Client Need: Safe and Effective Care Environment; Management of Care
Cognitive Level: Analysis
Concept: Health-Care System

7. **ANSWER: 2, 3, 4, 5, 1.**

Rationales:

2. **An outpatient clinic is a setting where secondary health care occurs (care that focuses on early detection and intervention to cure disease and minimize further impairment).**

3. **Acute care settings, such as hospitals, provide medical and surgical procedures to meet clients' immediate health needs.**

4. **After people have acute care needs met, they often are discharged earlier than in the past. As a result, these clients need skilled nursing care until, hopefully, they are capable of returning home.**

5. **Clients who are unable to return home after an experience in a skilled nursing facility usually are transferred to an intermediate care facility to meet their ongoing custodial needs.**

1. **As people reach the end of their lives, hospice care can provide supportive services for clients and their family members. Hospice provides palliative care so that clients can die with dignity and without pain.**

Content Area: Health-Care System
Integrated Processes: Nursing Process: Analysis
Client Need: Safe and Effective Care Environment; Management of Care
Cognitive Level: Analysis
Concept: Health-Care System

8. **ANSWER: 2.**

Rationales:

1. Although hospice care is less costly than a hospital in the provision of end-of-life care, it has not had as dramatic an impact as another setting in reducing overall costs of health care.

2. **Home care successfully provides a team approach to providing health care in the home, which is significantly less costly than providing the same care in a hospital or in a subacute unit in a long-term care facility.**

3. Although a rehabilitation facility can provide rehabilitation services less expensively than in the hospital setting, it is not the setting that has made the most impact in reducing overall costs of health care.

4. Although a skilled nursing facility provides skilled nursing care and subacute care for people in a less costly setting than a hospital, it is still more costly than another setting presented.

Content Area: Health-Care System
Integrated Processes: Nursing Process: Analysis
Client Need: Safe and Effective Care Environment; Management of Care
Cognitive Level: Knowledge
Concept: Health-Care System

9. **ANSWER: 1, 3.**

Rationales:

1. **Primary prevention focuses on maintaining an optimum level of wellness and preventing disease or disability; it involves activities such as providing immunizations, promoting safety in the workplace, and counseling about lifestyle modifications (e.g., exercise, smoking cessation, and healthy diets).**

2. Secondary prevention involves early detection and intervention to cure disease and minimize impairment. An elevated cholesterol level alerts the employee to seek medical supervision.

3. **Exercise programs promote an optimum level of wellness and decrease the risk of disease and disability, the focus of primary health-care services.**

4. Secondary prevention involves early detection and intervention to cure disease and minimize impairment. Yearly physicals and routine dental care, mammograms, colonoscopies, and bone density tests are examples of secondary prevention.

5. Tertiary prevention includes activities such as making environmental modifications (e.g., ramps, widening doorways) for people recovering from physiological changes or rehabilitation and maximizing abilities.

Content Area: Health-Care System
Integrated Processes: Nursing Process: Implementation
Client Need: Health Promotion and Maintenance
Cognitive Level: Application
Concept: Health-Care System

10. ANSWER: 3, 5.

Rationales:

1. Education about palliative care that supports comfort is an example of tertiary care.

2. A heart-healthy diet will help maintain an optimum level of wellness; this is an example of primary prevention.

3. Obtaining a client's blood glucose level is a diagnostic procedure that provides valuable information for the identification of hyperglycemia or hypoglycemia. Secondary health-care services are concerned with early detection and intervention to treat disease and minimize further impairment.

4. Teaching a client how to use a walker is concerned with tertiary prevention; the nurse is providing information that will assist the client to engage in the activities of daily living to live independently.

5. A client's vital signs provide significant data and are integral to the diagnostic process; they assist with the identification of an illness, which is a part of secondary prevention.

Content Area: *Health-Care System*
Integrated Processes: *Nursing Process: Implementation*
Client Need: *Physiological Integrity; Reduction of Risk Potential*
Cognitive Level: *Application*
Concept: *Health-Care System*

11. ANSWER: 1, 3, 4.

Rationales:

1. This is an example of tertiary prevention; it is concerned with helping a client to develop skills related to a chronic problem and become independent.

2. This is an example of primary prevention; exercise is an activity that can promote wellness.

3. This is an example of tertiary prevention. Down syndrome is a health problem caused by a genetic mutation. Lifelong interventions are required to maximize the child's abilities and support the parents.

4. This activity is an example of tertiary prevention. Colostomy irrigations may be a temporary or permanent requirement; regardless, it requires the learning of new skills to become independent for the length of time it exists.

5. This is an example of secondary prevention; it involves the identification of a health problem so that appropriate interventions can be implemented as early as possible to promote a desirable outcome.

Content Area: *Health-Care System*
Integrated Processes: *Nursing Process: Planning*
Client Need: *Physiological Integrity; Physiological Adaptation*
Cognitive Level: *Analysis*
Concept: *Health-Care System*

12. ANSWER: 2.

Rationales:

1. The nurse manager is not the person with the most appropriate expertise to assist the nurse with this client care situation.

2. A clinical specialist has the most appropriate nursing education and experience to assist the nurse with this
client care situation. A clinical nurse specialist has the knowledge and ability to care for clients with complex health-care needs.

3. A licensed vocational nurse does not have the educational or experiential background to best assist the nurse with this client care situation.

4. A primary health-care provider has a medical, not a nursing, educational and experiential background.

TEST-TAKING TIP: Identify the word in the stem that sets a priority. The word *best* in the stem sets a priority.

Content Area: *Health-Care System*
Integrated Processes: *Communication and Documentation; Nursing Process: Implementation*
Client Need: *Safe and Effective Care Environment; Management of Care*
Cognitive Level: *Application*
Concept: *Collaboration*

13. ANSWER: 4.

Rationales:

1. The client does not have the physical abilities to live in an independent care environment. The client needs assistance with most of the activities of daily living.

2. The client does not need skilled nursing care. The client needs assistance with the activities of daily living that can be provided by assistive nursing personnel.

3. The client is cared for in the morning by a home health aide and is competent to be alone for several hours until the daughter returns from work. An older adult day-care center will not meet the daughter's needs.

4. A respite care center provides services that relieve family members from the caregiving role. In this situation, the daughter may be capable of keeping her father in the home if she has periodic opportunities to obtain adequate rest and relief from the daily responsibilities of caring for her father.

Content Area: *Health-Care System*
Integrated Processes: *Communication and Documentation; Nursing Process: Planning*
Client Need: *Safe and Effective Care Environment; Management of Care*
Cognitive Level: *Analysis*
Concept: *Patient-Centered Care; Health-Care System*

14. ANSWER: 4, 2, 1, 5, 3.

Rationales:

4. Collaboration with health-care professionals involves people who have expertise in relation to the issue. Collaboration with women who personally have successfully dealt with this issue ensures that the discussion remains reality based.

2. Identification of the social system of the community and the social services available within the community are part of the assessment of the community. An assessment of the community also should include the physical environment and economic status of the community, the characteristics and status of its population, and the safety and transportation systems available.

1. After a problem is identified and explored with all significant people involved, then initiatives can be devised

and carried out. The people in the target population must be reached before they can be helped.

5. Plans of care must be individualized. Women must be involved in the planning process to ensure that they have input and vested interest in goal achievement. Women who are victims of domestic violence often feel overwhelmed, powerless, and helpless. Increasing self-esteem may be an initial step toward feeling empowered.

3. Once a plan is in place, then the appropriate community services should be made available to the woman, and every effort should be made to ensure that the woman is physical and emotionally supported.

Content Area: Legal and Ethical Issues
Integrated Processes: Caring; Communication and Documentation; Nursing Process: Analysis
Client Need: Safe and Effective Care Environment, Management of Care
Cognitive Level: Analysis
Concept: Violence

15. ANSWER: 2, 4.
Rationales:

1. This statement is related to functional nursing. Functional nursing is a task-oriented approach in which certain tasks are assigned to different people. It focuses on efficiency and productivity, but it can lead to fragmentation of care and failure to meet emotional needs of clients.

2. This statement is related to primary nursing. One nurse is responsible for the delivery of nursing care to a group of clients. This prevents numerous people being involved with the client and therefore minimizes the fragmentation of nursing care.

3. This statement is related to both functional nursing and team nursing, not primary nursing. In primary nursing, the nurse communicates laterally with nurses on the other shifts who are assigned to care for the client.

4. This statement is related to primary nursing. A registered nurse is responsible for assigned clients throughout their hospitalization, 7 days a week, 24 hours a day (primary nurse). The primary nurse does not deliver all care personally but is responsible for ensuring that comprehensive and individualized care is delivered.

5. This statement is related to team nursing. A registered nurse team leader makes assignments based on the abilities of each member of the team, such as registered nurses, licensed practical nurses, and unlicensed nursing assistants. Team members work together and share responsibility for the care of a group of clients. The team leader is responsible for coordinating the team, planning care, and collaborating with professionals in other disciplines and, therefore, often does not provide direct client care.

Content Area: Health-Care System
Integrated Processes: Nursing Process: Analysis
Client Need: Safe and Effective Care Environment; Management of Care
Cognitive Level: Knowledge
Concept: Health-Care System

16. ANSWER: 1, 2.
Rationales:

1. In this scenario, the nurse is functioning in the role of caregiver. Direct care is given to a client to meet physical, psychosocial, developmental, sociocultural, and spiritual needs.

2. In this scenario, the nurse is functioning in the role of caregiver. Assessment is essential to providing direct nursing care.

3. In this scenario, the nurse is functioning in the role of advocate. An advocate protects the client's personal and legal rights and supports and promotes the client.

4. In this scenario, the nurse is functioning in the role of leader/manager. A leader/manager influences others to achieve goals.

5. In this scenario, the nurse is functioning in the role of teacher. A teacher presents information, assists with changes in behavior, and teaches skills related to learning self-care.

Content Area: Health-Care System
Integrated Processes: Nursing Process: Implementation
Client Need: Safe and Effective Care Environment; Management of Care
Cognitive Level: Analysis
Concept: Professionalism

17. ANSWER: 4.
Rationales:

1. A master's degree nursing program prepares registered nurses with a baccalaureate degree in nursing for advanced practice, such as clinical nurse specialist, certified nurse midwife, nurse practitioner, nurse administrator, and nurse educator.

2. Continuing education programs generally offer credit hours applicable toward state requirements for renewal of a registered nurse license. These programs are offered by employers, colleges, professional nursing organizations, and professional journals. These programs ensure that nurses keep abreast of new technology, theory, and clinical practice.

3. In-service education programs are provided by employers and focus on such topics as new equipment, policies, or topics mandated by a state health department.

4. A general nursing program usually is a 2-year baccalaureate degree program for graduates of an associate degree nursing program. Generic nursing programs are 3- to 4-year programs for students entering as freshmen with a major in nursing.

TEST-TAKING TIP: Identify the word in the stem that sets a priority. The word *most* in the stem sets a priority. Identify the clang associations. The word *nursing* in the stem and in options 1 and 4 are clang associations. Examine options 1 and 4 carefully.

Content Area: Health-Care System
Integrated Processes: Communication and Documentation; Nursing Process: Planning
Client Need: Safe and Effective Care Environment; Management of Care
Cognitive Level: Application
Concept: Professionalism

18. ANSWER: 3.
    Rationales:
    1. An assisted living facility will not provide the level of skilled nursing care and medical attention needed by this client at this time. Assisted living facilities help people with hygiene and dressing and provide meals and activities. Some limited nursing care may be provided, such as assistance with taking medications.
    2. A hospice care program provides a medically directed, nurse-coordinated program for terminally ill clients and their family members. Generally, this service is provided once the client no longer seeks curative treatment and the client is predicted to have less than 6 months to live. Comprehensive palliative care and emotional support for the client and family members are provided. Grief support is also provided for family members and friends after the death of the client.
    3. This setting provides skilled nursing and medical attention during the recovery phase of an illness. It provides skilled nursing care for a person who is not sick enough to require hospital care but is unable to provide for his or her own needs at home (subacute care). In addition, subacute care services may help a client prevent frequent hospitalization.
    4. A day-care center does not provide the level of skilled nursing care needed by this client. A day-care center is designed to provide a safe environment for infants, children, and older adults who cannot be left alone at home. Interventions involving socialization, exercise and stimulation, and some noncomplex nursing care, such as help with medications, minor treatments, and counseling, may be provided.
    TEST-TAKING TIP: Identify the word in the stem that sets a priority. The word *most* in the stem sets a priority.
    Content Area: Health-Care System
    Integrated Processes: Nursing Process: Analysis
    Client Need: Safe and Effective Care Environment; Management of Care
    Cognitive Level: Application
    Concept: Health-Care System

19. ANSWER: 4.
    Rationales:
    1. A person with a changed marital status may experience several stressors but probably not be at as great a risk for developing an illness as a person in one of the other options.
    2. A teenage mother may experience several stressors but probably not be at as great a risk to develop an illness as a person in one of the other options.
    3. A single-parent family may experience several stressors but probably not be at as great a risk to develop an illness as a person in one of the other options.
    4. People living on the street most likely have a multiplicity of stressors in many different categories that places them at the greatest risk for developing an illness, for example, physiological (poor nutrition and sleep patterns), physical (exposure to heat and cold), psychological (fear of being a target for assault, robbery and abuse, lack of family support, and possible history

of mental or emotional illness), economic (inadequate or no income), developmental (inability to complete developmental tasks), chemical (dependence on drugs, alcohol, and cigarettes), and microbiological (exposure to pathogens from living on the street and not having access to adequate bathing and toileting environments).
    Content Area: Health-Care System
    Integrated Processes: Nursing Process: Analysis
    Client Need: Health Promotion and Maintenance
    Cognitive Level: Analysis
    Concept: Culture

20. ANSWER: 3.
    Rationales:
    1. The home setting traditionally was associated with the concept of community nursing. However, in the current health-care environment, the community includes such settings as schools, work environments, community centers, neighborhood clinics, and even mobile units that bring services directly to people in a neighborhood.
    2. Community-based health activities are designed to help individuals and groups across all economic levels and low-risk as well as high-risk groups.
    3. Community health nursing reaches out to people and groups outside of acute-care facilities. Services are provided in neighborhoods, which includes the home.
    4. Community-based nursing assists individuals and groups from one end of the health–illness continuum to the other, not just the health end of the continuum.
    TEST-TAKING TIP: Identify the word in the stem that sets a priority. The word *mainly* in the stem sets a priority. Identify the option with a clang association. The word *community* in the stem and in option 3 is a clang association.
    Content Area: Health-Care System
    Integrated Processes: Nursing Process: Analysis
    Client Need: Safe and Effective Care Environment; Management of Care
    Cognitive Level: Comprehension
    Concept: Health-Care System

21. ANSWER: 4.
    Rationales:
    1. Family members are encouraged to provide emotional support to clients in all settings.
    2. In all settings in which a nurse works, the nurse and the client ideally formulate realistic, achievable, measurable, and acceptable goals together, not in isolation.
    3. The nursing process is used in all settings in which the nurse works to identify and meet the actual and potential human responses to illness, disease, or injury.
    4. The nurse functions more independently in the home setting, whereas in the acute setting, resources are immediately available for consultation and support.

Content Area: Health-Care System
Integrated Processes: Nursing Process: Implementation
Client Need: Safe and Effective Care Environment;
Management of Care
Cognitive Level: Knowledge
Concept: Health-Care System

22. **ANSWER: 2.**
Rationales:
1. Intensive care areas are concerned with treatment, not prevention.
2. **Health care is moving from the hospital to the community in response to an increased emphasis on health promotion and illness prevention. The words in the stem *changed from treatment to prevention* directs the nurse to the trend in health care whereby people are cared for more in the community rather than in the acute care environment. Also, because of prospective hospital reimbursement, lengths of stay are decreasing as clients are discharged more quickly than in the past and must rely on community resources to make the transition safely.**
3. Evidence-based practice is associated with making decisions regarding nursing care based on some form of validation or demonstrated proof of superiority. Results of evidence-based practice research apply to all aspects of nursing care.
4. Primary health-care providers are more concerned about the pathophysiology of illness. Nursing practice, regardless of the setting, focuses on reacting to human responses.
Content Area: Health-Care System
Integrated Processes: Nursing Process: Analysis
Client Need: Safe and Effective Care Environment;
Management of Care
Cognitive Level: Comprehension
Concept: Health-Care System

23. **ANSWER: 3.**
Rationales:
1. The family is included in both acute care and community health care.
2. Individuals are included in both acute care and community health care.
3. **A characteristic of community health is that it focuses on the health status of people in an aggregate (people who, as a group, form a distinct population).**
4. Neither acute care nor community health care is geographically focused. People who are served may come from different geographic areas, and groups can be identified by a variety of factors, such as common interests (e.g., citizens concerned about air pollution) or similar problems (e.g., homelessness, single-parent families).
Content Area: Health-Care System
Integrated Processes: Nursing Process: Analysis
Client Need: Safe and Effective Care Environment;
Management of Care
Cognitive Level: Knowledge
Concept: Health-Care System

24. **ANSWER: 1.**
Rationales:
1. **Acute care is provided by institutions with highly skilled, intensive, specialized services that cannot be provided in the home.**
2. Respite care provides services so that caregivers can get relief from the stress of their responsibilities. Respite care can be provided in the home or nursing home setting.
3. Hospice care offers services that enable dying persons to stay at home with the support needed to die with dignity.
4. Restorative care, efforts that seek to reduce disability and reestablish function, is related to rehabilitation. Recovering lost functions or developing new compensating skills is commonly accomplished in the home setting.
TEST-TAKING TIP: Identify the word in the stem that indicates negative polarity. The word *not* in the stem indicates negative polarity.
Content Area: Health-Care System
Integrated Processes: Nursing Process: Analysis
Client Need: Safe and Effective Care Environment;
Management of Care
Cognitive Level: Knowledge
Concept: Health-Care System

25. **ANSWER: 1, 2, 5.**
Rationales:
1. **Obesity is one of the 10 leading health indicators identified in *Healthy People 2020* that, when addressed, may motivate people to take action toward health promotion and illness prevention. Obesity increases the risks of many diseases, such as hypertension, cardiac disease, diabetes, and osteoporosis**
2. **Tobacco use is one of the 10 leading health indicators identified in *Healthy People 2020* that, when addressed, may motivate people to take action toward health promotion and illness prevention. Smoking contributes to lung diseases, such as emphysema, bronchitis, asthma, and lung cancer.**
3. Heart disease is one of the 28 focus areas, not a health indicator, identified in *Healthy People 2020*.
4. Family planning is one of the 28 focus areas, not a health indicator, identified in *Healthy People 2020*.
5. **Physical activity is one of the 10 leading health indicators identified in *Healthy People 2020* that, when addressed, may motivate people to take action toward health promotion and illness prevention. People who engage in physical activity reduce the risks of conditions such as heart disease, depression, colon cancer, and diabetes; activity increases muscle tone, muscle strength, and weight loss and contributes to psychological well-being.**
Content Area: Health-Care System
Integrated Processes: Teaching/Learning; Nursing Process: Planning
Client Need: Safe and Effective Care Environment;
Management of Care
Cognitive Level: Analysis
Concept: Health Promotion

26. **ANSWER: 2.**

Rationales:

1. Although this is important, it is associated with meeting a client's need to feel accepted and to have self-esteem supported, third- and fourth-level needs, respectively, according to Maslow's hierarchy of needs. Lower-level needs must be met first before moving on to meeting higher-level needs

2. Helping a homeless person find a source of food is the priority. Meeting nutrition needs is a first-level need according to Maslow's hierarchy of needs.

3. Although this may be done, it is associated with preventing infection, which is related to safety and security, a second-level need according to Maslow's hierarchy of needs. A first-level need is the priority.

4. Day-care programs are not designed to care for homeless people. Day-care programs generally are designed to assist in meeting the needs of children and people who have emotional illnesses or older adults who need a sheltered environment during the day while family members are at work.

TEST-TAKING TIP: Identify the word in the stem that sets a priority. The word *most* in the stem sets a priority. Use Maslow's hierarchy of needs to help establish the priority.

Content Area: *Health-Care System*
Integrated Processes: *Caring; Nursing Process: Implementation*
Client Need: *Health Promotion and Maintenance*
Cognitive Level: *Application*
Concept: *Health-Care System*

27. **ANSWER: 1, 2.**

Rationales:

1. An epidemiologist performs these functions. Tracking illnesses, diseases, and death rates allows the community to assess and evaluate the morbidity and mortality rates within the community. These results reflect trends as well as permit a comparison to national statistics.

2. An epidemiologist implements surveillance monitoring activities to identify trends in health in addition to the presence of risk factors that have the potential to threaten the health of specific populations and the health of members of the general community.

3. This is the role of a nurse advocate, not an epidemiologist. In addition, the nurse working in the community functions as an advocate by assisting clients to work their way through the health-care system to obtain appropriate services.

4. This is the role of a nurse educator, not an epidemiologist.

5. This is the role of a nurse case manager, not an epidemiologist.

Content Area: *Health-Care System*
Integrated Processes: *Nursing Process: Implementation*
Client Need: *Health Promotion and Maintenance*
Cognitive Level: *Comprehension*
Concept: *Health-Care System*

28. **ANSWER: 4.**

Rationales:

1. Although vocational counseling should be discussed, this will not cure the client of tuberculosis.

2. Although the nurse may seek sources of financial assistance for the client, this will not cure the client of tuberculosis.

3. The client should not be setting outcome criteria for the plan of care independently. The nurse and client should identify outcomes and the plan to achieve the outcomes in a collaborative manner. Because tuberculosis is a communicable disease, outcomes have to be formulated that protect the public as well as the client. For example, "The client knows and implements at least 5 actions that will help reduce the risk of transmission of microorganisms to others or the environment." A client acting independently may not be capable of identifying this as an essential outcome.

4. It is essential that clients with infections receive appropriate anti-infective medication according to the plan of care. Anti-infectives associated with any infection must be taken consistently, as prescribed to be effective. Since tuberculosis is a communicable disease and a public health risk, it is essential that a plan be placed in effect if a client is at risk for not attending a treatment program. Home-care visits help to ensure that the treatment plan is being followed to meet the needs of the client and protect people in the community.

TEST-TAKING TIP: Identify the word in the stem that sets a priority. The word *most* in the stem sets a priority.

Content Area: *Health-Care System*
Integrated Processes: *Nursing Process: Implementation*
Client Need: *Safe and Effective Care Environment; Management of Care*
Cognitive Level: *Application*
Concept: *Health-Care System*

29. **ANSWER: 3.**

Rationales:

1. This information reflects the physical environment of the community.

2. This information is associated with the economic status of the community.

3. Morbidity and mortality rates reflect the health status of the members of the community.

4. This information is related to the social system of a community.

TEST-TAKING TIP: Identify the word in the stem that sets a priority. The word *most* in the stem sets a priority.

Content Area: *Health-Care System*
Integrated Processes: *Nursing Process: Implementation*
Client Need: *Health Promotion and Maintenance*
Cognitive Level: *Comprehension*
Concept: *Health-Care System*

30. **ANSWER: 2.**

Rationales:

1. This setting generally is at no greater risk for legal or ethical concerns than are other traditional settings. Health-care services generally are provided in mobile clinics when

meeting the health-care needs of migrant workers. However, these services present a unique challenge because workers and their family members move about the country according to the timing of harvests.

2. Telehealth services are at the highest risk for potential legal and ethical issues because they require data to be transmitted via the Internet, telephone, or fax to primary health-care providers and specialists for consultation. Questions such as the following arise: Who is responsible for the client? How is confidentiality maintained? Does the primary health-care provider have to be licensed in the state in which the client lives?

3. Faith-based settings generally are at no greater risk for legal or ethical concerns than are other traditional settings. Faith-based settings generally offer services in regulated settings, such as hospitals, nursing homes, and clinics. Educational programs generally are provided by licensed health-care workers. In addition, volunteers usually provide supportive nonprofessional assistance, such as transportation and companionship, only after the volunteer meets training and educational criteria.

4. Prison-based settings generally are at no greater risk for legal or ethical concerns than are other traditional settings. Prison-based care generally offers services in a regulated setting, such as a clinic or hospital-like unit within the prison. However, nurses working in a prison-based setting generally are required to meet special training to provide for their own safety.

TEST-TAKING TIP: Identify the word in the stem that sets a priority. The word *highest* in the stem sets a priority.

Content Area: *Health-Care System*

Integrated Processes: *Communication and Documentation; Nursing Process: Analysis*

Client Need: *Safe and Effective Care Environment; Management of Care*

Cognitive Level: *Analysis*

Concept: *Health-Care System*

Chapter 5

Leadership and Management

NURSING CONCEPTS

Collaboration
Communication
Health-Care System

Leadership and Management
Professionalism
Quality Improvement

KEY TERMS

Accountability—Assumption of liability for the consequences of one's own actions and the actions of subordinates

Authority—Power to direct the work of others

Change—Process of transforming, modifying, or making something different

Conflict—An antagonistic state between individuals that results from different points of view or opinions

Delegation—Transfer of responsibility for the implementation of a task to another while retaining accountability for its outcome

Leadership—Interpersonal process of motivating others in the accomplishment of a goal

Management—Process of ensuring that tasks are accomplished to meet organizational goals

Power—Authority to influence others or implement actions to achieve a goal

Responsibility—Obligation to perform an assigned role

I. Leadership

Leadership is an interpersonal process of motivating others in the accomplishment of a goal or change. It involves *assisting* others to develop a sense of control and purpose, *developing* a commitment to accomplish a desired outcome, and *helping* others meet the challenges that arise in the fast-paced, technologically advanced, constantly changing health-care environment.

A. Behavioral leadership styles

1. Behavioral leadership styles are associated with what a leader does.

2. A nurse should know various leadership styles because each style lends itself to different settings and different situations. For example, an emergency might require a nurse to decide and act quickly, whereas a complex problem might require reflective thinking about and thorough discussion of the alternatives with others before making a decision.

3. The most common behavioral leadership styles include the autocratic, democratic, and laissez-faire styles (Table 5.1).

Table 5.1 Comparison of Behavioral Leadership Styles

Leadership Style	Control	Decision Making	Influence of the Leader	Responsibility	Efficiency
Autocratic	Retained by leader	By leader	High	Retained by leader	High
Democratic	Shared	By leader or shared	High	Shared	Moderate
Laissez-faire	Little or no control by anyone	Shared or by no one	Low	Relinquished by leader	Low

MAKING THE CONNECTION

Autocratic Leadership Style and Clinical Practice

A nurse team leader identifies a small fire in a client lounge. The nurse removes a client who is in immediate danger and shuts the door to the dayroom. The nurse then instructs one employee to activate the fire alarm, two employees to close doors to all rooms on the unit as well as the fire cutoff doors, and two other employees to get ABC fire extinguishers. The nurse needed to use the autocratic behavioral leadership style in this situation because it required an immediate, efficient response. Therefore, the nurse team leader made decisions for the safety of clients and employees on the unit, gave direct orders to staff members, and assumed responsibility for the outcomes.

B. Transformational leadership theory
   1. Leaders motivate followers by communicating the importance of their vision (goal), inspiring commitment, and exciting others to participate in the achievement of the vision. The vision is noble and for the good of humanity.
   2. Transformational leaders often are characterized as being charismatic, energetic, optimistic, and courageous; having integrity; and being risk takers.

DID YOU KNOW?

Magnet certification is recognition given by the American Nurses Credentialing Center (ANCC), an affiliate of the American Nurses Association, to hospitals that meet criteria that indicate quality nursing care and support of professional nursing practice. Transformational leadership is essential to achieving Magnet certification because the criteria address the establishment of a collaborative culture that empowers nurses, promotes job satisfaction, advances nursing standards and practice, and provides quality client care.

C. Situational leadership theories
   1. Situational leadership theories propose that each circumstance may require a different leadership style because situations can be multifaceted and the individuals involved have different strengths and weaknesses.
   2. The ability to acclimate to a situation is the central premise of situational theories.
D. Quantum leadership theory
   1. *Quantum* is a "unit of radiant energy."
   2. Quantum leadership theory is based on the concept that the fast growth of new information requires people to experience change, even as it is identified; this concept limits the thoughtful design and cautious implementation that other theories advocate.
   3. It is based on the tenets of quantum physics.
      a. Leadership involves an interactive energy field between the leader and followers.
      b. Leadership cannot be estimated or structured.
      c. Leadership is not continuous.
      d. The impact depends on interaction (content and level) between the leader and followers.

II. Management

Management is the process of ensuring that tasks are accomplished to meet organizational goals. Managers are formally and authoritatively appointed to a position that inherently holds power and entitlement to implement and enforce decisions (Table 5.2).
A. Management activities
   1. Identifying problems and implementing new initiatives.
      a. Determining the significance of collected data and identifying trends that indicate a problem.
      b. Implementing projects based on results of evidence-based practice research, new technology, and new ideas.
   2. Planning: Developing goals and determining strategies that are most likely to achieve organizational goals.

Table 5.2 **Leadership Versus Management Traits**	
Leadership Traits	**Management Traits**
• *Strive to influence and guide others (assisting, developing, helping)* • *May or may not be a manager* • *Depend on a leadership style to generate power* • *Communicate effectively verbally and in writing* • *Collaborate effectively* • *Think critically* • *Are competent* • *Are credible* • *Are respectful of others* • *Are inspiring, motivating, and flexible* • *Use scientific problem-solving* • *Think outside the box* • *Are self-aware and can assess their own effectiveness truthfully and openly*	• *Strive to achieve organizational goals through influencing others (identifying, planning, organizing, directing, controlling)* • *Must possess strong leadership skills to be effective* • *Use power for influence* • *Have power and authority associated with their titles* • *Are committed to achievement of organizational goals* • *Are committed to excellence in nursing practice and ongoing quality improvement* • *Understand power and organizational politics* • *Understand economics, finances, and budgets* • *Have decision-making skills* • *Have delegation skills* • *Are organized* • *Are open to suggestions of subordinates* • *Are fair and equitable in dealing with subordinates* • *Are sensitive to the needs of subordinates* • *Are responsible and accountable* • *Are experts in clinical practice*

3. Organizing: Obtaining and managing human and economic resources to meet desired clinical and financial goals.
4. Directing: Motivating, guiding, and leading staff members in meeting organizational goals.
5. Controlling: Using outcome criteria to measure effectiveness in goal achievement, ensuring ongoing evaluation, and implementing corrective actions when necessary.

B. Management theories
 1. Scientific management.
   a. Focuses on the task component of the management of subordinates.
   b. Based on the concept that when jobs are evaluated, tasks are planned so that they are more efficient and workers are provided with adequate incentives so that productivity increases.
 2. Human relations–oriented management.
   a. Focuses on the interrelationship component of management.
   b. Includes two types of management styles.
     (1) *Theory X:* Managers believe that firm rules, continuous supervision, and fear of negative consequences produce effective, productive workers.
     (2) *Theory Y:* Managers believe that assistance, support, guidance, and rewards produce satisfied, inspired workers; managers work at addressing conflict and supporting mutual respect and understanding to ensure a setting in which individuals can be most effective and productive.

III. Nursing Management

Nurse managers are formally and authoritatively appointed to the position. Inherent in the position is the power and entitlement to implement and enforce organizational decisions. Actual responsibilities and activities depend on the specific position within the hierarchy of the organization in which a nurse manager works. To function in this role effectively, a nurse manager should have strong leadership traits.

A. Principles of management applicable to nursing
 1. Authority.
   a. **Authority** is the power to direct the work of others.
   b. Authority is expressed through leadership and management activities and is related to accountability and responsibility.
 2. Accountability.
   a. **Accountability** is the assumption of liability for the consequences of one's own actions and the actions of subordinates.
   b. Accountability is reflected in one's personal ethical integrity, support of the philosophy and objectives of the organization, standards of nursing practice, and elements of the state nurse practice act.
 3. Responsibility.
   a. **Responsibility** is the assumption of the obligation to accomplish a task or perform an assigned role.
   b. Responsibility is assumed for the management and supervision of subordinates, utilization of financial resources, communication of

information to and from subordinates, implementation of organizational policies and procedures, and achievement of organizational goals and objectives.

B. Levels of management in nursing
1. First-level managers.
   a. Are commonly responsible for managing daily activities associated with a specific group of people on a unit level, including delegating, supervising, and motivating staff to achieve organizational goals.
   b. Communicate staff and unit issues to unit-level managers, and communicate information from higher-level managers back to staff on the unit.
   c. May have such titles as:
      (1) Primary nurse.
      (2) Team leader.
      (3) Charge nurse.
      (4) Case manager.
2. Unit-level managers.
   a. Are commonly responsible for 24-hour operation of a nursing unit, including staffing schedules, budget management, supervision of staff, and ongoing quality improvement.
   b. Communicate information to middle-level managers and to first-level managers.
   c. May have such titles as:
      (1) Nurse manager.
      (2) Assistant nurse manager.
3. Middle-level managers.
   a. Are commonly responsible for supervising a number of unit-level managers and the overall functioning of areas, units, or departments for which they are responsible.
   b. Spend less time on day-to-day management issues and more time on departmental planning and interdisciplinary problem-solving.
   c. Function as liaisons between upper-level and unit-level managers.
   d. May have such titles as:
      (1) Nurse coordinator.
      (2) Supervisor.
      (3) Assistant director of nursing.
4. Upper-level (top-level) managers.
   a. Are commonly nurse executives who are responsible for determining organizational goals and developing strategic plans to achieve these goals.
   b. Are responsible for the overall management and practice of nursing within the organization.
   c. May have such titles as:
      (1) Director of nursing.
      (2) Vice president for nursing.
      (3) Chief nurse.
      (4) Associate administrator.
      (5) Assistant administrator.
      (6) Vice president for clinical care services (if also responsible for such areas as pharmacy and dietary).

C. Examples of activities of nurse managers
1. Recruiting, hiring, and firing staff.
2. Scheduling staff.
3. Formulating and managing a budget.
4. Establishing annual goals.
5. Monitoring achievement of standards of practice.
6. Supervising and counseling staff.
7. Participating in and engaging staff in ongoing quality improvement activities.
8. Providing for staff education.
9. Providing a communication link among clients, upper management, and subordinates.
10. Alerting administration to changing client and subordinate needs.
11. Problem-solving issues proactively or reactively.
12. Conducting regular staff meetings.
13. Making rounds with primary health-care providers and nursing team members.
14. Encouraging staff to participate in interdisciplinary facility-wide committees.
15. Encouraging staff to participate in nursing research.

IV. Power and Empowerment

Power involves having the authority and ability to influence others to achieve a goal even in the presence of resistance. Power relates to actions. **Empowerment** involves a personal sense of competence, self-determination, and/or entitlement. Empowerment relates to feelings. Nurse managers must understand these concepts and integrate them into their practice.

A. Sources of power
1. *Power of authority:* A person in a position of authority can mandate compliance as a result of the power of the position.
2. *Power of reward:* A manager can use incentives, such as pay increases or promotions, to influence others.
3. *Power of coercion:* A manager can use the threat of an undesirable performance evaluation or job termination to influence others; clients can return a less-than-satisfactory client satisfaction survey or complain about a staff member to a charge nurse.
4. *Power of expertise:* A nurse can gain power by obtaining an advanced degree in nursing, such as nurse practitioner, or extensive experience in a specialty area, such as in pediatric, oncology, or emergency nursing.

Power Versus Empowerment

Empowerment should not be confused with power. A person who has power might not *feel* empowered; to feel empowered, a person needs to feel confidence in his or her ability to do a good job, feel that individuals will listen, feel that the work is meaningful, and feel free to decide how work will get done. In contrast, a person can feel empowered without having power. For example, nurses may feel empowered when they are treated with respect, receive recognition for a job well done, are given a reasonable work assignment, are included in organizational decisions, and have their contributions heard and valued.

B. Empowerment
  1. Empowerment is a feeling of competence, a feeling of capability to influence another person, or a feeling of privilege or entitlement.
  2. Nurse managers must support and nourish positive feelings of growth, accomplishment, and independence in subordinates that facilitate feelings of empowerment.

V. Delegation

The American Nurses Association (2009) defines **delegation** as the process of "transferring responsibility for the performance of an activity or task while retaining accountability for the outcome." Many changes in health-care delivery (e.g., reengineering of hospital organizations and downsizing the professional nursing workforce as a measure of cost containment) have resulted in the need for nurses to delegate tasks to unlicensed personnel, requiring nurses to spend more time in supervisory roles. The profession of nursing is working to ensure that unlicensed personnel are used only in supportive roles and not as substitutes for licensed nurses.

A. Five Rights of Delegation (must be met when a nurse delegates aspects of nursing care)
  1. *Right task:* The task is appropriate for delegation.
  2. *Right circumstances:* The nurse considers the appropriateness of the client setting, available resources, and other relevant factors.
  3. *Right person:* The task is delegated to a person who is competent to perform the task within his or her legal scope of practice.
  4. *Right direction/communication:* The nurse provides a clear, concise description of the task, including what should be accomplished and how it should be accomplished.
  5. *Right supervision:* The delegator is responsible for monitoring and evaluating the performance of the task and providing feedback to the person performing the task.

B. Policy considerations associated with delegation
  1. A registered nurse (RN) is responsible for delegating and supervising care provided by unlicensed individuals in health-care environments.
  2. Each state has its own definitions, regulations, and directives regarding delegation.
  3. The following general policy matters are common to all states regarding delegation.
     a. State nurse practice acts delineate the legal boundaries of nursing practice.
     b. There is a need for capable and properly supervised nursing assistive personnel in the delivery of cost-effective, quality health care.
     c. An RN should assign or delegate tasks based on clients' needs and statuses, the risk of harm, constancy of a client's condition, intricacy of the task, likelihood of the outcomes, capabilities of the staff member to whom the task is delegated, and the circumstances of other client needs.
     d. All delegation decisions should be based on maintaining the safety and welfare of the public.
  4. A nurse must understand the nurse practice act and the regulations and directives regarding delegation in the state in which the nurse works as well its application to the setting in which the nurse works.
  5. Nurses are responsible for providing safe and effective nursing care over a range of care provided in various settings (e.g., hospital, nursing home, school, public health clinic, home-health agency).
  6. In each setting, nurses are generally the coordinators of the health teams, which comprise a variety of licensed and unlicensed caregivers.

C. Principles of delegation related to nursing
  1. A nurse may delegate elements of care but retains responsibility to answer for personal actions associated with the nursing process.

  🛑 2. Pervasive functions of assessment, planning, evaluation, and nursing judgment cannot be delegated.

  3. A nurse must take into account the education and skills of the person to whom the nurse delegates components of care.
  4. The decision to delegate should be based on the nurse's judgment regarding the condition of the client, the abilities of nursing team members, and the amount of supervision that is necessary for the task delegated.

  🛑 5. A nurse must follow the Five Rights of Delegation and use professional judgment when delegating a task to another nursing team member.

6. A nurse must communicate effectively and ensure that communication is a two-way process between the delegator and the subordinate.
7. Nursing administrators are responsible for ensuring that assessment of policies and procedures and the evaluation of competence requirements associated with delegation are regularly conducted.

D. Delegation of activities to unlicensed assistive personnel

🛑 1. **A nurse should delegate only those tasks permitted by the state nurse practice act and facility policies and procedures.**

2. A nurse must know which care can be performed by unlicensed assistive personnel. (see Table 5.3).

VI. Managing Change and Conflict

Change is the process of transforming, modifying, or making something different; it also can be defined as learning, growth, or progress. With the explosion of advances in technology and vast increases in knowledge, nurses must be able to incorporate new information into nursing practice to meet clients' needs. However, points of view and opinions about how something should be accomplished can cause conflict. Nurses must be willing to negotiate and compromise with other members of the health team to effect change.

A. Change theory (Lewin)
1. Proposes a process to plan and implement change in organizations.
2. Purports that effective change entails three steps.
   a. *Unfreezing*: The need for change is identified, various supportive and resistive solutions are explored, and group members are motivated to change.
   b. *Moving*: Group members agree that the current status is unacceptable. Change is implemented after careful planning and with input from group members.
   c. *Refreezing*: Change is integrated, stabilized, and incorporated into practice.

B. Planned change
1. A purposeful, intended, systematic effort by a person, group, or organization to alter its present state.
2. A nurse must identify factors relative to the change.
   a. What is the complexity of the change?
   b. What is the magnitude of the change (how many people/departments are involved)?
   c. Is there readiness for the change?

Table 5.3 Care That May Be Performed by Unlicensed Assistive Personnel	
Health-Related Functions (Illustrative and Not All Inclusive)	**Non-Nursing Functions (Illustrative and Not All Inclusive)**
• *Making occupied and unoccupied beds* • *Obtaining routine vital signs, including temperature, pulse, respirations, blood pressure, and body weights* • *Bathing clients* • *Providing routine skin care* • *Promoting mobility, including ambulation and range of motion* • *Assisting with meeting routine urine and fecal elimination needs* • *Obtaining and reporting information at the direction of the registered nurse such as intake and output*	**Housekeeping** • *Cleaning unit surfaces, such as overbed and bedside tables* • *Disposing of trash* • *Changing linens on beds and stretchers* • *Stocking supplies* **Clerical** • *Recording routine data, such as temperature, pulse, respirations, blood pressure, and lab results* • *Checking clothing and valuables* • *Answering telephones* **Transportation** • *Transporting non-acute clients to tests off the unit, bodies to the morgue, and discharged clients to exits* • *Delivering medications, supplies, linens, specimens, and blood products* **Dietary** • *Delivering routine and isolation meal trays and nourishments* • *Recording food and oral fluid intake* **Miscellaneous** • *Assisting with visitors* • *Ordering stock supplies*

Adapted from New York State Nurses Association. (2004). *Position Statement: Registered Professional Nursing's Utilization of Unlicensed Assistive Personnel.* Retrieved October 25, 2012, from www.nysna.org/practice/positions/position1_04.htm, with permission.

d. What is the pace of the change (is it urgent or can it be implemented slowly)?

e. What is the current stress level of participants?

f. Are there forces of resistance within the organization?

3. A nurse should follow a process, such as the nursing process.

a. Recognize the need for change.

b. Identify the problem.

c. Analyze possible solutions.

d. Choose a solution.

e. Plan for making the change (e.g., objectives, implementation steps, timetables, selection of individuals to implement the change, preparation to address resistance, and ways to stabilize the change).

f. Put the plan into effect.

g. Evaluate the outcomes of the change.

h. Stabilize the change (may be permanent).

C. Resistance to change

1. Effective change requires the cooperation of all participants.

2. Individuals might resist change for four major reasons:

a. Technical concerns, such as lack of experience using a computer system.

b. Psychosocial concerns, such as fear, anxiety, low tolerance to change, and impact on income.

c. Threats to power, such as position or influence.

d. Lack of knowledge or misunderstanding.

🛑 3. Nurse managers should identify and address issues that can contribute to resistance as early as possible.

4. Nurse managers need to identify and address resistive behaviors because they can undermine the effort to change.

a. Obvious resistive behaviors include refusing to be involved in the process, writing negative memos, and organizing resistance.

b. Passive-aggressive resistive behaviors include missing meetings and agreeing with the change but avoiding activities to implement the change.

5. Nurse managers should implement strategies for lowering resistance to change.

a. Be prepared for resistance before change is introduced.

b. Increase communication and information to overcome lack of knowledge and to correct misconceptions, which are often significant threats to change.

c. Involve a resistive participant in developing and implementing the change, incorporating as many suggestions as feasible to ensure a vested interest in the success of the project.

d. Reduce the anxiety and fears of participants by recognizing their competence, providing staff education programs that support new learning and personal growth, allowing time for learning and practice, providing a nonjudgmental climate where participants can express feelings, and expressing appreciation for each participant's contributions.

e. Assure participants, when possible, that no one will lose a job or position because of the change.

f. Make the organization's commitment to the project clear.

g. Identify the positive consequences of the change, including ways in which the change will benefit participants.

D. Conflict

1. **Conflict** is an antagonistic state between individuals that results from different points of view or opinions. It can occur in the workplace when there are differences about if or how something should be accomplished.

2. Strategies for managing conflict.

a. Recognize that health-care workers have differences (e.g., different ages, nationalities, cultures, income levels, genders, educational backgrounds, and lifestyles).

b. Recognize that each person has personal values, beliefs, habits, and experiences.

c. Understand that the clinical setting can be stressful, which can generate problems.

d. Identify occurrences of conflict, which can occur between two individuals (e.g., two nurses, nurse and family member), workers of different shifts (workers on the day shift versus the night shift), or different departments (nursing and physical therapy, nursing and dietary).

e. Address conflict in a constructive manner that leads to professional growth rather than rejection and anger.

f. Handle conflict in a way that enables each party to gain insight into the other person's point of view; it can stimulate individuals to work together in more constructive ways, leading to increased productivity and improved relationships.

🛑 g. Use a win-win approach to conflict resolution. For example, when possible, integrate a combination of suggestions from those offered from both sides of a conflict so that both sides gain some benefit.

h. Engage in informal or formal negotiation if conflict cannot be managed through problem-solving.

CASE STUDY: Putting It All Together

A director of nursing at a local community hospital believes that nurses not only should be involved in the traditional roles of nursing (e.g., caregiver, teacher, advocate) but also should expand their roles into other areas associated with professional nursing. Based on this belief, the director of nursing invites all the nurse managers to a meeting to discuss future nursing initiatives. After a length of time with input from many of the nurse managers, the director of nursing makes the following statement: "We have discussed numerous interesting projects. However, I would like for us to begin with just one initiative. Since I firmly believe that nurses should be performing evidence-based practice, I really liked the suggestion that we conduct a small research project on each unit. What do you think?" Another discussion among the members of the meeting occurs, and the majority of nurse managers are in favor of instituting this initiative. The director of nursing then says, "I am sure that this is going to be an exciting new venture. Each unit can make its own determination on how to accomplish this goal. We have money in the budget, and we can hire a nurse researcher to assist you with your projects." After the meeting, one nurse manager of a medical unit says to another nurse manager, "I can't believe we are now going to have to do research projects. Don't you think we do enough already? Let's talk with the other nurse managers and see if we can reverse this decision." This nurse manager holds a unit meeting and tells the staff nurses, "We are going to be conducting a research project on our unit. I am not thrilled about having to do this, but we have no choice. Because we had three clients fall last month, I think we should attempt to reduce falls. I decided we should conduct a fall assessment for every client, and for all clients at risk for falls, we should put a star over the bed and make them wear red socks. That way, the nursing staff will know who is at risk and hopefully ensure the safety of those clients. I expect you all to participate in this project, and if you don't, I will have to include that information in your next evaluation."

A month later, when the director of nursing calls another nurse manager meeting, three of the eight nurse managers did not attend; two said they were too busy, and the third took the day off to avoid the meeting.

Case Study Questions

A. What leadership style seems to be preferred by (1) the director of nursing and (2) the nurse manager of the medical unit. What evidence in the case study supports your conclusions?

1. _____

2. _____

B. What management style seems to be preferred by (1) the director of nursing and (2) the nurse manager of the medical unit? What evidence in the case study supports your conclusions?

1. _____

2. _____

C. What behaviors in the scenario reflect resistance? What evidence in the case study supports your conclusions?

1. _____

2. _____

3. _____

D. What types of power are exhibited in the scenario? What evidence in the case study supports your conclusions?

1. _____

2. _____

3. _____

REVIEW QUESTIONS

Be sure to read the Introduction for valuable test-taking tips.

1. Which actions are appropriate for the nurse to delegate to unlicensed assistive personnel (UAP)? **Select all that apply.**
   1. Obtaining routine weekly weights of clients in a nursing home
   2. Assisting a client with a prosthetic leg to ambulate to the bathroom
   3. Teaching a client with diabetes about the importance of eating an entire meal
   4. Helping a client to drink contrast media that was poured into a cup by a nurse
   5. Asking a client who recently had surgery about the intensity of pain being experienced

2. A nurse is in charge of a team consisting of a registered nurse (RN), a licensed practical nurse (LPN), and a nursing assistant (NA). Which tasks should the nurse delegate to the LPN for the **most** effective use of the expertise of staff members? **Select all that apply.**
   1. Take vital signs on a postoperative client one day after surgery.
   2. Obtain a blood glucose level on a client with unstable diabetes.
   3. Perform a bed bath for a client on contact precautions.
   4. Provide client education regarding a dressing change.
   5. Discontinue tubing that was used to administer blood.

3. A nurse on the day shift is annoyed with the nurse on the night shift and reports concerns to the nurse manager. The nurse on the day shift states that the nurse on the night shift often does not complete client assignments or provide for needed supplies, such as medication draws that are missing the next dose of medication and supplies that are not stocked for isolation rooms. In addition, specimens are not being collected as prescribed. What is the nurse manager's **best** response?
   1. "What do you think I should do to correct these problems?"
   2. "Which of these jobs can you assign to the nursing assistant on your team?"
   3. "Working nights is difficult, so do you think you can help the night shift staff when you can?"
   4. "When are you available so that I can arrange a meeting for the three of us to discuss these concerns?"

4. A nurse and a nursing assistant (unlicensed assistive personnel) are working together caring for a group of clients who recently had surgery. Which actions by the nursing assistant require immediate intervention by the nurse? **Select all that apply.**
   1. Asking a client about the characteristics of pain being experienced
   2. Reinforcing a dressing that is soiled with serosanguineous drainage
   3. Providing total assistance with a bed bath for a client who is disoriented
   4. Giving a cup of tea to a client whose diet was changed from NPO to clear liquid
   5. Assisting a client to the bathroom on the second day after the client had minor abdominal surgery

5. A charge nurse is delegating assignments to staff members working on a surgical unit. Which client should be assigned to a recently licensed RN rather than an experienced RN?
   1. A woman with a high temperature after surgery for an ectopic pregnancy
   2. A middle-aged client who had elective surgery for repair of an abdominal hernia
   3. A young adult who had a fractured femur as well as multiple soft tissue injuries from an automobile collision
   4. An older adult male who had a transurethral resection of the prostate who has cherry red drainage from the continuous bladder irrigation

6. A nurse manager of an emergency department of a trauma center receives notification of a domestic terrorist attack in the community and that multiple casualties are on route to the hospital. Which leadership style is **most** appropriate when the nurse manager responds to this event?
   1. Autocratic
   2. Democratic
   3. Laissez-faire
   4. Transformational

7. A nurse manager identifies that the nurse in charge on evenings needs additional in-service education about the legal roles of nursing staff members. Which assignments by the nurse in charge in the evenings influenced the nurse manager to come to this conclusion? **Select all that apply.**
   1. Nursing assistant to monitor vital signs and determine those that are significant
   2. Registered nurse to teach a client with a colostomy how to care for the stoma
   3. Licensed practical nurse to discontinue a central venous line
   4. Licensed practical nurse to change a sterile dressing
   5. Nursing assistant to bathe a client with dementia

8. A nurse is seeking a position in nursing management. The nurse reads a classified ad that indicates that the hospital is seeking a person who will spend less time on day-to-day management issues and more time on departmental planning and interdisciplinary problem-solving. Which level manager is this agency seeking?
   1. Unit-level manager
   2. First-level manager
   3. Upper-level manager
   4. Middle-level manager

9. Which activities are appropriate for an unlicensed nursing assistant to implement? **Select all that apply.**
   1. Collecting urine for a 24-hour urine test
   2. Measuring and recording a client's oral fluid intake
   3. Reviewing an 1,800-calorie diet with an obese client
   4. Placing a tube feeding pump on hold while bathing a client
   5. Helping with the insertion of a nasogastric tube by a primary health-care provider

10. Which are examples of independent nursing interventions? **Select all that apply.**
    1. Administering an enema
    2. Changing a soiled dressing
    3. Exploring a dying client's feelings
    4. Assessing the characteristics of a pressure ulcer
    5. Delegating the giving of a bath to a nursing assistant
    6. Assisting a client with a transfer from a bed to a wheelchair

11. A nurse manager of a client care unit is determining if the nursing team members of the unit are meeting organizational goals. Which should the nurse manager do **first**?
    1. Plan approaches to meet client needs.
    2. Identify trends that indicate a problem.
    3. Develop strategies to achieve objectives.
    4. Share the purpose of the unit with colleagues.

12. A nurse manager believes in theory X human relations–oriented management. What behavior can a newly hired nurse expect the nurse manager to exhibit? **Select all that apply.**
    1. Describing the continuous evaluation of nursing performance
    2. Explaining the agency's policies regarding the use of sick days
    3. Informing the nurse of the consequences for being late to work
    4. Ensuring the nurse that an orientation program will provide guidance
    5. Directing the nurse to seek assistance from another nurse when necessary

13. A nurse in charge of a client care unit is considering staff member assignments. Which criterion is **most** significant for the nurse to consider when delegating a task to another member of the nursing team?
    1. Who will ultimately be responsible for the client's care?
    2. Is the activity within the person's job description?
    3. How much experience does the person have?
    4. What is the acuity level of the client?

14. Which of the following is related to the statement, "Managers have authority in the workplace"?
    1. Managers have the power to direct the work of others.
    2. Managers are expected to maintain personal ethical integrity.
    3. Managers assume the obligation to accomplish tasks associated with the job description.
    4. Managers assume liability for the consequences of ones' actions as well as those of subordinates.

15. Which statement by a nurse coordinator at a staff meeting exemplifies the major focus of leadership?
    1. "Every staff member will be scheduled to attend an in-service program on this new procedure."
    2. "A committee is being formed to develop a policy and procedure for the nursing manual regarding this new procedure."
    3. "I know from your past performance with other procedures that you have the expertise to implement this new procedure."
    4. "I expect that each unit will meet the criteria established by the state department of health regarding this new procedure."

16. A nurse manager of an emergency department identifies that a more efficient triage process is necessary. What should the nurse manager do to limit resistance to this change? **Select all that apply.**
    1. Offer to transfer staff members to another unit if they do not support the new policies.
    2. Allow adequate time for understanding the change before implementing the change.
    3. Provide a nonjudgmental climate for people to voice their concerns.
    4. Explain that the organization is committed to this change.
    5. Assure participants that they will not lose their jobs.

17. A nurse manager is planning to implement a change in how administered medications are documented. Which is **most** important for the nurse manager to do to avoid resistance to change?
    1. Incorporate incentives to promote a commitment.
    2. Establish multiple short-term goals to promote motivation.
    3. Convey to the staff that administration is committed to the new policy and procedure.
    4. Ensure that the new policy and procedure is consistent with the beliefs and ethics of staff members.

18. A staff nurse is counseled by the nurse manager regarding excessive time taken for lunch and breaks. The nurse manager indicates that if this behavior continues, then the nurse will receive an undesirable performance evaluation. Which type of power did the nurse manager exhibit?
    1. Reward
    2. Coercion
    3. Expertise
    4. Competence

19. An upper-level manager is assessing the qualities of several nurses who demonstrate leadership abilities for a promotion to a first-level management position. Which ability is required of a nurse manager that is not a necessity for a leader?
    1. Thinks critically
    2. Understands budgets
    3. Collaborates effectively
    4. Demonstrates competence

20. A nurse manager endorses the theory Y human relations–oriented management style. Which interventions by the nurse manager reflect this style of leadership? **Select all that apply.**
    1. Reviewing periodically the consequences for not adhering to steps listed in an activity in the procedure manual
    2. Explaining that an interim performance evaluation may be necessary if standards of care are not maintained
    3. Offering help when a nurse is overwhelmed with work at the end of a shift
    4. Ensuring that staff members adhere to policies established by the agency
    5. Arranging meetings among staff members when conflicts arise

21. A charge nurse in a nursing home identifies that the weights of residents assigned to a particular nursing assistant are exactly the same as the week before. The nurse is concerned that the nursing assistant is not weighing residents and is falsifying the weights. Which should the nurse do **first?**
    1. Confront the nursing assistant responsible for taking the weights.
    2. Report the problem regarding the nursing assistant to the nursing supervisor.
    3. Reweigh the residents assigned to the nursing assistant who had duplicate weights for both weeks.
    4. Assign the nursing assistant to take the weight of another resident and observe if the weight is actually taken.

22. A nurse manager identifies that the number of clients with hospital-acquired *Clostridium difficile* has increased on the unit during the past 3 months. The nurse manager recognizes that this issue must be addressed and involves the entire nursing team on the unit. Place the following interventions in the order in which they should be performed.
    1. Stabilize the change.
    2. Identify the expected outcomes of change.
    3. Evaluate the actual outcomes of the change.
    4. Explore and choose a solution to the problem.
    5. Identify why the *C. difficile* rate has increased.
    6. Put the plan into effect and deal with resistance.
    Answer: _____

23. A nurse coordinator is orienting a new manager to the responsibilities associated with scheduling staffing and managing a budget. Which type of power is **most** associated with a nurse coordinator functioning as a mentor?
    1. Reward
    2. Coercive
    3. Expertise
    4. Authority

24. When considering leadership styles, "democratic" leadership is related to the word "consultative." Which word is related to the "autocratic" leadership style?
    1. Sharing
    2. Dictatorial
    3. Participative
    4. Collaborative

25. A nurse manager implements a corrective action plan when a unit goal is not achieved. Which management function is being implemented by the nurse manager?
    1. Planning
    2. Directing
    3. Organizing
    4. Controlling

26. A nurse manager, in conjunction with the nursing team members on the unit, is instituting a new policy regarding criteria for assigning clients to specific rooms on the unit. After 3 weeks, the nurse in charge and a primary nurse engage in an intense discussion about how clients have been assigned. The nurse manager speaks with the two nurses and reviews the assignment of clients during the past week. Each nurse's perspective on the room assignments is as follows:

Charge Nurse's Perspective:

I have been following the criteria we identified at the beginning of this initiative. I reviewed every client's physical and emotional status and compared it to the criteria we identified. I then considered if a private room was warranted and who the primary nurse was for the district in which the room was located. I think I have been consistent and fair to the nurses in my client room assignments.

Primary Nurse's Perspective:

I do not think that the client room assignments have been appropriate. It seems that I have been getting all of the clients who require the most work. Every day this week I have had a client with a crisis on top of having to provide or supervise care for the rest of the clients in my district. It is not fair.

Nurse Manager's Perspective:

A review of the clients' assigned rooms indicated that the nurse in charge did follow the criteria identified at the beginning of the initiative. A review of the primary nurse's district and the assigned clients revealed that the nurse had an equal number of clients when compared to the other primary nurses. However, several of the clients did have more complex health problems. The primary nurse's district had three private rooms compared to the other districts, which have only one each. What is the **best** intervention by the nurse manager?
1. Meet with the nurse in charge and agree that the criteria have been followed.
2. Remove one of the private rooms from the primary nurse's district and add it to another district.
3. Meet with the primary nurse and explain that they will continue with the initiative for another month.
4. Arrange for a meeting of the nursing team and reconsider the criteria that were established for room assignments.

27. A nurse manager identifies that several medication errors occurred on the unit during the past month. Which should the nurse manager do **next**?
1. Implement a plan of action.
2. Analyze factors involving the errors.
3. Choose a solution to address the issues.
4. Explore all possible strategies to prevent future errors.

28. A new float rotation schedule is to be implemented in the hospital. A staff nurse, in an exasperated tone, says to the nurse manager, "This new schedule is ridiculous." What is the nurse manager's **best** response?
1. "Do you really think that the schedule is unreasonable?"
2. "Share with me your concerns about this proposed new schedule."
3. "You need to work with the new schedule a little before being judgmental."
4. "I know that you are upset with the new schedule, but can you try to be more positive?"

29. A nurse is promoted to the role of nurse manager. Which activities can the nurse expect to be included in this new job description that are not included in the role of case manager? **Select all that apply.**
1. Evaluating quality of nursing care delivered
2. Making decisions regarding allocation of resources
3. Ensuring continuity of care with community resources
4. Ensuring that client needs are met in a timely manner
5. Overseeing a client's progress through the health-care system

30. A hospital has been instituting new initiatives in an attempt to receive Magnet status. What approach is **most** appropriate for a nurse manager in this hospital to utilize?
1. Transformational
2. Laissez-faire
3. Democratic
4. Autocratic

REVIEW ANSWERS AND RATIONALES

1. ANSWER: 1, 2.
Rationales:

1. Obtaining routine body weights and vital signs, such as temperature, pulse, respirations, and blood pressure, are within the scope of practice of unlicensed assistive personnel (UAP). Obtaining vital signs of unstable clients should be performed by a licensed nurse.
2. Assisting clients with activities of daily living (e.g., bathing, dressing, ambulating) is within the legal role of UAP.
3. Client teaching is within the legal scope of nursing practice because it requires in-depth knowledge about the content being presented and the principles of teaching/learning.
4. Contrast material is considered a diagnostic medication. Nursing care associated with medications is within the legal role of a licensed nurse, not UAP.
5. Client assessment is within the legal scope of nursing practice because it requires in-depth knowledge and an assessment skill set.

Content Area: Leadership and Management
Integrated Processes: Communication and Documentation; Nursing Process: Planning
Client Need: Safe and Effective Care Environment; Management of Care
Cognitive Level: Application
Concept: Leadership and Management

2. ANSWER: 1, 2.
Rationales:

1. Delegating obtaining vital signs of this client to an LPN is appropriate because the LPN has the knowledge to identify postoperative complications as they relate to the vital signs. More complex tasks should be delegated to the RN. The NA does not have the education to assess the vital signs of a client on the first day after surgery.
2. Delegating blood glucose monitoring of a client with unstable diabetes to an LPN, rather than an RN, is appropriate; the LPN has the knowledge and skill to perform this skill safely. An NA does not have the education to measure the blood glucose level of a client with unstable diabetes.
3. Delegating a bed bath for a client on contact precautions to an LPN is inappropriate in this situation because an NA is capable of caring for clients on contact precautions.
4. All client education must be performed by an RN.
5. Interventions concerning the administration of blood should be performed by at least one RN.

TEST-TAKING TIP: Identify the word in the stem that sets a priority. The word *most* in the stem sets a priority. Identify the central person in the question. Although the question includes an RN, an LPN, and an NA, the LPN is the central person in the question.

Content Area: Leadership and Management
Integrated Processes: Communication and Documentation; Nursing Process: Planning
Client Need: Safe and Effective Care Environment; Management of Care
Cognitive Level: Analysis
Concept: Leadership and Management

3. ANSWER: 4.
Rationales:

1. The response by the nurse on the night shift to this statement may be an action that is inappropriate or impossible to implement. The nurse manager is responsible for taking the initiative. The nurse manager should collect information, identify the problem, and implement an appropriate response.
2. This response suggests an intervention before collecting enough information to make an informed decision.
3. This response denies the feelings and concerns of the nurse on the night shift.
4. Conflict resolution is best approached by having the individuals involved discuss the concerns. This approach allows each person to explain a personal point of view as well as gain insight into the other person's point of view. Suggestions from both perspectives will help achieve a win-win resolution.

TEST-TAKING TIP: Identify the word in the stem that sets a priority. The word *best* in the stem sets a priority. Identify the option that denies the feelings and concerns of the nurse on the day shift. Option 3 denies the nurse's feelings and concerns. Identify the clang association. The word *night* in the stem and in option 3 is a clang association. Although options with clang associations often are the correct answer, the fact that this option denies the feelings and concerns of the nurse on the day shift eliminates it from further consideration.

Content Area: Leadership and Management
Integrated Processes: Communication and Documentation; Nursing Process: Implementation
Client Need: Safe and Effective Care Environment; Management of Care
Cognitive Level: Analysis
Concept: Collaboration

4. ANSWER: 1, 2.
Rationales:

1. Many factors influence the intensity and characteristics of pain. This action requires the educational background and judgment of a licensed nurse.
2. This action requires the educational background and judgment of a licensed nurse. Additionally, the nurse must assess the client further to ensure that the client is not hemorrhaging.
3. Providing a bed bath is an activity that is within the scope of practice of a nursing assistant.
4. Assisting clients with prescribed diets is an activity that is within the scope of practice of a nursing assistant.
5. This is within the scope of practice of a nursing assistant. Generally, on the second day after minor abdominal surgery, a client may need minimal assistance to ambulate safely. The nurse should assist a postoperative client to ambulate for the first time after surgery and then evaluate the client's response.

TEST-TAKING TIP: Identify the word in the stem that sets a priority. The word *immediate* in the stem sets a priority. Identify the central person in the question. Because the behavior of the nursing assistant is being evaluated, the nursing assistant is the central person in this question.

Content Area: Leadership and Management
Integrated Processes: Nursing Process: Evaluation

Client Need: Safe and Effective Care Environment; Management of Care
Cognitive Level: Analysis
Concept: Leadership and Management

5. ANSWER: 2.
Rationales:
1. A high temperature after an ectopic pregnancy may indicate peritonitis, which can be life threatening. This client should be cared for by a nurse more experienced than a recently licensed RN.
2. This client is less likely to experience a life-threatening complication than the possible complications associated with the other client situations. The other clients require more critical assessments that a more experienced nurse with a broader knowledge base and experiential background can draw upon when diagnosing, planning, and implementing nursing care.
3. A client who sustained multiple traumatic injuries may experience any number of serious, life-threatening complications, which include hemorrhage, fat emboli, or neurovascular deficits, as a result of the fractured femur. This client should be cared for by a nurse more experienced than a recently licensed RN.
4. A client who may be hemorrhaging should be cared for by a nurse more experienced than a recently licensed RN. Also, the client's continuous bladder irrigation flow rate should be managed so that clotting and tube obstruction are avoided.
TEST-TAKING TIP: Identify the central person in the question. The central person in this question is the recently licensed nurse.
Content Area: Leadership and Management
Integrated Processes: Communication and Documentation; Nursing Process: Planning
Client Need: Safe and Effective Care Environment; Management of Care
Cognitive Level: Analysis
Concept: Leadership and Management

6. ANSWER: 1.
Rationales:
1. The autocratic leadership style is most appropriate in an emergency. Control and responsibility are retained by the leader and decisions are made by the leader. This style is highly efficient and appropriate in an emergency situation, where quick decisions are required.
2. The democratic leadership style is not the most appropriate style in an emergency. The democratic leadership style is only moderately efficient in emergency situations because the leader and subordinates share control and responsibility.
3. The laissez-faire is the least appropriate leadership style in an emergency situation because there is little or no control by anyone.
4. Transformational is a leadership theory, not a leadership style. Transformational leaders motivate followers by communicating the importance of their vision, inspiring commitment, and exciting others to participate in achievement of the goal.
TEST-TAKING TIP: Identify the word in the stem that sets a priority. The word *most* in the stem sets a priority.

Content Area: Leadership and Management
Integrated Processes: Nursing Process: Implementation
Client Need: Safe and Effective Care Environment; Management of Care
Cognitive Level: Application
Concept: Leadership and Management

7. ANSWER: 1, 3.
Rationales:
1. Determining the results of vital signs monitoring is not within the legal role of a nursing assistant. Although a nursing assistant may collect vital signs, determining the significance of vital signs is dependent on the educational preparation of a registered nurse.
2. All teaching interventions require the expertise of a registered nurse.
3. Licensed practical nurses' scope of practice does not include discontinuing a central venous line, including peripherally inserted central catheters.
4. A licensed practical nurse is educationally prepared to change sterile dressings.
5. A nursing assistant is educationally prepared to bathe a client with dementia.
TEST-TAKING TIP: Identify the words in the stem that indicate negative polarity. The words *needs additional* indicate negative polarity. The question is asking, "Which actions should not be implemented by the person delegated the task?"
Content Area: Leadership and Management
Integrated Processes: Nursing Process: Evaluation
Client Need: Safe and Effective Care Environment; Management of Care
Cognitive Level: Analysis
Concept: Leadership and Management

8. ANSWER: 4.
Rationales:
1. Unit-level managers are often responsible for 24-hour operation of a nursing unit, including scheduling staffing, budget management, supervision of staff, and ongoing quality improvement. Titles may be assistant nurse manager or nurse manager.
2. First-level managers are responsible for managing the work of daily activities of a specific group of people on a unit level. Titles may include primary nurse, team leader, or charge nurse.
3. Upper-level (top-level) managers often are nurse executives who are responsible for determining organizational goals and developing strategic plans to achieve the goals. They are responsible for the management and practice of nursing within the organization. Titles may include vice president for nursing, associate administrator, or assistant administrator.
4. Middle-level managers are responsible for supervising a number of unit-level managers and for the overall functioning of their assigned areas, units, or departments. They spend less time on day-to-day management issues and more time on departmental planning and interdisciplinary problem-solving. Titles may include nurse coordinator, supervisor, or assistant or associate director of nursing.

Content Area: Leadership and Management
Integrated Processes: Nursing Process: Analysis
Client Need: Safe and Effective Care Environment;
Management of Care
Cognitive Level: Comprehension
Concept: Leadership and Management

9. **ANSWER: 1, 2.**
Rationales:
1. This is an activity that an unlicensed nursing assistant is capable of performing safely. Collecting urine for a 24-hour urine test does not require sterile technique. The collection container is set up by the nurse, and nursing staff members working with the client are instructed to add all of the urine voided by the client during the 24-hour period to the collection container.
2. Measuring and recording a client's oral fluid intake is a procedure that is within the scope of practice of unlicensed assistive personnel. It is a procedure that can be mastered without extensive educational preparation.
3. All activities related to client teaching are the responsibility of a registered nurse. The registered nurse has the educational background regarding teaching principles and knowledge about the topic being taught and is therefore the qualified person to engage clients in teaching activities, not an unlicensed nursing assistant.
4. Only a registered nurse or licensed practical nurse is permitted to place a feeding tube on hold.
5. Only a registered nurse or licensed practical nurse is permitted to assist a primary health-care provider with an invasive procedure. An unlicensed nursing assistant does not have the educational foundation to assist other health-care providers with an invasive procedure.
Content Area: Leadership and Management
Integrated Processes: Nursing Process: Implementation
Client Need: Safe and Effective Care Environment;
Management of Care
Cognitive Level: Application
Concept: Leadership and Management

10. **ANSWER: 3, 4, 5.**
Rationales:
1. An enema requires a prescription from a primary health-care provider and is a dependent function of a nurse.
2. Changing a soiled dressing requires a prescription from a primary health-care provider and is a dependent function of a nurse.
3. Providing emotional support, which includes exploring client feelings, is an independent function of a nurse.
4. Assessing clients' physical, emotional, and mental status is within the scope of practice of a nurse. Therefore, assessing the characteristics of a pressure ulcer is an independent function of a nurse.
5. Delegating responsibilities to nursing team members does not require a prescription from the primary health-care provider. Delegation activities are within the scope of practice of a registered nurse.

6. A prescription from a primary health-care provider is necessary before a nurse can transfer a client out of bed to a wheelchair.
Content Area: Leadership and Management
Integrated Processes: Nursing Process: Implementation
Client Need: Safe and Effective Care Environment;
Management of Care
Cognitive Level: Application
Concept: Leadership and Management

11. **ANSWER: 2.**
Rationales:
1. Planning occurs earlier in the management process. Effective planning should result in the attainment of organizational goals.
2. A nurse manager must engage in evaluation activities when determining if organizational goals are being met. Current outcomes must be compared to desired outcomes. When a problem occurs, it should be explored to determine if it is an isolated event or if it has occurred before. Problems that reoccur must be addressed to prevent continuation of the problem.
3. The development of strategies to achieve objectives occurs earlier in the management process. Effective strategies should result in the attainment of organizational goals.
4. Although sharing this information with colleagues promotes collaboration, it does not evaluate whether organizational goals are being met.
TEST-TAKING TIP: Identify the word in the stem that sets a priority. The word *first* in the stem sets a priority. Identify equally plausible options. Options 1 and 3 are equally plausible.
Content Area: Leadership and Management
Integrated Processes: Nursing Process: Evaluation
Client Need: Safe and Effective Care Environment;
Management of Care
Cognitive Level: Application
Concept: Quality Improvement

12. **ANSWER: 1, 2, 3.**
Rationales:
1. Managers who support theory X management principles believe that continuous supervision and evaluation produce productive workers.
2. Managers who support theory X management principles believe that firm rules and regulations ensure that people will conform to the culture of the organization.
3. Managers who support theory X management principles believe that the fear of negative consequences produces effective workers.
4. Managers who support theory Y management principles believe that guidance and support provide an atmosphere that produces effective workers.
5. Managers who support theory Y management principles believe that assistance and mutual respect produce productive workers.
Content Area: Leadership and Management
Integrated Processes: Communication and Documentation;
Nursing Process: Analysis

Client Need: Safe and Effective Care Environment; Management of Care
Cognitive Level: Analysis
Concept: Leadership and Management

13. ANSWER: 2.

Rationales:

1. The nurse who is delegating the task is ultimately responsible.

2. A nurse can delegate only those tasks permitted by the state nurse practice act and the policies and procedures within the agency. Legal parameters of practice are indicated in state nurse practice acts.

3. Although experience does broaden one's experiential background, each person within a job description must be minimally competent to perform required skills.

4. Although a client's acuity level is an important factor to consider, legal parameters of practice must be considered first.

TEST-TAKING TIP: Identify the word in the stem that sets a priority. The word *most* in the stem sets a priority.

Content Area: Leadership and Management
Integrated Processes: Nursing Process: Planning
Client Need: Safe and Effective Care Environment; Management of Care
Cognitive Level: Application
Concept: Leadership and Management

14. ANSWER: 1.

Rationales:

1. This statement is associated with the concept of authority. Managers have the authority to direct the work of others based on the power associated with a title.

2. This statement is associated with the concept of accountability.

3. This statement is associated with the concept of responsibility.

4. This statement is associated with the concept of accountability.

TEST-TAKING TIP: Identify the clang association. The word *work* in the stem and in option 1 is a clang association. Examine option 1 carefully.

Content Area: Leadership and Management
Integrated Processes: Nursing Process: Analysis
Client Need: Safe and Effective Care Environment; Management of Care
Cognitive Level: Comprehension
Concept: Leadership and Management

15. ANSWER: 3.

Rationales:

1. This statement reflects the use of the power of authority, which is related to management, not leadership.

2. This statement is associated with producing a product, which is a function of a manager, not a leader.

3. This statement is associated with the transformational leadership style. Empowering and inspiring others by recognizing and respecting their knowledge and abilities supports cooperation when implementing change.

4. This statement reflects the use of the power of authority, which is related to management, not leadership.

TEST-TAKING TIP: Identify the word in the stem that sets a priority. The word *major* in the stem sets a priority. Identify the unique option. Options 1, 2, and 4 focus on dogmatic actions related to implementation of a new procedure. Option 3 is the only option that empowers and inspires staff and recognizes past accomplishments. Option 3 is unique and unlike options 1, 2, and 4. Identify the option with a specific determiner. Option 1 contains the word *every*, which is a specific determiner.

Content Area: Leadership and Management
Integrated Processes: Communication and Documentation; Nursing Process: Implementation
Client Need: Safe and Effective Care Environment; Management of Care
Cognitive Level: Analysis
Concept: Leadership and Management

16. ANSWER: 2, 3, 4, 5.

Rationales:

1. This can be viewed by staff members as a threat.

2. Communication, information, and participation are essential precursors to change. An increase in knowledge and time to process the information may promote a willingness to participate in the change with a positive attitude.

3. Expression of concerns and feelings allows issues to be discussed with mutual respect. New information can be provided and misinformation corrected. In addition, feelings can be validated.

4. Organizational goals should be shared and clarified with the staff involved with the change. An organization committed to a change should provide the physical, emotional, and financial support necessary to successfully achieve the change.

5. This fact provides a sense of security and may lower resistance to change.

TEST-TAKING TIP: Identify opposites in options. Options 1 and 5, for all practical purposes, are opposites. People being transferred to another unit are in fact losing their present jobs. Identify options with a clang association. The word *change* in the stem and in options 2 and 4 are clang associations. More often than not, an option with a clang association is a correct answer.

Content Area: Leadership and Management
Integrated Processes: Communication and Documentation; Nursing Process: Implementation
Client Need: Safe and Effective Care Environment; Management of Care
Cognitive Level: Application
Concept: Collaboration

17. ANSWER: 4.

Rationales:

1. Although this may be planned, it is not the priority. Incentives may motivate people with an external locus of control but not staff members with an internal locus of control.

2. Although this may be planned because achievement of small steps is motivating, it is not the priority.

3. This is the use of the power of authority and a veiled threat via the use of the power of coercion.

26. ANSWER: 4.

Rationales:

1. Individual meetings may lead the other members of the team to be suspicious about what was said. Lines of communication should be kept open among all members of the nursing team. Also, team members should be informed that the nurse in charge was following the criteria identified at the beginning of the initiative.

2. This is an authoritative approach and is premature. The private rooms may or may not be the cause of the perceived imbalance in client room assignments.

3. This approach denies the primary nurse's concerns. This approach devalues the nurse at a time when the nurse should feel empowered. A month is unrealistic to wait.

4. The entire nursing team should be involved with new initiatives. When people are involved in the decision making, usually there is a vested interest in being successful.

TEST-TAKING TIP: Identify the word in the stem that sets a priority. The word *best* in the stem sets a priority.

Content Area: Leadership and Management
Integrated Processes: Communication and Documentation; Nursing Process: Implementation
Client Need: Safe and Effective Care Environment; Management of Care
Cognitive Level: Analysis
Concept: Collaboration

27. ANSWER: 2.

Rationales:

1. This action is premature.

2. The occurrence of medication errors indicates a need for change. The next step involves identifying the problem: What factors are associated with the errors?

3. This action is premature.

4. This action is premature.

TEST-TAKING TIP: Identify the word in the stem that sets a priority. The word *next* in the stem sets a priority. Identify the option with a specific determiner. The word *all* in option 4 is a specific determiner. More often than not, an option with a specific determiner is a distractor. Identify the option with a clang association. The word *errors* in the stem and in option 2 is a clang association. Examine option 2 carefully because more often than not, an option with a clang association is the correct answer.

Content Area: Leadership and Management
Integrated Processes: Nursing Process: Assessment
Client Need: Safe and Effective Care Environment; Management of Care
Cognitive Level: Application
Concept: Quality Improvement

28. ANSWER: 2.

Rationales:

1. Although repeating the nurse's message is an invitation to respond, the nurse could respond with a yes or no answer that would close communication.

2. This response encourages the nurse to elaborate on the statement, "This new schedule is ridiculous." It sends the message that the nurse manager is interested in the nurse's thoughts and feelings.

3. This response is confrontational and accuses the nurse of being judgmental. This response will cut off communication.

4. Although the first part of the statement is an attempt to validate feelings, the second part of the statement is confrontational because it implies that the nurse is being negative; this may shut off communication.

TEST-TAKING TIP: Identify the word in the stem that sets a priority. The word *best* in the stem sets a priority. Identify the options that are equally plausible. Options 1, 3, and 4 are confrontational; one intervention is no better than the other. Identify the option that is unique. Option 2 is the only option that communicates to the nurse that the manager is interested in the nurse's concerns.

Content Area: Leadership and Management
Integrated Processes: Caring; Communication and Documentation; Nursing Process: Implementation
Client Need: Safe and Effective Care Environment; Management of Care
Cognitive Level: Analysis
Concept: Collaboration

29. ANSWER: 1, 2.

Rationales:

1. A case manager is not responsible for evaluating the quality of nursing care delivered. A nurse manager is responsible for the quality of care delivered by the members of the nursing team working in the areas assigned to the nurse manager.

2. A case manager is not responsible for making decisions regarding allocation of resources. A nurse manager is responsible for making decisions regarding allocation of resources within the assigned budget.

3. Case managers are responsible for ensuring continuity of care for clients transitioning back to the community setting with assistance from community resources.

4. Nurse managers and case managers both are responsible for ensuring that client needs are met in a timely manner within their own area of responsibility.

5. Although a nurse manager ensures that the client's needs are met within the acute care facility, it is the case manager's responsibility to ensure that a client's needs are met through the entire health-care system.

TEST-TAKING TIP: Identify the words in the stem that indicate negative polarity. The words *not performed* in the stem indicate negative polarity. The question is asking, "What activity is not performed by a case manager?"

Content Area: Leadership and Management
Integrated Processes: Nursing Process: Analysis
Client Need: Safe and Effective Care Environment; Management of Care
Cognitive Level: Analysis
Concept: Leadership and Management

30. ANSWER: 1.

Rationales:

1. Transformational leaders motivate followers by communicating the importance of their vision. They inspire and excite others to participate in the achievement of goals. To achieve Magnet status, multiple complex goals must be accomplished. It requires the integrated effort of many. Magnet status recognizes health-care organizations for quality client care, nursing excellence, and innovations in professional nursing practice. It is considered the "gold standard" of nursing excellence.

2. Laissez-fare leaders do not provide enough direction to accomplish multiple complex goals by many people. The achievement of complex goals requires leadership, supervision, and guidance.

3. Although democratic leaders may share control and responsibility with members of a group attempting to achieve multiple complex goals, they may not create enough excitement, motivation, or supervision to reach the goals over time.

4. Autocratic leaders retain control and responsibility. Although this style is efficient and appropriate in emergency situations, it is not effective in involving many people in achieving multiple complex goals.

Content Area: *Leadership and Management*
Integrated Processes: *Nursing Process: Implementation*
Client Need: *Safe and Effective Care Environment; Management of Care*
Cognitive Level: *Application*
Concept: *Leadership and Management*

Essential Nursing Care Concepts

Chapter 6

Critical Thinking and the Nursing Process

NURSING CONCEPTS

Collaboration
Communication
Evidenced-Based Practice

Patient-Centered Care
Professionalism

KEY TERMS

Analysis—The examination of data and identification of client problems, nursing diagnoses, and/or needs; it is the second step of the nursing process

Assessment—The ongoing, systematic collection, validation, and documentation of data; it is the first step of the nursing process

Critical thinking—A cognitive strategy by which one reflects on and analyzes personal thoughts, actions, and decisions

Data—Collected information

Delegate—Transferring the authority to act to another while retaining accountability for the outcome

Evaluation—The comparison of planned expected outcomes with a client's actual outcomes to determine whether client needs have been met; it is the fifth step of the nurse process

Goal—A broad statement about the status one expects a client to achieve

Implementation—The organization, management, and implementation of planned nursing actions that involves thinking and doing; it is the fourth step of the nursing process

Nonverbal data—Observable behavior transmitting a message without words

Nursing Interventions Classifications (NIC) system—A standardized classification of nursing interventions

Nursing Outcomes Classification (NOC) system—A standardized classification of client outcomes that respond to nursing interventions

Nursing process—A critical thinking framework that involves assessing and analyzing human responses to plan and implement nursing care that meets client needs as evidenced by the evaluation of client outcomes; consists of assessment, analysis, planning, implementation, and evaluation

Objective data (also known as *signs*)—Overt, measurable assessments collected via the senses

Outcome—A specific desired change in a client's condition as a result of nursing interventions

Planning—The identification of goals and/or outcomes and nursing interventions that address client problems, nursing diagnoses, or needs; it is the third step of the nursing process

Priority—Something ranked highest in terms of importance or urgency

Subjective data (also known as *symptoms*)—Covert information, such as feelings, perceptions, thoughts, sensations, or concerns, that are shared by the client and can be verified only by the client

Verbal data—Spoken or written messages

I. Critical Thinking

Critical thinking involves mental strategies associated with problem-solving, decision making, use of the scientific method, and diagnostic reasoning. When critical thinking is applied to the practice of nursing, it is called the nursing process. Before one can employ the nursing process, consisting of assessment, analysis, planning, implementation/intervention, and evaluation, one must first have a better understanding of what is critical thinking. The helix of critical thinking schematically represents the concept of critical thinking (Fig. 6.1). The helix consists of cognitive and personal competencies (Fig. 6.2). The helix of critical thinking can be applied to the nursing process (Fig. 6.3).

A. Introduction to critical thinking

1. **Critical thinking** is a cognitive strategy by which you reflect on and analyze your thoughts, actions, and decisions; it requires internal cognitive and personal competencies (see Fig. 6.2).

2. Cognitive competencies.

   a. *Cognitive competencies* are the intellectual or reasoning processes used when thinking and include such skills as the ability to understand, analyze, interpret, correlate, investigate, compare and contrast, categorize, determine significance, query evidence, establish priorities, make inferences, and determine consequences, to name a few.

   b. The more internal cognitive competencies a person can bring to the thinking process, the more successful a person will be at thinking critically.

3. Personal competencies.

   a. *Personal competencies* are the attitudes and characteristics that are associated with successful critical thinkers, such as being an independent thinker, open-minded, imaginative, disciplined, committed, accountable, inquisitive, confident, reflective, objective, intuitive, rational, curious, honest, and moral, to name a few.

   b. The more personal competencies a person can bring to the thinking process, the more successful a person will be at thinking critically.

B. Maximize your critical thinking ability

1. Self-analysis: The competencies listed previously are just a few of the competences in each category. Make a list or your own competencies. This will enable you to identify additional skills and abilities that you need to work on acquiring.

2. Techniques to improve critical thinking.

   a. Study your textbooks and other resources. A strong knowledge base is essential to thinking critically.

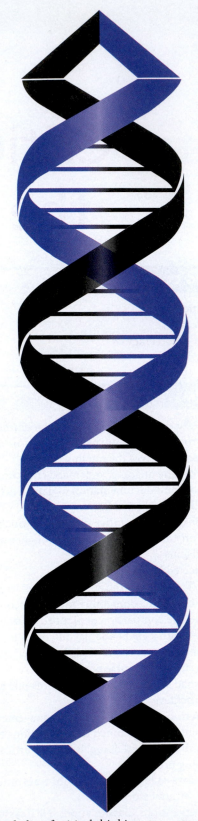

Fig 6.1 The helix of critical thinking. (From Nugent and Vitale [2015]. *Fundamentals success,* 4th ed. Philadelphia: F. A. Davis Company, with permission.)

Cognitive Competencies	Personal Competencies
Dissect	Tolerant of ambiguity
Modify	Think independently
Analyze	Perseverance
Interpret	Self-confident
Examine	Open-minded
Correlate	Accountable
Synthesize	Courageous
Recall facts	Imaginative
Investigate	Disciplined
Categorize	Committed
Summarize	Inquisitive
Understand	Motivated
Demonstrate	Risk taker
Self-examine	Confident
Translate data	Reflective
Query evidence	Objective
Make inferences	Authentic
Manipulate facts	Assertive
Present arguments	Intuitive
Establish priorities	Rational
Make generalizations	Creative
Compare and contrast	Humble
Determine significance	Curious
Determine implications	Honest
Determine consequences	Moral

Fig 6.2 The helix of critical thinking schematically elongated. (From Nugent and Vitale [2015]. *Fundamentals success,* 4th ed. Philadelphia: F.A. Davis Company, with permission.)

b. Reflect on your learning. Examine your performance: engage in post conferences, maintain a journal that objectively and subjectively explores your experience, ask faculty members to provide feedback on your progress and to make suggestions for improving critical thinking abilities.

c. Participate in a study group to dissect and examine information, work on case studies, and answer test questions and then identify rationales for right and wrong answers.

II. Introduction to the Nursing Process

The **nursing process** is a critical thinking framework that involves assessing and analyzing human responses to plan and implement nursing care that meets client needs as evidenced by evaluation of client outcomes. Nurses use critical thinking throughout the nursing process, which involves both "thinking" and "doing," to meet complex client needs.

A. Components of the nursing process
   1. Assessment.
   2. Planning.
   3. Analysis.
   4. Implementation.
   5. Evaluation.
B. Characteristics of the nursing process
   1. Is client-centered.
   2. Is interpersonal.
   3. Is collaborative.
   4. Is dynamic and cyclical.
   5. Requires critical thinking.

III. Assessment

Assessment, the first step of the nursing process, is the ongoing, systematic collection, validation, and documentation of data. **Data** are information. Nursing assessment should be comprehensive, holistic, and accurate so that it provides all the necessary information about a client. In addition, it should reflect the client's responses to a health problem and stressors, not disease processes. Adequate assessment depends on collecting data using various methods, collecting both subjective and objective data, verifying that data are accurate, and communicating information about assessments to other members of the health team.

A. Methods of data collection
   1. Physical examination: The use of inspection, auscultation, percussion, and palpation to collect data about a client's physical status. (See "Techniques of Physical Assessment Used by Nurses," in Chapter 14, Physical Assessment.)

Fig 6.3 The interactive nature of the helix of critical thinking within the nursing process. (From Nugent and Vitale [2015]. *Fundamentals success,* 4th ed. Philadelphia: F. A. Davis Company, with permission.)

2. Interviewing.
   a. Formal approach.
      (1) Used when collecting information in an arranged or official way, such as for a history and physical.
      (2) Usually involves direct rather than open-ended questions.
   b. Informal approach.
      (1) Used when collecting data in a casual and more relaxed manner, such as when exploring a client's feelings while providing other nursing care.
      (2) Usually involves open-ended questions.
   c. See also "Communication," "Therapeutic and Nontherapeutic Communication," and "Nursing Care Related to Communication" in Chapter 2, Communication, Collaboration, and Documentation.
3. Clinical record review.
   a. Involves monitoring information collected about the client in the clinical record.

   b. Gathers information about results of laboratory examinations, diagnostic procedures, consultations by other members of the health team, and progress notes.

B. Sources of data
1. Primary source.
   a. The client is the only primary source of data. The data include information such as feelings, physical and emotional perceptions, and beliefs.

   🛑 b. The client is the most valuable source because the data collected are most recent, unique, and specific to the client.

2. Secondary sources.
   a. These sources provide supplementary information about the client from some place other than the client but within the client's frame of reference.
   b. They include people other than the client (e.g., family members, friends, other health team members).

Application of Critical Thinking to the Nursing Process

Critical thinking is a cognitive strategy by which one reflects on and analyzes personal thoughts, actions, and decisions. It involves purposeful, goal-directed thinking (e.g., the nursing process); requires judgment based on facts and principles of science rather than conjecture or trial and error (e.g., evidence-based practice); and requires numerous cognitive and personal competencies. The helix of critical thinking (Fig. 6.1) demonstrates the interwoven relationship between cognitive competencies and personal competencies essential to thinking critically. Throughout the thinking process, there is constant interaction among cognitive competencies, among personal competencies, and between cognitive and personal competencies. The more cognitive competencies and personal competencies a person possesses, the greater the potential the person has to think critically (Fig. 6.2). Critical thinking has an interactive relationship with the nursing process. The nursing process is a dynamic, cyclical process in which each phase interacts with and is influenced by the other phases of the process. Critical thinking is an essential component within, between, and among the phases of the nursing process. Different combinations of cognitive and personal competencies may be used during the different phases of the nursing process (Fig. 6.3).

    c. A client's clinical record is also a secondary source, as it contains a vast amount of information about the client's physical, psychosocial, and economic history as well as information about the client's progress regarding physical and emotional responses to a health problem.

DID YOU KNOW?

Although a client's clinical record is a secondary source, laboratory and diagnostic procedure results are direct objective measurements of the client's status and are considered by some to be a primary source. The clinical record is a historical view of the client and, for that reason, is less current than data collected from the client.

    3. Tertiary sources.
      a. These sources produce data from outside the client's frame of reference.
      b. Examples include information from textbooks, surveys, medical and nursing journals, drug books, and policy and procedure manuals.

C. Types of data
    1. Objective data.
      a. **Objective data** (also known as *signs*), are overt, measurable assessments collected via the senses, such as sight, touch, smell, and hearing, and compared to an accepted standard.
      b. Examples include body temperature, pulse and respiratory rates, blood pressure, vomiting, distended abdomen, presence of edema, lung sounds, crying, skin color, and presence of diaphoresis.
    2. Subjective data.
      a. **Subjective data** (also known as *symptoms*) are covert information, such as feelings, perceptions, thoughts, sensations, or concerns that are shared by the client and can be verified only by the client.
      b. Examples include pruritus, nausea, pain, numbness, attitudes, beliefs, values, and perceptions of the health problem and life circumstances.
    3. Verbal data.
      a. **Verbal data** are spoken or written messages.
      b. Requires the nurse to listen to the pace of the communication pattern, tone of voice, vocabulary used, and presence of aggression, anxiety, or assertiveness.
      c. Allows for the assessment of difficulties such as slurring, lack of clarity, flight of ideas, difficulty finding the desired word, and inability to identify an item.
      d. Examples include statements made by the client or by a secondary source.
    4. Nonverbal data.
      a. **Nonverbal data** are observable behavior transmitting a message without words.
      b. Examples include client's appearance; facial expression; body language, such as posture, gestures, and eye contact or lack of eye contact.

D. Verifying collected data
    1. Data must be double-checked (verified) after they are collected.
    2. Ensures validity and accuracy.
    3. Ensures that the nurse does not come to a conclusion without adequate data to support the conclusion.
    4. Involves collecting additional information to support the initial data.
      a. If a client's pulse is increased above the expected range, the nurse should take the pulse again; if it is still increased, the nurse should collect other vital signs to supplement the original information.
      b. If a client says, "I feel that I am in a big, black hole," the nurse might use the communication technique of clarification to have the client explain in more detail what was meant: "Tell me more about this big, black hole that you feel you are in."

E. Communicating collected data
1. Outcomes of nursing assessments must be documented on correct forms and in appropriate places in the client's clinical record. Many forms are used to document data and are organized by topic or body systems.
2. Communicating data ensures that pertinent and current information relative to the client is shared with other members of the health team.
3. Data must be communicated in an objective and factual way and not be a summary of the nurse's interpretation of the data.
4. Value words, such as *good, bad, adequate, poor,* and *tolerated well,* should be avoided. For example, rather than saying that a client's appetite is poor, the nurse should document that the client ate half of a scrambled egg and a slice of toast. This manner of documentation communicates objective, measurable information about the client's appetite.
5. Value words related to a client's behavior, such as *lazy, difficult, stubborn, rude, uncooperative,* and *foolish,* should be avoided. These words reflect a value judgment made by the nurse that may be influenced by bias and personal values or beliefs. Nurses must always be nonjudgmental.
6. Subjective data should be documented in the exact words expressed by the client and put in quotation marks; this practice ensures that a client's meaning is not misinterpreted or inaccurately altered by words used by the nurse to describe an event.

IV. Analysis

Analysis, the second step of the nursing process, requires the nurse to use critical thinking strategies to scrutinize data. Activities associated with this step include clustering data, interpreting data, and identifying and communicating a client's nursing diagnoses, problems, or needs.

A. Clustering data
1. Involves grouping information into related categories, a beginning effort to organize and manage information.
2. Data can be clustered into general categories, such as physiological, sociocultural, psychological, and spiritual. Then each category may be further reduced into specific categories, such as nutrition, mobility, elimination, and oxygenation.
3. Data can be easy or difficult to cluster depending on the amount and variety of data collected.
4. Easy-to-cluster information commonly involves only one body system. For example, a client reports feeling low abdominal pressure, has not voided in 8 hours, and has abdominal distention

on palpation of the suprapubic area; these clinical indicators all relate to urinary elimination and lead to the interpretation that the client may have urinary retention.
5. Difficult-to-cluster information may at first seem unrelated because a variety of body systems are involved. For example, a client has a weak, thready pulse; decreased blood pressure; rapid respirations; pallor; and clammy skin; these clinical indicators cross body systems, but all are related to hypovolemic shock.
6. Inductive reasoning moves from the specific to the general. For example, if you identify that a client has a temperature and a wound with purulent drainage, you may come to the conclusion that the wound is infected.
7. Deductive reasoning moves from the general to the specific. For example, if you know that a newly admitted client has a wound infection, you might deduce that the client will have a temperature, purulent drainage, and a culture and sensitivity laboratory result identifying the causative agent.
8. Data must be clustered before it can be interpreted.
9. Established frameworks are available to provide structure for organizing clustered data.
    a. Abraham Maslow's hierarchy of human needs.
    b. Marjory Gordon's functional health patterns.
    c. NANDA International (formerly the North American Nursing Diagnosis Association) nursing diagnosis taxonomy.
10. Most health-care agencies have their own admission assessment forms, which commonly follow a systems approach to collecting and clustering data.

B. Interpreting data
1. Interpreting data requires identifying the significance of clustered data.
2. Determining significance requires a comparison of data collected with a wide range of standards and norms (e.g., expected vital signs and laboratory values, growth and development patterns and milestones, and cause-and-effect relationships). The nurse must then come to a conclusion about a specific identified pattern. It also involves querying evidence, exploring alternatives, and drawing initial conclusions.
3. Conclusions are drawn after the significance of data is determined. Conclusions are the opinions, perceptions, judgments, and inferences that result from the interpretation of data.
4. More data may be necessary to support an initial conclusion, thereby increasing validity and reliability.
    a. When a client has an increased blood pressure, pulse, and respiratory rate and is rubbing a

shoulder, the nurse makes an inference that the client is experiencing pain. To validate this conclusion, the nurse asks, "I noticed that you are rubbing your shoulder. Is it causing you discomfort?"

    b. If a client says, "I feel as though my bladder will burst," the nurse makes the inference that the client might be experiencing urinary retention. To validate this, the nurse should palpate the client's abdomen for distention. The nurse also can ask questions that clarify the client's statement.

5. Nurses should ask the following questions after arriving at conclusions.
    a. "Did I miss anything?"
    b. "What else do I need to know?"
    c. "Has the client's condition or situation changed since I initially assessed the client?"
    d. "Are there any inconsistent or conflicting data that require clarification?"
    e. "Is my data cluster complete, or do I need to collect additional data to better support my conclusion?"

C. Identifying nursing diagnoses

1. Introduction to nursing diagnoses.
    a. Nursing diagnoses are statements of specific health problems that nurses are legally allowed to independently identify, prevent, and treat.
    b. They convert an initial conclusion into a diagnostic statement.
    c. They logically link the assessment step to the planning, implementation, and evaluation steps of the nursing process.
    d. NANDA International provides a taxonomy of diagnostic labels and etiologies.
    e. Each nursing diagnosis in the taxonomy follows the same organization for the presentation of information.
       (1) Diagnostic label (title or name): A word or phrase that is based on a pattern of interconnected data. For example, *Impaired skin integrity*.
       (2) Definition: Explains the meaning of the diagnostic label, which differentiates it from similar nursing diagnoses. For example, *Altered epidermis and/or dermis*.
       (3) Defining characteristics: Identifies clinical indicators (signs and symptoms) that support the diagnostic label. For example, *Invasion of body structures, destruction of skin layers (dermis), disruption of skin surface (epidermis)*.
       (4) "Related to" factors: Situations, events, or conditions that precede, cause, affect, or are in some way associated with the diagnostic label. For example, *Related to physical immobilization*. The list of related factors in the taxonomy is not all-inclusive because it is impossible to list all possible factors.

DID YOU KNOW?

Although nursing diagnoses provide a framework for identifying a client's nursing problems using a standardized nomenclature or language, some professionals believe that they have become too complex and abstract to be useful in everyday practice. As a result, some areas of practice are moving away from using nursing diagnoses.

D. Communicating client nursing diagnoses, problems, or needs
1. Nurses communicate client nursing diagnoses, problems, or needs in a written plan of care.

MAKING THE CONNECTION

NANDA Taxonomy and a Nursing Diagnosis

A nurse is caring for a newly admitted client who has paralysis of the legs as a result of a spinal cord injury several years ago. The client sits in a wheelchair most of the day and lies in the supine position when sleeping. The nurse identifies that the client has a shallow, round, partial-thickness loss of dermis over the sacrum. The wound bed is red with no evidence of sloughing. The nurse identifies the nursing diagnosis: *Impaired skin integrity* (diagnostic label) *related to physical immobilization* (related to factor). Because the nurse understands that there can be more than one "related to" factor, the nurse includes all the causes of the client's impaired skin and develops this nursing diagnosis: *Impaired skin integrity related to physical immobilization, altered sensation, and pressure*. The nurse expands the nursing diagnosis to include "secondary to" information to make the etiology clearer. Often, "secondary to" information is a pathophysiological process or medical diagnosis. The nursing diagnosis is now: *Impaired skin integrity related to immobility, altered sensation, and pressure secondary to motor deficits*.

The nurse further expands the nursing diagnosis to include "evidenced by" information to make the etiology even more clear. Often, "evidenced by" information is the clinical indicators (signs and symptoms) included in the defining characteristics in the NANDA taxonomy. The final nursing diagnosis is: *Impaired skin integrity related to inactivity, altered sensation, and pressure secondary to motor deficits as evidenced by the inability to independently move the legs.*

2. The plan of care may be kept in a variety of places (e.g., client's clinical record, the medication administration record, and interdisciplinary clinical pathways).

V. Planning

Planning, the third step of the nursing process, provides direction for nursing interventions. It is concerned with identifying priorities, establishing goals and expected outcomes, and selecting nursing interventions that will help the client achieve those goals and expected outcomes. Planning begins when a client is admitted and is ongoing to meet the changing or emerging needs of the client. Effective planning includes collaboration with all appropriate health team members to facilitate continuity of care in a client-centered, individualized, and coordinated manner. Planning culminates in a document about the proposed plan of care that is communicated to all members of the health team.

A. Identifying priorities
   1. A **priority** is something ranked highest in terms of importance or urgency.
   2. A nurse must place a client's nursing diagnoses, problems, and needs in order of importance when confronted with a variety of client issues.
   3. A nurse must have a strong foundation of scientific theory, knowledge of the commonalities and differences in response to nursing interventions, and theories to determine the priority of a client's needs.
   4. Factors that promote the prioritization of care.
      a. Maslow's hierarchy of needs.
         (1) Needs are placed in order from the most basic needs to the highest-level needs.
         (2) Physiological is the first-level need, followed by safety and security, love and belonging, self-esteem, and self-actualization (see Fig. 7.3 in Chapter 7, Evidenced-Based Practice).
      b. Urgency of the health problem.
         (1) Ranks problems based on the degree of threat to the client's life. The nurse can use the ABCs of assessment (Airway, Breathing, Circulation) when determining priorities.
         (2) A high-priority problem poses the greatest threat and should be addressed first (e.g., an impaired airway).
         (3) A medium-priority problem follows a high-priority problem. It may be related to harmful physiological responses that are not an immediate threat to life (e.g., impaired mobility).

      (4) A low-priority problem should pose the least threat and be ranked last. It may require minimal support (e.g., nausea).
   c. Client's priorities.
      (1) Ranks client needs based on what is most important to the client.
      (2) Although a client's preference should always be taken into consideration, basic life-threatening needs require urgent interventions and override less important needs.
   d. Future impact of the client's condition.
      (1) Although a problem might not be life threatening and is not recognized by the client as important, the nurse may determine that it can cause future negative consequences if not addressed.
      (2) For example, a nurse identifies that a client newly diagnosed with type 1 diabetes has dirty feet and is wearing sandals instead of shoes that enclose the feet. The nurse knows that people with diabetes are at risk for foot problems secondary to impaired circulation to the lower extremities. Therefore, the client has a potential for skin breakdown, which can lead to infection and even amputation. The nurse ranks this issue as a priority and plans interventions to educate the client about foot care.

B. Identifying goals and expected outcomes
   1. Basic concepts.
      a. A **goal** is a broad statement about the status one expects a client to achieve.
      b. A goal generally is derived from the "diagnostic label" component of a nursing diagnosis. For example, if a client has the nursing diagnosis *Ineffective airway clearance related to excessive respiratory secretions,* the goal might be: "The client will maintain a patent airway."
      c. An **outcome** identifies a specific change in a client's condition as a result of nursing interventions. It is commonly influenced by the "related to" component of a nursing diagnosis. Also, it provides criteria to be used in the evaluation phase of the nursing process. For example, the outcome statement using the previously stated goal ("The client will maintain a patent airway") might be: "The client will expectorate respiratory secretions while hospitalized" (see Box 6.1, Nursing Outcomes Classification [NOC] System).
      d. Clients and nurses together should set goals and outcomes to ensure that these goals and outcomes are realistic, achievable, and in alignment with what the client and nurse want to achieve.

> **Box 6.1 Nursing Outcomes Classification (NOC) System**
>
> The **Nursing Outcomes Classification (NOC) system** is a standardized classification of client outcomes that respond to nursing interventions. Each NOC outcome has a label, indicators, and measurement scale. The advantages of the NOC system are that it uses language common to all health-care professionals, it is specific, and it identifies indicators with a measurement scale to allow nurses to evaluate client progress toward an outcome.
>
> Example of NOC outcomes with indicators for *Impaired skin integrity:*
> - *Tissue integrity: Skin and mucous membranes will be intact as evidenced by the following indicators: Skin intactness/ skin lesions/tissue perfusion/skin temperature.*
> - *Rate each indicator of tissue integrity: skin and mucous membranes: 1 = severely compromised, 2 = substantially compromised, 3 = moderately compromised, 4 = mildly compromised, 5 = not compromised.*

2. Criteria for goals and outcomes.
   a. Be client centered.
      (1) The client is the center of the health team; therefore, the client should be the subject of all goals and outcomes.
      (2) For example, "*The client* will transfer from the bed to a chair safely within 1 week." Some agencies believe that the words *the client* are understood and therefore do not include them when stating a goal.
   b. Contain an action verb.
      (1) The goal or outcome should identify the action that the client will learn, do, or express or the physical status the client will attain.
      (2) For example, "The client will *transfer* from the bed to chair safely within 1 week."
   c. Include performance criteria.
      (1) Actions must be specific and measurable. For example, "The client will transfer *from the bed to chair safely* within 1 week."
      (2) Conditions may be included to describe the kind of assistance or resources needed by the client. For example, "The client will transfer from the bed to chair safely *with a one-person assist* within 1 week."
   d. Include a time frame.
      (1) The goal must be achievable within a set time frame.
      (2) For example, "The client will transfer from the bed to chair safely *within 1 week.*" Additional examples of time frames include *by discharge, within 24 hours, at all times,* and *will maintain* (the word *maintain* implies continuously).

   e. Be realistic.
      (1) The performance criteria identified must be reasonable and feasible in light of the client's emotional and physical status.
      (2) Goals are realistic when the outcomes can be achieved in the indicated time frames.
      (3) Example of a realistic outcome for a client who had abdominal surgery is: "The client will exhibit bowel sounds within 3 days after surgery."
      (4) Example of an unrealistic outcome for a client with hemiplegia due to a brain attack is: "The client will perform active range-of-motion exercises independently within 1 week."

C. Identifying nursing interventions
   1. Selecting appropriate interventions depends on the accuracy and thoroughness of the data collected.
   2. Nursing interventions generally address the "related to" part (etiology) of the client's problem or nursing diagnosis. For example, if a person is *at risk for impaired skin integrity related to urinary incontinence and immobility,* the nursing interventions selected should keep the client clean and dry and relieve pressure.
   3. Nursing interventions should include nursing assessments, nursing care to avoid complications, administration of prescribed treatments and medications, and health promotion and illness prevention activities, as appropriate.
   4. Selected actions should have the greatest probability of achieving the desired goal/outcome with the least risk to the client. The nurse must consider:
      a. Cause: Planned action.
      b. Effect: Client's response.
      c. Risk: Potential for the client to have a negative consequence as a result of the planned action.
      d. Probability: Degree to which the client may have a positive consequence as a result of the planned action.
      e. Value of the consequences: Significance of results of the planned action to the client.
   5. Selected interventions should be based on evidence-based practice—that is, interventions that have been proven to be effective based on rigorous scientific evidence and clinical effectiveness studies rather than on tradition, intuition, or anecdotal information. Nursing practice based on evidence improves the quality of client care and justifies nursing interventions (see Box 6.2, Nursing Interventions Classification [NIC] System).

Nursing Interventions Classification (NIC) System

The **Nursing Interventions Classification (NIC) system** is a standardized classification of nursing interventions. It includes both physiological and psychosocial interventions that can be performed across all nursing disciplines. It consists of intervention labels. Each intervention label has a definition and a list of related nursing actions. The advantages of the NIC system are that it uses language common to all health-care professionals, it is specific, and it is based on evidence-based practice.

    Example of NIC interventions for pressure ulcer care:
- *Pressure ulcer care: Monitor color, temperature, edema, moisture, and appearance of surrounding skin; note characteristics of any drainage.*

D. Communicating the plan of care
  1. Plans of care promote communication and coordination among health team members, improving the continuity of client care.
  2. Information that should be included on a comprehensive plan of care includes:
      a. Client nursing diagnoses, problems, or needs and related independent and dependent nursing interventions.
      b. Activities of daily living (ADLs) and basic needs.
      c. Medical prescriptions and the nursing interventions required to implement them.
      d. Requirements to prepare the client for discharge, such as teaching, equipment, and services.
  3. Various types of care plans are used.
      a. Computer-generated care plans can be standardized or individualized. The nurse chooses a nursing diagnosis or health problem, and the computer presents potential goals/outcomes and nursing interventions. The nurse can then select interventions that are appropriate for the client. The computer then generates a written printout of the plan of care.
      b. Multidisciplinary care plans (collaborative care plans, critical or clinical pathways) sequence care that is to be delivered each day during a client's length of stay. Each day has a column and vertical boxes that address specific care that is to be delivered by each health-care discipline.
E. Modifying the plan of care
  1. Plans of care are dynamic and require modification to keep them current and relevant.
  2. The original plan of care may require changes because the original plan was inadequate or inappropriate or because additional assessments provide new information.

3. A plan of care may require modification after the evaluation step of the nursing process when it is identified that the client did not achieve an expected outcome or because the client's status improved.

VI. Implementation

Implementation, the fourth step of the nursing process, is the actual performance of nursing actions. It is the execution of the plan of care and involves thinking and doing. Therefore, nurses must have not only a strong knowledge base of the sciences, nursing theory, nursing practice, and legal parameters of nursing interventions but also the psychomotor skills to implement procedures safely. Nurses must implement only nursing actions that are described in their state's nurse practice act and conform to professional nursing standards of care.

A. Legal parameters of nursing interventions
  1. A nurse must know the legal parameters of nursing interventions, which include:
      a. Dependent nursing interventions.
          (1) Require a prescription from a primary health-care professional with prescriptive privileges (e.g., physicians, podiatrists, dentists, physician's assistants, nurse practitioners).
          (2) Nurses must ensure that prescribed interventions and medications are appropriate to meet the needs of a client. If a nurse implements an inappropriate intervention or prescription, the nurse can be held legally accountable as a contributor to the initial error made by the primary health-care provider. Nurses must question inappropriate prescribed interventions or prescriptions and not follow them blindly.
          (3) Examples of dependent nursing interventions include:
              (a) Administering medications or intravenous solutions.
              (b) Implementing activity prescriptions.
              (c) Inserting or removing a urinary retention catheter.
              (d) Providing a diet.
              (e) Implementing wound or bladder irrigations.
      b. Independent nursing interventions.
          (1) Registered nurses can legally plan and implement independent nursing interventions without supervision or direction from a person with a prescriptive license.
          (2) Each state's nurse practice act defines the scope of nursing practice within the state.

(3) Examples of independent nursing interventions include:
    (a) Assessing a client.
    (b) Diagnosing a client's nursing needs.
    (c) Planning, implementing, and evaluating nursing care.
    (d) Assisting with ADLs.
    (e) Teaching any subject associated with health promotion and illness prevention.
    (f) Counseling.
    (g) Advocating for a client.
    (h) Encouraging a client to express concerns and feelings.
    (i) Encouraging coughing and deep breathing.
    (j) Referring a client to community resources.
  c. Interdependent nursing interventions.
    (1) Nurses work in collaboration with primary health-care providers to implement dependent nursing interventions that have set parameters.
    (2) Some settings, such as intensive care units and birthing units, have standing protocols that delineate the parameters within which the nurse can implement a dependent nursing intervention.
    (3) Examples of interdependent nursing interventions include:
        (a) A prescription says, "Out of bed as tolerated." The nurse determines whether the client is tolerating an activity and therefore the amount of activity in which to engage the client.
        (b) A prescription for a pain medication states, "acetaminophen (Tylenol) 650 mg every 6 hours prn for mild lower back pain." The nurse assesses the level of the client's pain and then decides whether to administer the prescribed dose.
B. Types of nursing interventions
  1. Assisting with ADLs.
    a. Nurses assist clients with activities that people perform daily to promote comfort, health, and well-being.
    b. Problems interfering with these actions can be acute or chronic, temporary or permanent, and require teaching or assistance to restore function.
    c. Examples include helping a debilitated client eat, ambulating a client after surgery, providing range-of-motion exercises, turning and positioning a bed-bound client, and dressing and toileting a client.

2. Teaching.
   a. Nurses provide teaching in relation to the cognitive, psychomotor, and affective domains.
   b. Examples include conducting a class about the signs and symptoms of hyperglycemia (cognitive domain), teaching a client how to self-administer insulin (psychomotor domain), and facilitating a group session of adolescents discussing and role-playing how to say no when pressured to engage in alcohol or drug misuse (affective domain).
   c. See Table 8.1, "Understanding Learning Domains," in Chapter 8, Teaching and Learning, for more information about the various learning domains and related nursing strategies.
3. Responding to life-threatening events.
   a. Nurses use clinical judgment to identify and respond to life-threatening changes in a client's condition.
   b. The related interventions generally are associated with meeting a client's basic physiological needs.
   c. Examples include performing abdominal thrusts for a client who is choking, implementing cardiopulmonary resuscitation for a client who has no palpable pulse and is not breathing, and discontinuing a blood transfusion when a client has clinical indicators of a transfusion reaction.
4. Implementing health promotion and illness prevention activities.
   a. Nurses provide interventions that assist people to maintain health and avoid health problems.
   b. They aim to help people who are at an increased risk for illness because of their developmental level, such as neonates, young children, and dependent older adults. In addition, they help people who are at an increased risk for negative consequences of their behaviors, such as people who smoke, drink alcohol excessively, misuse drugs, have multiple sexual partners, or overeat. They also aim to help people limit exacerbations of illnesses and subsequent health problems as a result of an initial illness.
   c. Examples include administering a vaccine, teaching a class about healthy nutrition, promoting smoking cessation or weight reduction, using standard precautions, and turning and positioning an immobile client.
5. Performing technical skills.
   a. Nurses must competently perform technical psychomotor skills associated with a procedure.

b. The nurse should know the steps, principles, rationales, and expected outcomes relative to nursing procedures to implement them in the appropriate situation safely.

c. Examples include administering medications via various routes, suctioning a client's respiratory tract, changing a wound dressing, and irrigating a colostomy.

6. Employing psychosociocultural interventions.

a. Nurses use therapeutic interviewing techniques to encourage clients to express feelings and concerns. Once the nurse identifies a client's emotional needs, the nurse continues to support the client emotionally while exploring potential coping strategies. In addition, the nurse uses interpersonal interventions when working as an advocate for the client, coordinating health-care activities, and collaborating with others on the client's behalf.

b. Examples include using nondirective interviewing techniques, gently addressing a client's behavior, collaborating with a client to identify a goal, and explaining to family members that their loved one's angry behavior is associated with the anger stage of grieving in response to the diagnosis of cancer.

7. Delegating, supervising, and evaluating delegated nursing interventions.

a. **Delegation** is transferring the authority to act to another while retaining accountability for the outcome.

b. Nurses may delegate nursing care to:

(1) Unlicensed assistive nursing personnel.

(a) Uncomplicated, basic interventions.

(b) Examples: Bathing a bed-bound client, ambulating a stable postoperative client, obtaining vital signs from clients who are stable.

(2) Licensed practical nurse (LPN).

(a) Routine nursing care for clients who are stable and whose care is uncomplicated.

(b) Examples: Administering medications, changing a sterile dressing, instilling an enema.

(3) Registered nurse.

(a) Complex nursing interventions.

(b) Examples: Performing a physical assessment, teaching a client how to self-administer insulin, formulating a client's plan of care.

c. The nurse delegating care is responsible for:

(1) Assuming responsibility for the care that is delegated and its consequences.

(2) Ensuring that the person implementing the care is legally permitted to provide the delegated care, is knowledgeable, and is able to deliver the care safely.

(3) Ensuring that the care is implemented according to standards of care.

(4) Evaluating the client's responses to the interventions implemented.

(5) For additional information about delegation see "Delegation" in Chapter 5, Leadership and Management.

8. Reporting and documenting nursing interventions and client responses.

a. Nurses communicate information verbally and in writing to other members of the health team to provide continuity of client care. Written documentation also establishes a permanent legal record of the care provided and the client's response.

b. Examples include documenting vital signs on a client's graphic record, indicating the characteristics of a client's skin integrity on a pressure ulcer flow sheet, providing a verbal report regarding the status of clients to a nurse arriving for the next shift, and documenting the administration of medications and client responses to medications.

🛑 c. If interventions are not documented, they are considered not done.

VII. Evaluation

Evaluation, the fifth step of the nurse process, involves issues related to structure, process, and client outcomes. The nurse first reassess the client to identify client responses to interventions (actual outcomes) and then compares the actual outcomes with the planned outcomes (expected outcomes) to determine goal achievement. It is a continuous process that requires the plan of care to be modified as often as necessary either during or after care.

A. Components of evaluation

1. Structure.

a. Associated with the setting and effect of organizational features on the quality or excellence of nursing care.

b. Based on such things as policy and procedures, economic resources, available equipment, and the number, credentials, and experiential background of members of the nursing team.

c. Example of a structure goal against which the delivery of nursing care can be assessed: *A controller pump is used for administration of intravenous medication.*

2. Process.

a. Associated with evaluation of clinical performance of nursing team members.

b. Example of a process goal against which the care delivered by a nurse can be assessed: *The client's privacy is maintained by pulling the curtain and draping the client when assessing a client's wound.*

3. Client outcome.
   a. Associated with measurable changes in a client's status as a result of care implemented by a nurse.
   b. Example of an expected client outcome against which an actual client outcome can be assessed: *The client's skin will remain clean, dry, and intact.*

B. Types of evaluation activities
1. Routine evaluations.
   a. Occur at preset regular time frames.
   b. For example, obtaining clients' vital signs every shift; documenting intake and output every shift and every 24 hours.
2. Ongoing evaluations.
   a. Occur during and immediately after administering nursing care or after interacting with a client.
   b. For example, assessing a client's response to irrigation of a colostomy; determining whether a client understands the content in a teaching session.
3. Intermittent evaluations.
   a. Occur in specific situations.
   b. For example, obtaining daily weights to monitor a client receiving a diuretic; assessing the degree of pain relief after a client receives an analgesic.
4. Terminal evaluations.
   a. Occur in preparation for a client's discharge; health-care agencies generally have a comprehensive discharge form that provides structure and consistency within an agency.
   b. For example, evaluating a client's physical and emotional status; determining progress toward goal/outcome achievement; and formulating a plan of care to be implemented in the community setting, including topics such as medications, treatments, diet, and scheduled follow-up care.

C. Nursing interventions to ensure thorough evaluation of client responses to nursing care
1. Reassess the client to identify actual outcomes (client responses).
   a. The nurse must reassess the client to collect data, organize the data, and determine the significance of the data.
   b. Actual outcomes are then compared to the expected outcomes identified in the written plan of care to determine whether the client successfully achieved the goals/outcomes.

2. Compare an actual outcome with an expected outcome to determine goal achievement.
   a. If they are the same, then the nurse can infer that the nursing care was effective in assisting the client to achieve the expected outcome. In other words, a positive evaluation is indicated when an actual outcome meets the expected outcome.
   b. If they are not the same, then the nurse can infer that the nursing care was not effective in assisting the client to achieve the expected outcome. In other words, a negative evaluation is indicated when an actual outcome does not meet the expected outcome.
   c. Once it is determined that the expected outcome was not achieved, the nurse must analyze factors that may have affected the actual outcomes of care.
3. Analyze factors that may have influenced nonachievement of expected goals/outcomes.
   a. Each step of the nursing process must be examined to determine what contributed to the failure to achieve expected goals/outcomes. For example, the nurse must ask important questions such as:
      (1) Was the data cluster thorough and accurate?
      (2) Was the nursing diagnosis, problem, or need identified correctly?
      (3) Was the goal realistic and attainable?
      (4) Were the expected outcomes specific and measurable?
      (5) Did the planned interventions address all the etiological factors of the problem?
      (6) Were the nursing interventions consistently implemented as planned?
   b. The specific reason for not achieving a goal/expected outcome should be identified. A variety of reasons may have influenced the nonachievement of a goal/expected outcome. For example, the client might not have shared important information, the staff might not have completed all tasks as planned, the client might not have been motivated to participate adequately in the planned care, or the client's condition may have changed.

D. Modifying the plan of care
1. Plans of care are dynamic and require modification to keep them current and relevant.
2. The plan of care must be modified as soon as a nurse identifies that a plan of care is ineffective.
3. The plan will have to be modified when an expected goal/outcome is met. Goals and expected outcomes advance to address evolving needs as the client moves toward health on the health-illness continuum.
4. Once a new plan of care is implemented, the step of evaluation beings again.

CASE STUDY: Putting It All Together

A primary nurse is admitting an older adult to a surgical unit before surgery for prostate cancer. The primary health-care provider tells the nurse that the client was admitted early to ensure that the client is well hydrated and that electrolytes are within the expected range in preparation for surgery. The nurse assesses the client and collects the following information:

a. Skin is pale, dry, warm, intact, and tenting when pinched.
b. Capillary refill is delayed and nailbeds are pale.
c. Vital signs: apical pulse 95 beats/min, respirations 23 breaths/min with a slight expiratory wheeze; temperature 97.8°F using a temporal scanner thermometer (infrared sensor), and blood pressure 160/86 mm Hg.
d. Vesicular breath sounds are present.
e. Hyperactive bowel sounds are present.
f. Slight abdominal distention is present over the suprapubic area.
g. Tympany is noted on percussion of the abdomen.
h. No lower extremity edema is present.
i. Speech is rapid and at times tremulous.
j. Client appears clean and well groomed, with an absence of body and breath odor.

When the nurse interviews the client, the client's wife remains at the bedside at the client's request. The nurse documents the following information on the nursing admission history and physical:

The client told the nurse, "I've been taking Hytrin 2 mg at bedtime for the past six months because I was getting up so many times at night to urinate. I started to feel bloated and uncomfortable in the abdominal area several weeks ago and did not feel that I completely emptied my bladder after urinating. I finally went to the doctor, who ran tests and said I have prostate cancer." The client explained that his doctor then referred him to a urologist, who planned to do a total prostatectomy in the morning. The client stated, "Sometimes I need to go to the bathroom and I don't make it in time and I wet myself. It's embarrassing and I feel terrible. I'm afraid that I might become impotent and have incontinence after the surgery, but I trust the urologist and recognized that the surgery is necessary." The client asked many questions about what he can expect after surgery, which were answered. He said, "Having cancer puts a big monkey wrench into my retirement plans. I hope I'll live long enough to do a little traveling." The wife stated, "I don't care if we can't travel. I don't want him to die. Also, he forgot to tell you that he is always tired because he keeps getting up at night to go to the bathroom." During the interview, the client went to the bathroom and voided 200 mL of dark amber urine. A urine specimen was sent to the laboratory for a urinalysis. After the interview, the nurse obtained a drug handbook and reviewed the side effects of Hytrin.

Case Study Questions

A. Identify the objective data collected by the nurse.

1. _____

2. _____

3. _____

4. _____

5. _____

6. _____

7. _____

CASE STUDY: Putting It All Together   *cont'd*

_____ **Case Study Questions** _____

B. Identify the subjective data collected by the nurse during the client interview.

1. _____

2. _____

3. _____

4. _____

5. _____

6. _____

7. _____

C. Identify whether the client, wife, primary health-care provider, and nurse are primary, secondary, or tertiary sources of data.

1. _____

2. _____

3. _____

4. _____

REVIEW QUESTIONS

Be sure to read the Introduction for valuable test-taking tips.

1. Which activity is the nurse engaged in when identifying a nursing diagnosis?
   1. Discovering causes of diseases
   2. Documenting desired expected outcomes
   3. Planning care to meet nursing needs of a client
   4. Identifying human responses to actual or potential health problems

2. Which is the **most** important outcome of the nursing process?
   1. Meet the nursing needs of each client.
   2. Ensure that unit resources are allocated appropriately.
   3. Decrease the risk of an error regarding the admitting medical diagnosis.
   4. Reduce the risk of missing important data when collecting information about the client.

3. Which nursing actions are examples of the assessment step of the nursing process? **Select all that apply.**
   1. Administering pain medication for a headache
   2. Taking a client's blood pressure after ambulating
   3. Obtaining laboratory results performed in the emergency department
   4. Taking a client's apical pulse when the radial pulse obtained was irregular
   5. Determining if a client tolerated the change from a soft diet to a regular diet

4. Which actions are associated with the evaluation step of the nursing process? **Select all that apply.**
   1. A nurse takes the vital signs when a client reports chest pain.
   2. A nurse performs a physical assessment of a client just before discharge from a hospital.
   3. A nurse determines that a client is at risk for impaired skin integrity because of reduced mobility and malnutrition.
   4. A nurse and client decide that within 3 days the client will learn how to draw up and self-administer insulin safely.
   5. A nurse determines that further intervention is necessary when the client experiences sacral edema after being turned and positioned every 2 hours.

5. A client became short of breath and reported sudden chest pain while being transferred from the bed to a chair for the first time after surgery for a fractured hip. The nurse immediately returned the client to bed, raised the head of the bed, and started oxygen at 2 L via nasal cannula. Which step of the nursing process was **most** important in this scenario?
   1. Planning
   2. Assessing
   3. Evaluating
   4. Diagnosing

6. A 12-year-old child is transferred from the emergency department to the pediatric unit. The nurse on the pediatric unit reviews the emergency department summary note, performs an assessment, and interviews the child's mother. What must the nurse do **next**?
   1. Institute the oral rehydration protocol.
   2. Continue to monitor the child's vital signs.
   3. Formulate a plan of care to meet the child's needs.
   4. Cluster data that have a significant interrelationship.

Client's Clinical Record

Emergency Department Summary

A 12-year-old child arrived in the emergency department with her mother who states her daughter has had nausea and diarrhea for 2 days. Mother reports her daughter had an oral temperature of 100°F that increased to 101.2°F today, and she is thirsty but is afraid to drink fluids. Presently, the temperature is 101.4°F; pulse is 72 and regular; respirations are 22 breaths/min; blood pressure is 126/82 mm Hg. Child is lethargic, skin is pale and dry, and oral mucous membranes are dry. Stool specimen sent for culture and sensitivity. CBC and electrolyte panel pending. IV line inserted with normal saline infusing at 50 mL/hr. Institute oral rehydration therapy per hospital protocol.

Vital Signs on Admission to the Pediatric Unit

Temperature:	101.4°F, temporal
Pulse:	76 beats/min, regular
Respirations:	20 breaths/min, regular
Blood pressure:	130/78 mm Hg

Progress Notes

Mother states: "I can't believe how sick she got in such a short time. She's had nausea for several days, but the diarrhea started with a vengeance the day before yesterday. The diarrhea was so bad that she turned herself inside out. She's been afraid to drink anything because she doesn't want to throw up. I finally brought her to the hospital because I didn't know what to do for her."

7. A home-care nurse identifies that a home environment is dirty and the client's spouse appears tired and unkempt. The client and spouse are still in pajamas, even though it is 2:00 in the afternoon. The nurse determines that these cues may indicate caregiver role strain. Which type of reasoning has the nurse used?
   1. Socratic
   2. Intuitive
   3. Inductive
   4. Deductive

8. Which statements reflect deductive reasoning? **Select all that apply.**
   1. Research findings support a proposed theory.
   2. Specific information suggests a general conclusion.
   3. A suspicion moves toward identifying a clinical manifestation.
   4. Various nursing interventions are implemented until one is successful.
   5. A nurse obtains vital signs after inferring that the client has an infection.

9. A nurse understands that inadequate activity, dietary fiber, and/or fluid intake can result in constipation. As a result, the nurse asks a client who has hemiplegia as a result of a recent brain attack (cerebral vascular accident), "When was the last time you had a bowel movement?" Which type of reasoning has the nurse used when asking this question?
   1. Socratic
   2. Intuitive
   3. Inductive
   4. Deductive

10. A client is admitted to the emergency department with epigastric pain. The nurse asks the client to identify the intensity of pain using a scale of 0 to 10, with 0 being pain free and 10 reflecting excruciating pain. Which step of the nursing process does this action reflect?
    1. Analysis
    2. Planning
    3. Assessment
    4. Implementation

11. A nurse identifies that a client has dry skin and oral mucous membranes, lost 3 pounds in 2 days, and has dark amber urine. The nurse concludes that the client may be dehydrated. Which skill is the nurse using when coming to this conclusion?
    1. Intuitive thinking
    2. Inductive reasoning
    3. Scientific problem-solving
    4. Trial-and-error problem-solving

12. A nurse identifies the following desired outcome: "The client will walk 30 feet twice a day without exhibiting the signs and symptoms of activity intolerance." Which step of the nursing process does this statement reflect?
    1. Planning
    2. Assessing
    3. Evaluating
    4. Implementing

13. A nurse determines a client's flat neck veins, inadequate skin turgor, decreased blood pressure, and dry mucous membranes are a cluster of data that is significant. Which step of the nursing process is involved when the nurse comes to this conclusion?
    1. Analysis
    2. Evaluation
    3. Assessment
    4. Implementation

14. List the following nursing interventions in the order representing the steps of the nursing process beginning with the first step and progressing to the last step.
    1. Obtaining a list of the client's allergies
    2. Concluding that a client has a deficient fluid volume
    3. Administering a prescribed enema to a client who is constipated
    4. Assessing a client's level of pain after administering an opioid analgesic
    5. Identifying nursing interventions that should be implemented to meet a client's needs
    Answer: _____

15. A nurse is evaluating a client's response 30 minutes after administering morphine sulfate 10 mg Sub-Q. Which type of evaluation is the nurse implementing?
    1. Routine
    2. Ongoing
    3. Terminal
    4. Intermittent

16. A nurse identified the following expected outcome for a client: "The client will report incisional pain equal to or less than level 3 using a pain scale of 0 to 10 within 30 minutes of receiving acetaminophen (Tylenol)." Which step of the nursing process did the nurse complete?
    1. Planning
    2. Evaluation
    3. Assessment
    4. Implementation

17. A client says, "I asked to go to the hospital because I am seeing double and everything is very blurry." Which kind of data is the client describing?
   1. Objective data
   2. Subjective data
   3. Tertiary source of data
   4. Secondary source of data

18. The day after surgery, a client says to the nurse, "Since surgery yesterday, I have been having bloody urine." Which type of data is this information?
   1. Objective data
   2. Subjective data
   3. Tertiary source of data
   4. Secondary source of data

19. A nurse formulates the following goal with a client: "The client will ambulate in the hall without experiencing activity intolerance." Which statements address the status of this goal? **Select all that apply.**
   1. It is not measurable.
   2. It is not client-centered.
   3. It is missing a parameter.
   4. It is missing a target time.
   5. It is a correctly written goal.

20. Which nurses are demonstrating the planning phase of the nursing process? **Select all that apply.**
   1. A nurse who prioritizes a client's needs in order of importance
   2. A nurse who identifies a date when a goal should be achieved
   3. A nurse who collaborates with a client in designing a goal
   4. A nurse who observes that a client's urine is dark amber
   5. A nurse who identifies a cluster of data as significant
   6. A nurse who provides a backrub to induce sleep

21. A client reports to a nurse that an "accident" occurred and that the bed is wet with urine. Which step in the nursing process is associated with bathing the client and changing the linen?
   1. Planning
   2. Evaluation
   3. Assessment
   4. Implementation

22. A nurse is about to administer a medication to a client when the client states, "I really have a hard time getting that big pill down." The nurse responds, "How about if I crush it and mix it with applesauce?" Which step of the nursing process is associated with the nurse's response?
   1. Analysis
   2. Planning
   3. Assessment
   4. Implementation

23. A nurse assists a client to ambulate from the bed to the bathroom and back to a chair. Which step of the nursing process is associated with taking the client's vital signs 3 minutes later?
   1. Analysis
   2. Diagnosis
   3. Evaluation
   4. Assessment

24. A nurse is collecting a health history from a client newly admitted to the hospital. Which action associated with the data collection step of the nursing process is **most** important?
   1. Explaining to the client's spouse that the client's input is more significant than the spouse's input
   2. Communicating subjective data using the client's words
   3. Using only nondirective interviewing techniques
   4. Collecting primarily objective data

25. A nurse is assessing a client. Which information collected by the nurse reflects subjective information? **Select all that apply.**
   1. Clammy skin
   2. Agitated behavior
   3. Shortness of breath
   4. Numbness of the feet
   5. Coughing after a deep breath
   6. Feeling overwhelmed by a new diagnosis

26. Which statements reflect inductive reasoning rather than deductive reasoning? **Select all that apply.**
   1. Implementing various actions until one is successful
   2. Supporting the development of a theory with research
   3. Moving from specific information to a general conclusion
   4. Identifying a cue based on a suspicion or feeling without conscious analysis
   5. Concluding that a client with an irregular fast pulse may have a cardiac problem

27. A nurse is assessing a client. Which clinical manifestations experienced by the client are examples of objective, rather than subjective, information? **Select all that apply.**
   1. Crying
   2. Edema
   3. Heartburn
   4. Chest pain
   5. Bradypnea
   6. Lightheadedness

28. Which actions by a nurse are associated with the evaluation step of the nursing process? **Select all that apply.**
    1. Teaching Kegel exercises to a client to improve bladder control
    2. Monitoring a client's blood pressure who is receiving a diuretic drug
    3. Having a client use a voiding record to establish the pattern of elimination
    4. Exploring a client's degree of satisfaction related to urinary control interventions
    5. Securing a prescription for physical therapy for a client to increase strength and endurance
    6. Assessing an obese client's weekly weight to determine the extent of weight loss over time

29. A client has a prescription for levothyroxine 75 mcg by mouth once a day to treat hypothyroidism. The client's previous prescription was for 25 mcg by mouth once a day. The client wants to use up the previous tablets before filling the new prescription. The nurse teaches the client how many tablets of the previous prescription to take. How many tablets does the client have to take for the nurse to identify that the client understands the teaching? **Record your answer using a whole number.**

    Answer: _____ tablets

30. A nurse is assessing a client for objective and subjective data. Which information that the nurse documents in the client's clinical record is subjective information? **Select all that apply.**
    1. The client feels sad.
    2. The client is diaphoretic.
    3. The client has a headache.
    4. The client has a bounding pulse.
    5. The client states that the nausea is relentless.
    6. The client believes that the prescribed treatment plan will work.

REVIEW ANSWERS AND RATIONALES

1. ANSWER: 4.

Rationales:

1. Identifying the cause of disease is the responsibility of the primary health-care provider, not the nurse.

2. Identifying desired expected outcomes is part of the planning phase of the nursing process.

3. Proposed nursing interventions are associated with the planning phase of the nursing process.

4. Identifying human responses to actual or potential health problems is the definition of a nursing diagnosis. This is part of the analysis step of the nursing process.

Content Area: Critical Thinking and the Nursing Process
Integrated Processes: Nursing Process: Analysis
Client Need: Safe and Effective Care Environment; Management of Care
Cognitive Level: Comprehension
Concept: Patient-Centered Care

2. ANSWER: 1.

Rationales:

1. The nurse is responsible for identifying and meeting the nursing needs of each client. Nurses identify and treat human responses to disease, illness, or injury.

2. Ensuring that unit resources are allocated appropriately is the purpose of a client classification system that identifies the acuity of client needs for all the clients on a unit and the amount of resources needed to provide appropriate nursing care.

3. Determining the admitting medical diagnosis is the responsibility of the primary health-care provider, not the nurse. Nurses do not make medical diagnoses.

4. A classification system, such as Gordon's functional health patterns, is a framework used by a nurse to organize the collection of data about a client so that important information is not overlooked.

TEST-TAKING TIP: Identify the word in the stem that sets a priority. The word *most* in the stem sets a priority.

Content Area: Critical Thinking and the Nursing Process
Integrated Processes: Nursing Process: Evaluation
Client Need: Safe and Effective Care Environment; Management of Care
Cognitive Level: Comprehension
Concept: Patient-Centered Care

3. ANSWER: 3, 4.

Rationales:

1. Completing a nursing action, such as administering pain medication for a headache, is part of the implementation step of the nursing process.

2. Taking a client's blood pressure after ambulating is part of the evaluation step of the nursing process.

3. Monitoring results from laboratory tests, diagnostic procedures, and consultations by other members of the health team are all part of the assessment step of the nursing process.

4. The assessment phase of the nursing process includes verifying collected data to ensure validity and accuracy.

Also, collecting additional data provides more information to clarify or support previous data.

5. Determining a client's response to an intervention is part of the evaluation step of the nursing process.

Content Area: Critical Thinking and the Nursing Process
Integrated Processes: Nursing Process: Assessment
Client Need: Safe and Effective Care Environment; Management of Care
Cognitive Level: Application
Concept: Patient-Centered Care

4. ANSWER: 2, 5.

Rationales:

1. Taking a client's vital signs in response to a client's report of chest pain is an example of assessment.

2. Terminal evaluations (e.g., before a client's discharge from a facility), routine evaluations (e.g., vital signs every 8 hours), and intermittent evaluations (e.g., weekly body weights) are all conducted during the evaluation step of the nursing process. These evaluations collect information about a client's response to ongoing care.

3. Determining that a client is at risk for impaired skin integrity because of reduced mobility and malnutrition is associated with the analysis/diagnosis step of the nursing process. Making a nursing diagnosis is associated with identifying human responses and contributing factors to illness, disease, or injury.

4. Identifying a desired outcome is part of the planning step of the nursing process.

5. Revising a plan of care in response to a client not achieving a desired outcome (absence of signs and symptoms of pressure when turning and positioning a client every 2 hours) is part of the evaluation step of the nursing process.

Content Area: Critical Thinking and the Nursing Process
Integrated Processes: Nursing Process: Evaluation
Client Need: Safe and Effective Care Environment; Management of Care
Cognitive Level: Application
Concept: Patient-Centered Care

5. ANSWER: 3.

Rationales:

1. This scenario is not an example of the planning step of the nursing process. The planning step involves identifying goals, outcomes, and nursing interventions.

2. This scenario is not an example of the assessment step of the nursing process. Assessment is the systematic collection, validation, and documentation of data. The assessment step of the nursing process does not include the assessment that is done for the purpose of comparing actual outcomes to desired outcomes.

3. The nurse's actions were based on an evaluation of the client's response to the nursing care being delivered. The reassessment of the client and comparing the actual outcome to desired outcome is considered evaluation.

4. This scenario does not reflect the diagnosing step of the nursing process. However, eventually the nurse will have to progress to identifying an appropriate nursing diagnosis for this client's changed condition.

TEST-TAKING TIP: Identify the word in the stem that sets a priority. The word *most* in the stem sets a priority.
Content Area: Critical Thinking and the Nursing Process
Integrated Processes: Nursing Process: Evaluation
Client Need: Safe and Effective Care Environment; Management of Care
Cognitive Level: Analysis
Concept: Patient-Centered Care

6. **ANSWER: 4.**
Rationales:
1. Although instituting rehydration therapy should be done, there is something the nurse should do before this intervention.
2. Although the child's vital signs should be monitored, there is something the nurse should do before this intervention.
3. Although formulation of a plan of care should be done, this intervention is premature.
4. **The nursing process begins with the collection of data. The next step is to analyze the data and cluster significant information to arrive at the client's priority needs. A nursing assessment and analysis of data corroborates the assessment and plan of action of the medical members of the health team.**
TEST-TAKING TIP: Identify the word in the stem that sets a priority. The word *next* in the stem sets a priority.
Content Area: Critical Thinking and the Nursing Process
Integrated Processes: Communication and Documentation; Nursing Process: Analysis
Client Need: Safe and Effective Care Environment; Management of Care
Cognitive Level: Analysis
Concept: Patient-Centered Care

7. **ANSWER: 3.**
Rationales:
1. The nurse's conclusion does not rely on Socratic reasoning. Socratic reasoning is best used when searching for inconsistencies, examining multiple points of view, and separating what is known from what one believes.
2. The reasoning used by the nurse does not rely on intuition. Intuition is based on recognition of a pattern or cue based on clinical experience that supports a suspicion or feeling without using conscious reasoning.
3. **This scenario is an example of inductive reasoning. Inductive reasoning is used when certain information suggests an interpretation. It moves from specific information to a conclusion. If the nurse identifies a certain pattern of data and comes to a conclusion about the data, the nurse is using inductive reasoning. In this scenario, the nurse identified specific information (dirty environment, spouse appears tired and unkempt) that supported a general conclusion (caregiver role strain) moving from the specific to the general.**
4. Moving from a general premise to identifying data that supports the premise is an example of deductive reasoning. For example, if the nurse is concerned about caregiver role strain, the nurse should collect data to support this premise.

TEST-TAKING TIP: Identify the options that are opposites. Options 3 and 4 are opposites. Inductive reasoning moves from the specific to the general, whereas deductive reasoning moves from the general to the specific.
Content Area: Critical Thinking and the Nursing Process
Integrated Processes: Nursing Process: Analysis
Client Need: Safe and Effective Care Environment; Management of Care
Cognitive Level: Analysis
Concept: Patient-Centered Care

8. **ANSWER: 1, 5.**
Rationales:
1. **Deductive reasoning moves from a general premise to specific information. Research findings that support the development of a theory is an example of deductive reasoning.**
2. When a person identifies specific data and then arrives at a conclusion based on the data, the person is using inductive reasoning.
3. A suspicion moving toward identifying a clinical manifestation is an example of intuitive thinking.
4. Implementing various nursing interventions until one is successful explains the process of trial-and-error reasoning.
5. **Deductive reasoning moves from a general premise (e.g., the client may have an infection) to obtaining specific information to support the general premise (e.g., elevated temperature, pulse, and respirations support the premise that the client has an infection). In this scenario, even more information should be collected (e.g., inspection of a wound, culture and sensitivity testing of exudate).**
Content Area: Critical Thinking and the Nursing Process
Integrated Processes: Nursing Process: Analysis
Client Need: Safe and Effective Care Environment; Management of Care
Cognitive Level: Application
Concept: Patient-Centered Care

9. **ANSWER: 4.**
Rationales:
1. The question in the scenario does not rely on Socratic reasoning. Socratic reasoning is best used when searching for inconsistencies, examining multiple points of view, and separating what is known from what one believes.
2. The question in the scenario does not rely on intuition. Intuition is based on recognition of a pattern or cue based on clinical experience that supports a suspicion or feeling without using conscious reasoning.
3. The question in the scenario does not rely on inductive reasoning. Inductive reasoning moves from specific information to a generalized conclusion.
4. **Deductive reasoning moves from a general premise to seeking data to support the premise. The question asked in the scenario will elicit specific information as it relates to the general premise that constipation can be caused by reduced activity.**

TEST-TAKING TIP: Identify the options that are opposites. Options 3 and 4 are opposites. Inductive reasoning moves from the specific to the general, whereas deductive reasoning moves from the general to the specific.

Content Area: *Critical Thinking and the Nursing Process*
Integrated Processes: *Communication and Documentation; Nursing Process: Assessment*
Client Need: *Safe and Effective Care Environment; Management of Care*
Cognitive Level: *Analysis*
Concept: *Patient-Centered Care*

10. **ANSWER: 3.**
Rationales:
1. Analysis is the second step of the nursing process. Analysis of information occurs after information is collected during the first step of the nursing process, assessment.
2. A plan of care is formulated after nursing assessments are conducted and conclusions made about the information collected.
3. Assessment is the first step in the nursing process, which involves the collection of information.
4. Nursing care is implemented after a plan of care is formulated in the planning step of the nursing process.
Content Area: *Critical Thinking and the Nursing Process*
Integrated Processes: *Communication and Documentation; Nursing Process: Assessment*
Client Need: *Safe and Effective Care Environment; Management of Care*
Cognitive Level: *Analysis*
Concept: *Patient-Centered Care*

11. **ANSWER: 2.**
Rationales:
1. Intuitive thinking is a form of guessing based on a "feeling" about something. It does not use conscious reasoning or a scientific approach to arrive at a conclusion.
2. Inductive reasoning is used when certain information suggests a global interpretation. It moves from specific data to a generalized conclusion about the data.
3. Scientific problem-solving is a systematic seven-step process that starts with problem hypothesis; moves consecutively to data collection, hypothesis formation, plan of action, hypothesis testing, and interpretation of results; and ends with evaluation.
4. Trial-and-error problem-solving relates to the testing of multiple solutions until one is found to work for the identified problem.
Content Area: *Critical Thinking and the Nursing Process*
Integrated Processes: *Nursing Process: Analysis*
Client Need: *Safe and Effective Care Environment; Management of Care*
Cognitive Level: *Analysis*
Concept: *Patient-Centered Care*

12. **ANSWER: 1.**
Rationales:
1. Identifying desired outcomes and planning actions to assist the client in achieving the outcomes occurs in the planning step of the nursing process.

2. The assessment step includes the collection of data via physical assessment and interviewing.
3. Evaluation occurs when an actual client outcome is compared to an expected client outcome in an effort to determine if nursing actions have achieved the desired outcome.
4. The implementation step of the nursing process is when the nurse puts into action planned nursing interventions.
Content Area: *Critical Thinking and the Nursing Process*
Integrated Processes: *Nursing Process: Analysis*
Client Need: *Safe and Effective Care Environment; Management of Care*
Cognitive Level: *Analysis*
Concept: *Patient-Centered Care*

13. **ANSWER: 1.**
Rationales:
1. During the analysis step of the nursing process, data are critically analyzed and interpreted; cues and clusters of cues are compared to a theoretical knowledge base; inferences are made and validated; and goals and objectives are identified and prioritized.
2. The scenario in the stem does not reflect the evaluation step of the nursing process. Evaluation occurs when actual outcomes are compared to expected outcomes and establish whether the care provided reflects goal achievement or nonachievement.
3. The scenario in the stem does not reflect the assessment step of the nursing process. Assessment occurs when the nurse uses all the senses to collect data via interviewing, observation, auscultation, percussion, and palpation.
4. The scenario in the stem does not reflect the implementation step of the nursing process. The implementation step of the nursing process occurs when nursing care is delivered as planned.
Content Area: *Critical Thinking and the Nursing Process*
Integrated Processes: *Nursing Process: Analysis*
Client Need: *Safe and Effective Care Environment; Management of Care*
Cognitive Level: *Analysis*
Concept: *Patient-Centered Care*

14. **ANSWER: 1, 2, 5, 3, 4.**
Rationales:
1. Collecting data from the client is a form of assessment. Assessment is the first step of the nursing process.
2. Coming to a conclusion about collected data is part of the analysis step of the nursing process. Analysis is the second step of the nursing process.
5. Identifying nursing interventions that should be implemented is related to the planning step of the nursing process. Planning is the third step of the nursing process.
3. Administering an enema is the performance of a procedure. Procedures that require direct client care are part of the implementation step of the nursing process. Implementation is the fourth step of the nursing process.
4. Determining a client's response to a medication is part of the evaluation step of the nursing process. Evaluation of care is the fifth step of the nursing process.

Content Area: Critical Thinking and the Nursing Process
Integrated Processes: Nursing Process: Analysis
Client Need: Safe and Effective Care Environment;
Management of Care
Cognitive Level: Analysis
Concept: Patient-Centered Care

15. ANSWER: 2.
Rationales:
1. Routine evaluation is when a client's vital signs are monitored every shift. It is not in response to a specific nursing intervention.
2. Ongoing evaluations occur during and immediately after administering nursing care or after interacting with a client.
3. Terminal evaluations occur as the nurse implements the final evaluation just before discharge from a unit or facility. Health-care agencies generally have specific discharge forms that address an evaluation of the client's status (progress toward goal/outcome achievement) and standing medication prescriptions and treatments.
4. Intermittent evaluation occurs at a specific time; for example, daily weights in response to a specific health problem and weekly skin assessments in a long-term care facility.
Content Area: Critical Thinking and the Nursing Process
Integrated Processes: Nursing Process: Evaluation
Client Need: Safe and Effective Care Environment;
Management of Care
Cognitive Level: Application
Concept: Patient-Centered Care

16. ANSWER: 1.
Rationales:
1. This is an expected outcome included in a client's plan of care that involves the step of planning.
2. Evaluation is comparing a client's planned outcome to the actual outcome identified after nursing care is implemented; evaluation activities do not include the formulation of expected outcomes.
3. Assessment is the first step in the nursing process and mainly involves collecting data; assessment activities do not include the formulation of expected outcomes.
4. Implementation is when a nurse employs various nursing interventions to assist a client to achieve an expected outcome; evaluation activities do not include the formulation of expected outcomes.
Content Area: Critical Thinking and the Nursing Process
Integrated Processes: Nursing Process: Planning
Client Need: Safe and Effective Care Environment;
Management of Care
Cognitive Level: Analysis
Concept: Patient-Centered Care

17. ANSWER: 2.
Rationales:
1. The data in the statement are not objective data. Objective data are measurable, observable, or verifiable.
2. These are subjective data because only the client can report feelings and sensations.

3. A tertiary source of data refers to sources such as a textbook, policy or procedure manual, dictionary, or medical or nursing journals.
4. A secondary source is a person who provides supplemental information about a client.
TEST-TAKING TIP: Identify the options that are opposites. Options 1 and 2 are opposites. More often than not, one of these options is the correct answer. Examine options 1 and 2 carefully.
Content Area: Critical Thinking and the Nursing Process
Integrated Processes: Communication and Documentation;
Nursing Process: Assessment
Client Need: Physiological Integrity; Reduction of Risk
Potential
Cognitive Level: Analysis
Concept: Patient-Centered Care

18. ANSWER: 1.
Rationales:
1. Hematuria is objective information because it is measurable, observable, or verifiable.
2. Subjective data are information that only the client can report, such as feelings, sensations, or concerns.
3. A client is a primary, not tertiary source of information. Tertiary sources of data refer to sources such as a textbook, research studies, nursing journals, or policy or procedure manuals.
4. The client is a primary, not secondary source of data. A secondary source is someone other than the client, such as a family member or friend.
TEST-TAKING TIP: Identify the options that are opposites. Options 1 and 2 are opposites. More often than not, one of these options is the correct answer. Examine options 1 and 2 carefully.
Content Area: Critical Thinking and the Nursing Process
Integrated Processes: Communication and Documentation;
Nursing Process: Assessment
Client Need: Physiological Integrity; Reduction of Risk
Potential
Cognitive Level: Analysis
Concept: Patient-Centered Care

19. ANSWER: 1, 3, 4.
Rationales:
1. The words *activity intolerance* are vague. Although activity intolerance often is defined as a respiratory rate greater than 24 breaths/min and a pulse rate greater than 95 beats/min after 3 minutes of rest after activity, it is not included in the goal; for example, *as evidenced by a respiratory rate below 24 breaths/min and a pulse rate of less than 94 beats/min.* In addition, it does not identify how many feet the client should ambulate.
2. The goal is client-centered. It begins with: *The client will.*
3. The goal does not identify how many feet the client should ambulate; this is an important parameter that is missing in this goal.
4. The goal does not identify how many times a day the client should ambulate in the hall.

5. This goal is not correctly written. It should read, "The client will ambulate in the hall 50 feet three times a day without experiencing activity intolerance, as evidenced by a pulse rate below 94 beats/min and a respiratory rate below 24 breaths/min after 3 minutes of rest after ambulating."
Content Area: Critical Thinking and the Nursing Process
Integrated Processes: Nursing Process: Analysis
Client Need: Safe and Effective Care Environment;
Management of Care
Cognitive Level: Application
Concept: Patient-Centered Care

20. **ANSWER: 1, 2, 3.**
Rationales:
1. **The planning step of the nursing process provides direction for nursing interventions. Prioritizing a client's needs guides the nurse as to what should be done in order of importance.**
2. **The planning step of the nursing process includes identification of goals and the nursing care to be implemented to assist the client to achieve the goals. There are numerous components to a properly designed goal. One component must identify the time frame within which a goal should be achieved. Other components include the fact that a goal must be client centered, contain an action verb, include performance criteria and a time frame, and be realistic.**
3. **Identifying goals, outcomes, and planned interventions all are part of the planning step of the nursing process.**
4. Identifying urine as dark amber is part of the assessment phase; in addition, it may be part of the evaluation step of the nursing process if the assessment is made after providing care.
5. Determining the significance of data occurs during the analysis step of the nursing process.
6. Providing nursing care occurs in the implementation step of the nursing process.
Content Area: Critical Thinking and the Nursing Process
Integrated Processes: Nursing Process: Planning
Client Need: Safe and Effective Care Environment;
Management of Care
Cognitive Level: Application
Concept: Patient-Centered Care

21. **ANSWER: 4.**
Rationales:
1. Bathing a client and changing the linen are not part of the planning step of the nursing process. Planning involves identifying goals, outcomes, and interventions designed to meet client needs.
2. Bathing a client and changing the linen are not part of the evaluation step of the nursing process. Evaluation involves reassessing the client to identify the actual outcomes and then comparing them with the expected outcomes to determine whether outcomes are achieved.
3. Bathing a client and changing the linen are not part of the assessment step of the nursing process. Collecting data using various methods from various sources is what constitutes assessment activities.

4. **Bathing a client and changing the linen are associated with the implementation step of the nursing process. The implementation step of the nursing process is when the nurse carries out planned nursing care.**
Content Area: Critical Thinking and the Nursing Process
Integrated Processes: Nursing Process: Implementation
Client Need: Safe and Effective Care Environment;
Management of Care
Cognitive Level: Analysis
Concept: Patient-Centered Care

22. **ANSWER: 2.**
Rationales:
1. The analysis step of the nursing process includes analyzing data and identifying client problems.
2. **The nurse's response is the planning step of the nursing process. The nurse is collaborating with the client to design an intervention that facilitates ingestion of the prescribed medication.**
3. The assessment step of the nursing process includes the systematic collection, validation, and documentation of data.
4. The implementation step of the nursing process includes organizing, managing, and implementing planned nursing actions.
Content Area: Critical Thinking and the Nursing Process
Integrated Processes: Communication and Documentation;
Nursing Process: Planning
Client Need: Safe and Effective Care Environment;
Management of Care
Cognitive Level: Analysis
Concept: Patient-Centered Care

23. **ANSWER: 3.**
Rationales:
1. Taking a client's vital signs after the client rests for 3 minutes after activity is not the analysis step of the nursing process.
2. There is no step in the nursing process called diagnosis. However, during the analysis step of the nursing process, the nurse may diagnose a client's human response.
3. **Taking a client's vital signs after the client rests for 3 minutes after activity is associated with evaluation of the client's response to the activity. First, the client is reassessed to identify the client's actual outcome (response), which is then compared to the expected outcome to see if the expected outcome was achieved.**
4. Although the nurse is collecting data about the client, it is being done after a nursing intervention and therefore not considered part of the assessment step of the nursing process. The assessment step of the nursing process is concerned with collecting information to identify the client's health problems that can be treated by a nurse or provide information for the primary health-care provider.
Content Area: Critical Thinking and the Nursing Process
Integrated Processes: Nursing Process: Evaluation
Client Need: Safe and Effective Care Environment;
Management of Care
Cognitive Level: Analysis
Concept: Patient-Centered Care

24. ANSWER: 2.

Rationales:

1. This is an inappropriate comment to make to a family member. Although the client is the primary source of information, data provided by family members and friends may be extremely valuable.

2. Subjective data should be communicated in the words used by the client rather than those used by the nurse to avoid any unintentional change in meaning. Communicating collected information is part of the assessment step of the nursing process.

3. When collecting information associated with a health history, the nurse generally uses a combination of direct and open-ended questions.

4. Objective and subjective data are both important when collecting data for a health history. Subjective data involves data that only clients are able to provide, such as feelings, sensations, and concerns.

TEST-TAKING TIP: Identify the word in the stem that sets a priority. The word *most* in the stem sets a priority. Identify the option with a specific determiner. Option 3 has the word *only*, which is a specific determiner. Identify the unique option. Option 2 is unique because it is the only option that reflects a nursing action after the health history is completed. The other options include actions performed during the interview with the client.

Content Area: *Critical Thinking and the Nursing Process*
Integrated Processes: *Communication and Documentation; Nursing Process: Assessment*
Client Need: *Safe and Effective Care Environment; Management of Care*
Cognitive Level: *Application*
Concept: *Patient-Centered Care*

25. ANSWER: 3, 4, 6.

Rationales:

1. Clammy skin is objective information. It can be verified by someone other than the client.

2. Agitated behavior is objective information. It can be identified and verified by someone other than the client.

3. Shortness of breath cannot be measured. It is a feeling that one cannot catch the breath. This is subjective data that can be described only by the client.

4. Numbness of the feet is subjective information. Subjective data can be identified only by the client.

5. Coughing after a deep breath is observable and therefore objective information.

6. Feelings, attitudes, beliefs, values, and self-perceptions are all subjective information because they can be described only by the client.

Content Area: *Critical Thinking and the Nursing Process*
Integrated Processes: *Nursing Process: Assessment*
Client Need: *Physiological Integrity; Reduction of Risk Potential*
Cognitive Level: *Application*
Concept: *Patient-Centered Care*

26. ANSWER: 3, 5.

Rationales:

1. Implementing various actions until one is successful explains the process of trial-and-error reasoning.

2. When research is conducted to support a theory, thinking moves from the general to the specific; it uses deductive reasoning.

3. Moving from specific data to a general premise is an explanation of inductive reasoning.

4. Identifying a cue based on a suspicion or feeling, without conscious analysis, is an explanation of intuitive thinking.

5. Tachycardia and a pulse with an irregular rhythm are clinical manifestations that may indicate that the client may have a cardiac problem. Information moved from the specific to the general, which is reflective of inductive reasoning.

Content Area: *Critical Thinking and the Nursing Process*
Integrated Processes: *Nursing Process: Analysis*
Client Need: *Safe and Effective Care Environment; Management of Care*
Cognitive Level: *Analysis*
Concept: *Patient-Centered Care*

27. ANSWER: 1, 2, 5.

Rationales:

1. Crying can be observed by the nurse and therefore is objective information. However, the reason for the crying is subjective information.

2. Edema can be measured via observation using a parameter of 1+ to 4+ and is therefore objective information.

3. Heartburn is subjective information because it can be identified only by the client.

4. Chest pain is subjective information because it can be identified only by the client.

5. Bradypnea is a respiratory rate less than 12 breaths a minute. The respiratory rate can be counted by a nurse and therefore is objective information.

6. Lightheadedness is subjective information because it can be identified only by the client.

Content Area: *Critical Thinking and the Nursing Process*
Integrated Processes: *Nursing Process: Assessment*
Client Need: *Physiological Integrity; Reduction of Risk Potential;*
Cognitive Level: *Analysis*
Concept: *Patient-Centered Care*

28. ANSWER: 2, 4, 6.

Rationales:

1. Teaching is associated with the implementation step of the nursing process.

2. A client will often receive a diuretic to reduce an elevated blood pressure. By taking the blood pressure, the nurse is evaluating the effectiveness of the diuretic regimen.

3. Having the client complete a voiding record is associated with the implementation step of the nursing process. It involves teaching the client how to provide self-care.

4. Asking the client about the degree of satisfaction related to urinary control interventions is one way of assessing the outcome of care. Is the client satisfied or dissatisfied with the results of care? This is part of the evaluation step of the nursing process.

5. Seeking a prescription for physical therapy is associated with the implementation step of the nursing process.

6. Obtaining ongoing physical assessments while the client implements a weight-loss program is an example of the evaluation step of the nursing process. The client should lose weight if the interventions are successful.

Content Area: Critical Thinking and the Nursing Process
Integrated Processes: Nursing Process: Evaluation
Client Need: Physiological Integrity; Management of Care
Cognitive Level: Application
Concept: Patient-Centered Care

29. **ANSWER: 3.**

Rationale:

Solve the problem by using ratio and proportion.

$$\frac{\text{Desire 75 mcg}}{\text{Have 25 mcg}} = \frac{x\,\text{tablets}}{1\,\text{tablet}}$$

$$25x = 75 \times 1$$
$$25x = 75$$
$$x = 75 + 25$$
$$x = 3\ \text{tablets}$$

Content Area: Critical Thinking and the Nursing Process
Integrated Processes: Nursing Process: Evaluation
Client Need: Physiological Integrity; Pharmacological and Parenteral Therapies
Cognitive Level: Application
Concept: Medication; Safety

30. **ANSWER: 1, 3, 5, 6.**

Rationales:

1. Feeling sad can be described only by the client; therefore, this is subjective information.

2. Diaphoresis (sweating) is measured by observation and palpation and therefore is objective, not subjective, information.

3. Experiencing a headache is subjective information. Subjective data can be felt only by the client and cannot be measured or observed by another person.

4. A bounding pulse is objective information. A bounding pulse can be palpated by the nurse and is measurable.

5. Nausea and the perception that it is relentless are both subjection information. Only the client can indicate the presence of nausea and describe it as relentless. There is no objective way to assess nausea.

6. Client feelings, attitudes, and beliefs are subjective data. They can be described only by the client.

Content Area: Critical Thinking and the Nursing Process
Integrated Processes: Nursing Process: Assessment
Client Need: Physiological Integrity; Reduction of Risk Potential
Cognitive Level: Application
Concept: Patient-Centered Care

Chapter 7

Evidenced-Based Practice

NURSING CONCEPTS

Evidenced-Based Practice
Health Promotion

Patient-Centered Care
Professionalism

KEY TERMS

Continuing education—Acquisition of information that keeps nurses abreast of new technology, theories, and clinical practice

Evidenced-based practice—Use of research to prove the efficacy of a specific action

Framework—Broad, philosophical approach to a concept or idea

Health—As defined by the World Health Organization, "A state of complete physical, mental, and social well-being, and not merely the absence of disease or infirmity"

Health belief—Concept about health that a person considers or accepts as accurate

Illness—A state in which a person's status (e.g., physical, emotional, spiritual, developmental, intellectual, social) is diminished or impaired

Model—Symbolic representation of a concept or framework

Nursing certification—Voluntary endeavor to earn recognition for expertise in a specific area of nursing practice

Philosophy—Culturally determined system of beliefs, concepts, theories, or convictions

Theory—Organized set of ideas and concepts that assists one to find meaning in experiences

Value—Something that a person holds in high regard

Wellness—"A way of life oriented toward optimal health and well-being in which body, mind, and spirit are integrated by the individual to live more fully within the human and natural community," according to Myers, Sweeney, and Witmer (2000)

I. Definitions Related to Evidenced-Based Nursing Care

Nursing practice is based on a foundation of information that is viewed, organized, and utilized in accordance with professional and personal influences. A nurse's knowledge base includes theories, models, frameworks, and a philosophy of nursing. Personal influences impact both the client and nurse and include such components as values, health beliefs, stress, and the ability to respond to stress.

A. Evidenced-based practice
   1. **Evidenced-based practice** is the use of research to prove the efficacy of a specific action. Evidenced-based practice in the context of nursing is the performance of nursing interventions based on rigorous scientific evidence and clinical

effectiveness studies rather than tradition, intuition, or anecdotal information.
   2. Research collects data that identifies which interventions will most likely produce expected client outcomes.
   3. Nursing practice based on evidence improves the quality of client care, justifies nursing interventions, expands the foundation of nursing as a profession, and may contain health-care costs.

B. Theory
   1. A **theory** is an organized set of ideas and concepts that assists one to find meaning in experiences, organize thinking around a concept or idea, and develop new insight.
   2. Way of viewing, describing, predicting, and controlling phenomena.

C. Model
   1. A **model** is a symbolic representation of a concept or framework.
   2. Can be described in words or an illustration.
D. Framework
   1. A **framework** is a broad, philosophical approach to a concept or idea.
   2. Usually presented in an outline format.
E. Value
   1. A **value** is something (e.g., quality, practice, or behavior) that a person holds in high regard.
   2. Influenced by family, religion, school, culture, and governmental traditions.
   3. Influences the formation of beliefs and attitudes.
F. Health belief
   1. A **health belief** is a concept about health that a person considers or accepts as accurate.
   2. Influenced by social, cultural, and spiritual values.
G. Philosophy
   1. A **philosophy** is a culturally determined system of beliefs, concepts, theories, or convictions.
   2. Influences one's health practices (e.g., Jehovah's Witnesses do not accept blood transfusions, and Catholics do not accept abortion).

II. Theories of Nursing

Nursing theories identify and describe interrelated concepts that influence the practice of nursing. They provide a knowledge base that is broadly applicable to the variety of situations confronted by nurses. Each theory is unique, but they all include the client as the focus of the theory.

A. Self-care deficit theory of nursing—Dorothea Orem
   1. Self-care is a purposeful learned behavior in response to a need.
   2. Four concepts.
      a. *Self-care:* Self-initiated activities that a person performs to maintain life, health, and well-being.
      b. *Self-care agency:* An individual's ability to engage in self-care based on developmental level, experiences, and available resources.
      c. *Therapeutic self-care demand:* Comprehensive self-care actions required to meet personal self-care requisites.
      d. *Self-care requisites:* Actions directed to meeting universal needs common to all people, such as air, water, food, elimination, activity, rest, solitude/social interactions, safety, and promotion of human function.
   3. Nursing implications.
      a. Promotes nursing care, such as acting, doing for, guiding, teaching, supporting, and providing a supportive milieu that increases clients' self-care abilities.
      b. Increases clients' self-care activities to maintain life, health, and well-being.
B. Cultural care diversity and universality theory—Madeleine Leininger
   1. Transcultural care is a central and uniting feature of nursing.
   2. Focuses on cultural care that addresses:
      a. *Preservation:* Activities that help a client maintain health.
      b. *Accommodation:* Activities that promote ways a client adapts to and negotiates adjustments to health.
      c. *Repatterning:* Activities that help a client reconstruct life patterns to promote health.
   3. Nursing implications.
      a. Requires nurses to view nursing as a transcultural care profession.
      b. Requires nurses to provide culture-specific care that assists clients to achieve and maintain health.
C. Human caring theory—Jean Watson
   1. Care should be based on values of concern, kindness, love of self and others, and respect for the spiritual domain.
   2. Explains that nursing is an interpersonal process.
   3. Ten factors: The first three factors relate to the science of caring, and the rest relate to a focus of nursing practice.
      a. *Forming values.*
      b. *Instilling faith and hope.*
      c. *Cultivating sensitivity to self and others.*
      d. *Developing a helping-trusting relationship.*
      e. *Promoting and accepting expression of positive and negative feelings.*
      f. *Using problem-solving for caring processes.*
      g. *Promoting transpersonal teaching and learning.*
      h. *Providing supportive, protective, or corrective mental, physical, sociocultural, and spiritual environments.*
      i. *Assisting with meeting needs while preserving dignity and wholeness.*
      j. *Being open to dimensions of caring and healing that cannot be scientifically explained.*
   4. Nursing implications.
      a. Supports caring as the basis of all nursing interventions and differentiates nursing from medicine, which is more concerned with curing.
      b. Encourages nurses to treat clients with care, respect, and dignity so that clients feel accepted, supported, and protected.
D. Adaptation model—Sister Callista Roy
   1. A biopsychosocial adaptive system.
   2. Involves a feedback cycle of input and output of stimuli.

3. Pronounces that a person modifies and integrates human and environmental components to achieve adaptation that supports survival, continuity, and growth.
4. States that people respond in four modes.
   a. *Physiological-physical:* Relates to basic physiological issues (e.g., oxygenation, exercise, nutrition, elimination, fluid and electrolyte balance, and temperature regulation).
   b. *Self-concept:* Relates to the physical self (e.g., threats to bodily functions) or personal self (e.g., anxiety, guilt, and distress responses to physical or emotional stressors).
   c. *Role function:* Relates to a client's ability to adapt to physical and emotional stressors to maintain personal life roles.
   d. *Interdependence:* Relates to issues that interrupt a client's ability to maintain significant relationships.
5. Nursing implications.
   a. Promotes client adaptations in each of the four modes.
   b. Supports teaching about ways to alter internal and external environments to facilitate adaptations.
   c. Supports specific nursing care when adaptations are ineffective.
E. Functional health patterns—Marjory Gordon
1. Framework for organizing data.
2. Eleven health patterns.
   a. *Health perception-health management.*
   b. *Nutritional-metabolic.*
   c. *Elimination.*
   d. *Activity-exercise.*
   e. *Sleep-rest.*
   f. *Cognitive-perceptual.*
   g. *Self-perception.*
   h. *Role-relationship.*
   i. *Sexuality-reproductive.*
   j. *Coping-stress tolerance.*
   k. *Value-belief.*
3. Nursing implications.
   a. Facilitates the collection and organization of data.
   b. Promotes identification of interrelated information that assists nurses to determine clients' health needs and appropriate nursing care.
F. Science of unitary human beings—Martha Rogers
1. Abstract theory focusing on a person as a cohesive whole with a dynamic energy field that constantly interacts with environmental energy fields.
2. Fields are characterized by a pattern, universe of open systems, and dimensionality.
3. Nursing implications.
   a. Encourages nurses to focus on a person's wholeness.

b. Promotes interventions based on interaction between human and environmental energy fields, such as therapeutic touch and direct/redirect patterns of interaction to increase achievement of health.
c. Attempts to maintain an environment free from negative energy.

III. Theoretical Foundations Related to Concepts of Health, Wellness, and Illness

Health, wellness, and illness are terms used by people to reflect how they feel physically and/or emotionally. These terms, although used universally, are highly individualized, subjective, and influenced by a variety of factors. Theories have been developed to facilitate an understanding of the concepts and relationships between health, wellness, and illness.

A. Definitions of health
1. Is highly personal and subjective and is based on one's individual perception.
2. "A state of complete physical, mental, and social well-being and not merely the absence of disease or infirmity," according to the World Health Organization (1948).
3. "A dynamic state of being in which the developmental and behavioral potential of an individual is realized to the fullest extent possible," according to the American Nurses Association (1980).
4. "An experience that is often expressed in terms of wellness and illness, and may occur in the presence or absence of disease or injury," according to the American Nurses Association (2004).

B. Definition of wellness
1. "A way of life oriented toward optimal health and well-being in which body, mind, and spirit are integrated by the individual to live more fully within the human and natural community," according to Myers, Sweeney, and Witmer (2000).

C. Definition of illness
1. A state in which a person's status (e.g., physical, emotional, spiritual, developmental, intellectual, social) is diminished or impaired.
2. Not a disease but rather a response to a disease.

D. Health-illness continuum (Fig. 7.1)
1. The **health-illness continuum** is viewed along a continuum, with no distinct boundaries, that ranges from an excellent level of health to serious illness.
2. Placement on the continuum is determined by a person's self-perception and the perceptions of others; perceptions are influenced by many factors.

Fig 7.1 Health-illness continuum. (From Wilkinson and Treas [2016]. *Fundamentals of nursing*, Vol. 1, 3rd ed. Philadelphia: F.A. Davis Company, with permission.)

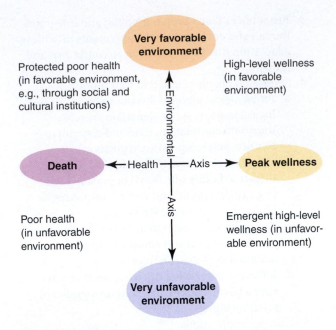

Source: U.S. Department of Health, Education and Welfare, Public Health Service. National Office of Vital Statistics.

Fig 7.2 High-level wellness grid. (From U.S. Department of Health, Education, and Welfare. Public Health Service. National Office of Vital Statistics.)

3. Placement on the continuum is dynamic and may change at any time.
4. Nursing implications.

🛑 a. **Requires nurses to explore their own perceptions about health and illness and not impose them on clients.**

   b. Assists nurses to identify where clients place themselves on the health-illness continuum because clients' health beliefs influence nursing care.

E. High-level wellness grid—H. L. Dunn (Fig. 7.2)
1. Allows a client's status to be plotted along an axis from peak wellness to death and against an intersecting axis from a very favorable environment to a very unfavorable environment.
2. Based on the intersection of the two axes, four quadrants of health and wellness are formed.
   a. *Protected poor health* (in favorable environment).
   b. *Poor health* (in unfavorable environment).
   c. *High-level wellness* (in favorable environment).
   d. *Emergent high-level wellness* (in unfavorable environment).
3. Examples of environments.
   a. Favorable: Health insurance to pay for health services; supportive, caring family members; clean, uncrowded home environment.
   b. Unfavorable: Indigence or poverty; role responsibilities that interfere with health-seeking behaviors; lack of family; dirty, crowded home environment.

4. Nursing implications.
   a. Allows nurses to identify environmental factors that influence a client's level of wellness.
   b. Facilitates prediction of whether clients' health will likely improve or decline on the basis of support or lack of support within the environment.

F. Wellness model—Anspaugh, Hamrick, and Rosato
1. To achieve health and wellness, a client must deal with features and dynamics within each of seven components of wellness.
   a. *Physical.*
   b. *Social.*
   c. *Emotional.*
   d. *Intellectual.*
   e. *Spiritual.*
   f. *Occupational.*
   g. *Environmental.*
2. Wellness requires working on all components of the model.
3. Nursing implications.
   a. Requires nurses to assess clients from seven perspectives.
   b. Facilitates a holistic approach to caring for clients because all components of wellness must be addressed.

G. Health belief model—Becker, Maiman, and Rosenstock
1. Addresses the relationship between an individual's beliefs and behaviors.

2. Three components.
   a. *Individual's perception of susceptibility to illness.*
   b. *Individual's perception of the seriousness of the illness.*
   c. *Individual's potential for action, which depends on benefits and barriers to taking action.*
3. Nursing implications.
   a. Facilitates an understanding of client behaviors.
   b. Provides a prediction of how clients might behave.
   c. Provides a basis for client teaching.
H. Role performance model
   1. Recognizes that all people generally fulfill a number of societal roles, such as parent, daughter or son, friend, and employee.
   2. People who are able to fulfill their roles are considered healthy even though they may have an illness or disability.
   3. Implies that people are unhealthy if they are unable to fulfill their roles.
   4. Nursing implications.
      a. Requires nurses to explore client perceptions about role performance versus the sick role to help plan and implement nursing care.
      b. Obligates nurses to foster independence when caring for clients who define their level of health by their ability to provide self-care.
I. Clinical or medical model
   1. Interpretation of health is based on the presence or absence of signs and symptoms of illness, disease, or injury; a narrow interpretation of health.
   2. A person is considered either healthy or sick; there is no continuum.
   3. The model is based on the perception that a person is a physiological system with associated functions.
   4. Nursing implications.
      a. Focuses on making nursing assessments in the physiological realm.
      b. Requires nurses to explore domains other than the physiological realm because this theory has a narrow interpretation of health.

IV. Theoretical Foundations of Nursing Practice

Nursing practice is an art and science that bases nursing care on information from a variety of disciplines (e.g., physical, social, and natural sciences) and related conceptual frameworks. A conceptual framework presents related ideas, statements, and concepts that address their significant interrelationships, providing an organized perspective to complex situations and problems. Theories that influence the discipline of nursing include those that present a framework reflective of growth and development, psychosocial issues, human needs, and grief and loss.

DID YOU KNOW?

Abraham Maslow introduced his five-stage hierarchy of needs model in the book *Motivation and Personality* (1954). The first four stages he identified as deficient, survival, or basic needs (physiological, safety, belonging, and self-esteem). These basic needs motivate people when they are unmet. The fifth stage he identified as a growth need (self-actualization). Self-actualization addresses the concept of achieving one's potential. This five-stage theory was expanded into seven- and eight-stage theories by other motivational psychologists who made inferences from Maslow's work. These expanded models include cognitive, aesthetic, and transcendence as separate additional stages. However, Maslow never identified these as distinct stages but rather to serve as illustrative aspects of self-actualization. Each one of these motivators (cognitive, aesthetic, and transcendence) concerns an area of self-development and self-fulfillment rooted in self-actualization. Maslow's five-stage hierarchy of needs theory remains the definitive classical representation of human motivation.

A. Hierarchy of basic human needs model—Abraham Maslow (Fig. 7.3)
   1. Human needs are arranged in a hierarchy of importance.
      a. *Physiological:* Includes basic needs essential to maintain life (e.g., air, water, food, elimination, rest, sleep, sex, and activity).
      b. *Safety and security:* Includes the need to be physically and emotionally protected from injury (e.g., performing hand hygiene, sterile technique, effective mobility, and activities that promote trust; ensuring that the call bell is within the client's reach, wheels are locked on equipment, and the bed is maintained in the lowest position; and explaining care before initiation).
      c. *Love and belonging:* Includes the need to give and receive love and acceptance and have a significant connection to family members, friends, and the community (e.g., treating clients with respect, ensuring privacy, and involving family members in care when appropriate).
      d. *Self-esteem:* Includes the need to have a positive self-regard, feel appreciated, and be independent and confident (e.g., encouraging independence, facilitating attainment of realistic goals, supporting roles, and accepting clients' values and beliefs).

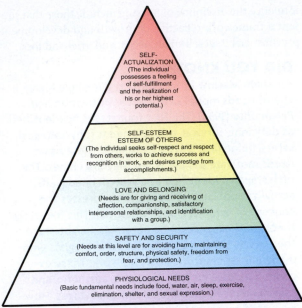

Fig 7.3 Maslow's hierarchy of basic human needs.

e. *Self-actualization:* Includes the need to achieve the highest potential within abilities (e.g., accepting clients as unique individuals, focusing on strengths, supporting hope, and teaching clients to be proactive in reaching their own potential).

2. Human needs motivate behavior.

3. Lower-level needs must be met to some degree before higher-levels needs are met.

B. Theory of psychosocial development—Erik Erikson

1. Based on interrelationships between emotional and physical variables rather than psychosexual stages.

2. Individuals at various stages of development cope with conflicts that may have a favorable or unfavorable outcome.

3. Extent of resolution of preceding stage influences subsequent stages.

4. Eight stages (Table 7.1).

Table 7.1 Erikson's Stages of Psychosocial Development

Stage	Signs of Successful Achievement	Behaviors That Support Achievement	Signs of Unsuccessful Achievement	Behaviors That Precipitate Unsuccessful Achievement
Trust versus mistrust Infant: Birth to 18 months	• Develops trust in others • Is optimistic	• Basic needs are met consistently • Supportive and affectionate care is received	• Mistrusts others • Withdraws • Is estranged from others	• Basic needs are not met • Impersonal and detached care is provided
Autonomy versus shame and doubt Toddler: 18 months to 3 years	• Is independent within abilities • Develops self-control • Begins to develop personal identity, body image, and self-esteem	• Choices are allowed • Ability to succeed or safely fail through experiences is allowed • Appropriate praise and encouragement are provided	• Has unnecessary dependence • Exhibits compulsive self-restraint • Has feelings of inadequacy • Is willful • Is defiant	• Overprotection occurs • Limited choices are offered • Shaming or insulting occurs • Excessive criticism is received • Harsh punishment is imposed
Initiative versus guilt Preschooler: 3 to 5 years	• Seeks new experiences • Is resourceful • Increases ability to provide basic self-care • Develops direction and purpose • Begins to establish a role identity and sexual identity	• Accomplishments are recognized • Creative activities are encouraged and supported • Questions are answered	• Is frustrated • Is hesitant to attempt new or challenging skills • Lacks self-confidence • Is pessimistic • Fears doing wrong • Blames self or feels guilty	• Creativity is limited • Experimentation with new roles is discouraged • Imagination and fantasy are stifled • Behavior is consistently labeled as "bad"
Industry versus inferiority School-aged child: 6 to 12 years	• Is eager to learn new skills • Thrives on realistic praise for accomplishments • Develops a sense of competency and self-confidence • Develops social skills	• Participation in activities that can be attained successfully within abilities is allowed • Realistic recognition for accomplishments is given	• Has feelings of inadequacy • Withdraws from peers and school	• Unrealistic expectations of the child are imposed by others • Unwarranted or harsh punishments are imposed

Table 7.1 Erikson's Stages of Psychosocial Development—Cont'd

Stage	Signs of Successful Achievement	Behaviors That Support Achievement	Signs of Unsuccessful Achievement	Behaviors That Precipitate Unsuccessful Achievement
Identity versus role confusion *Adolescent: 12 to 20 years*	• *Explores various roles* • *Plans activities based on abilities* • *Integrates childhood experiences into a coherent sense of self or personal identity* • *Develops devotion and fidelity to others, especially peers*	• *Assistance is provided with decision making* • *Encouragement to participate in family, school, and community endeavors is given* • *Socially responsible behavior is supported*	• *Has feelings of uncertainty about self* • *Is indecisive* • *Has difficulty making realistic plans*	• *Limited opportunities for decision making are offered* • *Adolescent's activities or plans for the future are criticized or disregarded by significant others*
Intimacy versus isolation *Young adult: 18 to 25 years*	• *Develops meaningful relationships with friends* • *Develops an intimate relationship with another person* • *Develops a commitment to work or career goal*	• *Relationships with others are supported* • *Exploration of career goals are encouraged and supported*	• *Has impersonal relationships* • *Is unable to develop an intimate relationship with another person* • *Fears commitment to work or career goals* • *Feels isolated and rejected*	• *Relationships are criticized* • *Disinterest in career goals by significant others*
Generativity versus stagnation *Middle-aged adult: 25 to 65 years*	• *Becomes a productive member of society* • *Performs activities that promote the growth of others, particularly those in the next generation* • *Establishes a family* • *Engages satisfactorily in an occupation*	• *Emotional support is provided* • *Activities, such as volunteerism, are supported*	• *Is self-indulgent* • *Lacks interests* • *Is unable to promote the growth of others, particularly those in the next generation* • *Regresses to an earlier level of coping*	• *Emotional support is lacking* • *Recognition and praise for accomplishments is lacking*
Integrity versus despair *Older adult: 65 years to death*	• *Views life as meaningful* • *Feels respected by others* • *Respects self*	• *Review of life experiences is encouraged and supported* • *Acceptance, appreciation, and respect are given by others*	• *Has sense of loss and regret* • *Views life as meaningless* • *Has inability to adjust to changes associated with aging (e.g., physical changes, retirement)*	• *Achievement of goals does not occur* • *Loss of a relationship with significant others occurs through isolation or death* • *Multiple physical and/or emotional problems occur*

5. Nursing implications.
   a. Helps nurses understand human behavior.
   b. Helps nurses identify clients' stages of development and extent of task achievement.
   c. Helps nurses assist clients to develop coping skills associated with each task.
C. Theory of cognitive development—Jean Piaget
   1. Thinking and reasoning develop through exposure to new experiences.

2. Four phases.
   a. *Sensorimotor:* Birth to 24 months; characterized by cognition, primarily through the senses and ability to process information on the physiological or emotional level.
   b. *Preoperational:* 2 to 7 years of age; characterized by an increasing ability to connect cognitively through language and actions.
   c. *Concrete operations:* 7 to 11 years of age; characterized by an increasing ability to organize

Theories and Nursing Implications

According to Maslow, human needs are arranged in a hierarchy of importance. Basic needs must be met to maintain life; then other needs emerge as previous needs begin to be met. Nurses can use this hierarchy to help identify client needs and prioritize care. Client needs must be considered within the context of a client's developmental level (related to theories by researchers such as Erikson [1963], Piaget [1952], and Havighurst [1971]) because certain needs become more dominant at different stages of development (e.g., adolescents concerned about peer acceptance may place a higher importance on self-esteem needs). A client's unique status (related to theories by researchers such as Roy [2003]; Gordon [1994]; and Anspaugh, Hamrick, and Rosato [2011]) must also be considered because personal factors can become more dominant when people are coping with illness (e.g., a woman who had a mastectomy might be more concerned about love and belonging needs or self-esteem needs than about physiological needs).

information and use logical thought, ability to solve concrete problems, and less egocentricity.

   d. *Formal operations:* 11 to 15 years of age; characterized by use of abstract thinking and deductive reasoning and ability to examine alternatives.

3. Movement through phases is based on inherited intellect and environmental impact.

4. Each phase developed through:

   a. *Adaptation:* Ability to adjust to and interact with the environment.

   b. *Assimilation:* Inclusion of new experiences and information within one's knowledge.

   c. *Accommodation:* Change in one's knowledge as a result of processing new experiences and information.

5. Nursing implications.

   a. Allows nurses to design nursing care, teaching plans, and activities that are appropriate for a child's developmental level.

   b. Helps nurses identify a child's developmental level and determine how far ahead to prepare the child for a procedure.

D. Developmental stages and tasks—Robert Havighurst

1. Each stage has a task requiring mastery.

2. Mastery of preceding tasks is essential for mastery of future tasks.

3. Six stages.

   a. *Infancy and early childhood: Birth to 6 years of age.*

   b. *Middle childhood: 6 to 13 years of age.*

   c. *Adolescence: 13 to 18 years of age.*

   d. *Early adulthood: 19 to 30 years of age.*

   e. *Middle adulthood: 30 to 60 years of age.*

   f. *Later maturity: 60 years of age and older.*

4. Nursing implications.

   a. Provides guidelines for supporting and evaluating task achievement.

   b. Facilitates identification of lack of task achievement, which requires interventions.

E. Psychoanalytic theory—Sigmund Freud

1. Childhood experiences form unconscious motivation for behavior.

2. The basis of the theory is the development of balance between pleasure-seeking instincts and the standards of society.

3. Sexual energy is centered in body parts at different ages.

   a. *Oral:* Birth to 12–18 months.

   b. *Anal:* 12–18 months to 3 years.

   c. *Phallic or oedipal:* 3 to 6 years.

   d. *Latency:* 6 to 12 years.

   e. *Genital:* Puberty through adulthood.

4. The personality has three parts.

   a. *Id* (sexual energy): Represents instinctual urges, pleasures, and gratification; dominant in infants and children.

   b. *Ego* (realistic part of self): Balances what is wanted (demands of the id) and what is possible in light of societal limitations; begins to develop at 4 to 6 months of age.

   c. *Superego* (conscience): Regulates and restrains behavior by balancing the demands of the id and pressures of society; begins to develop at 5 to 6 years of age.

5. Nursing implications.

   a. Helps nurses to understand human behavior.

   b. Allows nurses to develop a plan of care based on a client's psychosexual development and personality needs.

F. Theory of stages of moral development—Lawrence Kohlberg

1. Theory helps to explain the development of moral code.

2. Each stage builds on the previous stage and develops over time.

3. Based on the ability to think at a higher level as one matures.

4. Based on the study of boys; validity of application to females is criticized.

5. Six stages.

   a. *Obedience and punishment:* Motivation for behavior is fear of negative consequences (e.g., punishment, disapproval).

b. *Individualism and exchange:* Motivation for behavior is the desire for a positive consequence (e.g., good result, reward).

c. *Interpersonal relationships:* Motivation for behavior is based on pleasing others because it is what others expect.

d. *Maintaining social order:* Motivation for behavior is based on following rules.

e. *Social contract and individual rights:* Motivation for behavior is based on differing values, beliefs, and opinions but adheres to standards agreed upon by society.

f. *Universal principles:* Motivation for behavior is based on abstract reasoning, universal ethical principles (e.g., the "Golden Rule"), and principles of justice.

6. Nursing implications.

a. Increases nurses' understanding that client decision making is influenced by one's moral code.

b. Helps nurses examine their own moral code and not impose their moral orientation onto clients and their family members.

G. Faith development—James Fowler
Faith represents a set of beliefs and values that develop over time as a person ages. According to the faith development theory by James Fowler (1981), an individual progresses through six stages adding new patterns of values, beliefs, and ways of thinking as one ages from a preschooler to adulthood. (For more information associated with Fowler's theory on faith development, see "Faith Development—James Fowler" in Chapter 11, Diversity and Spirituality/Religion.)

H. Models of grieving

1. Engel's model of grief: See Chapter 13, Grief and Loss.

2. Kübler-Ross's stages of grieving: See Chapter 13, Grief and Loss.

V. The Profession of Nursing

Nursing is considered both a profession and a discipline. As a profession, it is based on technical and scientific knowledge; has members who are knowledgeable, competent, and evaluated by peers; and has a code of ethics. As a discipline, nursing has its own scientifically based body of knowledge involving both a theoretical foundation and a practical aspect in the form of clinical skills. In addition, nursing integrates knowledge and principles associated with other disciplines, such as anatomy and physiology, psychology, sociology, communication, and mathematics. A variety of nursing education programs, from those providing entry into practice through the doctoral level, prepare nurses to practice as professional nurses on various levels of nursing practice and in various health-care settings. Nursing organizations support the practice of nursing by activities such as publishing position statements on important issues affecting nursing, encouraging and supporting nursing scholarship and research, and identifying standards of nursing practice and codes directing nursing practice. In addition, they recognize expertise via certification of professional nurses who demonstrate proficiency in a specific area of nursing practice. Nurses should understand the educational programs available to continue personal growth and the services that nursing organizations provide to the profession of nursing.

A. Definitions of nursing

1. According to the International Council of Nurses (ICN) (2002), which represents nurses throughout the world, "Nursing encompasses autonomous and collaborative care of individuals of all ages, families, groups and communities, sick or well and in all settings. Nursing includes the promotion of health, prevention of illness, and the care of ill, disabled and dying people. Advocacy, promotion of a safe environment, research, participation in shaping health policy and inpatient and health systems management, and education are also key nursing roles."

2. According to the American Nurses Association (ANA), which represents nurses throughout the United States, "The protection, promotion, and optimization of health and abilities, prevention of illness and injury, alleviation of suffering through the diagnosis and treatment of human response, and advocacy in the care of individuals, families, communities, and populations" (2016).

B. Nursing organizations

1. American Nurses Association (ANA).

a. Mission: "Nurses advancing our profession to improve health for all."

b. National professional organization for nursing in the United States.

c. Involved in such activities as publishing standards of nursing practice; lobbying for professional, political, and economic issues impacting health care and nursing; and certifying expert nurses who meet experiential and testing criteria.

d. Online at www.nursingworld.org.

2. National League for Nursing (NLN).

a. Mission: "Promote excellence in nursing education to build a strong and diverse nursing workforce to advance the health of our nation and the global community."

b. Organization of individuals such as nurses, non-nurses, and agencies.

c. Involved in such activities as providing a voice for nursing education and advocates for nurse educator interests in academic, professional, and political arenas.

   d. Online at www.nln.org.

3. National League for Nursing Accrediting Commission (NLNAC).
   a. Mission: "Supports the interests of nursing education, nursing practice, and the public by the functions of accreditation."
   b. Involved in such activities as accrediting nursing education programs, both postsecondary and higher degree, that offer either a certificate, diploma, or recognized professional degree.
   c. Online at www.nlnac.org.

4. International Council of Nurses (ICN).
   a. Mission: "To represent nursing worldwide, advancing the profession and influencing health policy."
   b. Involved in such activities as representing the profession of nursing worldwide via a federation of national nursing associations and collaborating with other organizations to provide access to focused information and research on major nursing and health topics (e.g., International Center for Nursing Human Resources).
   c. Online at www.icn.ch\.

5. National Student Nurses' Association (NSNA).
   a. Mission: "To mentor students preparing for initial licensure as registered nurses, and to convey the standards, ethics, and skills that students will need as responsible and accountable leaders and members of the profession."
   b. Involved in such activities as representing student nurses; convening yearly conventions; and publishing *Image,* the official journal of the NSNA.
   c. Online at http://www.nsna.org.

6. Sigma Theta Tau International (STTI), the honor society of nursing.
   a. Mission: "Advancing world health and celebrating nursing excellence in scholarship, leadership, and service."
   b. Selects students in baccalaureate, masters, doctoral, and postdoctoral programs and practicing nurses for membership when they demonstrate excellence in nursing.
   c. Has a scholarly purpose rather than a social purpose.
   d. Involved in such activities as providing awards and grants supporting nursing research; conducting biennial conventions to address organizational business and programs; and supporting a leadership institute, nursing research library, and global initiatives.
   e. Online at www.nursingsociety.org.

C. Nursing education
1. Programs that prepare students to take the National Council Licensure Examination for Registered Nurses (NCLEX-RN).
   a. Diploma programs.
      (1) Were the most common nursing programs before the 1960s, when nursing education moved into community college and university settings; have dramatically declined in number.
      (2) Generally are under the sponsorship of a hospital and may provide college credit if associated with a community college.
      (3) Generally take 3 years to complete and focus on clinical experience.
   b. Associate degree programs, such as associate degree in nursing (ADN), associate of arts (AA), associate of science (AS), or associate in applied science (AAS).
      (1) Generally are 2-year programs offered by a community college or university; however, because many students are older with family and job responsibilities, may take 3 or more years of part-time study to complete.
      (2) Provide the basis for pursuing more advanced nursing education.
   c. Baccalaureate degree nursing programs, such as bachelor of science in nursing (BSN). Offer two courses of study.
      (1) Generic: Generally are 3- to 4-year programs for students entering as freshmen with a major in nursing.
      (2) General: Generally are 2-year programs for graduates of ADN programs or diploma programs with college credit; may offer a "fast track" option (1 to 1½ years of continuous classes).
   d. Master's entry program in nursing if the student earned a baccalaureate degree in another field.
   e. Doctoral entry program in nursing, which is similar to master's entry; has limited enrollment.

2. Licensed practical nurse or vocational nurse programs that prepare students to take the National Council Licensure Examination for Practical Nurses (NCLEX-PN).
   a. Prepare graduates to provide uncomplicated bedside nursing care under the supervision of an RN.
   b. Generally are 1 to 1½ years in length.

3. Programs that provide advanced degrees in nursing.
   a. Master's degree nursing programs, such as master of arts (MA), master of science (MS),

master of science in nursing (MSN), and master in nursing (MN).

   (1) Prepare RNs with a BSN degree for advance practice.

   (2) Prepare nurses to assume advanced roles in clinical practice, education, research, and administration, such as clinical nurse specialist (CNS), certified nurse midwife (CNM), certified registered nurse anesthetist (CRNA), nurse practitioner (NP), nurse administrator, and professor of nursing education.

   (3) Generally take 1½ to 2 or more years to complete.

  b. Doctoral programs in nursing, such as doctor of philosophy (PhD), doctor of nursing science (DNS, DNSc), and nursing doctorate (ND).

   (1) Prepare nurses with master's degrees in nursing for advanced practice.

   (2) Focus of programs varies, such as clinical practice, administration, education, and theory development; however, all emphasize research.

D. Nursing certification

  1. **Nursing certification** is documentation that recognizes and certifies the status, level of achievement, or expertise of a nurse in a specific area of nursing practice.

  2. Achieved in areas of practice, such as geriatrics, medical-surgical nursing, pediatrics, emergency nursing, nursing administration, nursing education, community health nursing, school nursing, and maternal-child nursing.

  3. Provided by the ANA or specialty nursing organizations.

E. Continuing education

  1. **Continuing education** is instruction received after leaving a formal educational system, generally consisting of short or part-time courses.

  2. Many states require a certain number of hours of ongoing education (e.g., 15 to 30 hours every 2 years) or completion of classes on a specific topic (e.g., infection control, child abuse) for RN licensure renewal.

  3. Classes ensure that nurses keep abreast of new technology, theories, and clinical practice.

  4. Programs are offered by employers, colleges, professional nursing organizations, and professional journals.

F. In-service education

  1. **In-service education** is instructions or educational programs provided by employers.

  2. Generally focus on new equipment, introduction of new policies or procedures, or topics mandated by a state health department, such as infection control and cardiopulmonary resuscitation.

CASE STUDY: Putting It All Together

Subjective Data

A 66-year-old woman is brought to a clinic by her female partner because of increasing shortness of breath and fatigue. The client was reluctant to come to the clinic, but her partner insisted. The client reports being diagnosed with emphysema 10 years ago and states, "I've been smoking since I was 15 years old, but I can't stop. The smoking finally got the best of me. I guess I should have stopped smoking when I was diagnosed with emphysema. If I had to do it over, I would do a lot of things differently. I have so much phlegm; I cough all the time. I can hardly breathe, and I'm exhausted all the time. My partner hates that I always smell like smoke, and my fingers and teeth have turned yellow."

Objective Data

Temperature:	100.2°F, orally
Pulse:	88 beats/min, regular
Respirations:	26 breaths/min
Blood pressure:	138/84 mm Hg

Case Study Questions

A. Which of the following concerns identified by the nurse is the client's primary problem, and why did you come to this conclusion? Why are the other concerns not the priority?

  1. Impaired oxygenation due to retained secretions _____

_____

_____

continued.

CASE STUDY: Putting It All Together *cont'd*

Case Study Questions

2. Potential for falls because of overwhelming fatigue _____

_____

_____

3. Impaired relationship with partner associated with changes in appearance _____

_____

_____

4. Diminished self-esteem related to an inability to stop smoking _____

_____

_____

B. What additional objective data should the nurse collect in relation to the client's respiratory status? Explain why each abnormal clinical indicator may have occurred by exploring its relationship to the client's respiratory problem.

1. _____

2. _____

3. _____

4. _____

5. _____

6. _____

7. _____

8. _____

C. What client statement indicates that the client is struggling with one of the age-related tasks associated with Erikson's and Havighurst's developmental theories? Explain your answer.

_____

D. Considering the concepts of the health belief model, what factors in the scenario indicate that the client may be ready to make behavioral changes? Explain your answer.

_____

REVIEW QUESTIONS

Be sure to read the Introduction for valuable test-taking tips.

1. Which activity associated with the National League for Nursing Accrediting Commission impacts on the quality of care directly provided by a nurse?
   1. Approving nursing education programs
   2. Publishing standards of professional nursing practice
   3. Lobbying economic issues impacting on the profession of nursing
   4. Mentoring the professional development of future registered nurses

2. Which actions are associated with third-level needs according to Maslow's hierarchy of needs? **Select all that apply.**
   1. Taking deep breaths after exercising
   2. Hanging a self-made painting in a senior center
   3. Treating clients with respect when providing care
   4. Receiving weekly phone calls from adult children
   5. Keeping a small light on in a bedroom during the night
   6. Removing scatter rugs after experiencing a fall in the home

3. Which statement by a nurse meets a second-level need according to Maslow's hierarchy of needs?
   1. "I see that you have applied makeup today for the first time since you had your surgery."
   2. "I am your nurse for the next 12 hours. You can use your call bell to page me."
   3. "Your family can visit every day between 10 in the morning and 8 at night."
   4. "A physical therapist will be in today to complete an evaluation."

4. A middle-aged adult fell in the driveway at home and came to the emergency department to ensure that he had not sustained a bone fracture. Which statement made by the client to the emergency department nurse indicates the developmental task of this age group?
   1. "If I get a cast, my fiancé will be furious because we're getting married next month and this will ruin the pictures."
   2. "I don't want you to call my place of employment about my health insurance coverage."
   3. "I must be out of here in a few hours because I have to coach my son's baseball team."
   4. "If my arm is broken, my friends will get another guy for our golf foursome."

5. Which nursing interventions meet a client's physiological needs according to Maslow's hierarchy of needs? **Select all that apply.**
   1. Closing the door to a client's room to reduce noise
   2. Wearing sterile gloves when changing a client's dressing
   3. Lowering the height of a client's bed to the lowest position
   4. Encouraging a parent to stay with a hospitalized child overnight
   5. Providing assistive utensils so that a client can eat independently

6. Dorothea Orem identified a theory of nursing. Which statement is associated with Orem's theory?
   1. Promotes nursing care that increases a client's self-care abilities
   2. Helps nurses provide culture-specific care that assists clients to achieve and maintain health
   3. Assists nurses to identify behaviors associated with various stages of coping with death and dying
   4. Facilitates identification of a child's stage of development so that appropriate interventions are planned

7. Which statement is accurate in relation to the concepts of health and wellness indicated in the presented theoretical framework?

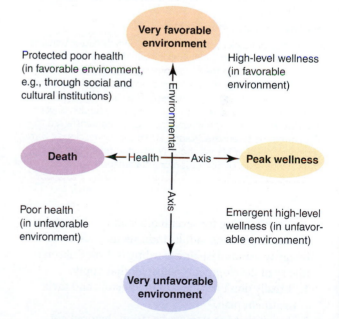

1. Implies that people are unhealthy if they are unable to fulfill their roles in society
2. Promotes meeting basic-level needs first and then progressing to higher-level needs
3. Supports teaching about how to alter internal and external factors to facilitate adaptations
4. Facilitates prediction of whether clients will likely improve in health or experience a decline based on level of support

8. A nurse is caring for a client newly admitted to the hospital because of altered mental state and to rule out a urinary tract infection (UTI) and brain attack. The nurse reviewed the client's clinical record and assessed the client. Based on the collected data, which nursing action addresses a second-level need according to Maslow's hierarchy of needs?
   1. Seek a prescription for oxygen via a nasal cannula.
   2. Encourage the client to increase oral fluid intake.
   3. Activate the bed alarm on the client's bed.
   4. Take vital signs every four hours.

Client's Clinical Record

Vital Signs

Temperature: 102°F, rectally
Pulse: 120 beats/min, irregular rhythm
Respirations: 26 breaths/min
Blood pressure: 150/88 mm Hg

Emergency Department Nurse's Progress Note

Client is a 75-year-old woman brought to the emergency department by her daughter, who found the client wandering in the neighborhood without a winter coat or shoes. Client recognizes the daughter and can state her name but is not oriented to time or place. This is a dramatic change in mentation since the previous 24 hours, when the client was alert and oriented. Daughter shared that yesterday her mother said she felt burning when she urinated. IVF 1,000 mL 0.45% NaCl at 125 mL/hour.

Nurse's Admission Progress Note

Client in semi-Fowler position. Upper side rails raised. Daughter sitting at bedside and quietly talking with her mother. Client is unable to verbalize the time or recognize that she is in a hospital. Client asks, "Why are these people in my house, and why can't I get up and cook supper?" The client's mucous membranes are dry, skin turgor is inadequate, and skin is warm and flushed. Client experienced dyspnea when transferred to the commode to urinate. Voided 200 mL of urine, cloudy with sediment. IV set at 125 mL/hour. IV site dry, intact, free from clinical indicators of infiltration or inflammation.

---

9. A nurse is caring for several older adults. Which statements by older adults indicate the conflict of ego integrity versus despair according to Erik Erikson's theory of development? **Select all that apply.**
   1. "I really don't trust any of my doctors and their treatment plan."
   2. "I wish that I took more vacations before I got too sick to travel."
   3. "I don't care what the doctor says; I will do it my way or no way."
   4. "I hope that in my next lifetime I get the chance to become a doctor."
   5. "I feel that I will never get better because nothing ever goes well for me."

10. A nurse is caring for an older adult male newly admitted to the hospital. The nurse understands the importance of organizing data and then prioritizing needs based on Maslow's hierarchy of needs. Place the following data collected by the nurse in order following Maslow's hierarchy of needs, progressing from first-level needs up to fifth-level needs.
    1. Reported that he has difficulty taking a deep breath
    2. Requested help with the telephone so that he can call his son
    3. Informed the nurse that he feels dizzy when he moves to a standing position
    4. Asked about his condition so that he can make realistic health-care decisions
    5. Stated that he feels foolish when he can't find the right words to express himself
    Answer: _____

11. A nurse identifies that clients are experiencing middle-adulthood developmental crises. Which information supports the nurse's conclusion? **Select all that apply.**
    1. Inability to carry a wanted pregnancy to term
    2. Failure to develop friendships with peers
    3. Demotion to a lesser position at work
    4. Powerless to postpone gratification
    5. Unable to discuss eventual death

12. Which nursing action supports a client's basic need for safety and security? **Select all that apply.**
    1. Positioning a commode next to a client's bed at night
    2. Teaching a client how to transfer from the bed to a chair
    3. Placing a client's dentures in a labeled denture cup in the bedside table
    4. Assessing a client's abdomen for clinical indicators of urinary retention
    5. Ensuring that a client with neutropenic precautions is provided a mask when being transported for an x-ray

13. An older adult is living in a nursing home because of multiple chronic health problems. Which nursing actions are appropriate to assist the older adult to achieve the task associated with Erikson's stage of integrity versus despair? **Select all that apply.**
    1. Engage the client in social activities.
    2. Encourage the client to reminiscence.
    3. Provide the client with opportunities to make choices.
    4. Teach the client the importance of balancing exercise and rest.
    5. Give the client recognition for accomplishments attained during life.

14. Which activity associated with the American Nurses Association has the **greatest** impact on the quality of care provided by a nurse at a client's bedside?
    1. Accrediting nursing education programs
    2. Publishing standards of professional nursing practice
    3. Lobbying economic issues impacting on the profession of nursing
    4. Mentoring the professional development of future registered nurses

15. A client is scheduled to have an amputation of the left arm near the shoulder because of a crushing injury sustained during an accident. According to Maslow's hierarchy of needs, which human need does the nurse expect to be **most** affected?
    1. Safety
    2. Security
    3. Self-esteem
    4. Self-actualization

REVIEW ANSWERS AND RATIONALES

1. **ANSWER: 1.**

Rationales:

1. Approving nursing education programs, a role of the National League for Nursing Accrediting Commission, ensures that schools of nursing provide students with classroom and clinical experiences necessary to be prepared to take the National Council Licensing Examination.

2. The American Nurses Association, not the National League for Nursing Accrediting Commission, establishes standards of nursing practice.

3. Lobbying economic issues impacting on the profession of nursing is one of the activities of the American Nurses Association, not the National League for Nursing Accrediting Commission.

4. The National Student Nurses Association, not the National League for Nursing Accrediting Commission, mentors the professional development of future registered nurses.

Content Area: Evidenced-Based Practice
Integrated Processes: Nursing Process: Analysis
Client Need: Safe and Effective Care Environment; Management of Care
Cognitive Level: Comprehension
Concept: Professionalism

2. **ANSWER: 3, 4.**

Rationales:

1. Taking deep breaths after exercising is an example of a first-level need: meeting a physiological need.

2. Hanging a self-made painting in a senior center is an example of a fourth-level need: need for self-esteem.

3. Treating clients with respect displays acceptance and a satisfactory interpersonal relationship between the client and the nurse, both of which are related to love and belonging needs according to Maslow. Love and belonging are third-level needs.

4. Receiving weekly phone calls from adult children is an example of a third-level need: need for love and belonging. Love and belonging needs have a significant connection to family members.

5. A small light on at night provides enough illumination so that walking from the bedroom to the bathroom is safer than ambulating in the dark. Safety and security is a second-level need according to Maslow.

6. Removing scatter rugs after experiencing a fall in the home is an example of a second-level need: need for safety and security.

Content Area: Evidenced-Based Practice
Integrated Processes: Nursing Process: Implementation
Client Need: Safe and Effective Care Environment; Safety and Infection Control
Cognitive Level: Analysis
Concept: Evidenced-Based Practice

3. **ANSWER: 2.**

Rationales:

1. Supporting a client's need for self-esteem is a fourth-level need according to Maslow.

2. Providing information to a client about who is providing care and who and how to call for help when necessary supports the need to feel secure and safe. This is a second-level need according to Maslow.

3. Explaining when family can visit helps meet love and belonging needs, a third-level need according to Maslow.

4. Meeting a physiologic need, such as activity, nutrition, elimination, or oxygenation, is a first-level need according to Maslow.

Content Area: Evidenced-Based Practice
Integrated Processes: Communication and Documentation; Nursing Process: Implementation
Client Need: Safe and Effective Care Environment; Safety and Infection Control
Cognitive Level: Application
Concept: Evidenced-Based Practice

4. **ANSWER: 3.**

Rationales:

1. This statement is unrelated to the task of generativity versus self-absorption associated with middle adulthood.

2. This statement is unrelated to the task of generativity versus self-absorption associated with middle adulthood.

3. This statement is related to the task of generativity versus self-absorption associated with middle adulthood. This task is associated with giving back to the community.

4. This statement is unrelated to the task of generativity versus self-absorption associated with middle adulthood.

Content Area: Evidenced-Based Practice
Integrated Processes: Communication and Documentation; Nursing Process: Analysis
Client Need: Health Promotion and Maintenance
Cognitive Level: Analysis
Concept: Evidenced-Based Practice

5. **ANSWER: 1, 5.**

Rationales:

1. Closing the door to a client's room to reduce noise supports the physiological needs of rest and sleep.

2. Wearing sterile gloves when changing a client's dressing protects against exposure to infectious microorganisms, which meets a client's safety and security needs.

3. Lowering a client's bed to the lowest position helps to prevent a fall, which provides for the safety needs of the client.

4. Encouraging a parent to stay with a hospitalized child overnight supports the child's need to feel safe and secure as well as loved; it does not meet a client's physiological needs.

5. Providing assistive utensils helps a client meet nutritional needs. In addition, it should support self-esteem needs because a client may feel more independent.

Content Area: Evidenced-Based Practice
Integrated Processes: Nursing Process: Analysis
Client Need: Physiological Integrity; Basic Care and Comfort
Cognitive Level: Analysis
Concept: Evidenced-Based Practice

6. **ANSWER: 1.**

Rationales:

1. This statement is related to Dorothea Orem's care deficit theory of nursing. Orem stated that self-care is a purposeful learned behavior in response to a need.

2. This statement is related to Madeleine Leininger's culture care diversity and universality theory. She believed that transcultural care is a central and uniting feature of nursing.
3. This statement is related to Elizabeth Kübler-Ross's theory on death and dying. She believed that clients have commonalities of responses when coping with the diagnosis of a terminal illness.
4. This statement is related to Jean Piaget's cognitive development theory. He believed that thinking and reasoning developed through exposure to new experiences.
TEST-TAKING TIP: Identify the clang association. The word *nursing* in the stem and in option 1 is a clang association.
Content Area: Evidenced-Based Practice
Integrated Processes: Nursing Process: Analysis
Client Need: Health Promotion and Maintenance
Cognitive Level: Knowledge
Concept: Evidenced-Based Practice

7. ANSWER: 4.
Rationales:
1. This statement is associated with the role performance model of health and wellness.
2. This statement is associated with Abraham Maslow's hierarchy of basic human needs model of health and wellness.
3. This statement is associated with Sister Callista Roy's adaptation model of health and wellness.
4. This statement describes the purpose of H. L. Dunn's high-level wellness grid theory of health and wellness.
TEST-TAKING TIP: Identify the clang association. The word *health* in the stem and in option 4 is a clang association.
Content Area: Evidenced-Based Practice
Integrated Processes: Nursing Process: Analysis
Client Need: Safe and Effective Care Environment; Management of Care
Cognitive Level: Analysis
Concept: Evidenced-Based Practice

8. ANSWER: 3.
Rationales:
1. Seeking a prescription for oxygen is associated with a physiological need, which is a first-level need, according to Maslow's hierarchy of needs. In addition, seeking a prescription for oxygen is premature. The nurse should collect additional data, such as a decreased oxygen saturation level, before arriving at the conclusion that the client has an oxygen problem.
2. Oral fluid intake is associated with a physiological need, which is a first-level need, according to Maslow's hierarchy of needs.
3. Meeting a client's safety and security needs is a second-level need according to Maslow's hierarchy of needs. The client is not oriented to time or place and may not understand the instruction to call for assistance when getting out of bed. A bed alarm will alert the nurse that the client is attempting to get out of bed, and a caregiver can assist the client immediately.
4. Taking the client's vital signs every 4 hours is associated with assessing a person's physiological status, which is a first-level need, according to Maslow's hierarchy of needs.

TEST-TAKING TIP: Identify the equally plausible options. Options 1, 2, and 4 are related to physiological needs and are equally plausible. Option 3 is related to a need other than meeting a physiological need.
Content Area: Evidenced-Based Practice
Integrated Processes: Communication and Documentation; Nursing Process: Implementation
Client Need: Safe and Effective Care Environment; Management of Care
Cognitive Level: Analysis
Concept: Patient-Centered Care; Evidenced-Based Practice

9. ANSWER: 2, 4.
Rationales:
1. This response indicates mistrust of others, which may be associated with unsuccessful achievement of the task of trust versus mistrust related to Erik Erikson's theory of development.
2. This statement expresses regret. Regrets often leave a person with a feeling of loss or despair. Integrity versus despair is the task of the older adult.
3. This response indicates willfulness, which may be associated with unsuccessful achievement of the task of autonomy versus shame and doubt.
4. Integrity versus despair is the task of the older adult. The person reviews life experiences and is either encouraged and views life as meaningful or has a sense of loss and regret. Nonachievement of a goal, such as becoming a doctor, may leave a person with a sense of loss or regret.
5. This response indicates pessimism, which may be associated with unsuccessful resolution of the task of initiative versus guilt.
Content Area: Evidenced-Based Practice
Integrated Processes: Communication and Documentation; Nursing Process: Analysis
Client Need: Health Promotion and Maintenance
Cognitive Level: Analysis
Concept: Evidenced-Based Practice

10. ANSWER: 1, 3, 2, 5, 4.
Rationales:
1. The need for oxygen is a physiological need. Physiological needs are first-level needs according to Maslow's hierarchy of needs.
3. A client who reports feeling dizzy when moving to a standing position is experiencing hypotension, which increases the risk of a fall. A risk of falls is a safety issue and is a second-level need according to Maslow's hierarchy of needs.
2. Wanting to talk to his son is related to love and belonging needs. The need to belong and feel loved is a third-level need according to Maslow's hierarchy of needs.
5. When a person expresses feeling foolish, it indicates a loss of self-esteem. The need for self-esteem is a fourth-level need according to Maslow's hierarchy of needs.
4. Making an informed and realistic health-care decision is characteristic of a self-actualized person. Self-actualization is a fifth-level need according to Maslow's hierarchy of needs.

Content Area: *Evidenced-Based Practice*
Integrated Processes: *Nursing Process: Planning*
Client Need: *Safe and Effective Care Environment;*
Management of Care
Cognitive Level: *Analysis*
Concept: *Evidenced-Based Practice*

11. ANSWER: 1, 3.
Rationales:
1. The developmental stage of generativity versus stagnation is associated with the middle-adult years (ages 25 to 65). During these years people establish a family and promote the growth of others, particularly those in the next generation.
2. Development of peer relationships is associated with the developmental tasks of 6- to 12-year-old children, not middle-aged adults.
3. Successfully fulfilling lifelong goals involving family, parenthood, employment, and role in society is associated with the developmental task of middle adulthood.
4. Inability to postpone gratification is associated with the developmental task of an 18-month-old to 3-year-old child, not a middle-aged adult.
5. Confronting eventual death is associated with the developmental task of an adult 65 years of age or older, not a person in middle adulthood.
Content Area: *Evidenced-Based Practice*
Integrated Processes: *Nursing Process: Analysis*
Client Need: *Health Promotion and Maintenance*
Cognitive Level: *Analysis*
Concept: *Evidenced-Based Practice*

12. ANSWER: 1, 2, 3, 5.
Rationales:
1. Positioning a commode next to a client's bed provides for safety and security. The client can easily transfer from the bed to the commode and avoid walking to the bathroom at night, which may precipitate a fall.
2. Teaching a client how to transfer from the bed to a chair includes actions that provide for safety. For example, teaching a client to sit on the side of the bed until the blood pressure adjusts to the change in position will minimize dizziness and the potential for a fall that may occur if the person stands up too quickly.
3. This action supports a client's safety and security needs. Placing a client's dentures in a labeled denture cup in the bedside table secures the dentures in a safe place with the client's name.
4. Assessing and implementing nursing actions to address urinary retention is associated with the basic physiological need of urinary elimination, not a safety and security need.
5. This action meets the safety and security needs of a client who has a low white blood cell count and is at risk for an infection. A mask will protect the client from exposure to microorganisms while being transported for an x-ray.
Content Area: *Evidenced-Based Practice*
Integrated Processes: *Nursing Process: Analysis*
Client Need: *Safe and Effective Care Environment; Safety and Infection Control*

Cognitive Level: *Analysis*
Concept: *Evidenced-Based Practice*

13. ANSWER: 2, 5.
Rationales:
1. Although engaging the client in social activities is important, it is not the intervention that will help the client achieve the major task associated with the older adult.
2. Acceptance of one's worth and viewing one's life as meaningful is the task of the older adult. Engaging the older adult in reminiscing enables the client to discuss his or her past life and develop a sense of satisfaction with the life that was lived. Additional tasks of this age group include adjusting to physical decline and losses, establishing new roles, and preparing for death.
3. Although providing the client with opportunities to make choices is important because it supports self-esteem, it is not the intervention that will help the client achieve the major task associated with the older adult.
4. Although teaching the client about balancing exercise, rest, and sleep is important, it is not the intervention that will help the client achieve the major task associated with the older adult.
5. Expressing appreciation for a client's life accomplishments allows the client to view the past life as meaningful. People often develop self-respect and a sense of integrity when respected by others. The developmental stage of the older adult is integrity versus despair.
Content Area: *Evidenced-Based Practice*
Integrated Processes: *Caring; Communication and Documentation; Nursing Process: Implementation*
Client Need: *Health Promotion and Maintenance*
Cognitive Level: *Application*
Concept: *Evidenced-Based Practice*

14. ANSWER: 2.
Rationales:
1. The National League for Nursing Accreditation Commission for Education in Nursing, American Association of Colleges of Nursing, and Commission on Collegiate Nursing Education are responsible for accrediting nursing educational programs, not the American Nurses Association.
2. The American Nurses Association establishes standards of nursing practice, which is the component of their responsibilities that has the greatest impact on a nurse's daily practice.
3. Although this is one of the activities of the American Nurses Association, another option has the *greatest* impact on the quality of nursing care delivered at the bedside.
4. The National Student Nurses Association mentors the professional development of future registered nurses, not the American Nurses Association.
TEST-TAKING TIP: Identify the word in the stem that sets a priority. The word *greatest* is the word in the stem that sets a priority.
Content Area: *Evidenced-Based Practice*
Integrated Processes: *Communication and Documentation; Nursing Process: Analysis*

Client Need: Safe and Effective Care Environment; Management of Care
Cognitive Level: Comprehension
Concept: Evidenced-Based Practice

15. ANSWER: 3.

Rationales:

1. Although clients who sustain an amputation of a limb may believe that they are less able to provide for their own safety, it is not the human need that the nurse should anticipate to be most affected.

2. Although clients who sustain an amputation of a limb may believe that they are less able to provide for their own security, it is not the human need that the nurse should anticipate to be most affected.

3. Self-esteem, self-concept, and body-image are interrelated. Body image is how people perceive the appearance and function of their bodies. It includes the value of the body part to a person, the importance of the body part in culture and society, and the degree to which the person's body resembles his or her ideal body. Loss of a body part, as with an amputation of a limb, often challenges a person's self-esteem and the way in which the *self* is viewed.

4. Although clients who sustain an amputation of a limb may believe that this event will interfere with their ability to achieve self-actualization, it is not the human need that the nurse should anticipate to be most affected.

TEST-TAKING TIP: Identify the word in the stem that sets a priority. The word *most* in the stem sets a priority. Identify the equally plausible options. Options 1 and 2 are equally plausible because both reflect Maslow's second-level needs, safety and security.

Content Area: Evidenced-Based Practice
Integrated Processes: Nursing Process: Analysis
Client Need: Psychosocial Integrity
Cognitive Level: Application
Concept: Evidenced-Based Practice

Chapter 8

Teaching and Learning

NURSING CONCEPTS

Cognition
Communication
Culture
Growth and Development

Health Promotion
Patient-Centered Care
Self
Sensory Perception

KEY TERMS

Affective domain (feeling)—Learning that deals with changes in feelings, beliefs, attitudes, and values

Auditory learner—A person who learns by hearing

Cognitive domain (thinking)—Learning that deals with acquiring, storing, and recalling information

External locus of control—A desire to achieve a goal because of recognition or reward outside the self

Goal—A desired outcome that is client-centered, realistic, measurable, and time bound

Internal locus of control—A desire from within the self to achieve a goal

Kinesthetic learner—A person who learns by touch and manipulation

Learning—An active process that involves assimilation of information that produces the acquisition of new attitudes, behaviors, or skills

Long-term goal—Desired outcome that can be obtained within weeks to months

Motivation—Driving force that produces an action or promotes the achievement of a goal

Psychomotor domain (doing)—Learning that deals with attaining a new skill that requires both mental and physical activity

Role playing—Acting out of a character in a protective environment to practice a response that can be used when confronted with a similar situation in real life

Short-term goal—Desired outcome that can be obtained within hours or days

Teaching—An interactive process that promotes acquisition of new information, attitudes, or skills

Visual learner—A person who learns by processing information with the eyes

I. Introduction

Teaching is an interactive process that promotes acquisition of new information, attitudes, or skills. It involves steps that mirror the steps of the nursing process (assessment, analysis, planning, implementation, and evaluation). **Learning** is an active process that involves assimilation of information that produces the acquisition of new attitudes, behaviors, or skills. These activities help to promote wellness, prevent illness, and facilitate the acquisition of coping strategies to restore health or function.

A. Purposes of teaching and learning
   1. Wellness promotion.
      a. Presents information and skills that support and develop health practices.
      b. Examples: Information about health, nutrition, exercise, and hygiene; prenatal and parenting classes.

2. Illness prevention.
   a. Presents information and skills that promote early detection or prevention of disease and disability.
   b. Examples: Information about risk factors of disease; dietary teaching to decrease the risk of cancer; information about immunizations, smoking cessation, and safe use of car seat restraining devices for infants and children.
3. Promotion of coping strategies.
   a. Presents information and skills that enable a client to better cope emotionally and physically with a new diagnosis, interventions, impaired function, or loss of a loved one.
   b. Examples: Information about using a walker safely, using an assistive device to eat, walking with a prosthesis, coping with role expectations, managing care for a loved one at home, coping with death and dying, administering a gastrostomy tube feeding, managing stress.
4. Restoration of health or function.
   a. Presents information and skills that enable a client to manage a current health problem, focusing on etiology, medical condition, treatment, and strategies to meet client needs.

   b. Examples: Information about self-injecting insulin, employing preoperative and postoperative interventions to prevent complications of surgery, and caring for a wound drain.
B. Learning domains
   1. People learn through three different domains.
      a. **Cognitive domain:** Thinking.
      b. **Affective domain:** Feeling.
      c. **Psychomotor domain:** Doing.
   2. Each domain requires the use of specific strategies that best promote learning. (See Table 8.1 for more information on learning domains and ways to tailor nursing strategies to those domains.)

II. Individual Factors That Influence Learning

People learn in different ways, such as by seeing, hearing, and touching. Learning is motivated by either an internal desire to achieve a goal (internal locus of control) or a desire to receive external recognition or a reward (external locus of control). In addition, people primarily use information-processing functions from either the left hemisphere (logical thinking) or right hemisphere (intuitive thinking) of the brain. The way in which learning occurs is never identical for two different people and is

---

Table 8.1 Understanding Learning Domains

Domain and Definition	Nursing Strategies

Cognitive (Thinking Domain)
• Deals with acquiring, storing, and recalling information
• Involves intellectual thinking that demonstrates increasing complexity:
  – Knowing, such as memorizing and recalling
  – Comprehending
  – Analyzing
  – Synthesizing
  – Applying and evaluating ideas
• Example outcome: Client is able to verbalize the differences between regular and NPH insulin
	• Lecture
	• Written material
	• Panel discussion
	• Audiovisual materials
	• Programmed instruction
	• Computer-assisted instruction
	• Case studies
	• Care plans
	• Evaluate learning by seeking oral or written feedback

Affective (Feeling Domain) • Deals with changes in feelings, beliefs, attitudes, and values • Involves increasing the depth of emotional response to tasks, receiving and responding to new ideas, demonstrating commitment to new ideas, and integrating new ideas into one's value system • Behavioral changes commonly emerge slowly after intellectual understanding is internalized • Example outcome: Client maintains a diabetic diet	• Panel discussion • Role modeling • One-to-one counseling • Support groups • Evaluate learning by observing behavioral changes that reflect beliefs, feelings, and values
Psychomotor (Skill Domain) • Deals with learning a new skill that requires both mental and physical activity • Involves sensory awareness of cues, imitation, and performance of new skills • Example outcome: Client is able to self-administer insulin, maintaining principles of asepsis	• Demonstration • Return demonstration • Audiovisual materials • Printed material with illustrations • Evaluate learning by seeking a return demonstration

not identical for one person in different situations. Therefore, nurses must consider these factors when engaged in the teaching/learning process.

A. Learning styles

1. **Visual learners.**
   a. Learn best by processing information with the eyes.
   b. Examples: Use of pictures, illustrations, photographs, models, and videos.

2. **Auditory learners.**
   a. Learn best by processing information by listening to words.
   b. Examples: Use of verbal instructions, discussions, and videos with verbal commentary.

3. **Kinesthetic learners.**
   a. Learn best when processing information by doing.
   b. Examples: Engage in physical activities and allow touching and handling of equipment.

B. Locus of control

1. **Internal locus of control.**
   a. Clients are motivated from within and hold themselves responsible for actions and consequences.
   b. Example: A person loses weight because of a desire to personally achieve the goals of improved health and appearance.

2. **External locus of control.**
   a. Clients are motivated by pressure or rewards from outside the self.
   b. Example: A person loses weight because a significant other places pressure on the client, such as praise, guilt, or rewards.

III. Principles of Teaching and Learning and Related Nursing Care

Implementing client education requires the nurse to assume the role of teacher. As a teacher, a nurse should use universal principles that guide client teaching, regardless of the content being taught or the personal factors of learners. However, when a client presents with specialized needs, these common universal principles should be augmented by individualized interventions that address the client's specific needs.

A. Learning takes place within the learner

1. Support learning because it is a continuous process of growth throughout life.

2. Understand that learning occurs when the need to learn is relevant to the learner.

3. Assess understanding of the health problem; build a teaching plan based on developing what is already known and then moving on to the unknown. Use examples to which the client can relate.

4. Recognize that the ability and speed at which one learns depends on the individual.

5. Match teaching strategies to the client's learning style and learning needs.

6. Accept that a teacher only facilitates learning.

B. Motivation facilitates learning

1. **Motivation** is the driving force that produces an action or promotes the achievement of a goal.

2. Identify behaviors that indicate the client's readiness to learn.
   a. Acknowledging a need and believing that the need can be met through learning.
   b. Demonstrating health-seeking behaviors, such as asking questions, attempting to participate in own care, and requesting reading material or referrals to support groups.
   c. Believing that the information to be learned has value.
   d. Believing that identified goals are attainable.

3. Identify behaviors that indicate the client's lack of readiness to learn.
   a. Exhibiting moderate to high anxiety: Identify level of anxiety and promote expression of feelings and concerns.
   b. Exhibiting behaviors that indicate avoidance, denial, or lack of participation in own care: Accept where the client is at and support the client emotionally until ready to participate in the teaching/learning process.
   c. Expressing presence of pain: Medicate the client to address pain before the teaching session or postpone the session because the client's physiological status can impede concentration and energy.

4. Begin teaching and learning activities as soon as the need is identified by the nurse or client and as soon as possible, such as on admission to the agency.

5. Formulate a learning contract with the client that includes both short- and long-term goals. **Short-term goals** are desired outcomes that can be obtained within hours or days **Long-term goals** are desired outcomes that can be obtained within weeks to months.
   a. **Goals** should be client centered, realistic, measurable, and time bound.
   b. Short-term goals provide more opportunities for achievement that supports motivation.
   c. Learning contracts support mutual respect and responsibility.

6. Provide prompt feedback.

7. Identify progress, and employ rewards and incentives for goal achievement.

8. Understand that discussing potential complications may provoke mild anxiety that can increase motivation.

🛑 9. Avoid using fear tactics (e.g., "Unless you stop smoking, you may get lung cancer") to motivate a client.

10. Identify and investigate the cause of nonachievement of goals. Recognize that nonadherence to a treatment regimen may be due to the presence of competing incentives rather than a lack of motivation; for example, learning new ways to achieve independence may be less important than the gains related to continuing in the sick role.

11. Modify the teaching plan according to the client's progress and changing needs.

MAKING THE CONNECTION

Client Behavior and the Reason for Behavior

Many health-care professionals report that a client is "noncompliant" or "uncooperative" when goals are not met. However, nonachievement of goals can be due to reasons other than the client ignoring the benefits of learning. For example, economics, lack of understanding, and negative side effects of therapy can all cause a client to not adhere to a treatment regimen. **All behavior has meaning,** and a logical connection exists between client behavior and the reasons for the behavior. To identify the true cause of failure to meet outcome goals, nurses must first identify client behaviors or statements that indicate nonadherence to a plan of care, and then they must explore the etiology of the nonadherence. In addition, the terms *noncompliant* and *uncooperative* should never be used when describing or documenting client behavior; failure to meet outcome goals should be described, and the reasons for the behavior should be explored and identified.

C. Teaching strategies must be appropriate for the client's developmental and cognitive levels
  1. According to Piaget, cognitive development progresses through three levels.
     a. Age 2 to 7 years: Find meaning through use of symbols and pictures.
     b. Age 7 to 11 years: Have logical thinking and understand relationships.
     c. Age 11 and older: Use abstract thinking and deductive reasoning.
  2. Use teaching strategies that are appropriate for the learner's gross and fine motor development when teaching psychomotor skills.
  3. Use teaching strategies that are appropriate for the learner's level of intellectual ability.
  4. Encourage participation in the teaching/learning process; recognize that adults prefer to be partners in this process.

5. Encourage independence; recognize that adults are more independent and self-directed than are children.
  6. Reinforce that one is never too old to learn; recognize that adults may believe that they are too old to learn, fear failure, or feel threatened and therefore resist change.
  7. Identify and build on positive past learning experiences; recognize that adults have previous life experiences that can hinder or enhance learning.
  8. Build repetition into the teaching plan; recognize that older adults might take longer to learn than younger adults do, but they *are* able to learn.

D. Teaching must be consistent with the client's cultural and religious beliefs
  1. Understand that culture and religion influence beliefs, values, and behaviors; identify factors, such as customs and taboos, that can influence content to be taught or teaching strategies to be used.
  2. Identify whether the client is the decision maker; be aware that, in some cultures, women are not allowed to make decisions, and therefore the decision maker in the family should be included in teaching sessions.
  3. Identify behaviors that may be culturally related, such as avoiding eye contact to demonstrate respect and smiling and nodding the head to indicate that teaching is understood, even if it is not, so as not to embarrass the nurse.
  4. Respect and accept a client's values and beliefs; incorporate them into the learning plan unless they are unsafe.

🛑 5. Use humor cautiously; the intended meaning may be lost in translation by a client from a different culture, or a client may consider the comment condescending rather than funny.

E. Learning occurs best in an environment that is physically and emotionally conducive to learning
  1. Schedule teaching so that it does not interfere with rest, meals, tests, and treatments; when appropriate, schedule sessions when a family member can be present to offer support and also learn what is being taught.
  2. Determine appropriate teaching session length and frequency on the basis of the client's condition, such as attention span or activity tolerance.
     a. Short, more frequent sessions are better than long, infrequent sessions.
     b. Enough time should occur between sessions so that information can be absorbed and applied.
  3. Provide an environment that is private, quiet, and free from distractions and interruptions.

4. Ensure that the environment is physically comfortable.
   a. Room temperature should not be too hot or too cold.
   b. Lighting should be adequate and free from glare.
5. Ensure that the environment is emotionally comfortable and provides privacy; close the door, pull the curtain, and drape the client appropriately when teaching personal physical skills.
6. Identify the client's level of anxiety; be aware that mild anxiety enhances motivation and learning, whereas moderate and higher levels of anxiety impede learning; teaching sessions may have to be shortened or postponed depending on the client's level of anxiety.
7. Emphasize what is most important to know first for a client who is very ill because fatigue shortens teaching sessions.
8. Address the client's fears and concerns before beginning teaching and learning activities.
F. Literacy, language, and communication are essential components of the teaching and learning process
   1. Commonalities of nursing care related to literacy, language, and communication.
      a. Use a variety of teaching strategies to present information; stimulate as many of the senses as possible, such as hearing, vision, and touch.
      b. Use short, simple words and sentences; speak clearly and slowly; use words the client understands; and avoid clichés, slang words, colloquialisms, medical jargon, abbreviations, and ambiguous words.
      c. Present information so that it progresses with increasing complexity, such as simple to complex and known to unknown.
      d. Pace teaching sessions so that learning is achieved before moving on to the next concept; identify whether teaching is too fast or too slow and modify the pace accordingly.
      e. Build repetition of information into the teaching plan; repetition reinforces learning.
      f. Provide written materials that have many drawings, photographs, and illustrations; avoid handouts with large amounts of written information.
      g. Document teaching interventions and learning progress; be aware that some facilities have teaching and learning activity forms that document progress and are signed by both teacher and learner.
   2. Nursing care specific to literacy.
      a. Understand that literacy involves the ability to use print and written information to function

in society to develop one's knowledge and potential and achieve one's goals.
      b. Never assume that a client is literate.

DID YOU KNOW?

Many illiterate adults in the United States hide the fact that they cannot read or write. However, illiteracy in the United States is widespread. Consider these facts: Sixty-three million adults older than age 16 do not read well enough to understand a newspaper story written at the eighth-grade level. An additional 30 million can read at only a fifth-grade level or lower. Forty-three percent of adults with the lowest literacy rates in the United States live in poverty.

      c. Assess a client's ability to read.
      d. Teach at the fifth-grade level, and move up levels as appropriate.
      e. Check the reading level of presented written materials and ensure that it is at the level of the client's ability; most educational materials are written at the high-school level, which can be challenging for some clients to read.
   3. Nursing care specific to language.
      a. Determine whether the client clearly understands English.
      b. Use a professional interpreter if the client does not understand English because clients have a right to be taught in a language that they understand. The Joint Commission mandates the use of interpreters for non–English-speaking clients.
         (1) Employ the use of a language line service, whereby a bilingual operator provides translation, if available.
         (2) Do not use family members as interpreters because information must be communicated accurately, objectively, and confidentially.
         (3) Talk to and look at the client when using an interpreter.
      c. Provide information in written and audio formats in the client's language.
   4. Nursing care specific to communication.
      a. Understand that teaching requires effective interpersonal verbal and nonverbal interaction.
         (1) Teaching can be formal or informal.
         (2) Teaching can be planned or spontaneous.
         (3) Teaching can be performed with an individual or with a group.
      b. Encourage the client to ask questions and to write down questions that arise between teaching sessions.

c. See "Nursing Care Related to Communication" in Chapter 2, Communication, Collaboration, and Documentation.

IV. Special Needs Populations Require Specific Teaching Strategies

A. Clients who have visual impairments.
1. Encourage use of prescription eyeglasses.
2. Provide written material in large print.
3. Provide special equipment or learning materials, such as prefilled or automatic-stop syringes, Braille learning materials, and audio learning materials.
4. See "Clients Who Are Visually Impaired" in Chapter 2, Communication, Collaboration, and Documentation.

B. Clients who have hearing impairments.
1. Encourage the use of hearing aids.
2. Talk toward the client's ear with the most acute hearing.
3. Speak slightly louder than normal, but do not yell.
4. Face the client when speaking; speak slowly and enunciate each word clearly, but do not overly enunciate each word because doing so can interfere with lip reading.
5. See "Clients Who Are Hearing Impaired" in Chapter 2, Communication, Collaboration, and Documentation.

C. Clients who have sensory or motor impairments.
1. Understand that sensory and motor impairments interfere with learning psychomotor skills.
2. Plan more practice time for clients with sensory or motor impairments, such as neuropathy or hemiplegia.
3. Teach clients to use assistive devices to facilitate psychomotor skills when appropriate.

V. Teaching Strategies

The selection of an instructional approach should be based on a client's educational needs and personal factors, the time available for teaching, and the resources available. Each instructional approach has advantages, disadvantages, and related specific nursing actions. To maximize learning, nurses should use a variety of teaching approaches.

A. Lecture
1. A *lecture* presents information verbally and may be accompanied by written material.
2. Advantages.
   a. Is cost effective.
   b. Is easy to use with large groups.
3. Disadvantages.
   a. Does not permit individualization of the material.

b. Is not effective in the psychomotor or affective domains.
c. Can be a challenging format for a person with impaired hearing as well as for visual learners unless additional teaching strategies are used.
4. Nursing care.
   a. Provide time for discussion at the end of the program.
   b. Provide time for additional questions and answers and to correct misconceptions.

B. One-to-one discussion
1. A *one-to-one discussion* allows the teacher and learner to talk about content to be learned without interference from another learner.
2. Advantages.
   a. Allows for development of a relationship with the learner.
   b. Is learner-centered.
   c. Allows time for frequent feedback.
   d. Is effective in all three learning domains.
3. Disadvantages.
   a. Can be labor intensive.
   b. Isolates the learner from others who may provide support.
4. Nursing care.
   a. Use for clients who have special learning needs, such as cognitive or sensory impairment, learning disability, mental illness, and activity intolerance.
   b. Individualize the program to meet the learner's needs.

C. Demonstration
1. A *demonstration* involves hands-on manipulation of equipment with time to practice a skill.
2. Advantages.
   a. Is effective for teaching psychomotor skills.
   b. Can be used with small groups.
3. Disadvantages.
   a. Is not effective with large groups.
   b. Is time consuming and labor intensive.
4. Nursing care.
   a. Demonstrate each step slowly and accurately; move on to the next step only after it is determined that the previous step is mastered via return demonstration.
   b. Allow adequate time to practice the skill within and between teaching sessions.

D. Groups (instructional and support)
1. A *group* consists of two or more individuals interacting, thereby enhancing learning with the exchange of information.
2. Advantages.
   a. Is effective when teaching in the affective domain.
   b. Promotes interaction among participants.

3. Disadvantages.
   a. Occurs in a less-structured environment that allows for unexpected responses by group members.
   b. Is not effective for the psychomotor domain.
4. Nursing care.
   a. Use when participant interaction is desired so that learners learn from each other; learners can share ideas, foster development of positive attitudes, solve problems, and offer solutions to each other.
   b. Function as a group facilitator to keep the group on task.

E. Role playing
1. **Role playing** is the acting out of a character in a protected environment to practice a response that can be used when confronted with a similar situation in real life.
2. Advantages.
   a. Offers a safe environment to rehearse and practice responses before being confronted with a real-life situation.
   b. Raises issues that can be pursued through discussion.
3. Disadvantages.
   a. May be uncomfortable for people who are too embarrassed or feel awkward engaging in role playing.
   b. May increase anxiety when emotionally charged areas are explored.
4. Nursing care.
   a. Set an example by demonstrating behaviors or attitudes that should be learned.
   b. Establish the situation so that participants involved in the role playing develop an understanding of the principles to be learned.
   c. Recognize when an increase in anxiety occurs and provide emotional support.

VI. Teaching Tools

The selection of a teaching tool should be based on a client's educational needs and personal factors, the time available for teaching, and the resources available. Each teaching tool has advantages, disadvantages, and related nursing care. To maximize learning, nurses should use a variety of teaching tools.

A. Printed materials
1. *Printed materials* present information in a written format; they support comprehension of complex concepts and relationships.
2. Include materials such as pamphlets, booklets, brochures, drawings, and charts.
3. Advantages.
   a. Allow for standardization of information.
   b. Can be read at learner's own pace.

   c. Are efficient.
   d. Can be provided in the client's first language.
4. Disadvantages.
   a. Cannot be used with clients who are illiterate.
   b. Cannot be used with clients who have visual impairments unless the materials are in large print or Braille.
5. Nursing care.
   a. Ensure that the learner is literate and able to see.
   b. Provide materials in the primary language of the learner.
   c. Use printed materials especially for clients who are visual learners.
   d. Ensure that printed materials are easy to read, current, and accurate.
   e. Use charts to present key points because charts provide easy retrieval of highly condensed information.

B. Programmed instruction
1. *Programmed instruction* presents information in a "frame" and requires a response before the learner can move onto the next frame; some programmed instructions are linear and some are branching.
2. Includes computer programs, programmed textbooks, and booklets.
3. Advantages.
   a. Allows learners to proceed at their own pace.
   b. Requires learners to be actively engaged in learning.
   c. Provides immediate feedback for right and wrong answers.
   d. Allows for efficient use of a teacher's time.
4. Disadvantages.
   a. Is not as stimulating as an audiovisual-type presentation.
   b. Requires a motivated, independent learner.
5. Nursing care.
   a. Teach the learner how to use the program.
   b. Explain that the program is a written sequential presentation of learning steps that actively engages the learner in the learning process.
   c. Teach that programmed instruction is designed so that the learner can proceed at his or her own pace as well as receive immediate feedback for right and wrong answers.

C. Audiovisual aids
1. *Audiovisual aids* present information that stimulates both the eyes and ears.
2. Include CD programs, computer apps, and videos.
3. Advantages.
   a. Stimulate the hearing and sight of the learner.
   b. Can be used with individuals or large groups.
4. Disadvantages.
   a. May require expensive equipment, such as computers and software.

b. Require participants to be able to hear or see material being presented.

c. Require a large room when being presented to a large group.

5. Nursing care.

   a. Ensure that all participants have adequate hearing and vision and are positioned to see and hear the material presented.

   b. Use audiovisual aids for all clients but especially for auditory learners or individuals with literacy issues.

   c. Use audiotapes for clients who have visual impairments.

D. Equipment and models

1. *Equipment and models* provide hands-on items that can be observed, touched, and sometimes utilized.

   a. Models provide a two- or three-dimensional representation of subject matter that can be observed and touched.

   b. A piece of equipment may be the actual apparatus that is the focus of the teaching session.

2. Includes materials such as a skeleton, heart model, manikin for CPR, simulation manikin used to mimic clinical situations, various catheters, and syringes.

3. Advantages.

   a. Are effective in teaching kinesthetic learners.

   b. Are effective when teaching psychomotor skills.

4. Disadvantages.

   a. Are expensive.

   b. Require storage.

5. Nursing care.

   a. Use for clients who are kinesthetic learners because it allows for manipulation of objects.

   b. Use for clients who are learning psychomotor skills to promote transfer of information from the brain (cognitive learning) to the hands (psychomotor learning).

   c. Use to provide visual reinforcement of verbally presented information.

   d. Employ to teach use of new equipment and related skills presented in continuing education or in-service programs for health-care professionals.

E. Internet

1. The *Internet* provides immediate access to a vast amount of information using a computer connected to the Internet.

2. Advantages.

   a. Is entertaining, informative, and convenient.

   b. Offers a diversity of resources, including electronic learning platforms, search engines, electronic libraries, content portals, and social networking such as chat rooms, bulletin boards, and blogs that offer sharing of information, counseling, and support.

3. Disadvantages.

   a. Exposes the learner to information that might not be accurate, reliable, or current and content that is unregulated.

   b. May require the learner to read above a fifth-grade reading level.

   c. Can be accessed without input from a knowledgeable health-care professional.

4. Nursing care.

   a. Ensure that the learner knows how to access the Internet.

   b. Teach the learner ways to evaluate the reliability of a site, such as by determining whether an author or organization is reputable and using readily available checklists to assess the quality of a Web site.

   c. Encourage the learner to access recommended, quality Web sites.

   d. Review the suitability of a site before making a client referral.

F. Computer-assisted instruction

1. *Computer-assisted instruction* works like a programmed text in that a frame requires a response before the learner moves to the next frame; however, has more capabilities than a linear approach and can branch to a multiple number of responses based on the learner's response and is therefore significantly more interactive and individualized.

2. Advantages.

   a. Allows the learner to proceed at his or her own pace.

   b. Usually includes interactive activities to engage the learner.

   c. Commonly includes pretests and posttests so that learning can be self-evaluated.

   d. Is convenient if the client has a personal computer.

   e. Allows the teacher to design a learning prescription and/or corrective action plan that addresses a learner's specific learning needs.

3. Disadvantages.

   a. Requires access to a computer.

   b. Client may not be computer literate.

   c. Can be costly for an agency if it provides the computers.

4. Nursing care.

   a. Teach the learner how to use the computer to access the learning program software.

   b. Use when a learner response pattern is desired to select future lessons.

CASE STUDY: Putting It All Together

A man who is unconscious is brought to the emergency department by his wife. The client has type 2 diabetes and has had the flu for a week. The client is diagnosed with ketoacidosis and is admitted to the hospital to correct fluid and electrolyte imbalances and receive insulin therapy. While being interviewed by the nurse after regaining consciousness, the client says repeatedly, "I can't believe I have to take insulin. No one in my family who has diabetes has to take insulin."

Later, the nurse has a discussion with the client about what he knows about diabetes and gives the client printed materials. The nurse meets with the client every day to discuss diabetes and to explore the client's feelings and concerns. Eventually, the nurse teaches the client how to perform self-blood glucose monitoring (SBGM) and how to perform a subcutaneous injection using a model of an abdomen. The nutritionist performs dietary counseling, and the nurse reviews the principles of a diabetic diet with the client at mealtimes. At discharge, the nurse schedules a follow-up visit with the diabetes counseling center.

The client misses this visit, so the nurse in the counseling center telephones him and schedules a new appointment. The client attends the appointment accompanied by his wife. He states, "My wife would kill me if I didn't come this time." When reviewing the client's self-care diary, the nurse identifies that the client takes the morning dose of insulin but is inconsistent with monitoring blood glucose levels and administering insulin during the day. When exploring these issues, the client says, "My wife doesn't let me out of the house unless I take the insulin. But I am not going to give myself insulin at work where everyone can see." The client's wife says, "He's had type 2 diabetes for several years, but he didn't take his pills consistently then and he doesn't take his insulin consistently now, never does the fingerstick test, and eats anything he wants. I make good meals at home, but I can't control what he does at work."

Most of the visit focuses on exploring the client's feelings and concerns. Eventually, the nurse reviews and demonstrates the procedures for SBGM and self-administration of a subcutaneous injection and has the client perform return demonstrations. At the end of the visit, the client tells the nurse, "I learn new things better if I can actually do what I am supposed to do." The nurse gives the client additional booklets with illustrations and a CD about these procedures. The nurse also recommends that the client attend a support group at the counseling center and gives the client a schedule of meetings.

Case Study Questions

A. What learning domains did the nurse address in the teaching sessions? Give examples.

1. _____

2. _____

3. _____

B. Identify and explore individual factors related to teaching and learning that the client exhibited in this scenario.

1. _____

2. _____

C. What data demonstrated that the client lacked readiness to learn?

1. _____

2. _____

3. _____

continued.

CASE STUDY: Putting It All Together

cont'd

Case Study Questions

D. What teaching and learning principles did the nurse use in this scenario?

1. _____

2. _____

3. _____

4. _____

E. What specific teaching strategies did the nurse use when teaching this client, and what were the advantages of these teaching strategies for this client?

1. _____

2. _____

3. _____

F. What teaching tools did the nurse use, and what are the advantages of each?

1. _____

2. _____

3. _____

_____

REVIEW QUESTIONS

Be sure to read the Introduction for valuable test-taking tips.

1. A nurse is evaluating client outcomes associated with managing a urinary retention catheter in the home. Which planned outcomes indicate learning in the cognitive domain? **Select all that apply.**
   1. Client demonstrates effective perineal care.
   2. Client accepts requiring a tube to empty his bladder.
   3. Client explains why a urinary retention catheter should be kept below the bladder.
   4. Client identifies three actions that help reduce the risk of a urinary tract infection.
   5. Client empties the contents of the collection bag without contaminating the entire system.

2. A nurse is planning to educate an adult client newly diagnosed with diabetes regarding self-blood glucose monitoring and performing an insulin injection. Which interventions are **most** helpful? **Select all that apply.**
   1. Show the client a video about self-blood glucose monitoring and then discuss the video with the client.
   2. Demonstrate self-blood glucose monitoring and then have the client perform a return demonstration.
   3. Provide a pamphlet that explains these skills and then discuss them.
   4. Have another client with this illness teach the client these skills.
   5. Use abstract statements while educating the client.

3. Which nursing intervention **best** promotes a client's adherence to a medication regimen?
   1. Instruct the client to take the medication as prescribed or the primary health-care provider will discharge the client from treatment.
   2. Provide information about the safety of the medication as indicated by the Food and Drug Administration.
   3. Warn that if the medication is not taken, the illness will get worse.
   4. Explain how the medication can reduce the client's illness.

4. A female nurse is assessing a client's readiness to learn a self-help skill. What client factors alert the nurse that the teaching session should be postponed? **Select all that apply.**
   1. Male gender
   2. 75-year-old adult
   3. High anxiety level
   4. Pain of 5 on a 0-to-10 scale
   5. Graduated only from grammar school

5. A nurse is caring for a client from Spain who experienced a hypertensive crisis while on vacation in the United States. The client knows only a few words of English. What is **most** important when planning an educational session about nutrients that are high in sodium?
   1. Providing a professional interpreter fluent in Spanish
   2. Securing written material in Spanish from the Internet
   3. Using the technique of demonstration when teaching information
   4. Showing pictures of foods that should be avoided to lower blood pressure

6. A nurse is evaluating client outcomes associated with learning about hypertension and self-care. Which outcomes indicate success in the psychomotor domain? **Select all that apply.**
   1. Client explains how to interpret the serving size on a food label to calculate the caloric value of the nutrient.
   2. Client is able to identify five foods high in salt that should be avoided when on a low sodium diet.
   3. Client is able to accurately obtain a blood pressure reading using a sphygmomanometer.
   4. Client can divide daily doses of multiple medications in a weekly pill dispensing box.
   5. Client adheres to a weight-reduction diet, as evidenced by a weekly 2-lb weight loss.

7. A client is admitted to an alcohol rehabilitation program. On admission, the client states, "I'm here because it is what I have to do to get my license back." What is motivating this client to participate in the rehabilitation program? **Select all that apply.**
   1. An internal locus of control
   2. An external locus of control
   3. A desire to achieve a personal goal
   4. The need to fulfill a legal requirement
   5. The desire to regain control over the problem

8. A nurse is evaluating the outcome of a teaching program presented to a client newly diagnosed with diabetes. Which outcomes indicate learning in the affective domain? **Select all that apply.**
   1. Maintains a diabetic diet
   2. Can safely draw up insulin into a syringe
   3. Verbalizes the difference between short- and long-acting insulin
   4. Identifies clinical indicators of hyperglycemia and hypoglycemia
   5. Believes that adhering to the plan to manage the diabetes is achievable

9. Which strategy increases the probability that learning essential information will be achieved?
   1. Postponing a teaching session if the client appears mildly anxious
   2. Using a formal rather than an informal approach to teaching
   3. Emphasizing information that is most important first
   4. Setting room temperature on the cool side

10. A nurse is to prepare a client who has a moderate intellectual disability for a procedure. Which approaches will be **most** effective for the nurse to plan to use with this client? **Select all that apply.**
    1. Demonstrate the procedure.
    2. Describe the procedure in writing.
    3. Use pictures to describe the procedure.
    4. Provide a preprinted booklet that accurately describes the procedure.
    5. Use group instruction with other clients who are going to have the same procedure.

11. A nurse is caring for a client who emigrated from a foreign country. The nurse teaches the client how to perform a wall-climbing exercise with the affected arm after a mastectomy. Later, the nurse sees the client attempting to perform the exercise, and a family member is attempting to hold her arm down. What might be the nurse's **most** accurate conclusion?
    1. Family member's place within the family system allows control over others.
    2. Family member thinks that the client is performing the exercise incorrectly.
    3. Family member's cultural beliefs may not conform to the exercise regimen.
    4. Family member has intimidated the client.

12. Place the following steps in the order in which they should be performed by a nurse when developing a teaching plan?
    1. Establish readiness.
    2. Select teaching tools.
    3. Determine motivation.
    4. Ascertain level of ability.
    5. Provide an appropriate environment.
    Answer: _____

13. A nurse is planning to teach a weight-loss diet to an adolescent who is obese. What concept related to adolescence is **most** important when attempting to motivate this client to learn how to lose weight?
    1. Enjoying praise
    2. Pleasing parents
    3. Improving health
    4. Enhancing appearance

14. A nurse is teaching an obese client how to lower the caloric content of the diet. Which statements indicate that the client understands the teaching? **Select all that apply.**
    1. "I will stop eating cake for dessert."
    2. "I will use cooking spray instead of butter."
    3. "I will eat three meals a day with no snacks."
    4. "I will keep a diary of how many calories I eat per day."
    5. "I will commit to losing approximately one pound a week."

15. A nurse is teaching a client who was recently diagnosed with type 2 diabetes about limiting carbohydrates in the diet. Which statements indicate that the client has learned in the cognitive domain? **Select all that apply.**
    1. "I have stopped adding sugar to my coffee."
    2. "It will be difficult to stop eating chocolate."
    3. "It has not been easy to stop drinking regular sodas."
    4. "I will read the labels on food before I decide to eat them."
    5. "I now understand the signs and symptoms of hyperglycemia and hypoglycemia."

16. A nurse is planning to teach a client with a newly created colostomy how to perform a colostomy irrigation. What client assessments indicate that the client is ready to learn? **Select all that apply.**
    1. Client keeps asking questions about the procedure.
    2. Client reports pain at a level of 6 on a scale of 0 to 10.
    3. Client requested reading material about the procedure.
    4. Client refused to look at the stoma during previous care.
    5. Client states experiencing the passage of intestinal gas 2 times in the last hour.

17. A nurse is facilitating a weight-reduction program for a group of employees of a business organization. Which statements by a participant indicate an external locus of control? **Select all that apply.**
    1. "I want to lose weight so that I live to a ripe old age."
    2. "I plan to lose weight so that I improve how I look to others."
    3. "I am going to lose weight because I believe it will make me feel better."
    4. "I need to lose weight because my children are embarrassed by how heavy I am."
    5. "I hope to lose weight because my company will give me a bonus if I reach my goal."

18. A nurse is assessing a client's motivation to follow an exercise and dietary regimen. What client statement has the **greatest** influence on whether the client will be successful?
    1. "I hope to reach my goals this time doing what I should be doing."
    2. "I believe that the changes I implement will make a difference."
    3. "I plan on keeping a daily diary of everything I eat."
    4. "I am going to join a gym in my neighborhood."

19. A client who has had type 2 diabetes for 15 years has become insulin dependent. A daily morning injection of insulin and insulin coverage a.c. and h.s. are prescribed. The nurse reviews the client's demographic information and past medical history and then interviews the client. What nursing statement is **most** appropriate before teaching the client about self-injection of insulin?
    1. "What were you thinking when you were told you had to use insulin?"
    2. "Which coping mechanisms did you use when confronted with past health problems?"
    3. "Which was more difficult to cope with, the mastectomy or the diagnosis of diabetes?"
    4. "What problems do you anticipate related to giving yourself an injection while living alone?"

Client's Clinical Record

Demographic Information

68 years old, divorced for 4 years
Lives alone in an apartment
High school English teacher; retired 3 years ago
Has health insurance, collecting a pension and social security

Past Medical History

Right mastectomy for cancer of the breast 5 years ago
Has had type 2 diabetes for 15 years
Has had stage 1 hypertension for 5 years (systolic BP between 140 and 159 mm Hg and diastolic BP between 90 and 99 mm Hg)
Taking Lasix 10 mg by mouth once a day

Client Interview

Client states that her husband left her because she had a mastectomy and diabetes. States she was bitter but has since made a life with her family and friends.

20. A nurse is planning to teach a 75-year-old adult how to change a surgical dressing before being discharged from the hospital. What strategy should the nurse use that takes into consideration the client's developmental level?
    1. Incorporate repetition into the teaching plan.
    2. Obtain a return demonstration of the procedure.
    3. Include a family member in the teaching sessions.
    4. Build on the client's past positive learning experiences.

21. A nurse is planning to educate a 13-year-old adolescent about future surgery. Which modality is **most** appropriate for the nurse to include in the teaching session?
    1. Providing a hospital brochure regarding the surgery
    2. Explaining in detail what the surgery entails
    3. Using pictures to reinforce verbal teaching
    4. Demonstrating the surgery using a doll

22. A client is to have abdominal surgery, and deep vein thrombosis prophylaxis is prescribed to be administered 12 hours before surgery. The prescription states, enoxaparin 40 mg subcutaneously 9:00 p.m. the night before surgery. The client demonstrates a subcutaneous injection using a teaching injection pad. The nurse gives the client a prefilled syringe of enoxaparin that states that there are 100 mg/1 mL. How much solution should the nurse teach the client to waste before self-injecting the solution? **Record your answer using 1 decimal place.**
    Answer: _____ mL

23. A nurse is caring for several clients who just had surgery for a variety of pathophysiological problems. Which client probably will benefit **most** from several teaching sessions that focus on demonstrations and return demonstrations?
    1. Adolescent who had a cast applied for a fractured femur
    2. Man who had a pacemaker inserted because of recurrent bradycardia
    3. Woman who had a vaginal hysterectomy because of multiple benign fibroids
    4. Older adult who had the creation of a colostomy because of cancer of the rectum

24. A client is prescribed a medication for infertility. The prescribed dose is 100 international units subcutaneous once a day for 7 days to be self-administered as part of the infertility protocol. The vial contains 150 international units and instructs the user to add 0.8 mL of diluent to yield 1 mL. The nurse teaches the woman how to reconstitute the medication and draw up the appropriate amount prescribed. To which line should the woman fill the syringe with the correct dose of the medication?
    1. A
    2. B
    3. C
    4. D

25. A nurse plans to teach a client how to self-administer insulin. The nurse identifies that the client is a kinesthetic learner. Which teaching strategy should the nurse use to **best** meet this client's learning style?
    1. Encourage the client to handle the equipment.
    2. Present information using a computer-assisted program.
    3. Supply written material that the client can review at an individual pace.
    4. Conduct the program in a group setting, supporting auditory exchange of information.

26. A nurse is designing a teaching plan on how to safely empty a portable wound drainage system for a client who has impaired hearing. Which nursing interventions are specific to enhance learning for this client? **Select all that apply.**
    1. Avoiding overly enunciating each word
    2. Planning more time to practice psychomotor skills
    3. Standing on the client's side with the more acute hearing
    4. Including the client in a group discussion about the topic
    5. Providing pictures with written material about the drainage system

27. A nurse is educating an obese client about a 1,500-calorie weight-reduction diet. Which statement by the nurse would be **most** effective in motivating adherence to the dietary regimen?
    1. "Just think how great you will look in a bathing suit next summer."
    2. "You can design your menu to include some of your food preferences."
    3. "If you lose weight, you will live long enough to see your grandchildren."
    4. "It is essential that you lose weight so that you reduce your blood pressure."

28. A nurse is preparing to educate a client regarding self-blood glucose monitoring. Place the following interventions in the order that they should be performed.
    1. Demonstrate for the client the skill of self-blood glucose monitoring.
    2. Give the client a brief overview of the information to be covered.
    3. Explain to the client the reasons for glucose monitoring.
    4. Have the client perform self-blood glucose monitoring.
    5. Determine the client's preferred learning style.
    6. Assess the client's cognitive abilities.
    Answer: _____

29. A client has an appointment in the department of ambulatory surgery to receive preoperative teaching from a nurse. Place the following interventions in the order that they should be performed by the nurse when communicating with the client.
    1. Summarize the goals and objectives of the meeting.
    2. Read the client's chart before meeting the client.
    3. Explain the purpose of the visit to the clinic.
    4. Verify the client's identification.
    5. Provide preoperative teaching.
    6. Introduce self.
    Answer: _____

30. A nurse is caring for a client who was admitted to the hospital for cardiac bypass surgery. What client statement indicates that the client has an internal locus of control? **Select all that apply.**
    1. "My future is in the hands of my health-care team."
    2. "Many people in my family have coronary artery disease."
    3. "I experienced the chest pain very suddenly out of nowhere."
    4. "I have decided to try cardiac rehabilitation after I am discharged."
    5. "It's time for me to give up smoking, since I don't want to go through this again."

REVIEW ANSWERS AND RATIONALES

1. ANSWER: 3, 4.
Rationales:
1. This outcome involves the performance of a skill that is associated with the psychomotor domain.
2. This outcome involves the affective domain because it reflects a willingness to receive and endure a particular intervention.
3. **This outcome is associated with the cognitive domain. It demonstrates knowledge about the catheter and how it functions via the principle of gravity.**
4. **This outcome is associated with the cognitive domain. It involves knowledge and recall of information.**
5. This outcome involves the performance of a skill that is associated with the psychomotor domain.

TEST-TAKING TIP: Identify the clang association. The word *urinary* in the stem and in options 3 and 4 are clang associations. Frequently, an option with a clang association is a correct answer. Assess options 3 and 4 carefully.
Content Area: Teaching and Learning
Integrated Processes: Teaching/Learning; Nursing Process: Evaluation
Client Need: Health Promotion and Maintenance
Cognitive Level: Application
Concept: Patient-Centered Care

2. ANSWER: 1, 2, 3.
Rationales:
1. **Using an educational video is an effective method of educating clients, especially when followed by a discussion.**
2. **Demonstration and return demonstration are effective methods of educating clients because they allow the nurse to perform a psychomotor skill and then observe the client's performance when implementing the same skill. Actions speak louder than words.**
3. **Providing printed material is an effective method of educating clients, especially when combined with a discussion between the nurse and client.**
4. Having a client educate another client is unacceptable because the client may teach inappropriate techniques.
5. The use of abstract statements is not the method of choice because abstract words are prone to misinterpretation. When educating a client, the nurse should use concrete terms and phrases to avoid the chance of client misinterpretation.

TEST-TAKING TIP: Identify the word in the stem that sets a priority. The word *most* in the stem sets a priority. Identify the clang associations. The words *self-blood glucose monitoring* in the stem and in options 1 and 2 are clang associations.
Content Area: Teaching and Learning
Integrated Processes: Teaching/Learning; Nursing Process: Planning
Client Need: Health Promotion and Maintenance
Cognitive Level: Analysis
Concept: Patient-Centered Care

3. ANSWER: 4.
Rationales:
1. This is an authoritarian approach and a threat.
2. Although this information may be shared with the client, it is not information personalized to the client. The more personalized the information, the more likely it will motivate a client.
3. This intervention is a threat. In addition, it focuses on the negative rather than the positive.
4. **Receiving information about how and why a treatment regimen is necessary and how it will improve the client's condition is empowering, which can motivate a person to adhere to the regimen.**

TEST-TAKING TIP: Identify the word in the stem that sets a priority. The word *best* in the stem sets a priority. Identify the client-centered option. Option 4 is client centered. It focuses on a positive outcome for the client. Identify the options that are opposites. Options 3 and 4 are opposites. Consider these options carefully.
Content Area: Teaching and Learning
Integrated Processes: Teaching/Learning; Nursing Process: Implementation
Client Need: Health Promotion and Maintenance
Cognitive Level: Application
Concept: Patient-Centered Care

4. ANSWER: 3, 4.
Rationales:
1. Being male or being of the opposite sex of the nurse should not be a reason to postpone client education.
2. Being 75 years old is not a reason to postpone client education. The nurse's role is to assess a client's cognitive abilities and to ensure the nurse is providing instruction where the "client is at."
3. **A high level of anxiety is a reason to postpone client education because people with high anxiety levels have a decreased ability to focus and concentrate.**
4. **Pain decreases a person's ability to focus and concentrate. The teaching session should be postponed until nursing interventions reduce the client's pain.**
5. A client's current education level is not a reason to postpone client education; however, the nurse should tailor teaching to the client's cognitive, emotional, and educational level.

TEST-TAKING TIP: Identify the words in the stem that indicate negative polarity. The words *teaching session should be postponed* indicate negative polarity. The question is asking "What factors *do not* indicate a readiness to learn?" Identify the option that contains a specific determiner. The word *only* in option 5 is a specific determiner. More often than not, options with specific determiners are distractors and can be eliminated.
Content Area: Teaching and Learning
Integrated Processes: Caring; Teaching/Learning; Nursing Process: Analysis
Client Need: Health Promotion and Maintenance
Cognitive Level: Application
Concept: Patient-Centered Care

5. ANSWER: 1.

Rationales:

1. The Joint Commission requires hospitals to provide professional interpreters or an interpreter service via a phone link so that clients clearly understand their condition, medical treatment, and the nursing plan of care. In addition, interpretive services must be provided when engaging a client in teaching and learning.

2. Although the nurse may obtain written material in Spanish from the Internet, it is insufficient to meet this client's learning needs. The client is unable to engage in a meaningful discussion about the topic and does not have the opportunity to ask questions and receive answers.

3. Information in the cognitive or affective domain cannot be taught via demonstration.

4. Although the nurse may show pictures of food, it is insufficient to meet this client's learning needs. The client is unable to engage in a meaningful discussion about the topic and does not have the opportunity to ask questions and receive answers.

TEST-TAKING TIP: Identify the word in the stem that sets a priority. The word *most* in the stem sets a priority. Identify the options with clang associations. The words *Spain* in the stem and *Spanish* in options 1 and 2 are clang associations. Examine options 1 and 2 carefully.

Content Area: *Teaching and Learning*
Integrated Processes: *Communication and Documentation; Teaching/Learning; Nursing Process: Planning*
Client Need: *Health Promotion and Maintenance*
Cognitive Level: *Application*
Concept: *Patient-Centered Care; Communication*

6. ANSWER: 3, 4.

Rationales:

1. This outcome is associated with the cognitive domain on a higher level than just recalling information. It involves comprehending and applying an idea in a situation, such as interpreting and using a food label to identify the caloric value of the food.

2. This outcome involves remembering and recalling information, which are associated with the cognitive domain (thinking domain).

3. This outcome involves the use of the hands to perform a skill, which is associated with the psychomotor domain (doing domain).

4. Placing a variety of medications in a weekly pill dispensing box is a psychomotor skill. It requires knowledge about what medications must be taken and at what times of day. That information then must be transferred from the "brain" to the "hands" to complete the skill of filling a weekly medication dispensing box.

5. Accepting limitations in life imposed by the medical diagnosis of hypertension and incorporating actions to support weight loss as evidenced by actual weight loss is associated with the affective domain (feeling domain).

Content Area: *Teaching and Learning*
Integrated Processes: *Teaching/Learning; Nursing Process: Evaluation*
Client Need: *Health Promotion and Maintenance*
Cognitive Level: *Application*
Concept: *Patient-Centered Care*

7. ANSWER: 2, 4.

Rationales:

1. The client's statement does not reflect an internal locus of control. A person with an internal locus of control is motivated from within and takes responsibility for actions and consequences.

2. The client's statement reflects an external locus of control. A person with an external locus of control is motivated by pressure or rewards from outside the self.

3. The client's statement does not reflect a personal goal; it is a goal set by the legal system.

4. The client's statement reflects the need to participate in the rehabilitation program to meet the requirements of the legal system.

5. The client's statement does not reflect any interest in resolving the dependence on alcohol.

TEST-TAKING TIP: Identify the options that are opposites. Options 1 and 2 are opposites. One of these is a correct answer and one is not.

Content Area: *Teaching and Learning*
Integrated Processes: *Communication and Documentation; Teaching/Learning; Nursing Process: Analysis*
Client Need: *Health Promotion and Maintenance*
Cognitive Level: *Analysis*
Concept: *Patient-Centered Care*

8. ANSWER: 1, 5.

Rationales:

1. To maintain a diabetic diet, the client has to emotionally accept the need to incorporate a diabetic diet into one's lifestyle. This requires a positive attitude and the need to value activities that promote health and wellness. Attitudes and values are associated with the affective domain.

2. Manipulating equipment to safely draw up insulin into a syringe is related to the psychomotor, not affective, domain. The psychomotor domain is related to handling equipment safely.

3. This outcome is related to learning in the cognitive, not affective, domain. The cognitive domain is associated with the acquiring of information, memorization, recall, intellectual thinking, and applying and evaluating ideas.

4. Learning the clinical indicators of hyperglycemia and hypoglycemia is associated with the cognitive, not affective, domain. Memorizing, recalling, and comprehending information are related to learning in the cognitive domain.

5. The affective domain is concerned with feelings, beliefs, attitudes, and values. Emotional commitment to the plan reflects the affective domain.

TEST-TAKING TIP: Identify the clang associations. The word *diabetes* in the stem is related to the word *diabetic* in option 1 and *diabetes* in option 5. Consider these options carefully.

Content Area: *Teaching and Learning*
Integrated Processes: *Teaching/Learning; Nursing Process: Evaluation*
Client Need: *Health Promotion and Maintenance*
Cognitive Level: *Application*
Concept: *Patient-Centered Care*

9. **ANSWER: 3.**

Rationales:

1. A teaching session does not have to be postponed because a person is mildly anxious. Research demonstrates that a mildly anxious person is alert and focused, which enhances learning.

2. Both formal and informal approaches are effective teaching methods.

3. This is an excellent teaching strategy. It ensures that critical content is addressed first in the event that additional learning must be postponed because the client becomes tired or experiences pain during the learning session.

4. Not all clients are comfortable in a cool environment. The temperature of the learning environment should be physically comfortable for the client. When physically comfortable, the client can focus on the content being learned rather than on being too cold or too hot.

TEST-TAKING TIP: Identify the word in the stem that sets a priority. The word *essential* in the stem sets a priority. Identify the obscure clang association. The word *essential* in the stem and the words *most important* in option 3 is a clang association. The words *essential* and *most important* basically have the same meaning. Examine options with a clang association carefully. More often than not, the option with a clang association is the correct answer.

Content Area: Teaching and Learning
Integrated Processes: Teaching/Learning; Nursing Process: Planning
Client Need: Health Promotion and Maintenance
Cognitive Level: Application
Concept: Patient-Centered Care

10. **ANSWER: 1, 3.**

Rationales:

1. Demonstrating the procedure is an effective method to educate a client with an intellectual disability because it allows for visual learning.

2. Describing the procedure in writing involves the use of abstract thought and symbolism, which a client with an intellectual disability may not possess.

3. Using pictures to describe a procedure is an effective method to educate a client with an intellectual disability because it allows for visual learning.

4. A preprinted book may not be an effective teaching approach because a client with an intellectual disability may not understand the written word, and this approach does not allow for questions.

5. Group instruction for a client who has an intellectual disability is not a method of choice because the person may feel overwhelmed in a group setting; in addition, HIPAA laws prevent discussion of a client's clinical condition with other clients without consent.

TEST-TAKING TIP: Identify the word in the stem that sets a priority. The word *most* in the stem sets a priority.

Content Area: Teaching and Learning
Integrated Processes: Teaching/Learning; Nursing Process: Planning
Client Need: Health Promotion and Maintenance
Cognitive Level: Application
Concept: Patient-Centered Care

11. **ANSWER: 3.**

Rationales:

1. Although this may be accurate, it is too specific an initial assumption.

2. If this were so, the nurse would expect the family member to be attempting to teach the client, not trying to restrain her arm.

3. Although the culture is unknown, there appears to be a reason why the client's arm is being restrained. The nurse should pursue this further because it may be related to cultural beliefs.

4. The client would have stopped the exercise if intimidated by the family member.

TEST-TAKING TIP: Identify the words in the stem that set a priority. The word *most* in the stem sets a priority. Identify the clang associations. The word *exercise* in the stem and in options 2 and 3 are clang associations. Examine options 2 and 3 carefully.

Content Area: Teaching and Learning
Integrated Processes: Teaching/Learning; Nursing Process: Analysis
Client Need: Psychosocial Integrity
Cognitive Level: Application
Concept: Culture

12. **ANSWER: 1, 3, 4, 2, 5.**

Rationales:

1. The nurse must first determine whether the client realizes that there is a need to learn more.

3. After readiness to learn is established, the nurse should verify motivation by recognizing health-seeking behaviors, such as requests to participate in own care, asking for written materials or referral to a support group, and belief that interventions will precipitate desired outcomes.

4. After determining client readiness and motivation to learn, the nurse must then establish the level at which the client is capable of learning, such as cognitive and developmental levels, physical ability, and need for repetition.

2. After the nurse determines the client's readiness and motivation to learn and after ascertaining the client's level of ability, the nurse selects teaching tools. The selection of teaching tools is based on the client's level of learning and capabilities, such as visual and auditory acuity, communication skills, language, and cultural differences.

5. The last step of the options presented is associated with providing an appropriate learning environment for this client. An environment conducive to learning, such as a quiet, private, comfortable place where lessons of appropriate time, length, and frequency are provided, enhances learning.

Content Area: Teaching and Learning
Integrated Processes: Teaching/Learning; Nursing Process: Planning
Client Need: Safe and Effective Care Environment; Management of Care
Cognitive Level: Analysis
Concept: Patient-Centered Care

13. **ANSWER: 4.**
    Rationales:
    1. Praise is not a motivating factor for a teenager. It is associated with school-aged children.
    2. Pleasing parents is not a motivating factor, since teenagers often are in conflict with their parents because of their struggle between dependence and independence.
    3. Improving health is not a motivating factor because teenagers believe they are immortal. They live in the present and generally are uninterested in the relationship between health and maintaining a positive lifestyle.
    4. Teenagers often are concerned with their appearances and use various methods of weight loss that are unhealthy, such as bulimia, fad diets, and excessive exercise. The teenager may be motivated to lose weight by appealing to the goal of enhancing appearance.
    TEST-TAKING TIP: Identify the word in the stem that sets a priority. The word *most* in the stem sets a priority.
    Content Area: *Teaching and Learning*
    Integrated Processes: *Teaching/Learning; Nursing Process: Analysis*
    Client Need: *Health Promotion and Maintenance*
    Cognitive Level: *Application*
    Concept: *Patient-Centered Care; Growth and Development*

14. **ANSWER: 4, 5.**
    Rationales:
    1. The chances of maintaining a diet decrease when depriving oneself of favorite foods. The calories for food preferences can be calculated into the total daily recommended caloric intake.
    2. Although this may lower the caloric count of the diet, it is not as tasty or satisfying as butter. A pad of butter can be calculated into the total daily intake of calories.
    3. Eating snacks between meals, provided the calories are within the recommended total intake, minimize hunger.
    4. Keeping a daily caloric intake diary is a motivating factor for staying within the recommended daily limits.
    5. Making a commitment indicates a vested interest in the dietary plan. Also, losing one pound a week is a realistic outcome goal associated with a diet that meets nutritional needs while reducing calorie intake.
    TEST-TAKING TIP: Identify the words in the stem and options that are clang associations. The words *caloric content* in the stem and *calories* in option 4 is a clang association. Examine option 4 carefully.
    Content Area: *Teaching and Learning*
    Integrated Processes: *Communication and Documentation; Teaching/Learning; Nursing Process: Evaluation*
    Client Need: *Health Promotion and Maintenance*
    Cognitive Level: *Application*
    Concept: *Patient-Centered Care; Nutrition*

15. **ANSWER: 4, 5.**
    Rationales:
    1. Adhering to a dietary regimen reflects the affective domain. Sugar may be added to coffee as long as it is calculated into the dietary regimen.

2. This comment reflects the affective domain (feelings, values, attitudes, and beliefs). Chocolate may be included in the diet as long as it is calculated into the dietary regimen.
3. This comment reflects the affective domain (feelings, values, attitudes, and beliefs), not the cognitive domain. Regular soda may be included in the diet as long as it is calculated into the dietary regimen.
4. The client is indicating comprehension by verbalizing the importance of knowing how many carbohydrates are included in packaged foods.
5. Understanding the signs and symptoms of hyperglycemia and hypoglycemia reflect learning in the cognitive domain, which is associated with acquiring, storing, and recalling information.
Content Area: *Teaching and Learning*
Integrated Processes: *Communication and Documentation; Teaching/Learning; Nursing Process: Evaluation*
Client Need: *Health Promotion and Maintenance*
Cognitive Level: *Application*
Concept: *Patient-Centered Care: Nutrition*

16. **ANSWER: 1, 3, 5.**
    Rationales:
    1. Asking questions indicates interest and a readiness to learn. The client wants answers.
    2. Pain can interfere with learning because the client may not be able to focus beyond coping with the pain. A client with moderate to severe pain should receive an analgesic to reduce the pain before a teaching session.
    3. Requesting information about a situation is a behavior that indicates a readiness to learn. The client wants more knowledge.
    4. A client who refuses to look at a colostomy may be in denial or unable emotionally or physically to learn how to care for a colostomy.
    5. Passing of intestinal gas is expected with a colostomy. It indicates that peristalsis has returned and the client may be physically ready for colostomy irrigation.
    Content Area: *Teaching and Learning*
    Integrated Processes: *Communication and Documentation; Teaching/Learning; Nursing Process: Assessment*
    Client Need: *Health Promotion and Maintenance*
    Cognitive Level: *Application*
    Concept: *Patient-Centered Care*

17. **ANSWER: 2, 4, 5.**
    Rationales:
    1. This statement indicates an internal locus of control. The client has the personal desire to prolong life by losing excess weight.
    2. This statement indicates that the person is influenced by what others think, which reflects an external locus of control.
    3. This statement indicates that the change in behavior is motivated by a desire from within, which reflects an internal locus of control.
    4. This statement indicates that the person wants to please or gain the respect of others, which reflects an external locus of control.

5. This statement indicates that the person is motivated by an external reward, which reflects an external locus of control.
Content Area: *Teaching and Learning*
Integrated Processes: *Communication and Documentation; Teaching/Learning; Nursing Process: Analysis*
Client Need: *Health Promotion and Maintenance*
Cognitive Level: *Analysis*
Concept: *Patient-Centered Care*

18. **ANSWER: 2.**
Rationales:
1. The statement *I hope to reach my goals this time* is less emphatic than *I will be successful*. Hope is related to a desirable expectation, but it takes more than just hope to accomplish a positive outcome. Also, the words *this time* indicate that the client may not have been successful in the past; past experiences can impact present experiences and repeat themselves.
2. If a client believes that interventions will produce a beneficial outcome, the client will more likely adhere to the proposed medical regimen. This is one of the major components of the health belief model. Also, the statement reflects an internal locus of control and thinking related to the affective domain.
3. Although it is helpful to track dietary intake, it does not ensure that the client will follow the prescribed diet.
4. Although this is beneficial, it does not ensure that the client will attend the gym and perform the prescribed exercises.
TEST-TAKING TIP: Identify the word in the stem that sets a priority. The word *greatest* in the stem sets a priority. Identify the options that are equally plausible. Options 3 and 4 are equally plausible because each relates to just one aspect of the regimen; one is no better than the other. These options can be deleted from consideration.
Content Area: *Teaching and Learning*
Integrated Processes: *Communication and Documentation; Teaching/Learning; Nursing Process: Analysis*
Client Need: *Health Promotion and Maintenance*
Cognitive Level: *Application*
Concept: *Patient-Centered Care*

19. **ANSWER: 1.**
Rationales:
1. This statement focuses on the change the client is experiencing and allows the client to address concerns from a personal perspective. The nurse should focus on the client's concerns before beginning teaching. The focus should be on the present situation, not the past.
2. This question focuses on the past, is premature, and addresses only one factor, past coping mechanisms. This question would be more helpful during a later session.
3. This question is too direct and focuses on the past. Also, this question centers on the negative rather than the positive. The client can answer this question with one word, and the conversation could end.
4. This statement focuses on the negative and suggests that the client should anticipate problems with self-administration of insulin.

TEST-TAKING TIP: Identify the option with a clang association. The word *insulin* in the stem and in option 1 is a clang association. Identify the options that are equally plausible. Options 2 and 3 are equally plausible; they both address issues of the past. Usually, equally plausible options can be eliminated from consideration for the correct answer.
Content Area: *Teaching and Learning*
Integrated Processes: *Communication and Documentation; Teaching/Learning; Nursing Process: Implementation*
Client Need: *Health Promotion and Maintenance*
Cognitive Level: *Analysis*
Concept: *Patient-Centered Care; Communication*

20. **ANSWER: 1.**
Rationales:
1. Information-processing speed declines with age, slowing learning and increasing the need for repetition.
2. A return demonstration is the primary method to evaluate a client's ability to perform a psychomotor skill; this strategy is not age dependent.
3. A family member may be included in a teaching session regardless of the age of the client. The involvement of a family member requires the client's consent.
4. Teaching should always progress from what the client knows to the unknown; this strategy is not age dependent.
TEST-TAKING TIP: Identify the word in the stem that is a clang association with a word in the options. The words *teach* in the stem and *teaching* in options 1 and 3 are clang associations. Consider options 1 and 3 carefully.
Content Area: *Teaching and Learning*
Integrated Processes: *Communication and Documentation; Teaching/Learning; Nursing Process: Planning*
Client Need: *Health Promotion and Maintenance*
Cognitive Level: *Application*
Concept: *Patient-Centered Care; Growth and Development*

21. **ANSWER: 3.**
Rationales:
1. Providing a hospital brochure may facilitate education but will not allow for questions by the adolescent.
2. Explaining in detail what the surgery entails may create anxiety because too much information can be confusing. It is a nurse's role to assess the cognitive and emotional levels of the client before teaching.
3. Using pictures to reinforce the spoken word will assist the adolescent to understand what is being taught. A 13-year-old adolescent may not have the ability to think abstractly.
4. Using a doll with an adolescent may be beneath the adolescent's cognitive abilities; the adolescent may feel childish or become bored.
TEST-TAKING TIP: Identify the word in the stem that sets a priority. The word *most* in the stem sets a priority. Identify the unique option. Option 3 is unique because it is the only option that does not include the word *surgery*. Identify the option with a clang association. The word *teaching* in the stem and in option 3 is a clang association. Examine option 3 carefully.
Content Area: *Teaching and Learning*
Integrated Processes: *Teaching/Learning; Nursing Process: Planning*

Client Need: Health Promotion and Maintenance
Cognitive Level: Application
Concept: Patient-Centered Care; Growth and Development

22. ANSWER: 0.6.
Rationale:
Use ratio and proportion to determine the desired mL
dose and then subtract this amount from the total mL
of solution in the syringe to arrive at the correct answer.

$$\frac{\text{Desire 100 mg}}{\text{Have 250 mg}} = \frac{x \text{ mL}}{5 \text{ mL}}$$

$$100x = 40 \times 1$$
$$100x = 40$$
$$x = 40 \div 100$$
$$x = 0.4 \text{ mL is the desired}$$
$$\text{dose}$$

The prefilled syringe contains 1 mL. Subtract 0.4 mL
from 1 mL, which yields 0.6 mL that has to be wasted.
The desired dose of 0.4 mg remains in the syringe.
Content Area: Teaching and Learning
Integrated Processes: Teaching/Learning; Nursing Process:
Planning
Client Need: Physiological Integrity; Pharmacological
and Parenteral Therapies
Cognitive Level: Application
Concept: Medication; Safety

23. ANSWER: 4.
Rationales:
1. A client who had a cast applied for a broken bone
will be taught to keep the cast clean and dry. There is
no complex care to be learned by the client.
2. A man who had a pacemaker surgically implanted may
require education regarding monitoring of the pulse and
the need for routine follow-up health-care supervision;
however, there is no need for learning complex self-care.
3. A woman who had a vaginal hysterectomy may require
some education regarding assessment of the vaginal discharge but will not be required to learn complex self-care.
4. A client with a colostomy will have to learn how to
apply, remove, and empty the colostomy bag and learn
how to irrigate the colostomy. Therefore, demonstration
and return demonstration will be the most effective
forms of teaching for this client.
TEST-TAKING TIP: Identify the word in the stem that sets a
priority. The word *most* in the stem sets a priority.
Content Area: Teaching and Learning
Integrated Processes: Teaching/Learning; Nursing Process:
Planning
Client Need: Health Promotion and Maintenance
Cognitive Level: Analysis
Concept: Patient-Centered Care; Growth and
Development

24. ANSWER: 3.
Rationales:
1. This is too small a dose. It is 0.4 mL.
2. This is too small a dose. It is 0.6 mL.

3. This is the correct dose. It is 0.7 mL.
Solve the problem by using ratio and proportion.

$$\frac{\text{Desire 100 international units}}{\text{Have 150 international units}} = \frac{x \text{ mL}}{1 \text{ mL}}$$

$$150x = 100 \times 1$$
$$150x = 100$$
$$x = 100 \div 150$$
$$x = 0.66 \text{ mL. Round}$$
$$\text{the number up}$$
$$\text{to 0.7 mL.}$$

4. This is too large a dose. It is 1.2 mL.
Content Area: Teaching and Learning
Integrated Processes: Teaching/Learning; Nursing Process:
Implementation
Client Need: Physiological Integrity; Pharmacological and
Parenteral Therapies
Cognitive Level: Analysis
Concept: Medication; Safety

25. ANSWER: 1.
Rationales:
1. Handling equipment best meets the learning style
of kinesthetic learners. Kinesthetic learners process
information by doing, engaging in physical activity,
and handling equipment.
2. Computer-assisted programs best meet the learning
styles of visual and auditory learners. Visual learners learn
by processing information with the eyes. Auditory learners
process information by listening to words.
3. Written material best meets the learning style of visual
learners. Visual learners learn by processing information
with the eyes.
4. Group discussion best meets the learning style of
auditory learners. Auditory learners process information
by listening to words.
TEST-TAKING TIP: Identify the word in the stem that sets a
priority. The word *best* in the stem sets a priority.
Content Area: Teaching and Learning
Integrated Processes: Teaching/Learning; Nursing Process:
Planning
Client Need: Health Promotion and Maintenance
Cognitive Level: Application
Concept: Patient-Centered Care

26. ANSWER: 1, 3, 5.
Rationales:
1. Overly enunciating each word should be avoided
because it interferes with lip reading.
2. This is unnecessary. Impaired hearing should not interfere with learning in the psychomotor domain. Demonstration and return demonstration are the most effective
ways to teach and evaluate learning in the psychomotor
domain.
3. Standing on the client's side with the more acute
hearing maximizes the transmission of the nurse's voice.
4. A person with impaired hearing may not be able to
follow (hear) the discussion among members of a group.
Clients who are hearing impaired learn best in a one-
to-one situation rather than in a group setting.

5. Written material with pictures will supplement the nurse's verbal discussion with the client.

TEST-TAKING TIP: Identify the clang associations. The word *hearing* in the stem and in option 3 and the word *drainage* in the stem and in option 5 are clang associations. Examine options 3 and 5 carefully.

Content Area: Teaching and Learning
Integrated Processes: Communication and Documentation; Teaching/Learning; Nursing Process: Planning
Client Need: Health Promotion and Maintenance
Cognitive Level: Application
Concept: Patient-Centered Care; Sensory Perception

27. **ANSWER: 2.**
Rationales:
1. Looking good in a bathing suit is a potential long-term outcome. Also, the nurse is making the assumption that this factor is important to the client.
2. This is an empowering statement because it gives the client some control over implementing the dietary regimen. It is client centered and focuses on the present and near future. The achievement of short-term goals is motivating.
3. Living long enough to see grandchildren is a potential long-term outcome. Also, the nurse is making the assumption that this factor is important to the client.
4. Reducing blood pressure is a long-term outcome. Also, the nurse is making the assumption that this factor is important to the client.

TEST-TAKING TIP: Identify the word in the stem that sets a priority. The word *most* in the stem sets a priority. Identify the unique option. Option 2 is unique. It is the only option that addresses the process of losing weight rather than a potential outcome. It is a short-term intervention rather than a long-term outcome. It focuses on the present rather than the future. Identify the clang associations. The word *weight* in the stem and in options 3 and 4 are clang associations. However, in this question, this tip is not helpful because options 3 and 4 are distractors. More often than not, but *not always*, a clang association is the correct answer.

Content Area: Teaching and Learning
Integrated Processes: Communication and Documentation; Teaching/Learning; Nursing Process: Implementation
Client Need: Health Promotion and Maintenance
Cognitive Level: Application
Concept: Patient-Centered Care; Communication

28. **ANSWER: 6, 5, 2, 3, 1, 4.**
Rationales:
6. The client's ability to intellectually handle the information must be assessed first. Also, this assessment will influence the level of verbal language and written materials required for this client.
5. Determining the client's preferred learning style is the second step. Information is best learned by a client if the information is presented in the client's preferred learning style (e.g., visual, auditory, or kinesthetic).

2. After the client's cognitive abilities and preferred learning style are assessed, the third step involves a brief overview of the teaching session which informs the client about what information will be covered. An outline helps to provide structure for the teaching session.
3. Explaining to the client the reasons for glucose monitoring occurs in the fourth step of the options presented. Information in the cognitive learning domain provides the foundation for learning in the psychomotor and affective learning domains.
1. After the cognitive and affective learning domains are addressed, the teacher can proceed to demonstrating the skill which is the fifth step of the options presented. It is important that the nurse demonstrate the skill, allow the client to manipulate the equipment, and have the client practice the skill.
4. After the nurse has completed the teaching of a skill and the client has had an opportunity to practice the skill, the client should perform a return demonstration of the skill. This allows the nurse to evaluate whether the client can perform the skill appropriately and is the last step of the options presented in the question.

Content Area: Teaching and Learning
Integrated Processes: Teaching/Learning; Nursing Process: Planning
Client Need: Safe and Effective Care Environment; Management of Care
Cognitive Level: Analysis
Concept: Patient-Centered Care

29. **ANSWER: 2, 6, 4, 3, 5, 1.**
Rationales:
2. Reading the client's chart before meeting the client is the first thing the nurse should do. This permits the nurse to gather significant information about the client before actually meeting the client.
6. Introducing one's self is the second thing that the nurse should do. Clients have a right to know who is providing care and the role that the person fulfills.
4. Verifying the client's identity is the third thing that the nurse should do. It is essential that the nurse verify the client's name with at least two qualifiers. This ensures that the nurse is sharing confidential information with the correct person.
3. Explaining the goals and objectives provides an orientation for the client regarding the remainder of the interaction and is the fourth step of the options presented in the question. It provides an initial exchange of information.
5. Preoperative teaching is the working phase of this relationship and is the fifth step of the options presented in the question. The nurse imparts information, provides teaching, explores client concerns, and evaluates the client's understanding.
1. Summarizing the goals and objectives of the teaching session is the last step of the options presented in the question. At the completion of the session, it is essential

that the nurse review what was achieved. This is best accomplished by briefly reviewing the desired outcomes of the preoperative teaching session.
Content Area: Teaching and Learning
Integrated Processes: Teaching/Learning; Nursing Process: Planning
Client Need: Safe and Effective Care Environment; Management of Care
Cognitive Level: Analysis
Concept: Patient-Centered Care; Communication

30. ANSWER: 4, 5.
   Rationales:
   1. The statement in option 1 assigns responsibility for future personal health to members of the health team. This statement reflects an external, not internal, locus of control.

2. The statement in option 2 is a statement of fact and is not assigning responsibility for future growth to others or to oneself (neither external nor internal locus of control).
3. The statement in option 3 is a statement of fact and is not assigning responsibility for future growth to others or to oneself (neither external nor internal locus of control).
4. The statement in option 4 accepts personal responsibility for one's future health status. This demonstrates an internal locus of control.
5. The statement in option 5 indicates a desire to change behavior, which indicates an internal locus of control.
Content Area: Teaching and Learning
Integrated Processes: Communication and Documentation; Nursing Process: Analysis
Client Need: Psychosocial Integrity
Cognitive Level: Analysis
Concept: Self

Chapter 9

Medication

Communication
Collaboration
Ethics
Fluid and Electrolyte Balance
Legal

Medication
Health Promotion
Patient-Centered Care
Safety

KEY TERMS

Adverse effect—Unintended, usually unpredictable harmful response to a medication that is more severe than a side effect

Allergic reaction—Response of a client's immune system to the presence of a substance that produces a hypersensitivity reaction

Biotransformation (metabolism)—Conversion (detoxification) of a medication to a less active form in preparation for excretion

Drop factor—The number of drops it takes for specific tubing to deliver 1 mL of fluid

Enteric-coated—Product that is encased in a substance that dissolves in the intestine

Idiosyncratic reaction—Resistance, overreaction, or unpredictable reaction to a medication that is different from the expected response

Parenteral—Other than the alimentary canal (gastrointestinal tract)

Peak blood level—Highest blood concentration of a medication

Pharmacodynamics—Study of the mechanisms of actions of a medication (e.g., biochemical and physiological) and the way in which it achieves its effects in the body

Pharmacokinetics—Study of the absorption, distribution, biotransformation (metabolism), and excretion of medications

Polypharmacy—Administration of many medications together

Potentiation—Interaction of two medications that result in an increase in the action of just one of the medications

Side effect—Common unintended response to a medication that generally is predictable and well tolerated

Sustained-release—Product that gradually is released, ensuring a constant blood level of the product

Synergistic effect—Combined effect of two medications is greater than when the effects of each are added together

Teratogenic effect—Effect of a medication that causes abnormal development of a fetus when taken by a pregnant woman

Therapeutic range—Dosage range or serum concentration of a medication usually expected to achieve the medication's desired effect

Time-release—Product that is further enclosed in smaller casings that release a dose over time

Tolerance—Decreased physiological response after repeated exposure to a medication

Toxic effect—Dangerous, harmful response to a medication

Trough blood level—Lowest blood concentration of a medication

Vial—Glass rubber-sealed container covered with a metal cap that contains a sterile parenteral solution

I. Pharmacodynamics

Pharmacodynamics is the study of how medications achieve their effects in the body. It takes into consideration how medication molecules interact with cells and tissues of the body as well as their biological responses, which influence the selection of specific medications for a therapeutic regimen. Medications have a variety of names, are classified by their characteristics, and have a primary reason for being administered (therapeutic effect). Because of the numerous medications available for use and their complexity of action, primary and secondary effects, and potential for interactions, nurses must know not only the commonly prescribed medications but also how to access information based on a medication's name or classification.

A. Medication names
1. *Chemical.*
   a. Describes a medication's chemical and molecular structure.
   b. Example: **2-(4-isobutylphenyl) propionic acid**: ibuprofen (Motrin, Advil).
2. *Generic (nonproprietary, official).*
   a. Simple name that is easier to pronounce.
   b. Begins with a lowercase letter.
   c. Example: 2-(4-isobutylphenyl) propionic acid: **ibuprofen** (Motrin, Advil).
3. *Trade (brand, proprietary).*
   a. Usually short and easy to recall.
   b. Begins with a capital letter.
   c. Registered by the U.S. Patent Office and approved by the FDA.
   d. Example: *2-(4-isobutylphenyl) propionic acid*: ibuprofen (**Motrin, Advil**).

B. Medication classifications
1. Medications are grouped together based on common characteristics.
2. Ways to classify medications.
   a. Effect on the body, such as central nervous system depressants.
   b. Therapeutic use, such as anticoagulants.
   c. Chemical characteristics, such as beta-adrenergic blocking agents.
3. Medications may fit into more than one classification because they have a broad range of effects.

MAKING THE CONNECTION

Medications and Their Effects on the Body

Medication molecules bind with cellular receptors within the body, thereby exerting their action (pharmacodynamics). Once a medication molecule binds with a site receptor, a pharmacological response occurs. A medication receptor complex can activate a further cellular reaction that promotes or hinders normal cellular function by such actions as altering intracellular enzymes, increasing or decreasing cellular metabolism, altering permeability of cell membranes, and liberating or deactivating neurohormones that influence physiological processes. The specific characteristics of a medication's constituents and receptor site characteristics influence the degree of medication action in the body. Nurses should understand how medications work in the body to better understand their resulting therapeutic and nontherapeutic effects.

C. Primary effects of medications (therapeutic effects)
1. Symptomatic (palliative).
   a. Used to relieve signs or symptoms of disease, not the disease itself.
   b. Example: Acetaminophen relieves fever.
2. Preventive.
   a. Used to avoid disease.
   b. Example: Measles vaccine prevents measles.
3. Diagnostic.
   a. Used to help diagnose the presence of disease.
   b. Example: Radiopaque dye outlines internal body structures.
4. Curative (chemotherapeutic).
   a. Used to eradicate a disease or destroy disease-producing pathogens or body cells.
   b. Examples: Antibiotics such as azithromycin (Zithromax) destroy bacteria, and antineoplastics such as cisplatin destroy cancer cells.
5. Health maintenance (substitutive).
   a. Used to support normal body function.
   b. Examples: Regular insulin (Novolin R) lowers serum glucose level in clients with diabetes; levothyroxine (Synthroid) replaces thyroid hormones in clients with hypothyroidism.
6. Contraceptive.
   a. Used to prevent pregnancy.
   b. Example: Combined oral contraceptives (estrogen and progestin) and progestin-only pills are prescribed to prevent pregnancy.
7. Antidote.
   a. Used to reverse the toxic effect of another medication.
   b. Examples: Vitamin K limits bleeding due to warfarin (Coumadin) and naloxone (Narcan) limits central nervous system depression due to opioids.

D. Secondary effects of medications (unintended effects) and related nursing care
1. Side effect.
   a. A **side effect** is a common unintended response to a medication that generally is predictable and well tolerated.
   b. Examples: Dry mouth, anorexia.

c. Nursing care.
    (1) Implement palliative independent and dependent measures to address side effects that are not serious.
    (2) Examples: Offering frequent mouth care for a client experiencing dry mouth; providing food preferences for a client with anorexia.

2. Adverse effect.
  a. An **adverse effect** is an unintended, usually unpredictable harmful response to a medication that is more severe than a side effect.
  b. Example: Bone marrow depression.
  c. Nursing care.
    (1) Notify the primary health-care provider of the client's status.
    (2) Discontinue the medication per the primary health-care provider's prescription (cessation of the medication generally is indicated).

3. Toxic effect.
  a. A **toxic effect** is a dangerous, harmful response to a medication.
  b. May result from a medication overdose, accumulation of a medication's ingredients due to impaired biotransformation or excretion (cumulative effect), or the body's abnormal sensitivity to a medication.
  c. Examples: Liver damage (hepatotoxicity), kidney damage (nephrotoxicity).
  d. Nursing care.
    (1) Assess the type and amount of over-the-counter (OTC) medications the client is using.
    (2) Teach clients how to examine medication labels to identify ingredients in OTC medications that can cause a cumulative effect when taken with another medication with the same ingredient (e.g., acetaminophen [Tylenol] for pain and an OTC cold remedy that contains acetaminophen; taken together they may exceed the recommended dose limit for acetaminophen).
    🛑 (3) Withhold the medication and notify the primary health-care provider if the client exhibits a toxic reaction to a medication.

4. Allergic reaction.
  a. An **allergic reaction** is the response of a client's immune system to the presence of a substance that produces a hypersensitivity reaction (e.g., medication).
  b. Certain classifications of medications frequently cause allergic reactions (Box 9.1).
  c. Example: Rash, breathing difficulty, circulatory collapse (anaphylaxis).

Box 9.1 Medications That Commonly Cause Allergic Reactions

- Analgesics: Codeine, morphine sulfate.
- Antiseizure medications: Phenytoin.
- Antibiotics: Penicillin.
- Iodinated contrast dye.
- Biological agents: Vaccines.
- Other medications: Quinidine, iodines, phenothiazines.

---

  d. Nursing care.
    (1) Collect information from the client and primary health-care provider about a history of medication and food allergies before administering prescribed medications.
    (2) Document the presence of allergies according to agency policy and procedure (e.g., in the nursing history and physical, on the medication administration record, and on the medication reconciliation form); have the client describe the clinical manifestations of the allergic response.
    (3) Secure an allergy alert band to the client's wrist to alert health-care team members of the client's history of allergies.
    (4) Check the client's clinical record, medication administration record, and wristband to ensure that the client has no allergies before administering medications.
    (5) Ensure that medication products that a client is susceptible to are not contained in a prescribed or OTC medication that the client will be taking.
    (6) Assess for clinical manifestations of an allergic response to medications, especially when administering a medication for the first time.
    🛑 (7) Implement emergency measures if a client experiences an anaphylactic response to a medication (e.g., initiate the rapid response team and prepare medications, such as epinephrine, that may be prescribed to support the client).
    (8) Teach a client who has a medication allergy how to examine medication labels to ensure that OTC medications do not contain offending allergens.

5. Idiosyncratic reaction.
  a. An **idiosyncratic reaction** is a resistant, overreaction, or unpredictable reaction that is different from the expected response to a medication.
  b. Example: An older adult becomes agitated or restless after receiving a sedative.

c. Nursing care.
   (1) Notify the primary health-care provider of the client's status.
   (2) Discontinue the medication per the primary health-care provider's prescription cessation of the medication generally is indicated.

6. Tolerance.
   a. **Tolerance** occurs when there is a decreased physiological response after repeated exposure to a medication.
   b. Example: A client receiving an opioid no longer experiences relief from pain.
   c. Nursing care.
      (1) Notify the primary health-care provider if tolerance occurs.
      (2) Implement the primary health-care provider's prescriptions, which may include discontinuation of the medication, an increase in the medication dose, or replacement of the medication with a different medication.

7. Teratogenic effect.
   a. A **teratogenic effect** occurs when a medication causes abnormal development of a fetus when taken by a pregnant woman, especially during the first trimester of pregnancy, when the organs of the fetus are developing (organogenesis).
   b. Medications are classified from category A (no risk to fetus) and progressively escalate in level of risk to category D (evidence of fetal risk but potential benefit to the mother may be acceptable).
   c. A separate category identified as X classifies medications that cause fetal abnormalities, for example, isotretinoin (Claravis) for severe acne and acitretin (Soriatane) for severe psoriasis.
   d. Examples: Classifications include diuretics, antiepileptics, analgesics, antihistamines, antibiotics, and antiemetics.
   e. Nursing care.

   🛑 (1) Ensure that the client is not pregnant when a medication that is teratogenic is prescribed.

      (2) Teach the client to abstain from sexual intercourse or use more than one contraceptive method during the course of therapy.

E. Medication interactions and related nursing care
   1. Synergistic effect.
      a. A **synergistic effect** occurs when the combined effect of two medications is greater than when the effects of each are added together.
      b. Example: Administration of either a diuretic or an antihypertensive to treat hypertension may

decrease the client's blood pressure by 10%; however, when administered together, the drugs may interact exceeding the combined effect of both drugs which may decrease the client's blood pressure excessively.
      c. Nursing care.
         (1) Assess resources to identify whether medications being administered concurrently have the potential for precipitating a synergistic effect.
         (2) Assess for clinical manifestations of an excessive response. If one occurs, withhold the next dose and notify the primary health-care provider of the client's status.

   2. Potentiation.
      a. **Potentiation** occurs when the interaction of two medications results in an increase in the action of just one of the medications.
      b. Example: Probenecid blocks the excretion of penicillin, increasing the blood level of penicillin and, therefore, its effectiveness.
      c. Nursing care.
         (1) Assess resources to identify whether medications being administered concurrently have the ability to precipitate a potentiation effect.
         (2) Assess for clinical manifestations of the expected therapeutic effects, particularly those related to the medication that is being maximized by the interaction of the two medications.

   3. Physical or chemical incompatibilities.
      a. **Physical or chemical incompatibilities** occur when two medications interact with each other resulting in an unintended effect.
      b. *Antagonistic relationship.*
         (1) One medication decreases the therapeutic effect of another medication.
         (2) Example: Loop diuretics can decrease the effects of nonsteroidal anti-inflammatory medications.
      c. *Chemical incompatibility.*
         (3) Two intravenous medications when combined can cause chemical deterioration of one or both medications (usually due to acid-base incompatibility), resulting in precipitate formation, color change, or gas development.
         (4) Example: Famotidine (Pepcid) and azithromycin (Zithromax) cannot be combined in one solution.
      d. Nursing care.
         (1) Assess resources to identify whether medications being administered concurrently are compatible or incompatible.

(2) Administer incompatible intravenous medications separately to maintain the integrity of each medication.

(3) Check mixed solutions before administration for changes in appearance that indicate a medication interaction (e.g., precipitate, color change, or gas development).

F. Commonalities of nursing care related to nontherapeutic reponses to medications

1. Check medication compatibility charts before administering medications being given concurrently to ensure that they are compatible.

2. Assess for therapeutic and nontherapeutic clinical manifestations of medication therapy.

⓵ 3. Withhold a medication when a client demonstrates a sign or symptom that is more serious than a side effect or if a medication-medication interaction occurs and report the finding to the primary health-care provider.

4. Teach the client about the medication regimen.
   a. The action of and rationale for the prescribed medication.
   b. Pertinent information regarding safe administration.
   c. Actions to take if a dose is accidentally omitted.
   d. Assessments to make to evaluate responses to the medication.
   e. Actions to take in the event of a nontherapeutic response.

5. Document consultation with the primary health-care provider regarding a client's nontherapeutic response to medication therapy and resulting interventions.

6. Document all information associated with medication administration and client responses to therapy.

⓵ 7. Implement emergency actions to support a client who has a serious nontherapeutic response until a primary health-care provider assumes responsibility for prescribing medical interventions; for example, activate the rapid response team, administer oxygen, elevate the head of the bed, and prepare for intubation and mechanical ventilation if a client is having difficulty breathing.

8. Implement measures based on standing prescriptions; for example, administer an antidote for an overdose or epinephrine for an anaphylactic reaction.

II. Pharmacokinetics

Pharmacokinetics is the study of the absorption, distribution, biotransformation (metabolism), and excretion of medications. Each of these factors is related to

the concentration of the medication in the body and can be viewed in relation to a time frame associated with the medication's pharmacological effects (Fig. 9.1). Nurses should understand these concepts as well as the factors that affect pharmacokinetics and related nursing care.

A. Elements of pharmacokinetics

1. Absorption.
   a. *Absorption* is the process of movement of a medication into the bloodstream.
   b. Rate of absorption depends on a number of factors.
      (1) Route of administration: Oral route requires time for medication absorption versus the intravenous route, which is distributed immediately.
      (2) Presence or absence of food in the stomach: Food in the stomach can delay absorption of medications and lengthen the time it takes for a medication to reach the small intestines, where most medications are absorbed.

2. Distribution.
   a. *Distribution* is the transport of a medication from the site of absorption to the site of medication action.
   b. Affected by such factors as degree of membrane permeability; protein binding capacity of the medication; and interruption in arterial blood supply to a tissue, organ, or extremity

Fig 9.1 Medication concentrations in the blood. (From Wilkinson and Treas [2016]. *Fundamentals of nursing*, Vol. 1, 3rd ed. Philadelphia: F. A. Davis Company, with permission.)

that limits delivery of a medication to the target site.

(1) Tightly packed endothelial cells prevent some medications from being distributed to the brain (blood-brain barrier).

(2) Only medications that are lipid soluble and are more loosely bound to plasma proteins can pass through the blood-brain barrier.

3. Biotransformation (metabolism).

a. **Biotransformation** is the conversion of a medication to a less active form (detoxification) in preparation for excretion.

b. Occurs mainly in the liver but also can occur in the kidneys, intestinal mucosa, lungs, or blood plasma.

c. Can be affected by disease states.

4. Excretion.

a. *Excretion* is the elimination of medications by the body.

b. Occurs primarily via the kidneys, where medications are eliminated from the body via urine but also can occur via feces, perspiration, saliva, breath, and breast milk.

c. Ability to excrete medications decreases with age, placing older adults at risk for medication accumulation and toxicity.

d. Kidney disease can interfere with excretion, thereby causing medication accumulation and toxicity.

B. Concepts associated with medication effectiveness and related nursing care

1. Duration.

a. **Duration** is the length of time a therapeutic blood concentration of a medication is maintained.

b. Nursing care.

(1) Assess the client's response, considering the medication's expected duration of action.

(2) Notify the primary health-care provider if an unexpected response occurs.

(3) Example: A client receiving a sedative is lethargic long after the effect of the medication should have dissipated, requiring a decrease in the dosage of the medication or discontinuation of the medication.

2. Half-life.

a. **Half-life** is the time needed to metabolize or inactivate one-half the amount of a medication.

b. Nursing care.

(1) Assess the client's response, considering the medication's half-life.

(2) Notify the primary health-care provider if an unexpected response occurs.

(3) Example: A client has pain before the next scheduled dose of an analgesic, indicating that the dose should be increased or the time between doses shortened.

3. Onset.

a. **Onset** is the length of time it takes the body to respond to a medication.

b. Nursing care.

(1) Assess the client's response to a medication at the time of the medication's expected onset.

(2) Example: Most oral analgesics have an onset of 20 to 30 minutes.

4. Peak blood level.

a. A **peak blood level** is the highest blood concentration of a medication (see Fig. 9.1).

b. Nursing care.

(1) Arrange for the client's blood to be drawn for a peak plasma level 30 to 60 minutes after medication administration.

(2) Example: Client's peak blood level for a medication exceeds the expected therapeutic level; withhold the medication and inform the primary health-care provider; a decrease in the frequency or dose usually is required.

(3) Seek a prescription for a decrease in the dose and/or frequency of administration.

5. Trough blood level.

a. A **trough blood level** is the lowest blood concentration of a medication (see Fig. 9.1).

b. Nursing care.

(1) Arrange for the client's blood to be drawn for a trough level just before the next scheduled dose.

(2) Example: Client's trough level for a medication is less than the expected therapeutic level; inform the primary health-care provider; an increase in the frequency or dose usually is required.

(3) Seek a prescription for an increase in the dose and/or frequency of administration.

6. Therapeutic range.

a. The **therapeutic range** is the dosage range or serum concentration of a medication usually expected to achieve the medication's desired effect.

b. Nursing care.

(1) Monitor serum peak and trough levels to ensure that levels fall within the established therapeutic window for the medication.

(2) Example: The peak level for gentamicin should not exceed 10 mcg/mL and trough levels should not be below 2 mcg/mL).

C. Factors affecting pharmacokinetics and related nursing care

1. Age.

a. Infants have immature body systems and are small in size.

b. Older adults experience decreased multiorgan functioning, which increases medication absorption and decreases biotransformation and excretion.

c. Nursing care.

(1) Ensure that medication doses are appropriate for body weight of infants and children.

(2) Assess infants, children, and older adults for clinical manifestations of medication toxicity. Clients may require a lower dose of the medication.

2. Body mass.

a. A person with a larger body mass may require a larger dose.

b. A person with a smaller body mass may require a lower dose.

c. Nursing care.

(1) Evaluate the response of obese clients to medications to ensure that a therapeutic response is achieved with the prescribed dose.

(2) Evaluate the response of a client with a small body mass to ensure that the dose prescribed is not excessive.

3. Diet.

a. The presence of food can delay the absorption of some medications.

b. Some medications can cause gastric irritation when not taken with food.

c. Some foods can alter the action of medications.

(1) Foods high in vitamin K should be consistently limited in clients receiving the anticoagulant warfarin (Coumadin) because vitamin K is the antidote for warfarin toxicity; in addition, inconsistent intake of vitamin K causes fluctuating prothrombin times and International Normalized Ratio (INR) levels.

(2) Tyramine-rich foods, such as aged cheese, pickled herring, yogurt, raisins, chicken liver, dried sausage, and sauerkraut, when taken with a monoamine oxidase (MAO) inhibitor, can precipitate a hypertensive crisis, intracranial bleeding, and death.

d. Some medications can alter nutrients or appetite.

(1) Quinolone antibiotics may extend the effects of caffeine.

(2) Lisdexamfetamine (Vivance) reduces appetite, contributing to weight loss.

e. Nursing care.

(1) Teach clients when a medication should be given with or without food.

! **(2) Teach clients about foods to ingest or avoid to prevent nontherapeutic effects of medications.**

4. Environment.

a. Hot environments cause peripheral vasodilation, intensifying the action of vasodilators.

b. Cold environments cause peripheral vasoconstriction, inhibiting the action of vasodilators while increasing the action of vasoconstrictors.

c. Noisy environments can interfere with the therapeutic effects of sedatives and analgesics.

d. Nursing care.

(1) Ensure a temperate (moderate, not excessive) environmental temperature when a client is receiving a vasodilator or vasoconstrictor.

(2) Ensure a quiet environment when a client is receiving a sedative or analgesic.

5. Gender.

a. Medication response discrepancies in men and women are attributable to body fat distribution, percentage of body fluid differences, and hormonal differences that affect medication absorption.

b. The majority of medication research is based on studies involving men; responses of women may be different from what is documented in medication literature.

c. Nursing care.

(1) Explore manufacturer-provided information to determine if research included women if the medication is to be administered to a woman.

(2) Assess for therapeutic and nontherapeutic responses in women.

6. Genetic, ethnic, and cultural factors.

a. Genes can cause liver metabolism to be slow or rapid, influencing medication metabolism.

b. Research demonstrates that a dose of medication may be therapeutic for individuals in a specific ethnic group and toxic for those in another group (e.g., opioids are metabolized at a slower rate by individuals of Asian descent).

c. Nursing care.

(1) Identify clients who are at risk for nontherapeutic effects of medication therapy because of genetic, ethnic, and cultural factors.

(2) Assess clients of Asian descent who are prescribed opioids for clinical manifestations of medication toxicity.

7. Illness and disease.
   a. Impaired gastrointestinal, liver, kidney, or cardiovascular function can alter a client's response to a medication because of altered absorption, transport, biotransformation, or excretion.
   b. Nursing care.
      (1) Assess clients with impaired gastrointestinal functioning to ensure that oral medications are effective; route may need to be changed when oral medications are ineffective.
      (2) Assess clients with impaired cardiovascular functioning to ensure that medications are effective; impaired cardiovascular functioning may not transport medications to desired site of action.
      (3) Assess clients with impaired liver or kidney functioning for signs of toxicity due to inadequate biotransformation or excretion of the medication.
8. Psychological factors.
   a. If a client believes that a medication will work, the client often has a more favorable therapeutic response.
   b. If a client mistrusts the value of a medication, this belief can interfere with the medication's effectiveness.
   c. Anxiety can interfere with the therapeutic effect of central nervous system depressants.
   d. Nursing care.
      (1) Explore the client's beliefs about the value of a medication regimen.
      (2) Clarify the client's misunderstandings about a medication to increase trust in the value of the regimen.
      (3) Employ nursing measures to reduce anxiety when a client is receiving central nervous system depressants.
9. Route of administration.
   a. The route influences the volume of medication absorbed into the circulation and its transport to the target site (e.g., oral medications require time to be absorbed and transported, whereas those administered via the intravenous route produce an immediate response).
   b. Nursing care.
      (1) Ensure that the route is appropriate for the client's situation. For example, if the client has gastric surgery, the oral route may not be appropriate; if the client is confused, the client may not understand that a troche should be held in the buccal cavity until dissolved.
      (2) Assess the client's response to medication based on the expected onset associated with the route used.

III. Medication Misuse

Many medications, particularly central nervous system stimulants and depressants, have a narrow therapeutic window. When medications are misused, the therapeutic window may be exceeded, resulting in numerous negative physiological and psychological consequences, including death. Nurses must teach clients how to use medications responsibly, assess clients for the clinical manifestations of medication misuse, and intervene to help clients who are struggling with the negative consequences of medication misuse.

A. Terminology related to medication misuse
   1. *Drug misuse*: Continual or periodic maladaptive use of a medication different from the recommended prescribed pattern, causing physical and/or emotional harm with a risk of disturbance of daily life.
   2. *Habituation*: Repeated misuse that causes a person to feel better than when not using the medication; the person generally can discontinue use without severe psychological or physical effects.
   3. *Illicit medications (street medications)*: Medications that are sold illegally.
   4. *Physiological dependence*: Need for a medication to avoid physical manifestations of withdrawal.
   5. *Psychological dependence*: Emotional need for a medication to maintain a feeling of well-being, satisfaction, or pleasure.
   6. *Tolerance*: Condition in which the body becomes accustomed to a medication and needs a larger dose to attain the desired effect or to prevent clinical manifestations of withdrawal.
   7. *Withdrawal syndrome*: Presence of specific physical and/or psychological signs and symptoms associated with cessation of a particular medication on which the client is dependent.

B. Nursing care related to medication misuse
   1. Assess for clinical manifestations of physiological dependence on a medication (e.g., signs and symptoms of withdrawal when the medication is not taken).
      a. Stimulants: Pressured speech, hyperactivity or hypoactivity, signs of central nervous system stimulation or depression, and requests for analgesics before the next scheduled dose.
      b. Opioids: Watery eyes, runny nose, dilated pupils, tremors, chills, fever, yawning, diaphoresis, nausea, vomiting, diarrhea, and abdominal cramps.
   2. Assess for clinical manifestations of psychological dependence on a medication (e.g., signs and symptoms of anxiety when the medication is not taken, compulsive behaviors associated with procuring and using a medication).

3. Assess for clinical manifestations of tolerance to a medication (e.g., request for a medication before the next scheduled dose, nonachievement of a therapeutic effect after receiving what is considered to be an adequate dose).

4. Assess for clinical manifestations of habituation to a medication (e.g., taking a laxative every day, using an antihistamine to promote sleep).

5. Use interviewing skills to determine insight into personal problems resulting from medication misuse and explore client concerns.

6. Teach nonpharmacological strategies to manage stress and anxiety.

🛑 7. Teach pregnant women to avoid unnecessary medications, alcohol, and nicotine because of the risk of fetal harm.

8. Reinforce efforts by the client toward stopping medication misuse.

9. Provide information about referrals to professionals or agencies that can assist the client with withdrawal.

IV. Herbal Supplements

Herbs are plants used for medicinal purposes. Many people take them to promote health and wellness, increase energy and performance, prevent and treat illnesses, or relieve depression. The use of herbal supplements has increased concurrent with the expanding interest in alternative therapies as people seek more "natural" therapies. Unfortunately, many people are misinformed of the facts about herbal supplements. Nurses must educate clients so that clients can make informed decisions about the use of herbal supplements.

A. Factual information about herbal supplements

1. Some herbal supplements may prevent, treat, and cure some illnesses through the use of plant substances.

2. Some manufacturers of herbal supplements claim benefits that are unproven.

DID YOU KNOW?

Many people believe that supplements are safe because they are advertised as being "natural." However, this is not necessarily the case. Also, herbal supplements are not regulated by the FDA for safety and efficacy, even though they are chemicals that have an influence on the body.

3. Some herbal supplements, when taken with prescribed or OTC medications, can cause serious medication-medication interactions or nontherapeutic responses.

4. Some clients do not share information regarding self-medication with herbal supplements because either they do not realize the importance of this information or they are embarrassed that they are self-medicating.

5. Information and research about herbal supplements can be obtained from a variety of sources.
   a. FDA official Website (www.fda.gov).
   b. Herb Research Foundation (www.herbs.org).
   c. American Botanical Council (www.abc.herbalgram.org).
   d. WebMD (www.webmd.com).

B. Herbal supplements and related nursing care

1. Know and understand information related to the most common herbal supplements.

2. Collect data about herbal supplement intake (including the name of each supplement and the amount, frequency, and reasons for its use), and share this information with clients' primary health-care providers. Also include this information on medication reconciliation forms.

3. Explore each client's understanding about herbal supplements being taken.

4. Assess for signs and symptoms of adverse reactions to herbal supplements.

5. Teach clients that herbal supplements can increase or decrease the effects of other medications and therefore must be avoided when taking certain prescribed or OTC medications.

6. Teach clients to avoid the ingestion of alcohol with many herbal supplements because of the risk of nontherapeutic interactions.

7. Teach clients about the risk of having an allergic reaction to herbal supplements and instruct them to discontinue intake if signs and symptoms occur.

8. Encourage clients to discuss benefits and risks of taking herbal supplements with their primary health-care providers.

🛑 9. Teach clients to stop the use of herbal supplements that have antiplatelet properties, such as garlic and gingko biloba, when scheduled for dental intervention or surgery.

🛑 10. Encourage women who are pregnant or trying to become pregnant to avoid all herbal supplements because little is known regarding teratogenic effects.

🛑 11. Encourage women who are breastfeeding to avoid taking herbal supplements because of unknown effects on infants.

12. Refer clients to reliable sources of information about herbal supplements.

13. See Table 9.1 for nursing care related to specific herbal supplements.

Table 9.1 Common Herbal Supplements and Related Nursing Care

Specific Herbs	Effect	Nursing Care
Echinacea	• Believed to increase white blood cells, spleen cells, and the activity of granulocytes, helper T cells, and cytokines. • Used for immune-enhancing properties to prevent and treat upper respiratory infections and the flu. • May decrease the effectiveness of immunosuppressants.	1. Encourage the client to avoid taking echinacea when receiving an immunosuppressant. 2. Teach the client to seek a primary health-care provider's attention when no improvement is noted after a few days of treating an upper respiratory infection or flu with echinacea.
Garlic *(Allium sativum)*	• Contains the amino acid allicin, which has antibacterial qualities. • Possesses antimicrobial, antitumor, antilipidemic, and antithrombolytic properties. • Used to prevent hypertension, hyperlipidemia, and cardiovascular disease. • Increases antiplatelet action in clients receiving an anticoagulant. • Decreases the effectiveness of antihypertensives. • Allergic reactions are common, such as contact dermatitis, asthma, rash, and diaphoresis. • Chronic use decreases hemoglobin level and causes lysis of red blood cells.	1. Monitor blood pressure if a client is concurrently taking an antihypertensive to ensure its effectiveness. 2. Assess a client who is concurrently taking an anticoagulant for bruising or bleeding. 3. Instruct the client to inform the primary health-care provider of the chronic use of garlic so that hemoglobin and red blood cell levels are monitored.
Gingko biloba	• Believed to increase cerebral and peripheral blood flow. • Used for memory impairment, dementia, tinnitus, leg cramping, pain caused by walking (intermittent claudication), vertigo, and impotence. • Can increase antiplatelet action of anticoagulants. • Can cause cerebral bleeding.	1. Teach the client to avoid taking Gingko biloba when also taking an anticoagulant. 2. Assess a client for bruising and bleeding when the client insists on concurrently taking an anticoagulant.
Ginseng	• Research demonstrates anti-inflammatory, antioxidant, analgesic, diuretic, and anticancer effects. • Used for improving a feeling of well-being, stamina, appetite, sleep pattern, memory, concentration, and energy. • Has nontherapeutic herb-medication interactions with MAO inhibitors, caffeine, and glaucoma medications. • American ginseng increases hepatic lipogenesis and storage of glycogen. • Panax ginseng has serious adverse effects. • Should not be taken by clients with cardiovascular disease, hypertension, or hypotension and those who are receiving steroid therapy because of herb-medication interactions with medications prescribed for these conditions.	1. Assess for signs and symptoms of ginseng toxicity: diarrhea, restlessness, nausea, vomiting, and headache. 2. If the client insists on taking ginseng, encourage taking American ginseng with meals to prevent inadvertent hypoglycemia in people who are not diabetic. 3. Assess a client who is diabetic more frequently for hypoglycemia until the response is determined. 4. Encourage a client taking an MAO inhibitor, glaucoma medication, or any form of caffeine to avoid ginseng because of nontherapeutic herb-medication interactions. 5. Encourage the client to avoid Panax ginseng because of adverse effects. 6. Instruct clients with hypertension or hypotension, those receiving steroids, and those with cardiovascular disease to discontinue ginseng due to interactions with medications prescribed for these conditions.
Saw Palmetto	• Has antiandrogenic, anti-inflammatory, and antiproliferative properties in prostate tissue. • Used to reduce the frequency of urination, urgency, hesitancy, and nocturia associated with benign prostatic hyperplasia. • May decrease prostate-specific antigen (PSA) levels, delaying prostate cancer diagnosis. • Contraindicated during pregnancy and breastfeeding.	1. Assess urinary function, such as force of urinary stream, dribbling, straining, urgency, hesitancy, feeling of incomplete bladder emptying, and dysuria. 2. Encourage the client to consult with a urologist to monitor the size and status of the prostate gland. 3. Instruct a woman who anticipates pregnancy or breastfeeding to discontinue saw palmetto.
St. John's Wort	• Believed to selectively inhibit serotonin, dopamine, and norepinephrine reuptake in the central nervous system. • Used for mild to moderate depression and sleep disorders. • Is safe if used alone. • Reduces therapeutic levels of oral contraceptives, anticoagulants, and antivirals. • Can cause photosensitivity.	1. Teach the client to avoid taking St. John's Wort when receiving an anticoagulant, antiviral, or oral contraceptive because it increases elimination of these medications. 2. Encourage the client to reduce sun exposure and teach the client to use sunscreen to protect from photosensitivity reactions.

V. The Rights of Medication Administration and Related Nursing Care

A nurse should focus on five elements when administering medications. These elements are called the Five Rights of Medication Administration and include the right client, right medication, right dose, right route, and right time. A nurse should consider these five elements when administering each medication because they have proven to be valuable in reducing medication errors.

A. *Right client*
1. Check the client's name against two verifiers, following agency policy. For example, ask the client to state his or her name and birth date and verify the name against the medication administration record (MAR) and client's wristband; if applicable, use a computer scanner to verify the client's wristband bar code.
2. Follow alert procedures when two clients have a similar last name (e.g., place them in different rooms, flag their MARs and the front of their clinical records, and place wristbands issuing the alert).

B. *Right medication*
1. Know the normal dose for commonly administered medications.
2. Check a resource about a medication for which you are unsure.
3. Verify the medication against the primary health-care provider's prescription.
4. Use a computer scanner to verify the medication package bar code.

C. *Right dose*
1. Ensure that the prescribed dose is appropriate for the client. Use a pediatric calculation formula for infants and children.
2. Calculate the dose carefully and double-check all math calculations.
3. Use a computer scanner to verify the medication package bar code.
4. Question the primary health-care provider about a dose outside the expected range.

D. *Right route*
1. Give the medication via the prescribed route.
2. Ensure that the route is safe for the client (e.g., rectal route is contraindicated in clients with rectal bleeding; oral route is contraindicated when a client is vomiting).

E. *Right time*
1. Give the medication at the prescribed time, ensuring that it is less than 60 minutes before or after the scheduled time (e.g., numerous clients receiving care from one nurse cannot all receive 10:00 medications at the same time).
2. Ensure that the medication is administered at the prescribed frequency (e.g., once a day, twice a day, three times a day).

DID YOU KNOW?

The Five Rights of Medication Administration are so effective in reminding a nurse of the significant elements to consider when preparing and administering medications that an additional five rights were identified. They include right education, right assessment, right to refuse, right evaluation, and right documentation. These additional five rights reflect the fact that medication administration is not just the physical process of preparing and administering a prescribed medication. Nursing responsibilities also include educating the client, ensuring that the medication is still appropriate for the client, evaluating client responses, maintaining legal records through documentation, and respecting that a client has a right to refuse a prescribed medication.

F. *Right education*
1. Provide the client with information about the medication, including its name, action, expected therapeutic response, and associated precautions.
2. Ask whether the client has any questions and correct misconceptions.

G. *Right assessment*
1. Implement all assessments required before medication administration (e.g., pulse rate and/or blood pressure for cardiac medications).
2. Administer medications based on parameters identified by the primary health-care provider that require a specific assessment (e.g., give a specific number of units of insulin to "cover" a particular blood glucose level).
3. Ensure that the medication is still appropriate for the client.

H. *Right to refuse*
1. Explore the client's reason for refusing to take a medication.
2. Implement teaching regarding the necessity of the medication and correct client misconceptions.
3. Accept the client's right to refuse to take a medication.
4. Document the client's stated reason for refusing a medication.
5. Notify the primary health-care provider of the client's refusal to take a prescribed medication.

I. *Right evaluation*
1. Reassess the client and compare the actual outcome with the expected outcome to determine medication effectiveness.
2. Be alert for nontherapeutic effects.
3. Notify the primary health-care provider of nontherapeutic effects and seek new prescriptions as needed.
4. Document the client's response to all medications in the clinical record.

J. *Right documentation*

1. Document all medications given in the MAR *after* they are given, never before.
2. Maintain appropriate legal documents concerning controlled medications.
3. Follow agency policy when a medication is not administered; for example, circle, initial, or highlight the dose on an electronic chart and document why the medication was not given (e.g., client refused medication, BP beyond parameters).
4. Complete an incident report if a prescribed medication was not administered properly, such as not on time, missed dose, or inaccurate dose.

VI. Medication-Dispensing Systems

The introduction of individual packaging of medications (unit-dose) and the use of a medication cart with a drawer for each client provided a better system to secure, store, prepare, and deliver medications to clients prior to the previous system of large bottles of stock medications, reducing medication errors. Automated dispensing systems have added an additional level of safety by requiring a user password and providing a computer database that records all pertinent information when a medication is administered. The most recent safety measure is the use of a computer sensor to scan a bar code to verify the client's name and the medication to be administered; it also documents the medications administered. Multiple checks and balances help to maintain client safety concerning medication administration.

A. Medication cart

1. Lockable, rolling cabinet that contains medications for clients on a specific unit.
   a. Must be locked whenever the nurse steps away.
   b. Can be opened only by a key/card or access code.
2. Should be wheeled to outside each client's room when administering medications and left locked outside an open doorway to a client's room when giving medications to a client.
3. Generally are stored in or near the nurse's station when not in use, although some facilities require them to be locked to the wall of the nurse's station or stored in a locked medication room.
4. Generally contains the following contents.
   a. Top of the cart provides a work surface and holds important equipment and supplies, such as the computer, pitcher of water, medicine cups, and pill crusher.
   b. A sharps container, trash container, and light may be built into the top or attached to the side of the cart.
   c. Handles are provided for steering and for holding equipment, such as a stethoscope.
   d. The top drawer may contain straws, tongue blades, gauze, alcohol wipes, and other supplies.
   e. Small drawers correlate to the room number and beds on the unit; they are labeled with clients' identification information and contain the medications that each client is to receive for 24 hours.
   f. A large drawer may contain bulkier items, such as bottles of liquids.
   g. Another large drawer may contain stock medications, such as aspirin, ibuprofen, acetaminophen, and docusate sodium.
   h. Another drawer with divided compartments may contain different-sized syringes and gauge needles.
5. Medications in drawers are restocked by a member of the pharmacy department.
6. Generally contain medications in unit-dose packages, with each package stating the medication name, dose, and expiration date.

B. Medication room

1. Generally, contains controlled medications in a locked cabinet or an automated medication-dispensing cabinet. For managing controlled drugs see Box 9.2.
2. Used to prepare intravenous solutions before transport to a client's room or preparation of subcutaneous (Sub-Q) or intramuscular (IM) injections, which are then capped and transported individually to each client.

Box 9.2 Managing Controlled Drugs

Management and administration of controlled drugs are highly regulated by federal law. Be aware of these nursing considerations when working with controlled drugs.

- *Store controlled drugs in a double-locked cabinet, medication room, cart, or computer-automated drug-dispensing system.*
- *Use a secure identification code to access computer-automated drug-dispensing systems.*
- *Count opioids and controlled drugs at specific times, such as at change of shift (a nurse completing a shift counts the controlled drugs together with a nurse coming on duty). If a computer-automated dispensing system runs a continuous count, manual counting at the end of a shift is unnecessary.*
- *Account for each dose of an opioid or controlled drug on a controlled substance record, which includes the name of the client, amount of drug used, time the drug was administered, name of the prescribing primary health-care provider, and name of the nurse administering the drug.*
- *Ensure that stock doses remaining equal the number of doses available on the controlled-drug record before preparing a controlled drug.*
- *Report a discrepancy in a controlled drug count immediately to an administrative nurse and the pharmacy department, depending on facility policy.*
- *Employ efforts to help identify the source of the discrepancy immediately.*
- *Have a second nurse act as a witness if all or part of a controlled drug needs to be discarded; both nurses must sign the controlled drug sheet.*

3. May have a refrigerator dedicated only for the storage of medications that must be kept cool, such as some vaccines and skin test agents.

C. Automated medication-dispensing systems
1. Computer access system that controls the distribution, management, and control of medications.
2. Usually contains controlled medications, but some agencies are moving toward using an automated medication-dispensing cabinet for all client medications.
3. Requires the password/card of the caregiver, requires the nurse to access a client's name and select a medication, dispenses the medication, and records the entire transaction.

VII. Medication Prescriptions

Administration of a medication requires a prescription by a primary health-care provider and is a dependent function of the nurse. The nurse must ensure that all components of a prescription are evident before administering the medication. Primary health-care providers can write various types of prescriptions, such as *standing, as needed (prn), single-dose, immediately (STAT),* and *now orders.* Nurses must know the policies and procedures associated with the communication of medication prescriptions, such as transcription of medication prescriptions and reception of verbal and telephone prescriptions. These legal requirements and policies and procedures are designed to ensure safety and reduce errors associated with the delivery of medications.

A. Parts of a medication prescription
1. Client's full name.
2. Date and time the prescription is written.
3. Name of the medication.
4. Dosage of the medication.
5. Route of administration.
6. Frequency of administration.
7. Situation (e.g., when an as-needed medication should be administered, parameters for when a medication should be held).
8. Primary health-care provider's signature.

DID YOU KNOW?

A nurse must call the primary health-care provider to discuss concerns if a medication prescription is incomplete, ambiguous, contraindicated, inappropriate, or unusual. A nurse should document in the clinical record that the primary health-care provider was called, including details about the discussion and response.

B. Types of medication prescriptions
1. Standing (routine).
   a. Medication prescription that is carried out until it is discontinued or the required number of days has lapsed.

b. Nursing care.
   (1) Know facility policies regarding automatic discontinuation of medications.
   (2) Be aware that standing prescriptions must be reordered after surgery or transfer to a different service.
   (3) Administer a medication as prescribed until it is discontinued, the number of prescribed days' lapses, or according to facility policy, such as 5 to 14 days for specific antibiotics.
   (4) Evaluate the client's response to the medication.
2. As needed (prn).
   a. Prescription for a medication to be given only when it is needed; must include circumstances in which the medication is to be given (e.g., morphine sulfate 2 mg IV prn *every 3 hours for incisional pain*).
   b. Nursing care.
      (1) Document assessments that indicated the need for the medication in the clinical record.
      (2) Check the MAR to identify when a medication was last given to ensure that adequate time has lapsed since the previous dose.
      (3) Document administration in the prn section of the MAR.
      (4) Evaluate the client's response to the medication.
3. Single-dose (one time only).
   a. Prescription for a medication to be given only once, such as a medication given before a diagnostic test or before surgery.
   b. Nursing care.
      (1) Administer the medication one time only.
      (2) Document administration of the medication in the single-dose section of the MAR.
      (3) Evaluate the client's response to the medication.
4. Immediately (STAT).
   a. Prescription for a single dose of a medication to be given immediately.
   b. Often prescribed in emergency situations.
   c. Nursing care.
      (1) Administer a STAT medication immediately.
      (2) Document administration in the single-dose section of the MAR.
      (3) Evaluate the client's response to the medication.

C. Communication of medication prescriptions
1. Written prescription: A primary health-care provider writes a prescription following the protocol established by the agency. It generally involves

a computer form that is electronically sent to the pharmacy.

   a. Ensure that prescriptions contain all required elements.

   b. Notify the pharmacy of the new prescription; this may be done manually, by fax, or automatically when it was initiated on the computer; computer prescriptions help to minimize errors by automatically notifying the pharmacy and generating an MAR.

   c. Transcribe to or verify prescriptions on the MAR; this may be done manually or by a computer; recheck it several times to ensure accuracy.

2. Verbal prescription: Prescription given by a primary health-care provider verbally in person.

   a. Accept only in emergency situations, when there is no time to put it in writing.

   b. Repeat the prescription back to the primary health-care provider for confirmation.

   c. Ensure that the primary health-care provider countersigns it as soon as possible and no later than 24 hours after the event.

3. Telephone prescription: Prescription given by a primary health-care provider via the telephone; generally used in emergency situations when a primary health-care provider is not present.

   a. Use only in situations in which a written or verbal prescription is not possible.

   b. Follow policy as to who can receive telephone prescriptions, such as a primary nurse or supervisor.

   c. Repeat the prescription back to the primary health-care provider for confirmation.

   d. Make sure that two nurses listen to the prescription and have both nurses countersign the prescription.

   e. Ensure that the primary health-care provider countersigns the prescription within 24 hours.

VIII. Nursing Care Related to Medication Administration

Preparing and administering medications involves more than just removing medication from a package and giving it to a client. It involves critical thinking throughout the process to ensure that the rights of medication administration are addressed as well as the general considerations associated with medication administration. When administering any medication, irrespective of the route, the nurse should follow guidelines to ensure that medications are prepared and administered safely. This process is complex and requires that the nurse remain focused without interruptions because it is too easy to become distracted and confused. Accuracy and client safety are the expected outcomes of medication administration.

A. General considerations when administering medications

1. Complete or review the medication reconciliation form, including prescribed medications, OTC medications, supplemental herbs, and vitamins, to ensure the client is receiving prescribed medications and help prevent nontherapeutic medication-medication interactions or an excess of medication intake.

2. Identify food and medication allergies and communicate them according to facility policies and procedures, such as on the MAR, on the front of the clinical record, on a wristband, in the plan of care, and by notification of the pharmacy. Doing so prevents allergic responses and ensures continuity of care.

3. Identify factors that impact medication therapy (e.g., age, disease, gender, body mass, diet) and perform a health history and physical examination as needed to ensure client factors are taken into consideration when determining the appropriateness of a medication.

4. Administer oral medications with food or between meals as indicated by the pharmacy and the medication manufacturer to facilitate absorption (e.g., taking ferrous sulfate [Feosol] with ascorbic acid [citrus juice] or taking certain medications, such as levothyroxine [Synthroid], on an empty stomach) and to help minimize gastric irritation for certain medications (e.g., ibuprofen [Advil, Motrin]).

5. Assess client understanding of prescribed medications and provide information to ensure accurate knowledge, including medication name; therapeutic action; nontherapeutic effects; parameters associated with the medication, such as pulse rate or BP; and actions to take in case of an adverse reaction or missed dose. Doing so ensures the client is knowledgeable about prescribed medications and supports participation in the medication regimen.

6. Assess pregnancy status if a prescribed medication is teratogenic to reduce the risk of injury to a developing fetus. Determine whether a mother is breastfeeding to reduce the risk of transfer of medication ingredients to a breastfeeding infant.

7. Perform (e.g., blood glucose monitoring) or review results (e.g., peak and trough levels) of diagnostic tests that impact medication administration to ensure administration of a safe dose of a medication.

8. Withhold a medication that indicates a peak level higher than the therapeutic level to ensure prevention of excessive medication levels.

9. Notify the primary health-care provider of medication levels outside the established parameters to ensure that the primary health-care provider can prescribe a corrective action if necessary.

B. Common nursing interventions when administering medications

1. Perform hand hygiene per policy and procedure, such as using soap and water or a hand sanitizer, to remove debris and minimize the number of microorganisms on the hands, thereby reducing the risk of infection.

2. Position the medication cart outside the client's room. Lock the cart when it is unattended and when away from the cart giving medications to a client to minimize contamination of the cart and prevent unauthorized access to medications.

3. Verify that the medication being prepared is prescribed for the client (right client and right medication), is the prescribed dose (right dose), is being administered via the prescribed route (right route), and is being given at the prescribed time (right time). This verification should be performed three times (triple check) to reduce the risk of medication errors. For example:
    a. *First check:* When removing the medication from a drawer.
    b. *Second check:* When preparing the medication, such as placing an unopened oral medication in a medicine cup, pouring a liquid, or filling a syringe.
    c. *Third check:* Just before opening the package of an oral medication at the bedside or just after preparation of a liquid or parenteral medication.

4. Verify the expiration date on a medication package and return the medication to the pharmacy if it is expired because expired medications can lose their potency.

5. Introduce yourself and state that you are there to administer medications. This supports a client's right to know who is providing care and what is to be done.

6. Ask the client to state his or her name and birth date and verify the response against the MAR and wristband; follow the verification policy and procedure of the facility (e.g., a medication package bar code must be verified against the bar code on the client's wristband).

7. Teach about the medications being administered and ask whether the client has any questions to ensure understanding about the medications being administered and support motivation to take the medication.

8. Establish whether a client's status is within prescribed or expected parameters before administering a medication (e.g., pulse rate greater than 60 beats/minute for digoxin or BP within parameters set by a policy or the primary health-care provider).

9. Withhold a medication and inform the primary health-care provider when a client's status does not meet set parameters to prevent an excessive level of the medication and promote an appropriate response by the primary health-care provider.

10. Assess for therapeutic and nontherapeutic responses to a medication before administering another dose (e.g., stools are not loose when receiving a stool softener or laxative.)

11. Withhold a medication if it is no longer appropriate or if an adverse response occurred to prevent client injury.

12. Notify the primary health-care provider if a nontherapeutic response occurs that is more serious than a minor side effect. Doing so ensures immediate attention to nontherapeutic responses that require medical intervention or a change in a medication prescription.

13. Assist the client into a comfortable position for the prescribed route, such as sitting or Fowler's for oral medications or side lying for IM injections. The upright position uses gravity to facilitate ingestion of oral medications; the side-lying position provides access to the dorsogluteal and ventrogluteal muscles for an IM injection.

14. Allow the client to self-administer medications when appropriate. Assist those who need assistance, such as with positioning, holding a cup, or inserting an oral medication into the mouth. Doing so supports independence, allows the client to set the pace, and facilitates medication ingestion.

15. Document administration of medications, only after medications are administered, in the clinical record or MAR or according to facility policy and procedure. Doing so ensures accurate and complete documentation of medication administration in a permanent record.

16. Document nonadministration of a medication in the MAR or the clinical record progress notes or according to facility policy and procedure. Doing so ensures documentation of the event.

C. Administering medications to clients at risk for complications

1. Introduction.
    a. A nurse must assess all clients to determine whether they are at risk for complications associated with medication administration.

For example, a nurse should assess the client's developmental level (particularly age) and health status (particularly the ability to swallow, presence of the gag reflex, and efficiency of kidney function).

  b. Once the potential for complications are identified, the nurse should implement additional interventions that specifically address the client's needs.

2. Older adults and related nursing care.
  a. May have difficulty swallowing tablets due to dry mouth.
    (1) Crush tablets that are crushable.
    (2) Give water before, during, and after medication administration.
    (3) Stroke under the chin to promote swallowing.
    (4) Seek a prescription for a liquid form of the medication.
  b. May process information more slowly, have slower physical movements, and/or experience decreased strength and reflexes.
    (1) Allow more time to provide information about medications.
    (2) Keep explanations simple.
    🛑 (3) Allow more time to administer medications; do not hurry the client.
    🛑 (4) Teach the client to avoid childproof safety tops on medication containers to facilitate easier handling of containers and to support independence if unable to open safety top containers. If children are in the home, then keep medications without safety tops in a locked cabinet.
    (5) Assess the client's ability to self-administer medications, such as eyedrops and injections.
    (6) Explore strategies for assistance, such as having a visiting nurse or family member assist with medication administration in the home.
  c. May be more forgetful, omitting doses or taking excessive doses of medications.
    (1) Construct a calendar of days and times medications are taken.
    (2) Instruct the client to place medications or signs in a prominent place in the home.
    (3) Teach the client how to use a divided pill container (e.g., if the morning section is empty in the evening, it confirms the morning medications were taken) to support the medication regimen and minimize errors.

  d. May have decreased visual acuity.
    (1) Write out the medication calendar in large letters or containers with raised letters.
    (2) Suggest using a large-labeled or braille divided pill container.
    (3) Suggest using a syringe that has a preset volume control feature to ensure an accurate dose when self-administering a parenteral medication.
  e. May not be able to afford prescribed medications.
    (1) Suggest that the primary health-care provider prescribe the generic form of the medication if available or a less costly medication.
    (2) Seek funding resources.

DID YOU KNOW?

Older adults are requesting primary health-care providers to write prescriptions for medications at twice the required dose. The client then divides the tablets into two doses in an effort to reduce the cost of prescribed medications. This practice is unsafe because the consistency of the dose may vary, and dividing doses increases the risk of contaminating the tablets. Nurses should teach clients why this practice is discouraged and assist clients to seek funding resources instead.

  f. Have decreased rate of medication metabolism and excretion, which increases the risk of toxicity.
    (1) Ensure that the prescribed dose takes into consideration the aging process to minimize the risk of an excessive dose.
    (2) Explore whether the client can manage with a lower dose than that for younger adults to avoid medication toxicity.
    (3) Assess for clinical indicators of medication toxicity.
    (4) Monitor blood levels of medications to ensure early identification of medication accumulation and promote early intervention to prevent toxicity.
    (5) Teach the client not to exceed the recommended doses of medications.
  g. Are at increased risk for medication interactions due to the intake of multiple medications (polypharmacy) necessary for treatment of chronic illnesses.
    (1) Assess for clinical indicators of medication interactions.
    (2) Encourage the primary health-care provider to periodically review the medication reconciliation form to promote discontinuation of unnecessary medications or to reduce a dose.

Polypharmacy and Aging

A nurse must understand the connection between the risks associated with the intake of multiple drugs and the factors related to aging. Because of the aging process, older adults are less able to metabolize and excrete medications, placing them at greater risk for drug toxicity. In addition, polypharmacy associated with the treatment of multiple chronic illnesses increases the risk of unfavorable drug interactions. According to the Centers for Disease Control and Prevention, by 2030, the number of U.S. adults age 65 years and older will double to about 71 million. That means, one out of every five people will be over the age of 65. Currently, 80% of older adults have one chronic illness and 50% of older adults have at least two chronic illnesses. Heart disease, cancer, brain attack (cerebrovascular accident, stroke), chronic obstructive pulmonary disease, and diabetes are among the most common causes of chronic illness in older adults. The essential challenge is to help older adults to remain healthy by preventing and/or minimizing these chronic diseases and their complications, thereby requiring fewer medications.

3. Infants and children and related nursing care.
   a. Infants and children vary in size, weight, and surface area and pass through various stages of growth and development.
      (1) Carefully calculate and recheck medication dosages using a pediatric calculation formula.
      (2) Assess developmental level and adjust interventions based on the child's physical, emotional, and cognitive levels.
   b. Infants and children are at risk for aspirating or choking on liquid medications.
      (1) Use a medication nipple for infants so that they can suck the medication; this is the safest method of administering a liquid medication to an infant because infants are familiar with breastfeeding or formula feeding.
      (2) Position the child in a sitting or semi-sitting position.
      (3) Use a needleless syringe or dropper.
      (4) Place the liquid between the lower gum and cheek.
      (5) Instill the medication slowly to avoid giving too much liquid at once.
      (6) Offer the child a choice of a spoon, needleless syringe, or dropper to support a sense of control.
   c. Young children may not be able to ingest tablets.
      (1) Crush tablets that are crushable and mix them with applesauce

      (2) Dissolve tablets that are dissolvable on a spoon with warm water.
      (3) Secure a liquid form of the medication.
   d. Young children are not moved by logic; saying, "This medication will make you feel better" will not work if the child does not like the taste.
      (1) Admit that the medication might not taste good, but that it will be followed with a nice-tasting juice to facilitate trust.
      (2) Give an ice pop just before giving an unpleasant tasting medication to numb the taste buds.
      (3) Avoid using an important food or liquid to mask the taste of a medication to prevent an unpleasant association and subsequent refusal of the important food or liquid.
   e. Children may be afraid of injections because they are associated with pain or the unfamiliar.
      (1) Awaken a sleeping child for an injection because doing so is less frightening and supports trust.
      (2) Admit that the injection might be uncomfortable, but that it will be over quickly to support trust.
      (3) Apply a topical anesthetic cream before an injection to minimize the discomfort of needle insertion.
      (4) Offer a toy to play with during and after the injection to distract the child.
      (5) Use the vastus lateralis muscle for children who are not walking yet because gluteal muscles are not fully developed.
      (6) Obtain the assistance of another health team member, rather than a parent, to restrain the child if necessary to avoid associating the parent with an unpleasant event.
      🛑 (7) Cuddle or have the parent cuddle the child after an injection to provide comfort.

4. Clients at risk for aspiration and related nursing care.
   a. The client may have difficulty chewing and swallowing or have an impaired gag reflex.
      (1) Assess the client's ability to swallow and cough and the presence of the gag reflex.
      (2) Place the client in an upright position if possible.
      (3) Thicken liquids or offer fruit nectars with oral medications to make fluid easier to control.
      (4) Avoid the use of a straw because fluid is harder to control when using a straw than when using a cup.

(5) Crush tablets that are crushable and mix them with a teaspoon of applesauce or secure a prescription for an alternate route.

(6) Allow the client to hold PO medications and a cup of water and to set the pace; do not hurry the client.

(7) Administer medications on the strong side of the mouth for a client with weakness of the oral cavity.

(8) Administer PO medications one at a time and ensure that each is swallowed before giving the next.

b. The client may have an altered level of consciousness.

(1) Seek a prescription for an alternate route for oral medications.

(2) Explain what is being done and why, with the assumption that the client hears and understands.

IX. Routes of Medication Administration and Related Nursing Care

The route of administration refers to where the medication enters the body. It is included as one of the parts of a medication prescription. The route of administration selected depends on such factors as the characteristics of the pharmacological product (e.g., insulin is destroyed in the gastrointestinal [GI] system and therefore is administered subcutaneously); the purpose of the medication (e.g., local or systemic effect); and client characteristics (e.g., client is unconscious, is vomiting, or has an impaired GI system). Routes of administration include oral, enteral tubes, oral mucous membranes (e.g., sublingual, buccal, swish and spit, swish and swallow), skin, eye, ear, rectum, vagina, upper or lower respiratory tract, and parenteral (e.g., intramuscular, subcutaneous, intradermal, and intravenous). Each route has its indications for use, advantages and disadvantages, and specific techniques that must be employed to deliver the medication appropriately to the client. Nurses must be knowledgeable about these issues and possess the necessary skills to administer medications safely via a variety of routes.

A. Oral
1. Introduction.
   a. Product is administered through the mouth or a tube into the stomach.
   b. Product is absorbed in the stomach or small intestine.
2. Types of oral medication preparations.
   a. Capsule: Product encased in a hard or soft container or gelatin shell that dissolves in the stomach.
   b. Caplet: Gelatin-coated tablet that is easy to swallow and dissolves in the stomach.

c. Tablet: Product molded into a disk or cylinder that is swallowed, chewed, or melted under the tongue (sublingual) and comes in different types.
   (1) **Enteric-coated:** Product encased in a substance that dissolves in the intestine.
   (2) **Sustained-release:** Product that is gradually released, ensuring a constant blood level of the drug.
   (3) **Time-release:** Product further enclosed in a smaller casing that releases a dose over time.

d. Liquid: Substance that flows readily.
   (1) Aerosol: Aqueous product that is delivered as a fine mist into the nose or mouth and absorbed in the upper airway.
   (2) Elixir: Product in a solution of alcohol containing glycerin or sweeteners.
   (3) Emulsion: Liquid product that is distributed as small droplets in another liquid.
   (4) Suspension: Powder or particle that is dissolved in a liquid when shaken vigorously.
   (5) Syrup: Product that is dispersed in a sugar liquid.

3. Advantages.
   a. Convenient.
   b. Comfortable for the client.
   c. Chewable forms that appeal to children.
   d. Seldom causes client anxiety.
   e. Easy to administer.
   f. Economical and cost effective; does not require expensive equipment.
   g. Can cause a local effect.
   h. Can cause a systemic effect.

4. Disadvantages.
   a. Slower action than other routes.
   b. Can irritate the oral and gastric mucosa, stain teeth, or have an objectionable taste.
   c. Contraindicated for some clients.
      (1) Clients who have impaired GI function.
      (2) Clients who are unconscious or cognitively impaired and cannot swallow.
      (3) Clients who are nauseated, vomiting, on nothing-by-mouth (NPO) status, or receiving gastric decompression.
      (4) Clients at high risk for aspiration.

5. Commonalities of nursing interventions specific to administering oral medications.
   a. Verify whether the client is receiving a restricted diet, is having intake and output (I&O) measured, or is on NPO status to ensure that fluid intake is permitted and should be documented.
   b. Assess the presence of contraindications for administering a medication via the oral route,

such as decreased level of consciousness, depressed gag reflex, presence of nausea or vomiting, and NPO status. Seek a prescription for an alternate route if any contraindications are present. Doing so ensures that the client can receive the medication via an alternate route without interruption of therapy.

c. Encourage the client to drink 5 oz of water with ingestion of the medication to facilitate dissolution and absorption of the medication.

d. Cut scored tablets with a cutting device or held within a tissue when splitting by hand. Ensure both halves of a tablet are equal in size to produce two equal doses (a cutting device is more effective than splitting tablets by hand) and to ensure an accurate dose.

e. Follow agency policy regarding using or discarding unadministered split tablets.

f. Crush crushable tablets and mix with applesauce when necessary to facilitate swallowing. Use only as much applesauce as necessary to mix with the medication to ensure ingestion of the entire dose.

g. Observe the client while he or she is ingesting the medication.

h. Inspect the mouth for "pocketed" medications (e.g., under the tongue or in the buccal cavity) after administration when ingestion is questionable, such as with difficulty swallowing, confusion, hoarding, or unilateral weakness, to ensure that the medication was ingested and reduce the risk of aspiration of an unswallowed medication.

🛑 i. Do not leave medications at the bedside to be taken later to prevent the medication from becoming lost, not being taken, being taken without supervision, or being hoarded for a nontherapeutic purpose.

6. Nursing interventions specific to administering enteric-coated, (delayed-release) and extended-release (sustained-release, time-release) medications.

a. Do not crush enteric-coated tablets to avoid deactivation by gastric juices and ensure delivery to the intestine, where it dissolves and is absorbed.

b. Do not crush extended-release medications to prevent the activation of the medication at one time, resulting in an excessive dose.

c. Notify the primary health-care provider if a client is unable to ingest a medication whole, necessitating a change in route.

d. Assess for the therapeutic effect of the medication over the length of time expected.

7. Nursing interventions specific to administering liquid medications (aerosols, elixirs, emulsions, suspensions, and syrups).

a. Follow the manufacturer's directions regarding whether a container should be vigorously shaken to ensure even distribution of constituents.

b. Place an opened top of a container on a surface with the inside lid facing up to prevent contamination of the inside of the lid and subsequent contamination of the bottle when the lid is returned and closed.

c. Measure oral liquids accurately.

(1) Measure oral liquids in a calibrated medication cup at eye level.

(2) Use a syringe without a needle to measure oral liquid volumes less than 5 mL and transfer them to a medication cup.

🛑 (3) Avoid keeping oral liquid medications in a syringe to prevent accidental administration of an oral liquid via the parenteral route.

d. Pour liquids with the label against the palm of the hand to prevent the liquid from dripping on and obscuring the label.

e. Wipe the outside rim of the bottle with a clean paper towel before replacing the top.

f. Use measures to make unpleasant tasting medications more palatable.

(1) Refrigerate unpleasant tasting liquids unless contraindicated to lessen objectionable taste and odor.

(2) Offer ice chips before giving unpleasant tasting medications to numb the taste buds.

(3) Use a needleless syringe to place unpleasant tasting medications on the back of the tongue to minimize unpleasant taste.

(4) Provide oral hygiene after administration of unpleasant tasting medications.

B. Gastrointestinal tubes

1. Introduction.

a. Tube inserted into the stomach or intestine.

b. Can be used to remove stomach secretions (gastric decompression) or intestinal secretions (intestinal decompression).

c. Can be used to deliver formula feedings to the stomach or small intestine to meet nutritional needs.

d. Can be used to deliver liquid, powder, or crushed medications even when the tube is being used for decompression or for formula feedings.

2. Types of GI tubes.

a. Nasogastric (NG).

(1) Tube passed through a nostril, the nasopharynx, and the esophagus with the distal end placed in the stomach.

(2) Used for clients who are unable to ingest substances through the mouth or esophagus due to impaired swallowing, an absent gag reflex, or recent head and neck surgery or for decompression after abdominal surgery.

b. Jejunostomy.
   (1) Tube passed through the nose, the esophagus, and the stomach with the distal end placed in the jejunum.
   (2) Used for clients with impaired gastric functioning so that formula feedings can enter the small intestine directly or to promote intestinal decompression in clients with a small bowel obstruction.

c. Percutaneous endoscopic gastrostomy (PEG) or percutaneous endoscopic jejunostomy (PEJ).
   (1) Tube surgically or laparoscopically inserted through the skin and abdominal wall into the stomach or jejunum and sutured in place to maintain placement. Also held in place by an internal retention balloon and flat external bumper.
   (2) Traditionally used for long-term (6 to 8 weeks or longer) nutritional support but now used more frequently for short-term support because of ease of insertion.

3. Advantages.
   a. Provide a route for administering medication that otherwise would need to be delivered parenterally.
   b. PEG tube considered the most comfortable feeding tube.

4. Disadvantages.
   a. Increased risk of aspiration that can lead to pneumonia, infection, abscess formation, and respiratory distress syndrome (RDS); risk is greater with an NG tube than with gastrostomy or jejunostomy tubes because an NG tube can curl up within the esophagus and enter the trachea and bronchi.
   b. Requires use of an enteral tube and a piston syringe for insertion of medication, which is more costly than most other routes.
   c. Requires shutting off a tube used for decompression for 30 minutes after medication administration to allow time for absorption.
   d. Does not permit administration of enteric-coated, time-release, or sustained-release medications because they would require crushing a tablet or emptying a capsule, which would expose the client to the entire dose at once.
   e. Requires more time for administration than do other routes.

5. Nursing interventions specific to administering medications via GI tubes.
   a. Administer liquid forms of medication when available to prevent clogging the tube.
   b. Crush crushable tablets into a fine powder and mix with 30 mL of warm water; avoid administering whole or undissolved medications to prevent clogging the tube.
   🛑 c. Identify placement of the tube in the stomach or intestine before medication administration. Doing so ensures that medication is administered into the appropriate place rather than into the respiratory system. (See "Ensure accurate placement of the tube using several methods" in the section "Nursing Care for Clients Receiving Enteral Nutrition" in Chapter 20, Nutrition.)
   d. Flush the tube with 15 to 30 mL of water before medication administration to ensure tube patency.
   e. Give each medication separately and flush with 15 to 30 mL of water between each and after the last medication. If necessary, modify the procedure if the client has a fluid restriction.
   🛑 f. Shut off a nasogastric tube used for decompression for 30 minutes after medication administration to enhance medication absorption and then reestablish decompression.

C. Oral mucous membranes (sublingual, buccal, swish and spit, swish and swallow)
   1. Introduction.
      a. The mucous membranes of the oral cavity line the entire cavity, including inside the lips, under the tongue (sublingual), between the gum and cheeks (buccal cavity), and the posterior oropharyngeal area, including the uvula and tonsils.
      b. Products for these routes are designed to dissolve or circulate in the mouth and produce either a local or a systemic effect.
      c. *Sublingual:* Tablet is dissolved under the tongue (e.g., nitroglycerine).
      d. *Buccal cavity* (Fig. 9.2): Troche or lozenge is dissolved between a cheek and the gum.
      e. *Swish and spit/swish and swallow:* Solution dispersed throughout the oral cavity and esophagus (when swallowed).
   2. Advantages.
      a. Same as oral route, plus information below.
      b. Sublingual.
         (1) Enters the blood, bypassing the liver, allowing for a quick effect.
         (2) Administered for a systemic effect.

Fig 9.2 Buccal route. (From Burton and Ludwig [2015]. *Fundamentals of nursing care: Concepts, connections & skill*, 2nd ed. Philadelphia: F. A. Davis Company, with permission.)

c. Buccal.
   (1) Dissolves slowly between the cheek and gum to affect the mucous membranes of the oral cavity.
   (2) Administered for a local effect.
d. Swish and spit/swish and swallow.
   (1) Solution circulated in the mouth and expelled or swallowed.
   (2) Administered for a local effect (e.g., mucous membranes of the mouth and esophagus if swallowed).
3. Disadvantages.
   a. Contraindicated for individuals who are unable to maintain a tablet in place until dissolved or unable to follow directions regarding dispersing a solution throughout the oral cavity.
   b. Sublingual: Must remain under the tongue until completely dissolved for best effect.
   c. Buccal: Must remain in the buccal cavity until completely dissolved for best effect and may cause irritation of the mucous membranes.
   d. Swish and spit/swish and swallow: Client may accidentally aspirate the solution or swallow the solution meant to be expelled.
4. Commonalities of nursing interventions specific to administering medications via oral mucous membranes.
   a. Ensure that the client is physically able and mentally aware of the need to keep the tablet, troche, or lozenge in place until dissolved to ensure that the medication dissolves in the mouth, minimizing the risk of aspiration.
   b. Inform the primary health-care provider if the client is unable to keep the medication in place until dissolved and seek a prescription for a route that can be tolerated.
   c. Teach the client not to chew or swallow the tablet.
   d. Assess the mucous membranes for irritation; inform the primary health-care provider if any occurs, and suggest a change in route.

5. Nursing interventions specific to administering medications via the sublingual route.
   a. Instruct the client to keep the tablet under the tongue until the medication dissolves.
   b. Assess for a therapeutic effect immediately to promote evaluation and documentation of the client's response (sublingual route has a quick absorption rate).
6. Nursing interventions specific to administering medications via the buccal route.
   a. Instruct the client to place the troche or lozenge against the mucous membrane of the cheek and gum until it dissolves.

   🛑 b. Ensure that the client stays awake until the troche or lozenge dissolves to reduce the risk of aspiration.

   c. Advise the client to alternate cheeks when taking additional doses to minimize the risk of mucosal irritation.
7. Nursing interventions specific to administering medications via swish and spit/swish and swallow.
   a. Instruct the client to keep the lips closed and puff the cheeks in and out to ensure that the solution is dispersed to all mucous membranes in the oral cavity.
   b. Instruct the client to expel the solution from the mouth for swish and spit to ensure that the solution is in contact with only the oral mucous membranes.
   c. Instruct the client to swallow the solution for swish and swallow to ensure that the solution is in contact with the mucous membranes of the oral cavity and the esophagus.

D. Skin
   1. Introduction.
      a. Skin is the largest organ of the body (integumentary system); it protects underlying tissue, helps to regulate body temperature, secretes sebum, transmits sensations through nerve endings, and produces and absorbs vitamin D.
      b. The product is designed to be absorbed through the skin and produce either a local or systemic effect.
         (1) *Topical:* Applied to the skin to provide a local or systemic effect, depending on the site, but usually used for a local effect.
         (2) *Transdermal:* Applied to the skin for a systemic effect.
   2. Types of preparations.
      a. Liniment: Alcohol, oil, or soapy emollient containing a medicated substance.
      b. Lotion: Medication in a liquid suspension often used to clean, cool, or protect the skin.
      c. Ointment (salve or cream): Semisolid substance containing a medication.

    d. Paste: Thick ointment that is absorbed slowly through the skin and generally is used for skin protection.

    e. Transdermal patch: Impregnated sheath that releases a controlled amount of medication to produce a systemic response.

3. Advantages.
   a. Topical.
      (1) Easy to apply.
      (2) Generally painless.
   b. Transdermal.
      (1) Provides a prolonged systemic effect (1 to 7 days, depending on the medication).
      (2) Convenient when used for 72 hours or longer.
      (3) Replaces daily administration of a medication.

4. Disadvantages.
   a. Topical.
      (1) Risk for fast absorption and a systemic effect in the presence of impaired skin integrity, such as excoriation or a break in the skin.
      (2) May irritate the skin.
      (3) May cause adverse systemic effects.
      (4) May leave oily matter on the skin that can soil clothing.
   b. Transdermal.
      (1) May require shaving of hair to facilitate adherence of the patch.
      (2) May cause skin irritation.

5. Commonalities of nursing interventions specific to administering medications via the skin.
   a. Follow standard precautions (e.g., don gloves) when applying topical medications to prevent exposure to the medication and contact with blood and body fluids.
   b. Maintain sterile technique if the client's skin lacks integrity to reduce the risk of infection.
   c. Assess for irritation at the site and report to the primary health-care provider if any occurs.

6. Nursing interventions specific to administering liniments, lotions, ointments, and pastes.
   a. Clean the skin before application to improve medication absorption.
   b. Place the lid of a container on a surface with the inside facing upward to prevent contamination of the inside of the lid.
   c. Use a separate sterile tongue blade each time when obtaining paste from a container to maintain the sterility of the inside of the container.
   d. Apply in a thin or thick layer, according to the manufacturer's directions.
   e. Apply onto the skin with the degree of rubbing recommended by the manufacturer.

7. Nursing interventions specific to administering medications via a transdermal patch.
   a. Follow standard precautions when administering a patch.
   (!) b. Remove the previous patch before applying a new one to minimize the risk of overdose.
   c. Contain and dispose of a used patch to protect others from exposure to the active substance still on the patch.
   d. Wash and dry the skin after removing a used patch. Doing so removes any lingering medication and minimizes the risk of overdose.
   e. Shave hair on the skin with the client's consent if the hair interferes with patch adherence.
   f. Apply the patch to a different location than the previous patch and gently compress the patch with a gloved hand for 10 seconds to facilitate adherence.
   g. Write the date, the time, and your initials on a patch.

E. Eye
1. Introduction.
   a. *Ophthalmic medications:* Medicinal substances administered into an eye.
   b. Ophthalmic medications produce a local effect.
2. Advantages.
   a. Provides medication directly to the desired site.
   b. Allows medication of one or both eyes.
3. Disadvantages.
   a. Difficult to self-administer, particularly if the client has impaired vision.
   b. Damage may occur to the eye if the tip of the dropper or tube touches the eye or drops fall directly on the cornea.
   c. Infection may occur if the tip of the dropper or tube touches the eye because this contaminates the medication container.
4. Nursing interventions specific to administering eye medications.
   a. Clean the eyelid and lashes with sterile normal saline solution–soaked cotton balls. Use a new one for each stroke, moving from the inner canthus to outer canthus. Doing so cleans the eye and reduces the risk of debris entering the lacrimal duct.
   b. Tilt the client's head slightly back and toward the eye being medicated to prevent the solution from flowing toward the other eye.
   c. Have the client look up to reduce the risk of blinking.
   d. Place a finger just below the lower eyelashes and exert gentle downward pressure over the bony prominence of the cheek to expose the conjunctival sac.

e. Hold the dropper close to the eye without touching it and administer the prescribed number of drops so they fall into the conjunctival sac and not on the eyeball.

f. Apply ointment along the edge of the lower conjunctival sac without touching the eye with the tube to maintain the sterility of the ointment tube.

g. Release the lower lid and instruct the client to close the eyes gently to prevent the medication from being squeezed out of the eye.

h. Apply gentle pressure over the inner canthus to prevent medication from flowing into the lacrimal duct.

i. Teach the client not to rub the medicated eye to avoid irritation and contamination of the hands, which may contaminate the other eye, surfaces in the environment, and other people.

F. Ear
1. Introduction.
   a. *Otic medications:* Medicinal substances administered into an ear.
   b. Otic medications produce a local effect.
2. Advantages.
   a. Provides medication directly to the desired site.
   b. Allows medication of one or both ears.
3. Disadvantages.
   a. May require removal of earwax (cerumen) for the medication to reach the involved tissue.
   b. May cause damage if drops fall directly onto the tympanic membrane.
4. Nursing interventions specific to administering ear medications.
   a. Warm the solution to room temperature by holding the container of medication in the palm of a hand for several minutes to minimize discomfort.
   b. Clean the external ear of drainage with normal saline solution–moistened cotton balls.
   c. Place the client in the side-lying position with the affected ear facing toward the ceiling to help retain the drops in the ear.
   🛑 d. Gently pull up and back on the cartilaginous part of the pinna for an adult and a child older than 3 years of age. Pull the cartilaginous part of the pinna down and back for an infant or child younger than age 3 years.
   e. Place the drops on the side of the ear canal so that the drops flow down the wall of the ear canal, but avoid touching the canal with the dropper to protect the dropper from contamination and avoid injury to the tympanic membrane.

f. Release the pinna and gently press on the tragus several times to move the medication along the canal to the tympanic membrane.

g. Maintain the client in the side-lying position with the affected ear facing the ceiling for 5 minutes after medication administration. Doing so uses gravity to ensure drug contact with the structures within the ear canal.

h. Loosely insert a cotton ball into the external canal, if prescribed, to prevent the drug from leaking out of the ear canal.

G. Rectum
1. Introduction.
   a. The rectum is the last 7 to 8 inches of the large intestine. The last inch of the rectum is called the *anal canal*, and the opening itself is called the *anus*.
   b. Products must be inserted through the anus and anal canal to reach the rectum.
   c. Products include creams that are inserted with an applicator or a cone-shaped, firm substance (suppository) that can be inserted with a gloved finger.
   d. Products are designed to dissolve and be absorbed through the mucous membranes of the rectum.
2. Advantages.
   a. Provides for a local or systemic effect, depending on the medication (e.g., laxative or anti-inflammatory for a local effect; sedative or analgesic for a systemic effect).
   b. Allows medication to be released at a slow, steady rate.
   c. Provides an alternate administration site when the client is vomiting or oral medication has an objectionable taste.
3. Disadvantages.
   a. Rates of absorption are unpredictable.
   b. Is contraindicated if the client had rectal surgery or has rectal bleeding.
   c. May be perceived by the client as unpleasant or cause client embarrassment.
   d. May soil or stain clothing.
4. Nursing interventions specific to administering medications via the rectum.
   a. Store foil-wrapped suppositories in a refrigerator to help the suppository retain its form for ease of insertion.
   b. Follow standard precautions, including donning gloves, to prevent exposure to body fluids.
   c. Close the door and pull the curtain around the bed to provide privacy.
   d. Position the client in the left-lateral position.
   e. Drape the client with a sheet, exposing only the perianal area to provide privacy.

f. Identify whether the client has a fecal mass in the rectum. If a mass is present, the product must be inserted between the fecal mass and the rectal wall to promote its effect.

⊘ g. Lubricate the suppository and the index finger of your gloved hand to facilitate insertion and prevent tissue trauma.

h. Direct insertion toward the umbilicus, using the full length of an index finger. Doing so ensures placement past the anal canal, anal sphincter, and anal-rectal ridge, which promotes retention of the suppository (Fig. 9.3).

i. Instruct the client to remain in the lateral or supine position for 10 to 20 minutes after insertion to keep the suppository in place, which facilitates absorption.

H. Vagina
1. Introduction.
   a. The vagina is a 3-inch long area (vaginal canal) extending from the cervix of the uterus to the vaginal opening (vaginal introitus).
   b. Products must be inserted through the vaginal introitus and be placed deep within the vaginal canal.
   c. Products include creams, foams, jellies, or tablets that are inserted with an applicator or a cone-shaped, firm substance (suppository) that can be inserted with a gloved finger.
   d. Products are designed to dissolve and be absorbed through the mucous membranes of the vagina.
2. Advantages.
   a. Provides a local effect.
   b. Provides an alternate route for a contraceptive other than oral or intradermal.

3. Disadvantages.
   a. May be perceived by the client as unpleasant or cause client embarrassment.
   b. May soil or stain clothing.
4. Nursing interventions specific to administering medications via the vagina.
   a. Store foil-wrapped suppositories in a refrigerator to help the suppository retain its form for ease of insertion.
   b. Follow standard precautions, including donning gloves to prevent exposure to body fluids.
   c. Have the client void before insertion of the medication to eliminate the pressure of a full bladder, which may cause discomfort during insertion.
   d. Close the door and pull the curtain around the bed to provide privacy.

⊘ e. Provide perineal care with soap and water before inserting the medication to remove debris and minimize the presence of microorganisms.

   f. Position the client in the dorsal recumbent position.
   g. Drape the client with a sheet, exposing only the vaginal area to provide privacy.

⊘ h. Lubricate the vaginal suppository and your gloved index finger with a water-soluble jelly or expel a small amount of vaginal cream at the tip of the applicator supplied by the manufacturer to facilitate insertion and limit tissue trauma.

   i. Direct insertion downward and backward using the full length of the applicator or index finger. Doing so follows the contour of the vaginal anatomy and ensures that the medication is inserted deep in the vaginal canal (Fig. 9.4).
   j. Use a rolling motion when inserting a cream with an applicator. Doing so spreads lubricant along the vaginal lining, easing insertion.

Suppository
Anal-rectal ridge
Anal sphincter
Rectum

Fig 9.3 Inserting a rectal suppository. (From Burton and Ludwig [2015]. *Fundamentals of nursing care: Concepts, connections & skills,* 2nd ed. Philadelphia: F. A. Davis Company, with permission.)

Fig 9.4 Inserting a vaginal suppository. (From Wilkinson and Treas [2016]. *Fundamentals of nursing,* Vol. 2, 3rd ed. Philadelphia: F. A. Davis Company, with permission.)

k. Fully compress the plunger of the applicator to ensure disbursement of the cream or placement of the tablet deep in the vaginal canal.

l. Remove the applicator slowly to prevent tissue trauma.

m. Instruct the client to remain in a supine position for 10 to 20 minutes after insertion to keep the medication in place, which facilitates absorption.

I. Upper and lower respiratory tracts

1. Introduction.

a. The upper respiratory tract consists of the nose, nasopharynx, sinuses, oropharynx, laryngopharynx, and larynx.

b. The lower respiratory tract consists of the trachea, all segments of the bronchial tree, and the alveoli.

c. Medications are introduced into the upper respiratory tract through the nose via drops or sprays.

d. Medications are introduced into the lower respiratory tract usually through the mouth via a fine spray, fog, powder, or mist.

e. Most medications are delivered to achieve a local effect, improving ventilation and oxygenation (e.g., bronchodilators, anti-inflammatory agents, antihistamines, and nasal decongestants).

f. Intranasal mists may be given for a systemic effect (e.g., flu vaccine, naloxone).

2. Types of respiratory tract medication delivery systems.

a. Upper respiratory tract.

(1) Drops: Drops of medicated solution are introduced into a nostril by a dropper.

(2) Nasal sprays: Sprays suspend droplets of medication that are propelled into the nose by depressing a cartridge adaptor or squeezing the container.

b. Lower respiratory tract (Fig. 9.5).

(1) *Metered-dose inhaler (MDI):* A pressurized container propels medication as a fine spray through a mouthpiece that is then inhaled into the lower respiratory tract.

(2) *Nonpressurized aerosol (handheld nebulizer):* Medication is changed to a fine mist or fog so that it can be inhaled deep into the lower respiratory tract; generally administered via a mouthpiece but can be delivered with a mask to infants or children or an adult who has difficulty using the mouthpiece.

(3) *Dry powder disk inhaler:* Multiple-dose disks deliver dry powder to the lower respiratory tract when inhaled through the mouth.

Fig 9.5 Types of inhalers: (A) An ultrasonic nebulizer delivers medication and humidity as a fine mist. (B) An MDI delivers measured doses. This one has a spacer. (C) A dry-powder inhaler (Turbuhaler). (D) A Diskhaler. (From Burton and Ludwig [2015]. *Fundamentals of nursing care: Concepts, connections & skill,* 2nd ed. Philadelphia: F. A. Davis Company, with permission.)

3. Advantages.

a. Lower respiratory tract delivery systems: Promote inhalation of medication deep into respiratory passages.

b. Have a rapid, efficient local effect due to the highly vascular nature of airways and alveoli.

c. Some can be administered to an unconscious client.

4. Disadvantages.

a. Requires sufficient inhalation flow rates to deliver inhaled medication to the lower respiratory tract.

b. Metered-dose and dry powder disk inhalers require coordination with device activation and inhalation.

c. May cause unwanted systemic effects (e.g., tachycardia and palpitations with some bronchodilators) or irritate the mucous membranes of the respiratory tract, depending on the medication.

d. Some delivery systems cannot be used for children and cognitively impaired persons who cannot follow directions.

e. Requires the use of special equipment that needs to be cleaned.

5. Commonalities of nursing interventions specific to administering mediations via the upper and lower respiratory tract.

a. Assess respiratory function.

(1) Rate, rhythm, and effort.

(2) Sounds: crackles, rhonchi, stridor, wheezing, diminished.

(3) Use of accessory muscles.

(4) Nasal flaring.

(5) Orthopnea.

(6) Pulse oximetry: 95% and higher is normal.

(7) Cough: Productive or nonproductive; characteristics.

(8) Secretions: Amount, color, odor, and consistency.

(9) Nasal congestion.

(10) Gross abnormalities of the visible mucosa, such as lesions, irritation, or inflammation.

b. Wear gloves if contamination is likely to prevent exposure to blood and body fluids.

🛑 c. **Encourage the client to blow the nose and cough up respiratory tract secretions. Doing so clears excess secretions from the respiratory tract and permits the medication to reach the mucous membranes.**

d. Position the client's head as indicated for the specific delivery system to facilitate distribution of the medication to the appropriate site.

e. Avoid sharing sprays, droppers, and inhalers to minimize the risk of cross-contamination.

f. Clean equipment after each use or weekly, based on the manufacturer's recommendations, to minimize the risk of bacterial contamination of equipment and prepare the equipment for the next dose.

g. Discard expired inhalers, sprays, and drops.

🛑 h. **Instruct the client to rinse the mouth after administration to remove any unpleasant taste, if present, and minimize the risk of candidiasis (with steroidal agents).**

6. Nursing interventions specific to administering medications via an MDI (Fig. 9.5B). Teach the client to:

a. Shake the canister before each depression to mix the propellant with the medication.

b. Attach the mouthpiece to the medication canister.

c. Exhale slowly and completely through pursed lips to ensure air is exhaled fully from the lower lobes of the lungs and prepare the lungs for full inhalation.

d. Hold the inhaler 2 cm from the mouth (open-mouth method) or insert the mouthpiece beyond the teeth and instruct the client to form a tight seal with the lips (closed-mouth method, Fig. 9.6).

e. Depress the device while inhaling slowly and deeply and hold the breath for 5 to 10 seconds at the height of inhalation. Doing so disperses the medication deep in the respiratory tract and prolongs contact of the medication with the respiratory mucosa.

f. Exhale slowly and completely through pursed lips to keep the smaller airways open during exhalation.

g. Use a spacer device for better results because the medication is released into the spacer and is then inhaled via a mouthpiece (Fig. 9.6). Doing so eliminates the need to coordinate inhalation with canister compression and promotes larger droplets to fall to the bottom of the spacer and increases the volume of smaller droplets reaching the lungs.

7. Nursing interventions specific to administering medications via a nasal spray. Teach the client to:

a. Insert the tip of the nasal device into one nostril while occluding the other by gently pressing on the nostril toward the midline. Doing so minimizes the aerosol from entering the other nostril.

b. Press the adapter cartridge or squeeze the container while inhaling through the accessed nostril to discharge a measured dose into the accessed nostril.

c. Exhale slowly through the mouth to help retain the medication in the nasal passage.

d. Insert the tip into the other nostril and, while breathing in slowly through the nose, squirt the spray into the nostril; do not occlude the first nostril. Doing so discharges one measured dose in the accessed nostril; occluding the first nostril may expel previously administered medication.

e. Exhale slowly through the mouth to help retain medication in the nasal passage.

f. Tilt the head backward to allow the spray to reach the back of the nose.

g. Wait 1 minute before administering a prescribed second dose to allow time for the first dose to take effect.

Fig 9.6 MDI with spacer. (From Wilkinson and Treas [2016]. *Fundamentals of nursing,* Vol. 1, 3rd ed. Philadelphia: F. A. Davis Company, with permission.)

h. Clean the outside of the container weekly according to the manufacturer's recommendations to minimize the risk of bacterial contamination of equipment.

🛑 i. **Avoid excessive use of OTC nasal decongestants; limit use to 7 days. Increased congestion can occur after the therapeutic effect subsides with excessive use (rebound congestion).**

8. Nursing interventions specific to administering medications via an aerosol handheld nebulizer (Fig. 9.5A). Teach the client to:
   a. Place the medication and a small volume of saline (if required) in a cup connected to a handheld nebulizer that has a mouthpiece. Doing so mixes the medication and saline, preparing it for aerosolization.
   b. Attach the nebulizer to wall oxygen or a nebulizer compressor to propel oxygen or air through the medication cup, changing the medication solution to a mist.
   c. Sit in an upright position to promote thoracic excursion by allowing the abdominal organs to drop by gravity.
   d. Insert the mouthpiece beyond the teeth and form a tight seal with the lips (Fig. 9.7) to ensure that the mist does not escape from the mouth.
   e. Inhale and exhale slowly and deeply through the mouth without removing the mouthpiece to deliver the medication deep into the small respiratory airways.
   f. Tap the side of the nebulizer occasionally to dislodge the solution from the sides of the cup down to where it can be misted.

🛑 g. **Continue for several minutes until the misting stops to ensure the entire dose is delivered.**

   h. Disassemble the nebulizer, mouthpiece, and cup; clean them with soap and water; and reassemble when dry to minimize the risk of infection.
9. Nursing interventions specific to administering medications via a dry-powder inhaler or diskhaler (Fig. 9.5 C and D). Teach the client to:
   a. Hold the disk horizontal in one hand throughout administration; put the thumb in the notch and push it away from the body until the mouthpiece appears. Doing so accesses the mouthpiece of the inhaler.
   b. Use a thumb to slide the lever away from the body until it clicks to ensure the medication is ready for delivery.
   c. Seal the lips around the mouthpiece and breathe in quickly and deeply through the mouth to move medication into the respiratory tract.

Fig 9.7 Handheld nebulizer. (From Williams and Hopper [2015]. *Understanding medical surgical nursing,* 5th ed. Philadelphia: F. A. Davis Company, with permission.)

   d. Remove the disk from the mouth and hold the breath for 5 to 10 seconds to lengthen the time the medication is in contact with the respiratory mucosa.
   e. Use the thumb to slide the notch back to shut the disk, preparing it for the next dose.
10. Nursing interventions specific to administering nose drops. Teach the client to:
    a. Hyperextend the head slightly (place a rolled towel behind the shoulders or place the head over the edge of the bed) to promote distribution of the solution over the surfaces of the nasal mucosa.
    b. Hold the dropper over the nostril without touching the nose to avoid contamination of the dropper.
    c. Apply the prescribed number of drops.
    d. Avoid swallowing the medication to ensure that the medication stays in contact with the nasal mucosa.
    e. Maintain the head tilt for a few minutes after insertion of drops to prevent the solution from exiting the nose via gravity.
    f. Return the dropper to the bottle and then close the bottle tightly to maintain the integrity of the medication and dropper.

J. Parenteral routes
1. Introduction.
   a. Parenteral: Means other than the alimentary canal (GI tract).
   b. Parenteral medications are administered intramuscularly, subcutaneously, intradermally, or intravenously.
2. Advantages.
   a. Avoids the GI tract when the GI tract is impaired, the medication is too irritating to the mucosa, or the GI tract inactivates the medication.
   b. Has more rapid onset than the oral route.

Fig 9.8 Parts of a syringe and safety needle. (From Burton and Ludwig [2015]. *Fundamentals of nursing care: Concepts, connections & skills,* 2nd ed. Philadelphia: F. A. Davis Company, with permission.)

c. Has more predictable results than other routes.

d. Can be administered to unconscious clients.

3. Disadvantages.

   a. Punctures the skin, increasing the risk of infection.

   b. May cause tissue injury if the solubility or pH of the medication is inappropriate for the tissue being accessed.

   c. Requires sterile equipment and is a more complex procedure than oral or topical medication administration (e.g., use of sterile technique, multiplicity of sites that can be used, safe disposal of equipment).

4. Characteristics of syringes and needles.

   a. Type of syringe.

      (1) Consists of a barrel, plunger, hub, needle (cannula, shaft), and safety device to prevent a needlestick injury; measurement calibrations are on the barrel (Fig. 9.8).

      (2) Generally packaged with an attached needle; however, the needle should be changed after drawing up a caustic drug or when a more appropriate needle gauge or length is desired.

      (3) Luer-Lok syringe: Marked in 0.1 (tenths); requires a special needle that twists on the tip of the syringe and locks into place.

      (4) Tuberculin syringe: Marked in 0.01 (hundredths) for doses less than 1 mL and has a very narrow barrel.

      (5) Insulin syringe: Marked in either 50 or 100 units and has a narrow barrel.

      (6) Prefilled single-dose syringe: May require a drug calculation before administering the correct dose; larger volumes of the drug than that which is prescribed may have to be wasted (Fig. 9.9).

   b. Volume of syringe (Fig. 9.10).

      (1) Sizes vary, with volumes, from 0.5 mL to 60 mL.

      (2) Syringes with volumes of 1 mL or less usually are used for subcutaneous (Sub-Q) injections.

      (3) Syringes with volumes of 3 mL usually are used for IM injections.

      (4) Syringes with volumes larger than 3 mL are used to administer intravenous (IV) medications, add solutions to IV bags, or irrigate tubes or wounds.

   c. Needle length (shaft).

      (1) Vary in length from ¼ to 3 inches.

      (2) Shorter needles (⅝, ½, and 1 inch) are used for infants, children, and thin adults and for subcutaneous injections.

      (3) Longer needles (1½ inch) are used for IM injections.

      (4) Needles longer than 1½ inches in length are used for obese clients and invasive procedures that require insertion of a needle, such as biopsies, paracentesis, and thoracentesis.

Fig 9.9 Prefilled single-dose syringe and three types of holders. (From Burton and Ludwig [2015]. *Fundamentals of nursing care: Concepts, connections & skill,* 2nd ed. Philadelphia: F. A. Davis Company, with permission.)

(A)

(B)

(C)

(D)

(E)

Fig 9.10 Syringe volumes: (A) U-100 insulin syringe marked in units, of which there are 100/mL. (B) 1-mL tuberculin syringe marked in 0.01 mL (1/100th of a milliliter) and minims (16 minims equals 1 mL). (C) 3-mL standard syringe marked in whole milliliters and 0.1 mL (1/10th of a milliliter). (D) 5-mL standard syringe marked in whole milliliters and 0.2 mL (2/10ths of a milliliter). (E) 10-mL standard syringe marked in whole milliliters and 0.2 mL (2/10ths of a milliliter). (From Burton and Ludwig [2015]. *Fundamentals of nursing care: Concepts, connections & skills,* 2nd ed. Philadelphia: F. A. Davis Company, with permission.)

(5) Needles in different size gauges and lengths are packaged in individual sterile sheaths or come attached to a packaged syringe.

(6) Syringe needles can be replaced with a different-gauge or -length needle as necessary.

d. Needle gauge (diameter of shaft).

(1) Gauge: Diameter of a needle; varies in size from #18 to #28 gauge.

(2) The smaller the needle gauge, the larger the diameter of the needle; the larger the needle gauge, the smaller the diameter of the needle.

(3) Larger gauge needles cause less tissue damage when inserted.

(4) Viscous solutions require a smaller gauge needle.

e. Needle bevel.

(1) Tips of needles are slanted (beveled) to create a narrow slit in the skin when inserted; when the needle is removed, the slit in the skin closes to prevent leakage of fluid.

(2) Long-beveled needles are more pointy and sharp; generally used for IM and Sub-Q injections.

(3) Short-beveled needles are used for intradermal injections because the risk of the bevel becoming occluded is less likely.

5. Commonalities of nursing interventions specific to administering medications via all parenteral routes.

a. Perform hand hygiene to prevent infection.

b. Select an appropriate-size syringe, needle gauge, and needle length to ensure that the medication is deposited at the correct tissue depth.

Fig. 9.11 Recapping a sterile needle. (From Wilkinson and Treas [2011]. *Fundamentals of nursing,* Vol. 2, 2nd ed. Philadelphia: F. A. Davis Company, with permission.)

Fig 9.12 Needle insertion angles. (From Wilkinson and Treas [2016]. *Fundamentals of nursing*, Vol. 1, 3rd ed. Philadelphia: F. A. Davis Company, with permission.)

c. Maintain sterile technique (the outside of the barrel and tip of the plunger can be touched but not the hub or the shaft of the plunger).

d. Aspirate the prescribed volume of solution.

e. Recap the sterile needle using a hands-free method (Fig. 9.11) to prevent a needlestick injury and maintain the sterility of the needle.

f. Close the door and curtain to provide privacy.

g. Put on clean gloves to prevent contact with blood and body fluids.

h. Select the injection site.

   (1) Check the MAR for the site of the last injection and select a new site; systematically rotate sites to minimize underlying tissue damage, which may decrease absorption.

   (2) Inspect the potential injection site for bruises, inflammation, edema, and signs of prior injections; avoid the area if any of these signs are present because they can interfere with absorption.

   (3) Use landmarks to select a site to minimize trauma to underlying structures, such as nerves and bones.

i. Assist the client into a comfortable position that permits access to the selected injection site.

j. Drape the client to expose only the injection site to provide for privacy.

k. Clean the injection site with an alcohol wipe in a circular motion from the center outward to minimize the risk of infection.

l. Pinch, spread, or move skin to the side, based on the injection type, to position the skin and underlying tissue for insertion of the needle into the correct tissue layer.

m. Insert the needle at a 15- to 90-degree angle to the skin, depending on the type of injection (Fig. 9.12).

n. Stabilize the syringe with your nondominant hand; use your other hand to depress the plunger smoothly and slowly to reduce discomfort and inject the medication into the tissue.

o. Aspirate or avoid aspiration, depending on the type of injection; see IM, Sub-Q, and intradermal injections for specifics regarding aspiration.

p. Move the nondominant hand away from the site slightly; apply pressure with an antiseptic swab but not too close to the needle; quickly but carefully withdraw the needle in one smooth motion along the line of insertion

---

Box 9.3 **Preventing Needlestick Injuries**

- *Use safety syringes that are designed to actively (A) or passively (B) cover used needles to protect the caregiver. Be aware that many facilities use needleless equipment (C).*

- *Dispose of ampules, needles, and sharps (e.g., broken glass, lancets, razors, and any other disposable sharp instruments) in a sharps container, which usually is positioned in strategic locations, such as on medication carts, in medication rooms, in client rooms, and in dirty utility rooms. Place a used syringe in an emesis basin to transport it to a sharps container if a sharps container is not easily accessible.*
- *Never place a used syringe in a pocket, in a wastebasket, or on a surface at the bedside.*

Photo credits: (From Wilkinson and Treas [2016]. *Fundamentals of nursing*, Vol. 2, 3rd ed. Philadelphia: F. A. Davis Company, with permission.)

Fig 9.14 Removing fluid from an ampule. Tilt the ampule for medication removal. (From Burton and Ludwig [2015]. *Fundamentals of nursing care: Concepts, connections & skills,* 2nd ed. Philadelphia: F. A. Davis Company, with permission.)

Fig 9.13 Removing fluid from an ampule. Invert the ampule and insert a sterile needle into the ampule, keeping the needle tip below the fluid level. (From Burton and Ludwig [2015]. *Fundamentals of nursing care: Concepts, connections & skills,* 2nd ed. Philadelphia: F. A. Davis Company, with permission.)

to minimize discomfort and reduce the risk of a needlestick injury.

q. Massage the area if directed by the medication's instructions to increase drug distribution and absorption and stimulate circulation. Avoid massaging when administering insulin or anticoagulants to limit bleeding and bruising.

r. Institute precautions to prevent a needlestick injury (Box 9.3).

s. Dispose of used gloves in an appropriate receptacle.

6. Withdrawing fluid from an ampule.
   a. Introduction.
      (1) Ampule: Characteristically shaped glass container that has a prescored, generally colored ring around a constricted neck.
      (2) Ampules generally hold a single dose of a drug but may hold up to 10 mL or more.
   b. Nursing interventions.
      (1) Flick the top of the ampule repeatedly if fluid is trapped to move the fluid below the constricted neck to ensure the entire dose is in the ampule for withdrawal.
      (2) Position a plastic ampule opener over the top of the constricted neck and snap off the top to protect the hands from injury.
      🛑 (3) Use a filter needle to aspirate the fluid into the syringe to prevent aspiration of glass particles.
      (4) Aspirate fluid into the syringe.
          (a) Invert the ampule, place the needle into the liquid, and aspirate the required volume (Fig. 9.13). Doing so allows surface

tension to hold the solution inside the ampule until the syringe's negative pressure pulls the solution into the syringe.
          (b) Place the ampule on a counter, insert the needle, and aspirate the solution (Fig. 9.14).
      (5) Change the filter needle to a needle suitable for the injection.
      (6) Dispose of the used ampule, glass top, and filter needle in a sharps container to prevent a puncture injury.

7. Withdrawing fluid from a vial.
   a. Introduction.
      (1) **Vial:** Glass rubber-sealed container covered with a metal cap that maintains sterility of the seal until the metal cap is removed.
      (2) Vials hold single or multiple doses.
      (3) Medication is supplied as a liquid or a powder that requires reconstitution because it is stable only for a short period of time when in solution.
   b. Nursing interventions.
      (1) Remove the metal cap that keeps the rubber seal sterile to provide access to the top seal of the vial.
      (2) Clean the rubber seal by wiping its surface with a 70% alcohol swab in a firm circular motion from the center, working outward when accessing a multiple-dose vial that has no metal cap, to ensure sterility of the seal.
      (3) Dissolve a medication supplied as a dry powder (reconstitution).
          (a) Instill fluid into the vial (diluent) with a syringe, following the manufacturer's instructions on the label of the vial for the type and amount of fluid in milliliters.
          (b) Remove the syringe and then gently roll the vial between the palms of the hands to prevent the formation of bubbles, which may result in withdrawal of an inaccurate dose.

(c) Indicate on the label of a multidose vial the amount of solution that provides a specific dose, along with the date, time, and your initials if you plan to use the vial again in the near future.

(d) Be aware that some reconstituted drugs must be given within 15 minutes of preparation to prevent degradation of the medication.

🛑 (e) Do not use a vial that has been reconstituted by another nurse. Only use vials that you have reconstituted to ensure that you know the accuracy of the dose per milliliter.

(4) Select an appropriate syringe and needle and draw air into the barrel to the calibration mark indicating the volume of desired medication. Doing so ensures that an equal volume of air is injected into the vial to ease removal of the same volume of medication.

(5) Insert the needle into the vial above the level of the solution and slowly inject the air to prevent turbulence that can cause bubbles.

(6) Invert the vial and gently pull on the plunger until the calibration mark indicates that the desired volume of medication is withdrawn; keep the tip of the needle below the surface of the solution to prevent air from being aspirated into the syringe.

(7) Remove the needle from the vial and replace it with an appropriate needle for the situation. Doing so provides a sharp, capped needle and eliminates medication on the outside of the needle that could irritate tissue along the needle tract during insertion.

(8) Administer the medication immediately to prevent errors and degradation of the medication if it was reconstituted.

8. Mixing two medications in one syringe.
   a. Introduction.
      (1) Two medications can be mixed in one syringe, if compatible, to limit the number of injections reducing the risk of infection.
      (2) Do not mix more than two drugs in one syringe to minimize the risk of medication incompatibility.

🛑 (3) Ensure medications are compatible by reading package inserts or consulting with a pharmacist, medication formulary, or textbook; administer drugs separately if compatibility is undetermined to prevent an incompatibility reaction.

   b. Commonalities of nursing interventions when mixing two medications in one syringe.
      (1) Determine the volume of each medication as well as the total volume to ensure that the right volume of each medication when added together equals the expected total volume of medication.
      (2) Maintain sterile technique throughout the procedure to reduce the risk of contaminating the medication and reduce the risk of infection.
      (3) Observe the combined solution in the syringe for cloudiness or precipitate formation, which indicates an incompatibility; discard the solution if this occurs and prepare the doses in separate syringes.
      (4) Recap the sterile needle using a safety capping device or a hands-free method to prevent a needlestick injury and maintain the sterility of the needle.
      (5) Administer the medication immediately to prevent drug degradation.

9. Preparing a dose from one multidose vial and one single-dose vial.
   a. Insert air into both vials to facilitate aspiration of the medication from the vials.
   b. Withdraw the required volume from the multidose vial first to prevent contamination of the multidose vial with medication from the single-dose vial.
   c. Withdraw the required volume from the single-dose vial last.

10. Preparing a dose from one multidose vial and an ampule.
    a. Withdraw the required volume from the multidose vial first. By drawing the solution from the multidose vial first, medication from the ampule will not contaminate the multidose vial.
    b. Withdraw the required volume from the ampule last.

11. Preparing a dose from two multidose vials (e.g., insulin, Fig. 9.15).
    a. Identify which medication should be in vial 1 and which should be in vial 2: Vial 1 is the medication that should not be diluted accidentally with medication from vial 2 (e.g., regular insulin is vial 1 and NPH insulin is vial 2).
    b. Instill air into the NPH insulin first and then the regular insulin.
    c. Withdraw the prescribed dose from the regular insulin first and then the NPH insulin.

Step 1	Step 2	Step 3	Step 4
Inject air (cloudy insulin vial).	Inject air (clear insulin vial).	Withdraw dose (clear vial).	Withdraw dose (cloudy vial).

Fig 9.15 Mixing insulin. (From Wilkinson and Treas [2016]. *Fundamentals of nursing*, Vol. 2, 3rd ed., Clinical Insight 23.5: Mixing two kinds of insulin in one syringe, p. 515, Philadelphia: F. A. Davis Company, with permission.)

K. Intramuscular (IM) injections
 1. Introduction.
   a. IM injection: Insertion of medication into a muscle below the subcutaneous layer.
   b. The volume of solution injected depends on the site being used and client characteristics (e.g., age, weight).
     (1) Up to 3 mL can be inserted in a large muscle, such as the ventrogluteal site, in a well-developed adult.
     (2) Divide the dose when more than 3 mL is prescribed.
     (3) Insert only 1 to 2 mL in less-developed muscles associated with children, older adults, and thin clients.
     (4) Insert only 0.5 to 1 mL in the deltoid muscle in an adult.
   c. The length of the needle depends on the site being used and the client's age and weight.
     (1) Adults: Use a 1-inch-length needle for the deltoid muscle and 1½-inch for all other intramuscular sites.
     (2) Obese adults: May have to use a 2-inch needle to pass through the layer of fatty tissue above the subcutaneous tissue to reach the muscle.
     (3) Infants and children: Generally use a ⅝- to 1-inch-length needle, depending on size and depth of the muscle at the selected site.
   d. The gauge of the needle depends on the viscosity of the solution (e.g., #20 for thick [viscid] solutions and #22 for thin solutions).

 2. Advantages.
   a. Can use two medications in one syringe.
   b. Allows rapid absorption because of more ample blood supply in the muscles than in the subcutaneous tissue.
 3. Disadvantages.
   a. Carries a risk of tissue injury if landmarks are not used to select the site.
   b. Is more painful than a Sub-Q injection because it uses a smaller gauge and longer needle.
   c. May cause fibrosis, abscess, nerve damage, pain, tissue necrosis, and muscle contraction.
   d. Has variable absorption depending on the adequacy of circulation at the injection site.
 4. Selection of an IM injection site depends on multiple variables (e.g., advantages, disadvantages, and client characteristics) (Table 9.2).
 5. Nursing interventions specific to administering an IM injection.
   a. Select the appropriate gauge needle to ensure the needle gauge is strong enough to pass through the tissue and reach the muscle.
   b. Select the appropriate needle length to permit passage through the tissue to penetrate a deep muscle.
   c. Alternate sites among the deltoid, vastus lateralis, and ventrogluteal muscles, when appropriate, to minimize tissue injury and facilitate absorption.
   d. Position the client in a comfortable, appropriate position and identify landmarks to ensure the needle is inserted into the muscle, avoiding undesirable body structures.
   e. Spread the skin taut between the index finger and thumb to facilitate needle insertion and minimize discomfort.
   f. Insert the needle at a 90-degree angle (Fig. 9.12) to ensure that the needle tip reaches muscle tissue.
   g. Aspirate by pulling the plunger back gently; check the manufacturer's instructions to determine whether aspiration is contraindicated.
     (1) If no blood appears, continue with the procedure because the needle is outside a blood vessel.
     🛑 (2) If blood appears, withdraw the needle because it is in a blood vessel; prepare a new syringe.
   h. Inject the medication.
     (1) Inject the medication quickly for a child or an infant to minimize client anxiety.
     (2) Inject the medication over 5 to 10 seconds for an adult to minimize discomfort and allow time for drug dispersal.

Table 9.2 **Intramuscular Injection Sites: Advantages, Disadvantages, and Nursing Care**

Advantages and Disadvantages	Nursing Care

Deltoid

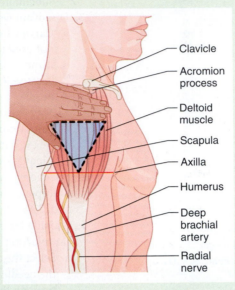

- Clavicle
- Acromion process
- Deltoid muscle
- Scapula
- Axilla
- Humerus
- Deep brachial artery
- Radial nerve

Advantage
- *Easily accessible.*

Disadvantages
- *Generally not used for infants and children because the deltoid is not well developed.*
- *Carries risk of injury to radial and ulnar nerves and brachial artery.*

1. *Position the client standing with the arm at the side; sitting with the lower arm on lap; or supine with the lower arm across the abdomen.*
2. ***Landmark:** Make an inverted triangle between two to three finger-widths below the acromion process and a line from the anterior to posterior axillary crease.*

Vastus Lateralis

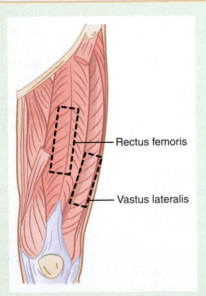

- Rectus femoris
- Vastus lateralis

Advantages
- *Lacks major nerves and blood vessels.*
- *Easily accessible.*
- *Used often for infants, toddlers, and children for immunizations until ventrogluteal muscles develop.*

Disadvantage
- *None.*

1. *Position the client supine with knee slightly flexed.*
2. *Determine the angle of insertion, which depends on the volume of subcutaneous tissue and needle length.*
3. ***Landmark:** The muscle extends from a handbreadth above the knee to a handbreadth below the greater trochanter of the femur on the anterior lateral aspect of the thigh.*

Table 9.2 Intramuscular Injection Sites: Advantages, Disadvantages, and Nursing Care—cont'd

Advantages and Disadvantages	Nursing Care
Ventrogluteal (VG) Gluteus Medius Muscle	

Advantages
- *Provides greatest muscle thickness.*
- *Is located away from major nerves and blood vessels.*
- *Carries a reduced risk of contamination from incontinent clients or infants.*
- *Is easily located by obvious bony landmarks.*
- *Is a deep, well-developed muscle even in older infants and children; is the preferred site for children 7 months of age and older and adults.*
- *Desirable for larger volume, more viscous, and irritating medications.*

Disadvantage
- *None.*

1. *Position the client laterally or on the back with knee and hip slightly flexed.*
2. **Landmark:**
   - *Place the heel of your hand over the greater trochanter with your wrist perpendicular to the client's femur; use your left hand for the right hip and right hand for the left hip.*
   - *Point your thumb toward the groin and index finger toward the anterior superior iliac spine.*
   - *Extend the middle finger back along the iliac crest toward the buttock.*
   - *The middle of the triangle between the middle and index fingers marks the injection site.*

Figure credits: (From Wilkinson and Treas [2016]. *Fundamentals of nursing*, Vol. 2, 3rd ed. Philadelphia: F. A. Davis Company, with permission.)

6. Nursing interventions specific to administering an IM injection via the Z-track method.
   a. Change the needle after drawing the medication into the syringe to prevent tissue irritation caused by the drug adhering to the outside of the needle.
   b. Use the ulnar side of the hand or thumb of the nondominant hand to pull the skin laterally 1 to 1.5 inches (2.5 to 3.5 cm) (Fig. 9.16); hold until the dominant hand injects the medication if there was no blood return on aspiration; remove the needle after 10 seconds and then release the skin. Doing so ensures that a zigzag path is established before needle insertion, which seals the needle track as the tissue planes slide across each other upon release, confining the drug in the muscle, minimizing irritation, and preventing tissue discoloration caused by some medications.

Fig 9.16 Z-track method. (From Burton and Ludwig [2015]. *Fundamentals of nursing care: Concepts, connections & skill*, 2nd ed. Philadelphia: F. A. Davis Company, with permission.)

L. Subcutaneous (Sub-Q) injections
1. Introduction.
   a. Sub-Q injection: Insertion of medication between the dermis and muscle.
   b. The volume of solution injected should be less than 1 mL.
   c. The length of the needle depends on the angle of needle insertion; for example, usually a ⅜- or ½-inch needle for a 90-degree angle and ⅝- or 1-inch needle for a 45-degree angle (Fig. 9.12).
   d. The gauge of the needle usually is #25 to #30.
   e. The type of syringe used depends on the type of medication (e.g., an insulin syringe should be used for insulin).
2. Advantages.
   a. Is more comfortable than an IM injection because it uses a larger gauge and shorter length needle.
   b. Is commonly used for drugs given multiple times daily, such as heparin and insulin.
   c. Allows slower absorption of drugs than IM route because of less-rich blood supply in subcutaneous tissue versus muscle.
3. Disadvantages.
   a. Allows administration of a maximum of only 1 mL of solution.
   b. Cannot be used for many drugs because they are irritating to subcutaneous tissue.
4. Selection of a Sub-Q injection site depends on multiple variables (e.g., advantages, disadvantages, and type of medication) (Table 9.3).
5. Nursing interventions specific to administering a Sub-Q injection.
   a. Select the appropriate gauge needle.
   b. Select the appropriate length needle (should be half the width of a pinched skinfold) to

Table 9.3 Subcutaneous Injection Sites: Advantages, Disadvantages, and Nursing Care	
Advantages and Disadvantages	**Nursing Care**
Abdomen	

Advantages
• *Has a large subcutaneous layer that allows for rotation of injections within one site.*
• *Allows medication to be absorbed more evenly than thighs and buttocks, which are affected by activity.*
• *Is the best site for insulin and anticoagulant administration because of a quicker absorption rate than other sites.*
Anterolateral and posterolateral abdominal wall ("love handles")
• *Best site for low-molecular-weight anticoagulants, such as enoxaparin (Lovenox), because of its deep subcutaneous layer.*
Disadvantages
• *None.*
	1. *Position the client in any position but prone.*
	2. ***Landmark***
	  • ***Abdomen:*** *Left and right of the umbilicus and below the umbilicus on the left, right, and middle; avoid 2 inches around the umbilicus to reduce the risk of bleeding. (See figure below, green dots.)*
	  • *"**Love handles**": Tissue around the midsection on the sides of the lower waist and lower back. (See figure below, red dots.)*
	  • ***Additional areas of subcutaneous tissue:*** *(See figure below, blue dots.)*

Outer, Posterior Aspect of Upper Arms; Anterior Thighs; and Upper Buttocks	
Advantage • *Have large subcutaneous tissue layers that allow for rotation of injections within one site.* **Disadvantages** • *Absorption may be uneven because areas are affected by activity.* • *Should not be used for low-molecular-weight heparin because of increased risk of bruising.*	1. *Position the client so that each site is accessible. (See figure below, blue dots.)*

2 inches away from the umbilicus

Figure credit: (Adapted from Vitale [2017]. *NCLEX-RN notes: Core review and exam prep*, 3nd ed. Philadelphia: F. A. Davis Company, with permission.)

ensure the drug is inserted into the subcutaneous layer.

c. Select the appropriate site.

d. Alternate the site from recent injections; use a body flow chart to identify various sites by number. Doing so minimizes tissue injury, facilitates absorption, and minimizes lipodystrophy and lipohypertrophy.

e. Position the client so the site is accessible and the client is comfortable to provide accessibility to the injection site and relax the client for needle insertion.

f. Pinch a fold of skin between your fingers and thumb to elevate subcutaneous tissue and insert the needle at a determined angle using a smooth movement. The angle depends on the volume of subcutaneous tissue and needle length.

   (1) If you can pinch 2 inches of tissue, use a 90-degree angle.

   (2) If you can pinch only 1 inch of tissue, use a 45-degree angle.

   (3) For obese adults, inject deep into the tissue fold to avoid injecting the medication into adipose tissue.

g. Release the pinch and hold the syringe steady with the nondominant hand to minimize discomfort. Push the plunger slowly with the dominant hand to limit tissue discomfort and damage (see the information below on anticoagulants regarding holding a pinch); aspiration is not necessary because piercing a blood vessel is rare.

🛑 h. Follow the drug manufacturer's instructions regarding massage of the site to limit local tissue trauma; do not massage for insulin and anticoagulants.

6. Nursing interventions specific to administering insulin.

🛑 a. Check the client's blood glucose level before administration to evaluate response to insulin therapy and guide the next dose.

b. Generally, use a large gauge, short needle to minimize trauma and discomfort (a larger gauge needle is less painful than a smaller gauge needle).

c. Check documentation of the previous site and rotate sites to support absorption and minimize the risk of lipodystrophy and lipohypertrophy.

d. Leave the needle in place for 5 seconds after the injection of solution to ensure disbursal of the solution prior to needle removal.

7. Nursing interventions specific to administering an anticoagulant (e.g., heparin, low-molecular-weight heparin).

a. Observe injection sites daily for signs of complications, such as bleeding, bruising, pain, swelling, and heat; withhold the medication and notify the primary health-care provider if any are present.

🛑 b. Check coagulation laboratory results, such as International Normalized Ratio (INR); notify the primary health-care provider if findings are outside the expected parameters.

c. Have protamine sulfate (antidote for heparin) readily available if the client is receiving heparin.

d. Add 0.2 mL of air when preparing the correct dose. Do not expel the air bubble in a prefilled syringe; allow the air bubble to follow the medication into the needle tract, which limits bleeding and bruising.

e. Select the appropriate site.

   (1) Heparin: Inject in the abdomen, level with the iliac crest, at least 2 inches from the umbilicus.

   (2) Low-molecular-weight heparin: Inject in the anterolateral and posterolateral abdominal wall ("love handles").

f. Hold the pinch throughout the procedure and insert the full length of the needle to ensure the solution enters the subcutaneous tissue; do not aspirate.

g. Inject solution slowly over 30 seconds, including the air bubble, to allow for drug dispersal and minimize pain and bleeding.

🛑 h. Leave the needle in place for 10 seconds after the injection of solution to ensure delivery and dispersal of the anticoagulant dose.

🛑 i. Keep the plunger depressed while removing the needle to ensure that the bubble stays in the needle track.

🛑 j. Do not massage the site to minimize trauma and bleeding.

k. Document the site used to promote rotation of sites.

l. Institute sharps precautions, such as avoiding the use of blade razors, to protect the client from injury.

m. Avoid giving and tell the client to avoid taking aspirin and other OTC drugs that can decrease platelet aggregation, causing bruising and bleeding.

M. Intradermal (ID) injections

1. Introduction.
   a. ID injection: Insertion of medication into the dermis, which is just below the epidermis and above the subcutaneous tissue.
   b. The volume of solution generally is 0.01 to 1 mL of solution.
   c. The length of the needle generally is ¼ to ⅝ inch.
   d. The gauge of the needle generally is #25 to #28.
   e. The type of syringe used generally is a 1-mL or tuberculin syringe.

2. Advantages.
   a. Avoids the need to use more invasive and risky anesthetic agents when used as a local anesthetic.
   b. Is less expensive than other methods for testing for TB or allergens.

3. Disadvantages.
   a. Local inflammatory response may be uncomfortable or painful.
   b. Can cause an anaphylactic reaction to allergens being injected.

4. Nursing interventions specific to administering an ID injection.
   a. Select a tuberculin syringe with a gauge of #25 to #28 and a needle length of ¼ to ⅝ inch to ensure the needle is inserted into the dermis.
   b. Select the appropriate site: Choose the inner aspect of the forearm, upper chest, or upper back; avoid pigmented areas or areas with excessive hair.
   c. Use your nondominant hand to stretch the skin over the site with your forefinger and thumb to facilitate needle insertion.
   d. Insert the needle slowly at a 10- to 15-degree angle no more than ⅛ inch below the surface of the skin with the bevel facing upward (see Fig. 9.12) to ensure the solution is injected upward within the dermis rather than down toward the subcutaneous tissue.
   e. Slowly inject the solution until a small bleb forms under the surface of the skin (Fig. 9.12), indicating the solution was deposited into the dermis.
   🛑 f. Do not massage the area; massage will disperse solution into local tissue, which may alter test results.
   g. Draw a circle around the site to identify the site for future analysis.
   h. Instruct the client to return to the primary health-care provider at the time indicated (usually 24 to 48 hours); measure the area of redness and induration in millimeters and document the results.

N. Intravenous (IV) medication administration (see "Administration of IV Solutions" in Chapter 21, Fluid, Electrolyte, and Acid-Base Balance.)

1. Introduction.
   a. IV medications are administered directly into a vein.
   b. Methods of administration.
      (1) Addition of a medication, such as potassium chloride or vitamins, to a large-volume bag of IV fluid that is running continuously.
      (2) *Bolus ("push")*: Single dose of a medication in a syringe or in a small amount of IV fluid administered through a primary IV line or a venous access device, such as a heparin or saline lock. Heparin or saline locks are used for intermittent IV medications to allow the client more freedom of movement.
      (3) *"Piggyback" infusion*: Single dose of medication mixed with a small volume of fluid in its own IV bag administered via secondary tubing attached to a current IV line (primary line).
         (a) May be administered concurrently through the primary line.
         (b) May interrupt the primary line solution while the medication solution is administered.
   c. Method of IV medication preparation.
      (1) Most large-volume bags of IV fluid that contain medication are prepared and labeled by the manufacturer or pharmacy.
      (2) Most piggyback infusions are prepared and labeled by the pharmacy.
      (3) Some piggyback infusions and bolus infusions are prepared by the nurse administering the medication.

2. Advantages.
   a. Is rapid acting, making it useful in an emergency.
   b. Used for clients who cannot take drugs via the oral route.
   c. Avoids barriers to drug absorption associated with other routes.
   d. Allows larger volumes to be administered than by IM or Sub-Q routes.
   e. Provides for slow administration of a drug when required.
   f. Is more comfortable than administering an irritating drug into a muscle or subcutaneous tissue.
   g. Provides for a continuous blood level of a drug.

3. Disadvantages.
   a. Carries a greater risk of adverse reactions because of rapid action and is difficult to

reverse if the client has an adverse reaction or received an excessive dose; bolus method is most dangerous because the medication is not diluted in a larger volume of solution.

b. May irritate the blood vessel, particularly with a bolus dose.

c. Carries a greater risk of complications, such as bleeding, infection, fluid overload, and extravasation, as well as phlebitis and thrombosis, which cause discomfort and pain. (See "Complications of intravenous infusions and related nursing care," Table 21.3 in Chapter 21, Fluid, Electrolyte, and Acid-Base Balance.)

4. Nursing interventions common to administering all intravenous medications.

🛑 a. Double-check all calculations to ensure accuracy and prevent dosage errors.

b. Assess the IV site for signs of infiltration, such as swelling and edema, and check whether the flow rate is accurate.

c. Assess the IV site for clinical indicators of phlebitis, such as redness, swelling, and heat.

5. Nursing interventions specific to administering medication via a large-volume infusion.

a. Spike the IV bag with appropriate tubing, flush the air out of the tubing (prime the tubing), and connect it to the venous access device. Doing so prepares the tubing and ensures that air is flushed from the tubing.

b. Ensure that the IV fluid is compatible with the medication to be added to prevent drug and fluid incompatibilities.

c. Prepare the syringe with the prescribed drug.

d. Wipe the IV additive port with an alcohol wipe to reduce the risk of infection.

e. Insert the needle or needleless syringe into the center of the IV additive port and inject the medication; then withdraw the syringe. Doing so allows the IV additive port to self-seal; using the sides of a port may produce leaks and cause fluid contamination.

f. Gently turn the IV bag end to end to mix the solutions without causing bubbles.

g. Attach the label with the client's name, medication, dose, date, time, and nurse's initials.

h. Hang the IV bag and open the roller clamp on the tubing to the prescribed rate of infusion if administered by gravity OR use an infusion pump and set the rate accordingly.

6. Nursing interventions specific to administering medication via a bolus infusion ("IV push").

a. Ensure that medication is administered by a registered nurse; do not delegate this procedure to a licensed practical nurse.

b. Determine the rate of solution administration by considering the volume of solution to be administered in relation to the amount of time the medication is to be given, such as 4 mL over 2 minutes (therefore, instill 0.5 minims every 30 seconds). Doing so ensures the medication is diluted slowly in the client's blood, preventing excessive intake in a short amount of time that may irritate the vein or cause an unwanted reaction.

c. Cleanse the insertion port with an alcohol wipe to limit the risk of infection.

d. Access the insertion port.

(1) Heparin or saline lock.

(a) Follow agency policy and procedure for identifying patency and flushing the venous access device before a bolus dose.

(b) Insert the syringe into the venous access device and instill the medication.

(c) Withdraw the syringe and follow agency policy and procedure for flushing the venous access device after the bolus dose to ensure that the entire dose is received and that the venous access device is free from medication.

(2) Currently running IV infusion (Fig. 9.17).

(a) Pinch the IV tubing just above the injection port closest to the venipuncture site to stop the flow of IV fluid from the IV bag temporarily, which allows the drug to be instilled toward the client rather than up the tubing.

(b) Insert the syringe into the port and aspirate until a slight amount of blood appears in the syringe or tubing to ensure that the device is in a vein and that the bolus will be injected into the vein.

(c) Inject the medication at the prescribed rate.

(d) Remove the syringe and release the pinch in the tubing to allow the primary solution to flow.

e. Dispose of the syringe in the nearest sharps container.

f. Monitor the client closely for adverse drug reactions.

7. Nursing interventions specific to administering a medication via an intermittent (piggyback) infusion.

a. Ensure the medication bag has a label with the client's name, medication, dose, time/frequency, date, and nurse's initials.

b. Attach the tubing to the medication bag; prime the tubing without losing

Fig 9.17 IV push. (From Burton and Ludwig [2015]. *Fundamentals of nursing care: Concepts, connections & skill,* 2nd ed.. Philadelphia: F. A. Davis Company, with permission.)

more than 1 drop of the solution. Doing so prepares the equipment for use, removes air from the tubing, and ensures that the client receives the entire dose.

   c. Wipe the insertion port with alcohol to prevent infection.
   d. Access the insertion port.
      (1) Heparin or saline lock: Attach the medication tubing directly to the venous access device or use a needleless piercing device.
      (2) Currently running IV (primary) line.
         (a) When a primary line is not interrupted to deliver a piggyback (Fig. 9.18): Use the tubing port closest to the insertion site; keep both bags at the same height; open the clamp on the medication bag; control the flow of solution from both bags using the clamp on the primary tubing.
         (b) When a primary line is interrupted to deliver a piggyback (Fig. 9.19): Use the tubing port farthest from the insertion site; drop the primary infusion bag lower than the medication bag; open the clamp on the medication tubing and control the flow using the clamp on the primary tubing. Doing so ensures that the primary infusion will flow (via gravity) after the medication bag is empty.
   e. Depending on the critical nature of the medication, use an infusion pump to ensure an accurate flow rate.
   f. Reestablish the prescribed flow rate of the primary infusion, if one is present, to maintain continuity of IV fluid administration.

Fig 9.18 Intermittent (piggyback) infusion. Tandem (secondary) setup. (From Wilkinson and Treas [2011]. *Fundamentals of nursing,* Vol. 1, 2nd ed. Philadelphia: F. A. Davis Company, with permission.)

Fig 9.19 Intermittent (piggyback) infusion. Piggyback setup. (From Vitale [2013]. *NCLEX-RN notes: Content review & exam prep,* 2nd ed. Philadelphia: F. A. Davis Company, with permission.)

8. Nursing interventions specific to administering IV medication via a volume-controlled infusion set (Fig. 9.20).
   a. Prepare a syringe with the prescribed medication.

Fig 9.20 Volume-controlled administration set. (From Wilkinson and Treas [2016]. *Fundamentals of nursing,* Vol. 2, 3rd ed. Philadelphia: F. A. Davis Company, with permission.)

b. Fill the set by opening the clamp between the set and main IV tubing until the desired volume of IV fluid enters the set and then clamp the main IV tubing.
c. Cleanse the injection port on the set with an alcohol wipe to reduce the risk of infection.
d. Inject the medication into the medication port of the set and gently mix the solutions to ensure even distribution of medication in the IV fluid and prevent formation of bubbles.
e. Open the clamp below the set, and adjust it to the prescribed flow rate (usually delivered over 30 to 60 minutes).

X. Medication Calculation Formulas

A. IV drop rate formula (Fig. 9.21)
  1. IV tubing drop factor: The number of drops it takes for specific tubing to deliver 1 mL of fluid.
  2. The **drop factor** is a component of the formula when calculating the IV flow rate when using a specific IV set.
  3. Drop factors are indicated on the tubing box. For example:
     a. Macro-drops: Drop factor of 10 delivers 10 drops/1 mL; drop factor of 15 = 15 drops/1 mL; drop factor of 20 = 20 drops/1 mL.
     b. Micro-drops: Drop factor of 60 = 60 drops/1 mL.
B. Conversion of pounds to kilograms (Kg) (Fig. 9.22)
C. Ratio and proportion formulas (Fig. 9.23)
D. Body surface area (BSA) method to calculate a pediatric dose for infants and children ≤12 years of age (Fig. 9.24)

• Multiply the numerators (total mL × drop factor).
• Multiply the denominators (1 hour × 60 minutes).
• Divide the numerator by the denominator to obtain the drops per minute.

$$\text{Drops per minute} = \frac{\text{total mL} \times \text{drop factor} \quad \text{(total volume in drops)}}{1 \text{ hour} \times 60 \text{ minutes} \quad \text{(total time in minutes)}}$$

Fig 9.21 IV drop rate formula. (From Vitale [2017]. *NCLEX-RN notes: Content review & exam prep,* 3rd ed. Philadelphia: F. A. Davis Company, with permission.)

• Solve for X by cross multiplying.
• Divide both sides of resulting equation by the number in front of the X.
• Reduce to lowest terms to achieve child's weight in kilograms (kg).

$$\frac{\text{child's weight in pounds}}{2.2 \text{ pounds}} = \frac{\text{X kg}}{1 \text{ kg}}$$

Fig 9.22 Conversion of pounds to kilograms (Kg). (From Vitale [2017]. *NCLEX-RN notes: Content review & exam prep,* 3rd ed. Philadelphia: F. A. Davis Company, with permission.)

- Ordered (prescribed) dose and dose on hand must be in the same unit of measure.
- Formulas 1 and 2: Solve for X by cross multiplying.
- Formula 3: Solve for X by multiplying the means and the extremes.
- For all three formulas, divide the resulting equation by the number in front of the X.
- For all three formulas, reduce to lowest terms to achieve the quantity of dose.

$$\text{\#1}\quad \frac{\text{desired}}{\text{have}} = \frac{\text{ordered dose}}{\text{dose on hand}} = \frac{\text{X quantity desired}}{\text{quantity on hand}}$$

$$\text{\#2}\quad \frac{\text{quantity on hand}}{\text{dose on hand}} = \frac{\text{X quantity desired}}{\text{ordered dose}}$$

$$\text{\#3}\quad \underset{\text{(extremes)}}{\text{dose on hand}} : \underset{\text{(means)}}{\text{quantity on hand}} : : \underset{\text{(means)}}{\text{ordered dose}} : \underset{\text{(extremes)}}{\text{X quantity desired}}$$

Fig 9.23 Ratio and proportion formulas. (From Vitale [2017]. *NCLEX-RN notes: Content review & exam prep,* 3rd ed. Philadelphia: F. A. Davis Company, with permission.)

$$\text{pediatric dose in mg} = \frac{\text{*child's BSA in square meters (m}^2\text{)}}{1.73\ m^2} \times \text{adult dose in mg}$$

- *Estimate the child's body surface area (BSA) in square meters (m^2) by using a BSA chart (nomogram).
- The BSA chart consists of three columns. The left column is height, the middle column is BSA, and the right column is weight. These numbers increase from the bottom to the top of each column.
- Draw a straight line from the child's height in the left column to the child's weight in the right column. The number found where the line crosses the middle column is the child's estimated BSA.
- The BSA should be used in the formula for the BSA method to calculate a pediatric dose.
- To access the nomogram: Vallerand, Sanoski, Deglin. (2015). *Davis's Drug Guide for Nurses,* 12th Ed., Appendix F, p. 402. Philadelphia: F. A. Davis Company.

Fig. 9.24 BSA method to calculate a pediatric dose for infants and children ≤12 years of age. (From Vitale [2017]. *NCLEX-RN notes: Content review & exam prep,* 3rd ed. Philadelphia: F. A. Davis Company, with permission.)

CASE STUDY: Putting It All Together

An 80-year-old man is admitted to the emergency department. He states that he has lived alone since his wife passed away a few years ago but that his son visits about once a month. He says, "I'm on a tight budget because my only income is Social Security. I hoped that I would get better and not have to pay for an emergency room visit. I finally came because I couldn't breathe, and my legs were very swollen." The client shares that, at times, he gets a little forgetful and does not remember to take his medication every day. The client brought all the containers of the medications that he takes daily. The nurse identified the following medications that the client is taking at home and why and documented the medications on the medication reconciliation form.

- Furosemide (Lasix) 20 mg PO, daily (diuretic)
- Docusate sodium (Colace) 100 mg PO, bid (stool softener)
- Famotidine (Pepcid) 20 mg PO, bid (antiulcer agent for gastroesophageal reflux disease)
- 1 Tab Centrum Silver for Men daily (multivitamin for men)
- Metoprolol (Toprol XL) 50 mg PO, daily (beta-blocker for hypertension)

The client states that he has a history of hypertension. His blood pressure on admission is 180/90 mm Hg. He says that he does not always take the Lasix when he has to go out in the morning to do errands because he has to stop so often to urinate. He also has some urinary frequency, urinary urgency, and nocturia because of an enlarged prostate. When talking, the client stops frequently to catch his breath. Respirations are 30 breaths/min, the client is using accessory muscles to breathe, and capillary refill is longer than 3 seconds. Oxygen saturation is 90%.

The primary health-care provider writes and signs the following prescriptions:
- I&O
- 2-g sodium diet
- OOB to chair every shift with assistance
- VS (vital signs) every 8 hours
- IV lock—flush with 10 mL NS every 8 hours
- 2 L oxygen via nasal cannula
- Furosemide (Lasix) 40 mg IVPB
- Famotidine (Pepcid) 20 mg bid
- Docusate sodium (Colace) 1 tab PO, bid
- Metoprolol (Toprol XL) 50 mg PO, daily

CASE STUDY: Putting It All Together

cont'd

After 6 hours, the client still has not voided, his abdomen is distended, and he says, "I feel a lot of pressure in my lower belly and I have to urinate, but I can't." The nurse calls the primary health-care provider, who prescribes the following interventions via a telephone prescription.

- Insert urinary retention catheter to bedside drainage
- Tamsulosin (Flomax) 0.4 mg PO, daily after a meal

Case Study Questions

A. Discuss the factors that place the client at risk for complications related to a medication regimen.

1. _____

2. _____

3. _____

B. What nursing interventions should the nurse implement to help the client manage his forgetfulness associated with his medication regimen?

1. _____

2. _____

3. _____

C. What medication prescriptions are incomplete? Also indicate what information the primary health-care provider must include to make the prescriptions complete.

1. _____

2. _____

3. _____

D. When taking the telephone prescription for the urinary retention catheter and Flomax, what procedural steps should the nurse implement to ensure accuracy?

1. _____

2. _____

3. _____

REVIEW QUESTIONS

Be sure to read the Introduction for valuable test-taking tips.

1. A nurse plans to administer an intramuscular injection to an obese client. What muscle should the nurse consider the least desirable site for an intramuscular injection in an obese adult?
   1. Vastus lateralis
   2. Rectus femoris
   3. Dorsogluteal
   4. Deltoid

2. An antibiotic 0.75 g IM is prescribed for a client with an infection. The vial of the medication contains 1 gram of the medication and it must be reconstituted. The vial has instructions to instill 1.8 mL of diluent to yield 2 mL of solution. How much solution should the nurse administer?

   1. A
   2. B
   3. C
   4. D

3. A nurse must administer a rectal suppository. Which should the nurse do when administering the suppository? **Select all that apply.**
   1. Explain the need to remain in the left lateral position for 15 to 20 minutes after insertion of the suppository to promote its retention in the rectum.
   2. Use the full length of a gloved, lubricated index finger, about 3 to 4 inches long, when inserting the suppository to ensure it is beyond the rectal sphincters.
   3. Take the suppository out of the refrigerator a half hour before insertion to allow it to warm to room temperature.
   4. Place the client in the supine position to allow easy access to the anus when inserting the suppository.
   5. Use an applicator to insert the suppository to ensure appropriate placement.

4. A nurse is interviewing a newly admitted client as part of a nursing history and physical. What information should be included in the medication reconciliation form? **Select all that apply.**
   1. Vitamins
   2. Drug allergies
   3. Food supplements
   4. Over-the-counter herbs
   5. Prescribed medications

5. A nurse must administer 3 mL of a distasteful liquid medication to a 3-year-old child. Which should the nurse do to promote ingestion of the medication?
   1. Dilute it in several ounces of the child's favorite fruit juice and then give it to the child.
   2. Use a needleless syringe and instill it all at the same time into the child's buccal cavity.
   3. Mix it in a glass of water and have the child sip the medication through a straw.
   4. Have the child eat an ice pop and then administer the medication to the child.

6. A nurse observed another nurse administering an injection via the Z-track technique. Which actions by the nurse indicated that the technique was performed correctly? **Select all that apply.**
   1. Changed the needle after drawing up the medication
   2. Massaged the site well after administration of the medication
   3. Obtained a syringe with a 25-gauge needle for the procedure
   4. Attached a needle with a 1-inch length after the medication was drawn into the syringe
   5. Pulled the skin laterally before insertion of the needle and removed the needle at the same angle of its insertion

7. A nurse is to administer eyedrops to a client. The nurse verifies the prescription, washes the hands, and collects the medication following the five rights and three checks associated with medication administration. The nurse places the client in a supine position with the head extended and then dons clean gloves. Place the following steps in the order in which they should be implemented.
   1. Instruct the client to look up toward the ceiling without moving the head.
   2. Direct the client to gently close the eyelids but avoid squeezing the eyes shut.
   3. Instruct the client to press firmly on the nasolacrimal duct for 30 to 60 seconds.
   4. Wash each eye from inner to outer canthus using a different moistened cotton ball for each swipe.
   5. Place a finger of the nondominant hand below the lower lid and gently pull the skin down to reveal the conjunctival sac.
   6. Place the dominant hand on the forehead, approach the eye from the side with the eye dropper 1 to 2 cm above the conjunctival sac, and instill the prescribed number of drops.

   Answer: _____

8. A nurse is to administer 1 mL of a liquid medication to a 3-month-old infant. Which is the **best** way to administer this medication?
   1. Use a needless syringe to instill the medication on the back of the infant's tongue.
   2. Use a dropper to insert the medication into the infant's buccal cavity.
   3. Use a medicine cup to allow the infant to sip the medication slowly.
   4. Use a medication nipple so that the infant can suck the medication.

9. A nurse is to administer one nose drop to each nostril of a school-aged child. Which actions should the nurse perform as part of this procedure? **Select all that apply.**
   1. Instruct the child to exhale through the mouth and then breathe though the mouth for a few minutes after the drop is inserted.
   2. Instruct the child to remain in the administration position for several minutes after insertion of the drops.
   3. Position the child in the supine position with the head tilted backward when inserting the drops.
   4. Position the tip of the medication dropper within the nasal opening when expelling the drop.
   5. Return the unused nose drops in the dropper to the medication bottle.

10. A nurse is to administer an intradermal injection for a tuberculin test to an adult. The nurse verifies the prescription, washes the hands, and collects the medication following the five rights and three checks associated with medication administration. The nurse then dons clean gloves. Place the following steps in the order in which they should be implemented.
    1. Draw a 1-inch circle around the wheal.
    2. Position the client with the forearm supinated.
    3. Stabilize tissue on both sides of the puncture site as the needle is quickly removed at the same angle of insertion.
    4. Clean the site with an alcohol wipe using a circular motion moving from the center outward and allow the site to dry.
    5. Inject the solution with slow, even pressure so that a small wheal (raised welt, bleb) of fluid becomes apparent under the skin.
    6. Insert a ¼- to ⅝-inch, 25- to 27-gauge needle with the bevel up just below the skin surface at a 10- to 15-degree angle until the bevel is no longer visible.

    Answer: _____

11. A nurse is caring for a client who was admitted to the hospital as a result of an accidental double dose of a prescribed medication. Which strategy should the nurse suggest that the client use to **best** prevent this from happening again?
    1. Teach the client how to use a medication organizer system.
    2. Set an alarm clock to ring at the time a drug is to be taken as a reminder.
    3. Suggest that a family member call to remind the client when to take medications.
    4. Hang a calendar in a significant place that indicates the drug name, dose, and time it is to be taken.

12. A nurse receives a prescription for a medication based on a child's weight from a primary health-care provider. The pediatric nurse identifies that the prescribed dose is for a child weighing 10 lb more than the weight of the child for whom the drug dose was prescribed. What should the nurse do?
    1. Call the primary health-care provider and discuss the excessive dose.
    2. Recalculate the dose using the actual weight and give the recalculated dose.
    3. Ask the pharmacist about the weight difference and whether it is necessary to change the dose.
    4. Notify the nurse manager and seek support to confront the primary health-care provider about the dose.

13. Which site is appropriate for the nurse to use for the administration of heparin?

1. A
2. B
3. C
4. D

14. Which nursing actions are indicated when administering a heparin injection? **Select all that apply.**
1. Aspirating before injecting the medication
2. Placing the needle just under the epidermis
3. Avoiding massage of the site after the injection
4. Spreading the skin during insertion of the needle
5. Cleaning the site with a disinfectant before the injection

15. A client with moderate dementia, who lives at home with a relative, insists on being as independent as possible. The client frequently forgets to take the prescribed morning medications. Which action should the nurse discuss with the client and relative?
1. The relative should verbally explain to the client which medications to take each morning.
2. A divided medication-dispensing system should be used for all of the client's medications.
3. A written list of the medications that must be taken should be left on the client's bedside table.
4. The relative should place the medications in a medication cup by the client's toothbrush in the bathroom each morning.

16. A nurse must administer 2 mL of a medication via the intramuscular route. Which syringe should the nurse use for this injection?

A

B

C

D

1. A
2. B
3. C
4. D

17. A nurse receives a telephone prescription from a client's primary health-care provider. What actions must the nurse take before hanging up the telephone? **Select all that apply.**
1. Insert the prescription into the client's clinical record.
2. Recite the prescription back to the primary health-care provider.
3. Confirm that the prescribed medication is available in the hospital pharmacy.
4. State that the primary health-care provider must sign the prescription within forty-eight hours.
5. Have another nurse listen to the prescription and countersign the prescription in the appropriate document.

18. A nurse receives a prescription for a medication to be administered every 6 hours prn. What should the nurse teach the client about this medication?
    1. "I will give this medication over 6 hours."
    2. "I can give you this medication every 6 hours if you need it."
    3. "I must wait 6 hours before administering this medication to you."
    4. "I have to give you this medication every 6 hours around the clock."

19. A client has a prescription for 2 drops of a medication to be placed into an eye. Which nursing actions are associated with this procedure? **Select all that apply.**
    1. Holding the dropper close to the eye without touching it
    2. Having the client look up while the eyedrops are inserted
    3. Instructing the client to close the eyes firmly after the eyedrops are administered
    4. Placing a finger on the top lid while simultaneously pulling the lid toward the forehead
    5. Cleansing the eye by wiping gently from the outer canthus to the inner canthus with a new cotton ball for each swipe

20. A nurse is caring for a client who is to be screened for tuberculosis. Which injection route should the nurse use to inject tuberculin purified protein derivative?

21. A nurse reconstituted and drew up a medication from a vial. Which nursing actions compromised the ability to withdraw an accurate dose? **Select all that apply.**
    1. Injected air into the vial with the bevel of the needle below the level of the solution
    2. Placed slightly more air into the vial than the volume of solution to be removed
    3. Shaked the vial in the palm of a hand after the diluent was added to the vial
    4. Wiped the rubber seal with alcohol before withdrawing the solution
    5. Instilled the diluent into the vial slowly

22. A nurse is to administer an intramuscular injection into the deltoid muscle. What bony landmark should the nurse use to help locate the appropriate site?
    1. Knee
    2. Greater trochanter
    3. Acromion process
    4. Anterior superior iliac spine

23. What should the nurse do to **best** prevent needlestick injuries when administering injections?
    1. Bend the needle of the syringe before disposal.
    2. Recap the needle while transporting it to a sharps container.
    3. Use a syringe with a device that automatically covers the needle after its use.
    4. Dispose of a syringe with its attached needle into the closest sharps container.

1. A
2. B
3. C
4. D

24. A client has a prescription for 22 units of NPH insulin and 8 units of regular insulin subcutaneously once daily at 8 a.m. The nurse teaches a client how to draw up and self-administer these insulins. Which amount of solution depicted in the illustration indicates that the client prepared the correct dose?

1. A
2. B
3. C
4. D

25. A client has an intravenous infusion running at 30 drops/minute by gravity. The nurse must administer hydromorphone IV push via an infusion port in this line. What should the nurse do to ensure that the client receives the full effect of the dose?
1. Use the port farthest from the insertion site.
2. Pinch the tubing above the port as the medication is instilled.
3. Double the flow rate of the solution for a half hour after the drug is given.
4. Shut the roller clamp off on the tubing before administering the medication.

26. A nurse is planning to piggyback an intermittent infusion of a medication (IVPB) into a primary infusion set that is delivering normal saline at 100 mL per hour. What steps should the nurse perform to administer this medication appropriately? **Select all that apply.**
1. Warm the bag of solution with the drug before administration.
2. Hang the secondary infusion bag lower than the primary infusion bag.
3. Wipe the port with alcohol before connecting the secondary infusion tubing.
4. Prime the secondary infusion line before attaching it to the primary infusion line.
5. Open the clamp on the secondary infusion tubing and use the clamp on the primary infusion tubing to control the flow.

27. A nurse is teaching a parent how to administer eardrops to a 2-year-old child with an ear infection. What instructions should the nurse give the parent? **Select all that apply.**
1. "Dispense the drops along the side of your child's ear canal."
2. "Tap gently on the tragus of the ear after instilling the drops."
3. "Keep the medication refrigerated until just before you are going to give your child the drops."
4. "Pull your child's pinna down and backward to straighten the ear canal before inserting the drops."
5. "Have your child lie with the ear facing the ceiling while inserting the drops and for five minutes after the drops are inserted."

28. A nurse is applying a transdermal patch to a client's upper arm. Which nursing actions are essential for every client to complete this procedure? **Select all that apply.**
1. Wear clean gloves when removing and applying a medicated patch.
2. Shave body hair in the area that the medicated patch is to be applied.
3. Wash and dry the area where the previous medicated patch was removed.
4. Compress the medicated patch against the skin for 10 seconds after it is applied.
5. Remove the previous medicated patch one hour after applying the new medicated patch.

29. A nurse is to administer an antibiotic capsule orally but first asks the client, "What is your name and date of birth?" What should the nurse do **next** after receiving this information?
    1. Give the client a glass of apple juice to take with the oral medication.
    2. Compare the response to the client's identification bracelet to verify the information.
    3. Raise the head of the client's bed to allow gravity to facilitate swallowing the oral dose.
    4. Check the client's allergy bracelet to ensure that the client is not allergic to the medication.

30. A nurse is preparing to administer a medication that is known to be teratogenic. What should the nurse say to the client before administering this medication?
    1. "Are you pregnant?"
    2. "Do you have an allergy to gluten?"
    3. "You must eat some food just before taking this drug."
    4. "I have to obtain blood for a culture and sensitivity test before you take this drug."

31. A client had multiple surgical procedures as a result of extensive injuries sustained in a motor vehicle collision. The client has type 1 diabetes and blood glucose monitoring before meals and at the hour of sleep with related insulin coverage is prescribed. The nurse obtains the client's blood glucose level, verifies the prescription for insulin coverage, and assesses the client. Which should the nurse do in this situation?
    1. Administer 2 units of regular insulin in the deltoid site.
    2. Administer 8 units of regular insulin into the vastus lateralis site.
    3. Administer 8 units of regular insulin several inches away from the stoma.
    4. Administer 2 units of regular insulin into the love handles on the right side.

▮ Client's Clinical Record

Blood Glucose Level

190 mg/dL

Primary Health-Care Provider's Prescriptions

Blood glucose monitoring before meals and hour of sleep with regular insulin coverage via subcutaneous route.
150 to 200 mg/dL—2 units regular insulin.
201 to 225 mg/dL—4 units regular insulin.
226 to 275 mg/dL—8 units regular insulin.
276 to 300 mg/dL—12 units regular insulin.
>300—notify primary health-care provider.

Progress Notes

Bilateral above-the-knee amputations with compression dressings; an abdominal incision that extends from the sternum to the symphysis pubis and a new colostomy in the left lower quadrant of the abdomen. Client lying in the low-Fowler position. Dependent edema 2+ noted. The client states, "There is no way anyone is going to give me another injection in my arms. I've had it!"

---

32. A nurse enters a client's room to administer a drug that is in the form of a tablet. The client states, "I am nauseated and feel like I am going to vomit." What should the nurse do **next** in relation to administration of the medication?
    1. Obtain a prescription for an alternate route of administration.
    2. Give the medication and hope that the client keeps it in the stomach.
    3. Obtain a liquid form of the prescribed medication and give it to the client.
    4. Withhold the medication for an hour and a half and then attempt to give it again.

33. A nurse is teaching a client about self-administering a medication via the buccal route. Which should the nurse instruct the client to do? **Select all that apply.**
    1. "Remain awake until the medication is dissolved."
    2. "Hold the medication under your tongue until it is absorbed."
    3. "Swish the medication around in your mouth and then swallow it."
    4. "Alternate cheeks when taking additional doses of the medication."
    5. "Hold the medication between your cheek and gum until it dissolves."

34. A client has a prescription for the insertion of a vaginal cream. Which steps should the nurse perform when administering this medication? **Select all that apply.**
    1. Have the client void before the procedure.
    2. Clean the perineal area before inserting the cream.
    3. Withdraw the applicator rapidly after the cream is inserted.
    4. Place the client in the supine position with the legs extended.
    5. Direct the insertion of the applicator upward toward the umbilicus.
    6. Press the plunger to expel a small amount of cream at the tip of the applicator before insertion.

35. A nurse is evaluating a client's ability to self-administer a medication to both nasal passages via a nasal spray. What action by the client indicates that the nurse must provide additional teaching?
    1. Compressing the other nostril while initiating the spray into the first nostril
    2. Exhaling slowly through the nose after initiating the spray
    3. Tilting the head backward after inhaling the spray
    4. Inhaling the spray while squeezing the container

36. A client with diabetes who is on insulin coverage has been receiving three to four injections of insulin a day. What is important for the nurse to do when administering these injections? **Select all that apply.**
    1. Use a 26- to 30-gauge needle.
    2. Alternate injection sites to minimize tissue injury.
    3. Pinch the skin to facilitate entry of the needle through the skin.
    4. Instill the medication over 5 seconds to promote absorption of the medication.
    5. Use a syringe with a needle that is 1½ inches long to ensure access of subcutaneous tissue.

37. A nurse receives a prescription for 1,000 mL of 0.9% sodium chloride with 20 mEq of KCl to be administered at 75 mL/hour to a client. The nurse finds only 250-mL bags of 0.9% sodium chloride on the unit. What should the nurse do in this situation?
    1. Use a 1,000-mL bag of dextrose 5% in water with 20 mEq of KCl until the appropriate bag of solution is obtained.
    2. Withhold starting the intravenous infusion until a 1,000-mL bag of the appropriate solution is obtained.
    3. Insert 20 mEq of KCl into a 250-mL bag of 0.9% sodium chloride and set it at 25 mL/hour.
    4. Insert 5 mEq of KCl into a 250-mL bag of 0.9% sodium chloride and set it at 75 mL/hour.

38. A nurse withdrew fluid from an ampule. What did the nurse do to ensure that the entire dose was withdrawn?
    1. Placed a plastic cover over the top of the ampule before snapping the constricted neck
    2. Changed the needle on the syringe after aspirating the solution from the ampule
    3. Flicked the ampule above the constricted neck several times
    4. Used a filter needle to aspirate solution from the ampule

39. In what section of the medication administration record should a nurse document a STAT drug given in an emergency?
    1. prn section
    2. Single-dose section
    3. Progress note section
    4. Standing drugs section

40. During report, a nurse is informed that an assigned client has diabetes mellitus with insulin coverage before meals and before going to sleep at night. The nurse tests the client's blood glucose level before lunch and identifies that it is elevated. Place the interventions in the order in which the nurse should perform them.
    1. Wash the hands with soap and water.
    2. Verify the prescription for insulin coverage.
    3. Don gloves and administer the prepared insulin.
    4. Draw up the prescribed amount of insulin to be administered.
    5. Compare the client's blood glucose level to the insulin prescription.
    Answer: _____

41. What is the **best** site for the nurse to inject a newborn with vitamin K?
    1. Deltoid muscle
    2. Dorsogluteal muscle
    3. Ventrogluteal muscle
    4. Vastus lateralis muscle

42. Which is the **best** resource when a nurse requires information concerning recall of a medication, safety alerts, new medications, and generic approvals?
    1. U.S. Food and Drug Administration
    2. American Nurses Association
    3. U.S. Pharmacopoeia
    4. National Formulary

43. A client is receiving a narcotic analgesic for pain associated with cancer of the pancreas. Several weeks after initiation of therapy, the client says to a nurse, "The medication does not control the pain as much as it did several weeks ago." What response to the medication should the nurse conclude this client is experiencing?
    1. Tolerance
    2. Potentiation
    3. Adverse effect
    4. Idiosyncratic reaction

44. A nurse is administering an oral antibiotic to a client who has an infected leg wound and a history of impaired peripheral circulation to the lower extremities. Which is the nurse's **most** important concern about this client's status when evaluating a response to the antibiotic?
    1. Competence to biotransform the medication
    2. Ability to move the medication around the body
    3. Potential to excrete the medication from the body
    4. Capacity to absorb the medication into the blood stream

45. A nurse is caring for a client who has impaired kidney function. For which process associated with pharmacokinetics should the nurse be **most** concerned when evaluating this client's response to an oral medication regimen?
    1. Biotransformation
    2. Distribution
    3. Absorption
    4. Excretion

46. A nurse is caring for a client who has a prescription for an opioid for pain every 4 hours prn. The client asks, "How long will it take for the medication to relieve my pain after I take the pill?" Which concept is **most** important for the nurse to explain to the client?
    1. Peak plasma level
    2. Duration
    3. Half-life
    4. Onset

47. A nurse is caring for a client who reports taking multiple over-the-counter herbal supplements. Which information about supplements should the nurse include when teaching this client about supplements? **Select all that apply.**
    1. Herbal supplements are safe to take.
    2. Herbal supplements are regulated by the FDA.
    3. Manufacturers' advertising of benefits is not supported with evidence.
    4. Some clients do not realize the importance of reporting supplement use.
    5. Alcohol should not be ingested with herbal supplements because of the risk of nontherapeutic interactions.

48. A nurse is explaining to a client the need to perform blood tests to determine if a medication the client is receiving is in the therapeutic range. Which statement should the nurse include in the discussion?
    1. "We need to draw your blood at the medication's half-life to determine if the dose needs to be adjusted."
    2. "We need to draw your blood just before the next dose to identify the lowest level of the medication in your blood."
    3. "We need to draw your blood two hours after administering the medication to determine the peak plasma level of the drug."
    4. "We need to draw your blood hourly to determine the duration of the therapeutic concentration of the medication in your blood."

49. A nurse is caring for a client who is receiving an antibiotic intravenously. The client asks, "Why are you drawing my blood so many times since I've started getting my antibiotic?" Which response by the nurse **best** answers the client's question?
    1. "We want to ensure that the dose is not so strong that it causes toxicity."
    2. "The results will reflect if the dose is being absorbed appropriately by your body."
    3. "We want to determine if the medication gets into your blood within thirty minutes."
    4. "The results will reveal if the blood level of the medication is being maintained within the therapeutic range."

50. A nurse is caring for a client who has a prescription for azithromycin (Zithromax) 500 mg by mouth once followed by 250 mg by mouth daily for 5 days. It is available in 250 mg tablets. How many tablets should the nurse administer to the client for the first dose? **Record your answer using a whole number.**

    Answer: _____ tablets

51. A nurse is unfamiliar with a new medication and reviews information about it in *Davis's Drug Guide for Nurses*. Which information will help the nurse identify the generic name of the medication?
    1. The chemical structure is described.
    2. The name begins with a lowercase letter.
    3. The name is easier to recall than other names.
    4. The medication is registered by the United States Patent Office.

52. A nurse is evaluating a client's response to a medication. Which is important for the nurse to recall about factors that impact on the efficacy of a medication?
    1. Environment has little effect on responses to medications.
    2. Most medications are best absorbed on a stomach that is empty.
    3. Medication response discrepancies occur between men and woman.
    4. Infants experience multiorgan slowdown, increasing the risk of medication toxicity.

53. A nurse who just came on duty is assigned to care for an older adult male who is receiving chemotherapy for cancer. The nurse reviews the client's clinical record. For which priority concern should the nurse assess the client for clinical indicators?
1. Infection
2. Hemorrhage
3. Medication toxicity
4. Deficient fluid volume

Client's Clinical Record

Primary Health-Care Provider's Prescriptions

CBC, basic metabolic panel daily.
Furosemide (Lasix) 40 mg IV push once daily in a.m. Withhold Lasix for systolic blood pressure <90 mm Hg and inform primary health-care provider.
Discontinue chemotherapy.
Strict I&O.
2 g Na, low-protein, low-potassium diet.
Daily weight.

Laboratory Results

BUN: 60 mg/dL.
Creatinine: 4.1 mg/dL.
Hb: 14.8 g/dL.
WBC: 5,500/mm³.
Platelets: 200,000/mm³.

Progress Notes

The client states feeling fatigued and drowsy. Pulse 88 beats/minute bounding; respirations 22 breaths/minute, bibasilar crackles; temperature 97.8°F; blood pressure 160/90 mm Hg. 1+ sacral edema noted. Intake last 24 hours: 2,400 mL IV and 800 mL PO. Urine output: 1,000 mL. Jugular venous distention noted. IV site dry, intact, free from signs and symptoms of infiltration and thrombophlebitis.

---

54. A nurse is evaluating a client's response to a medication and identifies a predictable, secondary effect of the medication. Which terminology should the nurse use when documenting the client's response?
1. Idiosyncratic reaction
2. Allergic reaction
3. Adverse effect
4. Side effect

55. A client in the emergency department tells the nurse, "I am allergic to penicillin." What should the nurse do **next**?
1. Ask the client about what kind of responses occurred.
2. Ask the client about the presence of other types of allergies.
3. List the allergy on an allergy alert band on the client's wrist.
4. List the allergy in the client's medication administration record.

56. A nurse is caring for a client with a diagnosis of deep vein thrombosis who is receiving warfarin. The client's INR is 2.5. Place the following statements in order based on the steps of the nursing process.
1. Administer 10 mg of warfarin as prescribed by the primary health-care provider.
2. The risk of hemorrhage is related to the effects of the anticoagulant warfarin.
3. Obtain a blood specimen before the next dose to assess the client's INR.
4. The client will not experience bleeding while receiving warfarin.
5. Left calf is pale, cool, and edematous.
Answer: _____

57. A nurse is caring for a client diagnosed with diabetes and who is receiving insulin. Which medication use category should the nurse include when discussing insulin with this client?
1. Curative
2. Preventive
3. Maintenance
4. Contraceptive

58. A nurse is concerned about a client's ability to metabolize a newly prescribed medication. Laboratory tests associated with which part of the body should the nurse monitor for functional performance because it is mainly associated with biotransformation of medication?
1. Liver
2. Lungs
3. Kidneys
4. Intestines

59. A nurse is caring for a middle-aged adult newly admitted to the hospital who has prescriptions for six different medications. Which nursing action is the priority before administering these medications to the client?
1. Verify that the medications are compatible.
2. Have the antidotes for medications easily available.
3. Teach the client the therapeutic action of the medications.
4. Ensure that these medications are included on the medication reconciliation form.

60. A nurse is caring for a client who is receiving a monoamine oxidase (MAO) inhibitor. Which food should the nurse teach the client to avoid when receiving this medication? **Select all that apply.**
1. Yogurt
2. Sausage
3. Chocolate
4. Chicken liver
5. Cream cheese

REVIEW ANSWERS AND RATIONALES

1. ANSWER: 3.

Rationales:

1. The vastus lateralis site is appropriate for an intramuscular injection in an obese individual as long as the amount of fluid injected is 3 mL or less.

2. The rectus femoris is an appropriate site for an intramuscular injection in an obese individual as long as the amount of fluid injected is 3 mL or less.

3. The dorsogluteal muscle has a thick fat layer, and an intramuscular injection will deposit the medication into subcutaneous tissue rather than a muscle.

4. The deltoid is an appropriate muscle for an intramuscular injection in an obese individual as long as the amount of fluid injected is 2 mL or less.

TEST-TAKING TIP: Identify the word in the stem that indicates negative polarity. The word *least* in the stem indicates negative polarity.

Content Area: Medication

Integrated Processes: Nursing Process: Planning

Client Need: Physiological Integrity; Pharmacological and Parenteral Therapies

Cognitive Level: Application

Concept: Medication; Safety

2. ANSWER: 3.

Rationales:

1. This is an inaccurate dose; it is only 0.5 mL, which is less than the prescribed dose.

2. This is an inaccurate dose; it is only 1 mL, which is less than the prescribed dose.

3. This is the accurate dose. The markings on the syringe indicate that it contains 1.5 mL of solution. Solve the problem by using ratio and proportion and then identify the place on the syringe that indicates 1.5 (1½) mL.

$$\frac{\text{Desire 0.75 grams}}{\text{Have 1 gram}} = \frac{x\ mL}{2\ mL}$$

$$1x = 0.75 \times 2$$
$$1x = 1.5$$
$$x = 1.5 \div 1$$
$$x = 1.5\ mL$$

4. This is an inaccurate dose; it is 2 mL, which exceeds the prescribed dose.

Content Area: Medication

Integrated Processes: Nursing Process: Planning

Client Need: Physiological Integrity; Pharmacological and Parenteral Therapies

Cognitive Level: Application

Concept: Medication; Safety

3. ANSWER: 1, 2.

Rationales:

1. The client should remain in the left lateral position for 15 to 20 minutes after insertion to allow the suppository to melt in the rectum, where the medication will be absorbed through the mucous membranes.

2. A gloved, lubricated index finger moves the suppository 3 to 4 inches into the rectum past the external and

internal rectal sphincters. Lubrication with a water-soluble jelly prevents trauma to the mucous membranes of the intestines.

3. A warm suppository will soften or melt and be impossible to insert into the anus. A suppository should be administered immediately after removal from the refrigerator while it is still firm.

4. The supine position will not allow access to the anus. The client should be placed in the left lateral position to permit access to the anus and allow the suppository to follow the contour of the rectum and sigmoid colon once inserted.

5. An applicator generally is used to insert a vaginal, not rectal, suppository.

TEST-TAKING TIP: Identify clang associations. The word *rectal* in the stem and in option 2 and *rectum* in option 1 are clang associations. Examine options 1 and 2 carefully.

Content Area: Medication

Integrated Processes: Nursing Process: Implementation

Client Need: Physiological Integrity; Pharmacological and Parenteral Therapies

Cognitive Level: Application

Concept: Medication; Elimination

4. ANSWER: 1, 2, 3, 4, 5.

Rationales:

1. Vitamins are a medication and should be included on a medication reconciliation form. An accurate list of all the drugs that a client is taking (including drug name, dose, route, and frequency) should be reconciled on admission and during transitions (e.g., transfer between units, when new medication administration records are implemented, and at discharge). This list should be compared to new medications prescribed and education provided to the client about each medication.

2. Most drug reconciliation forms contain a section that records drug allergies.

3. Food supplements are considered medications because they contain ingredients that may interact with medicinal products.

4. Over-the-counter herbs are considered medications because they contain ingredients that may interact with medicinal products.

5. Prescribed medications should be included on a medication reconciliation form.

TEST-TAKING TIP: Identify clang association. The word *medication* in the stem and the word *medications* in option 5 is a clang association. Examine option 5 carefully.

Content Area: Medication

Integrated Processes: Communication and Documentation; Nursing Process: Implementation

Client Need: Safe and Effective Care Environment; Management of Care

Cognitive Level: Application

Concept: Medication; Safety

5. ANSWER: 4.

Rationales:

1. Administering a distasteful medication in a child's favorite fruit juice should not be done because it may result in the child refusing to ingest the juice in the future.

2. Instilling 3 mL of medication at one time may over-whelm the child's ability to safely swallow the dose, resulting in aspiration. This is unsafe.

3. This is unsafe. Sipping liquid through a straw makes it difficult to control the flow of fluid being delivered to the back of the oral cavity. It is safer to drink out of a cup. Also, the child may not be able to ingest a full glass of water and would not receive a full dose of the medication.

4. An ice pop numbs the nerve endings in the taste buds of the tongue, limiting the experience of distasteful medication.

TEST-TAKING TIP: Identify the option with a specific determiner. Option 2 contains the word *all*, which is a specific determiner. Rarely is an option with a specific determiner the correct answer. Identify clang associations. The word *medication* in the stem and in options 3 and 4 are clang associations. Examine options 3 and 4 carefully.

Content Area: Medication
Integrated Processes: Nursing Process: Implementation
Client Need: Physiological Integrity; Pharmacological and Parenteral Therapies
Cognitive Level: Application
Concept: Medication; Comfort

6. **ANSWER: 1, 5.**
   Rationales:

1. The Z-track technique is used for medications that are known to irritate or discolor subcutaneous tissue. Therefore, the needle should be changed so that there is no medication residue on the needle during insertion.

2. A Z-tract site should not be massaged after drug administration because this may cause the medication to be moved above the muscle layer.

3. The Z-track technique is used for an intramuscular injection. A 25-gauge needle is too thin and fragile as well as too short (usually is ½ to 1 inch in length) for an intramuscular injection. In addition, medications administered via the Z-track technique are thick (viscous) and require a needle gauge of 18 to 22.

4. A 1-inch needle is used for subcutaneous injections. The Z-track technique is used for an intramuscular injection. Therefore, a needle length of 1½ inches should be used to ensure access to a muscle.

5. Pulling the skin and subcutaneous tissue to the side establishes a zigzag path before needle insertion; when the skin is released after insertion of the medication, the tissue planes slide across each other, confining the medication in the muscle and preventing it from flowing back up the needle track.

Content Area: Medication
Integrated Processes: Nursing Process: Evaluation
Client Need: Physiological Integrity; Pharmacological and Parenteral Therapies
Cognitive Level: Application
Concept: Medication; Tissue Integrity

7. **ANSWER: 4, 1, 5, 6, 2, 3.**
   Rationales:

4. Washing the eyes before administering eyedrops removes crusts and microorganisms and facilitates medication absorption. Using separate cotton balls for each eye and each swipe reduces the risk of cross-contamination, and wiping from the inner to outer canthus limits entrance of microorganisms into the lacrimal duct.

1. Looking upward helps reduce the likelihood of blinking or squinting during the procedure.

5. Exposing the conjunctival sac reduces the risk of touching the cornea with the dropper when instilling eyedrops.

6. Placing the dominant hand on the forehead stabilizes hand movement. Approaching the eye from the side minimizes blinking. Instilling the drop 1 to 2 cm above the conjunctival sac eliminates the danger of corneal injury by either a drop falling directly on the cornea or the dropper touching the cornea.

2. Gently closing the eyes spreads the medication over the eyeball. Squeezing the eyes shut should be avoided because this can cause injury to the eye and force the medication out.

3. Pressing firmly on the nasolacrimal duct for 30 to 60 seconds prevents the medication from draining out of the eye and to the nasopharynx. Also, it may help to prevent an unpleasant taste.

Content Area: Medication
Integrated Processes: Nursing Process: Planning
Client Need: Physiological Integrity; Pharmacological and Parenteral Therapies
Cognitive Level: Analysis
Concept: Medication; Sensory Perception

8. **ANSWER: 4.**
   Rationales:

1. Using a needleless syringe to instill medication on the back of the tongue is unsafe. The infant may be unable to manage liquid instilled in this location because it is so close to the trachea and it can result in aspiration of the medication.

2. Using a dropper to insert medication into the buccal cavity is more appropriate for a child rather than an infant; it is not the best method to administer a liquid medication to an infant because of the risk of aspiration.

3. A 3-month-old infant is unable to manage sipping fluid from a cup. This is unsafe.

4. Using a medication nipple is a method that is familiar to an infant. Infants obtain milk by sucking on a human nipple or a nipple of a bottle containing formula. They become proficient at sucking the milk at a rate that they can manage without causing aspiration of the liquid.

TEST-TAKING TIP: Identify the word in the stem that sets a priority. The word *best* in the stem sets a priority.

Content Area: Medication
Integrated Processes: Nursing Process: Implementation
Client Need: Physiological Integrity; Pharmacological and Parenteral Therapies
Cognitive Level: Application
Concept: Medication; Safety

9. **ANSWER: 1, 2, 3.**
   Rationales:

1. The child should be instructed to exhale through the mouth and then to breathe though the mouth for a few minutes after insertion to help keep the medication in contact with the nasal mucosa.

2. Remaining in the head-tilted-backward position facilitates absorption by moving the medication throughout the nasal passages rather than having the medication flow out of the nose by gravity.

3. Positioning the child in the supine position with the head tilted backward facilitates dispersing the medication to all of the nasal surfaces via gravity.

4. Positioning the tip of the medication dropper within the nostril violates an infection control practice. The tip of the dropper may touch the mucous membranes of the nose, contaminating the dropper. The tip of the dropper should be held just outside the opening to the nostril.

5. Returning the unused nose drops in the dropper to the medication bottle violates an infection control practice. The unused medication should be wasted and the empty dropper should be returned to the medication bottle.

TEST-TAKING TIP: Identify clang associations. The word *child* in the stem and in options 1, 2, and 3 are clang associations.

Content Area: Medication
Integrated Processes: Nursing Process: Implementation
Client Need: Physiological Integrity; Pharmacological and Parenteral Therapies
Cognitive Level: Application
Concept: Medication; Oxygenation

10. **ANSWER: 2, 4, 6, 5, 3, 1.**
    Rationales:

    2. The forearm allows for easier insertion of the solution into the dermis which is just below the epidermis and above the subcutaneous tissue. It is easily accessible and permits visualization of the client's response to the injection.

    4. Cleaning the site with an alcohol wipe decreases the presence of microorganisms.

    6. Using a small-gauge, short needle with the bevel up facilitates needle placement just below the epidermis.

    5. Slow, steady insertion of the medication allows time to stop the procedure if a systemic reaction occurs. The formation of a wheal (raised welt, bleb) confirms correct drug administration.

    3. Stabilizing the tissue on both sides of the puncture site as the needle is quickly removed minimizes the skin from dragging on the needle as it is removed. Removing the needle along the insertion angle prevents tissue trauma.

    1. Drawing a 1-inch circle around the wheal identifies the site for evaluation purposes. The site should not be massaged, and the client should be instructed not to rub the area.

Content Area: Medication
Integrated Processes: Nursing Process: Planning
Client Need: Physiological Integrity; Pharmacological and Parenteral Therapies
Cognitive Level: Analysis
Concept: Medication; Immunity

11. **ANSWER: 1.**
    Rationales:

    1. Many accidental drug overdoses result from a person forgetting that a medication was ingested and therefore taking another dose. A drug organizer has 7 horizontal rows of boxes and up to four vertical rows of boxes for 4 different times during the day (a.m., noon, afternoon, p.m.). Each box holds the tablets/pills that are to be taken on a particular day and at a particular time. This is a safe way to know if drugs prescribed for a particular day or time was taken. If the box is empty, they were taken. If the box is still full, they were not taken. Some clients may need assistance in filling the boxes on a weekly basis to ensure accuracy.

    2. Setting an alarm clock may help to take the medication initially, but it will not help if the client later has difficulty remembering if the drug was taken.

    3. Relying on a family member can be a burden for the family member. Also, it takes the responsibility away from the client, contributing to dependence.

    4. Making a calendar may help to take the medication initially, but it will not help if the client later has difficulty remembering if the drug was taken.

TEST-TAKING TIP: Identify the word in the stem that sets a priority. The word *best* in the stem sets a priority. Identify the clang association. The word *medication* in the stem and in options 1 and 3 are clang associations.

Content Area: Medication
Integrated Processes: Teaching/Learning; Nursing Process: Implementation
Client Need: Health Promotion and Maintenance
Cognitive Level: Application
Concept: Medication; Safety

12. **ANSWER: 1.**
    Rationales:

    1. The nurse is required to question prescriptions when they are outside normal, expected parameters. If the nurse blindly follows prescriptions and administers an excessive dose of a medication, the nurse compounds the initial error and also is liable for damages.

    2. Administering a medication is a dependent function of the nurse. It is not within the nurse's scope of practice to change the size of the dose without a prescription from a primary health-care provider.

    3. It is unnecessary to call the pharmacist because it is within the nurse's role to manage this situation.

    4. A nurse does not need to seek the support of a nurse manager to initially discuss an excessive dose of a medication with a primary health-care provider. It is wise to inform the nurse manager of the problem if the primary health-care provider refuses to adjust the prescription and the nurse in turn refuses to administer the excessive dose of the medication.

TEST-TAKING TIP: Identify the clang associations. The words *primary health-care provider* in the stem and in options 1 and 4 are clang associations. The word *weight* in the stem and in options 2 and 3 are clang associations. Using the test-taking tip, identify clang associations, does not help you to focus on a potential correct answer because all four options contain a clang association.

Content Area: Medication
Integrated Processes: Communication and Documentation; Nursing Process: Implementation

Client Need: Safe and Effective Care Environment; Management of Care
Cognitive Level: Application
Concept: Medication; Collaboration

13. **ANSWER: 3.**

Rationales:

1. This site is the vastus lateralis. This site is not recommended for the injection of heparin. It is used mainly for intramuscular injections. This is the second site after the ventrogluteal site for the injection of 1 mL or larger of solution. Also, it is used for newborns and infants who have not yet developed the gluteal or deltoid muscles.
2. This is the ventrogluteal site. This site is not recommended for the administration of heparin. It does not have a large area of subcutaneous tissue, and the legs have muscular activity that can hasten absorption of solution from a subcutaneous injection.
3. This site is the abdomen. It is the best site to inject heparin because the abdomen has a large subcutaneous layer under the skin and above the muscle. A subcutaneous injection into the abdominal area must avoid a 2-inch area around the umbilicus.
4. This site is the deltoid and is not recommended for the administration of heparin. It has a small subcutaneous layer and arm activity hastens absorption, which is not desired.

Content Area: Medication
Integrated Processes: Nursing Process: Implementation
Client Need: Physiological Integrity; Pharmacological and Parenteral Therapies
Cognitive Level: Analysis
Concept: Medication; Safety

14. **ANSWER: 3 , 5.**

Rationales:

1. Aspiration before inserting the medication is contraindicated because doing so may traumatize tissue and cause bruising.
2. Placing the needle just under the epidermis is the technique used for an intradermal injection. Heparin is administered via the subcutaneous route.
3. Massaging the site should be avoided after an injection of heparin. Massaging the site can cause bleeding and bruising because heparin is an anticoagulant.
4. Spreading the skin when administering a subcutaneous injection of heparin is contraindicated. Spreading the skin may permit the needle to enter a muscle rather than subcutaneous tissue.
5. The needle pierces the skin and enters subcutaneous tissue during an injection of heparin. A disinfectant, such as alcohol, will minimize microorganisms on the skin before the needle pierces the skin. This will limit the development of an infection at the site of the injection.

TEST-TAKING TIP: Identify the option with a specific determiner. Option 2 contains the word *just,* which is a specific determiner. Identify clang associations. The word *injection* in the stem and in options 3 and 5 are clang associations. Identify the unique option. Option 3 is unique because it

is the only option that identifies what should not be done. Examine options 3 and 5 carefully.

Content Area: Medication
Integrated Processes: Nursing Process: Implementation
Client Need: Physiological Integrity; Pharmacological and Parenteral Therapies
Cognitive Level: Application
Concept: Medication; Safety

15. **ANSWER: 4.**

Rationales:

1. Verbal interactions, particularly if they involve complex information or instructions concerning the future, may not be understood or remembered by a client who is cognitively impaired.
2. How to use a plastic box with multiple sections may not be understood by a client who is cognitively impaired.
3. Writing involves the use of symbols that may not be able to be read or understood by a client who is cognitively impaired.
4. Placing medications next to the client's toothbrush provides a reminder for the client to take them. It allows the person a sense of independence. Repetitive, routine activities that have been performed throughout life, such as brushing the teeth, usually can be performed by a person with moderate dementia.

TEST-TAKING TIP: Identify the option with a specific determiner. Option 2 contains the word *all,* which is a specific determiner. Identify clang associations. The word *relative* in the stem and in options 1 and 4 are clang associations. Examine options 1 and 4 carefully.

Content Area: Medication
Integrated Processes: Caring; Teaching/Learning; Nursing Process: Implementation
Client Need: Physiological Integrity; Pharmacological and Parenteral Therapies
Cognitive Level: Application
Concept: Medication; Health Promotion

16. **ANSWER: 4.**

Rationales:

1. This is a U 100 syringe marked in units, of which there are 100 per 1 mL. It has a needle that is ½ inch in length, which is not long enough to reach a muscle. This syringe is used for insulin injections.
2. This is a 1-mL tuberculin syringe marked in 0.01 mL (1/100th of a milliliter) and minims (16 minims = 1 mL). It has a needle that is ½ inch in length, which is not long enough to reach a muscle. This syringe is used for intradermal injections, such as instillation of allergens for allergy testing and purified protein derivative (PPD) to identify exposure to the pathogen causing tuberculosis.
3. This is a 3-mL standard syringe marked in whole milliliters and 0.1 mL (1/10 of a milliliter). It has a needle that is ⅝ inch in length, which is not long enough to reach a muscle. This syringe is used for subcutaneous injections.
4. This is a 5-mL standard syringe marked in whole milliliters and 0.2 mL (2/10 of a milliliter). It has a needle that is 1½ inches long, which is capable of reaching a muscle. This syringe is used for intramuscular injections.

Content Area: Medication
Integrated Processes: Nursing Process: Planning
Client Need: Physiological Integrity; Pharmacological and Parenteral Therapies
Cognitive Level: Analysis
Concept: Medication; Safety

17. **ANSWER: 2, 5.**
Rationales:
1. Inserting the prescription into the client's clinical record can be done after the telephone call.
2. Reciting the prescription back to the primary health-care provider is essential for safety. It repeats the message for the primary health-care provider and ensures that the prescription was understood correctly.
3. It is unnecessary to confirm that the medication is available in the hospital pharmacy before the telephone call is completed. The nurse can contact the primary health-care provider if the medication is unavailable.
4. A telephone prescription usually is required to be signed by the primary health-care provider within 24, not 48, hours.
5. Two nurses listening to the prescription confirms that the prescription was accurately heard by both nurses.
TEST-TAKING TIP: Identify clang associations. The words *primary health-care provider* in the stem and in options 2 and 4 are clang associations. Examine options 2 and 4 carefully.
Content Area: Medication
Integrated Processes: Nursing Process: Implementation
Client Need: Physiological Integrity; Pharmacological and Parenteral Therapies
Cognitive Level: Application
Concept: Medication; Safety

18. **ANSWER: 2.**
Rationales:
1. A direction instructing the nurse to deliver a medication over 6 hours usually is not indicated in a prescription. This information usually is included in directions from the pharmacist, in literature distributed by the manufacturer of the medication, or in a reputable drug book that includes the medication.
2. The letters *prn* mean *as needed* or *when necessary*. The prescription basically states that the medication may be taken by the client every 6 hours if needed. Frequently, additional parameters are stipulated by the primary health-care provider depending on the medication, such as every 6 hours prn for severe pain or every 6 hours prn for diarrhea.
3. The need to wait 6 hours before administering the mediation is not related to the client's prescription.
4. Administering a medication every 6 hours around the clock is information related to a standing (routine) prescription. A routine prescription might state, "Give aspirin 325 mg by mouth every 6 hours." This prescription is carried out by a nurse until it is discontinued by the primary health-care provider, a hospital policy stipulates that it should be discontinued, or a nurse determines that it is placing the client in jeopardy. The primary health-care

provider should be notified when a medication is discontinued or when a client is in jeopardy.
TEST-TAKING TIP: Although the word *every* in options 2 and 4 are specific determiners they should not be discarded, because the words *every 6 hours* in the stem is a clang with the words *every 6 hours* in options 2 and 4. Options 2 and 4 should be examined carefully.
Content Area: Medication
Integrated Processes: Teaching/Learning; Nursing Process: Implementation
Client Need: Physiological Integrity; Pharmacological and Parenteral Therapies
Cognitive Level: Application
Concept: Medication; Patient-Centered Care

19. **ANSWER: 1, 2.**
Rationales:
1. This prevents contamination of the dropper and trauma to the conjunctival sac or cornea.
2. The client should look up during insertion of eyedrops because this limits the risk of blinking.
3. Closing the eyes gently, not firmly, after insertion of eyedrops prevents the medication from being squeezed out of the eyes.
4. A finger should be placed just below the lower eyelashes while simultaneously exerting downward pressure toward the cheek.
5. Debris around the eye should be removed before medication insertion and excess medication removed after medication insertion by wiping from the inner to the outer canthus with a new cotton ball for each swipe.
TEST-TAKING TIP: Identify the options with a clang association. The word *drops* in the stem and *eyedrops* in options 2 and 3 are clang associations. The word *eye* in the stem and *eyedrops* in options 2 and 3, and *eye* in options 1 and 5 are clang associations. Examine options with a clang association carefully.
Content Area: Medication
Integrated Processes: Nursing Process: Implementation
Client Need: Physiological Integrity; Pharmacological and Parenteral Therapies
Cognitive Level: Application
Concept: Medication; Sensory Perception

20. **ANSWER: 4.**
Rationales:
1. This is the intramuscular route. The intramuscular route is not used to test for tuberculosis or allergies.
2. This is the subcutaneous route. The subcutaneous route is not used to test for tuberculosis or allergies. When a ½-inch or ⅝-inch needle is used to administer a medication via the subcutaneous route, the needle is inserted at a 90-degree angle to ensure that the medication is injected into subcutaneous tissue and not muscle.
3. This is the subcutaneous route. The subcutaneous route is not used to test for tuberculosis or allergies. When a 1-inch needle is used to administer a medication via the subcutaneous route, the needle is inserted at a 45-degree angle to ensure that the medication is injected into subcutaneous tissue and not muscle.

4. This is the intradermal route. It is used mainly for testing for tuberculosis and allergies.
Content Area: *Medication*
Integrated Processes: *Nursing Process: Implementation*
Client Need: *Physiological Integrity; Pharmacological and Parenteral Therapies*
Cognitive Level: *Analysis*
Concept: *Medication; Safety*

21. **ANSWER: 1, 3, 4.**
Rationales:
1. Injecting air with the bevel of the needle below the level of the solution will cause turbulence resulting in bubbles. Bubbles in the solution will result in the withdrawal of a dose less than the prescribed dose.
2. Instilling slightly more air into the vial than the amount of solution to be withdrawn will increase pressure within the vial, but it will not result in an inaccurate dose.
3. Shaking a vial after a diluent is added to the vial will cause turbulence resulting in bubbles. Bubbles in the solution will result in the withdrawal of a dose less than the prescribed dose.
4. Wiping the rubber seal with alcohol before withdrawing the solution removes debris and microorganisms from the surface of the rubber seal before the needle of a syringe pierces the rubber.
5. Instilling the solution slowly limits turbulence that causes bubbles.
TEST-TAKING TIP: Identify the word in the stem that indicates negative polarity. The word *compromised* in the stem indicates negative polarity. The question is asking, "What is an inappropriate action when withdrawing medication from a vial?"
Content Area: *Medication*
Integrated Processes: *Nursing Process: Evaluation*
Client Need: *Physiological Integrity; Pharmacological and Parenteral Therapies*
Cognitive Level: *Application*
Concept: *Medication; Safety*

22. **ANSWER: 3.**
Rationales:
1. The vastus lateralis site extends from one handbreadth above the knee to one handbreadth below the greater trochanter of the femur on the anterior lateral aspect of the thigh.
2. The greater trochanter is one of several bony landmarks used to locate the ventrogluteal site.
3. The deltoid is located by making an inverted triangle approximately 2 to 3 finger-widths below the acromion process and a line from the anterior to the posterior axillary crease.
4. The anterior superior iliac spine is one of several bony landmarks used to locate the ventrogluteal site.
Content Area: *Medication*
Integrated Processes: *Nursing Process: Implementation*
Client Need: *Physiological Integrity; Pharmacological and Parenteral Therapies*
Cognitive Level: *Application*
Concept: *Medication; Safety*

23. **ANSWER: 3.**
Rationales:
1. Bending the needle of a syringe is unsafe and could result in a needlestick injury.
2. A used needle should never be recapped, particularly when walking, because it may precipitate a needlestick injury.
3. Many syringes are designed to actively or passively cover used needles to protect the caregiver from needlestick injuries.
4. Although disposing of a used syringe with its needle attached into the closest sharps container should be done, it does not protect the nurse if the needle is not covered when walking from the client to the location of a sharps container.
TEST-TAKING TIP: Identify the word in the stem that sets a priority. The word *best* in the stem sets a priority.
Content Area: *Medication*
Integrated Processes: *Nursing Process: Implementation*
Client Need: *Physiological Integrity; Pharmacological and Parenteral Therapies*
Cognitive Level: *Application*
Concept: *Medication; Safety*

24. **ANSWER: 3.**
Rationales:
1. This is 8 units, which reflects the amount of solution required if just the regular insulin were to be administered. This is an inaccurate dose.
2. This is 22 units, which reflects the amount of solution required if just the NPH insulin were to be administered. This is an inaccurate dose.
3. This is the correct volume of solution (30 units) when the NPH insulin dose (22 units) is added to the regular insulin dose (8 units). These medications can be administered safely in the same syringe.
4. This volume of solution is 42 units, which exceeds the combined volume of the prescribed insulins.
Content Area: *Medication*
Integrated Processes: *Teaching/Learning; Nursing Process: Evaluation*
Client Need: *Physiological Integrity; Pharmacological and Parenteral Therapies*
Cognitive Level: *Analysis*
Concept: *Medication; Patient-Centered Care*

25. **ANSWER: 2.**
Rationales:
1. If the port farthest from the insertion site is used, some of the medication will mix with the larger volume of fluid in the tubing and will not reach the client for a longer period of time. The port closest to the insertion site should be used.
2. Pinching the tubing above the insertion port ensures that the medication being instilled flows toward the client rather than backward up the intravenous tubing; the port closest to the client should be used.
3. Increasing the flow rate is unsafe and not within the legal role of the nurse. The nurse should set the flow rate as prescribed. The administration of intravenous fluids is a dependent function of the nurse.

4. It is not necessary to shut the roller clamp off on the tubing before administering the medication.

TEST-TAKING TIP: Identify clang associations. The word *port* in the stem and in options 1 and 2 are clang associations. Examine options 1 and 2 carefully.

Content Area: Medication
Integrated Processes: Nursing Process: Implementation
Client Need: Physiological Integrity; Pharmacological and Parenteral Therapies
Cognitive Level: Application
Concept: Medication; Safety

26. **ANSWER: 3, 4, 5.**
    Rationales:
    1. Warming the solution is unnecessary; it can be administered at room temperature.
    2. When hanging an IVPB, the primary infusion bag must be hung lower than the secondary infusion bag. Hanging the secondary infusion bag lower than the primary infusion bag will cause fluid from the primary infusion bag to enter the secondary infusion tubing and bag. This occurs because the pressure in the primary infusion set is higher than the pressure within the secondary infusion set, and the secondary infusion set does not have a check valve that prevents fluid from flowing up the secondary tubing into the bag.
    3. Wiping the port with alcohol is a necessary infection control intervention. This is a sterile procedure because the port has direct access to the client's circulatory system.
    4. Priming the secondary line removes air from the tubing, which will prevent the introduction of air into the client's circulatory system.
    5. Opening the clamp on the secondary infusion tubing and using the clamp on the primary infusion tubing to control the flow ensures that the primary infusion will flow after the secondary infusion bag is empty.
    TEST-TAKING TIP: Identify the clang associations. The words *primary infusion* in the stem and in options 2, 4, and 5 are clang associations. Examine options 2, 4, and 5 carefully.
    Content Area: Medication
    Integrated Processes: Nursing Process: Implementation
    Client Need: Physiological Integrity; Pharmacological and Parenteral Therapies
    Cognitive Level: Application
    Concept: Medication; Safety

27. **ANSWER: 1, 2, 4, 5.**
    Rationales:
    1. Ear drops should be directed to the side of the canal so that the drops do not fall directly on the tympanic membrane. Drops directed to the center of the auditory canal may injure the tympanic membrane because of the pressure of falling drops.
    2. Tapping gently on the tragus of the ear after instilling the drops facilitates the flow of medication into the auditory canal.
    3. The medication should be administered close to body temperature. The nurse should hold the medication bottle

in a hand for several minutes until it is warm. Medication for the ear usually is stored at room temperature.
4. The pinna should be pulled down and backward to straighten the ear canal of a child younger than 3 years of age. The pinna should be pulled up and backward to straighten the ear canal of an adult or child older than 3 years of age.
5. Gravity will facilitate the flow of medication into the ear and retain it in contact with structures within the ear canal when the child is in a position with the ear facing the ceiling. A cotton ball can be placed gently into the external canal, if prescribed, to prevent the drug from leaking out of the ear canal when sitting up.

TEST-TAKING TIP: Identify the option with a specific determiner. Option 3 contains the word *just,* which is a specific determiner. An option with a specific determiner usually is an incorrect answer. Identify the clang associations. The word *ear* in the stem and in options 1, 2, 4, and 5 are clang associations. Examine these options carefully.

Content Area: Medication
Integrated Processes: Teaching/Learning; Nursing Process: Implementation
Client Need: Physiological Integrity; Pharmacological and Parenteral Therapies
Cognitive Level: Application
Concept: Medication; Patient-Centered Care

28. **ANSWER: 1, 3, 4.**
    Rationales:
    1. Gloves should be worn when removing and applying medicated patches to protect the nurse from being exposed to the medication.
    2. Shaving hair on the skin is necessary only if the hair is interfering with adherence of the patch. This action is not necessary for every client. The nurse must receive consent from the client when hair must be shaved.
    3. Washing and drying the skin after removing a used patch removes any drug lingering on the skin and minimizes the risk of an overdose.
    4. Compressing the medicated patch against the skin for 10 seconds after it is applied ensures that it is firmly adhered to the client's skin.
    5. An excessive amount of medication may be administered if both patches are on at the same time. The previous patch should be removed and the area cleansed at the time that a new patch is applied. The new patch should be applied to a different area.
    Content Area: Medication
    Integrated Processes: Nursing Process: Implementation
    Client Need: Physiological Integrity; Pharmacological and Parenteral Therapies
    Cognitive Level: Application
    Concept: Medication; Safety

29. **ANSWER: 2.**
    Rationales:
    1. Offering the client apple juice next to take with the medication is premature. Another action should be implemented first.

2. Administering a medication to the *right client* is one of the 10 rights of medication administration. Before administering a medication, the nurse should check the client's stated name and date of birth against an objective source of this information.

3. Although the head of the bed should be raised before administering oral medications to a client, this action is premature at this time.

4. Although checking the client's armband and medical record for allergies should be done before administering the antibiotic, checking for the client's allergies next in this scenario is premature.

TEST-TAKING TIP: Identify the word in the stem that sets a priority. The word *next* in the stem sets a priority.
Content Area: Medication
Integrated Processes: Communication and Documentation; Nursing Process: Implementation
Client Need: Physiological Integrity; Pharmacological and Parenteral Therapies
Cognitive Level: Application
Concept: Medication; Safety

30. **ANSWER: 1.**
Rationales:
1. A drug that is teratogenic may negatively affect a fetus, producing a congenital anomaly. Drugs that are known to be teratogenic should not be administered to pregnant women.
2. Gluten, the protein of wheat and other grains, is unrelated to drugs that are teratogenic.
3. Eating food before receiving a medication that is teratogenic is unnecessary. Food should be taken with medications that are known to be gastrointestinal irritants.
4. Obtaining a blood specimen for a culture and sensitivity test is required before administering an antibiotic so that the antibiotic does not influence the test results.

TEST-TAKING TIP: Identify the option with a specific determiner. Option 3 contains the word *just* which is a specific determiner.
Content Area: Medication
Integrated Processes: Communication and Documentation; Nursing Process: Implementation
Client Need: Physiological Integrity; Pharmacological and Parenteral Therapies
Cognitive Level: Analysis
Concept: Medication; Safety

31. **ANSWER: 4**
Rationales:
1. The deltoid site is the upper arm. The nurse can be sued for battery when performing an injection into a site against the client's wishes.
2. The vastus lateralis sites are beneath the compression dressings at the site of the amputations. They cannot be accessed for an injection. Also, the dose being administered is inaccurate.
3. Performing injections close to a new colostomy may be traumatic and should be avoided. Also, the dose being administered is inaccurate.
4. Two units of regular insulin is the accurate dose to be administered as per the primary health-care provider's

prescription (150 to 200 mg/dL—2 units regular insulin). The lateral sides of the waist just above the iliac crests (love handles) are alternate injection sites for a subcutaneous injection. The side opposite to the colostomy ensures that the injection will not traumatize the area around the colostomy. The ventral gluteal and scapular areas should not be used because of 2+ dependent edema. Dependent edema, when a client is in the low-Fowler position, will occur in the back and sacrum.

TEST-TAKING TIP: Identify duplicate facts in options. Options 1 and 4 have a duplicate fact (2 units) and options 2 and 3 have a duplicate fact (8 units). If you know the correct dose to be administered, you can reduce the options to be considered to just 2 options. By doing this, you increase your chances of selecting the correct answer from 25 to 50 percent.
Content Area: Medication
Integrated Processes: Communication and Documentation; Nursing Process: Implementation
Client Need: Physiological Integrity; Pharmacological and Parenteral Therapies
Cognitive Level: Analysis
Concept: Patient-Centered Care; Medication

32. **ANSWER: 1.**
Rationales:
1. Administering medication is a dependent function of the nurse. The nurse should notify the primary health-care provider of the client's status and obtain a prescription for an alternate route of administration.
2. Giving the medication and hoping that the client does not vomit is unsafe because it may precipitate vomiting.
3. Although substituting the liquid form of the drug for the tablet form of the drug is acceptable practice, in this instance, any form of the drug administered orally may precipitate vomiting and should be avoided.
4. Withholding the medication for an hour and a half and then attempting to give it again is outside the legal practice of nursing. Administering medications is a dependent function and a nurse cannot make this decision independently. A drug may be withheld for 1 hour because administering drugs 1 hour before or 1 hour after the prescribed time of administration is acceptable nursing practice. This practice is acceptable because all the medications due at a certain time cannot feasibly be administered to all the clients on a unit at the same exact time.

TEST-TAKING TIP: Identify the word in the stem that sets a priority. The word *next* in the stem sets a priority. Identify the option with a clang association. The word *administration* in the stem and in option 1 is a clang association. Identify the option that is unique. Option 1 is unique; it is the only option that does not contain the word *medication*.
Content Area: Medication
Integrated Processes: Communication and Documentation; Nursing Process: Implementation
Client Need: Safe and Effective Care Environment; Management of Care
Cognitive Level: Application
Concept: Medication; Collaboration

33. **ANSWER: 1, 4, 5.**
    Rationales:
    1. **Remaining awake until the medication dissolves completely reduces the risk of accidental aspiration of the medication.**
    2. Placing a medication under the tongue is called the sublingual route of administration.
    3. Swishing a solution around the oral cavity and swallowing it is called *swish and swallow*.
    4. **Alternating cheeks when taking additional doses of the medication will minimize irritation of the mucous membranes.**
    5. **The buccal cavities are the spaces between the cheek and gum on either side of the mouth. The mucous membranes in a buccal cavity are warm and moist and a tablet will melt slowly.**
    Content Area: Medication
    Integrated Processes: Teaching/Learning; Nursing Process: Implementation
    Client Need: Physiological Integrity; Pharmacological and Parenteral Therapies
    Cognitive Level: Application
    Concept: Medication; Safety

34. **ANSWER: 1, 2, 6.**
    Rationales:
    1. **An empty bladder limits the discomfort that may be experienced when the medication is inserted into the vagina.**
    2. **Cleaning removes debris and reduces the amount of microorganisms in the perineal area; this limits the risk of infection.**
    3. The applicator should be removed slowly to prevent tissue trauma.
    4. The supine position with the legs extended will not allow access to the vagina. The client should be placed in the dorsal recumbent (supine with hips and knees flexed) or Sims (side lying with the top hip and knee flexed) position to allow visualization of and access to the vagina.
    5. Inserting the applicator upward toward the umbilicus is unsafe; it will traumatize the delicate mucous membranes of the vagina. The applicator should be inserted downward and backward toward the cervix. Insertion of a catheter toward the umbilicus is the technique used when inserting a catheter to perform an enema.
    6. **Expelling a small amount of cream at the tip of the applicator will act as a lubricant to facilitate insertion of the applicator and limit tissue trauma.**
    Content Area: Medication
    Integrated Processes: Nursing Process: Implementation
    Client Need: Physiological Integrity; Pharmacological and Parenteral Therapies
    Cognitive Level: Application
    Concept: Medication; Safety

35. **ANSWER: 2.**
    Rationales:
    1. This is a correct technique. When administering a nasal spray to both nostrils, the client should compress the opposite nostril while administering the nasal spray into the first nostril; this prevents the medication from entering the other nostril. When instilling the nasal spray into the second nostril the client should not compress the first nostril; compressing the first nostril may expel the previously administered medication from the first nostril.
    2. **This is an undesirable practice. Exhaling through the nose will facilitate leakage of medication out of the nasal passage, minimizing its contact with the mucous membranes of the nose.**
    3. This is a correct technique. Tilting the head backward will help retain the medication in the nasal passage.
    4. This is a correct technique. Compressing the container discharges a dose and inhaling the spray ensures that it enters the nostril.
    TEST-TAKING TIP: Identify the words in the stem that indicate negative polarity. The words *provide additional teaching* indicate negative polarity. The question is asking, "What is *not acceptable* when self-administering a nasal spray?"
    Content Area: Medication
    Integrated Processes: Teaching/Learning; Nursing Process: Evaluation
    Client Need: Physiological Integrity; Pharmacological and Parenteral Therapies
    Cognitive Level: Application
    Concept: Medication; Patient-Centered Care

36. **ANSWER: 1, 2, 3.**
    Rationales:
    1. **A 26- to 30-gauge needle causes less tissue trauma because the diameter of the body of the needle is smaller than a lower-number gauge needle which has a larger diameter.**
    2. **The administration of numerous injections in one site may cause tissue injury, such as degradation of adipose tissue (lipodystrophy). Lipodystrophy is less of a problem since the advent of human insulin. The nurse should rotate sites and document them on the medication administration record so that there can be continuity of care among the nurses administering insulin to the client.**
    3. **Insulin is administered via a subcutaneous injection, which often involves pinching the skin while inserting the needle. Spreading the skin is done with an intramuscular injection.**
    4. Insulin does not have to be administered over 5 seconds. Usually, a dose of insulin is a small volume that can be instilled over 1 to 2 seconds. However, the needle should remain in place for 5 seconds after instillation to ensure dispersing of the solution.
    5. Insulin is administered via a subcutaneous injection. The needle should be ½ inch, ⅝ inch, or 1 inch in length. A 1½-inch needle is used for an intramuscular injection.
    TEST-TAKING TIP: Identify the clang association. The word *injections* in the stem and the word *injection* in option 2 is a clang association. More often than not, an option with a clang association is a correct answer. Examine option 1 carefully.
    Content Area: Medication
    Integrated Processes: Nursing Process: Implementation
    Client Need: Physiological Integrity; Pharmacological and Parenteral Therapies

Cognitive Level: Application
Concept: Medication; Tissue Integrity

37. **ANSWER: 4.**
    Rationales:
    1. This is unsafe and outside the legal role of the nurse. The administration of intravenous fluids is a dependent function of the nurse and the nurse should administer only the fluid prescribed by the primary health-care provider.
    2. This is unsafe. The time it takes to obtain the correct bag of solution will deprive the client of the prescribed therapy. The primary health-care provider prescribed intravenous fluids that the nurse should institute as soon as possible.
    3. This is an excessive dose of KCl and could harm the client. Excessive potassium can cause cardiac dysrhythmias.
    4. A 250-mL bag of 0.9% sodium chloride is ¼ of the solution prescribed (1,000 mL ÷ 250 mL = 4). Therefore, the nurse should divide the prescribed amount of KCl by 4 (20 mEq ÷ 4 = 5 mEq) to determine the amount of KCl to add to a 250-mL bag of solution.
    Content Area: Medication
    Integrated Processes: Nursing Process: Implementation
    Client Need: Physiological Integrity; Pharmacological and Parenteral Therapies
    Cognitive Level: Application
    Concept: Medication; Fluid and Electrolyte Balance

38. **ANSWER: 3.**
    Rationales:
    1. Placing a plastic cover over the top of the ampule before snapping the constricted neck protects the nurse's hands from injury; this action will not ensure that the prescribed dose was available for withdrawal.
    2. The filter needle must be changed to a needle suitable for the injection being given to the client; this action will not ensure that the prescribed dose was available for withdrawal.
    3. Flicking the top of the ampule moves solution in the top of the ampule to below the constricted neck of the ampule. This ensures that the entire dose is in the bottom of the ampule and ready for withdrawal.
    4. The use of a filter needle to aspirate solution from an ampule prevents the aspiration of glass particles that may have resulted from snapping the constricted neck of the ampule; this action will not ensure that the prescribed dose was available for withdrawal.
    Content Area: Medication
    Integrated Processes: Nursing Process: Implementation
    Client Need: Physiological Integrity; Pharmacological and Parenteral Therapies
    Cognitive Level: Application
    Concept: Medication; Safety

39. **ANSWER: 2.**
    Rationales:
    1. The "prn" section refers to a medication that is administered when a particular situation occurs; for example, morphine sulfate 2 mg IV every 3 hours prn for moderate incisional pain.

2. The "single-dose" section is used to document a medication given once. It may be a "STAT" (immediately) dose of a medication given in an emergency, a "one-time only" dose before a diagnostic test or before surgery, or a "now order" when a single dose is given quickly but not as quickly or emergent as a STAT prescription.
3. The "progress note" section generally is used to document why a medication was withheld, the client's nontherapeutic response to a drug, the reason for a client refusal, and whether a primary health-care provider was notified.
4. The "standing drug" section includes medications to be given until they are discontinued or the required number of days has lapsed, such as with antibiotics given for 7 to 14 days.
Content Area: Medication
Integrated Processes: Communication and Documentation; Nursing Process: Implementation
Client Need: Physiological Integrity; Pharmacological and Parenteral Therapies
Cognitive Level: Application
Concept: Medication; Communication

40. **ANSWER: 2, 5, 1, 4, 3.**
    Rationales:
    2. The administration of a medication is a dependent function of a nurse. The primary health-care provider's prescription must be verified by the nurse administering the medication.
    5. The client's blood glucose level must be compared to the insulin prescription to determine the exact dose to administer. Doses usually are on a sliding scale, with the dose increasing as the client's blood glucose increases.
    1. A nurse must always perform hand hygiene before preparing medication to avoid contaminating the medication, medication cart, and other equipment.
    4. After completing hand hygiene, the nurse should prepare the medication according to the prescription.
    3. A nurse must always wear gloves when there is potential for exposure to a client's blood or body fluids. An injection pierces the client's skin, increasing the risk of exposure to the client's blood or body fluids.
    Content Area: Medication
    Integrated Processes: Communication and Documentation; Nursing Process: Planning
    Client Need: Physiological Integrity; Pharmacological and Parenteral Therapies
    Cognitive Level: Analysis
    Concept: Medication; Safety

41. **ANSWER: 4.**
    Rationales:
    1. The deltoid muscle is too small to be used in infants and children.
    2. The dorsogluteal muscle is less well developed than the preferred muscle for an intramuscular injection in a newborn. The dorsogluteal muscle develops as the child begins to bear weight on the lower extremities.

3. The ventrogluteal muscle is less well developed than the preferred muscle for an intramuscular injection in a newborn. The ventrogluteal muscle develops as the child begins to bear weight on the lower extremities.

4. The vastus lateralis muscle is the best site for an intramuscular injection in a newborn because it is better developed than the gluteal muscles, which are poorly developed.

TEST-TAKING TIP: Identify the word in the stem that sets a priority. The word *best* in the stem sets a priority. Identify the unique option. Option 4 is unique because it has three words, and options 1, 2, and 3 have only two words. Examine option 4 carefully.

Content Area: Medication
Integrated Processes: Nursing Process: Implementation
Client Need: Physiological Integrity; Pharmacological and Parenteral Therapies
Cognitive Level: Application
Concept: Medication; Safety

42. ANSWER: 1.

Rationales:

1. The U.S. Food and Drug Administration is the best source of information regarding information about medications, medical devices, and food.

2. The American Nurses Association is not the best source for information about medications. However, it does publish standards of nursing practice regarding pharmacy and medication therapy.

3. Although the U.S. Pharmacopoeia lists medications and standards for their preparation, it is not the best all-inclusive source regarding recall of medications, safety alerts, new medications, and generic approvals.

4. Although the National Formulary lists officially recognized medications, including those not listed in the U.S. Pharmacopoeia, it is not the best source regarding recall of medications, safety alerts, new medications, and generic approvals.

TEST-TAKING TIP: Identify the word in the stem that sets a priority. The word *best* in the stem sets a priority.

Content Area: Medication
Integrated Processes: Nursing Process: Analysis
Client Need: Physiological Integrity; Pharmacological and Parenteral Therapies
Cognitive Level: Comprehension
Concept: Medication; Safety

43. ANSWER: 1.

Rationales:

1. Tolerance is indicated by a decreased physiological response to a medication after repeated exposure to the medication.

2. Potentiation occurs when an interaction between two medications results in an increase in the action of just one of the medications.

3. An adverse effect is an unintended, usually unpredictable, harmful response to a medication that is more severe than a side effect.

4. An idiosyncratic reaction happens when resistance, an overreaction, or an unpredictable reaction to a medication occurs that is different from the expected response.

Content Area: Medication
Integrated Processes: Communication and Documentation; Nursing Process: Evaluation
Client Need: Physiological Integrity; Pharmacological and Parenteral Therapies
Cognitive Level: Analysis
Concept: Medication; Safety

44. ANSWER: 2.

Rationales:

1. There are no data in the question that indicate a problem with the liver, which mainly detoxifies a medication to a less active form in preparation for excretion. Also, the question does not indicate that this client is an older adult who may have decreased liver function associated with aging.

2. The adequacy of the circulation to transport the medication to the target site is essential for eventual medication utilization. The question states that this client has "a history of impaired peripheral circulation to the lower extremities."

3. Most antibiotics are excreted via the kidneys. There are no data that indicate that this client has a problem with renal function. Also, the question does not indicate that this client is an older adult who may have decreased ability to excrete medication by-products because of reduced kidney function associated with aging.

4. There are no data in the question that indicate a problem with the ability to absorb medication, such as the presence of or lack of food in the stomach or any gastrointestinal problem that can interfere with absorption. Also, the question does not indicate that this client is an older adult who may have decreased gastrointestinal function associated with aging.

TEST-TAKING TIP: Identify the word in the stem that sets a priority. The word *most* in the stem sets a priority.

Content Area: Medication
Integrated Processes: Nursing Process: Evaluation
Client Need: Physiological Integrity; Pharmacological and Parenteral Therapies
Cognitive Level: Application
Concept: Medication; Perfusion

45. ANSWER: 4.

Rationales:

1. Biotransformation (metabolism) mainly takes place in the liver, where medications are detoxified into less active forms in preparation for excretion. There is no information in the question that indicates that this client has impaired liver function.

2. Distribution is involved with the transport of a medication from the absorption site to the site of medication action. There are no data in the question that indicate that this client is experiencing a problem with cardiovascular function.

3. Absorption is associated with the process of movement of a medication into the bloodstream. There is no information in the question that indicates that this client is having a problem with the gastrointestinal tract.

4. Most medications are excreted from the body in urine via the kidneys. Kidney disease can interfere with

medication excretion, thereby causing medication accumulation. The nurse should be most concerned about the potential for medication toxicity.

TEST-TAKING TIP: Identify the word in the stem that sets a priority. The word *most* in the stem sets a priority. Identify the obscure clang association. The words *kidney function* in the stem and *excretion* in option 4 is an obscure clang association.

Content Area: Medication
Integrated Processes: Nursing Process: Evaluation
Client Need: Physiological Integrity; Pharmacological and Parenteral Therapies
Cognitive Level: Comprehension
Concept: Medication; Elimination

46. ANSWER: 4.
Rationales:
1. A peak plasma level is associated with the highest blood concentration of a single medication dose, not how fast a person can anticipate pain relief after receiving an opioid.
2. Duration is associated with the length of time a therapeutic blood concentration of the medication is maintained, not how fast a person can anticipate pain relief after receiving an opioid.
3. Half-life is associated with the time needed to metabolize or inactivate one-half the amount of a medication, not how fast a person can anticipate pain relief after receiving an opioid.
4. Onset is associated with the time it takes for the body to respond to a medication—in other words, how fast a person can anticipate pain relief after receiving an opioid.

TEST-TAKING TIP: Identify the word in the stem that sets a priority. The word *most* in the stem sets a priority.

Content Area: Medication
Integrated Processes: Communication and Documentation; Nursing Process: Implementation
Client Need: Physiological Integrity; Pharmacological and Parenteral Therapies
Cognitive Level: Application
Concept: Medication; Perfusion

47. ANSWER: 3, 4, 5.
Rationales:
1. Herbal supplements are unsafe to take unless the primary health-care provider states that it is safe to take the supplements. Herbal supplements have active ingredients that can cause serious medication interactions with prescribed medications as well as cause serious nontherapeutic effects.
2. Herbal supplements are not regulated by the FDA for safety and efficacy. However, the FDA has an Office of Special Nutritionals in its Center for Food Safety and Applied Nutrition that documents herbal products' adverse effects reported to the FDA.
3. There are no regulations to hold manufacturers of herbal supplements accountable for the claimed benefits of their supplements.
4. Some clients do not report their use of supplements because they are embarrassed that they are self-medicating

or do not realize the importance of potential medication-supplement interactions.
5. An increased risk of nontherapeutic interactions is associated with alcohol ingestion.

Content Area: Medication
Integrated Processes: Teaching/Learning; Nursing Process: Planning
Client Need: Physiological Integrity; Pharmacological and Parenteral Therapies
Cognitive Level: Comprehension
Concept: Medication; Patient-Centered Care

48. ANSWER: 2.
Rationales:
1. The statement, "We need to draw your blood at the medication's half-life to determine if the dose needs to be adjusted," will provide no significant information concerning the therapeutic level of a medication.
2. The statement, "We need to draw your blood just before the next dose to identify the lowest level of the medication in your blood," describes the protocol for the determination of the lowest level (trough level) of a medication in the blood. The trough level of a medication should be at or more than the lowest value in the identified blood therapeutic range of the medication.
3. A peak plasma level is the concentration of a medication in a blood specimen drawn 30 to 60 minutes, not 2 hours, after the administration of a medication.
4. Blood specimens do not have to be drawn hourly to determine the therapeutic concentration of a medication in the blood.

TEST-TAKING TIP: Identify the options that are opposites. Options 2 and 3 are opposites. Option 2 is associated with a time frame before administration of the medication, and option 3 is associated with a time frame after administration of the medication. Review these options carefully.

Content Area: Medication
Integrated Processes: Communication and Documentation; Nursing Process: Implementation
Client Need: Physiological Integrity; Pharmacological and Parenteral Therapies
Cognitive Level: Application
Concept: Medication; Safety

49. ANSWER: 4.
Rationales:
1. Although wanting to ensure that the dose is not so strong that it causes toxicity is one of the reasons why a peak plasma level is monitored, an explanation including the words "too strong" and "causes toxicity" may cause anxiety. Another option answers the client's question is a more positive and less threatening tone.
2. Absorption is not a concern because the medication was administered directly into the intravascular compartment.
3. Determining if the medication gets into your blood within 30 minutes is inaccurate information. A medication that is administered via an intravenous line is immediately introduced into the blood, not 30 minutes later.
4. Stating that the results will reveal if the blood level of the medication is being maintained within the

therapeutic range best describes the purpose of the blood test, without using words that may precipitate anxiety.

TEST-TAKING TIP: Identify the word in the stem that sets a priority. The word *best* in the stem sets a priority. Identify the global option. Option 4 is the global option. The concept of therapeutic range includes peak and trough levels.
Content Area: Medication
Integrated Processes: Communication and Documentation; Nursing Process: Implementation
Client Need: Physiological Integrity; Pharmacological and Parenteral Therapies
Cognitive Level: Application
Concept: Medication; Safety

50. ANSWER: 2.
Rationale:
Solve the problem by using the formula for ratio and proportion.

$$\frac{\text{Desire } 500 \text{ mg}}{\text{Have } 250 \text{ mg}} = \frac{x \text{ tablets}}{1 \text{ tablet}}$$
$$250x = 500 \times 1$$
$$250x = 500$$
$$x = 500 \div 250$$
$$x = 2 \text{ tablets}$$

Content Area: Medication
Integrated Processes: Nursing Process: Planning
Client Need: Physiological Integrity; Pharmacological and Parenteral Therapies
Cognitive Level: Application
Concept: Medication; Safety

51. ANSWER: 2.
Rationales:
1. The chemical, not generic, name describes the chemical and molecular structure of a medication.
2. The generic name begins with a lowercase letter and is easier to pronounce than the chemical name.
3. The trade, not generic, name usually is short and easy to recall.
4. The trade, not generic, name of a medication is registered by the U.S. Patent Office and approved by the U.S. Food and Drug Administration.

TEST-TAKING TIP: Identify the clang associations. The word *name* in the stem and in options 2 and 3 are clang associations. Examine options 2 and 3 carefully.
Content Area: Medication
Integrated Processes: Nursing Process: Implementation
Client Need: Physiological Integrity; Pharmacological and Parenteral Therapies
Cognitive Level: Comprehension
Concept: Medication; Safety

52. ANSWER: 3.
Rationales:
1. The environment may affect the body's response to medications. A hot environment will intensify the action of vasodilators, a cold environment will inhibit the action of vasodilators while increasing the action of

vasoconstrictors, and a noisy environment may interfere with the therapeutic effect of a sedative or analgesic.
2. This is not an accurate statement for all medications. Vitamin C in citrus fruit juice aids the absorption of iron. In addition, many medications can irritate the gastrointestinal tract and should be taken with food.
3. Medication response discrepancies in men and women are attributable to body fat distribution as well as fluid and hormonal differences, which affect medication absorption. Also, the majority of medication research is based on studies involving men; responses of women may be different from what is documented in medication literature.
4. Older adults, not infants, experience multiorgan slowdown or impairment, causing greater medication absorption and decreased excretion, which increases the risk of medication toxicity.
Content Area: Medication
Integrated Processes: Nursing Process: Evaluation
Client Need: Physiological Integrity; Pharmacological and Parenteral Therapies
Cognitive Level: Comprehension
Concept: Medication; Sexuality

53. ANSWER: 3.
Rationales:
1. The client's white blood cell count is within the expected range of 4,500 to 11,000/mm³, indicating that the client has an adequate volume of white blood cells to protect the body from invading pathogens.
2. The client's platelet count is within the expected range of 150,000 to 350,000/mm³, indicating that the client will not hemorrhage due to a platelet deficiency.
3. The client is at risk for drug toxicity due to impaired renal function, resulting in an inability to excrete toxic substances from the body. Impaired renal function is indicated by a BUN count increased beyond the expected range of 8 to 21 mg/dL and a creatinine count increased beyond the expected range of 0.6 to 1.2 mg/dL. A BUN level higher than 100 mg/dL and a creatinine level higher than 7.4 mg/dL are critical findings.
4. The client is experiencing excess, not deficient, fluid volume. The BUN and creatinine levels are elevated, indicating impaired kidney function. Clinical indicators of excess fluid volume include a fluid intake greater than urine output, an elevated pulse rate, bounding pulse, bibasilar crackles, jugular venous distention, elevated systolic and diastolic blood pressures, and sacral edema.

TEST-TAKING TIP: Identify the word in the stem that sets a priority. The word *priority* in the stem sets a priority.
Content Area: Medication
Integrated Processes: Nursing Process: Evaluation
Client Need: Physiological Integrity; Pharmacological and Parenteral Therapies
Cognitive Level: Analysis
Concept: Patient-Centered Care; Medication

54. ANSWER: 4.
Rationales:
1. An *idiosyncratic reaction* is not a predictable, secondary effect to a medication. An idiosyncratic reaction is a

resistance, overreaction, or unpredictable reaction that is different from the expected response.

2. An *allergic reaction* is not a predictable, secondary effect to a medication. An allergic reaction is a client's immune system response to the presence of a medication.

3. An *adverse effect* is not a predictable, secondary effect to a medication. An adverse effect is an unintended, usually unpredictable harmful effect that is more severe than a side effect.

4. A *side effect* is a predictable, secondary effect to a medication. It is unintended but generally is well tolerated because the benefit is greater than the inconvenience of the side effect (e.g., drowsiness, dry mouth).

TEST-TAKING TIP: Identify the clang associations. The word *effect* in the stem and in options 3 and 4 are clang associations. Examine options 3 and 4 closely. More often than not, an option with a clang association is the correct answer.

Content Area: Medication
Integrated Processes: Communication and Documentation; *Nursing Process:* Evaluation
Client Need: Safe and Effective Care Environment; Management of Care
Cognitive Level: Knowledge
Concept: Medication; Communication

55. ANSWER: 1.
Rationales:
1. Asking about what kind of responses occurred is information that relates to the specific allergy identified by the client. The specific reaction to each allergy should also be determined as each allergy is identified.

2. Asking about the presence of other types of allergies is premature; it ignores the need for further exploration of the client's statement.

3. Placing an allergy alert wristband on the client is premature; additional allergies may need to be included.

4. Listing the allergy in the client's medication administration record is premature; additional information should be obtained from the client.

TEST-TAKING TIP: Identify options that are equally plausible. Options 3 and 4 are equally plausible. Both alert other health team members to the presence of the client's allergy to penicillin. Option 3 is no better than option 4. Eliminate both options from consideration. Identify the option that is unique. Option 1 is the only option that does not contain the words *allergies* or *allergy*.

Content Area: Medication
Integrated Processes: Communication and Documentation; *Nursing Process:* Implementation
Client Need: Safe and Effective Care Environment; Safety and Infection Control
Cognitive Level: Application
Concept: Medication; Safety

56. ANSWER: 5, 2, 4, 1, 3.
Rationales:
5. The first step of the nursing process is assessment. "Left calf is pale, cool, and edematous" are three classic clinical indicators of deep vein thrombosis.

2. The second step of the nursing process is analysis. The client is receiving warfarin (Coumadin) and therefore there is a risk of hemorrhage related to the effects of this anticoagulant.

4. Planning is the third step of the nursing process. It involves identifying an expected outcome. "The client will not experience bleeding while receiving warfarin (Coumadin)" is a measurable and realistic outcome. The second half of the planning step is identifying planned interventions. In this situation, warfarin (Coumadin) is prescribed, which the nurse plans to implement as prescribed.

1. The fourth step of the nursing process is implementation. Administering warfarin (Coumadin) as prescribed is implementation of a planned intervention.

3. The fifth step of the nursing process is evaluation. In this situation, the nurse must monitor the client's International Normalized Ratio (INR) level to ensure that it remains within the therapeutic range of 2.0 to 3.0 times the control.

Content Area: Medication
Integrated Processes: Nursing Process: Analysis
Client Need: Physiological Integrity; Pharmacological and Parenteral Therapies
Cognitive Level: Analysis
Concept: Medication; Patient-Centered Care

57. ANSWER: 3.
Rationales:
1. Insulin does not cure diabetes. An antibiotic is an example of a curative medication that eradicates a disease-producing pathogen.

2. Insulin does not prevent diabetes. A medication such as the measles vaccine is a preventative medication.

3. Insulin is considered a health maintenance medication. It supports normal body function and is prescribed to maintain health.

4. Insulin does not prevent conception. A medication that contains estrogen and progestin is a contraceptive medication.

Content Area: Medication
Integrated Processes: Communication and Documentation; *Nursing Process:* Planning
Client Need: Physiological Integrity; Pharmacological and Parenteral Therapies
Cognitive Level: Application
Concept: Medication; Metabolism

58. ANSWER: 1.
Rationales:
1. Metabolism (biotransformation) of medications occurs mainly in the liver. Liver function studies reflect the status of the liver.

2. Although metabolism of some medications may occur in the lungs, biotransformation mainly occurs in another organ of the body.

3. The kidneys are associated primarily with excretion, not metabolism, of medications in the body. Although metabolism of some medications may occur in the kidneys, biotransformation mainly occurs in another organ of the body.

4. Although metabolism of some medications may occur in the intestinal mucosa, biotransformation mainly occurs in another organ of the body. The intestines are more readily associated with excretion of medication via feces, although excretion of medications mainly is associated with the kidneys.

TEST-TAKING TIP: Identify the word in the stem that sets a priority. The word *mainly* in the stem sets a priority. Identify the unique option. Option 1 is unique because the liver is one organ. There are two lungs, two kidneys, and small and large intestines.

Content Area: Medication
Integrated Processes: Nursing Process: Assessment
Client Need: Physiological Integrity; Pharmacological and Parenteral Therapies
Cognitive Level: Comprehension
Concept: Medication; Safety

59. ANSWER: 1.
Rationales:

1. The priority is to ensure that the six medications are compatible. Medications when combined can cause chemical deterioration of one or more of the medications (usually due to acid-base incompatibility), resulting in precipitate formation, color change, or gas development. Also, one medication may interfere with the functioning of another medication by increasing or decreasing its effectiveness.

2. Although having the antidotes for medications easily available may be done, it is not the priority. Also, not all medications have an antidote.

3. Although teaching the client the therapeutic action of medications may be done, it is not the priority.

4. Although ensuring that medications are included on the medication reconciliation form may be done, it is not the priority.

Content Area: Medication
Integrated Processes: Nursing Process: Planning
Client Need: Physiological Integrity; Pharmacological and Parenteral Therapies
Cognitive Level: Application
Concept: Medication; Safety

60. ANSWER: 1, 2, 3, 4.
Rationales:

1. Yogurt contains a significant amount of tyramine and should be avoided by a client receiving an MAO inhibitor. An MAO inhibitor prevents the breakdown of tyramine. Too much tyramine leads to excessive epinephrine, causing a hypertensive crisis, which can precipitate an intracranial hemorrhage.

2. Sausage is high in tyramine and should be avoided by a client receiving an MAO inhibitor.

3. Chocolate is high in tyramine and should be avoided by a client receiving an MAO inhibitor.

4. Chicken liver is high in tyramine and should be avoided by a client receiving an MAO inhibitor.

5. Cream cheese and cottage cheese are two types of cheese permitted on a tyramine-restricted diet for a client receiving an MAO inhibitor because they are not high in tyramine.

Content Area: Medication
Integrated Processes: Teaching/Learning; Nursing Process: Implementation
Client Need: Physiological Integrity; Pharmacological and Parenteral Therapies
Cognitive Level: Analysis
Concept: Medication; Safety

Essential Psychosocial and Cultural Concepts

Development Across the Life Span

KEY TERMS

Cooperative (associative) play—Child engaging in group play without rigid rules

Egocentric—View of self as the center of the universe

Male menopause (manopause, andropause)—Decreased production of androgens, such as testosterone, that results in decreased vigor and sexual desire; usually occurs between ages 45 and 55

Menarche—Initiation of first menstruation

Menopause—Permanent cessation of menstruation in women; usually occurs between ages 45 and 50

Object permanence—Realization that objects moved out of sight still exist

Parallel play—Child playing alongside, not with, other children

Peer pressure—Intimidating, coercive behavior designed to persuade an individual to engage in activities in which the individual does not want to participate

Puberty—Interval when secondary sex characteristics emerge and the ability to sexually reproduce occurs

Separation anxiety—Child's infuriation, frustration, and fear precipitated by parental absence.

Stranger anxiety—Child's fear of people who are unfamiliar

Therapeutic play—Use of toys, crafts, puppets, and other tools to assist a child to express feelings or concerns or to learn something new

I. Infant

Infants are babies from 1 to 12 months of age. During this stage of development, babies experience dramatic physiological and psychosocial maturation as they begin to differentiate self from others. Newborns from birth to the end of the first month of age are called neonates.

A. Development
1. Physical.
   a. Weight triples.
   b. Chest measurement approaches head circumference.
   c. Has six to eight teeth.
   d. Turns from abdomen to back by 5 months and back to abdomen by 6 months.
   e. Sits by 7 months.
   f. Crawls, pulls self up, and uses pincer grasp by 9 months.
   g. Walks holding on by 11 months.
2. Psychosocial.
   a. Oral phase of psychosexual development; infants obtain pleasure from oral gratification through stimulation of mouth, lips, and tongue.
   b. Is confronted with resolving the conflict of trust versus mistrust that leads to faith and optimism; if basic trust is not satisfied, the infant becomes insecure, fearful, and mistrusting.
   c. Views self as the center of the universe (**egocentric**).
   d. Wants immediate gratification at 1 month; is able to tolerate some frustration and delay gratification at 8 months.
   e. Smiles and focuses on bright objects by 2 months.
   f. Laughs by 4 months.
   g. Has beginnings of **separation anxiety**, infuriation, frustration, and fear during parenteral absence, at 4 to 8 months.
   h. Fears strangers (**stranger anxiety**) by 6 to 8 months.
3. Cognitive.
   a. Sensorimotor phase; reflexes replaced by voluntary activity.
   b. Begins to understand cause and effect by 1 to 4 months.
   c. Realizes objects moved out of sight still exist (**object permanence**) by 9 to 10 months.
   d. Responds to own name and cries when reprimanded at 10 months.
   e. Uses and understands gestures, explores surroundings, throws kisses, gives hugs, may cling to security blanket or toy, and recognizes self as distinct from the environment by 12 months.
4. Language.
   a. Uses crying to signal displeasure during first 6 months.
   b. Babbles by 3 months.
   c. Imitates sounds by 6 months.
   d. Reacts to simple commands by 9 months.
   e. Says 1 word by 10 months; says 3 to 5 words and understands 100 words by 12 months.
5. Play.
   a. Plays alone (**solitary play**); revolves around own body.
   b. Play becomes more interactive and shows toy preferences by 3 to 6 months.
   c. Play involves sensorimotor skills by 6 to 12 months.
   d. Smiles at own image at 5 months.
   e. Enjoys peek-a-boo and bouncing in chairs at 7 months.
   f. Clutches soft objects at 8 months.
   g. Enjoys picture books at 10 months.
   h. Enjoys roughhouse play at 12 months.
6. Reaction to illness, hospitalization, and pain. For additional information see "Infants" in Table 15.1 "Developmental Variations Associated with Pain and Related Nursing Care" in Chapter 15, Pain, Comfort, Rest, and Sleep.
   a. Younger infant.
      (1) Recognizes pain, but is not emotionally traumatized by intrusive procedures.
      (2) Responses include high-pitched cry, irritability, tearing, stiff posture, fisting, brows lowered and drawn together, eyes tightly closed, mouth open, and difficulty sleeping and eating.
   b. Older infant.
      (1) Recognizes pain and may exhibit localized body response.
      (2) Responses include loud crying, facial expression of pain and anger, deliberate withdrawal of site and pushing away of external stimulus.

B. Nursing care
1. Assess developmental level.
2. Provide a consistent caregiver.
3. Meet needs immediately to increase trust.
4. Provide a pacifier for comfort and to meet oral needs, especially if the infant is on nothing-by-mouth status; provide a nipple dipped in sucrose solution during painful procedures.
5. Foster parent bonding with the infant; encourage rooming-in, if possible.
6. Communicate with the infant through auditory (talking, singing), visual (eye-to-eye contact), and tactile (touching, holding) stimulation.
7. Support the mother's decision to breastfeed or bottle-feed.

8. Teach parents to provide appropriate nutrition. For additional information see "Birth to 1 year" in Table 20.4 "Nutritional Variations Across the Life Span and Related Nursing Care" in Chapter 20, Nutrition.
   a. Provide adequate calories based on developmental needs.
   b. Introduce cereal and pureed foods around 5 to 6 months, progressing to chopped and then soft foods at 6 to 7 months, once dentition has begun.
   c. Provide finger foods to increase refinement of pincer grasp and hard crackers to provide pleasure and promote teeth eruption.
   d. Decrease volume of milk intake as more solid foods are ingested.
   e. Encourage weaning from bottle to cup progressively as readiness is demonstrated by improved hand-mouth coordination.
9. Teach parents to encourage age-appropriate play.
   a. Ensure play is interactive, recreational, and educational; rotate toys as developing skills progress.
   b. Encourage the infant to interact with self in mirror and with others to support social and creative growth.
   c. Provide a variety of toys because of short attention span to support cognitive growth.
   d. Provide black-and-white or brightly colored mobiles, stuffed animals, rattles, teething rings, push-pull toys, blocks, books with textures, and teething toys to support physical growth.
   e. Provide toys small enough to promote manipulation to develop fine motor skills, but larger than an adult's fist to prevent aspiration.
10. Teach parents ways to prevent injury. See reasons why infants are at risk for injury under "Age" in "Factors That Influence Client Safety" in Chapter 1, Safety.
    a. Suffocation and aspiration.
    🛑 (1) **Place in the supine position when sleeping.**
    (2) Avoid pillows, excessive bedding, tucked-in blankets, baby powder, bottle propping, latex balloons, buttons, plastic bags, and loose blind cords.
    (3) Avoid foods that can occlude the airway, such as nuts, grapes, hot dogs, hard candy, popcorn, and raisins.
    (4) Ensure that the distance between crib slats is no more than 2⅜ inches.
    b. Motor vehicle injuries.
    (1) Use a rear-facing car seat with five-point harness until the infant exceeds 20 pounds

or height and weight recommendations indicated by the manufacturer.

🛑 (2) **Do not leave an infant in a car unattended.**

c. Bodily harm.
   (1) Supervise the infant on raised surfaces.
   (2) Place gates at the tops and bottoms of stairs.
   (3) Use restraints on infant seats, high chairs, walkers, and swings.

🛑 (4) **Never shake a baby because it can lead to head injury *(shaken baby syndrome).***

d. Poisoning.
   (1) Store agents in locked cabinets.
   (2) Avoid secondhand smoke.
   (3) Remove lead paint from surfaces in the home.
   (4) Keep the poison control center number by the telephone.
e. Burns.
   (1) Set the home's hot water heater at 120°F.
   (2) Test water temperature before a bath and use a bathtub (not a sink) for baths.
   (3) Avoid excessive exposure to the sun.
   (4) Do not use a microwave to warm bottles or food.
   (5) Put inserts in electric outlets.
   (6) Install smoke detectors throughout the house.
f. Drowning.
   (1) Supervise the infant when in or near water, such as a bathtub, toilet, bucket, pool, or lake.
   (2) Keep bathroom doors closed and keep toilet lids down or use toilet seat guards.
g. Abduction.
   (1) Teach parents not to leave the infant unattended.
   (2) Complete a Child Identification Kit: fingerprints, body map for identifying body characteristics, current photograph, and kit to obtain and store a DNA sample.

II. Toddler

Toddlers are children 12 months to 36 months of age. Dramatic changes in growth and development during this stage promote the toddler's striving to differentiate self from others and attain independence.

A. Development
   1. Physical.
      a. Has a decrease in growth rate; birth weight quadruples by 2½ years.
      b. Anterior fontanel closes by 18 months.

c. Chest measurement is greater than head circumference.

d. Experiences a decrease in appetite (physiological anorexia), has 20 teeth, and has increased taste preferences.

e. Has a decrease in naps.

f. Achieves daytime bowel and bladder control at 2 to 3 years; nighttime control by 3 to 4 years.

g. Walks by 14 months; runs by 18 months.

h. Continues mastery of gross and fine motor movements.

2. Psychosocial.

a. Anal stage of psychosexual development; beginning development of independence with a focus on gaining control over excretory functions.

b. Is confronted with resolving the conflict of autonomy versus shame and doubt that leads to self-control; if unable to achieve autonomy, the child will have difficulty developing independence later in life.

c. Differentiates self from others; is able to separate from parents at 2½ years for short periods.

d. Notes sex role differences and explores own body.

e. Withstands short periods of delayed gratification; negativistic.

f. May have a security object or may suck thumb for comfort.

g. Needs routines.

h. May fear sleep, engines, and animals.

i. May experience sibling rivalry with a newborn.

3. Cognitive.

a. Continuation of sensorimotor phase.

b. Preconceptional thought by 2 to 4 years; beginning of memory.

c. Has increased sense of time.

d. Begins asking "why" and "how" by 2 years.

e. Engages in magical thinking (i.e., considers personal thoughts are all powerful).

f. Is egocentric and has increased concept of ownership ("mine").

g. Begins to develop a conscience.

h. May begin to develop fears.

4. Language.

a. Increased comprehension: 4 to 6 words by 15 months; more than 10 words by 18 months; and more than 300 words and understands simple commands by 2 years.

b. Uses words "no" and "mine" constantly.

c. Talks incessantly; uses sentences by 2 years.

5. Play.

a. Interactions: alone and with peers and adults; can amuse self for brief periods.

b. Plays alongside, not with, other children (**parallel play**).

c. Types of play: recreational, imitative, and educational.

d. Activities: quiet, active, structured, and unstructured.

e. Environments: home, park, and preschool.

6. Reaction to illness, hospitalization, and pain. For additional information see "Toddlers and preschoolers" in Table 15.1 "Developmental Variations Associated with Pain and Related Nursing Care" in Chapter 15, Pain, Comfort, Rest, and Sleep.

a. Fears punishment, the unknown, and separation.

b. Has increased stress in reaction to immobilization, isolation, and altered rituals.

c. Expresses pain in a word (e.g., "ow").

d. Clings to parent, cries, and regresses when in pain or anxious.

e. Experiences separation anxiety (Box 10.1).

MAKING THE CONNECTION

Knowledge of Growth and Development and the Nursing Role

A nurse working in an emergency department is completing a comprehensive assessment of a toddler who was brought to the hospital by his father. The toddler is self-splinting his left arm and cries when the arm is touched. The nurse suspects that the toddler has sustained a left upper extremity fracture and keeps the arm immobilized until the boy can be seen by the primary health-care provider. The father states, "My son is always being defiant. He says no to everything and refuses to share toys with his sister, and is constantly saying, 'It's mine, its mine.' I can't get him to behave. I only tried to make him sit in a corner for 10 minutes to learn to behave and he kept getting up." The nurse concludes that the father does not understand normal growth and development of toddlers. The nurse explains that a toddler constantly saying "no" and "mine" is an expected part of growth and development. The nurse also explains that the toddler's behavior reflects egocentricity and striving for autonomy, which are associated with the developmental task of toddlers. The nurse suggests that the toddler be removed from a situation and told to sit quietly in "time-out" for a length of time no longer than his age (1 minute per year). A longer period of time is unrealistic, excessively punitive, and counterproductive. In this situation, the nurse functioned as a caregiver to and advocate for the child as well as a teacher, resource person, and counselor for the father.

> **Box 10.1** **Phases of Separation Anxiety Associated With Separation From Parents Due to Hospitalization**
>
> **Protest**
> - *Lasts for a few hours to a few days*
> - *Inconsolable crying*
> - *Clinging to parents to prevent departure*
> - *Rejection of others*
>
> **Despair**
> - *Follows protest phase*
> - *Flat affect*
> - *Sadness*
> - *Passivity*
> - *Unresponsiveness to stimuli*
> - *Altered sleep*
> - *Decreased appetite*
> - *Moaning, rocking, thumb-sucking, and nose picking*
>
> **Detachment and Denial**
> - *Adjusts to the loss*
> - *Lack of preference for parents*
> - *Friendliness to all*
> - *Interest in surroundings*

B. Nursing care
   1. Assess developmental level.
   2. Provide a consistent caregiver.
   3. Stay with the child.
   4. Support routines.
   5. Encourage rooming-in and family participation in child care.
   6. Accept protest behaviors when toddler is separated from parents, and console the toddler when parents have to leave.
   7. Provide familiar objects (e.g., teddy bear) from home.
   8. Explain to the parents that the toddler's display of anger is healthy and expected.
   9. Encourage independence.
   10. Ignore regression, and praise appropriate behavior.
   11. Provide massage, distraction, medications, and thermotherapy as prescribed.
   12. Use the services of a child life specialist who is educated to provide age-appropriate activities to assist a child to cope with illness or hospitalization.
   13. Offer choices, avoid frustration, and provide for safety while ignoring tantrums.
   14. Supervise interaction with infant siblings, give individual attention, include toddler in newborn care, and provide a doll for imitative play.

15. Teach parents to provide appropriate nutrition. For additional information see "Toddlers and preschoolers" in Table 20.4 "Nutritional Variations Across the Life Span and Related Nursing Care" in Chapter 20, Nutrition.
    a. Provide finger foods and support use of utensils to encourage self-feeding.
    b. Avoid the desire to feed the toddler to complete the task.
    c. Avoid using foods, such as sweets, for rewards or punishments.
16. Teach the parents to encourage age-appropriate play.
    a. Provide a variety of play experiences.
    b. Encourage play with banging toys and musical instruments to help the toddler release aggression through play.
    c. Provide push-pull, pounding board, and pedal-propelled riding toys and large balls to support physical growth.
    d. Provide telephones, dolls, safe kitchen utensils, dress-up clothes, and trucks to support social and creative growth.
    e. Provide crayons, nesting blocks, finger paints, and clay to support fine motor skills.
    f. Provide simple puzzles, picture books, and appropriate television programs or videos to promote cognitive development.
17. Teach parents ways to prevent injury. See reasons why toddlers are at risk for injury under "Age" in "Factors That Influence Client Safety" in Chapter 1, Safety.
    a. Motor vehicles.
       (1) Use a forward-facing seat with a five-point harness for all children 2 years and older (20 to 40 pounds) and those who have exceeded height and weight recommendations for rear-facing seats according to the manufacturer.
       (2) Use a belt-positioning booster seat when the child exceeds height and weight recommendations (80 pounds) for forward-facing seats.
       🛑 (3) Do not leave the child in a car unattended.
    b. Drowning.
       (1) Supervise when in or near water.
       (2) Fence or cover pools and hot tubs; install lid locks on toilets.
       (3) Know cardiopulmonary resuscitation (CPR).
    c. Burns.
       (1) Turn handles of pots toward the back of the stove.
       (2) Use front guards on radiators, space heaters, and fireplaces.

(3) Keep appliance cords, candles, and irons out of reach.

d. Suffocation and aspiration.

🛑 (1) Avoid foods that can occlude the airway, such as hard, round, and sticky foods (e.g., marshmallows, peanut butter, nuts, grapes, hot dogs, hard candy, popcorn, and raisins).

DID YOU KNOW?

Children ages 1 to 3 years have the highest incidence of foreign body aspiration because the lumen of their airways is small. The right bronchus is the usual site of an obstruction because of its shorter length and straighter angle. Also, children of this age are just beginning to eat solid foods, and their chewing and swallowing may not be effective. Hot dogs, round candy, nuts, and grapes account for approximately 40% of all aspirated foods. The severity of the obstruction depends on what was aspirated, the location of the obstruction, and the extent of the obstruction.

(2) Keep garage door openers inaccessible.
(3) Avoid toy boxes with heavy hinged lids, clothing with drawstrings, and appliances that cannot be opened from the inside.

e. Bodily harm.
(1) Do not permit the child to run with objects in the mouth or to run and jump near doors or furniture with glass.
(2) Teach the child to hold pointed objects downward.
(3) Keep tools and firearms in locked cabinets.
(4) Keep the child away from lawnmowers and weed whackers.
(5) Lock windows or use window guards on windows on second story or higher buildings.

f. Poisoning.
(1) Store agents in locked cabinets.
(2) Avoid secondhand smoke.
(3) Keep the poison control center number by the telephone.

g. Abduction and abuse.
(1) Teach parents to not leave the child unattended.

🛑 (2) Teach the child never to go with a stranger or allow inappropriate touching.

III. Preschooler

Preschoolers are children between 3 and 5 years of age. Their growth and development supports their desire for direction and purpose and prepares them for entry into the school environment.

A. Development
1. Physical.
   a. Average increase in weight of 5 lb/year and increase in height of 2.5 to 3 inches/year.
   b. Increase in immune responses.
   c. Increase in strength.
   d. Refinement of gross and fine motor skills.
   e. Dresses and washes self.
   f. Goes up stairs with alternate footing at 3 years; skips and hops on one foot by 4 years; jumps rope and walks backward with heel to toe by 5 years.
   g. Ties shoes, uses scissors, and prints a few letters by 5 years.
   h. Achieves day and night bowel and bladder control usually by 3 to 4 years.
   i. Eruption of permanent dentition possible during 5th year.
   j. Visual acuity approaches 20/20 by 5 years; potential for amblyopia by 4 to 6 years.
   k. Most body systems are mature and stable and can adjust to moderate stress.
2. Psychosocial.
   a. Oedipal stage of psychosexual development; attaches to parent of opposite sex while identifying with same-sex parent, which encourages imitative and imaginative play.
   b. Confronted with resolving the conflict of initiative versus guilt, leading to direction and purpose, which encourages endeavors; if initiative is not supported, the child may develop a sense of guilt that limits further initiative.
   c. Is selfish and impatient and exaggerates.
   d. Takes pride in accomplishments.
   e. Is less defiant than a toddler and takes pride in manners and acting manly or womanly at 5 years.
   f. Begins to differentiate between right and wrong (morality).
   g. May have imaginary friend.
   h. Develops personality by 5 years.
3. Cognitive.
   a. Preoperational phase (two stages: preconceptual phase from 2 to 4 years and intuitive thought phase from 4 to 5 years), during which there is a shift from egocentricity to social awareness.
   b. Has increased readiness for learning and curiosity about immediate world.
   c. Considers others' views.
   d. Understands past, present, and future by 5 years.
   e. Begins to understand mathematical concepts.
   f. Questions parental rules by 5 years.

4. Language.
   a. Has totally intelligible speech.
   b. Knows 900 words by 3 years; 1,500 words by 4 years; and 2,100 words by 5 years.
   c. Language increases in complexity; uses all parts of speech and asks meaning of new words.
   d. Asks "who," "what," "where," "when," and "why."
   e. Stuttering and stammering common between 2 and 4 years.
5. Play.
   a. Begins to engage in group play without rigid rules (**cooperative, associative play**).
   b. Begins to notice group conformity; increases sharing by 5 years.
   c. Engages in physical, manipulative, imitative, and imaginary play of acting like an adult.
   d. Is at increased risk for pedestrian and motor vehicle accidents due to bicycle riding, running after balls into street, and crossing streets.
   e. May cheat to win in games.
6. Reaction to illness, hospitalization, and pain. For additional information see "Toddlers and preschoolers" in Table 15.1 "Developmental Variations Associated with Pain and Related Nursing Care" in Chapter 15, Pain, Comfort, Rest, and Sleep.
   a. Fears intrusive procedures, such as rectal temperature, injections, and ear examinations.
   b. Fears pain, punishment, rejection, bodily harm, castration, mutilation, and darkness.
   c. Is increasingly able to withstand temporary separation.
   d. Views death as temporary.
   e. Attempts to protect self from pain by crying, biting, hitting, and kicking.

B. Nursing care
1. Explain interventions and reasons for them in language the child can understand.
🛑 2. Engage the child in **therapeutic play** using visual aids and puppets; have the child handle appropriate equipment (e.g., stethoscope, needleless syringe, bandages) on a doll; encourage a presurgical visit to the hospital, if applicable.
3. Engage the services of a child life specialist.
4. Encourage initiative, praise accomplished tasks, ignore regressive behaviors, and encourage choices.
5. Encourage self-care regarding activities of daily living, but provide supervision to maintain safety; allow the child to progress at own pace.
6. Balance activity and rest.
7. Teach the child how to dial 911 in case of an emergency and to give his or her full name and location.
8. Allow the child to explore own body without fear of punishment; ignore masturbation.
9. Use distraction, thermotherapy, massage, and medications as prescribed.
10. Assess for nonbinocular vision (strabismus).
11. Prepare the child for a painful procedure several minutes before it is to be performed; reward attempts to cooperate.
12. Teach parents to provide appropriate nutrition. For additional information see "Toddlers and preschoolers" in Table 20.4 "Nutritional Variations Across the Life Span and Related Nursing Care" in Chapter 20, Nutrition.
    a. Encourage a variety of nutritious foods, capitalizing on color, flavor, and texture to expand the palate.
    b. Encourage nutritious snacks, such as fruits and vegetables.
    c. Encourage socialization during meals, including table manners.
    d. Avoid threatening, bribing, or forcing a child to eat.
13. Teach parents to encourage age-appropriate play.
    a. Arrange for preschoolers to play together.
    b. Encourage safe playground play and use of sports equipment and bicycles to support physical growth.
    c. Provide dress-up clothes and toys, puppets, and village sets to support social and creative growth.
    d. Provide construction sets, musical instruments (e.g., drums, tambourines), and craft projects to develop fine motor skills.
    e. Provide educational computer games (e.g., numbers, letters), simple board games, and activity books to support cognitive growth.
14. Teach parents ways to prevent injury. See reasons why preschoolers are at risk for injury under "Age" in "Factors That Influence Client Safety" in Chapter 1, Safety.
    a. Bodily harm.
       (1) Set examples for acceptable behavior by being a positive role model.
       (2) Teach the child to wear a helmet when engaging in activities that can result in head trauma (e.g., riding a bicycle, using a skateboard, skating).
       (3) Encourage the child to recognize dangerous situations (e.g., pools, kitchen knives).
       (4) Teach the child to "stop, drop, and roll" if clothing is on fire.
       (5) Encourage the child to follow parenteral rules and provide positive or negative feedback based on the child's adherence or nonadherence to rules.

b. Motor vehicles.
  (1) Use a forward-facing car seat until the child exceeds 40 pounds or height and weight recommendations as per the manufacturer.
  (2) Use a belt-positioning booster seat when the child is 40 to 80 pounds or exceeds height and weight recommendations for forward-facing seats according to the manufacturer.

  🛑 (3) Do not leave the child in a car unattended.

  (4) Teach the child to look both ways before crossing streets.
  (5) Encourage the child to play in yards or playgrounds instead of the street.
c. Abduction and abuse.
  (1) Teach parents not to leave child unattended.
  (2) Encourage parents to begin informal sex education.

  🛑 (3) Teach the child about stranger safety and recognition of unwanted touch; teach the child to report unwanted touch to a parent or other responsible adult.

IV. School-Aged Child

School-aged children are 6 to 12 years of age. Their world enlarges dramatically during this phase, and growth and development support their increasing ability to perform complex social, cognitive, and motor behaviors.
A. Development
  1. Physical.
    a. Average increase in weight of 4.5 to 6 pounds/year and height of 2 inches/year; girls pass boys in height and weight by 12 years.
    b. Beginning of permanent teeth with front teeth.
    c. Secondary sex characteristics emerge and the ability to sexually reproduce occurs (**puberty**); begins earlier in females (10 years) than in males (12 years).
    d. May be able to ride a bicycle and can print capital letters at 6 years.
    e. Develops good coordination and timing in motor activities by 9 years.
    f. Is skillful in most activities, such as skating, cycling, and skateboarding, and is able to use most tools skillfully and carefully by 10 years.
    g. Often appears awkward and lanky; may have difficulty coordinating muscle groups because of advancing bone growth at 11 years.
    h. Often overindulges in physical activity to point of exhaustion at 12 years.
  2. Psychosocial.
    a. Latent stage of psychosexual development; tranquil stage between oedipal stage of early childhood and the genital stage of adolescence.
    b. Is confronted with resolving the conflict of industry versus inferiority, which leads to personal and interpersonal competence; if standards, whether internal or external, are not met, feelings of inferiority will develop.
    c. Identifies with peers of same gender by 6 to 10 years; begins to become interested in opposite gender by 10 to 12 years.
    d. Needs group approval and is highly competitive at 10 years.
    e. Develops intrinsic motivation (mastery, self-satisfaction).
    f. Behaves according to set norms; has decreased egocentricity.
    g. Develops self-image and body image; is increasingly concerned with physical appearance, hygiene, and need for privacy at 12 years.
    h. Begins to hero worship.
    i. Has many worries.
  3. Cognitive.
    a. Develops concrete operations, inductive reasoning, and beginning logic by 7 to 11 years.
    b. Can count by multiples of 2, 4, 5, and 10 by 7 years.
    c. Classifies, serializes, tells time, and reads.
    d. Becomes more concerned about grades and failing at 9 years.
    e. Defines and understands abstract words, such as "peace" and "justice."
    f. Becomes more critical of own performance.
    g. Begins to think realistically about future and career by 11 years.
    h. Absorbs new information easily, shows interest in science and social studies, and is curious about people and places by 12 years.
  4. Language.
    a. Vocabulary and comprehension expand; all sounds mastered by 12 years.
    b. Adult speech well established by 9 to 12 years.
  5. Play.
    a. Has increased ego mastery, demands conformity in play, and is fanatic about rules.
    b. Is involved in peer relationships, such as team sports and clubs, and is highly competitive.
    c. Can play more complex board games.
    d. Is more selective about collections.
  6. Reaction to illness, hospitalization, and pain. For additional information see "School-aged children" in Table 15.1 "Developmental Variations Associated with Pain and Related Nursing Care" in Chapter 15, Pain, Comfort, Rest, and Sleep.
    a. Fears the unknown, decreased control, dependency, disfigurement, and death.
    b. Personifies death as "boogyman" but has realistic concept by 9 to 10 years.

c. Attempts to cooperate or stays rigid for procedures, but may cry, yell, or resist.

d. Clenches fists, grits teeth, closes eyes, and wrinkles forehead in response to pain.

e. Withstands some physical discomfort, but uses stall tactics to cope; self-image about reaction to pain is important.

f. Desires more complete explanation of disease processes and scientific rationales for procedures.

B. Nursing care

1. Place with an age-appropriate roommate, and support visits from peers.

2. Never belittle regression, resistance, or crying.

3. Recognize accomplishments; avoid comparisons.

4. Provide privacy; permit wearing underpants.

5. Provide concrete details of procedures, emphasizing basic scientific aspects.

6. Allow time for questions, and ask whether the child has any questions. Do not overwhelm the child with details, but provide honest, adequate answers. Reinforce that there is no such thing as a stupid question.

7. Encourage expression of feelings, concerns, and fears; use puppets or visual aids for expression of feelings if appropriate. Explain that expressing feelings of sadness, anger, and love is acceptable.

8. Allow manipulation of equipment, avoid procrastination, and praise attempts at cooperation.

🛑 9. Provide choices, and allow the child to be involved in some decisions about care (e.g., how long parents should stay).

10. Encourage diversional activities; seek assistance from a child life specialist.

11. Encourage completion of school work if the child is able; arrange for a tutor through the child's school.

12. Support appreciation of worthwhile heroes.

13. Help the child understand changes in body structure or appearance that make him or her different from peers.

14. Use a pain scale, distraction, guided imagery, thought stopping, soothing music, massage, thermotherapy, and medications as prescribed.

15. Teach parents to provide appropriate nutrition. For additional information see "School-aged children" in Table 20.4 "Nutritional Variations Across the Life Span and Related Nursing Care" in Chapter 20, Nutrition.

a. Teach principles of healthy nutrition (see the U.S. Department of Agriculture's MyPlate [*www.choosemyplate.gov*] and "MyPlate" in Chapter 20, Nutrition.).

b. Encourage intake of foods high in vitamin D and calcium for bone growth.

c. Encourage socialization during meals; avoid reprimands.

d. Adjust caloric intake based on level of physical activity.

e. Encourage intake of adequate breakfast at home or in a school nutrition program.

f. Involve the child in meal planning and trips to the supermarket.

DID YOU KNOW?

According to the Centers for Disease Control and Prevention, the definition of childhood obesity is a body mass index at or above the 95th percentile for children of the same age and sex. Using that criterion, approximately 17% (12.5 million) of children and adolescents ages 2 to 19 years of age are obese in the United States. Since 1980, obesity prevalence among children and adolescents has almost tripled, and there are significant ethnic/racial and economic disparities. For example, Hispanic boys (2 to 19 years) are significantly more likely to be obese than non-Hispanic white boys; non-Hispanic black girls are significantly more likely to be obese than non-Hispanic white girls; and 1 in 7 low-income, preschool-aged children is obese.

16. Teach parents to encourage age-appropriate play.

a. Encourage team sports and use of bicycles and skateboards to support physical growth.

b. Encourage participation in groups, such as boy scouts or girl scouts, to support social and creative growth.

c. Provide construction sets, musical instruments, and craft projects to support fine motor skills.

d. Provide computer games and increasingly complex board games, such as Monopoly, to support cognitive growth.

17. Teach parents ways to prevent injury.
See reasons why school-aged children are at risk for injury in the section "Age" under "Factors That Influence Client Safety" in Chapter 1, Safety.

a. Motor vehicles.

(1) Teach the child pedestrian skills (e.g., cross streets in a crosswalk or at a corner with the light).

(2) Encourage the child to play in a park rather than in the street.

(3) Use a belt-positioning booster seat when the child is 40 to 80 pounds or exceeds weight and height recommendations for forward-facing seats as per manufacturer; use a booster seat until the vehicle seatbelt fits properly (usually 4 feet, 9 inches in height, greater than 80 pounds and 8 years old); then use the vehicle-provided lap and shoulder seatbelts.

(4) Seat all children under the age of 13 in the rear seat.

b. Bodily harm.

(1) Teach the child to wear eye, mouth, and ear protection with sports.

(2) Avoid unsupervised gymnastics and climbing.

(3) Reinforce previous teaching about playground safety, 911 notification in case of an emergency, and "stop, drop, and roll" if clothes are on fire.

(4) Toxic substances: Practice role-playing to learn to say "no" to tobacco, drugs, and alcohol.

c. Gun safety.

(1) Recognize the presence of a gun.

(2) Interrupt any activity involving a gun.

(3) Do not touch the gun.

(4) Leave the area of the gun.

(5) Tell a parent or a person in authority about the presence of the gun.

d. Abduction and abuse.

(1) Teach parents to continue age-appropriate sex education.

🛑 (2) **Teach the child to never go with a stranger or allow inappropriate touching; tell the child to report physical, verbal, emotional, or cyber bullying, sexual harassment, or abuse to a parent, school nurse, teacher, or other responsible adult.**

V. Adolescent

Adolescents usually are between 13 and 20 years of age. Adolescence is divided into multiple levels, depending on when profound physical, psychosocial, and cognitive changes occur. It is a transitional stage between childhood and young adulthood.

A. Stages of adolescence

1. *Early adolescence* (as early as 11–14 years): Transitions through puberty (Table 10.1).

2. *Middle adolescence* (15–17 years): Transitions to peer group identification.

3. *Late adolescence* (18–19 years): Transitions to young adulthood.

B. Development

1. Physical.

a. Uncoordinated, as linear growth exceeds muscular growth.

b. Increased strength, especially in males.

c. Slouching in early-maturing females to hide tallness.

d. Overestimation of athletic ability in 16- to 18-year-olds, which increases the risk of accidents.

Table 10.1 Male Puberty Versus Female Puberty

Male Puberty	Female Puberty
• *Generally occurs at 12 to 16 years* • *Enlargement of scrotum, testes, and penis* • *Development of pubic, axillary, facial, and body hair* • *Initiation of nocturnal emissions and mature spermatozoa* • *Deepening of voice* • *Achievement of 95% of height by 15 to 16 years*	• *Generally occurs at 10 to 14 years* • *Development of breasts and pubic and axillary hair* • *Initiation of first menstruation (menarche)* • *Initiation of ovulation about 12 months after menarche* • *Achievement of 95% of height by menarche*

2. Psychosocial.

a. Genital stage; abundance of libidinal drives as sexual maturity progresses.

b. Is confronted with resolving the conflict of self-identity versus role confusion; strives to integrate self-concept and values with those of society; failure to achieve self-identity results in role confusion.

c. Feels omnipotent.

d. Engages in behaviors motivated by peers (**peer pressure**); increases risky behavior.

e. Is increasingly more confident and has increased interest in appearance.

f. Desires independence, but may avoid responsibility and resists enforcement of discipline.

g. Has increased interest in sex with experimentation; begins to form intimate relationships (opposite sex if heterosexual, same sex if homosexual).

h. Is able to make sacrifices for long-range goals at 16–19 years.

i. Is at increased risk for suicide and homicide (more frequently with males than females) related to bullying, economic deprivation, family dysfunction, availability of firearms, and mental illness.

j. May not seek medical care for sexually transmitted infections (STIs) due to lack of knowledge, guilt, shame, or fear.

DID YOU KNOW?

The Centers for Disease Control and Prevention reported that 41% of U.S. high school students surveyed had sexual intercourse in 2015. Thirty percent reported having sexual intercourse during the previous 3 months and of these:

• 43% reported not using a condom the last time they had sex.

- 14% reported not using any method to prevent pregnancy.
- 21% reported drinking alcohol or taking drugs before the last intercourse experience.
- 22% of all new HIV diagnoses in the U.S. in 2014 were people 13 to 24 years of age of which 80% were gay and bisexual males.
- 10 million new cases of sexually transmitted diseases reported in 2014 were among people 13 to 24 years of age.
- 250,000 babies were born to girls 15 to 19 years of age in 2014.

Adapted from: Centers for Disease Control and Prevention. (2016). Sexual risk behaviors: HIV, STD, & Teen Pregnancy Prevention. Retrieved November 23, 2016, from http://cdc.gov/Healthy Youth/sexualbehaviors/

3. Cognitive.
   a. Has formal operational thought; is capable of abstract, conceptual, and hypothetical thinking; and comprehends satire and double meanings.
   b. Has increased learning through inference versus repetition and imitation.
   c. Has difficulty accepting others' viewpoints; is idealistic.
   d. Is concerned with social, moral, and ethical issues.
   e. Develops a personal value system (value autonomy).
4. Language.
   a. Has increased vocabulary and reading comprehension.
   b. Experiments with language; uses jargon.
5. Play.
   a. Engages in individual and team sports for exercise; has increased social and personal development.
   b. Follows rules of complex games.
6. Reaction to illness, hospitalization, and pain. For additional information see "Adolescents" in Table 15.1 "Developmental Variations Associated with Pain and Related Nursing Care" in Chapter 15, Pain, Comfort, Rest, and Sleep.
   a. Similar to school-aged children, with increased need for independence, privacy, and body integrity.
   b. Has fear of disfigurement or decreased function.
   c. Has decreased need for parental visits, but separation from peers may be traumatic.
   d. Has realistic concept of death, but emotionally may be unable to accept it.
   e. Tolerates physical pain; stoicism important among males.

   f. Clenches fist or teeth, self-splints, and has decreased interest and concentration in response to pain.

C. Nursing care
   1. Encourage visits by peers.
   2. Talk to the adolescent directly, not through the parents, and show respect for level of knowledge.
   3. Allow time for a relationship to develop; do not force self on adolescent.
   4. Express an interest in the adolescent's life outside the hospital, especially hobbies, to aid communication.
   5. Encourage questions and the expression of feelings and concerns.
   6. Encourage participation in decision making, wearing own clothes, and performing own care.
   7. Explain reasons for sexual characteristics that are developing; encourage discussion of changing body image.
   8. Facilitate discussion about self-identify, role image, and goal direction.
   9. Encourage positive role models.
   10. Permit experience of competition, teamwork, and conflict resolution.
   11. Use distraction, music, massage, and medications as prescribed.
   12. Teach adolescents that pain does not have to be stoically tolerated; it is not a sign of weakness to express pain verbally or behaviorally; and to ask for medication to relieve pain.
   13. Teach parents to provide appropriate nutrition. For additional information see "Adolescents" in Table 20.4 "Nutritional Variations Across the Life Span and Related Nursing Care" in Chapter 20, Nutrition.
       a. Provide prescribed iron and B vitamins for increased muscle and tissue growth and red blood cell maturation, particularly in females following first menstruation (**menarche**).
       b. Teach the adolescent the importance of not following fad diets; encourage regular eating habits and avoidance of fast foods that are high in calories and salt.
       c. Provide nutritious between-meal snacks to meet increased caloric needs, physical growth, and emotional expenditure.
       d. Be alert for clinical indicators of an eating disorder, such as vomiting after meals, weight loss or gain, cachexia, and tooth decay.
   14. Teach parents to encourage age-appropriate play.
       a. Encourage participation in team sports and increasingly difficult sports, such as skiing and surfing, to support physical growth.

b. Encourage participation in school activities, such as theater and chorus, to support social and creative growth.

c. Provide musical instruments and advanced craft projects to support fine motor skills.

d. Provide computer games and increasingly complex board games, such as chess, to support cognitive growth.

15. Teach parents ways to prevent injury. See reasons why adolescents are at risk for injury under "Age" in "Factors That Influence Client Safety" in Chapter 1, Safety.

a. Motor vehicles.
(1) Assess the level of responsibility and ability to resist peer pressure; recognize that most accidents involving adolescent drivers result from distractions caused by passengers.
(2) Set limits on driving, and encourage wearing of lap and shoulder seatbelts.
(3) Encourage participation in a driver's education program; follow all laws regarding driving.
(4) Teach to avoid riding with a driver who is impaired; arrange for alternate transportation.

b. Sports.
(1) Encourage warming up and cooling down.
(2) Encourage playing within abilities.
(3) Encourage wearing protective gear.

c. Violence, abuse, suicide, and homicide.
(1) Assess risk due to frustration, deprivation, aggression, depression, bullying, and social isolation.
(2) Keep firearms in locked closets.
(3) Teach the adolescent to report bullying, sexual harassment, or abuse to a parent, school nurse, teacher, or other responsible adult.
(4) Discourage membership in gangs.

d. Sexually Transmitted Infections (STIs).
(1) Teach the adolescent sex education and STI prevention, such as engaging in abstinence, limiting number of partners, and using condoms.
(2) Engage the adolescent in role-playing to teach ways to resist peer pressure.

e. High-risk behaviors.
(1) Teach the adolescent to avoid body piercing, tanning beds, and tattoos.
(2) Teach the adolescent to avoid drug misuse, tobacco use, and alcohol.
(3) Teach the adolescent to check the depth of water before diving and to avoid swimming extended distances and in dangerous waters.

VI. Young Adult

Young adults are between the ages of 20 and 30 years. Young adulthood consists of multiple physical, psychosocial, and financial changes that involve decisions (e.g., intimate partner, career, high-risk behaviors) that can affect the quality and length of one's life.

A. Development
1. Physical.
a. At height of bodily vigor; period of peak sexual capacity for males.
b. Maximum level of strength, muscular development, height, and cardiac and respiratory capacity.

2. Psychosocial.
a. Is confronted with resolving the conflict of intimacy versus isolation; development of friendships and an intimate love relationship are imperative; failure to achieve feelings of affiliation and love inherent in relationships causes one to feel isolated and alone.
b. Has a vision of the future and imagines various possibilities for self; transfers an interest into an occupation.
c. Defines and tests what can be accomplished.
d. Seeks out a mentor to emulate as a guiding figure.
e. Experiments with and chooses a lifestyle.
f. Forms mature relationships with both males and females; may choose someone for a long-term relationship.
g. Learns to understand masculine and feminine aspects of self as well as an adult concept of roles.
h. Accepts responsibilities and pleasures of parenthood.
i. May not seek medical care for STIs due to lack of information, guilt, shame, or fear.
j. May continue to live with parents until financially solvent (increasing trend).

3. Cognitive.
a. At close to peak of intelligence, memory, and abstract thought.
b. Has maximum ability to solve problems and learn new skills.

4. Language: Has fully developed language.

5. Play.
a. May participate in or enjoy watching sports activities.
b. Engages in socialization with peers.
c. Enjoys playing with own children or with children of others.

6. Reaction to illness, hospitalization, and pain. For additional information see "Adults" in Table 15.1 "Developmental Variations Associated

with Pain and Related Nursing Care" in Chapter 15, Pain, Comfort, Rest, and Sleep.

a. May feel dependent and/or a lack of autonomy.

b. Chronic illness or prolonged hospitalization may interfere with establishment of intimacy and may result in isolation, loneliness, and withdrawal.

c. Frustration and isolation may occur when goals related to choice of occupation, life partner, and procreation are not attained.

B. Nursing care

🛑 1. Encourage participation in the plan of care and decision making; support independence and autonomy, especially when some aspect of physical, emotional, or financial dependence exists.

2. Foster feeling of acceptance and belonging.
3. Encourage expression of feelings and concerns.
4. Praise accomplishments and encourage initiative.
5. Assist with coping with unexpected alterations in body image, lifestyle, or long-term goals.
6. Teach to maintain appropriate nutrition. For additional information see "Adults," "Pregnant women," and "Lactating women" in Table 20.4 "Nutritional Variations Across the Life Span and Related Nursing Care" in Chapter 20, Nutrition.
   a. Limit caloric intake if lifestyle is more sedentary than it was during adolescence.
   b. Encourage a heart-healthy, balanced diet; discourage intake of foods high in carbohydrates, cholesterol, saturated fats, sugar, preservatives, and additives.
   c. Seek guidance from a nutritionist regarding nutrition during pregnancy and lactation.
7. Teach ways to prevent injury.
   See reasons why adults are at risk for injury in the section "Age" under "Factors That Influence Client Safety" in Chapter 1, Safety.
   a. Sports.
      (1) Encourage warm-up and cool-down before and after activities.
      (2) Encourage play within abilities.
      (3) Encourage wearing of protective gear.
   b. STIs.
      (1) Engage in abstinence, limit number of partners, and/or use condoms.
      (2) Learn signs and symptoms of STIs and the need to seek health care if they occur.

VII. Adult

Adults are between the ages of 31 and 45 years. During this time a realistic self-identify forms, concerns about

career are paramount, and interest in mentoring the next generation emerges.

A. Development
1. Physical.
   a. Still near peak in late 30s, but has gradual decline in biological functioning around 40 years.
   b. Peak sexual capacity for females occurs during mid-30s.
2. Psychosocial.
   a. Confronted with resolving the conflict of generativity versus self-absorption; inability to achieve generativity results in egocentricity and stagnation.
   b. Achieves a realistic self-identity.
   c. Accepts limitations while developing assets.
   d. Delays immediate gratification for future satisfaction.
   e. Struggles to establish a place in society; invests self in social structure, including work, family, and community.
   f. Has a stronger need to be responsible.
   g. Seeks advancement by becoming more creative and pursuing ambitions.

DID YOU KNOW?

Births to women ages 35 to 39 increased 47% from 1990 to 2008, and births to women ages 40 to 44 years increased 80% from 1990 to 2008. The main factor is related to women delaying marriage and/or motherhood as they seek attainment of higher education and establishment of a career. The advantages of delaying motherhood include financial security and fewer regrets. However, disadvantages include increased health risks for mother and baby, change in lifestyle, and fatigue associated with the physical care of a newborn due to the lower energy level associated with being older. The interesting impact is related to the delay of the developmental tasks of having and raising children, which is associated with the 20- to 30-year-old age-group. This, in turn, delays the achievement of the developmental task of generativity versus stagnation formerly associated with adulthood (31–45 years of age) as older first-time parents focus on family life and raising children.

3. Cognitive.
   a. Has perceptions based on reality.
   b. Takes longer to memorize, but still at peak in abstract thinking and problem-solving.
   c. Generates new levels of awareness; gives more meaning to complex tasks.
4. Language: Has fully developed language.
5. Play.
   a. May participate in or enjoy watching sports activities.

b. Engages in socialization with peers.

c. Enjoys playing with own children or with the children of others.

6. Reaction to illness, hospitalization, and pain. For additional information see "Adults" in Table 15.1 "Developmental Variations Associated with Pain and Related Nursing Care" in Chapter 15, Pain, Comfort, Rest, and Sleep.

   a. Illness can jeopardize job security, financial stability, and family cohesiveness, producing feelings of inadequacy.

   b. Illness heightens feelings associated with beginning bodily decline.

   c. Altered body image or function may interfere with solidification of a realistic self-identify.

   d. Chronic illness or prolonged hospitalization that stifles independence and creativity can lead to self-absorption and stagnation.

   e. Illness may interfere with sexual functioning.

B. Nursing care

1. Assess variables in the adult's environment that contribute to problems, such as economic, educational, health, and social variables.

2. Assess knowledge of self and influence of current illness on self-image.

3. Plan care so that the client can maximize self-expression.

4. Assist to establish goals for long-term health maintenance.

5. Help to maintain judgment and initiative when external pressures of job and family interfere with internal comfort.

🛑 6. Encourage family discussion of needs and concerns; facilitate decision making and supportive relationships.

7. Teach to maintain appropriate nutrition. For additional information see "Adults," "Pregnant women," and "Lactating women" in Table 20.4 "Nutritional Variations Across the Life Span and Related Nursing Care" in Chapter 20, Nutrition.

   a. Encourage intake of a heart-healthy, balanced diet.

   b. Teach to eat in an unhurried, pleasant atmosphere.

   c. Encourage participation in a weight-reduction program, if necessary.

8. Teach ways to prevent sports-related injury. See reasons why adults are at risk for injury under "Age" in "Factors That Influence Client Safety" in Chapter 1, Safety.

   a. Encourage warm-up and cool-down before and after physical activity.

   b. Encourage play within abilities.

   c. Encourage wearing of protective gear.

VIII. Middle-Life Adult

Middle-life adults are between the ages of 46 and 64 years. The decline in physical abilities becomes more apparent, particularly the senses of hearing and vision. Concern for the next generation continues and may include grandchildren.

A. Development

1. Physical.

   a. Has decreasing eyesight, especially close vision (may be one of the first signs of aging).

   b. Experiences gradual hearing loss; high-pitched sounds are impaired more readily than low-pitched sounds.

   c. Experiences gradual loss of taste buds in 50s and sense of smell in 60s.

   d. Has declining muscle strength because of decreased levels of estrogen and testosterone; takes longer to accomplish tasks.

   e. Experiences decreased lung capacity, which leads to decreased endurance.

   f. Skin begins to wrinkle due to decline in subcutaneous fat.

   g. Hair begins to turn gray because the follicles at the base of the hair shaft ceases to produce melanin.

   h. Experiences postural changes due to loss of calcium and reduced activity.

   i. Women experience a cessation of menstruation (**menopause**); usually occurs between the ages of 45 and 50.

   j. Men experience a decreased production of androgens, such as testosterone, that results in decreased vigor and sexual desire (**male menopause, manopause,** and **andropause**); usually occurs between the ages of 45 and 55.

2. Psychosocial.

   a. Continuation of resolving the conflict of generativity versus self-absorption.

   b. Middle years are rewarding if previous stages are fulfilled.

   c. Responsibility of raising children declines; less financial strain once childbearing expenses are completed.

   d. Often at height of career; may be leader in field.

   e. Self-realization generally achieved as evidenced by more inner direction, no longer feeling the need to please everyone, being less likely to compare self with others, and approval of self without being dependent on standards of others.

3. Cognitive.

   a. Begins to experience declining memory around 50 years.

b. Takes longer to learn new tasks and takes longer to perform old tasks.

c. Experiences increased practical judgment due to experiential background.

d. May tend to withdraw from mental activity or overcompensate by attempting the impossible.

4. Language: Has fully developed language.

5. Play.

a. May participate in or enjoy watching sports activities.

b. Engages in socialization with peers.

c. Enjoys playing with own children or grandchildren.

6. Reaction to illness, hospitalization, and pain. For additional information see "Adults" in Table 15.1 "Developmental Variations Associated with Pain and Related Nursing Care" in Chapter 15, Pain, Comfort, Rest, and Sleep.

a. Sensorimotor decline exaggerated by illness results in heightened feelings of aging.

b. Illness and recuperation may be prolonged due to reduced physiological and emotional adaptive capacity.

c. Illness occurring at this time of decreasing family responsibilities may lead to self-absorption and isolation.

d. Illness at height of one's career may promote denial and delay seeking medical attention; may produce resistance to hospitalization and curtail time necessary for recuperation.

B. Nursing care

1. Encourage expression of frustrations of attempting to meet life's goals and voicing of concerns about the meaning and purpose of the rest of one's life.

2. Assist with goal setting that is realistic and attainable.

3. Focus on individual strengths rather than weaknesses; support ego strengths.

4. Encourage productive communication with mate and close friends.

5. Help to identify areas of meddling in their children's or close friend's lives; assist development of ways of coping with concerns for others in an objective and positive manner.

6. Encourage reaching out to others and giving assistance rather than isolating self.

7. Encourage expression of feelings about the empty nest syndrome, if a concern.

8. Teach to maintain intake of appropriate nutrition. For additional information see Nursing Care number 7 under "Adult" in this chapter and "Adults" in Table 20.4 "Nutritional Variations Across the Life Span and Related Nursing Care" in Chapter 20, Nutrition.

9. Teach ways to prevent injury. See reasons why adults are at risk for injury under "Age" in "Factors That Influence Client Safety" in Chapter 1, Safety.

a. Sports: See Nursing Care number 8 under "Adult" in this chapter.

b. Falls.

(1) Avoid turning and altering position quickly due to a decline in sensorium and balance.

(2) Eliminate cluttered environment.

IX. Older Adult (Early Late Years)

Older adults (early late years) are between 65 and 79 years of age. Their physical abilities continue to decline, and they are beginning to address the issues of satisfaction or dissatisfaction with their past and contentment or fear of the future.

A. Development

1. Physical.

a. Continued decrease in vigor and capacity; more frequent aches and pains.

b. Seventy percent rate themselves as healthy, but likely to have at least one major illness.

c. Changes in vision, hearing, sensation (e.g., touch, taste, and smell), posture, muscle strength, cardiovascular and neurological functioning, and endurance as well as orthostatic hypotension may result in falls.

d. The ability to metabolize and excrete drugs decrease, increasing the risk of drug toxicity.

2. Psychosocial.

a. Confronted with resolving the conflict of ego integrity versus despair.

b. May be satisfied with life and able to accept personal strengths and weaknesses.

c. May be remorseful for what might have been, dissatisfied with the present, and fearful of the future, resulting in despair; reminisces.

d. Personality does not change, but may become more exaggerated.

e. May have intense feelings of aging and mortality when confronted with the reality of physical and mental changes.

f. Is adjusting to aging, decreased health, maintenance of quality of life, retirement, fixed income, death of spouse and friends, and change in residence.

g. May be more interested in utilizing own inner resources and less interested in obtaining rewards of society; feels a right to do what is important for self-satisfaction.

h. May become focused on bodily needs and comforts.

i. Feels sexual expression (e.g., love, touching, sharing, intercourse) is important and related to identity.

j. May provide moral support to grandchildren and be more tolerant of grandchildren than they were of own children.

k. Releases major authority of family to children while holding self in role of consultant.

l. Majority live in the community; increasingly more live in assisted living facilities.

3. Cognitive.
   a. IQ does not decrease, but mental acuity slows.
   b. Judgment and problem-solving remain intact, but processes may take longer.
   c. Long-term memory is better than short-term memory.

4. Language.
   a. Has fully developed language.
   b. May take longer to access words from memory.

5. Play.
   a. May engage in less physically demanding sports, such as golf, or watch sports activities.
   b. Engages in socialization with peers, although this declines as friends move away or die.
   c. May enjoy watching grandchildren play.

6. Reaction to illness, hospitalization, and pain. For additional information see "Older adults" in Table 15.1 "Developmental Variations Associated with Pain and Related Nursing Care" in Chapter 15, Pain, Comfort, Rest, and Sleep.
   a. Has longer recuperation from illnesses secondary to decreased adaptive capacity.
   b. Has increased feelings of inadequacy and mortality.
   c. May experience frustration, anger, depression, and self-pity due to illness that limits or interferes with deserved goals of retirement or enjoyment of "golden years."
   d. May react to unfamiliar environments with confusion, anxiety, or fear.
   e. May feel dependent or hopeless due to chronic illness, pain, or impending death.
   f. May have increased feelings of isolation and fear of death due to illness; may accept and prepare for death.

B. Nursing care
   1. Provide nursing care for older adults experiencing common problems associated with aging (Table 10.2).

Table 10.2 Common Problems Associated With Aging and Related Nursing Care	
Problem	**Related Nursing Care**
Dehydration	
• *Results from inadequate intake of fluid due to a decline in the thirst mechanism located in the hypothalamus.* • *Results from restricted fluid intake to minimize urinary frequency related to stress incontinence in women and prostate hyperplasia in men.*	• *Teach to drink the equivalent of eight glasses of fluid daily; may be consumed in smaller amounts at a time.* • *Explain the reason for and encourage intake of fluid despite urinary/toileting inconveniences; explain that deficient fluid volume can result in a urinary tract infection and systemic sepsis requiring hospitalization; systemic sepsis can be life-threatening.*
Bowel and Bladder Incontinence	
• *Incontinence is not part of the aging process.* • *It may be aggravated by decreased muscle tone of anal and urinary sphincters and prostatic hyperplasia.*	• *Ensure screenings for urinary tract infection and bladder or prostate cancer.* • *Assist with hygiene and skin care.* • *Institute bowel and bladder retraining.*
Adverse Drug Effects	
• *Multiple health problems require an increase in prescriptions (polypharmacy), commonly with decreased coordination among primary health-care providers.* • *Decreased hepatic and renal function can result in accumulation, drug toxicity, and increased paradoxical effects.*	• *Coordinate care among health-care team members.* • *Identify unnecessary or excessive doses of medications; explore medications that may be discontinued, changed to a lower dose, or substituted by a less-toxic drug.* • *Assess for adverse or toxic effects.* • *Teach the client to read over-the-counter drug labels to avoid accidental overdose when taking multiple products.*
Cognitive Impairment	
Not part of the aging process. • *Delirium: Acute decrease in cognition; potentially reversible; associated with acute illness.*	• *Provide a safe, nonstimulating, familiar environment with consistent routines and caregiver.* • *Use a calm, unhurried, nondemanding approach.*

Table 10.2 **Common Problems Associated With Aging and Related Nursing Care—cont'd**

Problem	Related Nursing Care
Clinical manifestations: Lability of mood; fear; delusions; increased pulse, respirations, and blood pressure; hallucinations; illusions; disorientation; dilated pupils; diaphoresis; sleep disturbance; tremors. • ***Dementia:*** *Chronic, progressive, irreversible disorder; progresses from mild to severe; ultimately requires total care.* *Clinical manifestations: Intellectual decline, such as decreased short-term memory, language, insight, and judgment; self-preoccupation; can be passive, as evidenced by flat affect and decreased spontaneity or irritability, as evidenced by sarcasm, decreased concern for others, and paranoia.* • ***Sundowning syndrome:*** *Thought to be associated with disturbance in circadian rhythms; associated with seasonal affective disorder and depression.* *Clinical manifestations: Agitation, confusion, and disorientation in late afternoon and evening.*	• *Consider the client's mood and easy distractibility when planning care.* • *Reorient to time, place, and person; use simple language and visual clues.* • *Promote independence within ability; assist with activities of daily living.* • *Encourage reminiscing about earlier years.* • *Identify events that increase agitation, such as environmental stimuli, altered routines, strangers, increased expectations, and "lost" items.* • *Involve in simple, repetitive tasks and one-on-one activities.* • *Promote involvement in therapy, such as music and pet therapy, and current events.* • *Support primary caregivers and encourage periodic respite care.*
Alcohol Misuse	
• *Develops secondary to depression, loneliness, and lack of social support.*	• *Explore effective coping strategies.* • *Refer the client to Alcoholics Anonymous.*
Risk of Suicide	
• *Occurs secondary to multiple losses, such as loss of loved ones and health, and lack of social support.* • *20% of older adults experience depression, feelings of hopelessness, and isolation.*	• *Assess for suicide risk.* • *Provide reality orientation, validation therapy, and reminiscence.* • *Support body image.* • *Encourage psychological counseling.* • *Obtain a prescription for an antidepressant.* • *Refer the client to social services for home-care services.*
Decreased Sexual Response and Erectile Dysfunction	
• *Sexual response takes longer due to decreased testosterone and estrogen, chronic health problems, and medications.* • *Can occur secondary to unavailable partner or cognitive impairment.*	• *Provide privacy, support dignity and nonjudgmental attitude.* • *Encourage expression of concerns.* • *Suggest lubricant, penile prostheses, or medication to promote erection, as applicable.*
Sexually Transmitted Infections	
• *Need for sexual expression continues.* • *Increased society recognition that sexual activity is natural and acceptable, even if single by choice or after death of spouse.*	• *Maintain a nonjudgmental attitude.* • *Teach about sexually transmitted infection prevention.*

2. Understand commonalities of aging, but approach each person as unique; avoid stereotyping because it denies uniqueness, decreases access to health care, and impacts negatively on the individual.

🛑 3. Encourage an older adult to express feelings about aging; facilitate feelings of pride in self-integrity.

4. Ensure access to health care and social services, especially in the home.

5. Encourage ongoing follow-up medical care and health promotion and illness prevention activities within the client's abilities; provide aggressive treatment for critical illnesses, if desired.

6. Assess for digestive or intestinal disturbances, such as gastric acidity and constipation, that occur with aging.

7. Encourage engagement in self-satisfying endeavors.

8. Encourage the client to seek harmony in relationships with significant others.

9. Encourage social involvement outside the home.

10. Accept an older adult's need for love and belonging and to have sexual needs met; provide for privacy, and encourage exploration of medications or devices to minimize dysfunction.

11. Help others to see that older adults deserve dignity and respect.

12. Teach to maintain appropriate nutrition. For additional information see "Older Adults" in Table 20.4 "Nutritional Variations Across the Life

Span and Related Nursing Care" in Chapter 20, Nutrition.

   a. Have multiple small meals or between-meal snacks to ensure adequate intake of calories.

   b. Use spices other than salt to compensate for a decline in taste and smell.

   c. Reduce caloric intake because metabolic and activity levels decline.

   d. Encourage daily dental hygiene and to visit a dentist regularly.

   e. If experiencing difficulty with shopping or cooking, seek assistance of community agencies that can help shop, serve, or deliver meals to the home; if on a limited income, apply for food stamps or seek assistance from community food banks.

   f. Maintain adequate intake of fiber and fluid and reduce intake of high-fat foods to promote fecal elimination; discourage use of laxatives and enemas because they can become habitual.

13. Teach ways to prevent injury.
See reasons why older adults are at risk for injury under "Age" in "Factors That Influence Client Safety" in Chapter 1, Safety.

   a. Falls.

     (1) Follow safety precautions, such as using grab bars, railings, and walkers; rising slowly; and keeping feet apart for a wide base of support.

     (2) Use ambulation assistive devices, as indicated.

     (3) Remove scatter rugs from the home environment.

   b. Motor vehicles.

     (1) Assess ability to drive (e.g., vision, hearing, sensation in feet, reflexes, judgment).

     🛑 (2) **Encourage the older adult to give up driving when impairment jeopardizes the safety of self or others; encourage family members to take away car keys if the individual is incompetent to drive.**

X. Older Adult (Later Years)

Older adults (later years) are 80 years and older. Their physiological abilities continue to decline and may progress to the point that they are frail, their psychosocial environment narrows significantly, and they begin to address the inevitability of death.

A. Development

  1. Physical.

    a. Experience additional sensory problems, including diminished sensation to touch and pain.

    b. Are at risk for falls due to diminished physical and sensorial abilities and orientation to space and sense of balance.

    c. Experience more acute and chronic health problems.

    d. May experience decreased control of urinary and anal sphincters, resulting in incontinence, due to illness.

  2. Psychosocial.

    a. Continuation of the conflict of ego integrity versus despair; continues to reflect on past life and comes to terms with self.

    b. Few significant relationships remain; death of friends, family, and associates and an increased inability to leave the home cause isolation.

    c. Dependence, hopelessness, and helplessness may occur in response to significant impairment of adaptive responses and structural and functional alterations associated with aging.

    d. May be preoccupied with immediate bodily needs and personal comforts; gastrointestinal tract frequently becomes a major focus.

    e. May provide others with an example of wisdom and courage.

    f. May be concerned with own mortality; may cope with process of dying and prepare for own death.

  3. Cognitive.

    a. Has better memory for past than present; repetition of memories occurs.

    b. May use confabulation to fill in memory gaps; forgetfulness may lead to safety problems.

    c. Increased arteriosclerosis may lead to mental illness, such as organic brain syndrome.

  4. Language.

    a. Has fully developed language.

    b. May take longer to access words from memory.

  5. Reaction to illness, hospitalization, and pain.
For additional information see "Older adults" in Table 15.1 "Developmental Variations Associated with Pain and Related Nursing Care" in Chapter 15, Pain, Comfort, Rest, and Sleep.

    a. May experience helplessness and despair because of multiple health problems and impairments causing dependence.

    b. May become egocentric due to a significant decline in physical and mental status, producing behavior that is demanding, inflexible, irritable, hostile, and suspicious.

    c. May experience confusion, disorientation, anxiety, and fear in response to hospitalization.

    d. May have feelings of relief that life is nearly over.

B. Nursing care

  1. Encourage independence with activities of daily living within abilities and assist as needed; praise accomplishments.

  2. Provide constant supervision as needed.

  3. Allow the client to proceed at own pace; support personal-care rituals.

4. Follow bowel and bladder routine or training, if appropriate.
5. Orient to time, place, and person as needed; keep a clock and calendar in view.
6. Ask questions about the past to foster reminiscence; avoid becoming annoyed when the client is repetitious.
7. Allow the client to explore the meaning of life and listen to expressed feelings in a nonjudgmental manner.
8. Provide for dignity, such as pulling curtains and draping the client when providing direct care.
9. Support dying individuals in accordance with desires, religious convictions, and beliefs.
10. Facilitate visits by a pastoral counselor of choice if desired by the client.
11. Support family members so that they are capable of helping a dying relative.
    See "Nursing Care for Family Members of a Client Who is Dying" in Chapter 13, Grief and Loss.
12. Teach to maintain appropriate nutrition.
    See Nursing Care number 12 under "Older Adult (Early Late Years)" in this chapter and "Older adults" in Table 20.4 "Nutritional Variations Across the Life Span and Related Nursing Care" in Chapter 20, Nutrition.

13. Teach ways to prevent injury.
    See reasons why older adults are at risk for injury under "Age" in "Factors That Influence Client Safety" in Chapter 1, Safety.
    a. Falls.
       (1) Use hand rails, shower seats, and raised toilets to support safety.
       (2) Use grab bars, railings, and a cane or walker as needed for ambulation.
       (3) Rise slowly.
       (4) Keep feet apart for a wide base of support; encourage wearing sturdy shoes.
       (5) Suggest bed or chair alarms, bed bolsters, or mattresses on floor next to bed, if necessary.
    b. Polypharmacy.
       (1) Consult with the primary health-care provider before taking over-the-counter medications.
       (2) Ensure that the primary health-care provider is notified of all medications prescribed by other primary health-care providers.
       (3) Take medications only for the length of time prescribed; discard unused medications.
       (4) Encourage the use of a pill box organizer to simplify taking medications and provide a visual cue when medications were not taken on time.

CASE STUDY: Putting It All Together

A public health nurse makes an initial home visit to assess the needs of a 75-year-old woman who was discharged after surgery for a fractured hip. She moved permanently into her daughter's home. The daughter has a 10-month-old infant who was born 6 weeks premature, a 3-year-old toddler, and a 5-year-old child. The daughter's husband works in another state and comes home every other weekend for 2 days. During the home visit, the public health nurse assesses all the children as well as the grandmother. The assessment findings are as follows:

Infant
• Turns from abdomen to back and from back to abdomen
• Is not sitting, crawling, or pulling self up to a standing position
• Is not using a pincer grasp
• Holds on to mother and refuses to go to nurse
• Reacts to simple commands
• Enjoys peek-a-boo

Toddler
• Has 14 teeth
• Has made no progress with daytime bladder and bowel control

• Sucks thumb while holding a security blanket
• Is fearful of loud noises
• Is always saying "mine" and "no"

5-Year-Old
• Needs help with dressing and undressing
• Climbs stairs using the right foot first for each step
• Hops on two feet, but not on one
• Is unable to tie shoes
• Does not print letters
• Takes pride in accomplishments
• Is difficult to understand when speaking
• Has a limited vocabulary
• Fears temperature and ear examinations

75-Year-Old Grandmother
• States that she is not as strong as she once was
• States "My groin is itchy."
• States that she is fearful of falling and is using a walker
• States that she has been depressed since her husband died 6 months ago and since losing her home

continued.

CASE STUDY: Putting It All Together   cont'd

Case Study Questions

A. Which assessments of the 10-month-old indicate that the infant is meeting developmental norms? Which assessments indicate a developmental delay?

Assessments that meet developmental norms include:

1. _____

2. _____

3. _____

4. _____

Assessments that indicate a developmental delay include:

1. _____

2. _____

3. _____

B. The nurse collects and analyzes the data related to the toddler. Which data are typically associated with toddlers and which are a cause for concern?

Data typically associated with toddlers include:

1. _____

2. _____

3. _____

Data that raise a cause for concern include:

1. _____

2. _____

C. Identify four clusters of data related to growth and development delays in the 5-year-old, and list nursing interventions planned to address each cluster.

1. _____

2 _____

3. _____

4. _____

D. Identify nursing interventions the nurse should implement to address the needs of the grandmother before leaving the home.

1. _____

2. _____

3. _____

4. _____

5. _____

6. _____

REVIEW QUESTIONS

Be sure to read the Introduction for valuable test-taking tips.

1. Preoperative teaching was performed for a 4-year-old child regarding elective surgery. Which is the **least** appropriate method to assess if the teaching was effective?
   1. Ask the child to repeat what the nurse said.
   2. Have the child write down what was learned.
   3. Provide a coloring book for the child to draw what was taught.
   4. Use role-playing so that the child can demonstrate what is going to be done.

2. A nurse is planning a health promotion program for a group of middle-aged adults. Which topic is **most** appropriate for this age-group?
   1. Stress management
   2. Importance of exercise
   3. Adequate nutritional intake
   4. Maintenance of a safe home environment

3. A nurse is caring for a chronically ill freshman college student who is 21 years old. The student experienced numerous hospital admissions over the years and long convalescent periods, delaying educational goals. Which personal characteristics of the client may interfere with the achievement of the developmental task associated with young adulthood? **Select all that apply.**
   1. Accepts limitations
   2. Delays gratification
   3. Occupied with self-absorption
   4. Concerned about an altered body image
   5. Struggling to establish a place in society
   6. Attempting to perform own activities of daily living

4. Which information should the nurse consider when planning and implementing nursing care for toddlers? **Select all that apply.**
   1. Friends are important.
   2. Dependency is desired.
   3. Rituals are comforting.
   4. Pain can precipitate regression.
   5. Organized group play is preferred.

5. Which educational intervention is **most** specific to teaching older adults?
   1. Teaching about safety precautions in the home environment
   2. Providing suggestions about maintaining a healthy diet
   3. Presenting strategies to avoid the empty nest syndrome
   4. Exploring actions that support a healthy lifestyle

6. A nurse is caring for an adolescent admitted to the hospital for multiple fractures in a lower extremity requiring a large external fixation device. Which nursing intervention is **most** important when planning care for this adolescent?
   1. Encourage expression of concerns about outcomes of the injury.
   2. Suggest playing a complex board game with another client.
   3. Allow as much self-care as possible.
   4. Cover the leg with a bedspread.

7. A nurse is caring for a 20-year-old college student who is scheduled for outpatient surgery to revise an unattractive scar on the arm. During preoperative teaching, the client shares having anxious feelings. From whom does the nurse anticipate the client will benefit **most** when the person is providing emotional support?
   1. Professor
   2. Friends
   3. Parents
   4. Sibling

8. A nurse is assessing the developmental level of a toddler. Which activities does the nurse determine are beyond this child's ability? **Select all that apply.**
   1. Tying shoelaces
   2. Riding a tricycle
   3. Completing multiple chores
   4. Beginning control of elimination
   5. Walking up steps without assistance

9. A nurse is assessing the developmental level of a preschool-aged child (3–5 years of age). Which behaviors can the nurse expect to identify? **Select all that apply.**
   1. Making change for small amounts of money
   2. Playing a game of catch with a small ball
   3. Using words within complete sentences
   4. Investing energy in having a collection
   5. Engaging in group play

10. A nurse is assessing the developmental level of an adolescent (12–18 years). What developmental changes can the nurse generally expect? **Select all that apply.**
    1. Feeling independent from parents
    2. Demonstrating concern for personal appearance
    3. Exploring interests that may evolve into a career plan
    4. Beginning determination of one's own beliefs and values
    5. Working toward developing a mature relationship with another person

11. A nurse is presenting a class on infant development and care to a group of adolescents who are learning to be babysitters. Which statements by participants indicate that further teaching is necessary? **Select all that apply.**
    1. "I can cuddle a baby if crying occurs when being put down to sleep."
    2. "I should burp a baby frequently when feeding a bottle."
    3. "I can allow an infant to bite on a spoon when teething."
    4. "I may gently shake a baby to get its attention."
    5. "I must place a baby on the back for sleeping."

12. A nurse is caring for a group of children ranging in age from infancy to adolescence. The nurse considers the psychosocial task associated with each child's developmental level. Place the nursing intervention specifically associated with each developmental level progressing from infancy through adolescence.
    1. Encourage independence.
    2. Recognize accomplishments.
    3. Support a positive self-concept.
    4. Provide activities within abilities.
    5. Meet physical needs immediately.
    Answer _____

13. An older adult who was hospitalized has been experiencing sundowning syndrome. What interventions should the nurse include in the client's plan of care? **Select all that apply.**
    1. Follow the preset daily routine.
    2. Hurry through direct client care.
    3. Provide a nonstimulating environment.
    4. Explain in detail what care will be performed.
    5. Use a motion sensor device on the client's bed.

14. A nurse is obtaining a health history and performing a physical assessment of an older adult. Which clinical manifestations associated with aging should the nurse expect? **Select all that apply.**
    1. Impaired balance
    2. Close vision impairment
    3. Diminished muscle strength
    4. Intermittent urinary incontinence
    5. Decreased hearing of low-pitched sounds

15. Which statement by an adult child about the adult child's 90-year-old father indicates ageism?
    1. "My father was always egocentric, but it has gotten worse as he has gotten older."
    2. "My father's physical status has progressively declined these last few years."
    3. "I am so tired of him constantly talking about past experiences."
    4. "I would rather die than reach the useless age of my father."

16. A nurse in the child health clinic is assessing a preschool-aged child. Which behaviors that may indicate a developmental delay should the nurse bring to the attention of the primary health-care provider? **Select all that apply.**
    1. Goes up and down stairs using both feet on each step
    2. Is unable to dress self without assistance
    3. Has imprecise fine motor skills
    4. Uses magical thinking
    5. Falls frequently

17. For which physical changes associated with aging should a nurse assess when assisting an older adult with a bath? **Select all that apply.**
    1. Increased sweat gland activity
    2. Decreased pigment cells in hair
    3. Decreased vascularity of the skin
    4. Increased sebaceous gland activity
    5. Increased collagen fibers in the dermis

18. A nurse identifies that a client is experiencing a developmental crisis specifically associated with middle adulthood. Which assessment identified by the nurse supports this conclusion?
    1. Inability to postpone satisfaction
    2. Incapable of facing one's mortality
    3. Problems maintaining peer relationships
    4. Difficulty achieving a sense of fulfillment

19. What safety instruction addresses a major cause of accidental death among people from all developmental levels?
    1. Resist pressure to engage in high-risk activities.
    2. Rise slowly to a standing position.
    3. Wear a seatbelt when in a car.
    4. Cut all food into small pieces.

20. A nurse is teaching a group of parents of school-aged children about motor vehicle accidents and child safety. Which information is **most** important for the nurse to include in this program?
    1. Front passenger seats can be occupied by children when they weigh more than 110 lb.
    2. Ensure that safety seats are appropriate for the height and weight of the child.
    3. Children 14 years of age should ride in the back seat of a vehicle.
    4. Children 4 to 10 years of age should use a booster seat.

21. A hospitalized older adult who has an allergy attack and diphenhydramine (Benadryl) 50 mg by mouth every 4 hours is prescribed. The client experiences extreme drowsiness and the nurse calls the primary health-care provider. The nurse is instructed to give one-half the present dose when the next dose is due. Since the diphenhydramine is in the form of a capsule that cannot be cut in half, the nurse acquires diphenhydramine elixir that states that there is 12.5 mg per 5 mL. How much solution should the nurse administer? **Record your answer using a whole number.**

Answer: _____ mL

22. A nurse is caring for an 18-month-old child. Which behaviors are expected when assessing the child playing? **Select all that apply.**
1. Amusing self for brief periods of time
2. Playing interactively with another child
3. Being fanatical about rules in a game
4. Unwilling to share a favorite toy
5. Cheating to win a game

23. A nurse is planning a health promotion program for school-aged children. Which information is **most** important for the nurse to include in this program?
1. Encouraging nutritious snacks
2. Demonstrating how to care for teeth
3. Reporting bullying to a responsible adult
4. Seeking medical care for sexually transmitted infections

24. An 19-year-old male college student goes to the local urgent care center on 4/8/2017. The student visited the center several times in the last year. The nurse reviews the student's clinic file, reviews the primary health-care provider's diagnosis and prescriptions for the present clinic visit, and interviews the student. Which statement by the nurse is **most** appropriate?
1. "If you are not worried about yourself, at least think about your partner."
2. "I will have to notify local health authorities about your infection."
3. "Let's talk about how you can protect yourself in the future."
4. "Consider what this is doing to your future health."

Client's Clinic File

9/10/2016: Greenish-yellow penile discharge, swollen painful testes; gonorrhea; single dose ceftriaxone (Rocephin) 250 mg IM
11/2/2016: Thick yellow penile discharge, burning on urination; gonorrhea; single dose ceftriaxone (Rocephin) 250 mg IM

Primary Health-Care Provider: Diagnosis and Prescriptions

Client has chancre on shaft of penis; enlarged, nontender lymph node in right groin; primary syphilis; single dose of benzathine penicillin G 2.4 million units IM.

Client Interview

Now that I am away from home, I can do what I want. I've been having a good time. I love girls; the more the merrier. Last time, the nurse said I could have complications from an infection, but I'm healthy and that is not going to happen to me. I don't know what the big deal is. If I get an infection, it can be cured with a shot.

25. A public health nurse is visiting an 80-year-old widow who recently was discharged from a rehabilitation center after recovering from a fall. The woman shares that her three children and their families live several states away. The nurse identifies that the client looks fatigued, uses a walker to get around the house, and lives independently in her own home. She receives a little help from the community in the way of supermarket deliveries and a cleaning person who comes every other week. Which should the nurse identify as the main concern?
1. Risk for falls
2. Potential for loneliness
3. Decline in distant memory
4. Hopelessness regarding the situation

26. A nurse must perform a physical assessment of a 5-year-old child. What is the **best** way to prepare the child for the assessment?
1. Answer all of the questions asked by the child.
2. Show the child a video of another child having an examination.
3. Have one parent explain to the child what will be done during the examination.
4. Let the child play with the equipment that will be used during the physical assessment.

27. A nurse is teaching new parents about care of their newborn. What should the nurse teach them to do to prevent the leading cause of accidental death in infants?
    1. "Give your infant toys that are bigger than an adult's clenched fist."
    2. "Place your infant in a five-point infant seat when in an automobile."
    3. "Support your infant when placed on an elevated surface."
    4. "Position your infant on the back when sleeping."

28. A school nurse is planning a class about safety precautions for a group of parents who have children between the ages of 7 and 10 years. What information should the nurse include in the teaching plan? **Select all that apply.**
    1. "Supervise stretching exercises before your child engages in physical activities."
    2. "Check your child's toys to ensure that they are larger than a clenched fist."
    3. "Select activities that are appropriate for your child's developmental level."
    4. "Provide a five-point safety seat for your child when in the car."
    5. "Ensure that your child wears a seat belt when in the car."

29. A nurse is teaching a class on home safety to a group of parents of children younger than 4 years of age. Which interventions should the nurse include in the class? **Select all that apply.**
    1. Cut up firm foods into half-inch pieces.
    2. Install toilet lid locks on all toilets in the home.
    3. Ensure that crib slats are greater than three inches apart.
    4. Supervise balloon play and discard burst balloons immediately.
    5. Use a forward-facing car seat when body weight exceeds the recommendation for a rear-facing seat.

30. A nurse is planning a class about safety precautions for a group of parents who have toddlers. What information should the nurse include in the teaching plan? **Select all that apply.**
    1. Position them on the back when sleeping.
    2. Attend toddlers when on elevated surfaces.
    3. Use a rear-facing car seat until 4 years of age.
    4. Keep plastic inserts in unused electrical outlets.
    5. Turn pot handles toward the back of stove when cooking.

31. A nurse educator is preparing a health curriculum for high school students. Which content should be included in the program that addresses the leading cause of physical injury during adolescence?
    1. Driver education
    2. Anger management
    3. Alcohol and drug use
    4. Irresponsible water safety

32. A nurse is preparing a health promotion and illness prevention class for a group of parents of young school-aged children. Which information should the nurse include in the program to help prevent sensory disturbances in children in this age-group? **Select all that apply.**
    1. Obtain rubella, mumps, and measles vaccinations at recommended ages.
    2. Discourage sports that use sticks, such as hockey and lacrosse.
    3. Seek regular eye examinations to screen for eye problems.
    4. Allow use of pointed scissors only when sitting at a table.
    5. Encourage the use of sunglasses with UV protection.

33. A school nurse is teaching a group of high school students about safety precautions. What should the nurse include in the teaching session that addresses the leading cause of accidental deaths in adolescents?
    1. Use a seatbelt when riding in a car.
    2. Engage in sports that are within your physical abilities.
    3. Wear a life preserver when engaging in water-related activities.
    4. Resist peer pressure to participate in experimenting with illegal drugs.

34. A nurse is preparing a safety program for parents about accidental poisoning. What information should the nurse include concerning what to do in the event a toddler ingests a poison?
    1. Have the child drink salt water.
    2. Administer ipecac immediately.
    3. Take the child to an emergency department.
    4. Seek guidance from a poison control center.

35. A school nurse is teaching a third-grade class about safety precautions. What should the nurse include in the teaching session? **Select all that apply.**
    1. Run in the opposite direction if approached by a stranger to go someplace.
    2. Take a bicycle safety course when you get a two-wheeled bicycle.
    3. Get instructions before using equipment for the first time.
    4. Use a regular car seatbelt when you reach fifty pounds.
    5. Stop, drop, and roll if your clothes are on fire.

36. A nurse is preparing a program regarding health promotion for healthy individuals who are middle-aged adults. Which information is important to include regarding the prevention of injury? **Select all that apply.**
    1. Avoiding alcohol when planning to drive
    2. Doing warm-up exercises before engaging in sports
    3. Maintaining an exercise program to increase endurance
    4. Assisting with setting challenging and demanding goals
    5. Encouraging instillation of grab bars in bathrooms to assist rising to a standing position

37. A nurse is teaching a health promotion class for a group of recently retired older adults. Which information should be included to help reduce the risk of the major cause of physical injury in older adults?
    1. Remove throw rugs from the home.
    2. Look both ways before crossing a street.
    3. Do warm-up exercises before engaging in sports.
    4. Read the label of an over-the-counter drug before taking it.

38. A nurse is teaching a group of children about the importance of firearm safety because of the severity of unintentional firearm injuries involving children. Place the steps in the order that children should take when they see a gun.
    1. Tell an adult.
    2. Don't touch it.
    3. Leave the area.
    4. Stop the activity.
    5. Identify the presence of a gun.
    Answer _____

39. A nurse is teaching a class to parents of toddlers about how to reduce the risk of suffocation, asphyxiation, or drowning. What information should the nurse include in this program? **Select all that apply.**
    1. Ensure that slats of cribs are less than 2⅜ inches wide.
    2. Provide toys that are at least 2 inches in diameter.
    3. Avoid toy boxes with heavy hinged lids.
    4. Keep venetian blind cords out of reach.
    5. Use only light blankets when sleeping.

40. A nurse is teaching a group of older adults about safety precautions. What instruction should the nurse give them to prevent the leading cause of injuries in older adults?
    1. Have your vision evaluated yearly.
    2. Limit drinking alcohol to one glass a day.
    3. Rise slowly when moving from a sitting to a standing position.
    4. Wash your hands with an antimicrobial soap several times a day.

REVIEW ANSWERS AND RATIONALES

1. **ANSWER: 2.**

   Rationales:

   1. A 4-year-old child probably will be able to repeat what was taught. However, the nurse should assess the child further to determine understanding, not just recall.

   2. A 4-year-old child does not have the manipulative or cognitive skills to write down what was learned.

   3. Using a coloring book to assess knowledge is an appropriate intervention. A child of this age can manipulate a crayon and is probably familiar with this type activity.

   4. Role-playing is an appropriate intervention. A child of this age likes to imitate others.

   TEST-TAKING TIP: Identify the word in the stem that indicates negative polarity. The word *least* in the stem indicates negative polarity.

   Content Area: *Development Across the Life Span*
   Integrated Processes: *Teaching/Learning; Nursing Process: Evaluation*
   Client Need: *Health Promotion and Maintenance*
   Cognitive Level: *Application*
   Concept: *Growth and Development*

2. **ANSWER: 1.**

   Rationales:

   1. Middle-aged adults are faced with many stresses, including earning a living, supporting a family, paying for children's educational expenses, saving for retirement, and, for many middle-aged adults, caring for aging parents.

   2. Although learning about exercise is important for middle-aged adults, another option is more appropriate.

   3. Although learning about nutrition is important for middle-aged adults, another option is more appropriate.

   4. Maintaining a safe home environment is more appropriate for families with young children and for older adults who are more prone to falls than middle-aged adults.

   TEST-TAKING TIP: Identify the word in the stem that sets a priority. The word *most* in the stem sets a priority.

   Content Area: *Development Across the Life Span*
   Integrated Processes: *Teaching/Learning; Nursing Process: Planning*
   Client Need: *Health Promotion and Maintenance*
   Cognitive Level: *Application*
   Concept: *Health Promotion; Growth and Development*

3. **ANSWER: 3, 4.**

   Rationales:

   1. Accepting limitations enables a person to be realistic about career choices. This should not interfere with the developmental tasks associated with young adulthood.

   2. The ability to delay gratification is a responsible behavior and should not interfere with the resolution of the conflict of intimacy versus isolation, the conflict associated with young adulthood.

   3. Self-absorption may interfere with establishing an intimate relationship with another person, which is one of the developmental tasks of this age-group.

   4. When clients have concerns about altered body image, they may believe that they are no longer desirable. If this

belief is held by a young adult, the person may withdraw in an effort to protect the ego.

   5. Struggling to establish a place in society is expected in this age-group. It is part of the process of confronting the conflicts associated with young adulthood.

   6. Attempting to perform personal activities of daily living is responsible behavior expected of a young adult. This will not interfere with resolving the conflict of intimacy versus isolation associated with young adulthood.

   Content Area: *Development Across the Life Span*
   Integrated Processes: *Nursing Process: Analysis*
   Client Need: *Health Promotion and Maintenance*
   Cognitive Level: *Application*
   Concept: *Growth and Development*

4. **ANSWER: 3, 4.**

   Rationales:

   1. Socialization with peers is just beginning during the preschool years of 3 to 6. School-aged children 6 to 12 years of age learn to play in groups and develop special friendships, and adolescents 12 to 18 years of age are concerned with establishing close relationships with peers where they feel valued and accepted.

   2. Toddlers struggle for autonomy and independence, not to be dependent.

   3. Toddlers feel most comfortable with structured routines that are expected (e.g., a bedtime routine that the toddler can anticipate: having a bath, putting on pajamas, brushing the teeth, listening to a story, singing a song, and giving and receiving hugs and kisses). Knowing what to expect reduces anxiety.

   4. Hospitalization and pain are perceived as threats by toddlers. Toddlers often regress to earlier behaviors, such as clinging to a parent or using a pacifier, to help them cope with these stressors.

   5. Organized group play takes on significance for school-aged children 6 to 12 years of age.

   Content Area: *Development Across the Life Span*
   Integrated Processes: *Caring; Nursing Process: Planning*
   Client Need: *Health Promotion and Maintenance*
   Cognitive Level: *Application*
   Concept: *Growth and Development*

5. **ANSWER: 1.**

   Rationales:

   1. As older adults physically decline, they are prone to falls and accidents in the home environment. Prevention of falls and a safe home environment are essential to explore when teaching older adults.

   2. Maintaining a healthy diet is not specific to older adults. A healthy diet should be an educational focus for all age-groups.

   3. Presenting strategies to avoid the empty nest syndrome generally is specific to the late-middle-adult age-group as children leave home to pursue their educations or live independently. In addition, not everyone has children.

   4. Exploring actions that support a healthy lifestyle is not specific to older adults. Leading a healthy lifestyle should be an educational focus for all age-groups.

   TEST-TAKING TIP: Identify the word in the stem that sets a priority. The word *most* is the word in the stem

that sets a priority. Identify the equally plausible options. Options 2 and 4 are equally plausible. One is no better than the other because option 4 includes the concept in option 2.
Content Area: Development Across the Life Span
Integrated Processes: Teaching/Learning; Nursing Process: Planning
Client Need: Health Promotion and Maintenance
Cognitive Level: Application
Concept: Patient-Centered Care; Safety

6. ANSWER: 1.
Rationales:
1. Encouraging expression of feelings is critical in this age-group. Adolescents are concerned about body image and generally fear disfigurement or decreased function.
2. Although engaging the client in diversional activities is important, it is not the priority.
3. Although it is important to support independence, it is not as important as the action in another option.
4. A bedspread may be too heavy to rest on top of an external fixation device. If the client feels self-conscious about the apparatus, the nurse can place a draw sheet over a bed cradle to provide for privacy.
TEST-TAKING TIP: Identify the word in the stem that sets a priority. The word *most* in the stem sets a priority. Identify the clang association. The word *injury* in the stem and in option 1 is a clang association. Examine option 1 carefully.
Content Area: Development Across the Life Span
Integrated Processes: Caring; Communication and Documentation; Nursing Process: Planning
Client Need: Health Promotion and Maintenance
Cognitive Level: Application
Concept: Growth and Development

7. ANSWER: 2.
Rationales:
1. A professor is not the person who generally affords the most benefit when providing emotional support to a young adult. Professors are often placed in the same group as parents by young adults because they are seen as authority figures.
2. Friends are most important to a young adult. Generally, a young adult will benefit most from the emotional support provided by peers.
3. Young adults are beginning to separate from parents as they seek independence. Young adults are more likely to rely on a person identified in another option rather than parents.
4. More likely, the young adult will seek support from a person identified in another option rather than a sibling.
TEST-TAKING TIP: Identify the word in the stem that sets a priority. The word *most* in the stem sets a priority.
Content Area: Development Across the Life Span
Integrated Processes: Nursing Process: Analysis
Client Need: Health Promotion and Maintenance
Cognitive Level: Application
Concept: Growth and Development

8. ANSWER: 1, 3.
Rationales:
1. Toddlers do not have the fine motor skills necessary to tie shoelaces. This activity is beyond the ability of a toddler and usually accomplished by preschool-aged children (3 to 5 years of age).
2. Riding a tricycle is within the expected range of motor development for a toddler 12 to 36 months of age.
3. Completing multiple chores is beyond the developmental activities of a toddler. This behavior is associated with school-aged children 6 to 12 years of age.
4. Beginning control of elimination is within the expected physiological development of a toddler.
5. Walking up steps without assistance is within the expected range of motor development of a toddler.
TEST-TAKING TIP: Identify the words in the stem that indicate negative polarity. The words *beyond this child's ability* in the stem indicate negative polarity. The question is asking, "What activity is a toddler unable to do?"
Content Area: Development Across the Life Span
Integrated Processes: Nursing Process: Assessment
Client Need: Health Promotion and Maintenance
Cognitive Level: Application
Concept: Growth and Development

9. ANSWER: 3, 5.
Rationales:
1. Making change for small amounts of money is within the expected psychosocial development of a school-aged, not preschool-aged, child.
2. Throwing and catching a small ball is within the expected motor development of a school-aged, not preschool-aged, child.
3. Increasing vocabulary and using words in complete sentences are within the range of expected psychosocial development for a 3- to 5-year-old child (preschooler).
4. Having a collection or hobby is within the expected psychosocial development of a school-aged, not preschool-aged, child.
5. Preschool-aged children engage in group play (cooperative play, associative play) without rigid rules.
Content Area: Development Across the Life Span
Integrated Processes: Communication and Documentation; Nursing Process: Assessment
Client Need: Health Promotion and Maintenance
Cognitive Level: Application
Concept: Growth and Development

10. ANSWER: 2, 3, 4.
Rationales:
1. Feeling independent from parents occurs during young adulthood, not adolescence. Young adults demonstrate emotional, social, and economic responsibility for their own lives.
2. Adolescents generally are concerned about their personal appearance. Hair style, clothing, and skin care are important factors associated with adolescents as they search for self-identity.
3. Adolescents explore areas for their own learning as well as those that may interest them as a potential career.

4. Adolescents examine their values, beliefs, standards, and morals. They may discard those adopted from parents for those that they believe are more appropriate for themselves.

5. Developing a mature relationship with another person occurs during young adulthood, not adolescence. According to Erikson, the developmental task of young adulthood is intimacy versus isolation.

Content Area: Development Across the Life Span
Integrated Processes: Nursing Process: Assessment
Client Need: Health Promotion and Maintenance
Cognitive Level: Application
Concept: Growth and Development

11. ANSWER: 3, 4.

Rationales:

1. Cuddling and rocking will comfort a crying infant. Additional measures to comfort a crying infant include swaddling, finding the most comfortable position, and positioning the infant in a baby swing or vibrating chair.

2. An infant may swallow air when feeding, when sucking too quickly, or when having allergies. Frequent burping may help minimize associated abdominal/intestinal discomfort.

3. A spoon can cause injury and /or gagging if placed in the mouth of an infant. Only special objects designed for teething should be placed in the mouth of a teething infant.

4. An infant or young child should never be shaken, even gently, for any reason. Shaken baby syndrome (SBS) can cause a whiplash that may result in severe brain injury, especially in infants. Blindness, spinal cord damage, cerebral damage, subdural hematoma, and neurological impairments can occur.

5. Sleeping in the supine position is desirable. Research demonstrates that positioning an infant on the back, not prone, greatly decreases the risk of sudden infant death syndrome (SIDS).

TEST-TAKING TIP: Identify the words in the stem that indicate negative polarity. The words *further teaching* indicate negative polarity. The question is asking, "What should not be done when caring for an infant?"

Content Area: Development Across the Life Span
Integrated Processes: Teaching/Learning; Nursing Process: Evaluation
Client Need: Health Promotion and Maintenance
Cognitive Level: Application
Concept: Health Promotion; Growth and Development

12. ANSWER: 5, 1, 4, 2, 3.

Rationales:

5. The task of infancy is the development of trust. When basic physiological needs are met immediately, the infant feels safe and secure and develops trust.

1. The task of toddlerhood is the development of autonomy. Personal decision making and having independence (within parameters of safety) help to promote autonomy.

4. The task of preschoolers is the development of initiative. Successful completion of activities within one's abilities promotes motivation and initiative.

2. The task of school-aged children is industry. Learning new information and skills promotes being productive.

3. The task of adolescence is the development of a self-identity. Recognition from others and internal satisfaction with personal accomplishments help to promote a positive self-concept.

Content Area: Development Across the Life Span
Integrated Processes: Caring; Nursing Process: Analysis
Client Need: Safe and Effective Care Environment; Management of Care
Cognitive Level: Analysis
Concept: Growth and Development

13. ANSWER: 1, 3, 5.

Rationales:

1. Daily routines provide structure and repetition that limit the unknown. Clients are more in control and less anxious if they know what to expect regardless of the time of day, but particularly late afternoon or evening.

2. The opposite is true; an unhurried routine is less demanding and less likely to precipitate anxiety.

3. Fewer stimuli are better than a stimulating environment. Excessive stimuli precipitate confusion, increase anxiety, and exacerbate the sundowning syndrome.

4. Simple communication (e.g., declarative statements, short sentences with one noun and one verb) with just the essential information is less confusing.

5. A motion sensor will alarm if a client attempts to get out of bed. The alarm will alert the nurse so that supervision can be provided.

Content Area: Development Across the Life Span
Integrated Processes: Communication and Documentation; Nursing Process: Planning
Client Need: Health Promotion and Maintenance
Cognitive Level: Application
Concept: Cognition

14. ANSWER: 1, 2, 3.

Rationales:

1. Impaired balance is associated with aging because the spinal column begins to deteriorate and vertebral fractures and loss of cartilage between the vertebrae occur; these changes alter the center of gravity and body alignment, resulting in difficulty maintaining balance.

2. Close vision impairment (presbyopia) occurs because the lens becomes less elastic and is no longer able to accommodate to close objects.

3. Diminished muscle strength occurs because body and bone mass decrease. The effects of decreased joint mobility inhibit the ability to exercise to the extent possible when younger.

4. Urinary incontinence is not associated with aging; it is associated with urinary tract infections and decreased tone of the muscles in the pelvis. This can occur at any age, especially in women.

5. Decreased hearing of high-pitched sounds (presbycusis), not low-pitched sounds, occurs with aging because the hair cells in the cochlea deteriorate with aging.

Content Area: Development Across the Life Span
Integrated Processes: Nursing Process: Assessment
Client Need: Health Promotion and Maintenance
Cognitive Level: Application
Concept: Growth and Development

15. **ANSWER: 4.**
Rationales:
1. This may occur as people age and is referred to as an exacerbation of a person's premorbid personality. This statement does not reflect ageism.
2. All systems of the body gradually decrease in size and function as one ages (e.g., decreased mass and strength in both bones and muscles, decreased joint mobility, impaired balance and coordination). This statement does not reflect ageism.
3. The adult child may be frustrated by the father's behavior, but the adult child's statement is not a reflection of ageism.
4. This comment reflects ageism because it assumes older adults are useless. Ageism is negative attitudes and beliefs about older adults that include stereotyping, prejudice, or discrimination against people based on their age.
Content Area: Development Across the Life Span
Integrated Processes: Communication and Documentation; Nursing Process: Analysis
Client Need: Health Promotion and Maintenance
Cognitive Level: Application
Concept: Growth and Development

16. **ANSWER: 1, 2, 5.**
Rationales:
1. Climbing up and down steps using alternate feet, not using two feet on each step, is expected by 3 years of age.
2. A preschool-aged child should be able to don clothing without assistance, except for back-closing garments.
3. Imprecise fine motor skills are still obvious during the preschool-aged years (3 to 5 years of age) and the school-aged years (6 to 12 years).
4. Magical thinking is commonly associated with 3- to 5-year-old children.
5. Falling frequently is expected by a toddler, not a preschool-aged child.
TEST-TAKING TIP: Identify the words in the stem that indicate negative polarity. The words *behavior* and *developmental delay* are the key words in the stem that indicate negative polarity. The question is asking, "Which behaviors are not expected of a preschool-aged child?"
Content Area: Development Across the Life Span
Integrated Processes: Communication and Documentation; Nursing Process: Assessment
Client Need: Safe and Effective Care Environment; Management of Care
Cognitive Level: Application
Concept: Growth and Development

17. **ANSWER: 2, 3.**
Rationales:
1. Sweat gland activity decreases, not increases, with aging.
2. Hair turns white or gray because pigment cells in hair decrease as a person ages.
3. Decreased vascularity of the skin occurs with aging, causing coolness and pallor.
4. Sebaceous gland activity decreases, not increases, with aging.
5. Collagen and elastin in the dermis deteriorate with aging, causing the skin to become wrinkled.

TEST-TAKING TIP: Identify the equally plausible options. Options 1, 4, and 5 all refer to physiological processes that increase with aging. Options 2 and 3 refer to physiological processes that decrease with aging. Since aging is associated with a decline in many physiological processes, give special consideration to options 2 and 3 when attempting to answer this question.
Content Area: Development Across the Life Span
Integrated Processes: Nursing Process: Assessment
Client Need: Health Promotion and Maintenance
Cognitive Level: Application
Concept: Growth and Development

18. **ANSWER: 4.**
Rationales:
1. Children between the ages of 18 months and 3 years are concerned with learning how to delay satisfaction, not middle-aged adults.
2. Coping with death is one of the developmental tasks of older adults, not middle-aged adults.
3. Developing peer relationships is a developmental task of children who are 6 to 12 years of age as well as adolescents, not middle-aged adults.
4. The most important developmental task of middle adulthood is successfully achieving goals that involve family, career, and society. A developmental crisis occurs when a middle-aged adult has difficulty achieving these goals.
Content Area: Development Across the Life Span
Integrated Processes: Nursing Process: Analysis
Client Need: Health Promotion and Maintenance
Cognitive Level: Analysis
Concept: Growth and Development

19. **ANSWER: 3.**
Rationales:
1. Instructing a person to resist high-risk activities is most appropriate for adolescents who are vulnerable to peer pressure because they want to be accepted and belong.
2. Instructing a person to rise slowly to a standing position is most appropriate for older adults because their voluntary and autonomic reflexes have declined and made them vulnerable to orthostatic hypotension and falls.
3. The leading cause of accidental death in infants, toddlers, preschoolers, school-aged children, adolescents, and adults is motor vehicle accidents. Motor vehicle accidents are one of the leading causes of injuries in older adults after falls. Seatbelts reduce the incidence of morbidity and mortality.
4. Many foods are small or soft and do not need to be cut into small pieces. Although cutting food into small pieces is advisable for everyone, it is most significant in infants and toddlers. Risk for choking is the greatest between 6 months and 3 years of age.
TEST-TAKING TIP: Identify the option with a specific determiner. Option 4 contains the word *all*, which is a specific determiner. An option that contains a specific determiner rarely is the correct answer.
Content Area: Development Across the Life Span
Integrated Processes: Nursing Process: Implementation

Client Need: *Safe and Effective Care Environment; Safety and Infection Control*
Cognitive Level: *Analysis*
Concept: *Patient-Centered Care; Safety*

20. **ANSWER: 2.**

Rationales:
1. Children 12 years of age or younger, regardless of weight, should ride in the back seat of a vehicle. This action is associated with a 30% reduction in the risk of a fatal injury in a vehicular accident.
2. Age-, height-, and weight-appropriate automobile safety seats are essential to protect infants and children when in a motor vehicle accident.
3. This option does not indicate the weight of the child. If the child is 14 years of age and weighs greater than 110 pounds, the child may sit in the front seat. Children 12 years of age or younger and children older than 12 years of age but weighing less than 110 pounds should ride in the back seat of a vehicle.
4. Booster seats are safer than a seatbelt alone for average-size children 4 to 8 years of age, not 4 to 10 years of age. Children who are older than 4 years of age should not transition to a booster seat until they outgrow the criteria for using a five-point harness safety seat.
TEST-TAKING TIP: Identify the word in the stem that sets a priority. The word *most* in the stem sets a priority. Identify the unique option. Option 2 is unique because it is the only option that does not have a number. Identify the global option. Option 2 is global in that it is broad and all encompassing. Examine global options carefully.
Content Area: *Development Across the Life Span*
Integrated Processes: *Teaching/Learning; Nursing Process: Planning*
Client Need: *Safe and Effective Care Environment; Safety and Infection Control*
Cognitive Level: *Application*
Concept: *Health Promotion; Safety*

21. **ANSWER: 10.**

Rationale:
The ability to metabolize and excrete drugs decreases in older adults. Medications may require a reduction in the size of the dose to prevent toxicity. Solve the problem using ratio and proportion.

$$\frac{\text{Desire 25 mg}}{\text{Have 12.5 mg}} = \frac{x \text{ mL}}{5 \text{ mL}}$$
$$12.5\,x = 25 \times 5$$
$$12.5\,x = 125$$
$$x = 125 \div 12.5$$
$$x = 10 \text{ mL}$$

Content Area: *Development Across the Life Span*
Integrated Processes: *Nursing Process: Planning*
Client Need: *Physiological Integrity; Pharmacological and Parenteral Therapies*
Cognitive Level: *Application*
Concept: *Medication; Safety*

22. **ANSWER: 1, 4.**

Rationales:
1. Children between the ages of 12 to 36 months can amuse themselves for brief periods of time. They become involved in recreational, imitative, and educational play until they get bored.
2. Children between the ages of 12 and 36 months do not engage in interactive play. They play next to, not with, their peers.
3. Rigidity about rules of a game is associated with the play of children between the ages of 6 to 12 years of age.
4. Children 12 to 36 months of age (toddlers) are egocentric. They frequently use the word "mine" and are reluctant to share favorite toys without encouragement.
5. Cheating to win a game is associated with children 3 to 5 years of age when they engage in cooperative play (associative play).
Content Area: *Development Across the Life Span*
Integrated Processes: *Nursing Process: Assessment*
Client Need: *Health Promotion and Maintenance*
Cognitive Level: *Application*
Concept: *Growth and Development*

23. **ANSWER: 3.**

Rationales:
1. Although teaching about nutritious snacks is important because of the increased incidence of obesity in children, it is not the priority for school-aged children.
2. Although teaching about care of the teeth is important, this is not as high a priority as another option.
3. This is the priority from among the options presented. Being the target of bullying is extremely damaging to the ego. Children who are bullied are known to commit suicide or may resort to extreme violence in retaliation.
4. Information about sexually transmitted infections should be explored in a health promotion program for adolescents, not school-aged children.
TEST-TAKING TIP: Identify the word in the stem that sets a priority. The word *most* in the stem sets a priority.
Content Area: *Development Across the Life Span*
Integrated Processes: *Teaching/Learning; Nursing Process: Planning*
Client Need: *Health Promotion and Maintenance*
Cognitive Level: *Application*
Concept: *Health Promotion; Violence*

24. **ANSWER: 3.**

Rationales:
1. This is a judgmental response that may cut off communication.
2. Although this is a true statement, it may be perceived as a threat by the client. It is a confrontational statement that may cut off further communication.
3. The client does not perceive a benefit in changing his behavior because the consequence is insignificant to him. The client stated, "I do not know what the big deal is. If I get an infection, it can be cured with a shot." The client should be taught how to consistently use safe sex practices (e.g., condoms, uninfected sex partner) to prevent the acquisition and transmission of sexually transmitted infections.

4. This statement will have no impact on the client. The client has stated, "Last time the nurse said I could have complications from an infection, but I am healthy and that is not going to happen to me." This statement indicates that the client does not perceive that he is at risk for complications; he is in denial.

TEST-TAKING TIP: Identify the word in the stem that sets a priority. The word *most* in the stem indicates a priority.
Content Area: Development Across the Life Span
Integrated Processes: Communication and Documentation; Teaching/Learning; Nursing Process: Implementation
Client Need: Health Promotion and Maintenance
Cognitive Level: Analysis
Concept: Patient-Centered Care; Sexuality

25. ANSWER: 1.
Rationales:
1. **Risk for falls is the priority. The client is fatigued, uses a walker, lives alone, and has a history of a fall; these are risk factors for a future fall.**
2. Although this is a concern, it is not as important as another option.
3. Older adults generally experience a decline in recent, not distant, memory.
4. No data in the stem indicate that the client feels hopeless.

TEST-TAKING TIP: Identify the word in the stem that sets a priority. The word *main* in the stem sets a priority. Identify the word in the stem that is clang association. The word *fall* in the stem and in option 1 is a clang association. Examine option 1 carefully.
Content Area: Development Across the Life Span
Integrated Processes: Nursing Process: Analysis
Client Need: Safe and Effective Care Environment; Management of Care
Cognitive Level: Application
Concept: Safety

26. ANSWER: 4.
Rationales:
1. Although this may be done, the child may not know what questions to ask.
2. A video is a passive activity and only stimulates the senses of vision and hearing.
3. An explanation is a cognitive intervention that does not permit the visualization and handling of equipment.
4. **This is an interactive way to introduce the child to the equipment that will be used. It provides visual, auditory, and kinesthetic stimulation. Anxiety usually is reduced during an assessment when familiar objects are used.**

TEST-TAKING TIP: Identify the word in the stem that sets a priority. The word *best* in the stem sets a priority. Identify the option that contains a specific determiner. Option 1 contains the word *all,* which is a specific determiner. Identify the clang association. The words *physical assessment* in the stem and in option 4 is a clang association.
Content Area: Development Across the Life Span
Integrated Processes: Teaching/Learning; Nursing Process: Implementation
Client Need: Health Promotion and Maintenance
Cognitive Level: Application
Concept: Growth and Development

27. ANSWER: 2.
Rationales:
1. Avoiding small objects and providing toys that are bigger than a clenched fist help prevent airway obstruction accidents. Although the risk for choking is the greatest between 6 months and 3 years of age, it is not the leading cause of accidental deaths in infants.
2. **The leading cause of death in infants is motor vehicle accidents. A five-point infant car seat provides the necessary support to help limit injuries during a motor vehicle accident. The seat should be placed in the back seat of the car with the infant facing the rear of the car.**
3. Although supporting an infant when placed on an elevated surface will help limit injuries from falls, falls are not the leading cause of accidental deaths in infants.
4. Placing an infant on the back to sleep helps prevent sudden infant death syndrome; however, this is not the leading cause of accidental death in infants.

TEST-TAKING TIP: Identify the word in the stem that sets a priority. The word *leading* in the stem sets a priority.
Content Area: Development Across the Life Span
Integrated Processes: Teaching/Learning; Nursing Process: Implementation
Client Need: Health Promotion and Maintenance
Cognitive Level: Application
Concept: Health Promotion; Safety

28. ANSWER: 1, 3, 5.
Rationales:
1. **School-aged children become more involved in physical activities and team sports as they progress through school. Stretching exercises before physical activities help to limit musculoskeletal injuries.**
2. Checking that toys are larger than a clenched fist is appropriate for infants, toddlers, and preschoolers. The risk for choking is greatest between 6 months and 3 years of age.
3. **Children's physical skills vary depending on the developmental age and individual abilities; these factors must be considered before engaging in activities such as skiing, bicycle riding, and skate boarding.**
4. A five-point safety car seat is appropriate for infants, toddlers, and preschoolers. School-aged children usually transition to using a booster seat or a regular car seatbelt.
5. **Motor vehicle collisions are the highest cause of accidental deaths in school-aged children. Wearing a seatbelt in a car helps to reduce morbidity and mortality.**

TEST-TAKING TIP: Identify options that are opposites. Options 4 and 5 are opposites. More often than not, a correct answer is one of the opposites.
Content Area: Development Across the Life Span
Integrated Processes: Teaching/Learning; Nursing Process: Planning
Client Need: Safe and Effective Care Environment; Safety and Infection Control
Cognitive Level: Application
Concept: Health Promotion; Safety

29. ANSWER: 2, 4, 5.

Rationales:

1. Food should be cut up into tiny, not half-inch, pieces. Food items are the main cause of nonfatal choking events in children younger than 4 years of age.

2. Toilet lid locks prevent a toddler from accidently falling head first into a toilet and drowning. In addition it may prevent expensive visits from a plumber to remove small toys that a young child may throw into a toilet.

3. Crib slats should be less than 2⅜ inches (6 cm) apart and the mattress should fit the bed frame snuggly. This prevents an infant or child from getting the head caught between slats, which could cut off the airway, or from suffocating between the mattress and bed frame.

4. Balloon play should be supervised. Latex balloons and plastic bags are the main cause of suffocation deaths in young children.

5. A rear-facing car seat should be used until a child's weight exceeds the manufacturer's recommendation (usually 20 lb.) and then the child should be placed in a forward-facing seat. A forward-facing car seat should be used until a child's weight exceeds the manufacturer's recommendation (usually 40 lb.)

Content Area: Development Across the Life Span
Integrated Processes: Teaching/Learning; Nursing Process: Implementation
Client Need: Safe and Effective Care Environment; Safety and Infection Control
Cognitive Level: Application
Concept: Health Promotion; Safety

30. ANSWER: 2, 4, 5.

Rationales:

1. Positioning on the back when sleeping is recommended for infants, not toddlers, because it decreases the risk of sudden infant death syndrome. Toddlers have the ability to change position and turn from front to back and back to front when in bed.

2. Toddlers can be rambunctious and lack judgment because of limited experiences; their position should be guarded/supported when on elevated surfaces (e.g., changing tables, playground equipment) to prevent falls.

3. Toddlers can transition to forward-facing car seats when they are 20 pounds or they reach the maximum height and weight specified by the car seat manufacturer.

4. Electrical outlets stimulate the curiosity of toddlers; plastic inserts keep toddlers from inserting fingers or objects into outlets.

5. Toddlers like to role play the activities of adults; reachable pot handles may result in accidental burns.

TEST-TAKING TIP: Identify the clang association. The word *toddler* in the stem and in option 2 is a clang association.

Content Area: Development Across the Life Span
Integrated Processes: Teaching/Learning; Nursing Process: Planning
Client Need: Safe and Effective Care Environment; Safety and Infection Control
Cognitive Level: Application
Concept: Health Promotion; Safety

31. ANSWER: 3.

Rationales:

1. Motor vehicle accidents are the leading cause of death, not injury, during adolescence.

2. Although a class in anger management is important, anger is not the leading cause of physical injury in adolescence.

3. Alcohol and drug use is the root cause of most physical injuries that occur in adolescence. Alcohol and drugs impair judgment, leading to reckless driving (leading cause of death in adolescence); fuels anger, which can lead to homicide (second leading cause of death in adolescence), and irresponsible behavior regarding water sports (drowning and paralysis).

4. Although a class about responsible water safety is important, drowning and diving incidents are not the leading cause of injury in adolescence.

TEST-TAKING TIP: Identify the word in the stem that sets a priority. The word *leading* in the stem sets a priority. Identify the unique option. Option 3 is unique. It is the only option with two parts separated by the word *and*.

Content Area: Development Across the Life Span
Integrated Processes: Teaching/Learning; Nursing Process: Planning
Client Need: Health Promotion and Maintenance
Cognitive Level: Application
Concept: Health Promotion; Safety

32. ANSWER: 1, 3, 5.

Rationales:

1. Rubella, mumps, and measles can cause hearing loss. Children should be immunized against these diseases.

2. Children can engage in sports that involve sticks if they are taught the proper use of sports equipment and wear protective gear (e.g., helmets, eye shields).

3. Regular eye examinations help identify problems early so that they can be treated.

4. Young school-aged children always should use round-tipped, not sharp, scissors.

5. Sunglasses with UV protection help avoid damage from ultraviolet rays. In addition, the nurse should encourage parents to teach their children to never look directly into the sun.

TEST-TAKING TIP: Identify the specific determiner in an option. The word *only* in option 4 is a specific determiner. Rarely are options with specific determiners correct answers. Eliminate option 4 from further consideration.

Content Area: Development Across the Life Span
Integrated Processes: Teaching/Learning; Nursing Process: Planning
Client Need: Health Promotion and Maintenance
Cognitive Level: Application
Concept: Health Promotion; Safety

33. ANSWER: 1.

Rationales:

1. Motor vehicle accidents are the leading cause of death in the adolescent age-group. Many adolescents believe that they are invincible and do not wear seatbelts when riding in a car. Seatbelts do limit morbidity and mortality associated with motor vehicle accidents.

2. Although it is appropriate advice to engage in sports that are within one's physical ability, sports-related injuries are not the leading cause of accidental deaths in adolescents.

3. Although wearing a life preserver when engaging in water-related activities is advisable, water-related accidents are not the leading cause of accidental deaths in adolescents.

4. Although it is excellent advice to resist peer pressure to participate in experimenting with illegal drugs, the use of illegal drugs is not the leading cause of accidental deaths in adolescents. In addition, role-playing appropriate behaviors is more beneficial than giving advice.

TEST-TAKING TIP: Identify the word in the stem that sets a priority. The word *leading* in the stem sets a priority.
Content Area: Development Across the Life Span
Integrated Processes: Teaching/Learning; Nursing Process: Implementation
Client Need: Health Promotion and Maintenance
Cognitive Level: Application
Concept: Health Promotion; Safety

34. ANSWER: 3.
Rationales:

1. Salt water induces vomiting. The ingested poison may cause additional damage to the esophagus and mouth if vomiting is induced.

2. Ipecac is an emetic that induces vomiting. The ingested poison may cause additional damage to the esophagus and mouth if vomiting is induced.

3. Poison control centers provide immediate instructions regarding what to do for the specific poison ingested. Never employ a home remedy without directions from a poison control center.

4. Taking the time to transport a child to an emergency department could delay an immediate response that may help minimize a negative consequence.

TEST-TAKING TIP: Identify the clang association. The words *poisoning* and *poison* in the stem and the word *poison* in option 4 are clang associations. Examine an option with a clang association carefully.
Content Area: Development Across the Life Span
Integrated Processes: Teaching/Learning; Nursing Process: Planning
Client Need: Safe and Effective Care Environment; Safety and Infection Control
Cognitive Level: Application
Concept: Health Promotion; Safety

35. ANSWER: 1, 2, 3, 5.
Rationales:

1. Children tend to be naive and trustful of others, including strangers. They should be taught about self-protection and what to do if approached by a stranger.

2. School-aged children develop gross motor skills and balance and progress from a three-wheeled bicycle to a two-wheeled bicycle. Learning to ride a two-wheeled bicycle should include instruction about safety precautions, physical support, and practice.

3. School-aged children are less fearful than infants and preschoolers, which results in an increase in risk-taking behaviors with inadequate information to perform the

skills safely. Students should be reminded to get directions before using new equipment.**

4. School-aged children should transition to using regular car seatbelts when they reach 80 pounds, are at least 4 feet 9 inches in height, and at least 8 years of age. School-aged children should sit in the back seat until 13 years of age.

5. These interventions help limit the amount of oxygen feeding the base of the flames, which helps to put out the fire.
Content Area: Development Across the Life Span
Integrated Processes: Teaching/Learning; Nursing Process: Implementation
Client Need: Health Promotion and Maintenance
Cognitive Level: Application
Concept: Health Promotion; Safety

36. ANSWER: 1, 2, 3.
Rationales:

1. Motor vehicle accidents, often linked to alcohol use, are the leading cause of death and injury to middle-aged adults. This is the reason why this topic is most important to include in a discussion of injury prevention.

2. Because middle-aged weekend athletes have an increased risk of sports injures, it is important to encourage doing warm-up exercises before engaging in sports.

3. Discussing a daily exercise program to increase endurance will help minimize the barely perceptible physical decline of aging during middle adulthood.

4. Goals should be realistic and attainable, not challenging and demanding, which may exceed the ability of a middle-aged adult.

5. Healthy middle-aged adults do not need grab bars in the bathroom to assist with rising to a standing position. Older adults who have a decline in health may require grab bars in the bathroom to assist with rising to a standing position.
Content Area: Development Across the Life Span
Integrated Processes: Teaching/Learning; Nursing Process: Planning
Client Need: Health Promotion and Maintenance
Cognitive Level: Application
Concept: Health Promotion; Safety

37. ANSWER: 1.
Rationales:

1. Falls are the major cause of injury in this age-group. Removing throw/scatter rugs minimizes the risk of a fall.

2. Although most older adults experience a decline in hearing and vision and may be victims of pedestrian accidents, this type of accident is not the major cause of injury in this age-group.

3. Although older adults engage in sports, such as golf and bowling, and may experience a sports injury because of an inadequate *warm-up*, it is not the major cause of injury in this age-group.

4. Polypharmacy is a concern because older adults may take several prescription drugs plus over-the-counter drugs, placing them at risk for toxicity and drug interactions; however, injury from these chemical stressors are not the major cause of injury in this age-group.

Content Area: *Development Across the Life Span*
Integrated Processes: *Teaching/Learning; Nursing Process: Implementation*
Client Need: *Health Promotion and Maintenance*
Cognitive Level: *Application*
Concept: *Health Promotion; Safety*

38. ANSWER: 5, 4, 2, 3, 1.

Rationales:

5. Recognizing that a gun is present is the first step in preventing accidental firearm injuries.
4. Stopping what one is doing immediately interrupts the activity; it gives the child time to remember the next three steps that should be implemented to provide for one's own safety and the safety of others.
2. If the gun is not touched, it cannot be fired accidentally.
3. Leaving the vicinity places distance between the child and the gun in the event another person touches the gun.
1. Reporting the presence of the gun to an adult enables the adult to intervene and secure the gun in a locked area so that it cannot be accessed.

Content Area: *Development Across the Life Span*
Integrated Processes: *Teaching/Learning; Nursing Process: Planning*
Client Need: *Safe and Effective Care Environment; Safety and Infection Control*
Cognitive Level: *Analysis*
Concept: *Health Promotion; Safety*

39. ANSWER: 1, 3, 4.

Rationales:

1. Slats of cribs should be less than 2⅜ inches in width to prevent a toddler's head from becoming wedged between the slats of a crib.
2. Toys should be much larger than 2 inches in diameter. Toys should be larger than the closed fist of an adult to minimize the risk of aspirating a toy.
3. Toy boxes with heavy hinged lids can fall on a child or a child can become trapped inside the box and not be strong enough to lift the lid to escape.

4. Keeping venetian blind cords out of reach of children is essential to protect a child from accidentally causing self-strangulation.
5. Toddlers should be placed in a blanket sleeper and not under even a light blanket when sleeping to prevent the risk of suffocation.

TEST-TAKING TIP: Identify the word in the stem that sets a priority. The word *essential* in the stem sets a priority. Identify the option with the specific determiner. The word *only* in option 5 is a specific determiner. Rarely are options with a specific determiner the correct answer.

Content Area: *Development Across the Life Span*
Integrated Processes: *Teaching/Learning; Nursing Process: Implementation*
Client Need: *Safe and Effective Care Environment; Safety and Infection Control*
Cognitive Level: *Application*
Concept: *Health Promotion; Safety*

40. ANSWER: 3.

Rationales:

1. Although having vision evaluated yearly is advisable, diminished vision is not the leading cause of falls in older adults.
2. The influence of alcohol is not the leading cause of falls in older adults.
3. The leading cause of injuries in older adults is falls that usually occur when moving from sitting to standing or when transferring from a bed to a chair.
4. Washing the hands with an antimicrobial soap helps prevent infections, not injuries.

TEST-TAKING TIP: Identify the word in the stem that sets a priority. The word *leading* in the stem sets a priority.

Content Area: *Development Across the Life Span*
Integrated Processes: *Teaching/Learning; Nursing Process: Implementation*
Client Need: *Health Promotion and Maintenance*
Cognitive Level: *Application*
Concept: *Health Promotion; Safety*

Chapter 11

Diversity and Spirituality/Religion

NURSING CONCEPTS

Culture
Evidenced-Based Practice
Family Dynamics
Growth and Development
Health-Care System

Patient-Centered Care
Self
Sexuality
Spirituality

KEY TERMS

Culturally appropriate—Care based on knowledge of the cultures and ethnicities of individuals for whom care is provided

Culturally competent—Care that addresses the overall context of the client's condition in a culturally appropriate manner

Culturally sensitive—Respect for the cultures and ethnicities of individuals for whom care is provided

Culture—Nonphysical traits, beliefs, attitudes, values, and customs common to a group and handed down from one generation to the next

Discrimination—Unequal treatment of people or groups on the basis of race, ethnicity, gender, social class, sexual orientation, or other characteristics

Ethnicity—Group within a social system that has common traits or characteristics, such as language or religion

Ethnocentric—Belief that one's own culture is better than the cultures of others

Prejudice—Negative belief that is generalized to all members of a group; also called *racism*

Race—Classification of individuals based on physical characteristics or genetic indicators, such as skin color, hair texture, features, and bone structure

Religion—System of beliefs associated with the worship of a superior being and the nature and purpose of the universe

Socialization—Process of being nurtured within a culture and assimilating the features and uniqueness of the group

Spirituality—The essence that integrates a person's biopsychosocial journey through life

Stereotyping—Presuming that all people of a group are alike, commonly unrelated to reality and precipitated by racism or discrimination

Transcultural nursing—Learning and exploring different cultures in relation to cultural norms, health beliefs, and health practices with the objective of delivering health care within the framework and perspective of the client's culture

I. Culture

Nurses are encountering increasing diversity among the populations for whom they provide care. To be culturally sensitive, appropriate, and competent, nurses must understand the characteristics, customs, and rituals common to various cultures. Nurses also must understand that, despite having cultural commonalities, no two people within a culture are likely to have identical views. Therefore, nursing care must always be individualized.

A. Characteristics of culture
  1. **Culture** is values, beliefs, practices, and traditions that are shared by members of a group; it provides an identity; may reflect individual variations.
  2. Culture is complex and is reflected in many aspects of life and on many levels, such as art, literature, attire, language, customs, rituals, and practices (socialization). (See "Common Beliefs of Different Cultural Groups," Table 11.1.)
  3. Culture is taught and learned through life experiences, such as traditions, encounters with individuals within the culture, and food preferences (socialization). (See "Common Food Preferences of Selected Cultural Groups and Related Nursing Care," Table 20.3 in Chapter 20, Nutrition.)
  4. Culture affects communication; for example:
     a. Different cultures may have different languages or dialects of the same language that pose a challenge not only for the client but also for health-care providers.
     b. American culture is associated with assertive, self-determined independence.
     c. Asian cultures value group harmony, show respect to elders and family leaders, consider direct eye contact disrespectful or aggressive, and engage in ambiguous communication, such as using incongruent agreeing statements rather than saying "no," which is considered disrespectful. The nurse must seek feedback to ensure that agreeing statements actually reflect understanding or consent.
  5. Cultures are organized on the basis of family relatedness and status within a family or society, such as gender, age, and education; for example:
     a. A Korean mother is subject to the authority of her husband and to the oldest son in the absence of the father.
     b. In many African cultures, the woman is the leader and decision maker of the family.
     c. In some cultures, men have a higher status than women and receive care before women.
  6. Culture influences physical placement when communicating with others and is related to personal space and territoriality; for example:
     a. North Americans tend to stand 18 inches apart when communicating with one another.
     b. People from Arab cultures stand closer than 18 inches when communicating.
  7. Culture influences time orientation regarding whether a person is past, present, or future oriented; for example:
     a. North Americans tend to be future oriented.
     b. Latinos tend to be present oriented.
  8. Cultures observe life events with traditions and/or religious rituals; for example:
     a. Female circumcision is practiced in some African cultures.
     b. Religious rites of passage may occur at puberty, such as a Bat or Bar Mitzvah in the Jewish faith or confirmation in Catholic and Protestant faiths.
     c. Females must participate in a ritual bath after each menstruation and before resuming intimate relations with a spouse in the Orthodox Jewish, Islamic, and Hindu cultures.
     d. Various cultures have specific attitudes and beliefs about cremation, organ donation, and autopsy because of the belief that the dead must face the creator with the body undesecrated.
  9. Culture affects health beliefs and practices; for example:
     a. Some cultures have folk healers (e.g., shaman, herbalist, medicine man) and folk practices to help restore health, such as religious healing rituals, amulets or talismans worn to ward off evil, and energy to restore balance.
     b. Asian Americans may tolerate pain stoically because they view pain as something that cannot be controlled.
  10. **Ethnicity** refers to belonging to a group that has common characteristics, such as language or religion.

B. Cultural diversity
  1. Population trends in the United States.
     a. The United States is a multicultural society, consisting of dissimilar cultural and ethnic groups. In 2014, 13.3% of the population were foreign born, an increase of 11% from 2013 to 2014. People with Latino/Hispanic and Asian heritage account for the largest groups.
     b. Minorities account for 37% of the population, and it is predicted that it will increase to 57% by 2060. By 2043, no group will make up a majority of the U.S. population.
     c. In 2013, 25 million people in the United States reported limited English proficiency, an increase

| Table 11.1 | Common Beliefs of Different Cultural Groups |

Culture	Common Beliefs
African American/ Black	• Are generally a matriarchal culture • Are present oriented rather than future oriented • May distrust others • May consume a diet high in fat • May believe illness is due to disharmony and that healing is spiritual • Generally believe in prayer, use of herbs, laying on of the hands, magic rituals, and Voodoo • May oppose abortion due to religious, moral, or cultural beliefs • May refuse advance directives • May be enthusiastically vocal when grieving
Amish	• Are patriarchal; women have status and respect; includes several generations in the nuclear family • Not outwardly demonstrative; quiet, modest manner; stoical toward suffering and grief • Prefer that birth and death occur in the home; neighbors provide physical and emotional support • Need permission from the church to seek care in a hospital • Accept anesthesia, surgery, blood transfusions, blood products, dental care, and organ transplantation other than the heart (heart transplantation is unacceptable because Amish believe that the heart is the soul of the body) • Avoid health insurance because it demonstrates lack of faith • Generally are afraid of disability but not death • Limit end-of-life care so that assets are used for the living
Asian American	• Generally include several generations in the nuclear family and may include extended family members • Have respect for elders • May avoid eye contact out of respect • Are subordinate to authority; ensure client understands information because individual may report he or she understands to show respect or avoid loss of face • Value self-respect and self-control; may stoically cope with disability, pain, and grief • Believe health is a state of balance of the physical and spiritual • Believe illness is disharmony of yin and yang • Have a rich history of Eastern medicine that includes herbs, diet, application of hot or cold, acupressure, and acupuncture to reestablish balance • Females may accept health care only from a person of the same gender
European American/ non-Hispanic white	• Value independence, individuality, and autonomy; emphasize achievement, youth, and beauty • Future oriented but balance the past with the present • Maintain direct eye contact; generally will readily disclose personal information • Believe that health is a balance in emotional and physical well-being • Accept health care in a variety of settings and care based on the newest technologies and approaches • Supplement traditional medical care with alternative therapies, such as acupuncture, spinal adjustment, massage, herbal therapy, aromatherapy, and naturopathy
Hispanic/ Latino	• Generally have extended family members living together; emphasis is on the group • Celebrate a girl's coming of age on 15th birthday (Quinceanera) • Believe in faith and spirituality • Fatalistic but believe in prayer, miracles, wearing religious medals or amulets; use herbs; engage in rituals • Believe health is a gift from God, a reward, or good luck • Believe illness is an imbalance in hot and wet, hot and dry, cold and dry, and/or cold and wet • Treat the body with respect • May consider illness to be a punishment • May be enthusiastically vocal when grieving
Native American	• Original inhabitants of North America; often prefer name specific to their cultural heritage (e.g., Navajo Indians, the largest tribe) • Most tribes are matrilineal; family unit is a nuclear family and among female relatives • Respect elders • Present rather than future oriented; punctuality not important • Avoid eye contact; comfortable with silences • Tend not to share thoughts and feelings with people outside the tribe • Believe in a spiritual power, acceptance of nature, tradition, and sharing • Treat the body with respect • Believe health is living in harmony with nature (Mother Earth); illness is associated with disharmony or evil spirits • Believe illness is a concern of the family, extended family, and tribe • Believe in folk medicine; engage in rituals, ceremonies, chanting, exorcisms, dancing, sand painting, meditation, wearing amulets, and use of herbs to treat illness

of 80% since 1990. In 2014, 20.9% of the population reported speaking a language other than English in the home.

d. Adults 65 years and older accounted for 13% of the population in 2010 and 14.5% in 2014. It is predicted that the number of adults ≥65 years of age will double between 2012 and 2060.

2. Inequalities in health, illness, and death rates correlate with racial and ethnic groups; however, social, economic, cultural, health-care access and quality, and other interrelated factors may influence these disparities rather than race or ethnic group.

a. In 2014, the U.S. Census Bureau reported that 14.8% of the U.S. population live in poverty.

b. Racial and ethnic groups in the United States have made gains in infant death rates, number of females who smoke, and numbers of uninsured, but disparities continue in obesity, caesarean births, and dental care.

   (1) Hispanic children ages 2 to 19 years have the highest rate (21.9%) of obesity in the United States.

   (2) Black African American women have the highest percentage (29.9%) of low-risk caesarean births in the United States.

   (3) Hispanic adults aged 18 to 64 years have the highest rate (15.7%) of those who went without needed dental care.

c. People from minority groups experience higher rates of illness and death than white (non-Hispanic) individuals in the United States.

   (1) Non-Hispanic Black African American mothers have the highest rate of infant mortality (11 per 1,000) associated with a live birth.

   (2) Black African American men and women have the highest rate of dying from cancer than any other group.

   (3) People diagnosed with HIV are disproportionately higher among racial/ethnic minorities than among whites: 47% Black African American, 28% Asian, and 21% American Indian/Alaska Native.

   (4) Preventable hospitalization rates increase as economic level decreases. In addition, there are large disparities in preventable hospitalizations in racial/ethnic groups.

   (5) Disparities in smoking and alcohol consumption exist among American Indians and Alaska Natives despite overall declines in other groups.

   (6) Eighty-five percent of individuals newly diagnosed with tuberculosis are reported to be individuals from racial or ethnic minority groups.

d. The Affordable Care Act has helped reduce health disparities in the United States by increasing health insurance coverage and access to health care. It remains to be seen how this will change after the 2017 presidential inauguration.

e. *Healthy People 2020* identifies national health promotion guidelines.

   (1) Two overarching goals include increasing quality and years of healthy life and eliminating health inequalities based on gender, ethnicity, education, income, disability, geographic location, and sexual orientation.

   (2) For more information about *Healthy People 2020,* see "Healthy People 2020" in Chapter 4, Health-Care System, and www.healthypeople.gov.

3. Nurses are challenged with meeting the needs of a culturally diverse population.

a. The National Council of State Board of Nursing reported that in 2013, 83 percent of nurses are white (non-Hispanic); numerous private and public, and national and state initiatives are aimed at increasing diversity of students applying for nursing educational programs.

b. Nurses will be caring for ever-increasing numbers of individuals with different cultural and ethnic backgrounds, educational preparation, financial status, disabilities, genders, and sexual orientation and who come from different geographic locations.

c. Conflicts in health-care delivery are commonly related to cultural misunderstandings.

C. Culturally competent nursing care

1. **Transcultural nursing:** Learning and exploring different cultures in relation to cultural norms, health beliefs, and health practices with the objective of delivering health care within the framework and perspective of the client's culture.

2. **Culturally competent:** Care that addresses the overall context of the client's condition in a culturally appropriate manner.

3. **Culturally sensitive:** Respect for the cultures and ethnicities of individuals for whom they are providing care.

4. **Culturally appropriate:** Care based on knowledge of the cultures and ethnicities of individuals for whom they are providing care.

5. Barriers to cultural competency.

a. **Prejudice:** Negative belief that is generalized to all members of a group; also called *racism.*

b. **Discrimination:** Unequal treatment of people or groups on the basis of race, ethnicity, gender, social class, sexual orientation, or other characteristics.

c. **Ethnocentric:** Belief that one's own culture is better than the cultures of others.

d. **Stereotyping:** Presuming that all people of a group are alike, commonly unrelated to reality and precipitated by racism or discrimination.

D. Nursing care to meet a client's cultural needs

1. Study and learn about cultures and religions that are different from their own.

2. Explore their true feelings about various cultures, and identify their own personal biases and prejudices if any exist.

(!) 3. Provide nonjudgmental nursing care that is accepting and respectful of a client's culture, beliefs, and rituals.

4. Involve a client's significant other who has authority within the family to be involved in decision making with the client's request and consent.

5. Ensure modesty when providing nursing care; assign a caregiver of the same gender as a client if requested; support a client's desire to wear clothing that is more modest than a hospital gown.

II. Spirituality/Religion

Since nurses care for the whole client, meeting physical, physiological, and emotional needs, care would be incomplete without also focusing on the spiritual/religious dimensions of clients. By identifying spiritual strengths or distress, the nurse can assist the client to explore concerns and formulate a plan that helps the client achieve identified goals. To be better able to accomplish this, nurses must understand the tenets and beliefs of the common religions.

A. Faith development—James Fowler

1. Faith is a force of knowing that gives meaning to life.

2. It develops from interaction between a person and the environment.

3. New patterns of values, beliefs, and ways of thinking are added with each stage.

4. Contains six stages.

a. *Intuitive-projective:* 3- to 7-year-old children imitate parental behaviors without thorough understanding.

b. *Mythic-literal:* School-aged children may accept the concept of God and appreciate the perception of others.

c. *Synthetic-conventional:* Adolescents begin to examine life-guiding beliefs, values, and personal religious practices.

d. *Individuative-reflective:* Older adolescents and young adults assume responsibility for their own commitments, beliefs, and attitudes about faith.

e. *Conjunctive:* Individuals integrate other viewpoints into their own understanding and identify personal conceptual realities in the context of faith development in others.

f. *Universalizing:* Individuals achieve a universal perspective with absolute love and justice for humankind regardless of the religion or faith involved; this stage rarely is achieved.

5. Nursing implications.

a. Increases nurses' understanding that spirituality is essential to providing holistic nursing care.

b. Helps nurses to examine their own faith and not impose their own commitments, beliefs, and attitudes about faith onto clients and their family members.

B. Spirituality

1. **Spirituality** is the essence that integrates a person's biopsychosocial journey through life.

2. Issues include faith, hope, and love.

3. Expresses a person's meaning, fulfillment, and satisfaction with one's life providing strength and significance.

C. Religion

1. **Religion** is faith or belief in and worship of a God or higher power; contains organized attitudes, beliefs, and practices (Table 11.2).

MAKING THE CONNECTION

Clients' Religious Beliefs and Practices and the Provision of Nursing Care

Dying and death customs and rituals associated with the Jewish faith include having a family member or representative present while a client is actively dying and remaining with a body until it is buried. This practice fulfills the desire to provide a constant presence for the person who is dying and for the body until burial. The body is washed with warm water by a member of the family or a member of the Chevra Kaddisha society, and then men are wrapped in a prayer shawl, while women are wrapped in a white burial shroud. The body is placed in a simple pine box and buried as soon as possible, often within 24 hours after death. Additional rituals include tearing an article of clothing to symbolize the loss, covering mirrors, and mourning for seven days (Shiva), when community members bring food to the family and reminisce about the deceased.

To support these customs and rituals, the nurse should provide privacy for the dying client and significant others. A lounge chair or bed should be provided for the person staying with the client who is dying. Discuss with the family whether the body can be touched after death or if arrangements should be made for a member of the Chevra Kaddisha society to care for the body. Obtain from the family the name of a funeral establishment that conforms to Jewish customs and rituals and arrange for removal of the body.

Table 11.2 Common Beliefs of Different Religions

Religion	Common Beliefs
Buddhist	• Admire Buddha (Enlightened One) as a way of life • Believe in avoiding evil, being moral and pure, calming the mind so as to observe rather than react, and doing good by helping others • Believe in multiple cycles of birth, life, death, and rebirth until a person is no longer involved with desire and the self; goal is to achieve eternal life without further reincarnation (nirvana) and achievement of liberty and freedom from distress and suffering • Do not engage in formal ceremonies; however, observe the birthday of Buddha • Consider illness part of life and therefore do not offer prayers for healing • Accept modern medicine, surgery, and technology • Read the Tibetan Book of the Dead on the seventh day after death to liberate the person's soul from the netherworlds (Tibetan Buddhists)
Catholic	• Believe in the Father, Son, and Holy Spirit and that redemption comes through the blood of Jesus, the Son of God • Priests administer the sacraments, which include Baptism, Reconciliation, Eucharist, Anointing of the Sick, and Matrimony. Bishops administer the sacraments of Holy Orders and Confirmation • A member of the faith can baptize in an emergency if a priest is unavailable • Participate as a congregation at a religious service called the Holy Sacrifice of the Mass, where bread and wine is transformed (transubstantiation) into the body and blood of Christ and then distributed in the form of bread wafers (Eucharist) and sips of wine • Engage in penance and acts of good work during Advent (time period before Christmas) and Lent (time period before Easter Sunday) to prepare for the celebration of the birth of Christ and Christ's resurrection after death on the cross respectively • Do not ingest meat on certain days, such as Fridays during Lent • Accept the rhythm method as the only acceptable form of birth control • Prohibit sterilization, suicide, euthanasia, and abortion
Christian Scientist	• A unique form of Christianity that teaches a dependence on God and not the medical establishment for health care • Do not smoke tobacco or drink alcohol and may not drink coffee or tea • Believe that illness is due to lack of knowledge, fear, or sin and that a person will recover when the circumstance is corrected • Engage in Christian Science health-care remedies and prayer to alleviate illness • Denounce drug therapy and surgery but do permit setting of a fracture • May require the U.S. court system to intervene on behalf of infants and children when parents refuse life-saving treatments
Hindu	• Believe in Brahman, the underlying universal life force; may revere several gods or goddesses • Believe the aim in life is relief from the karmic cycle of death and reincarnation; leading a good life will lead to a higher status in the next life • Observe Mahashivarathri, a celebration of Lord Shiva • Believe family members are important to each other • Believe in the tenets of astrology • Pray and meditate after bathing; prefer to wash in water that is free flowing • If female, wear saris that cover the body except for the arms and feet • Are vegetarians, eat sweets and yogurt at all meals, and use large amounts of spices • Eat with only the right hand because the left hand is used for toileting activities • May wear a religious thread around the wrist or body • Believe illness may be caused by actions in a past life • Believe that illness is due to supernatural causes that imbalance bile, phlegm, and wind (body humors) • Believe that pain is due to the anger of a higher power and therefore one must bear the condition and situation • Accept health care only from a person of the same gender • Use birth control, participate in organ donation, and receive blood transfusions • Do not accept abortion, circumcision, suicide, and euthanasia • Cremate the body within 24 hours after death because doing so is believed to release the body from connection with the earth

Table 11.2 **Common Beliefs of Different Religions—cont'd**

Religion	Common Beliefs
Islam	• Most Arabs are Muslims and are united by the Islam faith; there is no separation of church and state • Believe in six terms of faith: one must follow Allah; one must follow the Qur'an, Torah, and Psalms; each person has two angels appointed to them; Muhammad (the greatest prophet) is used to deliver Allah's messages; believe in life after death and hell; and Allah has power over everything • Believe in five pillars of faith: following Allah and Muhammad, praying facing Mecca five times a day, helping poor and impoverished people, fasting between sunup and sundown during the month of Ramadan (unless ill), and making a pilgrimage to Mecca at least once during one's lifetime • Do not eat pork • Men are the decision makers; do not permit women to make autonomous health-care decisions • May prefer same-sex caregivers, may wear a small leather bag around the neck containing a locket with religious writings, and may cover their body with clothing so that only the face or the eyes are exposed • May not practice birth control (strict Muslims) but may allow abortions for health reasons • May request that the body or head be positioned facing toward Mecca when dying • May request that a family member or representative provide a ritual bath after death
Jehovah's Witness	• Live according to the commandments in Old and New Testaments • May drink alcohol, but drunkenness is unacceptable • Do not permit use of tobacco and recreational drugs • Do not eat food with blood (animals must be bled according to custom to be acceptable, and some members do not eat any meat) • Allow birth control, autopsy, and cremation • Forbid blood transfusions and blood products but may use artificial blood expanders • Do not permit sterilization, abortion, and organ transplantation • May require the U.S. court system to intervene on behalf of infants and children when parents refuse life-saving treatment
Jewish	• Believe that there is only one God who is everywhere and that people have a free will and are responsible for their choices and actions • Believe in the Torah and Old Testament to show them how to worship and treat others • Consist of Orthodox, Conservative, and Reformed congregations; Orthodox congregations follow Jewish law more strictly than Conservative and Reformed congregations • Observe the Sabbath on Saturday and holy days such as Yom Kippur, Rosh Hashanah, and Passover • May wear a head scarf or a wig and clothing that is modest and covers the arms and most of the legs to show respect to God (Orthodox Jewish women) • Orthodox and Conservative members may follow strict laws of Kashrut (kosher diet). Prohibit pork but permit meat from animals that are cloven footed and cud chewing; do not ingest dairy at the same meal as meat; require two separate sets of dishes, pots, and utensils to ensure that meat and dairy products are maintained separately; can eat fish with scales and nonpredatory birds • Practice sexual self-denial during menstruation and a ritual bath afterward (a husband cannot touch his wife until after the ritual bath) • Practice rituals, such as hand washing, scripture reading, using prayer beads, meditation, praying before and after meals, and lighting candles on the Sabbath • Engage in a ceremony called a bris 8 days after birth, in which a Jewish male is circumcised by a mohel and named; infant females are named during a ceremony in the synagogue on the first Sabbath after the birth • Engage in a religious rite of passage called a Bat Mitzvah (females) or Bar Mitzvah (males) at puberty • Do not consider neonates to be human until birth of the head or after three-quarters of the body is born • Cherish health and life to the degree that no intervention is permitted to alleviate pain and suffering if it hastens death • Generally do not consider psychiatric care helpful • Believe that a person should be with the client when death occurs and with the body until burial, which should occur within 24 hours; burial society volunteers (Chevra Kaddisha) wash the body, close the eyes, wrap it in a linen shroud, and may lay it on the floor until burial • After death of a loved one, observe a mourning period (sit Shiva) during which people gather to pay respect and focus on the memory of the deceased • Prohibit tattoos, suicide, euthanasia, embalming, and cremation

Continued

Table 11.2 Common Beliefs of Different Religions—cont'd

Religion	Common Beliefs
Mormon (Church of Jesus Christ of Latter-day Saints)	• *Believe in Jesus and one God and the sacred writing of the Book of Mormon (believed to have been given to Joseph Smith by an angel)* • *Wear a sacred undergarment that is removed only for bathing and can be removed for surgery but must be treated with respect* • *Follow a strict health code that advises healthful living* • *Forbid alcohol, coffee, cola, tea, and overeating, and observe monthly fasting* • *Permit circumcision, organ transplantation, and autopsy* • *Permit cremation only if required by law* • *Forbid abortion, sterilization, drug misuse, and smoking* • *Provide a subsidized welfare system and financial assistance for congregants who are ill*
Protestant	• *Denominations include Lutheran, Presbyterian, Baptist, Episcopal, and Methodist* • *Believe that Jesus is the mediator between man and God and that Jesus' death redeems and with God's grace makes redemption possible* • *Believe in the authority of the scriptures in the Holy Bible and Books of Doctrine particular to specific religions, such as Lutheran, Baptist, and Methodist* • *Believe that individuals are prominent over the authority of a minister, priest, or pastor* • *May attend services, receive Communion, and celebrate Easter Sunday and Christmas* • *May fast in preparation for certain religious celebrations, such as Easter Sunday*
Seventh-day Adventist	• *Believe in infallibility of Scripture; that salvation comes through faith in Jesus Christ* • *Hold the Sabbath on Saturday and spend the day worshiping and resting* • *Follow kosher dietary laws, and most are vegetarians* • *Accept birth control for married couples* • *Forbid tattoos, body piercings, alcohol, opioids, stimulants, and caffeine* • *Believe that praying and anointing with oil will promote healing* • *Allow abortion when medically necessary* • *Prohibit euthanasia but accept stopping medical support* • *Consider death to be like sleep; believe that the body and soul remain together until Christ comes again*

2. Based on theories about God, sacred writings, rituals, and ceremonies.
3. Embrace concepts about salvation (Judeo-Christian religions), enlightenment (Eastern religions), and/or doctrines in relation to a soul and its relationship to death, judgment, and eternal life (Western concepts).

D. Nursing care to meet a client's spiritual/religious needs
1. Explore a client's spiritual beliefs and/or religious affiliation and steps that can be taken to better support spiritual and religious needs.
2. Respectfully handle religious articles, such as the Bible, the Koran, rosary beads, prayer beads, religious jewelry, medals, amulets, icons, and totems, and nonjudgmentally accept tattoos that have a religious, spiritual, or special meaning to the client.
3. Arrange for a dietitian to collaborate with a client who has specific dietary preferences, such as people who follow a kosher diet, do not eat pork, eat only vegetables, or avoid meat on certain days of the week.
4. Help clients explore their feelings if a health-care intervention that they desire is prohibited by their religion (e.g., a client who wants a blood transfusion whose religion prohibits the administration of blood or blood products).
5. Explore and document refusal of care related to religious beliefs to ensure that it is the client's desire and communicate the information to other health-care team members.
6. Arrange for a spiritual advisor or leader to visit or perform religious rituals.
7. Provide time and privacy for rituals, and provide extra seating for participants.
8. Avoid bathing the client for several hours if a ritual involved anointing with oils.

CASE STUDY: Putting It All Together

A 65-year-old devout Muslim woman diagnosed with an end-stage brain tumor is admitted to a hospice facility when the family felt that they could no longer provide adequate care to manage pain control. Family members, including her husband and two daughters, are attentive and are taking turns being with her because they don't want her to die alone. The client minimally interacts and most of the time is quiet and peaceful. The husband tells the nurse, "I try to get my wife to talk with me about all our happy times together, but she just closes her eyes and takes a deep breath and ignores me." The nurse reviews a resource about the Muslim culture and Islamic faith to better formulate a plan of care for this client and her family members.

Case Study Questions

A. Formulate a response to the husband's statement, "I try to get my wife to talk with me about all our happy times together, but she just closes her eyes and takes a deep breath and ignores me."

_____

_____

B. Identify at least five nursing interventions to meet the cultural and spiritual needs of this dying client.

1. _____

2. _____

3. _____

4. _____

5. _____

C. Identify at least five nursing interventions to meet the needs of family members of this dying client.

1. _____

2. _____

3. _____

4. _____

5. _____

REVIEW QUESTIONS

Be sure to read the Introduction for valuable test-taking tips.

1. A nurse is caring for a client who is from a Hispanic culture and is dying. What might the nurse expect from the client's family? **Select all that apply.**
   1. Have numerous family members at the bedside
   2. Desire for time for reflection in a peaceful and quiet environment
   3. Request that a religious representative care for the body after death
   4. Expression of happy thoughts to facilitate the dying person's journey
   5. Loud moaning and expressions of grief during the client's last hours

2. A nurse is caring for a client who was admitted for cardiac care. The client is Native American and believes in the benefit of a medicine man with healing powers (shaman). What should the nurse do when planning care for this client? **Select all that apply.**
   1. Ensure privacy for the performance of healing religious rituals.
   2. Recognize that feelings may not be shared with health-care workers.
   3. Check meal trays to verify that meat is not served with dairy products.
   4. Consult with a dietitian to ensure that the client receives a vegetarian diet.
   5. Accept the decision that a heart transplant violates the belief that the heart is the body's soul.

3. A nurse is planning care for a client who is a Jehovah's Witness. Which nursing actions are appropriate? **Select all that apply.**
   1. Position the bed so that the client's head is facing Mecca.
   2. Verify with certainty that the client does not want a blood transfusion.
   3. Assign a female nursing assistant to help the client with activities of daily living.
   4. Obtain a prescription for a shower so that the client can bathe in free-flowing water.
   5. Consult with the dietitian to ensure that the client's dietary preferences are respected.

4. An older adult shares, "I am a member of the Amish community and have been using herbs and receiving treatment from my community's practitioner for abdominal pain. After 6 months, the pain increased and my skin turned yellow. I received permission from my elders to come to the hospital." After multiple diagnostic tests, the client is diagnosed with inoperable pancreatic cancer and the primary health-care provider indicates that the situation is terminal. Which statement by the nurse is **most** appropriate when discussing discharge plans with the client?
   1. "When the time comes, would you like to receive hospice care?"
   2. "What can we do for you that will help keep you in your own home?"
   3. "What do you plan to do, since your community does not permit chemotherapy?"
   4. "Would you prefer to be discharged to a nursing home where you can receive skilled nursing care?"

5. A nurse notes on a male client's medical record that the client is Catholic. Which statements by the nurse show sensitivity for the client's religious practices? **Select all that apply.**
   1. "Would you like me to give your name to the priest who is distributing the Eucharist?"
   2. "I will let the dietary department know not to send dairy on the same tray as meat."
   3. "I will assign a male nursing assistant to help you with your bath this morning."
   4. "Are there any sacraments you would like to receive while hospitalized?"
   5. "Can I remove your sacred undergarment when I give you a bath?"

6. A nurse is caring for a woman who is a member of the Church of Jesus Christ of Latter-day Saints (Mormon). Which statements by the nurse demonstrate a lack of sensitivity for the client's religious related practices? **Select all that apply.**
   1. "I am assigning a male nursing assistant to help care for you tonight."
   2. "You have to remove your head covering so that I can wash your hair."
   3. "You cannot wear your sacred undergarment while hospitalized."
   4. "I will ensure that you get coffee with your dinner tonight."
   5. "I prayed last night for you that you would get well."

7. Which nursing intervention is related to providing sociocultural comfort to a hospitalized client?
   1. Arrange furniture so clients have a view from their rooms.
   2. Respect each client as a unique individual.
   3. Provide for basic physiological needs.
   4. Ensure continuity of care.

8. A preoperative client who is wearing a small religious medal around the neck is being prepared for surgery. The client states, "I never take this medal off because it is very important to me." Which is the appropriate action by the nurse?
   1. Ensure that the medal is kept close to the client during surgery.
   2. Ask the client to make an exception and give the medal to a family member.
   3. Remove the medal after the client is under anesthesia and replace it after the surgery.
   4. Explain that clients are not permitted in the operating room with a medal or jewelry of any kind.

9. A school-aged child is hit by a motor vehicle while crossing the street and is brought to the hospital where the child dies. The crying mother vehemently exclaims, "Why did God let this happen? I'll never go back to church again. God can go to hell!" The woman then falls into her husband's arms crying. Which is the nurse's **best** response?
   1. "Unfortunately, it was just an accident."
   2. "Now is when you need your God the most."
   3. "You need to do what it takes to help you cope."
   4. "I am going to give you some time to cry together privately."

10. A nurse is caring for a client who practices Buddhism. Which should the nurse do that is supportive of the client's religion?
    1. Accept the client's belief that illness is caused by actions in the past.
    2. Support the client's decision to have a blood transfusion.
    3. Provide the client privacy for religious rituals.
    4. Pray for healing with the client.

11. A nurse is interviewing a traditional Asian woman who is being admitted to the hospital for surgery. Which information and behaviors should the nurse determine relate to her culture? **Select all that apply.**
    1. Avoids eye contact
    2. Refuses to take pain medication
    3. Gets acupuncture treatments monthly
    4. Avoids eating pork and other meat products
    5. Lives with her husband, children, and parents

12. Clients who practice which of the following religions should a nurse anticipate may be reluctant to provide consent for a blood transfusion? **Select all that apply.**
    1. Church of Jesus Christ of Latter-day Saints
    2. Seventh-day Adventist
    3. Christian Scientist
    4. Jehovah's Witness
    5. Jewish

13. A nurse is obtaining a health history for a woman who is proud of her African American culture. Which assessments reflect the dominant attitudes of people with this cultural heritage? **Select all that apply.**
    1. Male-dominant family
    2. Distrustful of others
    3. Spiritual orientation
    4. Stoical about death
    5. Present focused

14. A nurse is caring for female clients with diverse religious beliefs. The nurse should ensure that female caregivers be provided for clients who practice which religions? **Select all that apply.**
    1. Islam
    2. Hinduism
    3. Catholicism
    4. Protestantism
    5. Christian Scientist

15. A nurse plans to provide for a client's comfort in relation to a sociocultural need. Which nursing action is an appropriate intervention?
    1. Administering a prescribed analgesic
    2. Using effective communication skills
    3. Dimming the lights in the room at night
    4. Encouraging a parent to stay with a hospitalized child

16. Which values in European American/white cultures make it difficult for these clients to cope with self-esteem and health issues? **Select all that apply.**
    1. Present orientation
    2. Significance of wealth
    3. Emphasis on youth and beauty
    4. Rejection of new technologies
    5. Reluctance to disclose personal information

17. A female client tells the nurse, "My religion prefers that I take a shower rather than a tub bath." Which religion is the client's affiliation that obliges the nurse to obtain additional client preferences regarding bathing?
1. Judaism
2. Hinduism
3. Buddhism
4. Mormonism

18. A recent female immigrant from Haiti is admitted to the hospital for surgery because of cancer. The nurse reviews the client's personal information on the admission document and notes that the client identifies her religion as Voodoo. The nurse obtains information from the Internet about the Voodoo religion and interviews the client. What should the nurse do based on this information and the conversation with the client?
1. Inform the client that a Voodoo ritual cannot be performed within the facility.
2. Notify the nursing supervisor of the client's intention to receive a Voodoo ritual.
3. Refer the situation about having a Voodoo ritual in the hospital to the Ethics Committee.
4. Ask the client what can be done to facilitate the Voodoo ritual to be performed by the priest.

19. A nurse is caring for a female married client who is a member of an Orthodox Jewish congregation. Which of the following should the nurse anticipate the client will perform? **Select all that apply.**
1. Wear a head scarf
2. Follow a kosher diet
3. Use the left hand for toileting activities
4. Wear a religious thread around the wrist
5. Engage in acts of good work during Advent

20. A nurse is caring for several clients from Hispanic/Latino cultures. Which beliefs can the nurse expect these clients to reflect? **Select all that apply.**
1. Prayer can result in miracles
2. The family is the most important group.
3. Health is living in harmony with nature.
4. The body should be treated with respect.
5. Illness is an imbalance between yin and yang.

■ Client's Admission Document

Gender: Female

Age: 36
Marital status: Married
Children: 1 female (age 10) and 1 male (age 12)
Religion: Voodoo

Information About Voodoo (Vodou) Religion

The Voodoo religion was brought to Western coasts by slaves from Africa. It recognizes one Supreme Being (known as Bondye) who is too remote for a personal relationship. Therefore, lesser deities and ordained clergy (priests) provide guidance for worshippers. There is no standardized dogma, but worshippers navigate daily life through presentation of offerings, devotional objects, and elaborate ceremonies or rituals of music, dance, and spirit possession. These ceremonies or rituals are a concentrated intent to affect a specific outcome, such as healing. The Voodoo religion is not a cult, black magic, or devil worship, and it is not a practice intended to hurt or control others. These views are a result of sensational movies from Hollywood.

Client Interview

Client worried about her diagnosis and its prognosis. Client stated, "My priest is coming tomorrow to perform a Voodoo ritual to help me heal. I hope it will cure me of this terrible disease." Client states that her husband also practices the Voodoo religion and supports her need for healing.

REVIEW ANSWERS AND RATIONALES

1. ANSWER: 1, 5.
Rationales:

1. People from Hispanic/Latino cultures value family relationships. Often, they have extended family members living together.

2. Amish people, not Hispanic people, generally prefer a quiet and peaceful environment when a person is actively dying. Most often, Amish people prefer to die at home, not in a hospital.

3. Some Jewish sects, not Hispanic people, permit only a specific religious representative to touch or prepare the body for burial.

4. People of the Hindu culture, not Hispanic people, believe that expressions of happy thoughts facilitate the dying client leaving the earth and traveling on his or her journey.

5. Loud moaning and expressions of grief with chanting is common in Latino and African American cultures.

TEST-TAKING TIP: Identify the clang associations. The word *family* in the stem and in option 1 and the word *client's* in the stem and option 5 are clang associations. Identify the options that are opposites. Options 1 and 2 are opposites. More often than not, one of the opposite options is the correct answer.
Content Area: Diversity and Spirituality/Religion
Integrated Processes: Caring; Culture and Spirituality; Nursing Process: Assessment
Client Need: Psychosocial Integrity
Cognitive Level: Application
Concept: Culture

2. ANSWER: 1, 2.
Rationales:

1. Native American tribes believe in purifying and healing chants, dances, exorcisms, and body painting performed at the bedside; they believe that it helps ward off evil spirits and promotes healing.

2. Generally, people from Native American cultures do not readily share thoughts and feelings with people outside the family or tribe. They tend to be comfortable with silences, avoid eye contact, and respect their elders.

3. People who are Jewish follow a kosher diet and do not consume meat and dairy products at the same meal.

4. People who are Native Americans are permitted to eat meat. People who are Buddhists and Hindu primarily are vegetarians.

5. People who are Amish believe that the heart is the body's soul.

TEST-TAKING TIP: Identify the clang association. The word *healing* in the stem and in option 1 is a clang association.
Content Area: Diversity and Spirituality/Religion
Integrated Processes: Caring; Culture and Spirituality; Nursing Process: Planning
Client Need: Psychosocial Integrity
Cognitive Level: Application
Concept: Culture

3. ANSWER: 2, 5.
Rationales:

1. People who follow the Islam faith believe that the head or body should be positioned facing toward Mecca.

2. A person who is a Jehovah's Witness is permitted to use only artificial blood expanders because blood and blood products are prohibited. The nurse should verify with certainty that no blood products or transfusions are desired by the client and not make the assumption that this is the client's desire.

3. There is no rule in the Jehovah's Witness religion that prohibits a person from receiving care from a person of the opposite gender.

4. People who follow the Hindu faith prefer to wash in water that is free flowing, pray and meditate after bathing, and use only the left hand for "dirty" activities such as toileting.

5. People who follow the Jehovah's Witness faith do not eat food with blood (animals must be bled according to custom to be acceptable), and some members do not eat any meat.
Content Area: Diversity and Spirituality/Religion
Integrated Processes: Caring; Communication and Documentation; Culture and Spirituality; Nursing Process: Implementation
Client Need: Psychosocial Integrity
Cognitive Level: Application
Concept: Spirituality

4. ANSWER: 2.
Rationales:

1. This statement is premature. This service probably will not be requested by the client or family members. Family members and other members of the Amish community usually prefer to meet their loved one's needs when dying. Also, it may increase the client's anxiety.

2. People from the Amish community are committed to caring for its members in their homes, including when giving birth, coping with an illness, and dying.

3. People from the Amish culture are permitted to receive chemotherapy.

4. There is no indication that the client needs skilled nursing care. Pain management can be provided in the home. Also, this may increase the client's anxiety.

TEST-TAKING TIP: Identify the word in the stem that sets a priority. The word *most* in the stem sets a priority. Identify the options that are opposites. Options 2 and 4 are opposites. In option 2, the client goes home, and in option 4, the client stays in a health-care facility.
Content Area: Diversity and Spirituality/Religion
Integrated Processes: Caring; Communication and Documentation; Culture and Spirituality; Nursing Process: Implementation
Client Need: Psychosocial Integrity
Cognitive Level: Application
Concept: Culture

5. ANSWER: 1, 4.
Rationales:

1. Catholics believe that a priest can transform bread and wine into the body and blood of Jesus Christ (transubstantiation); it is distributed in the form of bread wafers (Eucharist) and sips of wine.

2. This is one of the tenets of a kosher diet that is associated with the Jewish religion.

3. Catholicism does not require its male or female members to receive care from caregivers of the same gender.

4. People who are baptized Catholic believe in a variety of sacraments. The sacraments of Reconciliation, Eucharist, Matrimony, and Anointing of the Sick can be performed in a health-care setting.

5. Mormons, members of the Church of Jesus Christ of Latter-day Saints, wear a sacred undergarment that is removed only for bathing and possibly surgery. When removed, it must be treated with respect.

Content Area: Diversity and Spirituality/Religion
Integrated Processes: Caring; Communication and Documentation; Culture and Spirituality; Nursing Process: Implementation
Client Need: Psychosocial Integrity
Cognitive Level: Analysis
Concept: Spirituality

6. **ANSWER: 3, 4.**
   Rationales:

1. Caregivers of the opposite gender are permitted in the Church of Jesus Christ of Latter-day Saints. Women who follow the Hindu or Islam religions require caregivers to be the same gender.

2. Head coverings are not worn by women in the Church of Jesus Christ of Latter-day Saints. However, they do wear a sacred undergarment that is removed only for bathing. Orthodox Jewish women wear a head scarf or a wig. Arab, Muslim, and Islamic women generally wear some form of head covering (hijab).

3. The statement is not true and shows a lack of respect for the client's beliefs. People who are members of the Church of Jesus Christ of Latter-day Saints (Mormon) wear a sacred undergarment that is removed only for bathing but can be removed for surgery if treated with respect.

4. Coffee, cola, tea, and alcohol are forbidden in the Church of Jesus Christ of Latter-day Saints.

5. This statement demonstrates sensitivity for the client's religious beliefs because people who are Mormons believe in prayer. This is an insensitive statement for a person who follows Buddhism because they do not engage in prayers for healing; they believe that illness is part of life.

Content Area: Diversity and Spirituality/Religion
Integrated Processes: Caring; Communication and Documentation; Culture and Spirituality; Nursing Process: Implementation
Client Need: Psychosocial Integrity
Cognitive Level: Application
Concept: Spirituality

7. **ANSWER: 2.**
   Rationales:

1. Although arranging furniture so clients have a view from their rooms is a caring intervention, it is unrelated to psychocultural comfort.

2. No two people are alike. Viewing each client as a unique individual is basic to all interactions with a client. The nurse should view each client as a distinct individual with personal distinguishing characteristics and plan and implement nursing care accordingly.

3. Although providing for a client's basic physiological needs is important, it is related to providing physical comfort, not psychocultural comfort.

4. Although providing for continuity of care is important, it is related to safety and security, not psychocultural comfort.

Content Area: Diversity and Spirituality/Religion
Integrated Processes: Caring; Culture and Spirituality; Nursing Process: Implementation
Client Need: Psychosocial Integrity
Cognitive Level: Application
Concept: Culture

8. **ANSWER: 1.**
   Rationales:

1. A client cannot wear a metal object in the operating room because of the use of various equipment that conducts electricity. A religious medal can be kept near the client.

2. This is not a client-centered action; it does not meet the spiritual/emotional needs of the client.

3. A deceptive act violates the trusting relationship that is essential between the client and nurse.

4. This is not a client-centered response; it does not meet the spiritual/emotional needs of the client.

TEST-TAKING TIP: Identify the options that deny the client's feelings and concerns. Options 1 and 4 deny the client's feelings and concerns. Eliminate these options from further consideration.

Content Area: Diversity and Spirituality/Religion
Integrated Processes: Caring; Communication and Documentation; Culture and Spirituality; Nursing Process: Implementation
Client Need: Psychosocial Integrity
Cognitive Level: Application
Concept: Spirituality

9. **ANSWER: 3.**
   Rationales:

1. This statement denies the client's feelings.

2. This is a judgmental response and denies the client's feelings.

3. This is a nonjudgmental response and recognizes that the client is attempting to cope with a difficult situation. The decision not to go to church gives the client a sense of control in an uncontrollable situation.

4. This response abandons the parents, and it may be perceived by them as being judgmental.

TEST-TAKING TIP: Identify the options that deny client feelings, needs, or concerns. Options 1 and 2 deny the client's feelings. Identify the clang association. The word *God* in the stem and in option 2 is a clang association. In this item, the test-taking technique "Identify a clang association" will not help the reader in selecting the correct answer. Often *but not always*, a clang association will help the test-taker focus on a potential correct answer. Option 2 in this item is an incorrect answer.

Content Area: Diversity and Spirituality/Religion
Integrated Processes: Caring; Communication and Documentation; Culture and Spirituality; Nursing Process: Implementation
Client Need: Psychosocial Integrity

Cognitive Level: Application
Concept: Spirituality

10. **ANSWER: 2.**
Rationales:
1. The belief that illness is caused by actions in the past is a belief associated with Hinduism, not Buddhism.
2. People who practice Buddhism accept modern medicine, surgery, and technology.
3. People who practice Buddhism do not engage in formal ceremonies or rituals.
4. People who practice Buddhism consider illness part of life and therefore do not offer prayers for healing.
Content Area: Diversity and Spirituality/Religion
Integrated Processes: Caring; Culture and Spirituality; Nursing Process: Implementation
Client Need: Psychosocial Integrity
Cognitive Level: Application
Concept: Spirituality

11. **ANSWER: 1, 2, 3, 5.**
Rationales:
1. People within the Asian culture respect authority and their elders. They may avoid eye contact out of respect and as a demonstration of deference.
2. People within the Asian culture value self-respect and self-control. As a result, they may stoically cope with pain, disability, and grief.
3. People within the Asian culture believe in Eastern medicine, including acupuncture, acupressure, herbs, and applications of heat or cold.
4. Asian cultures do not forbid the ingestion of pork or other meat products.
5. People within the Asian culture respect elders and other family members. The nuclear family frequently includes extended family members.
Content Area: Diversity and Spirituality/Religion
Integrated Processes: Culture and Spirituality; Nursing Process: Assessment
Client Need: Psychosocial Integrity
Cognitive Level: Application
Concept: Culture

12. **ANSWER: 3, 4.**
Rationales:
1. People who participate in the Church of Jesus Christ of Latter-day Saints (Mormon) allow blood transfusions. They forbid abortion and sterilization.
2. People who participate in the Seventh-day Adventist church allow blood transfusions. They forbid euthanasia and the use of opioids and stimulants.
3. Generally people who practice the Christian Scientist religion are reluctant to agree to a blood transfusion because they regard transfusions as conflicting with their reliance on the spiritual means of healing. However, some people who practice the Christian Scientist religion have no objection to a blood transfusion, particularly for children, as long as a primary health-care provider considers it an essential treatment.
4. People who follow the Jehovah's Witness faith forbid transfusions of blood and blood products.

5. People who practice Judaism are not opposed to using medical technology. They are opposed to suicide, euthanasia, embalming, and cremation.
Content Area: Diversity and Spirituality/Religion
Integrated Processes: Culture and Spirituality; Nursing Process: Analysis
Client Need: Psychosocial Integrity
Cognitive Level: Application
Concept: Spirituality

13. **ANSWER: 2, 3, 5.**
Rationales:
1. African American families generally are female-dominant (matriarchal), not male-dominant, families.
2. Many people who are African American are distrustful of others because of a history of mistreatment.
3. Most people who are African American have a spiritual orientation. They believe in God, prayer, laying on of the hands, magic rituals, and Voodoo.
4. Most people who are African American are not quietly tolerant of dying and death. They frequently are enthusiastically vocal when grieving.
5. Most people who are African American are present, not past or future, focused. They feel the past is over, and they feel uncertain about the future. Therefore, they focus on today, preferring short-term benefits and immediate results.
Content Area: Diversity and Spirituality/Religion
Integrated Processes: Communication and Documentation; Culture and Spirituality; Nursing Process: Assessment
Client Need: Psychosocial Integrity
Cognitive Level: Application
Concept: Culture

14. **ANSWER: 1, 2.**
Rationales:
1. Women who practice Islam prefer female caregivers. They are forbidden to expose their bodies to or be touched by any man other than their husbands.
2. Women who practice Hinduism accept health care only from a person of the same gender. Also, they wear clothing that covers the body except for the arms and feet.
3. Women who practice Catholicism can have either male or female caregivers. They may have a personal preference for a female caregiver, and that preference should be respected.
4. Women who practice Protestantism (e.g., Lutheran, Presbyterian, Baptist, Episcopal, and Methodist) can have either male or female caregivers. They may have a personal preference for a female caregiver, and that preference should be respected.
5. Women who are Christian Scientists can have either male or female caregivers. They are not permitted to receive blood or blood products.
Content Area: Diversity and Spirituality/Religion
Integrated Processes: Culture and Spirituality; Nursing Process: Analysis
Client Need: Psychosocial Integrity
Cognitive Level: Application
Concept: Spirituality

15. ANSWER: 4.

Rationales:

1. Administering an analgesic relieves pain, which is related to a physical, not sociocultural, need.

2. Using effective communication skills, including active listening, addresses psychological, not sociocultural, needs.

3. Dimming lights in the room at night limits a noxious stimulus, which is related to an environmental, not sociocultural, need.

4. A parent staying with a hospitalized child addresses the sociocultural needs of both child and parent; interrelationships are significant.

Content Area: *Diversity and Spirituality/Religion*
Integrated Processes: *Caring; Communication/Documentation; Culture and Spirituality; Nursing Process: Planning*
Client Need: *Physiological Integrity; Basic Care and Comfort*
Cognitive Level: *Analysis*
Concept: *Culture*

16. ANSWER: 2, 3.

Rationales:

1. People in European American/white cultures are future oriented but balance the past with the present; they are not present oriented.

2. The emphasis on a high financial status is rampant in these cultures. The majority of people who have difficulty receiving health care are living in the culture of poverty.

3. These cultures place value on youth, beauty, and being thin. People who are older, not beautiful, and overweight or obese struggle with self-esteem and access to nonjudgmental health care.

4. People in European American/white cultures accept health care in a variety of settings and care based on the newest technologies and approaches.

5. People in European American/white cultures readily share personal information. Native Americans and Amish people tend not to share personal information, thoughts, and feelings with people outside their culture.

Content Area: *Diversity and Spirituality/Religion*
Integrated Processes: *Culture and Spirituality; Nursing Process: Assessment*
Client Need: *Psychosocial Integrity*
Cognitive Level: *Application*
Concept: *Culture*

17. ANSWER: 2.

Rationales:

1. The Jewish religion does not have beliefs concerning free-flowing water when bathing. However, those who are members of orthodox congregations expect women to perform a ritual bath after menstruation.

2. People who follow Hinduism prefer to bathe in free-flowing water. If that is not possible, the nurse should use a pitcher during a bed bath so that the water can be free flowing. Also, they use their right hand for eating and their left hand for toileting activities, and they pray and meditate after bathing.

3. The Buddhism religion does not have beliefs concerning free-flowing water when bathing.

4. The Mormon religion (Church of Jesus Christ of Latter-day Saints) does not have beliefs concerning free-flowing water when bathing.

Content Area: *Diversity and Spirituality/Religion*
Integrated Processes: *Culture and Spirituality; Nursing Process: Assessment*
Client Need: *Psychosocial Integrity*
Cognitive Level: *Application*
Concept: *Spirituality*

18. ANSWER: 4.

Rationales:

1. Religious rituals can be performed in a hospital setting. The only restriction may be the use of an open flame on a hospital unit. If an open flame is part of the ritual, an arrangement can be made for an appropriate location for the ritual.

2. Notifying the nursing supervisor is not necessary. The nurse caring for the client can manage this situation.

3. This is not a situation that is an ethical dilemma. An ethical dilemma is a complex situation that involves a conflict between moral imperatives, in which to permit one would result in violating the other.

4. Clients have a right to practice their religion. Facilitating the visit by the priest is a nonjudgmental response that supports the client's self-identified need to receive a healing ritual.

TEST-TAKING TIP: Identify options that are opposites. Options 1 and 4 are opposites.

Content Area: *Diversity and Spirituality/Religion*
Integrated Processes: *Caring; Communication and Documentation; Culture and Spirituality; Nursing Process: Implementation*
Client Need: *Psychosocial Integrity*
Cognitive Level: *Analysis*
Concept: *Patient-Centered Care; Spirituality*

19. ANSWER: 1, 2.

Rationales:

1. Orthodox Jewish women wear a head scarf or wig and clothing that is modest and covers the arms and most of the legs. These practices show respect to God, and because hair is considered to have sexual potency, only a husband can see his wife's hair. Synthetic wigs can be worn because they are considered inanimate and do not contain sexual potency.

2. Orthodox Jewish individuals follow strict laws of Kashrut (kosher diet). It prohibits pork and certain shellfish but permits meat from animals that are cloven footed and cud chewing, fish with scales, and nonpredatory birds. They do not ingest dairy at the same meal as meat and require two sets of dishes, pots, and utensils to ensure that meat and dairy products are maintained separately.

3. Using the left hand for toileting activities and the right hand for eating are practices associated with the Hindu religion.

4. Wearing a religious thread around the wrist is associated with Hinduism. Each color (e.g., white, black, yellow, red, and orange) has a specific purpose and meaning. For example, red promotes long life and protection from enemies, and yellow is worn by married women.

5. Engaging in acts of good work during Advent is associated with the Catholic religion.
Content Area: Diversity and Spirituality/Religion
Integrated Processes: Culture and Spirituality; Nursing Process: Assessment
Client Need: Psychosocial Integrity
Cognitive Level: Application
Concept: Spirituality

20. **ANSWER: 1, 2, 4.**
    Rationales:
    1. People from Hispanic/Latino cultures believe in faith and spirituality. They believe in miracles through prayer, wearing religious medals, and engaging in rituals.
    2. People from Hispanic/Latino cultures place an emphasis on the group, particularly the family. Generally, people from Hispanic/Latino cultures have extended family members living together.

3. Native Americans believe that health is living in harmony with nature. People from the Hispanic/Latino culture believe that health is a gift from God, a reward, or good luck.
4. People from Hispanic/Latino cultures value health and believe that it can be maintained by respecting the body.
5. People from Asian cultures believe that illness is disharmony of yin and yang. People from Hispanic/Latino cultures believe that illness is an imbalance in hot and wet, hot and dry, cold and dry, and/or cold and wet.
Content Area: Diversity and Spirituality/Religion
Integrated Processes: Culture and Spirituality; Nursing Process: Assessment
Client Need: Psychosocial Integrity
Cognitive Level: Application
Concept: Culture

Chapter 12

Psychosocial Health

Addition and Behaviors
Cognition
Evidence-Based Practice
Family Dynamics
Growth and Development
Neurologic Regulation
Mood

Patient-Centered Care
Safety
Self
Sexuality
Spirituality
Stress
Violence

KEY TERMS

Adaptation—Disturbance in the human system in response to an event or stimulus

Affect—Observable, outward expression of mood

Aggression—Hostile verbal, symbolic, or physical behavior that intimidates others

Anger—Emotion precipitated by extreme displeasure

Anxiety—Unpleasant emotional state that spans the range of mild to severe with escalation of uncomfortable physiological and motor responses

Behavior—Physical mannerisms that can be observed by others

Body image—Subjective mental image of one's physical appearance and functioning

Cognition—Intellectual operations, such as the capacity to think, reflect, and reason

Coping (adaptation)—Use of healthy and effective choices to reduce stress

Defense mechanisms—Mainly unconscious mental processes used to protect the self from anxiety precipitated by external threats or internal tensions

Delusion—False belief despite evidence to the contrary

Depression—Feeling sad, powerless, or hopeless; related to low self esteem, anxiety, and various psychiatric disorders

External locus of control—Motivation generated from outside the self

General attitude—Manner of acting that demonstrates one's temperament

Hallucination—False sensory perception without an external stimulus

Hyperactivity—Increased motor activity and speech, impulsivity, inattention; and expansive or irritable mood

Impulse control—Ability to resist urges, drives, temptations related to action that may harm self or others

Insight—Ability to understand the causes and significance of one's attitudes, emotions, moods, and behaviors

Internal locus of control—Motivation generated from within the self

Judgment—Ability to formulate a rational opinion or make a conventional decision based on information

Labile—Rapid changes or swings in emotion or mood

Maladaptive coping—Occurs when unhealthy and ineffective choices are used to reduce stress

Mood—Continued emotion that has a significant impact on a person's view of the world

Perception—Recognition and interpretation of stimuli

Personal identity—Person's view of the self as a unique, separate, and distinct individual

Pressured speech—Rapid talking

Self-concept—Totality of a person's perception of the physical and psychological self

Self-esteem—Degree to which a person believes others view him or her as well as how one views oneself

Continued

Sensory status—Ability to receive, discern, and react to seeing, feeling, hearing, or sensing aromas

Stress—External or internal event (stressor) that precipitates a response in an individual.

Suicidal ideation—Thoughts of suicide or self-injurious acts expressed verbally or symbolically

Suicide—Self-inflicted death

Suicide attempt—Self-directed act that may result in minor or major injury by a person who intended to die

Suicide gesture—Self-directed act that results in minor injury

Suicide threat—Expression of intent to commit suicide without action

Thought processes—Processes associated with cognitive activities, including thinking, reasoning, reflecting, conceiving ideas, conceptualizing, and having opinions; attention, concentration, and expectation; orientation, level of consciousness, and memory

I. Psychosocial Health

Psychosocial health begins within the self in relation to self-concept ("Who am I?"). Self-concept is a complex construct composed of self-esteem, body image, personal identity, personal strengths, and role performance. It is constantly evolving as a result of gender, parental and social influences, growth and development, socioeconomic status, personal motivational resources, successes or failures, and health-related stressors (e.g., illness, disability, and aging). Nurses must understand the influence of this information, the theories that relate to the development of self-concept, and the general concepts related to stress and coping (adaptation) to be prepared to help clients maintain psychosocial health.

A. Self-concept
  1. Overview.
     a. **Self-concept** is the totality of a person's perception of the physical and psychological self.
     b. Frame of reference from which an individual identifies and interrelates with the environment and others.
     c. Dynamic process that changes throughout life as one is exposed to different experiences and when one compares oneself to others.
  2. Components of self-concept.
     a. Self-esteem.
        (1) **Self-esteem** is the judgment of one's own worth.
        (2) May reflect personal admiration or respect for self in relation to the totality of the ideal self or a certain part of the self (e.g., appearance, intellect, accomplishments).
        (3) Based on one's view of the self in relation to personal standards or standards set by others; also by how others view the person.
     b. Body image.
        (1) **Body image** is the subjective mental image of one's physical appearance and functioning.
        (2) Can be altered by an abrupt loss or change over time of a body part or function, disfigurement, or developmental changes.
           (a) Change in the body can negatively affect a person's self-concept, health, and health-seeking behaviors.
           (b) Sudden change in the body, such as paraplegia or amputation of an extremity, generally is more traumatic than a gradual change due to aging.
           (c) Change in the body's appearance or function may precipitate denial, anger, despair, and depression.
     c. Personal identity.
        (1) **Personal identity** is a person's view of the self as a unique, separate, and distinct.
        (2) Influenced by culture and socialization, beginning in childhood when a person identifies with parents and extended family members and then by teachers, friends, and other people.
        (3) Remains relatively stable over time.
        (4) Characteristics of a person with a strong personal identity.
           (a) Values own viewpoints, perceptions, and contributions.
           (b) When faced with a crisis, is more likely to work hard to address the challenge.
        (5) Characteristics of a person with a weak personal identity.
           (a) May not value own viewpoints and perceptions or view contributions in a positive frame of reference.
           (b) Is more likely to compare self with others and be influenced by others.
           (c) When faced with a crisis, is more likely to limit activities or blame illness or disability on others.

d. Personal strengths.
   (1) **Personal strengths** are components within a person that one draws upon to manage stressful situations in life, such as a positive mental attitude, talents, pride in life achievements, and positive coping skills.
   (2) Can be drawn upon to manage stress.
e. Role performance.
   (1) **Role performance** is the characteristic social behaviors of a person in relation to a group or society (e.g., child, parent, spouse, sibling, grandparent, employee, and so on).
   (2) People tend to view themselves in light of the roles that they are expected to fulfill and whether they can fulfill them successfully.
   (3) Health and developmental challenges due to aging can affect how well one is able to meet role expectations.
   (4) Role changes in life require transition.
       (a) Can be situational, such as death of a spouse or child, divorce, job termination, and relocation.
       (b) Can be developmental, such as commencement of a career, marriage, parenthood, retirement, and so on.
   (5) People with a strong self-concept are better able to draw upon personal strengths to adjust to changes in role than people with a weak self-concept.
3. Factors affecting self-concept.
   a. Developmental level.
      (1) As people age, self-concept is less affected by others.
      (2) Adults generally view inadequacies and faults less as confirmation of incompetence and see them more as difficulties common to all people.
   b. Gender.
      (1) Women tend to place a higher value on teamwork and cooperation and have a higher self-concept for verbal and social competence than do men.
      (2) Men tend to place a higher value on personal achievement and have a higher self-concept for mathematical and physical dimensions than do women.
   c. Socioeconomic status.
      (1) Socioeconomic status (social class) is related to one's level of income and ability to support oneself.
      (2) The higher the social class, generally the stronger the self-concept.

d. Family and peer relationships.
   (1) Social identity is facilitated by interactions between infants and parents and expands as the child ages through relationships with siblings, grandparents, aunts, uncles, and cousins.
   (2) As children age, they are less influenced by family and more influenced by peers.
e. Personal motivational resources.
   (1) **Internal locus of control:** People are motivated from within and believe that their actions can exert control over their lives; they take responsibility for their actions and are more able to handle unanticipated adverse situations in a more optimistic light.
   (2) **External locus of control:** People are motivated from outside of the self and believe that control of situations is attributable to external factors, other people, organizations, or a superior being; they are more likely to blame others for a situation or seek recognition from others for motivation.
f. History of success or failure.
   (1) History of success contributes to a positive self-concept; multiple experiences resulting in success encourages a person to seek new challenges, especially if the person has a strong support system.
   (2) History of failure contributes to a negative self-concept; multiple experiences resulting in defeat or failure may predispose a person to expect failure in the future or even to avoid opportunities for growth because of the fear of failure.
g. Illness, disability, and aging.
   (1) The United States is a youth-oriented society in which physical attractiveness, vitality, health, and youth are valued.
   (2) Body disfigurement; chronic illness; loss of a body part; and wrinkles, loss of hair, and other signs of aging may pose a serious threat to a person's self-concept.
4. Characteristics of a person with a positive self-concept.
   a. Has a clear understanding of self and others.
   b. Finds productive ways of finding meaning in life.
   c. Relates to others in a fulfilling manner.
   d. Can manage problems using effective coping strategies.
   e. Is more willing and able to take action to improve health.

5. Characteristics of a person with a negative self-concept.
   a. Does not value oneself.
   b. May become stalled in the ability to find meaning in life.
   c. May have difficulty engaging in respectful relationships.
   d. May resort to ineffective or destructive ways of coping.
   e. May be unwilling, unable, or lack the energy to engage in activities to improve health.
   f. Can be challenged or negatively impacted by health problems, such as illness, disability, or disfigurement.
      (1) Clients may not have personal strengths to manage change in a positive way.
      (2) Clients may react with ineffective coping, such as anger, depression, and even suicide. (See "Nursing Care to Support Psychosocial Health" later in this chapter for nursing interventions to support clients who are angry, depressed, or suicidal.)
   g. Can be improved through nursing interventions that help a client to view oneself more positively, use positive strategies to improve relationships with others, employ more effective and positive coping strategies, and accept a change or deterioration in health and quality of life.
B. Theories related to the development of self
   1. See "Theoretical Foundations of Nursing Practice" in Chapter 7, Evidenced-Based Practice, for a variety of theories that relate to development of the self.
   2. Coopersmith's four components of self-esteem.
      a. Identifies critical components in the development of positive self-esteem that occur during childhood and adolescence.
      b. Consists of four critical components.
         (1) *Acceptance and worthiness:* A person cultivates a sense of self based on the quality and quantity of care and concern received from others.
         (2) *Power and control:* Toddlers learn power and control of the environment through exploration and learning the cause and effect of behavior; initiative continues to develop, especially in school-aged children as they learn the difference between a leader and a follower in team sports and competitive activities.
         (3) *Moral worth and virtue:* Morals and values of parents and other important individuals in a child's life are internalized by preschool- and school-aged children and

are integrated into behavior in an attempt to please significant others.
         (4) *Competence and mastery:* As developmental milestones are reached, a growth in abilities leads to task achievement and feelings of competence and mastery.
   c. Understanding of this theory helps direct nursing interventions that support growth and development associated with each component of self-esteem development.

II. Stress and Adaptation

A. Stress
   1. **Stress** is an external or internal event (stressor) that precipitates a response in an individual.
      a. Examples of an external stressor: Hot environment, physical trauma.
      b. Examples of an internal stressor: Fever, fluid imbalance.
   2. Can be positive or negative; usually perceived as a threat to physical or psychological functioning.
      a. Examples of a positive stressor: Wedding, promotion at work.
      b. Examples of a negative stressor: Death of a significant other, an illness.
B. Types of stressors
   1. *Situational stressors* are unpredictable and may occur anytime in the life span (e.g., divorce, illness, accident).
   2. *Psychological stressors* arise from events or in response to stressors (e.g., exposure to physical or emotional abuse, history of separation from parents, rejection by peers, mental illness, disfigurement, and impaired family dynamics).
   3. *Developmental stressors* are associated with a predictable event that occurs at an expected time in a person's life (e.g., beginning school, puberty, marriage, parenthood, pregnancy, commencement of a career, midlife crisis, family responsibilities, menopause, caring for parents, physical changes of aging, and retirement).
   4. *Microbiological stressors* include bacteria, viruses, and fungi (e.g., sexually transmitted diseases, methicillin-resistant *Staphylococcus aureus*, *Clostridium difficile*).
   5. *Chemical stressors* are toxic substances that can precipitate physiological or psychological changes within an individual (e.g., smoking, drug or alcohol misuse, habitual misuse of prescribed or over-the-counter drugs).
   6. *Physical stressors* are stimuli from outside the individual that change the structure and function within the body (e.g., surgical incision, extremes in environmental temperature, amputation).

7. *Physiological stressors* are stimuli from inside the body that change the structure or function within the body (e.g., pain, paralysis, loss of vision or hearing, impaired function of an organ).

C. Adaptation (coping)

1. An **adaptation** or ability to **cope** is a change that occurs within an individual in response to a stimulus.
2. Adaptive coping occurs when healthy and effective choices are used to reduced stress.
3. **Maladaptive coping** occurs when unhealthy and ineffective choices are used to reduce stress; multiple concurrent stressors, a high intensity of a stressor, and/or a prolonged exposure to a stressor can exhaust a person's ability to adapt.
4. Personal factors that influence adaptation.
   a. Perception of the stressor (e.g., the extent to which the person's view of it is realistic or exaggerated).
   b. General health (e.g., chronic illness can decrease a person's ability to adapt effectively).
   c. Extent of support system (e.g., family, friends, neighbors, and religious groups).
   d. Other factors (e.g., age, success of previous coping, and life experience).
   e. Personal approaches to coping.
      (1) Actions that remove or change the stressor, such as resigning from an excessively demanding job, using stairs instead of an elevator if one is claustrophobic.
      (2) Defense mechanisms help people to adapt to stress (Table 12.1).
         (a) Mainly unconscious mental processes used to protect the self from anxiety precipitated by external or internal stressors.
         (b) Are adaptive because they protect a person from anxiety through the release of tension; however, when extreme, they become maladaptive.
   f. Psychological reactions to stress include feelings, thoughts, and behaviors that are expressed, such as anxiety, fear, anger, aggression, depression, embarrassment, guilt, paranoia, hopelessness, helplessness, powerlessness, forgetfulness, disorganization, resistance to authority, and use of defense mechanisms.
   g. Physiological responses to stressors begin with generalized responses (see Table 14.1, "Stages of the General Adaptation Syndrome and Related Nursing Care," in Chapter 14, Physical Assessment; and "Inflammatory Response: Local Adaptation Syndrome" in Chapter 16, Inflammation, Infection, Immunity, and Wound Care). If adaptation is unsuccessful, then pathophysiological responses (diseases) occur.

Table 12.1 Defense Mechanisms

Defense Mechanism	Example
Compensation: Increased capabilities in one area to make up for deficiencies in another.	Nonathletic student joins the debate team.
Denial: Ego unable to accept painful reality.	Client assumes false cheerfulness or fails to seek medical help when needed.
Displacement: Directing anger toward less threatening substitute.	Client yells at a significant other after being diagnosed with cancer.
Intellectualization: Situation dealt with on cognitive, not emotional, level.	Client discusses all test results but avoids focusing on fears and feelings.
Projection: Attaching to others feelings that are unacceptable to self.	Preoperative client says to wife, "Don't be scared."
Rationalization: Attempt to logically justify or excuse unacceptable behaviors.	Parent of a latchkey 10-year-old says, "He needs to learn to be self-sufficient."
Reaction formation: Opposite reaction to the way one feels.	A person does not like a neighbor but is overly friendly.
Regression: Retreat to an earlier, more comfortable developmental age.	Adolescent has a temper tantrum when told not to do something.
Repression: Unconscious blocking of unacceptable thoughts from the conscious mind.	A female adult has no recollection of her father's sexual abuse.
Suppression: Conscious blocking of thoughts from the mind.	Client states, "I'll worry about that after my test tomorrow."
Undoing: Actions or words cancel previous actions or words to decrease guilt.	A man gives a woman a gift after abusing her.
Freud's theory of psychosocial development includes that the use of defense mechanisms protects ego integrity.	

From Vitale (2017). *NCLEX-RN Notes: Content Review and Exam Prep.* 3rd ed. Philadelphia: F. A. Davis Company. With permission.

III. Mental Health Assessment

A mental health assessment is an important component of a comprehensive health assessment. Various stressors, whether they are situational, physical, physiological, developmental, psychological, microbiological, or chemical, impact a person's mental and emotional functioning. Keep in mind that humans have a biopsychosocial connection as well as a holistic response to stressors. Therefore, adaptations to stressors may be reflected in a person's appearance, general attitude, behavior, activity, sensory and cognitive status, thought processes, judgment, insight, mood, affect, speech pattern, self-concept, self-esteem, body image, perception, ability to control one's impulses, potential for violence, level of anxiety, and use of defense mechanisms to protect the ego. Before the nurse can identify a plan of action to address a client's mental and emotional needs, the nurse must first collect, cluster, and determine the significance of data reflective of the client's mental and emotional status.

A. Stressors
   1. Assess for internal stressors.
   2. Assess for external stressors.
B. Appearance
   1. Outward aspects of an individual.
   2. Note the client's grooming and hygiene, posture, eye contact, and clothing.
   3. Determine whether the client's appearance is congruent with his or her developmental stage and age.
C. General attitude
   1. **General attitude** is the manner of acting that demonstrates one's temperament.
   2. Assess whether the client responds in a positive adaptive manner or in a maladaptive manner.
   3. Assess whether the client is friendly or distant, hostile or aloof, open or defensive, passive or aggressive, guarded, suspicious, or resistive.
D. Behavior
   1. **Behavior** is physical mannerisms that can be observed by others and it includes intensity of activity and quality or quantity of actions.
   2. Note mannerisms, such as gestures.
   3. Identify whether the client is rigid or relaxed and has tremors or tics.
   4. Determine whether the client is restless, agitated, hyperactive, or calm.
   5. Identify whether activity and behavior are congruent with feelings.
E. Sensory status
   1. **Sensory status** is the ability to receive, discern, and react to seeing, feeling, hearing or sensing aromas.
   2. Assess ability to receive visual stimuli.
   3. Assess ability to receive auditory stimuli.

4. Assess ability to receive olfactory stimuli.
5. Assess ability to receive tactile stimuli.
F. Cognition and thought processes
   1. **Cognition** and **thought processes** are associated with intellectual operations, such as the capacity to think and reason; conceiving ideas, concepts, and opinions; attention and concentration; orientation; level of consciousness; and memory.
   2. Assess whether thinking is organized, rapid, slow, or repetitious.
   3. Determine the length of the client's attention span.
   4. Assess level of consciousness, such as level of alertness.
   5. Assess orientation to time, place, and person.
   6. Assess memory, such as recall, recent, and remote.
   7. Assess ability to concentrate.
   8. Assess content of cognition (e.g., delusional, suicidal, obsessive, paranoid, phobic, or expressing religiosity or magical thinking).
G. Judgment
   1. **Judgment** is the ability to formulate a rational opinion or make a conventional decision based on available information.
   2. Assess decision-making, problem-solving, and coping abilities.
H. Insight
   1. **Insight** is the ability to understand the causes and significance of one's attitudes, emotions, moods, and behaviors.
   2. Assess ability to understand cause and effect.
I. Mood
   1. **Mood** is a continued emotion that has a significant impact on a person's view of the world.
   2. Assess whether the client is depressed, apathetic, sad, anxious, fearful, irritable, happy, guilty, despairing, angry, ashamed, proud, content, or confident.
   3. Assess whether the client is experiencing rapid swings in mood or emotion (**labile**) or has the potential for precipitating harm to self or others.
J. Affect
   1. **Affect** is an observable, outward expression of mood.
   2. Assess the client's ability to vary emotional expression.
   3. Identify whether the client's affect is congruent with mood or is flat, blunted, diminished, or inappropriate.
K. Speech pattern
   1. Vocalization of sounds and words that reflect elements of speech.
   2. Assess verbal communication, such as tone, volume, rate of speech, fluency, and enunciation and its congruency with the client's feelings and behavior.
   3. Assess for rapid talking (**pressured speech**).

4. Assess for impaired ability to communicate through speaking, writing, or behaviors (*aphasia*). Determine whether the client is having difficulty receiving a message (*receptive aphasia*) or sending a message (*expressive aphasia*).
5. Assess the fluency of speech, such as whether the client is hesitant, is mute, or exhibits a latent response.

L. Perception
1. **Perception** is the recognition and interpretation of stimuli.
2. Determine whether the client has a history of hallucinations (command or auditory), delusions, or illusions.
3. Determine whether the client has a history of feeling detached or separated from oneself or feeling that one is being treated as an object rather than a person (depersonalization).

M. Impulse control
1. **Impulse control** is the ability to resist urges, drives, or temptations related to an action that may cause harm to self or others.
2. Assess whether the client exhibits disinhibition, aggression, hyperactivity, hypersexuality, or other inappropriate social behavior.
3. Assess whether the client has the potential for precipitating harm to self or others.

N. Potential for violence
1. Likelihood of the use of force or physical compulsion to abuse or cause injury to oneself or others.
🛑 2. Assess for progressive behaviors that indicate an increasing risk of violence toward others (e.g., increased muscle tension, pacing, use of profanity, verbal and physical aggression).
🛑 3. Assess for progressive behaviors that indicate an increasing risk of violence toward self (e.g., depression, suicidal ideation, suicide threat, suicide gesture, suicide attempt).

O. Family and social systems
1. Identify significant others and resources that influence the client.
2. Assess ability to attain and maintain interpersonal relationships.
3. Assess the extent of the client's support system.

P. Spiritual status
1. Belief in a relationship with a higher power, divine being, or infinite source of energy in an effort to discern meaning in life.
2. Identify client's level of comfort with beliefs, values, and spiritual/religious beliefs.
3. Identify whether the client has an affiliation with a religious organization.

Q. Level of anxiety
1. **Anxiety** is an unpleasant emotional state that spans the range of mild to severe with accompanying escalation of uncomfortable physiological and motor responses; may promote or hinder function and learning depending on the level of anxiety. (See "Clients who are anxious" later in this chapter for more information about anxiety.)
2. Assess the client's level of anxiety (Table 12.2).

R. Defense mechanisms
1. **Defense mechanisms** mainly are unconscious mental processes used to protect the self from

Table 12.2 Levels of Anxiety and Related Signs and Symptoms

Factor	Mild	Moderate	Severe	Panic
Perception	Broad, alert	Narrowed, focused	Greatly narrowed, selective attention	Feeling of unreality or depersonalization, fear of losing control, fear of dying
Motor activity	Slight muscle tension	Increased muscle tension, tremors	Extreme muscle tension, increased motor activity	Erratic behavior, combative or withdrawn
Communication	Questioning	Pitch changes, voice tremors	Difficulty communicating	May be incoherent
Mood	Relaxed, calm	Energized, nervous	Irritable, extremely upset	Panicky, angry, terrified
Physiological responses	Normal vital signs (VS)	Slight increase in pulse and respirations	Fight-or-flight response: Increased VS, dilated pupils, hyperventilation, headache, diaphoresis, nausea, diarrhea, urgency, frequency	Palpitations, diaphoresis, trembling, shortness of breath, feelings of choking, chest pain, nausea or abdominal distress, lightheadedness, chills or heat sensations, paresthesias
Learning	Enhanced, uses learning to adapt	Impaired, focuses on one issue, selective attention	Greatly diminished, improbable, decreased concentration, increased distractibility	Impossible, unable to learn

From Vitale (2017). *NCLEX-RN Notes: Content Review and Exam Prep.* 3rd ed. Philadelphia: F. A. Davis Company. Adapted with permission.

anxiety precipitated by external threats or internal tensions

2. Assess for use of defense mechanisms (Table 12.1).
3. Identify whether defense mechanisms being used are adaptive or maladaptive.

IV. Nursing Care to Support Psychosocial Health

Stress is a part of everyday living. However, stress can multiply when a person is confronted with additional consequences associated with illness and disease. Nurses should implement actions that address needs common to all people adapting to stress. In addition, nurses should know how to meet the specific needs of clients who are exhibiting maladaptive coping behaviors, such as clients who are anxious, depressed, suicidal, angry, aggressive, or hyperactive and those who are experiencing delusions or hallucinations. This section discusses these common and specific nursing interventions.

A. Commonalities of nursing care that support psychosocial health
   1. Introduce yourself and explain what you are going to do and why.
   2. Address the client by name and always speak in a respectful manner.
   🛑 3. **Recognize that all behavior has meaning.**
   4. Actively listen to the client's message.
   5. Maintain a safe, supportive, and nonjudgmental environment; emphasize honesty and consistency.
   6. Use interviewing techniques to encourage expression of feelings; do not deny or approve feelings. (See "Therapeutic Communication Techniques and Related Nursing Care" in Table 2.1 in Chapter 2, Communication, Collaboration, and Documentation.)
   7. Maintain eye contact and use touch appropriately.
   8. Provide privacy when performing procedures or discussing something of a personal or sensitive nature.
   9. Accept and respect the client as an individual; provide choices, when able, to promote independence.
   10. Do not talk about the client to others in front of the client.
   11. Set simple, fair, consistent expectations and limits about behavior; address inappropriate behavior immediately.
   12. Help the client to test new interpersonal skills.
   13. Encourage activities that involve the client in recovery.
   14. Include family members, with the client's consent.
   15. Implement actions that support spiritual needs, such as supporting religious rituals and arranging for visits with a spiritual advisor.
   16. Recognize that sexual needs persist throughout life; maintain nonjudgmental acceptance of the client's need to meet sexual needs and provide privacy when client engages in meeting sexual needs.
   17. Discuss sexual concerns with the client, especially when the client has a physical illness or change in body image that impacts self-esteem and self-concept.

B. Nursing care to promote a client's self-concept and self-esteem
   1. Help the client develop and achieve realistic goals.
   2. Help the client identify past achievements and personal strengths.
   3. Discourage self-criticism and negative self-talk; teach the client to substitute positive self-talk.
   4. Be supportive and use positive, affirming language.
   5. Support personal preferences and previous routines when able.
   6. Encourage involvement in activities that offer opportunities for success.
   7. Help the client to cope with dependency needs associated with illness or the aging process.
   8. Encourage the client to be as independent as possible; include the client in planning care.
   9. Refer the client to self-help groups as needed.

C. Nursing care to promote a client's positive body image
   1. Ensure that one's body language and facial expressions do not reflect revulsion, fear, or rejection.
   2. Reinforce the client's personal strengths.
   3. Encourage the client to express feelings regarding the illness, surgery, or trauma that caused the altered body image and explore options associated with living with the altered change in body image.
   4. Support the client through the various stages of loss, and explain to the client that anger, crying, and depression are expected responses.
   5. Urge the client to be kind to oneself; point out when the client is being unrealistically critical about his or her body and to try to look at strengths to support personal identity.
   6. Suggest that the client identify what is liked about his or her body and refer to it when the client "feels down."
   7. Encourage acceptance of positive comments from others about appearance.
   8. Practice role playing, allowing the client to respond to negative comments from others about his or her appearance.
   9. Encourage the client to surround him- or herself with positive, upbeat people who are not critical.

10. Assess the response of family members and intervene if they are negatively affecting the client.
11. Provide for interaction with people who have comparable body changes.
12. Help identify all available resources.

D. Nursing care to promote a client's role enhancement
1. Help the client to differentiate between ideal and actual role performance; help the client to recognize that it is acceptable not to be perfect.
2. Help the client to identify current and future roles; encourage reminiscence by older adults.
3. Discuss expectations and modification of roles in light of the client's lifestyle, family, and specific health changes.
4. Help the client to focus on positive and supportive change.
5. Facilitate alteration in roles among family members, such as redistribution of responsibilities and behaviors in expanded roles as a result of the client's health problem.

E. Clients who are anxious
1. Introduction.
   a. Anxiety is a feeling of uneasiness and apprehension that occurs in response to a nonspecific, vague threat to the client's physical, emotional, or social integrity that activates the autonomic nervous system.
   b. Anxiety ranges from mild to severe.
   c. Mild to moderate anxiety supports motivation and may encourage a person to take positive action.
   d. Severe anxiety interferes with a person's ability to focus and communicate, causes one to be easily distracted, increases motor activity, and consumes energy because all behavior is directed toward seeking relief.
2. Nursing care for a client who is anxious.
   a. Assess level of anxiety (See "Levels of Anxiety and Related Nursing Care," Table 12.2).

   🛑 b. **Stay with the client during a panic attack and provide for safety.**

   c. Provide a single room and decrease environmental stimuli.
   d. Validate somatic complaints, but do not call attention to them.
   e. Assist with relaxation techniques, such as deep breathing and muscle relaxation, to decrease anxiety.
   f. Help the client identify and avoid anxiety-producing situations.
   g. Postpone teaching when anxiety reaches higher than a moderate level.

   🛑 h. **Intervene when acting-out impulses may harm self or others.**

   i. Administer an anxiolytic if prescribed. (See "Anxiolytics, Sedatives, and Hypnotics and Related Nursing Care," Table 15.8 in Chapter 15, Pain, Comfort, Rest, and Sleep.)

F. Clients who are depressed
1. Introduction.
   a. **Depression** generally is described as feeling sad, powerless, or hopeless and is related to low self-esteem, anxiety, and various psychiatric disorders.
   b. Depressed people tend to retreat from people and reality.
   c. Depression theories include chemical imbalance due to hormonal, neurological, or genetic factors; loss and emotional detachment; negative thinking; ineffective family and interpersonal relationships; socioeconomic factors; and loss of function, illness, and disability.
   d. Clinical indicators of depression: Anger, anxiety, guilt, sadness, tearfulness, regression, restlessness, withdrawal, self-blame, blaming others, preoccupation with loss, anorexia or overeating, headache, backache, chest pain, constipation, hopelessness, and powerlessness.
      (1) Hopelessness is when a person lacks the psychic energy to seek or comprehend alternatives because of a distressed emotional state.
      (2) Powerlessness is described as verbalizing a lack of control or influence over a situation and is externally based; a person can feel powerless but still have hope.
   e. Failure to address a depressive episode early can lead to major depressive disorder, described by the American Psychiatric Association as a depressed mood or decreased pleasure for more than 2 weeks, plus four or more of the following:
      (1) Increased or decreased weight.
      (2) Psychomotor changes (agitation or retardation).
      (3) Altered sleep (insomnia or hypersomnia).
      (4) Decreased concentration.
      (5) Fatigue.
      (6) Feelings of worthlessness or inappropriate guilt.
      (7) Recurrent thoughts of death or suicide.
2. Nursing care for a client who is depressed
   a. Accept feelings of worthlessness, hopelessness, and powerlessness as real to the client.

   🛑 b. **Monitor for risk of suicide, especially as depression lifts and energy increases.**

   c. Sit quietly next to the client and then encourage one-to-one interaction.

d. Spend time with the client to support worthiness; provide realistic praise.

e. Accept, but do not reward, dependence; provide simple choices.

f. Encourage self-care.

g. Minimize isolation; involve the client in simple, repetitive activities.

h. Assist the client to identify and replace self-deprecating thoughts with positive thoughts through cognitive restructuring.

i. Avoid false reassurance and excessive cheerfulness.

j. Implement measures to support self-esteem.

k. Administer an antidepressant if prescribed.

G. Clients who are suicidal

1. Introduction.

a. Risk of suicide is associated with stress, loss, depression, hopelessness, helplessness, serious illness, substance abuse, social isolation, young adults and adolescents, single older adults (higher in men), mood disorders, sexual identity crisis, and history of previous attempts.

b. Levels of suicidal behavior.

(1) **Suicidal ideation:** Thoughts of suicide or self-injurious acts expressed verbally or symbolically.

(2) **Suicide threat:** Expression of intent to commit suicide without action.

(3) **Suicide gesture:** Self-directed act that results in minor injury.

(4) **Suicide attempt:** Self-directed act that may result in minor or major injury by person who intended to die.

(5) **Suicide:** Self-inflicted death.

2. Nursing care for a client who is suicidal

a. Provide constant observation and a safe environment, such as no sharps, belts, and shoelaces and assignment to a two-bed room.

b. Identify the client's behaviors, involving giving away possessions or putting affairs in order, as precursors to a suicide attempt.

c. Ask the client whether he or she has a plan and the means to carry out suicide.

DID YOU KNOW?

A no-suicide contract, an agreement that outlines what a person should do if feelings of suicide occur (e.g., a statement it is not okay to die by suicide, ways for the client to get help, identification of where to keep the contract, and the client's signature), is no longer advocated as an appropriate intervention. Evidence indicates that when clients violate the contract, attempt suicide, and are rescued, they have enormous feelings of failure and guilt.

d. Identify factors that precipitated or contributed to the suicide crisis and address them.

e. Encourage exploration of feelings about wanting to die and about death.

f. Assist with problem-solving; prioritize problems and focus on one at a time.

g. Focus on strengths rather than weaknesses.

h. Help the client write a list of sources of support and community resources and ways to ask for help.

i. Ensure that family members are aware of the need to maintain safety because most suicides occur within 90 days after hospitalization.

H. Clients who are angry or aggressive

1. Introduction.

a. **Anger** is an emotion precipitated by extreme displeasure; it can progress to acting out behavior, such as aggression.

b. **Aggression** is hostile verbal, symbolic, or physical behavior that intimidates others.

c. Anger and aggression are associated with delirium, dementia, substance misuse, mania, paranoid schizophrenia, and conduct disorders. They may be a response to a reality-based stimulus or associated with the defense mechanism of displacement.

d. Clinical indicators include a clenched fist, furled brow, glaring eyes, tense mouth, clenched teeth, flushed face, and raised or lowered voice.

e. Signs of anger escalation include disproportionate anger, pacing, agitation, suspiciousness, throwing objects, and verbal and physical threats.

2. Nursing care for a client who is angry or aggressive

a. Assign the client to a single room.

b. Use nonthreatening body language and a calm approach; respect the client's personal space and do not touch; even gentle touch may be perceived as a threat.

c. Monitor for frustration, irritation, increasing anxiety, or distorted thinking that may precede violence.

d. Anticipate needs to decrease stress that can cause anger.

e. Assist the client to express anger in acceptable ways, such as using words, writing a list of grievances, engaging in physical exercise, and using assertiveness; provide positive reinforcement for acceptable behavior.

f. Teach the client to interrupt aggressive patterns, such as counting to 10 or removing self from the situation.

g. Always position oneself between the client and the door to provide an escape route.

h. If behavior becomes aggressive, request assistance from other staff members and use short command sentences such as, "John, calm down."

🛑 i. **Follow policies and procedures for progressively managing aggressive clients if verbal interaction is ineffective, such as removing the client from the situation and vicinity of others, offering an as-needed medication, using seclusion, and applying restraints.**

I. Clients who are hyperactive
1. Introduction.
   a. **Hyperactivity** is characterized by increased motor activity and speech, impulsivity, inattention, and an expansive or irritable mood.
   b. It is associated with attention deficit hyperactivity disorder or a manic episode associated with a psychiatric disorder, such as bipolar disorder.
2. Nursing care for a client who is hyperactive
   a. Provide a safe, nonstimulating environment.
   b. Approach the client in a calm, nonargumentative manner.
   c. Channel hyperactivity into safe, controlled activities.

🛑 d. **Use easy distractibility to redirect inappropriate behavior.**

   e. Keep activities simple, repetitive, and of short duration.
   f. Use rewards, such as tokens or praise, to support appropriate behavior.
   g. Balance energy expenditure and rest.
   h. Provide high-protein and high-calorie handheld foods.

J. Clients who experience delusions or hallucinations
1. Introduction.
   a. A **delusion** is a fixed, false belief despite evidence to the contrary.
   b. A **hallucination** is a false sensory perception without an external stimulus; person sees, hears, smells, tastes, or feels something that is not there.
2. Nursing care for a client who experiences delusions or hallucinations.
   a. Recognize and accept that delusions and hallucinations are real to the client; stay with the client because delusions and hallucinations increase with isolation.

🛑 b. **Identify commands that direct the client to commit an act of violence that may harm the self or others (command hallucination).**

   c. Distract from delusions by encouraging the client to listen to music or walk and talk with the nurse.
   d. Point out reality, but do not reason, argue, or challenge delusions or hallucinations.
   e. Focus on meaning and feelings rather than content after a command hallucination has been ruled out.
   f. Praise reality-based perceptions.
   g. Identify factors that can exacerbate sensory and perceptual disturbances, such as reflective glare, lights, and television and computer screens.
   h. Teach self-coping for delusions, such as recreational activities and diversionary activities.
   i. Teach self-coping for hallucinations, such as exercising; listening to music; saying, "Stop; go away!"; and engaging in structured activities.
   j. Administer an antipsychotic if prescribed.

CASE STUDY: Putting It All Together

A nurse is caring for a 42-year-old man who was admitted 7 days ago to the burn unit with partial-thickness burns on his neck, hands, and lower arms and patches of deep partial-thickness burns of his face, chest, and anterior upper arms. The nurse received report from the night nurse, completed a physical assessment, and interviewed the client.

Night Nurse Report
Client admitted 7 days ago after sustaining partial-thickness burns of his neck, hands, and lower arms and patches of deep partial-thickness burns of his face, chest, and anterior upper arms. Vital signs are slightly elevated and client is experiencing dyspnea at times. Voiding straw-colored urine greater than 50 mL/hr.

Ringer's lactate, 100 mL/hour, infusing as prescribed
Urinary retention catheter, monitoring hourly urine outputs
Nasal oxygen at 2 L/min; oxygen saturation 95%
Electrolytes within expected range at this time; basic metabolic panel every a.m.
Intake and output in balance at this time
Tracheostomy set and suction apparatus on unit
Vitamin C 500 mg PO daily
Cefazolin (Ancef) 1 g IVPB every 8 hours
Pantoprazole (Protonix) 40 mg IVPB every 24 hours
PCA: Hydromorphone (Dilaudid) 1 mg/hr with 0.2 mg/15 min lockout, not to exceed 7.2 mg in 4 hours

continued.

CASE STUDY: Putting It All Together *cont'd*

Physical Assessment

Vital signs	
Respirations:	28 breaths/min, dyspnea
Pulse:	110 beats/min, regular
Temperature:	99.8°F, rectal
Blood pressure:	146/88 mm Hg

Partial-thickness burns (erythema and blanching with pressure) on the neck, hands, and lower arms, involving more than 12% of body and patches of deep partial-thickness burns (erythema, moist blebs, and blisters) on face, chest, and anterior upper arms, involving 5% of body.

Singed hair on the forehead and sides of the head, absence of eyebrows and eyelashes, singed nostril hair, and sooty sputum noted.

Client demonstrating an increase in muscle tension, rapid talking when discussing the event, a hoarse voice with tremors when talking, and restless behavior, evidenced by nervously moving about in bed and shaking a lower leg.

Alert and oriented to time, place, and person.

Client Interview

Client is able to recall the accident. He explained that he was home alone when the fire started. His three children were in school. Client stated that he cares for his three children alone: "It's just me and the kids now, with a little help from my neighbors, since my wife took off with another man a year ago. I'm a baggage handler at the airport at night and was doing a few chores before I went to sleep when the fire occurred. I tried to put the flames out myself, but they spread too quickly. The entire kitchen, ceiling, and bedroom over the kitchen were heavily damaged. My children are staying with neighbors temporarily so that they can go to their school until I can make other arrangements. I'm worried about money, but I have homeowner's insurance and health insurance with my job. I am not sure what will be covered or how many sick days I have. You just get a little bit ahead—a house, no big bills, and a little breathing room. This is really going to set me back, but I'm not going to worry about that now." Client states that he has not seen his children since the accident but spoke to them a few times on the phone. He said, "I'm worried that my face will scare the kids, and I don't know how my coworkers will react when they see me. People will be horrified because I look like a monster. I think I'll have to get another job that doesn't require me to leave the house so I don't scare others." He went on to say, "I have been able to deal with what life has tossed at me because I always want to do right by my kids, but this is more than I can handle. Maybe it would be better for the kids if I just killed myself." Client is open and willing to share concerns and feelings while maintaining eye contact most of the time. Occasionally, he used hand gestures that were congruent with expressed feelings, such as shaking his head, shrugging his shoulders, and drawing his hand across his neck, as if he were cutting his throat when talking about killing himself. He spoke in a sad tone, had a sad facial expression and slumped posture, and avoided eye contact when discussing the financial and emotional setback of this event. Client's speech was hesitant at times when he became emotional. However, he put on a big smile and said, "Basically, God has been good to me. I have great kids who give me no trouble. I told them that they had to 'be strong.'"

Case Study Questions

A. Identify specific examples of stressors that the client is experiencing or is at risk for experiencing grouped in relation to the types of stressors.

1. Situational

   a. _____

   b. _____

   c. _____

   d. _____

CASE STUDY: Putting It All Together   *cont'd*

_____ **Case Study Questions** _____

2. Psychosocial

   a. _____

   b. _____

   c. _____

   d. _____

   e. _____

   f. _____

3. Developmental

   a. _____

   b. _____

4. Microbiological

   a. _____

   b. _____

5. Physiological

   a. _____

   b. _____

B. Identify data collected in the following areas when making a mental health assessment of the client.

   1. Stressors _____

   2. Appearance _____

   3. General attitude _____

   4. Activity and behavior _____

   5. Sensory and cognitive status _____

   6. Thought processes _____

   7. Judgment and insight _____

   8. Mood _____

   9. Affect _____

  10. Speech _____

  11. Self-concept and self-esteem _____

  12. Perception _____

  13. Impulse control _____

continued.

CASE STUDY: Putting It All Together   *cont'd*

Case Study Questions

14. Potential for violence _____

15. Family and social systems _____

16. Spiritual status _____

17. Signs and symptoms of anxiety _____

18. Use of defense mechanisms _____

C. Which information indicates the priority problem, and why did you come to this conclusion?

_____

_____

D. Identify at least 10 specific nursing interventions that the nurse should implement to help the client achieve the following nursing outcome: "The client will remain safe from self-injury."

1. _____

2. _____

3. _____

4. _____

5. _____

6. _____

7. _____

8. _____

9. _____

10. _____

REVIEW QUESTIONS

Be sure to read the Introduction for valuable test-taking tips.

1. A nurse is assigned to care for a client who is admitted for an abortion. Abortion is against the religious beliefs of the nurse. There is no other nurse to whom the client can be assigned. What should the nurse do?
   1. Care for the client in a nonjudgmental manner.
   2. Provide just basic physiological care for the client.
   3. Arrange to have the client moved to another unit within the hospital.
   4. Explore with the client the reason for the procedure, including alternatives.

2. Many people who are independent and perform all of their activities of daily living become dependent and demanding when physically ill and hospitalized. Which defense mechanism should the nurse conclude they are exhibiting?
   1. Denial
   2. Regression
   3. Compensation
   4. Reaction formation

3. A 57-year-old woman who had a mastectomy, radiation, and chemotherapy 6 years ago for breast cancer is admitted to the hospital because of metastasis to the lung. The client had no respiratory symptoms, and the metastasis was identified on a chest x-ray during a routine physical. The nurse reviews the client's diagnostic test results, obtains the client's vital signs, and interviews the client. Which nursing intervention is the priority based on this information?
   1. Maintaining a patent airway
   2. Providing emotional support
   3. Monitoring serum electrolytes
   4. Supporting the limbs when changing the client's position

Client's Clinical Record

Vital Signs

Temperature: 99.4°F orally
Pulse: 90 beats/min, regular
Respirations: 24 breaths/min, regular rhythm
Blood pressure: 138/84 mm Hg

Diagnostic Test Results

Oxygen saturation: 97%
Serum sodium: 142 mEq/L
Serum potassium: 4.2 mEq/L
Chest x-ray reveals a lesion in the left lower lobe
Dual x-ray absorptiometry test to measure bone density: T score +1

Client Interview

Client is crying and angrily states, "I can't believe it came back. I went through so much. I had surgery, radiation, and chemo, and I've been taking medication ever since. My whole life changed 6 years ago. I gave up wine, I don't eat a lot of fatty foods, and I eat only vegetables that have antioxidants. By doing all this, I thought I had it beat."

4. The spouse of a client who is dying tells the nurse, "Even though I want to visit, I can come only once a week because I work and have a dog that I need to walk and feed." Which defense mechanism does the nurse identify the spouse is using?
   1. Projection
   2. Sublimation
   3. Compensation
   4. Rationalization

5. What is psychosocial development **most** influenced by?
   1. Food
   2. Society
   3. Alcohol
   4. Genetics

6. A client stands 6 inches from the nurse and begins to talk to the nurse in a loud voice. The nurse feels uncomfortable with this behavior. What is the **most** appropriate response by the nurse?
   1. "I would like to talk to you, but you are standing too close to me."
   2. "If you come closer to me, you will have to stay in your room."
   3. "You are much too close to me; you must step back."
   4. "Please step back because you are scaring me."

7. A client with terminal cancer is projecting unwarranted and excessive anger onto a friend who is visiting. The friend approaches the nurse crying and states, "I do not know what is wrong with my friend." What is the **most** appropriate response by the nurse?
   1. "It is your friend's true personality coming out."
   2. "Do not take what your friend is saying personally."
   3. "Your friend is attempting to cope with a serious illness."
   4. "Although your friend's anger is directed at you, it is not your fault."

8. A nurse is assisting a moderately cognitively impaired client with morning care. What is the nurse's **most** appropriate verbal intervention to help the client get dressed?
   1. "Would you like to put on brown pants or blue pants before you go to breakfast?"
   2. "Here are your clothes. Would you rather get dressed before or after you have breakfast?"
   3. "The brown pants look good on you. Put them on and go to the dining room for breakfast."
   4. "Pick the outfit you would like to wear today and then go to the dining room for your breakfast."

9. A nurse is caring for a client with low self-esteem. What can the nurse do to promote the client's self-esteem? **Select all that apply.**
   1. Provide simple choices.
   2. Assist with setting achievable goals.
   3. Teach the client relaxation techniques.
   4. Point out the client's past achievements.
   5. Help the client to identify personal strengths.

10. Which interventions are examples of nursing actions designed to support psychosocial coping? **Select all that apply.**
    1. Reviewing health-care options with parents of a child with an intellectual disability
    2. Taking a client's vital signs just before implementation of a procedure
    3. Discussing strategies about how to live with a diagnosis of cancer
    4. Providing names of supportive agencies in the community
    5. Changing a client's dressing 3 days after surgery

11. Which response by the nurse is **most** effective when attempting to reduce a client's hostility about an event?
    1. "I am here to help you."
    2. "You need to calm down now."
    3. "What can I do now to help address this situation?"
    4. "Do you think that you can be objective at this time?"

12. A nurse is caring for an unconscious client who sustained a brain injury. What should the nurse include in a stimulation program? **Select all that apply.**
    1. Rub lotion on the extremities.
    2. Perform range-of-motion exercises.
    3. Explain thoroughly everything that is done.
    4. Keep a radio on in the background at all times.
    5. Provide mouth care using a mint-flavored agent.

13. A client with a blood glucose level of 550 mg/dL is diagnosed with type 1 diabetes and is admitted to the hospital for further diagnostic testing and treatment. The next day, the client says to the nurse, "They told me I have diabetes and I will have to give myself shots of insulin and test my glucose several times a day. What is this all about?" What is the nurse's **best** initial response?
    1. "I will give you some pamphlets that explain everything you need to know about diabetes."
    2. "Although it sounds overwhelming at first, eventually you'll learn these skills."
    3. "It must be difficult for you to have a serious chronic disease."
    4. "Let's talk a little bit about what it means to have diabetes."

14. A nurse is caring for a client who experienced numerous panic attacks. Place the following nursing interventions in the order that they should be performed when caring for this client.
    1. Identify which nursing interventions reduce the client's anxiety level.
    2. Maintain a nonjudgmental approach when caring for the client.
    3. Stay with the client when the client is having a panic attack.
    4. Explore own feelings about people who have panic attacks.
    5. Assess the client's level of anxiety.
    Answer: _____

15. A nurse is attempting to meet the psychosocial needs of a client. Place the following steps in the order in which they should be performed.
    1. Use interviewing techniques and do not deny feelings.
    2. Identify client needs and involve the client in recovery.
    3. Introduce yourself and explain what you are going to do.
    4. Address the client by name and speak in a respectful manner.
    5. Listen to the client and recognize that all behavior has meaning.
    Answer: _____

16. A nurse is assessing a client's level of anxiety. Which level of anxiety is the client exhibiting when the client is irritable, displays increased motor activity, and exhibits selective attention?
    1. Mild
    2. Panic
    3. Severe
    4. Moderate

17. A nurse is caring for a client who states, "I hear voices that keep telling me what to do." What is the nurse's **best** response?
    1. "Do you find them frightening?"
    2. "How often do you hear the voices?"
    3. "Is there anything I can do for you?"
    4. "What are the voices saying to you?"

18. A nurse is assessing a recently admitted client's mental status, particularly thought processes. Which should the nurse assess? **Select all that apply.**
    1. Is the client happy versus sad?
    2. What is the client's level of consciousness?
    3. Are the client's emotional expressions stable?
    4. Is the client oriented to person, place, and time?
    5. What is the length of the client's attention span?
    6. What is the client's ability to exhibit disinhibition?

19. Three days after a stressful event, a person can no longer remember what there was to worry about. What defense mechanism should the nurse conclude that the person may be using?
    1. Regression
    2. Repression
    3. Displacement
    4. Intellectualization

20. A nurse is caring for a group of clients with a variety of psychosocial problems. Which interventions are appropriate regardless of a client's problem? **Select all that apply.**
    1. Sit quietly next to the client.
    2. Treat the client with respect.
    3. Encourage expression of feelings.
    4. Maintain a nonjudgmental attitude.
    5. Position self between the client and the door.

21. A nurse is caring for a client who is hyperactive. Which are appropriate approaches to use with this client? **Select all that apply.**
    1. Redirect inappropriate behavior.
    2. Plan a variety of challenging activities.
    3. Provide a nonstimulating environment.
    4. Encourage the client to rest several times a day.
    5. Suggest that the client engage in a game of chess.
    6. Arrange for high-protein, high-calorie handheld foods.

22. A nurse identifies that a client who will have surgery in the morning is exhibiting mild anxiety. What behaviors exhibited by the client supported this conclusion by the nurse? **Select all that apply.**
    1. Client had increased muscle tension and kept focusing on one topic.
    2. Client was extremely upset and had difficulty concentrating.
    3. Client had flight of ideas and exhibited erratic behavior.
    4. Client was alert and was asking numerous questions.
    5. Client was relaxed and calm.

23. A client is exhibiting severe anxiety associated with a 3-year struggle with colon cancer. Gabapentin (Neurontin) 100 mg PO three times a day is prescribed. The primary health-care provider indicates that the oral solution form of the drug be dispensed because the client has difficulty swallowing tablets. The gabapentin solution states that there are 250 mg/5 mL. How much solution should the nurse administer? **Record your answer using a whole number.**
    Answer: _____ mL

24. A nurse identifies that clients are experiencing developmental stressors. Which information about the clients supports this conclusion? **Select all that apply.**
    1. Entering kindergarten
    2. Going through menopause
    3. Taking multiple medications
    4. Displaying signs of a vitamin deficiency
    5. Engaging in altercations with family members

25. A client is admitted to an alcohol rehabilitation unit. Which statement by the client indicates an internal reward to achieve a goal?
    1. "I'm going to get sober for my kids."
    2. "I need to get my life back on track."
    3. "My wife is constantly on my back to give up drinking."
    4. "The judge said I can have visitation with my kids if I go to rehab."

1. ANSWER: 1.
   Rationales:
   1. There are times when a nurse may have to care for a person whose personal values are different from the nurse's own. In these instances, the nurse should care for the client in a nonjudgmental manner based on the standards of nursing practice.
   2. This care is inadequate; the client has both physiological and emotional needs.
   3. This option is unrealistic and places the needs of the nurse before the needs of the client.
   4. The client has made the decision to proceed with the abortion. The nurse's role is to support the client's right to self-determination.
   TEST-TAKING TIP: Identify the client-centered option. Option 1 is client centered.
   Identify the option that contains a specific determiner. Option 2 contains the word *just*, which is a specific determiner. Rarely are options with a specific determiner the correct answer.
   Content Area: Psychosocial Health
   Integrated Processes: Caring; Nursing Process: Implementation
   Client Need: Psychosocial Integrity
   Cognitive Level: Application
   Concept: Patient-Centered Care

2. ANSWER: 2.
   Rationales:
   1. Clients may use denial during an illness, but this generally will not make them dependent and demanding.
   2. During a crisis, one may regress to a stage that provokes less anxiety in an attempt to cope with an unacceptable situation. Regression to a childlike, demanding stage can occur under stress.
   3. Compensation is a mechanism that is used to make up for a lack in one area by emphasizing capabilities in another.
   4. Reaction formation is used when a client acts in a way opposite to internal feelings.
   Content Area: Psychosocial Health
   Integrated Processes: Nursing Process: Analysis
   Client Need: Psychosocial Integrity
   Cognitive Level: Analysis
   Concept: Stress

3. ANSWER: 2.
   Rationales:
   1. In this scenario, the client is experiencing no respiratory symptoms, and the client's oxygen saturation is 97%. There are no data that indicate an inability to manage respiratory secretions or that the airway is compromised. Adequate oxygenation of cells occurs when the oxygen saturation is between 95% and 100%.
   2. The client is in Kübler-Ross's stage of grieving known as *anger*. The client is asking, "Why me?" The nurse must encourage the client to express feelings and provide emotional support.
   3. The client's serum electrolytes are within the expected range. The expected range for serum sodium is 135 to 145 mEq/L, and the expected range for serum potassium is 3.5 to 5.0 mEq/L.
   4. A T score is measured in the number of standard deviations from the level expected in a young adult. The client's bone density T score of +1 is within the acceptable range of +1 to –1 standard deviation from the expected young adult score. T scores between –1 and –2.5 standard deviations indicate osteopenia, and T scores of less than –2.5 standard deviations indicate osteoporosis.
   Content Area: Psychosocial Health
   Integrated Processes: Communication and Documentation; Nursing Process: Planning
   Client Need: Psychosocial Integrity
   Cognitive Level: Analysis
   Concept: Patient-Centered Care; Grief and Loss

4. ANSWER: 4.
   Rationales:
   1. Projection is the denial of emotionally unacceptable feelings and the attribution of traits to another person.
   2. Sublimation is the substitution of a socially acceptable behavior for an unacceptable feeling or drive.
   3. Compensation is making up for a perceived deficiency by emphasizing another feature perceived as an asset.
   4. Rationalization is offering a socially acceptable or logical explanation to justify an unacceptable feeling or behavior.
   Content Area: Psychosocial Health
   Integrated Processes: Communication and Documentation; Nursing Process: Analysis
   Client Need: Psychosocial Integrity
   Cognitive Level: Analysis
   Concept: Stress

5. ANSWER: 2.
   Rationales:
   1. Food is only one aspect of a society and its culture; the primary purpose of food is to meet physiologic needs.
   2. A person's cultural environment, which includes the family and the community, has the greatest impact on psychosocial development.
   3. Although alcohol meets some individuals' psychological needs and is served in social situations, it is not the factor that most influences psychosocial development.
   4. Although some theorists identify genetics as a factor related to personality and behavior, it is not the most influential factor in psychosocial development.
   TEST-TAKING TIP: Identify the word in the stem that sets a priority. The word *most* in the stem sets a priority. Identify the option with a clang association. The word *psychosocial* and the word *society* in option 2 is an obscure clang association. *Society* is closely related to *psychosocial*. Carefully consider option 2. More often than not, an option with a clang association is the correct answer.
   Content Area: Psychosocial Health
   Integrated Processes: Culture and Spirituality; Nursing Process: Analysis
   Client Need: Psychosocial Integrity
   Cognitive Level: Comprehension
   Concept: Culture

6. ANSWER: 1.

Rationales:

1. This statement demonstrates interest in the client while setting limits on behavior.
2. This statement is inappropriate and threatening.
3. This statement sets limits but does not validate the client.
4. This statement sets limits but does not validate the client. The nurse's statement about being scared may give the client the message that the nurse cannot keep the situation safe.

TEST-TAKING TIP: Identify the word in the stem that sets a priority. The word *most* in the stem sets a priority.

Content Area: Psychosocial Health
Integrated Processes: Communication and Documentation; Nursing Process: Implementation
Client Need: Psychosocial Integrity
Cognitive Level: Application
Concept: Communication

7. ANSWER: 4.

Rationales:

1. This is an inaccurate and inappropriate response. The way people respond to stress is not necessarily indicative of their true personality.
2. Although this response is somewhat helpful, it is not the best response to meet this visitor's needs.
3. Although this statement reflects reality, it is not the best response in this situation.
4. This statement is most appropriate because it validates the friend's concerns and supports the friend.

TEST-TAKING TIP: Identify the word in the stem that sets a priority. The word *most* in the stem sets a priority.

Content Area: Psychosocial Health
Integrated Processes: Caring; Communication and Documentation; Nursing Process: Implementation
Client Need: Psychosocial Integrity
Cognitive Level: Analysis
Concept: Family Dynamics

8. ANSWER: 1.

Rationales:

1. This statement provides the client with a simple choice and adequate direction.
2. This statement does not give the moderately cognitively impaired client enough guidance. The concept of before versus after may not be understood.
3. This statement takes control away from the client.
4. The client may not have the cognitive ability to make this decision. Receiving two directions at once may be overwhelming.

TEST-TAKING TIP: Identify the word in the stem that sets a priority. The word *most* in the stem sets a priority. Identify the option that denies the client's feelings, concerns, or needs. Option 3 makes a decision for the client and is not a client-centered option.

Content Area: Psychosocial Health
Integrated Processes: Communication and Documentation; Nursing Process: Implementation
Client Need: Psychosocial Integrity
Cognitive Level: Application
Concept: Cognition

9. ANSWER: 2, 4, 5.

Rationales:

1. This approach is not necessary for a client with low self-esteem. This approach is more appropriate for people who are depressed and do not have the emotional energy to make decisions.
2. When goals are attained, it promotes motivation and positive feelings of achievement. These in turn promote a positive self-esteem.
3. Learning relaxation techniques will not directly influence self-esteem. Learning relaxation techniques directly relates to reducing anxiety in people who are anxious or experiencing a panic attack.
4. Past achievements are accomplishments that promote positive feelings, which promote a positive self-esteem.
5. Reviewing personal strengths accentuates the positive. Personal strengths provide a foundation on which to build future strengths.

Content Area: Psychosocial Health
Integrated Processes: Caring; Nursing Process: Implementation
Client Need: Psychosocial Integrity
Cognitive Level: Application
Concept: Self

10. ANSWER: 1, 3, 4.

Rationales:

1. This intervention assists parents in making decisions about a child. Coping is associated with restoring homeostasis (balance, equilibrium) and involves thinking processes and behaviors designed to deal with stressors. Nursing interventions can help clients develop adaptive (effective) coping mechanisms or to recognize maladaptive (ineffective) coping as the first step in correcting unhealthy coping behaviors.
2. Taking a client's vital signs is a physical assessment, not an intervention to support coping.
3. Discussing strategies about how to live with a diagnosis of cancer is designed to help a client effectively adapt (cope) to the devastating emotional toll of living with a life-threatening disease.
4. Providing this information can lead a client and family members to agencies that can facilitate coping (physically and emotionally) with home-care health promotion and illness prevention.
5. Changing a client's dressing is the provision of physical care. It is not designed to assist a client with thinking processes and behaviors that support coping.

TEST-TAKING TIP: Identify the word in an option that is a specific determiner. The word *just* in option 2 is a specific determiner. An option with a specific determiner usually is not a correct answer.

Content Area: Psychosocial Health
Integrated Processes: Caring; Communication and Documentation; Nursing Process: Intervention
Client Need: Psychosocial Integrity
Cognitive Level: Application
Concept: Stress

11. ANSWER: 3.

Rationales:

1. Although this response conveys a desire to help, it does not move toward what should be done next.

2. This response is confrontational and may escalate the client's hostility.

3. This is the best response because it indicates that the nurse is ready to do something immediately and asks the client to participate in making a suggestion.

4. This response is confrontational; it is a judgmental statement regarding the client's hostility.

TEST-TAKING TIP: Identify the word in the stem that sets a priority. The word *most* in the stem sets a priority. Identify the options that are equally plausible. Options 2 and 4 are equally plausible because they are confrontational responses. Identify the client-centered options. Options 1 and 3 are client centered. Consider these options carefully. Identify the option that is unique. Option 3 is unique because it is the only response that actively attempts to move forward to explore a solution to the problem.

Content Area: Psychosocial Health
Integrated Processes: Caring; Communication and Documentation; Nursing Process: Implementation
Client Need: Psychosocial Integrity
Cognitive Level: Application
Concept: Communication

12. ANSWER: 1, 2, 5.

Rationales:

1. Rubbing lotion on the extremities stimulates tactile sensation. Sensory stimulation helps to foster brain recovery by awakening the reticular activating system.

2. Range-of-motion exercises prevent contractures as well as stimulate kinesthetic sensation and foster brain recovery.

3. A client with a brain injury should have interventions explained in simple, concrete terms. A thorough explanation may be too extensive to process and respond to for a person with a brain injury.

4. A radio should not provide constant background stimulation. Constant auditory stimulation may lead to sensory overload. Stimulation interventions should be implemented in a quiet environment so that the client can focus on the particular sense being stimulated.

5. Using a mint-flavored mouth-care agent causes gustatory stimulation, which fosters brain recovery.

TEST-TAKING TIP: Identify the option with a specific determiner. Option 4 contains the word *all,* which is a specific determiner. Generally, options with specific determiners are distractors.

Content Area: Psychosocial Health
Integrated Processes: Nursing Process: Planning
Client Need: Psychosocial Integrity
Cognitive Level: Application
Concept: Sensory Perception

13. ANSWER: 4.

Rationales:

1. By giving the client pamphlets regarding diabetes and not engaging the client in verbal and other modalities of teaching, the nurse is assuming that the client can learn by

reading. The most effective way to educate clients is to use multimodality methods (e.g., verbal, visual, tactile).

2. This response by the nurse assumes that the client is overwhelmed with being diagnosed with diabetes and that the client will eventually learn the skills necessary to monitor and treat the diabetes. Nurses should never make assumptions.

3. This response by the nurse is nontherapeutic because it assumes the client will find having diabetes difficult and does not allow the client to express self-identified concerns related to having diabetes. Nurses should never make assumptions.

4. This response by the nurse offers a broad opening that allows the client to discuss self-identified specific concerns regarding diabetes. It is important that questions and emotional needs be addressed before teaching psychomotor skills.

TEST-TAKING TIP: Identify the word in the stem that sets a priority. The word *best* in the stem sets a priority. Identify the clang associations. The word *diabetes* in the stem and in options 1 and 4 are clang associations. Examine options 1 and 4 carefully.

Content Area: Psychosocial Health
Integrated Processes: Caring; Communication and Documentation; Nursing Process: Implementation
Client Need: Psychosocial Integrity
Cognitive Level: Application
Concept: Health Promotion

14. ANSWER: 4, 2, 5, 3, 1.

Rationales:

4. Nurses must understand their own feelings before they can provide appropriate, nonjudgmental nursing care to others.

2. Nurses must not impose their own feelings and beliefs onto clients. When nurses are nonjudgmental, they provide an accepting attitude that promotes trust and further development of the nurse-client relationship.

5. Assessment is the first step of the nursing process. Although there are commonalities of nursing care for all the levels of anxiety, there are specific nursing interventions associated with different levels of anxiety. The client's level of anxiety will direct the nurse toward appropriate nursing interventions.

3. If the nurse identifies that a client is in the panic stage of anxiety, it would be unsafe to leave the client unattended. The client could harm self or others.

1. This action reflects the evaluation step of the nursing process. Evaluation involves assessing a client's status after nursing care is provided.

Content Area: Psychosocial Health
Integrated Processes: Caring; Nursing Process: Planning
Client Need: Psychosocial Integrity
Cognitive Level: Analysis
Concept: Stress

15. ANSWER: 3, 4, 1, 5, 2.

Rationales:

3. First, clients have a right to know who will be providing care and what is going to be done.

4. After introducing yourself, address the client by name and be respectful; these actions focus on the client as an individual and promote trust.

1. After the introductory phase, interviewing techniques invite the client to converse with the nurse. Accepting the client's feelings promotes a nonjudgmental approach and validates the client's feelings, both of which foster communication.

5. When a client speaks, the nurse must listen actively to really hear what the client is saying overtly and covertly; also, the nurse must recognize that there is a reason for all behavior because it is meeting a need of the client.

2. After data are collected, the client and nurse must work together to identify needs and implement interventions to progress toward recovery.

Content Area: Psychosocial Health
Integrated Processes: Caring; Communication and Documentation; Nursing Process: Planning
Client Need: Psychosocial Integrity
Cognitive Level: Analysis
Concept: Communication

16. **ANSWER: 3.**
Rationales:
1. A person with mild anxiety will be alert and calm and will exhibit slight muscle tension and curiosity.
2. A person in a state of panic will be erratic, combative, or withdrawn and be incoherent and scattered.
3. **A person experiencing severe anxiety will have perception that is narrowed, resulting in selective attention. In addition, the person will exhibit increased motor activity and extreme muscle tension, irritability, decreased concentration, increased distractibility, and signs of the fight-or-flight mechanism (e.g., increased respirations, dilated pupils, and diaphoresis).**
4. A person experiencing moderate anxiety will exhibit increased muscle tension, voice tremors and pitch changes, energized mood, increased respirations, and an impaired ability to focus on more than one issue.

Content Area: Psychosocial Health
Integrated Processes: Nursing Process: Analysis
Client Need: Psychosocial Integrity
Cognitive Level: Analysis
Concept: Stress

17. **ANSWER: 4.**
Rationales:
1. Although this statement focuses on feelings, focusing on feelings is not the priority at this time.
2. This information is not the priority at this time.
3. Although the nurse may eventually ask this question to focus on client-identified needs, it is not the priority at this time.
4. **The nurse must identify the content of the hallucinations to ensure that they are not command hallucinations that are directing the client to do something that will harm self or others.**

TEST-TAKING TIP: Identify the word in the stem that sets a priority. The word *best* in the stem sets a priority. Identify options with clang associations. The word *voices* in the

stem and in options 2 and 4 are clang associations. Examine options 2 and 4 carefully.

Content Area: Psychosocial Health
Integrated Processes: Caring; Communication and Documentation; Nursing Process: Implementation
Client Need: Psychosocial Integrity
Cognitive Level: Application
Concept: Cognition

18. **ANSWER: 2, 4, 5.**
Rationales:
1. Being happy or sad relates to mood. Other examples of mood include depressed, anxious, fearful, irritable, euphoric, guilty, angry, ashamed, proud, and so on.
2. **When assessing thought processes, it is important to determine the client's level of consciousness. Clients with a lowered level of consciousness generally are cognitively impaired. They may be confused and disoriented and be unable to think, concentrate, or communicate in a coherent, rational manner.**
3. Emotional expressions relate to affect, not thought processes.
4. **Assessment of orientation to person, place, and time is part of a mental assessment. The ability to recognize the self and where one is in relation to a time continuum is a cognitive function.**
5. **When assessing thought processes, it is important to determine the length of a person's attention span. An adequate attention span permits a reasonable amount of time for organized thinking.**
6. Inhibition and disinhibition are related to impulse control, not thought processes.

Content Area: Psychosocial Health
Integrated Processes: Nursing Process: Assessment
Client Need: Psychosocial Integrity
Cognitive Level: Analysis
Concept: Cognition

19. **ANSWER: 2.**
Rationales:
1. There is nothing that demonstrates regression, a return to an earlier, more comfortable developmental level.
2. **The person's inability to recall is an example of repression, which is the unconscious and involuntary forgetting of painful events, ideas, and conflicts.**
3. There is nothing that demonstrates displacement, the shifting of feelings from an emotionally charged situation to a relatively safe substitute (usually someone or something perceived as less powerful).
4. There is nothing that demonstrates intellectualization, the use of thinking, ideas, or intellect to avoid emotions.

Content Area: Psychosocial Health
Integrated Processes: Nursing Process: Analysis
Client Need: Psychosocial Integrity
Cognitive Level: Analysis
Concept: Stress

20. **ANSWER: 2, 3, 4.**
Rationales:
1. Sitting quietly with the client is most appropriate for clients who are depressed. It sends the message that the client is worthy of the nurse's time and attention.

2. All people have value; therefore, every client deserves to be treated with respect.

3. All clients should be encouraged to express feelings and concerns. When a client explores feelings and concerns, the nurse collects valuable information that will assist the nurse in meeting the client's emotional needs. It also may help to reduce the client's anxiety.

4. A nonjudgmental attitude by the nurse is an appropriate approach to be used with all clients. A nonjudgmental attitude provides an environment where clients feel accepted; this will promote a positive nurse-client relationship.

5. This action is appropriate if the client is angry or aggressive.

Content Area: Psychosocial Health
Integrated Processes: Caring; Communication and Documentation; Nursing Process: Implementation
Client Need: Psychosocial Integrity
Cognitive Level: Analysis
Concept: Communication

21. **ANSWER: 1, 3, 6.**
    Rationales:
    1. **Hyperactive people tend to have short attention spans and can be easily distracted. Inappropriate behavior should be redirected in safe, appropriate behavior.**
    2. A variety of challenging activities will be too stimulating and will exacerbate the hyperactivity.
    3. **This client is extremely active and easily distracted by factors in the environment. The environment should be kept calm, quiet, and nonstimulating.**
    4. Although a laudable approach, this is unrealistic. Advocating rest periods will be ineffective because a hyperactive client has too much energy that must be expended.
    5. The client has too much energy to engage in a quiet activity that requires focus.
    6. **Hyperactive clients may not have the ability to sit and eat a meal. High-protein, high-calorie foods provide the nutrients for the expenditure of energy and handheld foods allow the client to eat "on the run."**

    TEST-TAKING TIP: Identify the options that are opposites. Options 2 and 3 are opposites. One of these options is among the correct options.
    Content Area: Psychosocial Health
    Integrated Processes: Nursing Process: Implementation
    Client Need: Psychosocial Integrity
    Cognitive Level: Application
    Concept: Stress

22. **ANSWER: 4, 5.**
    Rationales:
    1. Increased muscle tension and keeping focused on one topic are signs associated with moderate, not mild, anxiety. The sympathetic nervous system responds to a perceived moderate-level threat by stimulating the release of adrenaline and norepinephrine, causing these moderate fight-or-flight responses.

2. Being extremely upset and having difficulty concentrating are signs associated with severe, not mild, anxiety. The sympathetic nervous system responds to a perceived severe-level threat by stimulating a greater release of adrenaline and norepinephrine than when faced with a moderate-threat level, causing these severe fight-or-flight responses.

3. Flight of ideas and exhibited erratic behavior are signs associated with a panic level of anxiety. The sympathetic nervous system responds to a perceived panic-level threat by stimulating a greater release of adrenalin and norepinephrine than when faced with a severe threat, causing these panic-level fight-or-flight responses.

4. Being alert and asking questions support the conclusion that the client may be experiencing mild anxiety. The sympathetic nervous system responds to a mild-level threat by stimulating a mild release of adrenalin and norepinephrine, causing these signs. Clients experiencing mild anxiety also may exhibit a slight increase in respirations and muscle tension.

5. Being relaxed and calm support the conclusion that the client may be experiencing mild anxiety. When mildly threatened, the sympathetic nervous system is only mildly stimulated, thereby allowing the client to remain relaxed and calm. With moderate anxiety, the client is energized and nervous. With severe anxiety, the client is irritable and extremely upset. When the client is experiencing a panic level of anxiety, the client is panicky, angry, and terrified. Responses associated with the various levels of anxiety are caused by increasing levels of adrenalin and norepinephrine in the blood.

Content Area: Psychosocial Health
Integrated Processes: Nursing Process: Analysis
Client Need: Psychosocial Integrity
Cognitive Level: Analysis
Concept: Stress

23. **ANSWER: 2.**
    Rationale:
    Solve the problem by using ratio and proportion.

$$\frac{\text{Desire } 100 \text{ mg}}{\text{Have } 250 \text{ mg}} = \frac{x \text{ mL}}{5 \text{ mL}}$$
$$250x = 100 \times 5$$
$$250x = 500$$
$$x = 500 \div 250$$
$$x = 2 \text{ mL}$$

Content Area: Psychosocial Health
Integrated Processes: Nursing Process: Planning
Client Need: Physiological Integrity; Pharmacological and Parenteral Therapies
Cognitive Level: Application
Concept: Medication; Safety

24. ANSWER: 1, 2.

Rationales:

1. Entering kindergarten is the beginning of the school-age years, a developmental milestone and a stressor for the child.

2. Menopause is a developmental stressor associated with a woman who no longer menstruates. Menopause generally occurs at approximately age 50.

3. Medications are chemical, not developmental, stressors.

4. A vitamin deficiency is a physiological, not a developmental, stressor.

5. Impaired family dynamics is a psychosociocultural, not a developmental, stressor.

Content Area: Psychosocial Health

Integrated Processes: Nursing Process: Analysis

Client Need: Health Promotion and Maintenance

Cognitive Level: Application

Concept: Stress

25. ANSWER: 2.

Rationales:

1. This statement reflects an external locus of control. The client is going to rehabilitation for his children, not himself.

2. This statement reflects an internal locus of control. The client is going to rehabilitation because he personally desires to regain control of his life.

3. This statement reflects an external locus of control. The client is going to rehabilitation for his wife, not himself.

4. This statement reflects an external locus of control. The client is going to rehabilitation to meet legal requirements.

TEST-TAKING TIP: Identify who is the central person in the question. Option 2 focuses on the client. Options 1, 3, and 4 focus on the kids, wife, and judge, respectively.

Content Area: Psychosocial Health

Integrated Processes: Communication and Documentation; Nursing Process: Analysis

Client Need: Health Promotion and Maintenance

Cognitive Level: Application

Concept: Addiction and Behaviors

Chapter 13

Grief and Loss

NURSING CONCEPTS

Culture
Ethics
Evidenced-Based Practice
Family Dynamics
Grief and Loss

Health-Care System
Legal
Patient-Centered Care
Spirituality

KEY TERMS

Grief—Overall physical, emotional, cognitive, spiritual, and behavioral response to loss or bereavement
Anticipatory grief—Experienced before the actual loss
Complicated (dysfunctional) grief—Occurs over an extended length of time (more than 2 years) or involves excessive intensity of emotion or maladaptive responses
Uncomplicated grief—Expected (normal) grieving
Hospice—Interdisciplinary services that focus on maintaining comfort and quality of life of dying individuals and providing supportive care to grieving family and support persons

Loss—Unwanted change, removal, or reduction of worth of a valued object, person, or situation; can be actual or perceived, physical, or psychological
Mourning—Social and cultural expressions that convey feelings of sadness and grief
Palliative care—Care focused on supporting comfort and quality of life

I. Introduction

Although feelings of loss and grief can occur with any situation in which a person experiences a change or reduction in a valued object, situation, or ability, they usually are related to the death of a significant other or oneself. The experience of death is universal because death is inevitable. Every human being will die. Coping with loss and grief occurs not only during the process of dying but also after the death of a significant other.

A. Loss
1. **Loss** is an unwanted change, removal, or reduction of worth of a valued object, person, or situation.
2. Can be actual, such as death of a spouse or amputation.
3. Can be perceived, such as loss of stamina or feeling less womanly after a hysterectomy.

B. Grief
1. **Grief** is the overall physical, emotional, cognitive, spiritual, and behavioral responses to a loss.
2. Factors affecting grief include the importance of the loss, amount of psychosocial support, unresolved conflict at the time of the loss, anticipated or unexpected loss, and number of losses experienced in a short period.
3. **Uncomplicated grief** is expected (normal) grieving.
4. **Complicated (dysfunctional) grief** occurs over an extended length of time (more than 2 years) or involves excessive intensity of emotion or maladaptive responses, such as severe depression or addictive behaviors.
5. **Anticipatory grief** is grief experienced before the actual loss; generally it occurs when a person is

caring for another person with a chronic, deteriorating illness, such as Alzheimer's disease.

C. Mourning
   1. **Mourning** is the social and cultural expressions that convey feelings of sadness and grief.
   2. Manifested by behavioral responses, religious rituals, burial practices, and expression of condolence.

D. Hospice and palliative care
   1. **Hospice** provides holistic care to clients with a terminal illness and their family members; hospice care can be provided at home or in hospitals, long-term care facilities, or freestanding hospice agencies.
   2. **Palliative care** focuses on supporting comfort and quality of life.

E. Legal rights and ethical issues related to end-of-life care (See "Legal Rights and Ethical Issues Related to End-of-Life Care" in Chapter 3, Legal and Ethical Issues.)

II. Models of Grieving

Models of grieving provide frameworks that reflect the ways in which people generally cope with dying and death. These models provide nurses with information that can help identify a client's progression toward death, which allows the nurse to formulate a plan of care that addresses individualized needs during specific stages of dying.

A. Engel's model of grief
   1. Consists of six phases.
      a. *Shock and disbelief:* A person is in denial or intellectually, but not emotionally, accepts the loss.
      b. *Developing awareness:* Reality of the loss is internalized, and psychological pain is experienced.
      c. *Restitution:* Process of mourning that includes funeral, religious practices, and rituals.
      d. *Resolving the loss:* Grieving person centers energy on thoughts and beliefs about the deceased.
      e. *Idealization:* All negative thoughts and feelings about the deceased are initially repressed; as time passes, the person incorporates some unique characteristics of the deceased into his or her own personality.
      f. *Outcome:* Psychological dependence on the deceased lessens, the person begins to focus on moving forward, and the person begins to seek new relationships.

B. Kübler-Ross's stages of grieving
   1. Classic theory for health-care professionals to help guide client-centered care to those who are dying.
   2. Has five stages (Table 13.1).
   3. Not all people move through every stage; progression through stages is not contingent on completing the previous stage.
   4. Movement through stages may be nonsystematic and may not be linear; the person may be in two stages at the same time; and, after completion of one stage, the client may regress back to a previous stage.
   5. Nurses should encourage expression of feelings regarding the stage the client is in and should not attempt to move clients to subsequent stages because doing so depends on the client's readiness and coping abilities.

Table 13.1 Kübler-Ross's Stages of Grieving

Stage and Responses	Nursing Care
Denial: "Not me"; unable to believe loss; may exhibit cheerfulness	• *Explore own feelings about death and dying.* • *Accept, but do not strengthen, denial.* • *Encourage communication.*
Anger: "Why me?"; questioning; resists loss with hostility and anger	• *Recognize anger is a form of coping.* • *Do not abandon the client or become defensive.* • *Help others to understand the client's anger.*
Bargaining: "Yes, me, but . . ."; barters for time and may express guilt for past behavior	• *Assist with expression of feelings, such as guilt, fear, sadness.* • *Help with unfinished business if appropriate.*
Depression: "Yes, me"; realizes full impact; grieves future losses; may talk, withdraw, cry, or feel extremely lonely	• *Convey caring; use touch; sit quietly with the client.* • *Acknowledge sad feelings.* • *Accept and support grieving.*
Acceptance: "OK, me"; accepts loss; may have decreased interest in activities and people; may be quiet or peaceful	• *Support completion of personal affairs.* • *Support family participation in care.* • *Do not abandon the client and family.* • *Help family members to understand and allow the client's withdrawal.*

DID YOU KNOW?
People have similar responses when coping with the diagnosis of a terminal illness or death and dying. Progression might not be linear; people might not go through every stage or might experience several stages at the same time. In addition, some people never reach the stage of acceptance.

III. Nursing Care Related to Grief and Loss

A. Nursing care for a client who is dying
1. Answer questions honestly.
2. Meet spiritual needs expressed by the client.
3. Encourage independence and offer choices, such as "Who do you want in the room with you now?" and "What can we do to help you go peacefully?" Acknowledge that the client has control over the plan of care and goals.
4. Support social needs; recognize that the client may want to mend a strained relationship or spend time with particular people or family members.
5. Assist with final arrangements, such as persons to notify, funeral arrangements, and completion of any last wishes when possible.
6. Balance activity and rest.
7. Implement measures to maintain hygiene, grooming, and skin integrity.
8. Provide for physical needs, such as elimination, nutrition, and oxygen.
🛑 9. Provide for adequate pain control. Also, accept an informed decision not to be medicated so that interaction with family members can be maintained.
10. Advocate for the client when the client and family members are at different stages of grieving.
11. Assess for signs and symptoms of preactive dying.
    a. Withdrawal from social interactions.
    b. Increased lethargy and periods of sleep.
    c. Decreased fluid and food intake.
    d. Increase in abnormal breathing patterns.
    e. Reports seeing people who have already died.
    f. Desires to complete unfinished business.
    g. Increase in agitation and restlessness.
12. Assess for signs and symptoms of active dying.
    a. Difficult to arouse, becomes unresponsive.
    b. Unable to swallow.
    c. Severely altered breathing patterns (e.g., longer periods of apnea, alternating slow breathing with fast breathing, and "death rattle" as fluid collects in respiratory tract).
    d. May experience severe agitation and even hallucinations.
    e. Significant decrease in blood pressure.
    f. Cold, mottled skin of the extremities; may report feeling cold and no longer able to feel hands and feet.
13. Provide care for an unconscious client.
    a. Continue to talk to as if hearing is intact.
    b. Wet the client's lips and mouth.
    c. Use artificial tears to keep eyes moist.
    d. Turn the client on his or her side and raise the head of the bed if respirations are congested and noisy (death rattle).
14. Understand that some clients wait for a specific date to die or until family members arrive; others wait until loved ones leave so as not to die in their presence.

B. Nursing care for family members of a client who is dying
1. Be aware of age-related reactions to the concepts of illness, dying, and death (see "Reaction to Illness and Hospitalization" under "Toddler, School-Aged Child, and Adolescent" in Chapter 10, Development Across the Life Span.).
2. Explain the stages of death and dying to family members so that they understand their loved one's behavior, and explain that dying clients may interact minimally with family members.
3. Involve family members in direct client care if that is the client's and their wishes.
4. Encourage family members to ensure their own needs are met (e.g., food and rest); provide chairs or recliners so that family members can stay near.
5. Encourage family members to continue to occasionally talk to a dying unconscious client.
6. Keep family members informed about physical signs that indicate active dying, such as falling blood pressure; diaphoresis; and mottled, cold skin.
7. Explain that moaning and grunting are common behaviors when death is near and may not mean that the client is uncomfortable.
8. Refer to the Ethics Committee when family members are having conflicts regarding end-of-life care for a client who is unconscious or unable to make informed decisions.

IV. Nursing Care When Death Occurs

Nursing care of the client and family continues after death occurs. Although a client's body is cared for respectfully after death, the major focus of care shifts to the needs of the family. Also, the nurse must arrange for an appropriate health-care provider to pronounce death.
A. Certification of death
1. Consider any legal issues related to postmortem care (Box 13.1).

Box 13.1 Legal Issues Related to Postmortem Care

Certification of Death

- *U.S. laws mandate that a death certificate be completed and filed with the local health department or other government office for every person who dies.*
- *Certificates of death also are necessary for legal matters and insurance purposes.*

Organ Donation (Upon Death)

- *All states have accepted the Uniform Anatomical Gift Act for organ donation.*
- *Generally, a person carries an organ or tissue donor card that stipulates all or specific organs and tissues that a person wishes to donate upon death; some states use a section of the driver's license as a donor card.*
- *Documents no longer require a witness to the person's signature or a family member's consent.*
- *An organ procurement team member may approach family members about organ donation in the absence of a donor card.*

Postmortem Examination (Autopsy)

- *An autopsy is an examination of a body to establish the cause of death.*
- *It is required in the event of an unexpected, suspicious, or violent death.*
- *Family member must give consent for an autopsy unless it is ordered by the court.*
- *The legal system may seek a court order for an autopsy in some situations.*

2. Be aware that death generally is pronounced by a primary health-care provider or coroner; however, some states grant advanced practice nurses and nurses working in long-term care facilities, home-health care, and hospice agencies the authority to pronounce death.

3. Quantifying death by primary health-care providers is guided by two sets of criteria:
   a. The President's Commission for the Study of Ethical Problems in Medicine and Biomedical and Behavioral Research (1981) defines death as "Absence of respiration and circulation; irreversible absence of all brain functions, including the brain stem."
   b. The Harvard Medical School Criteria of Death consists of five components:
      (1) Unreceptive and unresponsive to stimuli.
      (2) No movements.
      (3) No breathing.
      (4) No reflexes.
      (5) Flat electroencephalogram.

B. Nursing care for family members of a client who has died
   1. Do not impose on family members at the moment of death; accept family members' behaviors, such as picture taking and lying next to or hugging the body; allow family members as much time as they need to be with the body; stay near and wait quietly until they are ready to move away from the body.
   2. Remove any tubes or lines attached to the client (unless an autopsy is required) according to policy and procedure; straighten bedcovers; and make client look as natural as possible for viewing by family members.
   3. Take family members to view the body when they arrive, if they wish.
   4. Transfer the body after family members have viewed the body or stated a preference not to view the body.
   5. Offer support by saying, "I am sorry for your loss." Avoid efforts to minimize loss by saying, "She is in heaven now" or "You still have your children." Ask family members "How can I help?" or "What would you like me to do?"

C. Postmortem care
   1. After a person is pronounced dead and family members have left, prepare the body or delegate the task to unlicensed assistive personnel, as appropriate.
   2. Respect cultural and spiritual preferences, noting that some cultures require family members to wash the body.
   3. Follow facility policies and procedures regarding hygiene, grooming, and dressing changes.
   4. Remove tubes and lines unless an autopsy is scheduled.
   5. Provide postmortem care per facility policy.
      a. Secure a postmortem set, which contains items such as a plastic sheet called a *shroud*, identification tags, soft gauze, and padding.
      b. Position the body in functional alignment.
      c. Position a pillow under the head and shoulders to reduce the risk of settling blood, which can cause discoloration.
      d. Place dentures in the mouth.
      e. Close the eyes.
      f. Tie soft gauze under the chin and around the head to keep the mouth set in a natural position.
      g. Pad and tie the wrists together gently to hold the arms close to the body.
      h. Place an identification tag on the client's toe or ankle.
      i. Enclose the body within a shroud and place an identification tag on the shroud.
   6. Arrange to have the body transported to the morgue or removed by funeral home personnel. Be aware that most facilities have a special stretcher to transport a body to the morgue; it looks like a regular stretcher, but the body is enclosed below so that it is not visible to visitors and other clients.

CASE STUDY: Putting It All Together

A 76-year-old client was brought to the emergency department by ambulance. The client was conscious and alert to time, place, and person; was able to speak; and the gag reflex was intact but he had right hemiplegia. The vital signs were

- BP 190/89 mm Hg
- Pulse 120, bounding and regular
- Respirations 24 breaths/min
- Oxygen saturation 90%

A head CT confirmed a left cerebral brain attack, and a systemic tissue plasminogen activator was administered. Two days later, the client demonstrated slight improvement in the ability to move the right upper and lower extremities.

A nurse on a medical unit was assigned to care for the client. The nurse found the client in bed in the contour position with pillows and a trochanter roll maintaining the right arm and leg in functional alignment. The nurse addressed the client by name. The client appeared sad, and he responded slowly and said, "I am Mr. Jones." The nurse asked the client what brought him to the hospital. The client explained that when making breakfast, he suddenly became very weak and fell down. He said that he could not move his right arm and leg and immediately activated his medical alert device. He started to cry as he shared that he lost his wife to cancer 3 years ago. He said that he goes to the cemetery every day and has left the house just as it was the day she passed away. He said, "I miss her so much and can't go through her clothes or change anything in the house." He indicated that because of the stroke he will have to move into an assisted living facility. He said, "I can't believe that I can't take care of myself or walk. People even have to help me with going to the bathroom. It is so humiliating." After sitting quietly for a few minutes, he continued, "My daughter is getting married in 4 months, and I will not be well enough to walk her down the aisle." He continued to cry and said, "I am so lonely and sad."

Case Study Questions

A. Which type of grief (normal grief, complicated grief, or anticipatory grief) is the client experiencing regarding the loss of his wife, and what data supports this conclusion?

_____

_____

_____

_____

B. Based on Kübler-Ross's stages of grieving, which stage (denial, anger, bargaining, depression, acceptance) is the client experiencing regarding his brain attack, and what data supports this conclusion?

_____

_____

_____

C. Identify at least five past and/or future losses for which the client is grieving.

1. _____

2. _____

3. _____

4. _____

5. _____

REVIEW QUESTIONS

Be sure to read the Introduction for valuable test-taking tips.

1. A nurse is caring for an older adult who is in the last stage of dying. A family member keeps trying to get the father to ingest some soup. Which response by the nurse is **most** appropriate?
   1. "Nourishment is not necessary unless your father asks for it because vital organs are in decline."
   2. "Applying a protective lip balm on the lips supports comfort rather than encouraging eating."
   3. "You have been very attentive in trying to get your father to take some nourishment."
   4. "Ice chips or wetting the lips with a small amount of water is all that is necessary."

2. Place the following statements in order of Kübler-Ross's stages of grieving.
   1. "I will write my daughter a long letter about how much I will miss the milestones in her life."
   2. "I can't seem to get a decent meal in this hospital. They are either bland, cold, or dried out."
   3. "I don't think that I have a brain tumor. My imbalance is just due to an inner ear infection."
   4. "I hope that I can spend more time with my family than with my job, like I did in the past."
   5. "I am not going to make it to my son's wedding. I am so sad and cry all the time."
   Answer: _____

3. The spouse of a client who is dying has been at the bedside for the last 2 days and says that she wants to be in the room when her husband dies. It is lunch time, and the wife asks the nurse, "Should I go to lunch now or wait awhile?" The husband is experiencing Cheyne-Stokes respirations and is profusely diaphoretic. What is the **best** response by the nurse?
   1. "I think that you will have time to run down and get a quick lunch in the cafeteria."
   2. "You have time for lunch because he is not demonstrating signs that death is near."
   3. "I have an extra fruit platter in the pantry. I will bring it to the room for you."
   4. "Go to lunch, and if his condition deteriorates, I will call you immediately."

4. A nurse is caring for a client whose adolescent son recently died. The mother states, "Nothing is worse than losing a child. I wake up each morning and I feel as though I have been hit by a bus. I feel his loss in every bone in my body." Which stage of Engel's model of grief is the client experiencing?
   1. Developing awareness
   2. Shock and disbelief
   3. Resolving the loss
   4. Idealization

5. A client expired in the early morning hours, and the nurse immediately called the daughter, who has been very attentive to the father. Which is the **best** response by the nurse upon the daughter's arrival on the unit?
   1. "Is there anyone else in the family that you would like me to call for you?"
   2. "Do you want me to call a spiritual advisor to pray with you?"
   3. "Would you like to stay awhile with your father?"
   4. "I am very sorry for the loss of your father."

6. A nurse is caring for a man who is in the final stage of dying. The son appears alarmed and reports to the nurse that the father is making unusual sounds when breathing. What should the nurse do **first**?
   1. Explain that this is called death rattle.
   2. Wipe the mouth of secretions.
   3. Suction respiratory passages.
   4. Raise the head of the bed.

7. An elderly woman who lost her husband suddenly due to a massive heart attack one week ago came back to the emergency department to thank the nurses for being so kind to her husband. The woman stated, "I am very lonely and can hardly believe that he is gone." Which is an appropriate response by the nurse?
   1. "I am sure that you have many loving memories that will help when you feel sad."
   2. "The senior center has various programs to join so you are involved with others."
   3. "You will be experiencing feelings of grief and loss as you journey forward."
   4. "Take one day at a time because things will get better as time goes on."

8. Place the following statements in order according to Engel's model of grief.
   1. "Each morning, I awaken with this horrible empty feeling in the middle of my body."
   2. "I am going on a trip to visit some of my old friends who I have not seen in a while."
   3. "We are planning to spread my son's ashes on the lake. I know he would like that."
   4. "My son was always so kind. I am going to try to do one kind deed each day."
   5. "He was such a good son. I keep reliving each stage of his life."
   6. "It was so sudden. I just can't believe that my son is dead."
   Answer: _____

9. After several years of caring for his wife who has Alzheimer's disease, a man admits his wife to a nursing home because he no longer is able to provide the level of care that she needs. When visiting his wife, he begins to cry softly and makes the following comment to the nurse: "I always thought that we would have time to enjoy retirement, but I spent the last few years caring for my wife who no longer knows who I am. I worry about my wife, who is slowly dying, but I am very tired and need some relief." What type of grief is the man experiencing?
   1. Normal grief
   2. Anticipatory grief
   3. Complicated grief
   4. Dysfunctional grief

10. An emergency department nurse is caring for parents whose 15-year-old daughter, while walking to school, was killed by a hit-and-run driver. Identify statements made by the nurse that are based on principles of therapeutic communication. **Select all that apply.**
   1. "I am so sorry for your loss."
   2. "Losing a child is awful. It is okay to cry."
   3. "Maybe we can talk a little bit about how you are feeling."
   4. "I hope that the police find the driver and that justice is served."
   5. "You have to believe that God wanted her close to Him as an angel in heaven."

11. A nurse is caring for a client who has no family and has been battling ovarian cancer for 5 years. The client is now in the terminal stage of the disease and is told that there are no viable curative care options left and is offered a referral to a hospice facility. The nurse sits with the client after the primary health-care provider leaves. Which statement by the nurse is **most** appropriate after exploring the client's feelings?
   1. "It is unfortunate that there no longer are any medical therapies that can be done."
   2. "Let's explore what we can do together to control your pain and make you comfortable."
   3. "You'll find that the staff members at the hospice agency will become like family to you."
   4. "The agency the doctor suggested is excellent, and the people who work there are very supportive."

12. A nurse working in a nursing home is caring for a client whose wife died several years ago. The nurse believes that the client is experiencing dysfunctional grieving. Which of the following clinical manifestations by the client specifically support dysfunctional grieving rather than normal grieving?
   1. Focuses on little else but the death of his wife
   2. Focuses excessively on memories of his wife
   3. Feels that there is nothing to live for
   4. Feels sad at the thought of his wife
   5. Feels tired

13. A nurse is caring for a man with terminal pancreatic cancer. The wife is upset because her husband is quiet and withdrawn and is always suggesting that she go to the cafeteria to get something to eat. Which response by the nurse is therapeutic?
   1. "Maybe he just wants to sleep, and it is his way of asking you to leave so it is quiet."
   2. "Would you like the dietary department to bring you something during meal times?"
   3. "Why don't you bring a bag lunch tomorrow so that he sees that you are not missing a meal?"
   4. "Try not to take it personally because people who are dying often interact minimally with loved ones."

14. A nurse is caring for a client who is dying. The client is withdrawn and quiet. What should the nurse do? **Select all that apply.**
   1. Avoid talking unnecessarily.
   2. Engage in cheerful dialogue.
   3. Provide constant reassurance.
   4. Encourage interaction with family.
   5. Sit quietly by the bedside periodically.

15. An emergency department nurse is caring for a client who dies unexpectedly. Which of the following should the nurse understand when advising a family member about an autopsy? **Select all that apply.**
   1. It can be performed only with the consent of a family member.
   2. It is an examination of a body to establish the cause of death.
   3. It is necessary before a certificate of death is issued.
   4. It is mandatory in the event of a suspicious death.
   5. It is required in the event of a violent death.

16. A nurse is caring for a client who has just expired. Family members are on their way to the hospital in response to being informed of the death. What should the nurse do in preparation for the visit by family members? **Select all that apply.**
    1. Place the client in the supine position, and place the top linen across the shoulders.
    2. Remove as much medical equipment as possible from the room.
    3. Remove all tubes and IV lines unless an autopsy is expected.
    4. Remove the identification band from the client's wrist.
    5. Remove the pillow from under the client's head.

17. A family member maintaining a bedside vigil until the loved one dies asks the nurse, "How do I know that death is imminent?" What information should the nurse include in a response to this question? **Select all that apply.**
    1. Flushed, dry skin
    2. Mottled extremities
    3. Decreased temperature
    4. Decreased urine output
    5. Constant swallowing of secretion

18. A middle-aged adult had a leg amputated after being hit by an automobile. Which nursing intervention is **most** specific to help the client develop a positive body image?
    1. Encourage the client to explore future roles.
    2. Assist the client to identify past achievements.
    3. Support the client through various stages of loss.
    4. Help the client to avoid anxiety-producing situations.

19. A 26-year-old downhill skier who is preparing for the world championships has a terrible accident on the slopes, resulting in paraplegia. He makes numerous statements to the nurse with the same theme: "I don't understand how this happened to me. I am the strongest, best person out there." The nurse concludes that the client is in what stage of Kübler-Ross's stages of grieving?
    1. Anger
    2. Denial
    3. Bargaining
    4. Depression

20. A client dies, the family has left the bedside, and an autopsy will not be performed. What should the nurse do while performing postmortem care? **Select all that apply.**
    1. Tie soft gauze under the chin and around the head.
    2. Tie an identification tag on the right wrist.
    3. Position the body in functional alignment.
    4. Place a pillow under the shoulders.
    5. Pad and tie the wrists together.

REVIEW ANSWERS

1. ANSWER: 1.

Rationales:

1. The nurse functions as a client advocate as well as a teacher when explaining to a family member that nourishment is unnecessary at this stage of dying. In addition, forcing nourishment on a dying person when the person is not interested in eating or drinking may be uncomfortable and even painful. Lack of appetite is difficult for family members of a dying person to understand, especially when food is associated with caring. The nurse should convey this information in a nonjudgmental and gentle manner.

2. Although this statement explains that applying a protective lip balm on the lips supports comfort, it does not explain why food is unnecessary when organs are failing.

3. Although this statement acknowledges the caring demonstrated by the family member, it does not explain why food is unnecessary when organs are failing. By not intervening in the family member's behavior, the nurse failed to meet the needs of the client.

4. Although this statement states that ice chips or wetting the lips with a small amount of water is all that is necessary, it does not explain why food is unnecessary.

TEST-TAKING TIP: Identify the word in the stem that sets a priority. The word *most* in the stem sets a priority. Identify the options that are opposites. Options 1 and 3 are opposites. Option 1 is saying that nourishment is unnecessary, and option 3 supports the family member's effort to get the father to ingest soup. Identify the options with clang associations. The word *father* in the stem and in options 1 and 3 are clang associations. Carefully examine options 1 and 3.

Content Area: Grief and Loss
Integrated Processes: Caring; Communication and Documentation; Nursing Process: Implementation
Client Need: Psychosocial Integrity
Cognitive Level: Application
Concept: Grief and Loss

2. ANSWER: 3, 2, 4, 5, 1.

Rationales:

3. This statement indicates denial, the first stage of Kübler-Ross's stages of grieving. This is the "Not me" stage. The person is unable to believe what is happening.

2. This statement indicates anger, the second stage of Kübler-Ross's stages of grieving. This is the "Why me?" stage. The person resists loss with anger and hostility.

4. This statement indicates bargaining, the third stage of Kübler-Ross's stages of grieving. This is the "Yes, me, but . . ." stage. The person barters for more time and may express guilt for past behavior.

5. This statement indicates withdrawal, the fourth stage of Kübler-Ross's stages of grieving. This is the "Yes, me" stage. The person realizes the full impact of the loss. The person grieves future losses, may talk, withdraw, cry, or feel very lonely.

1. This statement indicates acceptance, the fifth stage of Kübler-Ross's stages of grieving. This is the "OK, me" stage. The person accepts the loss, may have decreased interest in activities and people, and may be quiet or peaceful.

Content Area: Grief and Loss
Integrated Processes: Communication and Documentation; Nursing Process: Implementation
Client Need: Psychosocial Integrity
Cognitive Level: Analysis
Concept: Grief and Loss

3. ANSWER: 3.

Rationales:

1. The client is diaphoretic and is experiencing Cheyne-Stokes respirations, which indicate that death is near. There may not be time to go to the cafeteria for lunch if the spouse wants to be present when the husband expires.

2. Diaphoresis and Cheyne-Stokes respirations indicate that death is near. If the spouse wants to be present when the husband expires, it is not good advice to suggest leaving the bedside to go for lunch at this time.

3. The presence of diaphoresis and Cheyne-Stokes respirations indicate that death is near. The wife expressed a desire to be present when the husband expires. By providing lunch, the nurse enables the spouse to stay at the bedside.

4. The client's condition is deteriorating. Diaphoresis and Cheyne-Stokes respirations indicate that death is near. It is not good advice to suggest leaving the bedside at this time.

TEST-TAKING TIP: Identify the word in the stem that sets a priority. The word *best* in the stem sets a priority. Identify the option that is unique. Option 3 is the only option that does not advise leaving the bedside of her dying husband. Identify the client-centered option. Option 3 is client centered because it enables the client to stay at the bedside of her spouse. Identify the central person in the question. The *wife* is the central person in the question.

Content Area: Grief and Loss
Integrated Processes: Caring; Communication and Documentation; Nursing Process: Implementation
Client Need: Psychosocial Integrity
Cognitive Level: Application
Concept: Grief and Loss

4. ANSWER: 1.

Rationales:

1. This statement indicates the stage of developing awareness according to Engel's model of grief. Reality of the loss is internalized, and psychological pain is experienced.

2. This scenario does not depict the stage of shock and disbelief according to Engel's model of grief. In the stage of shock and disbelief, a person is in denial or intellectually, but not emotionally, accepts the loss.

3. This scenario does not depict the stage of resolving the loss according to Engel's model of grief. In the stage of resolving the loss, the person centers energy on thoughts and beliefs about the deceased.

4. This scenario does not depict the stage of idealization according to Engel's model of grief. In the stage of idealization, all negative thoughts and feelings about the deceased are initially repressed; as time passes, the person incorporates some unique characteristics of the deceased into his or her own personality.

Content Area: Grief and Loss
Integrated Processes: Communication and Documentation;
Nursing Process: Implementation
Client Need: Psychosocial Integrity
Cognitive Level: Application
Concept: Grief and Loss

5. **ANSWER: 4.**
   Rationales:
   1. Although the nurse may offer to call another person, it is not the priority.
   2. Although the nurse may offer to call a spiritual advisor to visit with the daughter, it is not the priority. Also, to suggest that the daughter may want to pray with a spiritual advisor is an assumption and is inappropriate.
   3. This response does not acknowledge the death of the father. Also, this question is unnecessary because the fact that the daughter immediately came to the facility indicates a desire to be present.
   4. Stating, "I am very sorry for the loss of your father," is client centered because it acknowledges the loss and demonstrates caring.
   TEST-TAKING TIP: Identify the word in the stem that sets a priority. The word *best* in the stem sets a priority. Identify the clang associations. The word *father* in the stem and in options 3 and 4 are clang associations. Examine options 3 and 4 carefully. Identify the client-centered option. Option 4 is client centered. It is the only option that acknowledges the loss and expresses caring. Identify the option that is unique. Option 4 is the only option that is not a question.
   Content Area: Grief and Loss
   Integrated Processes: Caring; Communication and Documentation; Nursing Process: Implementation
   Client Need: Psychosocial Integrity
   Cognitive Level: Application
   Concept: Grief and Loss

6. **ANSWER: 4.**
   Rationales:
   1. It is unnecessary to explain that the breathing sounds heard near death are called *death rattle*. This information may be frightening to grieving people who are maintaining a vigil at the beside of a person who is dying.
   2. Although excessive secretions can be wiped from the mouth with a soft, moist cloth, another action should be implemented first.
   3. Suctioning the respiratory passages of a person who has excessive respiratory secretions and is in the final phase of dying rarely helps and is not recommended.
   4. Raising the head of the bed may facilitate breathing, thereby reducing the sound known as *death rattle*. The sounds are due to accumulated secretions in the pharynx and upper respiratory passages. The dying person may lose the ability to swallow saliva or cough up secretions, causing a gurgling or rattling sound as air passes through accumulated secretions. Minimizing the occurrence of a death rattle can reduce anxiety about difficulty breathing and suffering as grieving family members maintain a bed-side vigil of their loved one who is dying.

Content Area: Grief and Loss
Integrated Processes: Caring; Communication and Documentation; Nursing Process: Implementation
Client Need: Psychosocial Integrity
Cognitive Level: Application
Concept: Grief and Loss

7. **ANSWER: 3.**
   Rationales:
   1. This response denies the woman's feelings. Also, it is an assumption that the woman has loving memories of her husband.
   2. This response denies the woman's feelings and offers a suggestion that is unrealistic at this time. The woman is in the shock and disbelief stage of grieving and most likely is not ready to become involved with new social groups.
   3. This response acknowledges that the woman is grieving. Also, it focuses on the journey moving forward, subtly indicating a future without her husband.
   4. This response is false reassurance. Although it is best to take things one day at a time, things may not get better as time goes on.
   TEST-TAKING TIP: Identify the options that deny client feelings, needs, or concerns. Options 1, 2, and 4 deny client feelings, needs, or concerns. Identify the client-centered option. Option 3 is the only option that acknowledges that the client is grieving and therefore is a client-centered option.
   Content Area: Grief and Loss
   Integrated Processes: Caring; Communication and Documentation; Nursing Process: Implementation
   Client Need: Psychosocial Integrity
   Cognitive Level: Application
   Concept: Grief and Loss

8. **ANSWER: 6, 1, 3, 5, 4, 2.**
   Rationales:
   6. This statement reflects shock and disbelief, the first phase of Engel's model of grief. The person is in denial or intellectually, but not emotionally, accepts the loss.
   1. This statement reflects developing awareness, the second phase of Engel's model of grief. The reality of the loss is internalized, and psychological pain is experienced.
   3. This statement reflects restitution, the third phase of Engel's model of grief. This phase involves the process of mourning that includes funeral, religious practices, and rituals.
   5. This statement reflects resolving the loss, the fourth phase of Engel's model of grief. In this phase, the grieving person centers energy on thoughts and beliefs about the deceased.
   4. This statement reflects idealization, the fifth phase of Engel's model of grief. In this phase, all negative thoughts and feelings about the deceased are initially repressed; as time passes, the person incorporates some unique characteristics of the deceased into his or her own personality.

2. This statement reflects outcome, the sixth phase of Engel's model of grief. In this phase, the psychological dependence on the deceased lessens, the person begins to focus on moving forward, and the person begins to seek new relationships.

Content Area: Grief and Loss
Integrated Processes: Caring; Communication and Documentation; Nursing Process: Analysis
Client Need: Psychosocial Integrity
Cognitive Level: Analysis
Concept: Grief and Loss

9. **ANSWER: 2.**
   Rationales:
   1. The husband is not experiencing normal grief. The grief experienced by the client's husband not only reflects components of normal grief but also includes components that are associated with another type of grief.
   2. The husband is experiencing anticipatory grief. The wife is still alive, and the husband is grieving for goals that were not accomplished as well as what will come in the future. Anticipatory grief often includes depression, worrying about the dying person, preparing for the death, and beginning adaptation to changes that will be caused by the future death.
   3. The husband is not experiencing complicated (dysfunctional) grief. Complicated grief is associated with excessive intensity of emotion or maladaptive responses for more than 2 years.
   4. The husband is not experiencing dysfunctional (complicated) grief. Dysfunctional grief is associated with excessive intensity of emotion or maladaptive responses for more than 2 years.
   TEST-TAKING TIP: Identify the options that are equally plausible. Options 3 and 4 are equally plausible. The terms *complicated grief* and *dysfunctional grief* are interchangeable and have the same definition. Options 3 and 4 can be eliminated from consideration.
   Content Area: Grief and Loss
   Integrated Processes: Communication and Documentation; Nursing Process: Assessment
   Client Need: Psychosocial Integrity
   Cognitive Level: Application
   Concept: Grief and Loss

10. **ANSWER: 1, 2, 3.**
    Rationales:
    1. Stating "I am so sorry for your loss" acknowledges the loss and demonstrates caring.
    2. This statement acknowledges the loss and indicates that it is alright to express feelings. This statement communicates caring and nonjudgmental acceptance of behavior related to grieving.
    3. An open-ended statement offers an opportunity for the parents to discuss their feelings. It is a valuable therapeutic communication technique that allows the parents to direct the conversation.
    4. This statement is nontherapeutic. The focus should be on the parents and their feelings of loss. The parents are the central clients in this situation.

5. This statement is nontherapeutic and is a barrier to communication. It cuts off communication by implying that the parents have to accept the loss of their daughter because God wanted her close to Him as an angel. Also, it is inappropriate to assume that the parents believe in God.
TEST-TAKING TIP: Identify client-centered options. Options 1, 2, and 3 focus on the feelings of the parents. Identify options that deny client feelings, needs, or concerns. Option 4 avoids feelings of the parents and cuts off communication. Option 5 cuts off communication by encouraging optimism and assumes that the parents believe in God.
Content Area: Grief and Loss
Integrated Processes: Caring; Communication and Documentation; Nursing Process: Implementation
Client Need: Psychosocial Integrity
Cognitive Level: Application
Concept: Grief and Loss

11. **ANSWER: 2.**
    Rationales:
    1. This statement focuses on the fact that nothing more can be done and is a nonsupportive approach in this situation.
    2. This statement is therapeutic because it offers hope and empowers the client to participate in a plan to control pain and support comfort.
    3. This statement is an assumption that places an emphasis on the staff members of the hospice agency rather than on the client.
    4. This statement shifts the focus away from the client and the client's needs.
    TEST-TAKING TIP: Identify the word in the stem that sets a priority. The word *most* in the stem sets a priority. Identify the client-centered option. Option 2 is client centered. Once the client's feelings are explored, the focus should be on empowering the client to be in control by having opportunities to make choices regarding future care. Identify options that deny client feelings, needs, or concerns. Option 1 focuses on what cannot be done, which is not helpful. Options 3 and 4 direct attention away from the client and focus on convincing the client that the hospice agency provides excellent care.
    Content Area: Grief and Loss
    Integrated Processes: Caring; Communication and Documentation; Nursing Process: Implementation
    Client Need: Psychosocial Integrity
    Cognitive Level: Application
    Concept: Grief and Loss

12. **ANSWER: 1, 2, 3.**
    Rationales:
    1. Focusing on little else but the death of a love one over a long period of time (2 or more years) supports the inference that the client is experiencing dysfunctional grieving.
    2. Although focusing on memories of a loved one is a component of normal grieving, when it becomes extreme over a long period of time (2 or more years), it supports the inference that the client is experiencing dysfunctional grieving.

3. Thoughts of having nothing to live for after the death of a loved one can precipitate feelings of suicide ideation. These thoughts can occur with normal as well as dysfunctional grieving. However, such thoughts indicate dysfunctional grieving if they are still present years after the loss of a loved one.

4. Sadness at the thought of a loved one is consistent with both normal and dysfunctional grieving.

5. Feeling tired is associated with normal as well as dysfunctional grieving.

TEST-TAKING TIP: Identify the clang associations. The word *wife* in the stem and in options 1, 2, and 4 are clang associations. Examine these options carefully. Options 1 and 2 are correct answers.

Content Area: Grief and Loss
Integrated Processes: Caring; Nursing Process: Analysis
Client Need: Psychosocial Integrity
Cognitive Level: Analysis
Concept: Grief and Loss

13. ANSWER: 4.
Rationales:

1. This response is not therapeutic because it does not focus on the underlying reason for the husband's behavior. Also, it places the wife on the defensive by subtly saying that her presence is interfering with the husband's attempts to sleep.

2. This response is not therapeutic because it does not focus on the underlying reason for the husband's behavior.

3. This response is not therapeutic because it does not focus on the underlying reason for the husband's behavior. Also, it is confrontational and may shut off communication.

4. This response focuses on the underlying reason for the husband's behavior. Withdrawal is very common as the person works on the emotional-spiritual-mental process of dying. There is a tendency to sleep more and talk less, and there is a *letting go* of interest in surroundings and loved ones. This is the dying person's effort to let go of life and to get prepared for death.

TEST-TAKING TIP: Identify the option that is unique. Option 4 is unique. It is the only option that explains the underlying reason for the husband's behavior. Identify the options that are equally plausible. Options 2 and 3 are equally plausible. One is no better than the other. Eliminate both from consideration. Identify the client-centered option. The focus of the question is on the needs of the wife. Option 4 is client centered because it explains the husband's behavior to the wife. Identify options that deny client feelings, needs, or concerns. Options 1, 2, and 3 do not address the underlying concern of the wife, which is that the husband is quiet, withdrawn, and is rejecting her presence.

Content Area: Grief and Loss
Integrated Processes: Caring; Communication and Documentation; Nursing Process: Implementation
Client Need: Psychosocial Integrity
Cognitive Level: Application
Concept: Grief and Loss

14. ANSWER: 1, 5.
Rationales:

1. The client is in the phase of withdrawal. Unnecessary talking distracts the dying person from necessary preparation for letting go and should be avoided. Allowing time for silence conserves the client's energy for focusing on dying.

2. Cheerful dialogue is not therapeutic. The client is in the withdrawal phase of dying and requires only interaction necessary to meet needs.

3. Reassurance does not need to be constant. A quiet presence demonstrates to the dying person that the nurse is available when needed.

4. Encouraging interaction with family is not therapeutic. It does not meet the needs of a dying person who is in the phase of withdrawal. Unnecessary family interaction distracts the dying person from focusing on preparation for letting go.

5. Sitting quietly by the bedside lets the client know that someone cares and that the client is not alone. It demonstrates respect for the dying client who needs to focus on dying.

TEST-TAKING TIP: Identify the option that is unique. Option 1 is unique because it is the only option that begins with a negative word—an action that should not be implemented. Options 2, 3, 4, and 5 begin with words that are *positive* action verbs: *engage, provide, encourage,* and *sit.* Identify options that deny client feelings, needs, or concerns. Options 2, 3, and 4 do not recognize the need for the dying person to interact minimally as the client prepares for death.

Content Area: Grief and Loss
Integrated Processes: Caring; Communication and Documentation; Nursing Process: Implementation
Client Need: Psychosocial Integrity
Cognitive Level: Application
Concept: Grief and Loss

15. ANSWER: 2, 4, 5.
Rationales:

1. This is not true. The legal system may seek a court order for an autopsy in some situations.

2. This is the correct definition of autopsy.

3. In many situations, such as when the person who dies is under the care of a primary health-care provider for a specific life-threatening illness, an autopsy does not have to be performed. A certificate of death must be completed and filed with the local health department or other government office for every person who dies. This certificate is necessary for legal and insurance purposes.

4. When a death is suspicious, an autopsy is always done.

5. When a death is the result of violence, an autopsy is always done.

TEST-TAKING TIP: Identify the option with a specific determiner. The word *only* in option 1 is a specific determiner. Rarely is an option with a specific determiner a correct answer. Delete option 1 from consideration.

Content Area: Grief and Loss
Integrated Processes: Communication and Documentation;
Nursing Process: Implementation
Client Need: Psychosocial Integrity
Cognitive Level: Application
Concept: Grief and Loss

16. **ANSWER: 1, 2, 3.**
    Rationales:
    1. **The supine position is functional alignment, and the sheet covers the body but keeps the face uncovered in a natural manner.**
    2. **Removing medical equipment from the room provides for a more pleasant environment and reduces exposure of family members to equipment that may have unpleasant memories.**
    3. **Removing tubes and IV lines allows the family to view their family member in a more natural manner. This may help to make the viewing less traumatic for family members.**
    4. The identification band should remain on the client's wrist. It is important that the client's identity be secured as postmortem care is provided and the body is moved to the morgue or undertaker's premises.
    5. It is not necessary to remove the pillow from under the client's head.
    Content Area: Grief and Loss
    Integrated Processes: Caring; Nursing Process:
    Implementation
    Client Need: Psychosocial Integrity
    Cognitive Level: Application
    Concept: Grief and Loss

17. **ANSWER: 2, 4.**
    Rationales:
    1. The skin will become cool and clammy, not flushed and dry, as the client experiences cardiogenic shock.
    2. **Mottled extremities occur in response to the body's diversion of circulation to the vital organs.**
    3. The body temperature increases, not decreases, with impending death. This is probably the result of dehydration due to reduced oral intake and effects on the thermoregulatory center of the brain by altered metabolic processes.
    4. **As kidney function declines, urine output also declines. In addition, less fluid is ingested, and the client will become dehydrated with a concomitant decrease in urine output.**
    5. A client who imminently is dying experiences a loss of the swallowing reflex.
    Content Area: Grief and Loss
    Integrated Processes: Communication and Documentation;
    Nursing Process: Implementation
    Client Need: Psychosocial Integrity
    Cognitive Level: Application
    Concept: Grief and Loss

18. **ANSWER: 3.**
    Rationales:
    1. This intervention is premature. It is appropriate when the client is ready to focus on positive, supportive change.

2. Identifying strengths, weaknesses, and past achievements assists a client to develop a more positive self-image, not a positive body image.
3. **A change in body image usually precipitates feelings of loss of "what was" and "what will never be." An exploration of these feelings will promote movement toward acceptance of a change in body image.**
4. This intervention is more appropriate for clients who are anxious.
TEST-TAKING TIP: Identify the word in the stem that sets a priority. The word *most* in the stem sets a priority.
Content Area: Grief and Loss
Integrated Processes: Caring; Nursing Process:
Implementation
Client Need: Psychosocial Integrity
Cognitive Level: Application
Concept: Grief and Loss

19. **ANSWER: 1.**
    Rationales:
    1. **The client is in the stage of anger. He is asking, "Why me?" despite the fact that he is the "strongest, best person out there."**
    2. The client is not in denial. The client is intellectually and emotionally aware of his loss.
    3. The client is not in the stage of bargaining. He is not bartering for time or expressing feelings of guilt or regret.
    4. The client is not in the stage of depression. He has not realized the full impact of his loss. He is still coping in the present.
    Content Area: Grief and Loss
    Integrated Processes: Communication and Documentation;
    Nursing Process: Analysis
    Client Need: Psychosocial Integrity
    Cognitive Level: Analysis
    Concept: Grief and Loss

20. **ANSWER: 1, 3, 5.**
    Rationales:
    1. **Tying soft gauze under the chin and around the head keeps the mouth set in a natural position.**
    2. Identification tags should be placed on a toe or ankle of the body and on the outside of the shroud. Placing an identification tag on the right wrist may cause tissue trauma that may be seen if the client is viewed in an open casket.
    3. **Functional alignment keeps the body in a natural position.**
    4. Placing a pillow under the shoulders will cause hyperextension of the head and neck. A pillow should be placed under the shoulders and head to keep them in functional alignment.
    5. **The wrists should be padded and tied together gently to keep the arms close to the body. Padding the wrists prevents tissue trauma.**
    Content Area: Grief and Loss
    Integrated Processes: Nursing Process: Implementation
    Client Need: Psychosocial Integrity
    Cognitive Level: Application
    Concept: Grief and Loss

Essential Physiological Concepts

Chapter 14

Physical Assessment

NURSING CONCEPTS

Cognition
Collaboration
Communication
Evidenced-Based Practice
Growth and Development
Mood
Neurologic Regulation

Oxygenation
Patient-Centered Care
Perfusion
Sensory Perception
Sexuality
Thermo-regulation

KEY TERMS

Apical pulse—Number of times the ventricles of the heart contract in 1 minute when seen, felt, or auscultated over the apex of the heart

Auscultatory gap—A temporary loss of sound that occurs when a blood pressure cuff pressure is high, followed by the return of sounds at a lower level

Blood pressure—Indirect measurement of the force of blood against arterial walls during cardiac contraction and cardiac relaxation

Body temperature—The result of the amount of heat produced by the body and the amount of heat lost from the body

Bradycardia—Heart rate less than 60 beats/minute

Bradypnea—Respiratory rate less than 12 breaths/minute

Cardiac output—Volume of blood that is pumped from the heart in 1 minute (about 5.6 L)

Dyspnea—Difficulty breathing

Dysrhythmia—Irregular heart rate

Eupnea—Normal respiratory rate of 12 to 20 breaths/minute

Febrile—Presence of a fever

Fever (pyrexia)—Core body temperature more than a person's normal body temperature (usually 100°F orally or 101°F rectally) that is provoked by an increase in the body's temperature set point

General adaptation syndrome—Generalized, nonspecific response of the body that is the same and predictable regardless of the type of stress

Hyperpyrexia—Core body temperature of 105.8°F (41°C) or more

Hypertension—Systolic blood pressure more than 140 mm Hg or diastolic blood pressure more than 90 mm Hg on two separate occasions

Hyperthermia—Core body temperature more than the person's normal body temperature without a change in the body's temperature set point

Hypotension—Systolic blood pressure less than 100 mm Hg

Hypothermia—Body temperature less than 98.6°F (36°C)

Hypoxemia (hypoxia)—Deficient oxygen in the blood

Orthopnea—Dyspnea relieved by assuming an upright position

Orthostatic (postural) hypotension—A 10- to 20-mm Hg decrease between lying down and sitting blood pressures and/or a 10- to 20-mm Hg decrease between sitting and standing blood pressures caused by peripheral vasodilation without a compensatory increase in cardiac output

Peripheral pulse—Rhythmic expansion of an artery that is palpated when a surge of blood occurs in response to contraction of the heart

Peripheral vascular resistance—The amount of friction between blood flow and vessel walls

Pulse (heart rate)—Reflects the waves of pressure throughout the arterial vessels generated by

Continued

KEY TERMS—cont'd

contractions of the ventricles of the heart that occur within 1 minute

Pulse deficit—Difference between apical and radial pulse rates

Pulse pressure—Difference between systolic blood pressure and diastolic blood pressure

Respiration—The movement of gases into and out of the lungs, promoting an exchange of gases between the atmosphere and the capillary beds in the alveoli

Severe hypothermia—Body temperature less than 82.4°F (28°C)

Shortness of breath—Feeling of not being able to catch one's breath

Stroke volume—Amount of blood that exits the left ventricle with each contraction of the heart (about 70 mL in a healthy adult)

Tachycardia—Heart rate more than 100 beats/minute

Tachypnea—Respiratory rate more than 20 breaths/minute

Vital signs—Essential clinical indicators of the physiological status of a client; include body temperature, pulse, respirations, blood pressure, oxygen saturation, and pain

I. Overview of Physical Assessment

Physical assessment is a major component of data collection. It is used during the initial comprehensive health assessment, routinely at periodic intervals, and when assessments are focused on a particular potential problem or emergency situation. Before performing a client assessment, the nurse should understand developmental considerations, collect all the necessary equipment that will be used, and prepare the client for the procedure.

A. Types of physical assessment
1. Initial comprehensive health assessment (database).
   a. Conducted during the initial interaction with a client.
   b. Obtains baseline data that are global in their focus.
   c. Includes:
      (1) *Subjective data:* Data identified only by the person affected (e.g., sensations, feelings, attitudes, beliefs, and perceptions).
      (2) *Objective data:* Data that are measurable against a standard (e.g., data obtained by accessing body systems, monitoring vital signs, obtaining physical measurements, and monitoring laboratory values).
2. Ongoing assessment (reflects client's progress).
   a. Conducted on a repetitive routine.
   b. Required because people are dynamic, not stagnant.
   c. Includes VS as well as focused assessments that center on a particular topic, body system, or functional ability, such as weight, blood glucose level, and oxygen saturation level.
3. Focused assessment.
   a. Conducted when a risk factor or problem requires an in-depth assessment.
   b. Obtains information specific to a body part or system, functional ability, or topic; required for actual, potential, or suspected problems.
   c. Examples include assessing for clinical indicators that meet discharge criteria from a postanesthesia care unit, identifying rehabilitation needs as part of discharge planning, monitoring cardiac and respiratory function when a client reports chest pain, and using a weekly pressure ulcer assessment form to evaluate the progression of a pressure ulcer.
4. Emergency assessment.
   a. Conducted when a rapid assessment is required during a life-threatening situation.
   b. Typically focuses on the ABCs (**A**irway, **B**reathing, and **C**irculation).
   c. During a psychosocial crisis, focuses on identifying the client's perception of the crisis, immediate safety needs, and coping skills.

B. Times to perform physical assessment
1. On admission to a health-care agency to provide a baseline of the client's status and functional abilities against which to measure future change.
2. On an ongoing basis to assess progress.
3. When accepting responsibility for a client at a change of shift and when a client is transferred from an emergency department, postanesthesia care unit, or another unit within an agency.
4. When a client's status changes.
   a. An acute onset of new signs or symptoms; for example, when a client reports chest pain, shortness of breath, or dizziness.
   b. When signs or symptoms return or increase in intensity (exacerbation).

c. When signs or symptoms subside or decrease in intensity (remission).

d. When signs and symptoms persist for 6 months or more (chronicity).

5. To identify an issue or risk factor that may contribute to a problem.

6. When evaluating the effectiveness of medical/surgical therapy and nursing interventions; for example, level of pain relief after a client receives an analgesic, extent of wound healing during a dressing change, intake and output (I&O) and fluid balance of a client who is receiving a diuretic, and degree of client comfort after administration of hygiene and a back rub.

7. When a nurse has an intuitive belief that *something is wrong;* for example, when a nurse instinctively identifies a subtle variation in a client's condition.

C. Developmental considerations and nursing care related to age groups

1. The basic techniques of physical assessment are the same regardless of the client's age; however, the way in which the nurse approaches a client and the additional focused assessments that should be performed vary based on the client's age/developmental level.

2. A variety of factors must be considered, such as physical changes associated with aging, cognitive level, experiential background, and age-associated health problems. (Some age-related differences specific to physical assessment are presented here, but more details about growth and development are contained in Chapter 10, Development Across the Life Span.).

3. Infants/Toddlers.
   a. Have a parent hold an infant or toddler against the chest or have a toddler sit on the parent's lap.

   🛑 b. Place an infant or toddler on a padded examination table, but continually stay at the side of the table to prevent a fall.

   c. Convert pounds to kilograms if the childhood weight chart is expressed in kilograms. (1 kilogram is equal to 2.2 pounds. Divide the child's weight in pounds by 2.2 to determine the child's weight in kilograms.)

4. Preschoolers and school-aged children.
   a. Provide opportunities to make choices; for example, ask the child whether he or she prefers to sit in a parent's lap or to sit on the examination table.

   🛑 b. Involve the parent and child in the assessment; encourage the child to handle instruments because these actions support a sense of control that reduces anxiety.

c. Allow the child to wear underpants when this part of the body is not being assessed.

d. Start with the least invasive assessments, move to the more invasive assessments, and hold the most uncomfortable assessments until last; for example, examine the ear canal and oral cavity before auscultating the chest and palpating the abdomen.

e. Provide reassurance and compliment children on how helpful they are because these actions support participation.

5. Adolescents.

   🛑 a. Ask parents to remain outside the examining room unless the adolescent prefers that the parents remain. An adolescent is more likely to ask a sensitive question or give an honest answer to a sensitive question if the assessment is conducted in private.

   b. Provide privacy by pulling the curtain and draping the adolescent; recognize that adolescents are going through puberty and may be embarrassed about associated physical changes.

6. Adults.
   a. Consider the client's developmental age, physical condition, energy level, and mobility when planning a physical assessment.

   b. Schedule extra time because the aging process may compromise energy and comprehension, requiring longer for the client to process information and formulate an answer.

7. Older adult.
   a. Schedule physical assessments into several blocks of time so as not to exhaust a client who is low in energy or is physically, physiologically, emotionally, or mentally compromised.

   b. Pace care and provide rest periods if needed.

   c. Modify approaches to positioning because an older adult may have arthritic joints and stiff muscles; support functional alignment with pillows.

   d. Ensure the client wears prescribed hearing aids and eyeglasses; seek feedback to ensure that communication is understood.

   🛑 e. Use a comprehensive assessment format to identify problems common in older adults, such as the SPICES acronym.

   (1) Sleep disorders.
   (2) Problems with eating or feeding.
   (3) Incontinence.
   (4) Confusion.
   (5) Evidence of falls.
   (6) Skin breakdown.

f. Assess intake of substances, such as alcohol, laxatives and cathartics, pain medications, and over-the-counter medications and supplements, because these substances commonly are misused by older adults.

D. Equipment used for physical assessment and related nursing care
1. Ensure that equipment is clean or sterile.
2. Verify that equipment is working properly before use.
3. Use common equipment such as a drape, personal protective equipment (e.g., gloves, gown, face mask) if exposure to blood or body fluids is anticipated, penlight, tape measure, tongue depressor, lubricant, stethoscope, thermometer (e.g., oral, rectal, electronic, disposable, infrared sensor), sphygmomanometer or aneroid manometer, pulse oximeter, ultrasound (Doppler), scale (e.g., chair, bed, stretcher, cradle scale for infants, standing scale for weight and height), otoscope, and ophthalmoscope.
4. Clean or dispose of equipment or instruments after use. For example, use a separate alcohol swab to clean the diaphragm and each ear pod of a stethoscope, and place a disposable thermometer in an appropriate trash container.
🛑 5. Dedicate equipment to be left in a room when a client is receiving transition-based precautions to reduce the risk of cross-contamination; ensure terminal cleansing of equipment when a client is no longer in need of a device and before it is returned to general use.

E. Client preparation
1. Conduct assessments when the client is amenable. If possible, avoid physical assessments when a client is anxious, tired, hungry, or experiencing pain.
2. Respect the preference for a same-gender caregiver because of cultural or religious beliefs.
3. Identify yourself and the client; explain what you are going to do and why because doing so reduces anxiety, facilitates the client's assistance, and is a client right.
4. Encourage the client to void, especially when planning to palpate the abdomen; an empty bladder supports comfort and facilitates accurate examination of the abdomen.
5. Allow a family member to remain present to meet developmental, cultural, or psychological needs if requested by the client and if not detrimental to the client.
6. Draw the bed curtain and drape the client to avoid unnecessary exposure and to provide warmth.
7. Explain each assessment before touching the client because doing so educates and prepares the client, promotes rapport, and supports the development of trust.
8. Position the client, especially infants, children, and older adults, considering their developmental age, physical condition, energy level, and mobility. Organize interventions so that several assessments are conducted during each position to reduce the number of times the client is repositioned; use pillows to maintain functional alignment to avoid unnecessary stress and strain on muscles, joints, ligaments, and tendons.
9. Limit the amount of time a client has to assume an uncomfortable or embarrassing position to support comfort and dignity.

II. General Survey

A general survey begins when the nurse meets the client. The nurse makes initial observations regarding the client's overall characteristics, gathering basic impressions of the client's appearance, physical presence, mental status, and ability to communicate as well as generalized, nonspecific responses of the body that are the same regardless of the type of stress. The general survey provides information on the overall state of the client and provides a bridge to the next stage of the physical assessment, the measurement of vital signs.

A. Appearance
1. Identify the overall personal hygiene of the client.
   a. Is the client clean and well groomed?
   b. Does the client have body or breath odor?
   c. What is the client wearing and is it appropriate for the weather?
2. Understand that appearance can deteriorate as a result of issues such as immobility, fatigue, pain, depression, and impaired cognition.

B. Physical presence
1. Assess the client's overall weight, height, body type, posture, strength, symmetry, and gait.
2. Compare height and weight to appropriate charts to determine whether findings are outside the norm.
   a. Deviations from expected norms may indicate a problem with body systems, such as the gastrointestinal (GI) or neuromusculoskeletal system.
   b. Being underweight, overweight, or obese; issues may include an inability to procure, prepare, or chew food; a physiological problem, such as an inability to absorb adequate nutrients, resulting in malnutrition; or an emotional problem, such as depression or anorexia nervosa, resulting in either an inadequate or excessive nutrient intake.

C. Mood and behavior
1. Determine whether a client's behavior is appropriate for developmental age.
2. Determine the client's mood. Do the client's behavior and statements indicate that the client is happy, sad, pensive, depressed, fearful, anxious, or manic?

D. Cognitive status
1. Identify the client's level of consciousness.
2. Identify whether the client is lethargic, confused, or irritable.
3. Identify the client's ability to interact appropriately.
4. Identify the client's ability to recall short- and long-term events.

E. Speech pattern
1. Identify whether speech is logical, appropriate, and understandable.
2. Identify whether a language barrier exists. If necessary, seek the assistance of a professional translator to ensure that the client's rights are met.
3. Identify whether speech is rapid (pressured speech), which may indicate anxiety or hyperactivity associated with conditions such as hyperthyroidism, the manic phase of a mental disorder, or attention deficit-hyperactivity disorder.
4. Identify whether speech is slow, which is common with depression, neurological disorders, hypothyroidism, and excessive sedation.
5. Identify whether the client has a speech problem, such as hesitancy, stuttering, or aphasia (e.g., expressive, receptive, or global) or an inability to articulate words because of impaired enervation of the structures of speech or larynx.

F. The general adaptation syndrome
1. Stress causes wear and tear on the body that can be internal or external, physical or emotional, helpful or harmful, and realistic, exaggerated or unrealistic.
2. The **general adaptation syndrome** occurs when stress causes a generalized, nonspecific response of the body that is the same and predictable regardless of the type of stress.
3. The extent of the response depends on the type of stress, the severity of the stress, the duration of stress, and the multiplicity of the stressors.
4. The sympathetic nervous system and endocrine system play primary roles in the body's response to stress.
5. The general adaptation syndrome involves three stages (Table 14.1).

Table 14.1 **Stages of the General Adaptation Syndrome and Related Nursing Care**		
Stage	**Physiological Reactions**	**Changes That Nurses Can Assess**
Alarm reaction (fight or flight)	• Cerebral cortex perceives a stress. • Cerebral cortex stimulates the sympathetic nervous system. • Hypothalamus releases corticotropin-releasing hormone and endorphins. • Posterior pituitary releases endorphins and antidiuretic hormone. • Anterior pituitary releases adrenocorticotropic hormone. • Adrenal cortex releases cortisol and aldosterone. • Adrenal medulla releases epinephrine and norepinephrine.	1. Blood pressure increases as vasoconstriction brings more blood to vital centers. 2. Heart rate increases to increase cardiac output. 3. Respirations increase in rate and depth as bronchioles dilate to bring more oxygen to body cells. 4. Pupils dilate to improve vision. 5. Mental activity increases to maintain alertness. 6. Urinary output decreases to help increase the circulating blood volume. 7. Blood glucose levels increase to provide for energy expenditure.
Resistance or adaptation	• Parasympathetic nervous system activity balances sympathetic nervous system activity. • Hormonal levels return to normal. • Psychological defense mechanisms assist with coping.	1. Blood pressure, heart rate, and respirations return to normal. 2. Individual adapts and returns to homeostasis.
Exhaustion	• Physiological responses associated with the alarm reaction continue. • Energy level decreases. • Ability to adapt is exceeded. • Injury, illness, or death ensues.	1. Heart rate remains elevated. 2. Respiratory rate remains elevated. 3. Blood pressure decreases due to vasodilation. 4. Adaptations to stress diminish. 5. Exhaustion is evident.

Adapted from Selye (1936). Syndrome produced by diverse nocuous agents. *Nature*, 138(3479), 32.

III. Measurement of Vital Signs

Vital signs are referred to as "vital" because they provide essential information about a person's physical status. They are the most common measurements obtained by health-care professionals because they provide data about the effectiveness of the body's circulatory, respiratory, and neuroendocrine functions. Traditionally, temperature, pulse, respirations, and blood pressure were considered vital signs. Now, many health-care professionals view arterial blood oxygen saturation and the presence of pain as additional vital signs. When and how often vital signs should be obtained and the legal and ethical responsibilities of the nurse in relation to obtaining vital signs are significant issues for nurses to understand.

A. When a nurse should assess vital signs
1. When a client is admitted or discharged to an agency or service.
2. At the start of every shift.
3. Before, during, and after an invasive procedure (e.g., surgery, liver biopsy, or paracentesis).
4. Before and after a nursing intervention (e.g., ambulating a client for the first time after a period of bedrest).
5. Before administering a medication that may influence a vital sign (e.g., a client's pulse rate must be 60 beats per minute or higher to administer a prescribed antidysrhythmic; a client's blood pressure must be higher than a specified systolic or diastolic rate as indicated by the primary health-care provider to administer a prescribed antihypertensive).
6. After administering a medication that may influence a vital sign that is desired or result as a side effect (e.g., blood pressure after administering a diuretic or antihypertensive; temperature after administering an antipyretic; pulse rate and rhythm after administering an antidysrhythmic; respiratory rate, depth, and characteristics after administering a bronchodilator; and blood pressure and respiratory rate after administering an opioid).
7. Whenever a client's condition changes (e.g., when a client reports chest pain or dizziness, suddenly is short of breath, or falls).

B. How often a nurse should assess vital signs
1. Every shift or every 8 hours in an acute care facility or according to agency policy.
2. Every 4 hours if the client has an acute problem; more frequently if the client is unstable.
3. As often as prescribed by a primary health-care provider (e.g., "BP every 2 hr").

4. As often as indicated in a protocol (e.g., vital signs every 5 minutes for the first 15 minutes, then in 30 minutes, and then every hour when a client is receiving a blood transfusion; hourly if a client is receiving treatment with a temperature management blanket).
5. As frequently as necessary according to the nurse's professional judgment when a client's vital signs vary from the expected norm or varies from the client's baseline; every 5 to 15 minutes may be necessary until the client's vital signs return to the baseline.

C. Commonalities of nursing care related to vital signs
1. Perform hand hygiene before collecting equipment and before and after the procedure.
2. Ensure that equipment to be used is clean, intact, and charged if an electronic device; return electronic equipment to charging station after use.
3. Identify yourself, identify the client, and explain what you are going to do and why.
4. Provide privacy by closing the door, pulling the curtain, and draping the client to expose only the site being accessed.
5. Position the client so that the site of measurement is accessible.
6. Use anatomical landmarks to locate the specific site being accessed; ensure that the site being accessed is not contraindicated.
7. Use assessment devices (e.g., thermometers, sphygmomanometers, pulse oximetry sensors) according to manufacturer directions.
8. Implement medical aseptic techniques.
   a. Don clean gloves just before the procedure if exposure to body fluids is a risk.
   b. Use a sheath or probe cover (e.g., plastic, electronic, and tympanic thermometers) for each site being assessed and between clients.
   c. Prevent contamination of equipment (e.g., ensure coils from machine to probe and straps of equipment do not touch client or client's environment).
   d. Clean equipment that touches client or client's environment according to manufacturer directions.
   e. Discard probe covers, disposable equipment, and used gloves in appropriate receptacle.
9. Delegate routine ongoing assessments of vital signs to unlicensed assistive personnel only if a client is stable and not experiencing an acute or chronic condition that can affect vital signs; request an immediate report if a vital sign is outside the expected range.

🛑 10. Assess the client who is reported by an unlicensed nursing assistant to have a vital sign that is outside the expected range immediately because interpreting and determining the significance of unexpected results require the knowledge and judgment of a registered nurse.

11. Respond to an unexpected vital sign appropriately (e.g., raise the head of the bed and provide oxygen for a client experiencing a respiratory problem or a dysrhythmia, provide a prescribed as-needed antipyretic for a client with a fever).
12. Initiate the rapid response team and notify the primary health-care provider if vital signs are outside the normal range and are considered dangerous.
13. Document vital signs accurately on required forms, such as a graphic sheet, hourly flow record, and/or medication administration record; include the measurement and all related characteristics.

IV. Measurement of Body Temperature

Body temperature is the result of the amount of heat produced by the body and the amount of heat lost from the body. *Core body temperature* is the temperature of the deeper tissues of the body, such as the heart, brain, and other internal organs. The expected core body temperature of an adult is 98°F (more or less 1°F) (37°C more or less 0.6°C). Physiological, developmental, and environmental factors as well as gender all influence core body temperature. A nurse measures a client's body temperature to obtain baseline information, to assess the progression of an illness, and/or to monitor a response to therapy. Measuring a client's temperature requires the use of an instrument (thermometer) placed somewhere in or on the body. Nurses must understand the commonalities of nursing care for all routes and the differences for specific routes when obtaining a temperature. The result of this measurement may be within or outside the expected range of body temperature. Therefore, an understanding of thermoregulatory states is necessary to perform an accurate focused assessment and provide nursing care appropriate for an increase or decrease in body temperature.

A. Physiology related to temperature
1. Factors that promote heat production
   a. Basal metabolic rate (BMR).
      (1) *BMR* is the rate of energy used by the body to maintain crucial physiological activities, such as breathing.
      (2) Factors that increase the BMR include metabolism, activity, and certain hormones.
   b. Muscle activity.
      (1) Activity and exercise increase metabolic rate. Vigorous exercise can increase body temperature to as high as 104°F.

      (2) Shivering, an involuntary physiological trembling caused by the contraction of muscles, can increase the rate of heat production by four times normal.
         (a) Shivering also is associated with the onset of a fever and is a response to fear.
         (b) Contraction of the *arrector pili* muscles cause hair to rise above the skin (pilo-erection, also known as *gooseflesh* or *goosebumps*) and occurs in response to cold exposure, but it is not a significant heat-preserving process in humans.
         (c) During the first few months of life, infants are unable to shiver and instead metabolize brown fat to produce heat.
   c. Thyroxine production.
      (1) Thyroxine, a hormone of the thyroid gland, increases cellular metabolism, which in turn increases BMR; an increased BMR increases heat production.
      (2) Hyperthyroidism, an excessive production of the hormone thyroxine, increases cellular metabolism, metabolic rate, and body temperature.
   d. Epinephrine, norepinephrine, and the stress response.
      (1) Epinephrine and norepinephrine are hormones that quickly increase when the sympathetic nervous system is stimulated by emotional stress, excitement, or anxiety (fight-or-flight response), which increases cellular metabolism, metabolic rate, and body temperature.
      (2) Generally, a significantly stressed or highly anxious client may have an increased body temperature.
   e. Progesterone secretion by women during ovulation increases body temperature 0.5°F to 1°F when measured rectally.
2. Factors that promote heat loss
   a. Conduction.
      (1) *Conduction* is the transfer of heat from a warm surface to a cooler surface via direct contact.
      (2) For example, a body is placed in a tub of cool water or on a cool operating room table.
   b. Radiation.
      (1) *Radiation* is the transfer of heat from a warm surface to a cooler surface/air without direct contact; this is responsible for nearly 50% of body heat loss.
      (2) For example, body heat is lost via the skin in a room that is cooler than the skin.

c. Convection.
   (1) *Convection* is the transfer of heat via air or water by movement of heated elements to a cooler area of air or water.
   (2) For example, body heat is transferred to the air closest to the body and the air surrounding the body is continually replaced by circulating cooler air.

d. Evaporation).
   (1) *Evaporation* is the process by which water changes from a liquid to a gas or vapor (vaporization). As moisture on the skin or in the breath on exhalation evaporates, heat loss occurs. If the humidity in the environment is high, less evaporation and heat loss occur.
      (a) Insensible water loss is loss of moisture via vaporization.
      (b) Insensible heat loss is heat loss associated with insensible water loss.
   (2) For example, perspiration that results from a hot environment.

3. Factors that affect both heat production and heat loss
   a. Age.
      (1) Metabolic rate is higher in a younger person and decreases with age.
      (2) Infants and older adults are less able to manage extreme environmental temperatures.
      (3) Infants.
         (a) The normal range of body temperature in infants is 98.6°F to 99.8°F.
         (b) Thirty percent of heat loss occurs through the head of an infant, which is proportionally larger than the rest of the body when compared to an adult.
         (c) Infants and children should wear hats and adequate clothing when the environment is cool or cold. Hats are placed on the heads of newborns in a hospital to help retain body heat.
      (4) Older adults.
         (a) Have range of body temperature difference 0.3°F to 1.2°F less than younger adults, depending on the site of measurement.
         (b) Have problems maintaining body heat because they experience decreased thermoregulatory efficiency and have less subcutaneous fat, slower metabolism, and decreased vasomotor control.
   b. Circadian rhythms (diurnal variations).
      (1) *Circadian rhythms* are cyclical repetitions of various physiological processes throughout

24 hours; body temperature may increase or decrease by as much as 1.8°F throughout this time frame.
      (2) The highest temperature is between 4 and 6 p.m.; the lowest temperature is between 4 and 6 a.m.
   c. Environment.
      (1) Increased environmental temperature: High environmental temperature, high humidity, and a hot bath or immersion in a hot tub can cause an increase in body temperature.
      (2) Decreased environmental temperature: Lack of adequate clothing, lack of shelter, submersion in cold water, or an illness that prevents the body from physiologically raising the body temperature when cold can lead to hypothermia. A cold environmental temperature compounded by a strong air current can cause greater heat loss than that which is expected based on the environmental temperature alone; this is called the wind chill factor.

B. Types of thermometers with advantages, disadvantages and related nursing care (Table 14.2)

C. Routes for obtaining a temperature with advantages, disadvantages, and related nursing care (Table 14.3)

MAKING THE CONNECTION

The Hypothalamus and Regulation of Body Temperature

Body temperature remains stable within a relatively narrow expected range of 97°F to 100.8°F (36.1°C to 38.2°C) when heat production and heat loss are in balance (Fig. 14.1). The hypothalamus is the integrator of the body that controls core body temperature by responding to sensors in the skin that identify an increase or decrease in body temperature. The hypothalamus precipitates an increase in body temperature by stimulating shivering and discharging epinephrine, which increase cellular metabolism that results in heat production, and by stimulating vasoconstriction, which shunts blood away from peripheral blood vessels, minimizing the transfer of heat from the body to the environment. The hypothalamus precipitates a decrease in body temperature by stimulating sweating, which promotes evaporation and peripheral vasodilatation that permits transfer of heat from the body to the environment. These physiological responses make a person aware of being cold or hot. Awareness precipitates behavioral responses that alter body temperature—for example, putting on more clothing to keep warm and removing clothing or turning on a fan to keep cool.

C / F

C	F	
46	114.8	Irreversible cell damage and death
45	113	
44	111.2	
43	109.4	Hyperpyrexia
42	107.6	
41	105.8	
40	104	Pyrexia
39	102	
38	100.4	
37	98.6	Normal
36	96.8	
35	95	
34	93.2	
33	91.4	
32	89.6	Hypothermia
31	87.8	
30	86	
29	84.2	
28	82.4	
27	80.6	Severe hypothermia
26	78.8	
25	77	
24 and below	75.2	Cessation of cardiac and respiratory functions; cell still viable; death possible

Above thermometer range

Below thermometer range

Fig 14.1 Ranges of body temperature. (From Wilkinson and Treas [2016]. *Fundamentals of nursing*, Vol. 1, 3rd ed. Philadelphia: F. A. Davis Company, with permission.)

D. Decreased body temperature and related nursing care
1. **Hypothermia:** A body temperature less than 98.6°F (36°C).
2. **Severe hypothermia:** A body temperature less than 82.4°F (28°C).

3. When body temperature decreases to less than 77°F (25°C), cardiac and respiratory functions cease, cells may still be viable, and death is possible.
4. Clinical indicators of hypothermia: Shivering initially; decreased, irregular pulse; decreased respirations; hypotension; reports of feeling cold and chilly; pale, cool skin; oliguria; reduced muscle coordination; disorientation; and decreased level of consciousness progressing to coma.
5. Nursing care.
   a. Monitor vital signs.

   🛑 b. Monitor pulse oximetry, but do not apply a pulse oximeter probe to an appendage (e.g., finger, toe, ear lobe) that exhibits vasoconstriction because the result will be inaccurately low and may compromise skin integrity.

   c. Increase the environmental temperature.
   d. Ensure that clothing and linen are dry.
   e. Cover the client with warm blankets, and put a hat on the client.
   f. Position extremities close to the body.
   g. Provide warm oral fluids as prescribed.
   h. Administer warm IV fluids as prescribed.
   i. Administer procedures as prescribed.
      (1) Examples: Provide a warm bath, apply an electric blanket, or position a temperature management blanket over and/or under the client.

   🛑 (2) Avoid using an electric blanket or temperature management blanket if the client has severe hypothermia because it may burn skin that has peripheral vasoconstriction.

(Text continued on page 380)

Table 14.2 Thermometers: Advantages, Disadvantages, and Related Nursing Care

Thermometer Type	Advantages	Disadvantages	Related Nursing Care
Paper strip thermometer **A** Oral strip **B** Skin strip	• Easy to use; some go under the tongue or axillae, others are topical (forehead or abdomen). • Disposable. • Inexpensive.	• Less accurate than other thermometers; should not be used if very accurate monitoring of temperature is essential. • Indicates only body surface temperature. • Results may be difficult to read for some people.	1. *Oral strips (A): Read results immediately after removal* because colors change quickly when removed from the mouth. 2. *Skin strips (B): Ensure that the skin is dry before placement;* hold the strip firmly against the skin for 15 to 60 seconds, according to the manufacturer's instructions.

Continued

Table 14.2 Thermometers: Advantages, Disadvantages, and Related Nursing Care—cont'd

Thermometer Type	Advantages	Disadvantages	Related Nursing Care
Plastic non-mercury thermometer Glass thermometers with mercury should not be used due to risk of exposure to mercury if broken. **A** Oral **B** Rectal	• Accurate. • Can be used for oral, rectal, or axillary temperatures. • Easily cleaned and disinfected. • Less costly than electronic thermometers.	• Takes 3 to 8 minutes to provide results, depending on the site. • Results may be difficult to read for some people.	1. Use an appropriate probe for the route: – Oral/axillary thermometer has an elongated tip and is indicated by a blue dot on the opposite end (A). – Rectal thermometer has a bulb at the tip and is indicated by a red dot on the opposite end (B). 2. Use a new plastic sheath between uses. 3. *Shake the temperature down below 95°F before use.* 4. Leave in place for length of time recommended for route. 5. Read at eye level while rotating the device until marks are visible; each short line is two-tenths of a degree; use the higher degree if the mark is between two lines. 6. Clean with soap and water and soak it in a disinfectant according to the manufacturer's instructions; if it is dedicated to a specific client, clean, dry, and store it in a thermometer case in the client's bedside table.
Temporal scanner thermometer (infrared sensor) 	• Easy to use and read. • Provide results within 2 to 5 seconds. • Noninvasive, comfortable. • Unaffected by eating, drinking, smoking, and oxygen administration. • Can be used for infants and clients who have difficulty breathing.	• Expensive to purchase. • Less accurate than glass, plastic, or electronic thermometers. • Requires recharging of batteries and regular maintenance to guarantee accuracy. • Must be cleaned between clients. • Influenced by perspiration and head coverings, hair, or temporal area against a mattress or pillow that retains surface heat, resulting in inaccurately high results.	1. Ensure that the machine is charged before use, and return the device to the charger after use. 2. *Clean the probe before and after use.* 3. *Avoid this route if the area has been covered by a hat or hair or if the client's temporal area has been against a mattress or pillow.* 4. Press and hold the button while the probe is placed flat on the forehead between the eyebrow and hairline and slide laterally across the forehead to the opposite hairline. 5. Continue to hold the button and touch probe just below the mastoid behind the ear lobe. 6. Release the button and read the result.

Table 14.2 Thermometers: Advantages, Disadvantages, and Related Nursing Care—cont'd

Thermometer Type	Advantages	Disadvantages	Related Nursing Care
Tympanic thermometer (infrared sensor)	• Convenient. • Provide results within 3 seconds. • Unaltered by eating, drinking, smoking, and oxygen administration. • Can be used for infants and clients who have difficulty breathing.	• Expensive to purchase. • Can be uncomfortable. • Requires a new probe cover for each client to prevent cross-contamination. • Requires recharging of batteries and regular maintenance to guarantee accuracy. • Contraindicated for clients with an ear infection or ear surgery. • Ear wax (cerumen), incubators, and radiant heaters can influence results.	1. Ensure that the machine is charged before use, and return the device to the charger after use. 2. *Use a new probe cover for each ear;* discard the cover in an appropriate receptacle. 3. Point the probe gently and firmly directly at the tympanic membrane for an accurate result; be cautious with the small ear canals of children. 4. Straighten the ear canal in children younger than age 3 years by pulling the lobule of the ear down and back. 5. Straighten the ear canal of older children and adults by pulling the auricle up and back.
Electronic thermometer	• Convenient and easy to use. • Can be used for oral, rectal, and axillary temperatures. • Provides results within 2 to 60 seconds.	• Expensive to purchase. • Requires a new probe cover for each client to prevent cross-contamination. • Requires recharging of batteries and regular maintenance to guarantee accuracy. • Affected by intake of hot and cold foods or liquids, smoking, and oxygen administration if the oral route is used.	1. Ensure that the machine is charged before use, and return the device to the charger after use. 2. *Use an appropriate probe for the route:* blue probe for an oral or axillary temperature; red probe for a rectal temperature. 3. *Use a new probe cover for each client;* eject the probe cover into an appropriate receptacle. 4. Hold the probe in the client's mouth so that the client does not touch it and contaminate the probe; hold a rectal probe in the client's rectum to prevent trauma if the client should move; clean the handle of the probe if touched by the client and after use.

Photo credits: Wilkinson and Treas (2016). *Fundamentals of nursing*, Vol. 1, 3rd ed. Philadelphia: F. A. Davis Company, with permission; Burton (2015). *Fundamentals of nursing care: Concepts, connections, and skills*, 2nd ed. Philadelphia: F. A. Davis Company, with permission; Image of electronic thermometer provided by Covidien. FILAC is a trademark of Covidien AG. ©Covidien. All rights reserved.

Table 14.3 Routes for Obtaining a Temperature: Advantages, Disadvantages, and Related Nursing Care

Route and Normal Range	Advantages	Disadvantages	Related Nursing Care
Oral 97.5°F to 99.5°F 	• Easily accessible. • Reflects rapid change in core body temperature faster than rectal route. • Can be used for those who have rectal problems or severe diarrhea.	• Thermometer can be broken if bitten. • Cannot be used for children younger than age 3 years or for clients who are confused or at risk for a seizure. • Influenced by hot and cold food or liquids, smoking, oxygen therapy, and bradypnea. • Requires the client to keep lips sealed around the thermometer. • Contraindicated in clients with a problem with the oral cavity and mouth breathers. • Carries risk of caregiver exposure to body fluids, requiring use of gloves if client has excessive oral secretions.	1. Ensure that the client has not smoked or ingested hot or cold foods or liquids for 9 minutes before measurement and is capable of sealing lips around the thermometer. 2. Insert the thermometer under the tongue in the posterior sublingual pocket and instruct the client to seal his or her lips around the thermometer, but avoid biting down on the thermometer. 3. Hold the thermometer in place until temperature is obtained: several seconds for an electronic thermometer; 3 to 5 minutes for a plastic thermometer.
Rectal 98.5°F to 100.5°F 	• Most reliable for measuring core body temperature. • Can be used for clients who are unable to follow instructions, such as clients who are confused, disoriented, or unconscious.	• Inconvenient. • Risk of caregiver exposure to body fluids, requiring use of gloves. • Requires lateral positioning with knees flexed or Sims' position. • Stool may interfere with accuracy. • Lags behind core body temperature during rapid changes in temperature. • May embarrass the client; requires privacy. • Contraindicated for newborns; clients with clotting disorders, severe diarrhea, hemorrhoids, or a fragile rectal mucosa; and those who have had colon or rectal surgery. • Contraindicated for clients with heart conditions because it can stimulate the vagus nerve, slowing heart rate.	1. Draw the curtain and position the client in a lateral position with knees flexed or in Sims' position to access the anus. 2. Wash hands, and then don clean gloves. 3. *Lubricate the tip of the thermometer with a water-soluble gel.* 4. Raise the upper buttock with one hand, and instruct client to take a deep breath while inserting the thermometer into the anus beyond the rectal sphincter: 1 to 1.5 inches for an adult; 0.5 to 0.9 inches for a child; and 0.5 inches for an infant. 5. *Hold the thermometer in place until it is time for removal:* several seconds for an electronic thermometer; 3 to 5 minutes for a plastic thermometer. 6. Remove any gel from the client's perianal area after thermometer removal. 7. Remove and discard gloves in an appropriate trash receptacle; wash hands.
Axillary 96.5°F to 99°F 	• Noninvasive. • Easily accessible.	• Not as accurate as the rectal route; lags behind core body temperature during rapid temperature changes. • Risk of caregiver exposure to body fluids, requiring the use of gloves.	1. Draw the curtain and drape the client so that only an axilla is exposed. 2. *Dry the axilla if moist.* 3. Place the thermometer in the middle of the axilla and position the arm close to the body, with the forearm across the chest.

Table 14.3 Routes for Obtaining a Temperature: Advantages, Disadvantages, and Related Nursing Care—cont'd

Route and Normal Range	Advantages	Disadvantages	Related Nursing Care
			4. *Hold the thermometer in place until it is time for removal: seconds for an electronic thermometer; 8 minutes for a plastic thermometer.*
Tympanic 97°F to 100.4°F Adult Up and back **A** Auricle Probe tip Auditory canal Tympanic membrane **B**	• *Easily accessible.* • *Provides results within several seconds.* • *Reflects core body temperature.* • *Is unaltered by eating, drinking, smoking, and oxygen administration.* • *Can be used for infants, people who are unconscious, and those who have difficulty breathing.*	• *Can be uncomfortable.* • *Contraindicated for clients with an ear infection or ear surgery.* • *Earwax (cerumen) may cause an inaccurately low result.* • *Incubators and radiant heaters may cause inaccurately high results.*	1. *Position the client's head slightly to the side and straighten the ear canal: Pull the auricle up and back for an adult (A); pull the lobule down and back for a child younger than 3 years of age (auditory canal in a child is curved upward).* 2. *Insert the probe into the ear canal firmly but gently, aiming it toward the tympanic membrane, not against the wall of the ear canal because the wall is not as warm as the tympanic membrane (B).* 3. *Push the button to take the temperature.* 4. *Remove the device when it beeps, which takes seconds.* 5. *Eject the probe cover into an appropriate trash receptacle.* 6. *Repeat procedure for the other ear using a new probe cover if results are outside the expected range.* 7. *Return the device to the battery charger.*
Temporal Artery 97.4°F to 100°F **A** **B**	• *Easily accessible.* • *Provides results within several seconds.* • *Is more accurate than the tympanic route.* • *Is unaffected by eating, drinking, smoking, and oxygen administration.* • *Can be used for infants, people who are unconscious, and those who have difficulty breathing.*	• *Head covering, hair, or temporal area against a pillow or mattress can cause inaccurately high results.* • *Influenced by perspiration.*	1. *Determine that the site is not influenced by hair, a hat, or lying on a pillow or mattress.* 2. *Dry the site if perspiration is present.* 3. *Ensure the device is charged.* 4. *Remove the protective cap and clean the probe following the manufacturer's instructions.* 5. *Place probe with gentle pressure on the center of forehead, halfway between the hairline and eyebrows.* 6. *Depress and hold the start button while dragging the probe laterally across the forehead to the opposite hairline (A).* 7. *Continue to depress the start button and touch the probe behind the ear lobe on the soft area below the mastoid (B).* 8. *Release the button and read the result.* 9. *Clean the probe and return the device to the charger.*

Continued

Table 14.3 Routes for Obtaining a Temperature: Advantages, Disadvantages, and Related Nursing Care—cont'd

Route and Normal Range	Advantages	Disadvantages	Related Nursing Care
Skin *Forehead skin temperature usually is 2°F to 4°F less than core body temperature.* 	• *Easily accessible: Forehead or abdomen.* • *Available in disposable strips.*	• *Less accurate and reliable than other routes; should not be used if accurate monitoring of temperature is essential.* • *Indicates body surface temperature only.* • *Perspiration interferes with measurement.*	*1. Draw the curtain and position the client if the abdomen, rather than the forehead, is being used.* *2. Ensure that the skin is dry.* *3. Place the strip directly on skin, holding its edges firmly to the skin so that the entire strip is in contact with the skin.* *4. Observe for color changes as the strip reacts to the skin temperature.* *5. Read the result while the strip is still in contact with the skin.* *6. Remove the strip from the skin and discard it in an appropriate trash receptacle.* *7. Use another type of thermometer if the result is not within the normal range.*

Photo credits: Wilkinson and Treas (2016). *Fundamentals of nursing*, Vol. 2, 3rd ed. Philadelphia: F. A. Davis Company, with permission.

E. Increased body temperature and related nursing care
  1. Hyperthermia.
     a. **Hyperthermia** occurs when the core body temperature is more than the person's normal body temperature; however, the body's temperature set point does not change. Usually, this term is used to describe increases more than 105°F (40.5°C).
     b. *Heat exhaustion:* Condition caused by excessive environmental heat and dehydration; indicated by weakness, muscle aches, headache, syncope, nausea, vomiting, paleness, dizziness, diaphoresis, and a temperature usually between 98.6°F to 103°F.
     c. *Heat stroke:* Condition generally caused by exercise in hot weather; indicated by flushed, hot, dry skin; throbbing headache; rapid, strong pulse; and a temperature of 103°F or more, progressing to impaired judgment, dizziness, delirium, unconsciousness, and seizures.
  2. Fever (pyrexia).
     a. **Fever** occurs when the core body temperature is more than a person's normal body temperature (usually 100°F [37.8°C] orally or 101°F [38.3°C] rectally) that is provoked by an increase in the body's temperature set point.
     b. The higher set point is the body's attempt to establish an environment that inhibits pathogen replication. Fevers up to 102°F enhance the immune response, promote phagocytosis, hinder reproduction of many pathogens, and therefore should be permitted to achieve its objective.
     c. **Hyperpyrexia:** Core body temperature of 105.8°F (41°C) or more; extremely dangerous condition requiring medical intervention to avoid cell damage especially to delicate brain tissues. Clinical indicators include agitation, confusion, stupor, and coma.
     d. Stages of a fever.
        (1) *Onset (cold or chill phase).*
            (a) Body temperature increases, gradually or suddenly, but does not yet achieve the new set point.
            (b) Clinical indicators: Chilly feeling; increased pulse rate; increased respiratory rate and depth; pale, cold skin; absence of sweating; gooseflesh; shivering; and cyanotic nail beds.
        (2) *Course (plateau phase).*
            (a) Body temperature achieves the set point.
            (b) Clinical indicators: Flushing; warm, dry skin; increased pulse and respirations; thirst; mild to severe dehydration; absence of chills; glassy-eyed appearance; weakness; lethargy; and aching muscles.
        (3) *Defervescence (fever abatement, flush phase).*
            (a) Temperature begins to return to normal range.

MAKING THE CONNECTION

Fever and Invading Foreign Elements

A fever is caused by foreign elements (e.g., bacteria, viruses, fungi, and allergens) that enter the body and stimulate the production of phagocytes, which are specialized white blood cells (WBCs). Phagocytes consume the invaders and release pyrogens. Pyrogens stimulate the secretion of prostaglandin hormones that reset the hypothalamic thermostat to an increased temperature, called the *set point*. The body then attempts to increase the core temperature to the new set point.

      (b) Clinical indicators: Warmth and flushing due to vasodilation; diaphoresis (promotes heat loss through evaporation); possible dehydration.

  e. Types of fevers.

    (1) Constant (sustained) fever.

      (a) Temperature always is higher than the normal range.

      (b) Temperature may increase or decrease by 1°F.

    (2) Intermittent fever.

      (a) Temperature is higher than the normal range.

      (b) Temperature then decreases to a normal or subnormal temperature regularly, at least once a day.

    (3) Remittent fever.

      (a) Temperature is always above the normal range.

      (b) Temperature varies by 3.6°F or higher during a 24-hour time period.

    (4) Relapsing (recurrent) fever.

      (a) Temperature in the normal range lasting for 1 to 2 days.

      (b) Followed by 1 or 2 days where the temperature is higher than the normal range.

  3. Nursing care.

    a. Monitor vital signs.

    b. Assess skin temperature, color, degree of moisture, and other clinical indicators of fever.

    c. Monitor laboratory results and I&O for clinical indicators of infection and dehydration.

    d. Provide frequent oral care to maintain moist mucous membranes.

    e. Cover the client with blankets and limit drafts when the client reports feeling cold or when shivering (shivering increases body temperature); remove blankets when the client feels warm.

    f. Encourage rest to reduce BMR.

    g. Encourage nutritional intake to meet energy needs because a fever increases BMR.

    h. Encourage oral fluid intake, and administer prescribed IV fluids.

    i. Provide dry clothing and linens when the client is diaphoretic during the defervescence phase.

    j. Use tepid water when providing a bath for hygiene purposes to increase heat loss through the principle of conduction; administer tepid sponge baths as prescribed by the primary health-care provider. Avoid causing shivering because shivering increases body temperature.

    k. Avoid rapid lowering of body temperature because doing so causes vasoconstriction and a delay in decreasing the core temperature.

    l. Administer prescribed antipyretics, generally for a fever higher than 102°F. Antipyretics are prescribed to prevent a fever from becoming dangerously high and/or to minimize discomfort.

  🛑 m. Teach the client and family members interventions to prevent negative consequences from hot environmental temperatures.

    (1) Teach people, especially older adults, to drink adequate fluids, avoid alcohol and caffeine, take cool showers or baths, and use a fan or stay in an air-conditioned space.

    (2) Encourage family members to check on older adult family members and neighbors at least twice a day to ensure that they are safe.

V. Measurement of Pulse

A **pulse** (heart rate) reflects the waves of pressure throughout the arterial vessels generated by contractions of the ventricles of the heart that occur within 1 minute. In addition to rate, the characteristics of a pulse also are identified. These assessments provide information about the status of the heart and circulatory system. Nurses measure a client's pulse to obtain baseline information, to assess the progression of an illness, and/or to monitor a response to therapy. Measuring a client's pulse requires the use of the fingers, a stethoscope, or an instrument that magnifies sounds (Doppler). Nurses must understand the commonalities of nursing care for all sites of assessment and the differences for specific sites when obtaining a pulse. The site selected for measurement requires nursing judgment because the pulse rate is influenced by such factors as characteristics of the site, method used to obtain the pulse, as

well as the client's developmental level and pathophysiological condition.

A. Physiology related to pulse

1. **Apical pulse:** Central pulse auscultated over the
   apex of heart; reflects heart rate.
2. **Peripheral pulse:** Rhythmic expansion of an
   artery that is palpated when a surge of blood
   occurs in response to contraction of the heart;
   reflects heart rate and adequacy of circulation
   to a part of the body beyond the heart, such as
   an extremity.
3. **Pulse deficit:** Difference between apical and radial
   rates (apical rate minus radial rate).
4. **Stroke volume:** Amount of blood that exits the left
   ventricle with each contraction of the heart; about
   70 mL in a healthy adult.
5. **Cardiac output:** Volume of blood that is pumped
   from the heart in 1 minute; about 5.6 L/min; it is
   the product of the stroke volume multiplied by
   the heart rate per minute.

B. Factors that affect the pulse

1. Age.
   a. As age increases, heart rate gradually decreases.
   b. Variations by age.
      (1) Newborns: 120 to 160 beats/minute.
      (2) 1 to 2 years of age: 90 to 120 beats/minute.
      (3) 3 to 18 years of age: 80 to 100 beats/minute.
      (4) Adults: 60 to 100 beats/minute.
2. Gender: After puberty, the heart rate of males
   generally is slightly slower than the heart rate
   of females.
3. Circadian rhythm (diurnal variations).
   a. Rate is slowest from predawn to dawn hours.
   b. Rate progressively increases toward evening.
4. Blood volume.
   a. Increased blood volume *(hypervolemia)*.
      (1) Pulse is full and bounding; rate may
          increase.
      (2) Commonly caused by fluid volume excess
          or excess IV fluids.
   b. Decreased blood volume *(hypovolemia)*.
      (1) Pulse is weak or thready; rate increases
          to transport more oxygen to body cells.
      (2) Commonly caused by decreased fluid vol-
          ume related to dehydration or hemorrhage.
5. Body temperature.
   a. Increased body temperature: With a fever, each
      degree of Fahrenheit increases the heart rate
      by 10 beats/minute to compensate for the
      decreased blood pressure associated with
      vasodilation and increased BMR.
   b. Decreased body temperature: When the body
      cools, each degree of Fahrenheit decreases
      the heart rate by 10 beats/minute because
      BMR slows.

6. Exercise.
   a. Heart rate increases because of the increase
      in the metabolic rate and the increased
      demand for oxygen and nutrients at the
      cellular level; stroke volume and cardiac
      output increase.
   b. Increase in heart rate in athletes may be less
      than the average adult because of larger car-
      diac size, strength, efficiency, and endurance.
7. Rest, sleep, and biofeedback activities: These
   activities decrease the body's metabolic rate and,
   subsequently, the heart rate.
8. Stress, emotions, and hormones.
   a. Sympathetic nervous system releases epineph-
      rine and norepinephrine, resulting in constric-
      tion of peripheral blood vessels and an
      increase in the metabolic rate, force of cardiac
      contractions, and heart rate.
   b. Increased thyroid hormones (hyperthyroidism)
      increase the heart rate and decreased thyroid
      hormones (hypothyroidism) decrease the
      heart rate.
9. Medications.
   a. Some medications increase the heart rate
      (e.g., epinephrine, theophylline, and atropine).
   b. Some medications decrease the heart rate
      (e.g., digoxin, antihypertensives, and opioids).
10. Ingested or inhaled substances.
    a. Ingestion of food increases the heart rate
       slightly for several hours.
    b. Caffeine, nicotine, and illegal drugs, such
       as cocaine, increase the heart rate.
11. Pathological processes.
    a. Any condition that influences cardiac, respira-
       tory, or neurological functioning may alter the
       heart rate.
    b. For example, obstructive pulmonary diseases
       and hypoxia increase the heart rate; increased
       intracranial pressure (ICP) decreases the heart
       rate and may make it irregular; cardiovascular
       disease may increase or decrease the heart rate
       or make it irregular.

C. Sites for obtaining a pulse and related nursing care

1. Apical pulse.
   a. Auscultate over the apex of the heart, known as
      the *point of maximum impulse* (Fig. 14.2).
      (1) Find the angle of Louis (bump below the
          sternal notch where the manubrium and
          sternum meet) and slide your finger into
          the second intercostal space on the left side
          of the sternum.
      (2) Place one finger in each intercostal space,
          moving down to the fifth intercostal space.
      (3) Slide your finger to the midclavicular line
          over the apex of the heart.

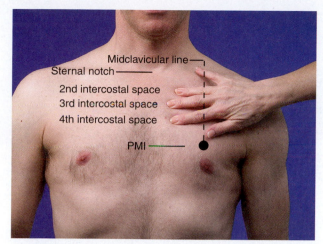

Fig 14.2 Technique to identify point of maximum impulse. (From Wilkinson and Treas [2011]. *Fundamentals of nursing*, Vol. 2, 2nd ed. Philadelphia: F. A. Davis Company, with permission.)

b. Place the diaphragm of a stethoscope over the site and count the rate of heart contractions for 1 minute.

c. Adjust the client's position or stethoscope placement if apical beats are difficult to hear because of large pectoral muscles or large or dense mammary tissue. Have the client tilt forward while in a sitting position; turn the client to the left-lateral position and move the stethoscope to the fifth or sixth intercostal space in the left midaxillary line.

d. Use the apical pulse to assess heart rate, particularly in children younger than age 3 years of age and clients with a cardiac problem.

2. Peripheral pulse sites.

a. Identify the site to be palpated by using anatomical landmarks (Fig. 14.3 and Table 14.4).

b. Apply gentle pressure to compress the artery between the fingers and an underlying bone.

c. Count each pulsating, tapping, or throbbing sensation as one beat; assess the presence and characteristics of the pulsations.

d. Perform assessment with a Doppler ultrasound machine if difficult to assess pulse via palpation.

e. Used to assess heart rate (e.g., radial), assess circulation to a body part (e.g., dorsalis pedis, posterior tibial), and identify a site for blood pressure measurement (e.g., brachial, popliteal).

D. Characteristics of a pulse and related nursing care

1. Rate.

a. Identify the number of beats of a pulse within a specific time frame.

(1) Apical rate: Count the number of heart beats while auscultating over the point of

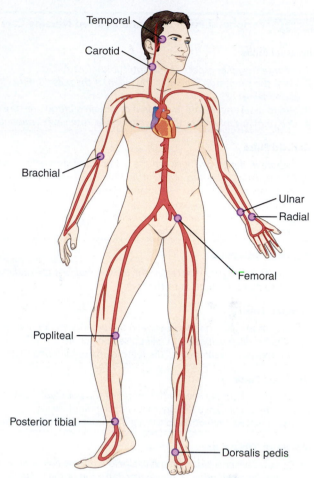

Fig 14.3 Peripheral pulse sites. (From Wilkinson and Treas [2016]. *Fundamentals of nursing*, Vol. 1, 3rd ed. Philadelphia: F. A. Davis Company, with permission.)

maximum impulse; two sounds, *lub* and *dub* together, are counted as one beat. Count the number of beats for a full minute.

(2) Peripheral rate: Count each pulsating, tapping, or throbbing sensation as one beat when palpating over an artery. Count the pulsations for at least 30 seconds and multiple the result by 2; some advocate counting the beats for 15 seconds and multiplying by 4, but this results in less accurate counts. An irregular rate should be counted for a full minute.

b. Assess distal peripheral pulses, such as the dorsalis pedis and posterior tibial, for their presence and quality rather than their rate because this assessment is done to assess the presence of circulation to the feet rather than assess the heart.

c. Determine the significance of the rate obtained in an adult.

(1) Expected rate for adults: 60 to 100 beats/ minute; for additional heart rates by age,

Table 14.4 Peripheral Pulse Sites and Related Nursing Care

Brachial Pulse

1. Palpate the inner aspect of the antecubital fossa.
2. Have the client turn the palm downward if the pulse is difficult to obtain because doing so moves the brachial artery over a bony prominence.
3. Use to assess heart rate in children or obtain a blood pressure measurement.
4. Use to assess infants, birth to 1 year of age, receiving cardiopulmonary resuscitation (CPR).

Carotid Pulse

1. Palpate in the groove between the trachea and sternocleidomastoid muscle.
2. Palpate gently to avoid obliteration of the pulse, which decreases blood flow to the brain or stimulates the carotid bodies, precipitating a decrease in heart rate and blood pressure.
3. Never palpate both arteries at the same time.
4. Use to assess adults and children older than 1 year of age receiving cardiopulmonary resuscitation (CPR) or when assessing the presence of circulation to the brain.

Dorsalis Pedis Pulse

1. Palpate in the groove between the big toe and first toe and move toward the top of the foot.
2. Use to assess circulation to the foot.

Femoral Pulse

1. Palpate the groin halfway between the anterosuperior iliac spine and the symphysis pubis.
2. Requires deep palpation to feel pulse in an adult.
3. Use to assess circulation to the leg; may be used during CPR.

Popliteal Pulse

1. Palpate behind the knee in the center of the popliteal fossa.
2. Flex the client's knee slightly to facilitate palpation.
3. Use to assess circulation to the leg or obtain a thigh blood pressure measurement.

Posterior Tibial Pulse

1. Palpate the inner side of the ankle below the medial malleolus.
2. Avoid deep palpation to prevent obliteration of the pulse; however, may be necessary to use deeper palpation in some people.
3. Use to assess circulation to the foot.

Radial Pulse

1. Ensure the arm is in a resting position, such as flexed across the chest or lying on the bed or table to eliminate muscle contraction that can interfere with accurate assessment.
2. Palpate in the groove on the thumb side of the wrist over the radial artery.
3. Begin with light pressure and increase pressure until pulse is felt.

Temporal Pulse

1. Palpate over a temporal bone on the side of the face, lateral and superior to the eye.
2. Use for infants.

---

see "Factors That Affect the Pulse, Age" in this chapter.

    (2) **Bradycardia:** Pulse rate less than 60 beats/minute.

    (3) **Tachycardia:** Pulse rate more than 100 beats/minute.

2. Rhythm.

  a. Identify rhythm by comparing the intervals between beats.

  b. Determine the significance of the intervals obtained.

    (1) Regular rhythm: Intervals are equal in length.

    (2) Irregular rhythm (**dysrhythmia**): Intervals vary in length.

  c. Identify the pattern of an irregular rhythm.

    (1) Regularly irregular: Lengths of intervals between beats are repetitive and predictable (e.g., short delay after every third beat).

    (2) Irregularly irregular: Lengths of intervals between beats are unpredictable (e.g., delays after beats with no identifiable pattern).

  🛑 d. Count the number of beats for a full minute when an irregular rhythm is identified.

3. Quality of volume.

  a. Assess the force produced by blood surging through the artery (pulse volume).

Table 14.5 Quality of Pulse Volume Rating Scale

Rating Scale	Description of Pulse
3+ Bounding	• Feels strong and full. • Not obliterated with moderate pressure. • Easily detected and counted.
2+ Strong	• Feels strong. • Obliterated with moderate pressure. • Easily detected and counted.
1+ Weak	• Feels weak. • Obliterated with slight pressure.
Thready Feeble	• Feels very weak. • Obliterated with slight pressure. • Difficult to detect; may require use of a Doppler ultrasound machine.
0 Absent	• Not detectable via palpation or use of a Doppler ultrasound machine.

b. Recognize that the rating scale is somewhat subjective (Table 14.5).

c. Assess adequacy of contractions and arterial circulation.

   (1) Adequate strength of contractions of the heart produces a palpable pulse with a rating scale of bounding (3+) or strong (2+).

   (2) Inadequate strength of contractions of the heart or impaired arterial circulation to the site produces a palpable pulse with a rating scale of weak (1+) or thready or an absent pulse (0). These indicate inadequate perfusion, resulting in decreased oxygen and nutrients to body cells adjacent to and distal to the pulse site.

d. Assess next proximal pulse site in the extremity when a distal peripheral pulse volume is 1+ or absent.

e. Perform additional peripheral vascular assessments when pulses are 1+, thready, or absent to assess circulation to the site.

4. Symmetry of characteristics.

   a. Determine whether all pulse characteristics are equal bilaterally by comparing results of unilateral assessments; assessments may be done concurrently or one after the other.

   b. Perform focused assessments, such as neurovascular assessments (see Table 14.11 in this chapter), electrocardiogram, and cardiac enzymes if unequal results are identified.

VI. Measurement of Respirations

Respiration involves the movement of gases into and out of the lungs, promoting an exchange of gases between the atmosphere and the capillary beds in the alveoli of the lung. The measurement of respirations involves observing and counting the number of cycles of inhalations (breathing in) and exhalations (breathing out) within a specific time frame. Although breathing usually is an involuntary act, people can actively control respirations. Therefore, nurses must know how to perform accurate assessments. Assessment of respirations also includes the characteristics of respirations, including depth, rhythm, and effort. (See Chapter 19, Oxygenation, for details about the structures and functions of the respiratory system, factors that influence respiratory functioning, breathing patterns, and auscultation of breath sounds.)

A. Physiology related to respirations

   1. Respiration involves the movement of gases into and out of the lungs.

   2. An exchange of gases occurs between the atmosphere and the capillary beds in the alveoli (*external respiration*).

   3. An exchange of gases occurs in the systemic blood capillaries and body cells (*internal respiration*).

   4. Respirations are under both involuntary and voluntary control.

      (a) Involuntary: The respiratory center in the brain stem regulates ventilation via levels of carbon dioxide, oxygen, and hydrogen ion concentration in the arterial blood.

      (b) Voluntary: An individual can consciously decide to take a breath overriding the respiratory center in the brain stem.

B. Assess respirations discreetly

   1. Assess respirations without the client's awareness to ensure that the respirations counted are under involuntary control.

      a. Position the client's arm across the diaphragm and palpate over the client's radial pulse site at the same time respirations are being assessed. The client will assume you are obtaining a pulse and not feel self-conscious and voluntarily alter the respiratory rate.

      b. Observe the rate and characteristics of respirations while the client is resting or sleeping.

C. Count the respiratory rate

   1. One respiration consists of one inhalation and one exhalation.

   2. Observe them by the rise and fall of the chest or abdomen or palpate them with the palm of the hand on the chest, diaphragm, or abdomen.

   3. Count respirations for a minimum of 30 seconds and multiply the result by 2.

   4. Assess the respiratory rate.

      a. **Eupnea:** Normal respiratory rate of 12 to 20 breaths/minute.

      b. **Bradypnea:** Less than 12 breaths/minute.

      c. **Tachypnea:** More than 20 breaths/minute.

D. Identify the depth of respirations
1. Depth refers to the observed amount of chest expansion; it is directly related to the volume of air inhaled.
2. Depth can be described as shallow, normal, or deep; this is a somewhat subjective observation by the nurse.
3. Amount of air inhaled in one breath usually is between 300 and 500 mL *(tidal volume)*.

E. Identify the rhythm and pattern of respirations
1. Rhythm is determined by identifying the length of intervals between respirations.
    a. Regular rhythm: Evenly spaced intervals between respirations.
    b. Irregular rhythm: Unevenly spaced intervals between respirations.

🛑 2. Assess irregular rhythms for a full minute.

3. Assess irregular rhythms further to identify patterns associated with Cheyne-Stokes, Biot, and Kussmaul respirations. (See "Breathing Patterns" in Table 19.1 in Chapter 19, Oxygenation)

F. Identify the degree of respiratory effort
1. Respiratory effort is the amount of work required to breathe.
2. The act of breathing should be effortless.
3. **Dyspnea** is difficulty breathing that can be observed by another.
4. **Shortness of breath** is the feeling of not being able to catch your breath; a subjective symptom that only the client can describe.
5. Clinical indicators of respiratory distress (see "Assess Breathing Patterns" in Chapter 19, Oxygenation, for more information about respiratory distress).
    a. *Use of accessory muscles of respiration:* Use of intercostal, trapezius, and abdominal muscles help to expand the thoracic cavity.
    b. *Retractions:* Sinking of intercostal, supraclavicular, and subcostal tissues during inspiration.
    c. *Nasal flaring:* Widening of the nares during inhalation to reduce resistance to airflow; occurs more often in infants and children.
    d. *Grunting or moaning:* A closed glottis immediately before exhalation results in grunting or moaning; a closed glottis promotes exchange of gases in alveoli.
    e. *Pursed-lip breathing:* Exhaling through the mouth with lips shaped like a small O to lengthen exhalation; helps keep airways open and prevents trapping of air in the alveoli.
    f. *Startled look:* Wide-eyed look or other signs of fear related to an inability to breathe.

    g. **Orthopnea:** Dyspnea relieved by assuming an upright position.
    h. *Orthopneic position:* Leaning forward while in a sitting position to improve breathing.

VII. Measurement of Blood Pressure

Blood pressure is an indirect measurement of the force of blood against arterial walls during cardiac contraction and cardiac relaxation. Numerous factors influence blood pressure, including physiological factors, such as cardiac output, blood volume, peripheral vascular resistance, and viscosity of the blood, and personal factors, such as age, activity, body weight, medications, and lifestyle behaviors. To obtain accurate blood pressure measurements and analyze measurement results, a nurse must not only know how to perform the skill of obtaining a blood pressure measurement but also understand the physiological and personal determinants that influence blood pressure.

A. Physiology related to blood pressure
1. **Blood pressure** is the force of circulating blood against the walls of blood vessels.
2. **Systolic blood pressure** (SBP) is the maximum arterial pressure that occurs during a contraction of the left ventricle.
3. **Diastolic blood pressure** (DBP) is the minimum arterial pressure that occurs between contractions of the heart.
4. Cardiac output.
    a. **Cardiac output** is the volume of blood that is pumped from the heart in 1 minute (about 5.6 L).
    b. It increases as a result of an increase in heart rate, an increase in heart contractility, and an increase in circulating blood volume.
5. Blood volume.
    a. **Blood volume** is the amount of blood within the intravascular compartment.
    b. When the amount of circulating blood increases within the intravascular compartment, the pressure in that space also increases because the blood exerts more pressure against the vessel walls.
    c. As the amount of circulating blood decreases, blood pressure decreases.
6. Peripheral vascular resistance.
    a. **Peripheral vascular resistance** is the amount of friction between blood flow and vessel walls.
    b. It is influenced by the thickness of the blood (viscosity), elasticity of arterial walls, and width of arterial lumens.
    c. Decreased elasticity of arterial walls, decreased width of arterial lumens, and increased blood viscosity all increase blood pressure.

d. Increased elasticity of arterial walls, increased width of arterial lumens, and decreased blood viscosity all decrease the blood pressure.

B. Factors that affect blood pressure

1. Age.
   a. Infants have a mean systolic blood pressure (SBP) of approximately 75 mm Hg.
   b. Blood pressure increases with age and arrives at the expected adult values at puberty; continues to rise slightly during adulthood.
   c. Both systolic and diastolic blood pressures increase in older adults because of decreased arterial wall elasticity.

2. Gender.
   a. After puberty, women tend to have lower blood pressures than men of the same age.
   b. After menopause, blood pressure may increase due to a decrease in estrogen.

3. Diurnal rhythms.
   a. Blood pressure usually is lowest in the morning, increases during the day, and is highest in the late afternoon or evening.
   b. These changes are related to the body's metabolic rate.

4. Race.
   a. Evidence, based on men in the United States, supports the fact that people of specific ethnicities may have a higher or lower risk of developing certain illnesses; whether this difference is caused by some genetic component or due to cultural circumstances is unclear.
   b. For example, some believe that the higher rate of hypertension among men of African American heritage (43%) versus men of white European heritage (27.8%) may be due to a genetically based salt sensitivity. In addition, men of African American heritage have a higher rate of kidney disease, which can increase blood pressure. American men of Asian or Pacific Islander heritage have a 9.7% rate of hypertension. These statistics hold constant across independent research, suggesting a genetic component.

5. Exercise: Activity increases metabolic rate and cardiac output, thereby increasing blood pressure.

6. Stress.
   a. The sympathetic nervous system response to stress increases cardiac output and constricts blood vessels; therefore, blood pressure increases.
   b. Acute pain increases blood pressure; however, chronic pain might not.

7. Obesity: An additional vascular supply is necessary to perfuse excessive body mass, resulting in increased peripheral resistance; thus, blood pressure increases.

8. Lifestyle behaviors: Excessive dietary sodium, smoking tobacco, and three or more alcoholic beverages a day may increase the blood pressure.

9. Medications.
   a. Blood pressure may decrease with use of opioids, antihypertensives, antidysrhythmics, and diuretics.
   b. Blood pressure may increase with use of some over-the-counter medications, herbal preparations, and illicit drugs.

10. Diseases: Any condition that affects the circulatory system or any major organ of the body (e.g., kidneys, thyroid gland, and brain) may affect the blood pressure.

11. Body position: Blood pressure is higher when a person is standing rather than sitting or lying; when the arm being used for measurement is held higher than the heart; when sitting, when the feet are dangling rather than on the floor; and when the legs are crossed at the knees when sitting.

C. Nursing care when obtaining a blood pressure measurement

1. Collect appropriate equipment for measuring blood pressure (BP).
   a. Sphygmomanometer: May have a dial that registers the BP by a pointer attached to a spring or an electronic machine that can detect either sounds or pressure waves as blood flows through an artery and registers a measurement.
      (1) Blood pressure cuff: The width and length of the bladder of the cuff being used must be appropriate for the limb used and the client's size (Fig. 14.4)
      (2) Width of bladder: Should cover about two-thirds of the length of the person's upper arm.
      (3) Length of bladder: Should encircle 80% of the upper arm.
      (4) If the cuff is too small, the BP result will be inaccurately high. If the cuff is too large, the BP result will be inaccurately low.

Fig 14.4 Blood pressure cuff. (Adapted from Wilkinson and Treas [2016]. *Fundamentals of nursing*, Vol. 1, 3rd ed. Philadelphia: F. A. Davis Company, with permission.)

Fig 14.5 Stethoscope. (From Wilkinson and Treas [2016]. *Fundamentals of nursing*, Vol. 1, 3rd ed. Philadelphia: F. A. Davis Company, with permission.)

b. Stethoscope: The diaphragm or bell of a stethoscope may be used to auscultate the sounds associated with a BP (Fig. 14.5). Clean each area of the stethoscope (e.g., bell, diaphragm, and ear pieces) with a separate alcohol wipe before and after use.

DID YOU KNOW?

Most nurses use the diaphragm of a stethoscope to auscultate BP. However, evidence-based practice supports the use of the bell rather than the diaphragm because diastolic pressure (low-pitched sounds) can be heard more accurately using the bell.

2. Ensure that equipment is working properly, and charged if it is an electronic device, before using it with a client.
3. Introduce yourself, identify the client, explain what you are going to do, and provide privacy by closing the door or pulling the curtain.
4. Identify the site to be used and position the client accordingly.
   a. Arm.
      (1) Contraindications for obtaining a BP in an arm include presence of an intravenous infusion or renal dialysis shunt; presence of a cast, brace, or dressing; amputation, trauma, or surgery of the arm being considered; and mastectomy or therapy to the breast on the side of the arm being considered.
      (2) Place the client in the low-, semi-, or high-Fowler position or sitting position; support the arm at the level of the heart.
      (3) Place the cuff above (proximal) the antecubital fossa (area opposite to the elbow) when auscultating over the brachial artery or around the forearm when auscultating over the radial artery.

Fig 14.6 Placement of a blood pressure cuff on the thigh. (From Wilkinson and Treas [2016]. *Fundamentals of nursing*, Vol. 2, 3rd ed. Philadelphia: F. A. Davis Company, with permission.)

   b. Thigh.
      (1) Contraindications for obtaining a BP in a thigh include upper or lower amputation of the extremity, presence of edema, capillary refill more than 3 seconds, and any inflammation, infection, lesions, or trauma in the leg.
      (2) Place the client supine with the leg in a slightly flexed position.
      (3) Place the cuff just above the knee around the thigh while auscultating over the popliteal artery in the popliteal fossa (area behind the knee) (Fig. 14.6).
5. Determine systolic blood pressure (SBP) by palpation.
   a. A palpable pulse provides an indication of the approximate level of the SBP.
   b. This technique prevents erroneously underestimating the SBP by beginning the BP measurement during an auscultatory gap.
      (1) An **auscultatory gap** is the temporary loss of sound when the cuff pressure is high followed by the return of sounds at a lower level.
      (2) It occurs more often in clients with excessively high BPs.
   c. Palpating BP can be done when BP is difficult to hear; however, it reveals only the SBP.
   d. Palpate the artery, inflate the cuff rapidly to 80 mm Hg, and continue to inflate the cuff in 10 mm Hg increments until the pulse can no longer be felt. Note the level of the SBP.
   e. Deflate the cuff and wait 2 minutes before obtaining the auscultated BP.
6. Determine the systolic and diastolic BP by auscultation.
   a. Place the bell or diaphragm of the stethoscope over the artery without touching the cuff and ensure that the tubing of the stethoscope and sphygmomanometer are not touching anything; these actions eliminate interfering sounds.

b. Inflate the cuff 30 mm Hg above the level of the palpated SBP. This ensures that the first sound associated with a BP will be heard accurately.

c. Release the pressure within the cuff slowly (2 to 3 mm Hg per second) to allow the return of blood flow to the arm. As blood begins and continues to flow through the artery, listen for a variety of sounds (Korotkoff sounds) (Table 14.6).

⚠ 7. Wait 2 minutes before reinflating a cuff if a second assessment is necessary to prevent a falsely elevated diastolic result due to venous congestion.

8. Analyze BP measurement results.
   a. *Normal blood pressure:* SBP <120 mm Hg and a DBP <80 mm Hg.
   b. **Hypotension:** SBP less than 100 mm Hg.
   c. **Orthostatic (postural) hypotension:** A 10- to 20-mm Hg decrease between lying down and sitting and/or a 10- to 20-mm Hg decrease between sitting and standing; results from peripheral vasodilation without a compensatory increase in cardiac output.
   d. *Prehypertension:* SBP 120 to 139 mm Hg or DBP 80 to 89 mm Hg.
   e. **Hypertension:** SBP 140 mm Hg or higher or DBP 90 mm Hg or higher on two separate occasions.
      (1) High blood pressure—Stage I: SBP 140 to 159 or DBP 90 to 99 mm Hg.
      (2) High blood pressure—Stage II: SBP ≥160 mm Hg or DBP ≥100 mm Hg.
   f. *Hypertensive crisis:* SBP higher than 180 mm Hg or DBP higher than 110 mm Hg.

g. **Pulse pressure:** Difference between SBP and DBP; reflects the volume of blood exiting the left ventricle; should be no more than one-third the SBP.

9. Document the BP measurement in the client's clinical record and report results outside the expected range that are dangerous.
   a. Adult: The SBP is the first sound heard; the DBP is the last sound heard.
   b. Child: The SBP is the first sound heard; the DBP is when the sound becomes muffled (fourth sound heard).
   c. Some advocate recording the level of three sounds: the first sound heard, the muffling of the sound, and the last sound heard.
   d. Initiate rapid response team and notify primary health-care provider of dangerous results.

VIII. Measurement of Arterial Oxygen Saturation

An arterial oxygen saturation level provides vital information about a person's cardiopulmonary status and, therefore, is now considered one of the vital signs. *Pulse oximetry* is a noninvasive technique that estimates the percentage of hemoglobin molecules carrying oxygen in circulating red blood cells (RBCs). It detects the presence of deficient oxygen in the blood (**hypoxemia**) before visible signs develop. Nurses must understand factors that affect oxygen saturation results, factors indicting the need for monitoring oxygen saturation, clinical manifestations of alterations in oxygen saturation, and ways to perform pulse oximetry to assess blood oxygen saturation.

A. Physiology related to oxygen saturation
1. Oxygen entering the body binds with hemoglobin in RBCs and is transported via the circulation to body cells.
2. Expected normal values of oxygen saturation are between 95% and 100%.

B. Factors that affect oxygen saturation
1. Amount of RBCs/hemoglobin: Oxygen saturation measurement will be within the normal range when the circulating hemoglobin is fully saturated. However, if the client has a low RBC count (anemia), all the hemoglobin may be saturated, but the client may have inadequate oxygen reaching body tissues.
2. If circulation under the sensor is impaired, then the reading will be inaccurately low.
3. Excessive movement, tremors, or shivering interferes with accurate readings.
4. Acrylic nails and dark nail polish interfere with an accurate assessment.
5. Excessive perspiration and oils on the skin can interfere with accurate readings.

Table 14.6 **Korotkoff Sounds**	
Sound	**Description**
First	• This is the systolic blood pressure in adults and children. • Faint, clear, rhythmic tapping sounds that gradually increase in intensity. • First sound heard as blood begins to flow through artery as compression of the artery is released.
Second	• Represent turbulent blood flow through the somewhat compressed artery. • Soft, swishing, whooshing sounds.
Third	• Sharper, crisper, rhythmic, and more intense sounds, but not as intense as first sounds.
Fourth	• This is the diastolic blood pressure in children. • Soft, rhythmic, muffled sounds. • Compression of the artery is lessening.
Fifth	• This is the diastolic blood pressure in adults. • Last sound heard. • Followed by silence.

C. Factors indicating the need for monitoring oxygen saturation
1. Acute or chronic impaired respiratory or cardiac functioning.
2. Recovery from any type of anesthesia or conscious sedation.
3. Any trauma, including surgery.
4. Ventilatory dependency.
5. Receipt of supplemental oxygen.

D. Clinical manifestations of altered oxygen saturation
1. Altered respiratory rate, depth, or rhythm.
2. Dyspnea and use of accessory muscles of respirations. (See "Assess Breathing Patterns" in Chapter 19, Oxygenation.)
3. Adventitious breath sounds. (See "Distinguishing Abnormal Breath Sounds" in Table 19.3 in Chapter 19, Oxygenation.)
4. Pallor or cyanosis of the lips, mucous membranes, nail beds, and skin.
5. Restlessness, irritability, confusion, and decreased level of consciousness.

E. Measurement of pulse oximetry and related nursing care
1. Obtain measurement intermittently or continuously as indicated by client's status; indicate parameter of room air or oxygen administration.
2. Select site for application of sensor.
   a. Finger, toe, ear lobe, or forehead.
   b. Remove dark nail polish from finger nail or toe nail or select an alternate site.
   c. Avoid appendages with thickened nails, edema, or if capillary refill is more than 3 seconds or more than 5 seconds in an older adult.
   d. Use ear lobe or forehead rather than finger or toe if the client has excessive activity or is shivering.
3. Clean the site with an alcohol swab to remove perspiration or skin oils before placing the sensor.
4. Set alarm parameters for pulse rate and oxygen saturation measurement.
🛑 5. Assess the skin under the sensor every 2 hours if monitoring is continuous to ensure tissue integrity; rotate the site of a clip-on probe every 2 hours and an adhesive probe every 4 hours.
6. Document results in the client's clinical record; evaluate measurements in light of client's laboratory results for red blood cell count and hemoglobin level.
7. Initiate the rapid response team and notify the primary health-care provider if measurements outside the preset parameters are dangerous.

IX. Measurement of Pain

Pain is an unpleasant, emotional or sensory experience related to potential or actual tissue damage. It is a physiological compensatory mechanism that signals that something is not right with the body, and therefore, it is now considered one of the vital signs. Although pain is a universal phenomenon, the experience of pain is unique to each individual. It is a subjective symptom that only the client can describe—*pain is what and where the client says it is.* Therefore, a thorough comprehensive assessment of pain must be conducted when a client reports feeling pain. (See Chapter 15, Pain, Comfort, Rest, and Sleep, for a thorough discussion of pain, including measurement of pain and related nursing care.)

X. Techniques of Physical Assessment Used by Nurses

After performing a general survey of the client and obtaining vital signs, the nurse should perform a comprehensive physical assessment. Before performing this assessment, the nurse must understand information specific to the techniques of physical assessment and must also understand that the techniques used should progress from least invasive to most invasive so as not to influence subsequent assessments. These techniques should begin with inspection and progress to auscultation, percussion, and finally palpation.

A. Inspection
1. Use of the naked eye to visually observe and examine the client.
2. Performed first because it is the least invasive physical assessment technique.
3. Also involves using the sense of smell.
4. Principles of inspection.
   a. Begin inspection immediately on visual contact with the client and continue while conducting the general survey; move to a focused inspection when you identify a specific problem.
   b. Provide adequate lighting to ensure that the colors of the curtains and walls do not influence visual assessments.
   c. Use equipment to enhance vision, such as a penlight to examine pupil reaction to light or to examine the oral cavity and an otoscope to examine inside the nose, ear canals, and tympanic membranes.
   d. Position and drape the client appropriately to ensure that the part of the body being inspected can be seen in its entirety.
   e. Examine the body for size, shape, symmetry, position, movement, and color.
   f. Compare one side of the body with the other side to determine whether they are the same (symmetry) or different. For example, one leg may be pink

and the other pale, indicating impaired circulation to the pale leg, or the client may be able to move one side of the body but not the other side, indicating a neurological problem.

B. Auscultation
1. Use of the ears to listen for sounds produced by the body.
2. Performed after inspection because it is more invasive than inspection and before percussion and palpation because these steps can alter the results of auscultation.
3. Principles of auscultation.
   a. Listen to sounds.
      (1) Directly: Use unaided ears for audible sounds, such as burping, passing flatus, snoring, loud wheezing, and a grating sound when moving a joint.
      (2) Indirectly: Use a device (e.g., stethoscope, electronic Doppler) to magnify the sound when sounds are not audible outside the body.
      (3) To detect sounds in different parts of the body: Lungs (e.g., normal and adventitious breath sounds), heart (e.g., rate, rhythm, murmurs, rubs, or gallops), intestines (e.g., bowel sounds [*borborygmi*]), uterus (e.g., fetal heart rate and blood flowing through uterine arteries of a pregnant woman [*soufflé*]).
   b. Assess the characteristics of the sounds heard.
      (1) Pitch: Quality of a sound based on its frequency.
         (a) High-pitched sounds have more vibrations per minute.
         (b) Low-pitched sounds have fewer vibrations per minute.
      (2) Intensity: Amplitude of the sound (e.g., loud or soft).
      (3) Quality: Characteristics of the sound (e.g., musical, gurgling, or grating).
      (4) Duration: Length of time the sound is heard (e.g., short, medium, or long).
      (5) Precipitating factors: Sound caused by or associated with some condition (e.g., pleural friction rub heard at the height of inspiration, wheezes heard on exhalation).
      (6) Relieving factors: Factors that minimize or eliminate the sound (e.g., bowel sounds decrease after flatus is expelled).

C. Percussion
1. Use of fingers to strike a client's body part directly to elicit a sound or vibration.
2. Performed after auscultation because it is more invasive than auscultation and before palpation because palpation can alter the results of percussion.
3. Can involve the use of a small rubber-tipped hammer (e.g., for assessment of deep tendon reflexes).
4. Principles of percussion.
   a. Use the middle finger of one hand to firmly and rapidly strike the middle finger of the other hand that is placed in direct contact with the client's skin to elicit a sound or vibration (Fig. 14.7).
   b. Assess the sounds produced to determine the location, dimension, or density (e.g., solid, hollow, filled with air) of underlying body structures.
      (1) Flatness: Dull sound generated by very dense tissue, such as bone and muscle.
      (2) Dullness: Thud-like sound generated by dense tissue, such as the liver, heart, or spleen; fluid-filled abdominal cavity *(ascites)*; or distended bladder.
      (3) Resonance: Hollow sound generated by a normal lung.
      (4) Hyperresonance: Abnormal booming sound heard when percussing a lung of a client with emphysema.
      (5) Tympany: Musical sound associated with air in the stomach or intestines.

D. Palpation
1. Use of the fingers or hands to apply pressure to the external surface of the body to feel for deviations in the skin or determine underlying structures below the skin.
2. Performed last after percussion.
3. Principles of palpation.
   a. Keep fingernails short.
   b. Perform hand hygiene and warm the hands before touching the client.
   c. Palpate tender or painful areas last; observe for grimacing, response to initiation or release of pressure, and reports of discomfort or pain.

Fig 14.7 Percussion. (From Wilkinson and Treas [2016]. *Fundamentals of nursing*, Vol. 2, 3rd ed. Philadelphia: F. A. Davis Company, with permission.)

d. Assess all four quadrants of the abdomen.

e. Light palpation depresses the skin 1 to 2 cm; for example, assessing extent of edema (see Fig. 21.8 in Chapter 21, "Fluid, Electrolyte, and Acid-Base Balance"), bladder distention, and a peripheral pulse.

f. Deep palpation depresses the skin 3 to 5 cm; performed only by a skilled practitioner because excessive pressure can injure an organ; not usually done during a routine nursing assessment.

4. Assessment sites.

a. Assess the status of the skin for texture, turgor, moisture, and temperature; use the back of the fingers where skin is thinner to assess for surface temperature (Fig. 14.8). Assess both legs at the same time for symmetry.

b. Assess the rate and quality of arterial pulses.

c. Assess the status of muscle relaxation or rigidity (e.g., tense muscles indicate muscle contraction, board-like abdomen, or compartment syndrome).

d. Assess for the presence of fluid (e.g., distention of the urinary bladder, indicating retention of urine, or distention of the abdomen, indicating ascites).

e. Assess the location and characteristics of pain in response to pressure (e.g., pain associated with appendicitis that occurs in response to pressure applied to McBurney's point, located in right lower quadrant of the abdomen halfway between the anterior iliac crest and

Fig 14.8 Assessing skin temperature. (From Dillon [2016]. *Nursing health assessment: The foundation of clinical practice*, 3rd ed. Philadelphia: F. A. Davis Company, with permission.)

the umbilicus) or tensing of abdominal muscles or pain that occurs when moderate pressure is applied to the abdomen, held, and then quickly released (*rebound tenderness*).

XI. Performance of a Physical Assessment

After performing a general survey of the client and obtaining vital signs, the nurse should assess the client's physical status in more detail. Physical assessment should follow a systematic, thorough, and consistent approach. For this discussion, assessment is performed in relation to the systems of the body (e.g., neurological, integumentary, respiratory, cardiovascular, gastrointestinal, genitourinary, and so on).

A. Neurological system

1. The anatomy of the nervous system includes the brain (cerebrum, cerebellum, brain stem, and cranial nerves), spinal cord and spinal tracks, and spinal nerves. There are 31 pairs of spinal nerves that arise from the spinal cord and exit at each intervertebral foramen (vertebrae include 8 cervical, 12 thoracic, 5 lumbar, and 5 sacral).

2. Assessment involves mental status, level of consciousness, reflexes, cranial nerves, sensory function, and motor function.

3. Assess mental status: Indicates functioning of the cerebrum.

a. Language: Ability to send and receive messages in verbal, written, or behavioral forms.

(1) *Expressive aphasia:* Inability to express oneself by verbal or written words or behavioral signs.

(2) *Receptive aphasia:* Inability to comprehend spoken or written words or behavioral signs.

b. Orientation: Ability to identify time, place, and person.

(1) Time: Knows the year, month, day of the week, or time of day. Ask, "What day is it?"

(2) Place: Knows location. Ask, "Where are you?"

(3) Person: Knows own name and recognizes or knows names of significant others. Self-identity remains the longest when there is dysfunction with time, place, and person. Ask, "What is your name?"

c. Memory: Ability to recall information.

(1) *Immediate recall:* Remembers information given seconds before tested. State three numbers and immediately have client recall the numbers.

(2) *Recent memory:* Remembers information within hours and days. Ask, "What did you have for breakfast?"

(3) *Long-term memory:* Remembers information within months to years. Ask, "Where were you born?"

d. Cognitive skills: Ability to focus on a mental task. Ask, "How much is three plus three?" or "Start with the number 100 and count backward in intervals of five."

4. Assess level of consciousness.
a. Determines the client's level of arousal.
(1) *Alert:* Follows commands.
(2) *Lethargic:* Is drowsy, drifts off to sleep.
(3) *Stuporous:* Requires vigorous stimulation for a response.
(4) *Comatose:* Does not respond to verbal or painful stimuli.
b. Use a stimulus to precipitate a response from the client. Progressively move to the next type of stimulus if the previous stimulus does not evoke a response.
(1) *Verbal:* Responds to spoken stimulus. State, "Open your eyes."
(2) *Tactile:* Responds to touch. Gently shake the client's shoulder or stroke the arm.
(3) *Painful stimulus:* Responds to uncomfortable stimulus (e.g., pressure, pain). Press on the sternum or over a fingernail bed or squeeze the trapezius muscle.
c. Use a standard reference for assessing level of consciousness when assessing a client with a

head injury; decreasing level of consciousness is one of the first indications of increased intracranial pressure (ICP).
(1) Glasgow Coma Scale: Assesses client's eye response, motor response, and verbal response to stimuli.
(2) Full Outline of UnResponsiveness (FOUR) score: Assesses the client's respirations, brain stem reflexes, eye response, and motor response to stimuli.

DID YOU KNOW?
Evidence-based practice indicates that the FOUR score is a good predictor of the prognosis of critically ill clients and has important advantages over the Glasgow Coma Scale. In addition to assessing eye response and motor response, the FOUR score also assesses respirations and brain stem reflexes.

5. Assess reflexes:
a. A *reflex* is an automatic response to a stimulus that does not require conscious thought.
b. Indicate the integrity of sensory and motor pathways of the reflex arc and spinal cord segments.
c. Superficial reflexes: Abdominal, anus, cremasteric, and plantar (Table 14.7); result graded as positive or negative.

Table 14.7 Evaluating Superficial Reflexes

Reflex	Expected Response	Deviation
Abdominal Stroke each abdominal quadrant toward the umbilicus.	• *Positive: Umbilicus moves toward stimulus.*	• *Negative: No response indicates problem involving T8, T9, or T10.*
Anus Touch the side of the anus with a gloved finger.	• *Positive: Anus puckers.*	• *Negative: No response indicates problem involving S3, S4, or S5.*
Cremasteric Stroke the inner aspect of a male's thigh.	• *Positive: Elevation of testes.*	• *Negative: No response indicates problem with L1 or L2.*
Plantar (Babinski) With a thumb or dull instrument, stroke the sole of the foot from the heel up the lateral side toward and then across the ball of the foot to the great toe.	• *Negative: All toes curl downward or no response; positive response is normal until age 2 years.*	• *Positive: Dorsiflexion of great toe with or without fanning of other toes indicates problem with upper motor neurons.*

Photo credits: Dillon (2016). *Nursing health assessment: The foundation of clinical practice,* 3rd ed. F. A. Davis Company, with permission.

Table 14.8 Evaluating Deep Tendon Reflexes

Reflex	Expected Response	Deviation
Biceps Support the client's elbow with your thumb over the biceps tendon and strike the percussion hammer on your thumb.	• *+2; feel biceps contract under your thumb; observe slight flexion of the elbow.*	• *Increased or decreased response indicates problem with C5 or C6.*
Triceps Abduct the client's shoulder; flex the elbow, letting the arm hang down; and strike the triceps tendon 1 to 2 inches above the olecranon process.	• *+2; observe and feel extension of the elbow.*	• *Increased or decreased response indicates a problem with C7 or C8.*
Brachioradialis Rest the arm on the client's leg, strike 1 to 2 inches above the bony prominence of the wrist on the side by the thumb.	• *+2; observe flexion of the elbow and supination of the forearm.*	• *Increased or decreased response indicates a problem with C5 or C6.*
Patellar Place the client in a sitting position with the legs dangling, strike the patellar tendon just below the patella.	• *+2; observe extension of the knee.*	• *Increased or decreased response indicates a problem with L2, L3, or L4.*
Achilles Strike the Achilles tendon 2 inches above the heel.	• *+2; observe plantar flexion of the foot.*	• *Increased or decreased response indicates a problem with S1 or S2.*

d. Deep tendon reflexes: Biceps, triceps, brachioradialis, patellar, Achilles (Table 14.8); results graded as 0 = no response, +1 = diminished, +2 = normal response, +3 = increased but not pathologic, +4 = hyperactive or involuntary contraction and relaxation of skeletal muscle.

6. Assess the cranial nerves.
   a. The 12 cranial nerves are peripheral nerves that arise from the brain rather than from the spinal cord.
   b. They control numerous sensory and motor functions (Table 14.9).

7. Assess sensory functions.
   a. Assess the client's ability to perceive sensations of light touch, pain, and temperature while the eyes are closed.
      (1) Use a wisp of cotton; use the sharp end of a toothpick or paper clip (do not use an object, such as a needle, that will break the skin); use test tubes filled with hot and cold water.
      (2) Assess distal areas first and then proximal areas; if the distal area is intact, you need not test the proximal area. If pain sensation is intact, you need not test for temperature because these stimuli are transmitted along the same spinal tracks.
      (3) Monitor for expected client responses: client should feel light touch, pain, and temperature variations in all extremities; assess for symmetry.
      (4) Monitor for deviations from expected responses; dysfunction will relate to areas innervated by specific spinal nerves *(dermatomes).*
         (a) *Hyperalgia:* Increased pain sensation.
         (b) *Analgesia:* No pain sensation.
         (c) *Paresthesia:* Numbness and tingling.
   b. Assess ability to identify an object via touch *(stereognosis):* Have the client close the eyes, place a familiar object in the client's hand, and then have the client identify the object (e.g., key, coin, paper clip). Abnormal finding indicates problem with sensory cortex or posterior column of spinal cord.
   c. Assess ability to identify the position or movement of the body *(kinesthesia):* Move a client's finger from one position to another, and ask the client to describe the direction of movement. An abnormal finding indicates damage to peripheral nerves or the posterior column of the spinal cord.
   d. Assess for human responses to both sensory deprivation and sensory overload (e.g., irritability, confusion, reduced attention span, drowsiness, decreased problem-solving ability).
      (1) Assess for adaptations specific to sensory overload (e.g., fatigue, inability to concentrate, disorientation, anxiety, increased muscle tension).

Table 14.9 **Assessment of Cranial Nerves**

Cranial Nerve (CN) and Assessment Technique	Expected Response	Significant Deviations
I: Olfactory—Sense of smell		
• Have the client discriminate between odors (e.g., orange, peanut butter, coffee).	• Ability to discriminate odors.	• Impaired or absent ability to discriminate odors.
II: Optic—Sense of sight		
• Test far vision with a Snellen chart.	• Visual acuity of 20/20.	• Inability to read Snellen chart accurately.
• Test near vision with a Rosenbaum chart.	• Ability to read Rosenbaum chart.	• Inability to read Rosenbaum chart accurately.
• Ask the client to describe boundaries of visual field while eyes are in a fixed forward position.	• Peripheral vision of 50° in superior field, 70° in inferior field, 60° in nasal field, and 90° to 110° in temporal field.	• Limited peripheral vision (tunnel vision).
III: Oculomotor—Movement of eyeballs, position of lids, and constriction of pupils **IV: Trochlear—Moves eyeball downward and laterally** **VI: Abducens—Moves eyeball laterally**		
• Have the client follow your finger moving through all fields of gaze (up-down, left-right, at an angle up right to lower left, and at an angle up left to lower right).	• Movement of eyes through all fields of gaze equally.	• Lack of eye symmetry when moving through fields of gaze; rapid involuntary rhythmic eye movements (nystagmus).
• Place your finger 12 inches in front of the client's eyes and move toward the eyes.	• Pupils constrict and both eyes turn inward toward the nose as the person focuses on the finger.	• Failure of one or both pupils to accommodate or slow accommodation.
• Inspect location of lids.	• No lid lag.	• Drooping of eyelid (ptosis).
• Shine light on pupil.	• Pupils **e**qual, **r**ound, **r**eactive to **l**ight and **a**ccommodation (PERRLA).	• Slow pupil constriction or lack of constriction.
V: Trigeminal—Muscle strength, facial sensation, corneal reflex		
• Have the client clench the jaw while your hands are on the sides of the face.	• Firm and symmetrical muscle tone.	• Deviation of jaw to one side; unco-ordinated twitching of muscles.
• Touch the side of the face at the scalp, cheek, and chin with the point of a paperclip, alternating with a wisp of cotton; do not follow a predictable pattern.	• Ability to distinguish between the sharp versus light sensation.	• Inability to distinguish between the sharp versus light sensation.
• Touch a wisp of cotton to the cornea (usually not performed on a conscious client).	• Symmetrical blink reflex.	• Absent blink reflex or asymmetrical blink reflex.
VII: Facial—Facial expression, muscle strength, and taste		
• Have the client smile, wrinkle the forehead, puff out the cheeks, purse the lips, squeeze the eyes shut, and bare the teeth.	• Symmetrical facial movements.	• Asymmetrical facial movements (e.g., mouth droops, nasolabial fold flattens, or lower eyelid sags).
• Test taste by placing various foods on the anterior two-thirds of the tongue (e.g., sugar—sweet; lemon juice—sour; table salt—salty).	• Ability to distinguish among sweet, sour, and salt stimuli.	• Difficulty with or inability to distinguish among sweet, sour, and salt stimuli.
VIII: Auditory—Hearing acuity, sound conduction, and equilibrium		
• Stand behind the client and whisper or place a ticking clock by the client's ear.	• Ability to hear the voice or ticking clock.	• Diminished or absent ability to hear voice or ticking clock.
• Place a vibrating tuning fork on the top of the client's head (Weber test).	• Sound heard equally in both ears.	• Sound louder in an impaired ear with conductive hearing loss and louder in an unaffected ear if sensorineural hearing loss is present.

Continued

Table 14.9 **Assessment of Cranial Nerves—cont'd**

Cranial Nerve (CN) and Assessment Technique	Expected Response	Significant Deviations
• Place a vibrating tuning fork on the mastoid bone (Rinne test) and record the length of time it takes the client to no longer hear the sound; then place the fork next to the ear and again have the client indicate when the sound is no longer heard.	• The length of time that sound is heard via air conduction is twice as long as sound heard by bone conduction.	• Sound heard longer by air conduction with sensorineural hearing loss and sound heard longer by bone conduction with conductive hearing loss.
• Assess equilibrium by having the client stand with feet together and arms at the sides; done with eyes open and then closed (Romberg test).	• Maintenance of balance with minimal swaying.	• Swaying or loss of balance.

IX: Glossopharyngeal—Taste, swallowing, gag reflex, tongue movement, and secretion of saliva
X: Vagus—Swallowing, movement of vocal cords, peristalsis, digestive secretions, sensory in cardiac, respiratory, and blood pressure reflexes

• Listen to the client speak.	• Strong, clear voice.	• Hoarseness.
• Assess ability to swallow.	• Swallowing with ease.	• Impaired ability to swallow.
• Assess ability to cough.	• Coughing with ease.	• Impaired ability to cough.
• Depress the tongue with a tongue blade and observe the soft palate while the client says "ah."	• Symmetrical rising of uvula and soft palate.	• Asymmetrical movement of uvula and soft palate.
• Touch the back of the pharynx with a tongue blade.	• Elicits gag reflex.	• Absence of gag reflex.
• Test taste by placing sweet, sour, and salty foods on posterior one-third of tongue.	• Ability to distinguish among sweet, sour, and salt stimuli.	• Difficulty with or inability to distinguish among sweet, sour, and salt stimuli. May be diminished in older adults.

XI: Accessory—Head movement and elevation of shoulders

• Have the client turn the head from side to side against resistance.	• Full range of symmetrical movement without pain.	• Asymmetrical movement, limited or absent movement, or pain.
• Place your hands on the client's shoulders and ask the client to raise the shoulders against resistance.	• Ability to raise shoulders symmetrically.	• Asymmetrical movement, limited or absent movement, or pain.

XII: Hypoglossal—Tongue movement

• Have the client protrude the tongue and move it from side to side.	• Ability to move the tongue easily.	• Limited ability to move the tongue.
• Ask the client to say "l, t, d, n."	• Ability to articulate letters easily.	• Difficulty articulating letters.

(2) Assess for adaptations specific to sensory deprivation (e.g., depression, preoccupation with somatic ailments, delusions, hallucinations).

8. Assess motor functions.
   a. The cerebellum helps coordinate muscle movement, posture, equilibrium, and body positioning.
   b. Assess coordination; all movements should be smooth and rhythmical.
      (1) Have the client extend the arms out to the side and then alternately touch each index finger to the nose with the eyes closed.
      (2) Have the client touch the thumb to each fingertip in rapid sequence.
      (3) Place the client in the supine position and, with the ball of the client's foot in your hand, ask the client to repeatedly tap your hand with the foot.

   c. Assess balance.
      (1) Have the client perform the Romberg test (see Table 14.9, cranial nerve VIII).
      (2) Have the client stand on one foot with the eyes closed and the arms at the side; should maintain balance for ≥5 seconds with just slight swaying.
      (3) Have the client walk a straight line, alternating the feet while placing the heel of one foot directly in front of the toes of the other foot.
   d. See "Assessment of client mobility" in Chapter 17, Mobility.

B. Cardiovascular system
   1. The anatomy of the cardiovascular system consists of the heart, great vessels (e.g., aorta, superior and inferior vena cava, pulmonary arteries, and pulmonary veins), and peripheral circulation (e.g., arteries, capillaries, and veins).

2. Assessment involves determining the BP; rate and rhythm of heart contractions; rate, volume, and symmetry of peripheral arteries; and inspection of veins and condition of peripheral tissues.
3. Assess BP (see "Measurement of Blood Pressure" earlier in this chapter).
4. Auscultate heart sounds using a systematic progression; begin at the aortic area and end at the mitral area.
   a. Apical pulse: See "Measurement of Pulse" and Fig 14.2 for description about assessing the apical pulse.
   b. Auscultate over cardiac auscultation sites (Fig. 14.9).
      (1) Aortic valve: Second intercostal space (ICS) at right sternal border.

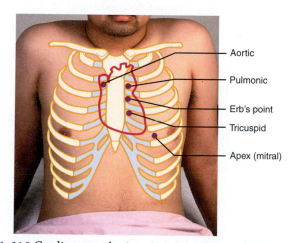

   (2) Pulmonic valve: Second ICS at left sternal border.
   (3) Tricuspid valve: Fourth ICS at left sternal border.
   (4) Mitral valve: Fifth ICS at midclavicular line.
   c. Heart sounds (Table 14.10).
   d. Identify the presence of a heart murmur.
      (1) A soft, muffled, swooshing prolonged heart sound rather than a clear S_1 or S_2.
      (2) Caused by turbulence of blood flow through a heart valve that does not close completely.
      (3) Aortic murmurs are best heart over Erb's point.
   e. Identify the presence of pericardial friction rub.
      (1) A short, scratchy, grating sound.
      (2) Caused by roughened pericardial membranes rubbing against each other; specific for pericarditis.
      (3) Heard at the apex, left of the sternum.
5. Assess the carotid arteries.
   (1) Auscultate over the artery to identify the presence of a whooshing sound due to narrowing of the lumen *(bruit)*.
   (2) Palpate the artery lightly if a bruit is auscultated to identify vibrations from turbulent blood flow *(thrill)*.

🛑 (3) Do not palpate both carotid arteries at the same time because doing so can impair cerebral blood flow.

6. Assess the external jugular veins.
   (1) Return blood flow from the brain to the superior vena cava and then the heart.

Fig 14.9 Cardiac auscultation sites. (Adapted from Wilkinson and Treas [2016]. *Fundamentals of nursing*, Vol. 2, 3rd ed. Philadelphia: F. A. Davis Company, with permission.)

Table 14.10	Heart Sounds		
Heart Sound	**Location**	**Physiology**	**Description**
First: S_1	Mitral and tricuspid areas while sitting.	• Beginning of systole.	• *lub:* Dull, low-pitched sound.
Second: S_2	Aortic and pulmonic areas while sitting.	• Closure of valves between the ventricles and the arteries exiting the heart (semilunar valves).	• *dub:* Higher in pitch and shorter in length than S_1.
Third: S_3	Apical site with client in left-lateral position.	• Early in diastole. • Immediately after S_2. • Produced by rapid ventricular filling.	• *ee:* Gallop tempo when combined S_1 and S_2: lub-dub-ee. • Disappears when client is sitting. • Failure to disappear when sitting indicates hypervolemia or heart failure.
Fourth: S_4	Apical site with client in left-lateral position.	• Late in diastole. • Immediately before S_1. • Produced by rapid ventricular filling.	• Presystolic gallop that has a rhythm like the word *FLOrida*. • Heard in some athletes and older adults. • Associated with hypertension, coronary artery disease, and pulmonic stenosis.

(2) Reflect functioning of the right side of the heart and circulating fluid volume.

(3) Place the client in the semi-Fowler (45° angle) position and then inspect for distention of the veins.

(a) No neck vein distention expected.

(b) Distended veins suggest a condition such as hypervolemia, right-sided heart failure, and tricuspid stenosis.

7. Assess peripheral circulation (Table 14.11).

8. Auscultate the abdomen for vascular sounds.

a. Listen over major blood vessels in the abdomen (Fig. 14.10).

b. Listen for the presence of a whooshing sound due to turbulent blood flow; associated with narrowing of the lumen (*stenosis*) or dilation of a lumen (*aneurysm*). Immediately notify the primary health-care provider if you identify this whooshing sound because it indicates a life-threatening situation.

C. Male genitourinary and reproductive systems

See Chapter 22, Urinary Elimination, for a thorough review of the anatomy and physiology of the urinary system, factors affecting urinary function, characteristics of normal and abnormal urine, and nursing assessments related to urinary status.

1. The male genitourinary system includes the structures of the urinary system and the reproductive system. The reproductive system has both internal and external structures (Fig. 14.11).

Fig 14.10 Auscultation of abdomen for vascular sounds. (From Wilkinson and Treas [2016]. *Fundamentals of nursing*, Vol. 2, 3rd ed. Philadelphia: F. A. Davis Company, with permission.).

2. Inspect and palpate external genital structures while wearing gloves and with the client standing, followed by the supine position.

a. Pubic hair: Assess distribution, amount, and characteristics.

(1) Normal findings: Triangular distribution of thick hair above the penis, spreading up toward the abdomen and possibly extending onto the thighs.

(2) Deviations: Thin texture; sparse or absent hair; presence of parasites.

b. Penis: Assess the shaft, glans, and urethral meatus.

(1) Normal findings: Color similar to client's skin; skin intact, slightly wrinkled. Absence

---

Table 14.11 Peripheral Neurovascular Assessments

Assessment	Expected Response	Deviations in Circulation
Volume of arterial pulses	• *Strong.* • *Obliterated with moderate pressure.*	• *Weak, thready, or absent.* • *Bounding (see Table 14.5).*
Capillary refill	• *Blanching on compression of nail bed or tip of toe.* • *Return of usual skin color in ≤3 seconds (up to 5 seconds in an older adult) when compression is released, as capillaries refill with blood.*	• *Return to original color in >3 seconds (5 seconds in older adults).*
Color and texture of nails	• *Variation of pink.* • *Translucid.*	• *Yellow, thick, and brittle.*
Color, texture, and temperature of skin	• *Similar in color to skin on rest of body.* • *Smooth and supple texture.* • *Warmth to touch.*	• *Arterial: Color pale, mottled, or dependent rubor; texture rough and dry; temperature cool to touch; ulcers of toes or heels.* • *Venous: Brownish discoloration due to breakdown of hemoglobin and deposition of ferrous sulfate; distended, tortuous, and palpable veins; edema; venous stasis ulcers around ankles and calves.*
Sensation	• *Ability to distinguish dull and sharp stimuli (e.g., cotton ball versus pointed object).*	• *Diminished or absent ability to distinguish dull and sharp stimuli.*
Mobility	• *Ability to move joints through full range of motion.*	• *Limited ability to move joints through full range of motion.*

Symphysis pubis

Ductus deferens

Urinary bladder

Corpus cavernosum

Corpus spongiosum

Cavernous urethra

Glans penis

Prepuce

Scrotum

Testis

Epididymis

Membranous urethra

Anus

Bulbourethral gland

Prostate gland

Ejaculatory duct

Seminal vesicle

Rectum

Opening of ureter

Sacrum

Fig 14.11 Male genitourinary and reproductive systems. (From Scanlon [2015]. *Essentials of anatomy and physiology*, 7th ed., Fig. 20-3, p. 503. Philadelphia: F. A. Davis Company, with permission.).

of foreskin if circumcised and presence of foreskin if uncircumcised; ability to retract foreskin, revealing small amount of thick white material *(smegma)*. Smooth and semifirm shaft. Absence of discharge from urethral meatus at tip of glans if gently compressed.

(2) Deviations: Presence of lesions, nodules, pimples, warts, rash, ulceration, or thickening; tenderness; inability to retract foreskin *(phimosis)*; urethral meatus on underside of shaft *(hypospadias)* or upper side of shaft *(epispadias)*; white, green, or yellow discharge from urethral meatus, possibly indicating a sexually transmitted infection (if present, obtain specimen for examination).

c. Scrotum: Assess condition, size, position, and symmetry.

(1) Normal findings: Intact skin, numerous wrinkles *(rugae)*, and darker in color than client's skin. Size and shape varies but in proportion to penis; smooth, rubbery, and free of nodules; symmetrical but left scrotal sac usually lower than the right.

(2) Deviations: Discolorations; tightening of skin with few rugae, possibly indicating edema, fluid, infection, torsion, or a mass; small, hard lump; rash caused by fungal infection *(tinea cruris)*.

d. Inguinal area: Assess the inguinal canal while the client bears down or coughs.

(1) Normal findings: Area free from bulges and swelling.

(2) Deviations: Bulge, possibly indicating an enlarged lymph node or a hernia if felt while client bears down.

e. Anus: Assess the anus and perianal skin for color, intactness, and presence of lesions.

(1) Normal findings: Color slightly darker than color of buttocks. Intact skin that is coarser and moister than perianal skin. Absence of

lesions. Puckering of anus when touched with gloved finger (*anal reflex*).

(2) Deviations: Fissures, lesions, warts, hemorrhoids, bleeding, rectal prolapse, or lack of anal tone.

D. Female genitourinary and reproductive systems
See Chapter 22, Urinary Elimination, for a thorough review of the anatomy and physiology of the female urinary system, factors affecting urinary function, characteristics of normal and abnormal urine, and nursing assessments related to urinary status.

1. The female genitourinary system includes the structures of the urinary system and the reproductive system. The reproductive system has both internal and external structures (Fig. 14.12).

2. Inspect and palpate the external genital structures while wearing gloves and with the client in the lithotomy position (Fig. 14.13).

   a. Pubic hair: Assess distribution, amount, and characteristics.
      (1) Normal findings: Triangular shaped, course, full, symmetrical over pad of fatty tissue over symphysis pubis (*mons pubis*); may extend toward inner thighs.
      (2) Deviations: Sparse, asymmetrical, or excessive; presence of parasites.

   b. Labia (consist of external folds [*labia majora*] and internal folds [*labia minora*]). Assess color, condition of skin, symmetry, and presence of discharge.
      (1) Normal findings: Color similar to client's skin; intact skin; symmetrical; no discharge.
      (2) Deviations: Presence of erythema, ecchymosis, swelling, rash, lesions, firm mass, and warts; asymmetrical; and presence of discharge.

   c. Clitoris: Inspect for size and position.
      (1) Normal findings: 2 cm long and 0.5 cm wide; no redness, swelling, or lesions.
      (2) Deviations: Enlargement may be due to excess androgen; swelling may be due to trauma or inflammation; absence may be due to female circumcision (ritual associated with some African countries and some Muslim groups).

   d. Urethral meatus: Assess color, shape, size, and position.
      (1) Normal findings: Slit-like opening midline below clitoris and above vagina; pink; moist.
      (2) Deviations: Displacement of urethral meatus; erythema; swelling; lesions; presence of discharge.

   e. Vaginal introitus: Assess color, shape, and size.
      (1) Normal findings: Pink; moist with clear to white odorless discharge; patent with no bulging or tenderness when the client bears down.
      (2) Deviations: Pale and dry, possibly caused by aging or topical steroids; any color discharge with a foul odor, possibly indicating a sexually transmitted infection; fissures, swelling, and ecchymosis, possibly

Fig 14.12 Female genitourinary and reproductive systems. (From Scanlon [2015]. *Essentials of anatomy and physiology*, 7th ed. Philadelphia: F. A. Davis Company, with permission.)

Fig 14.13 Female external genitalia. (From Scanlon [2015]. *Essentials of anatomy and physiology,* 7th ed. Philadelphia: F. A. Davis Company, with permission.)

indicating trauma or abuse; bulging of anterior vaginal wall *(cystocele)*; bulging of posterior vaginal wall *(rectocele)*.

    f. Anus: Same as for male genitourinary system.

3. Inspection and palpation of internal structures such as cervix, vaginal wall, uterus and ovaries should be performed only by an experienced practitioner.

E. Assessment of the breasts

1. The breasts of both males and females consist of glandular, fibrous, and adipose tissue. Glandular and lymphatic tissue in women is concentrated in the upper outer quadrant and extends into the axilla *(tail of Spence)* (Fig. 14.14).

2. Individuals who perform breast self-examination should do so monthly: premenopausal—several days after menstruation; postmenopausal—same date each month.

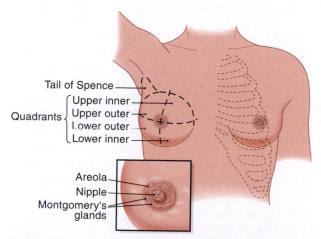

Fig 14.14 Female breast. External breast structures and quadrants. (From Dillon [2016]. *Nursing health assessment: The foundation of clinical practice,* 3rd ed. F. A. Davis Company, with permission.)

3. Assess the breasts via inspection for size, shape, symmetry, color, and condition of skin.

    a. View breasts with the client standing or sitting with arms at the sides, followed by pressing hands down on hips, pressing palms of hands together with elbows flexed, holding arms over head, and leaning forward.

        (1) Normal findings: Size and shape vary depending on individual; symmetrical, but one breast may be slightly larger than the other; skin color lighter than exposed skin surfaces; smooth skin texture; male breast even with chest wall.

        (2) Deviations: Swelling, edema, and erythema, possibly indicating infection; asymmetry, puckering, lesions, and dimpled skin texture *(peau d'orange),* possibly indicating cancer; enlargement of breasts in males *(gynecomastia),* possibly due to obesity, hormone imbalances, cancer, or estrogen therapy.

    b. Assess nipples and areolae for size, shape, position, direction, symmetry, discharge, and masses.

        (1) Normal findings: Symmetrical size, shape, position, and direction; darker color than breast tissue; nipples may be flat, point outward (eversion), or point inward (inversion) since puberty; no discharge or masses.

        (2) Deviations: Asymmetrical size, shape, position, direction, and color; recent inversion or eversion of one or both nipples; discharge unrelated to pregnancy or lactation; presence of a mass; more than two nipples *(supernumerary nipples).*

    c. Assess axillae for hair distribution, skin condition, and masses.

        (1) Normal findings: Hair growth begins at puberty and may decrease in older adults; intact skin with no masses.

        (2) Deviations: Rashes, redness, or unusual pigmentation, possibly related to infection or allergy to deodorants.

4. Palpate the breasts.

    a. Place the client in the supine position with a wedge under the shoulder on the same side as the breast being palpated; abduct the client's arm with the hand behind the head.

    b. Hold three fingers together and make a rotary motion with the finger pads while gently pressing down on the breast; ensure inclusion of the tail of Spence. Use a systematic method to palpate the breast, such as the vertical strip method (Fig. 14.15A, preferred method), pie wedge method (Fig. 14.15B), or concentric circles method (Fig. 14.15C). Palpate the nipple and areola for masses and gently squeeze the nipple to determine the presence of a discharge.

(1) Normal findings: Soft, nontender breast; elastic, nontender nipples; no masses or discharge from nipples.

(2) Deviations: Thickening, lump, or mass; loss of elasticity or discharge from nipple; tenderness. If you identify a mass, collect the following additional information.

   (a) Location: Distance from the nipple and distance from the tail of Spence; use a clock position to identify the location of the deviation around the nipple.

   (b) Size: Approximate width, length, and thickness in centimeters.

   (c) Shape: Regular, irregular, round, or oval.

   (d) Consistency: Hard or soft.

   (e) Mobility: Mobile or fixed.

Fig. 14.15A Patterns for breast palpation. Vertical strip method. (From Dillon [2016]. *Nursing health assessment: The foundation of clinical practice*, 3rd ed., F. A. Davis Company, with permission.).

Fig 14.15B Patterns for breast palpation. Pie wedge method. (From Dillon [2016]. *Nursing health assessment: The foundation of clinical practice*, 3rd ed. F. A. Davis Company, with permission.)

Fig 14.15C Patterns for breast palpation. Concentric circles method. (From Dillon [2016]. *Nursing health assessment: The foundation of clinical practice*, 3rd ed. F. A. Davis Company, with permission.)

   (f) Nipple: Normal or displaced, retracted; color of discharge (e.g., bloody, serous, purulent, and gray).

   (g) Tenderness: Level of discomfort when palpated.

5. Palpate the axillae.

  a. Place the client in the sitting position while abducting the arm on the side the breast is being assessed; support the client's arm on your forearm.

  b. Use flattened fingertips of four fingers to palpate all lymph nodes around the breast, above the clavicle, tail of Spence, and upper part of the arm (see Fig. 14.14).

   (1) Normal findings: Nonpalpable nodes; nontender.

   (2) Deviations: Enlarged, tender nodes, usually indicating infection; enlarged nontender nodes, usually malignancy.

DID YOU KNOW?

Research has not demonstrated a clear benefit of routine clinical breast exams by health-care professionals or monthly breast self-examination by women. Therefore, the American Cancer Society no longer advocates these routine assessments. However, women are advised to be familiar with how their breasts look and feel. The society believes that the most effective way to detect cancer of the breast early is through mammography. They make the following recommendations regarding mammograms for women with average risk of breast cancer: yearly between the ages of 40 and 44 in conjunction with medical advice, yearly 45 to 54 years, and every 2 years after 55 years of age if the woman is in good health.

F. Assessment of the eyes

1. Assess acuity of near vision and far vision, and boundaries of peripheral vision (see Cranial Nerve II in Table 14.9 in this chapter).

2. Assess fields of gaze, accommodation, and pupillary reaction to light (see Cranial Nerves III, IV, and VI in Table 14.9 in this chapter).

3. Assess color perception: Have the client identify the color bars on the Snellen Eye Chart or distinguish colors using Ishihara cards.

  a. Normal findings: Color perception is intact.

  b. Deviations: Inability to distinguish colors; be aware that some older adults have difficulty distinguishing pastels and purples.

4. Assess external structures via inspection (Fig. 14.16).

  a. Eyes for size, alignment, and protrusion.

   (1) Normal findings: Symmetrical size; clear and bright; parallel alignment; no protrusion beyond frontal bone.

Labels on figure:
Eyebrow
Iris
Pupil
Lateral canthus
Lower eyelid
Upper eyelid
Eyelash
Caruncle
Lacrimal punctum
Medial canthus
Sclera covered by bulbar conjunctiva
Palpebral conjunctiva covers lids

Fig 14.16 External structures of the eye. (From Wilkinson and Treas [2016]. *Fundamentals of nursing,* Vol. 1, 3rd ed. Philadelphia: F. A. Davis Company, with permission.)

(2) Deviations: Unequal size and alignment; glazed eyes, possibly indicating excessive tearing or fever; sunken appearance related to dehydration or a decrease in periorbital fat associated with older adults; eyes protruding out of the orbit *(exophthalmos)* is associated with hyperthyroidism; visible sclera between iris and upper lids *(sunset eyes)* is associated with hydrocephalus.

b. Eyelids for shape, position, and movement and distribution of eyelashes.
   (1) Normal findings: Symmetrical opening between margins of upper and lower lids; no lid lag; ability to open and close lids; even distribution of eyelashes.
   (2) Deviations: Asymmetry of lids; drooping lid *(ptosis)* due to malfunction of cranial nerve III; ptosis of one lid may indicate brain attack and ptosis of both lids may indicate myasthenia gravis; absence of eyelashes, possibly reflecting alopecia.

c. Conjunctivae for color, moisture, and lesions.
   (1) Normal findings: Clear; pink; moist; smooth; no lesions.
   (2) Deviations: Redness, swelling, drainage, and tenderness, possibly indicating infection *(conjunctivitis)*; pale pink color, possibly indicating anemia.

d. Sclerae for color, moisture, and lesions.
   (1) Normal findings: White; glistening; smooth with no lesions. Dark-skinned clients may have sclera with a yellowish cast in the periphery.

(2) Deviations: Redness ("bloodshot" appearance), indicating inflammation of the sclera; yellow, indicating jaundice *(icterus)*.

e. Iris for color, shape, and symmetry.
   (1) Normal findings: Uniform color (e.g., blue, brown, green, or a combination of these colors); round and symmetrical.
   (2) Deviations: Pigment deterioration in older adults; partial or total absence of iris, a congenital anomaly.

f. Cornea (colorless portion of eye covering the pupil and iris) and lens for clarity, texture, and moisture. Shine a light at an angle to the eye while the client looks straight ahead.
   (1) Normal findings: Clear, smooth, and glistening cornea and lens.
   (2) Deviations: Rough or irregular appearance to surface of cornea, which may indicate corneal abrasion or ulcer; cloudy lens appearance, which may indicate a cataract.

5. Assess internal structures via inspection with an ophthalmoscope. Note that this is an advanced assessment technique that should be conducted in a darkened room.
   a. Assess for red light reflex: Have the client look straight ahead, stand about 1 foot from the client at a 15° angle, and shine a light on one pupil while looking through an ophthalmoscope.
      (1) Normal findings: Positive red reflex caused by light illuminating the retina (red eyes sometimes seen in photographs when the flash of a camera illuminates the retina).
      (2) Deviations: Opacity of the lens; hemorrhage into vitreous humor.
   b. Assessment of other internal structures (e.g., retina, choroid, optic nerve disc, macula, fovea centralis, and retinal vessels) is not conducted by most nurses. These structures can be assessed by advanced practice nurses.

G. Assessment of the ears
1. Assess hearing acuity, sound conduction (Weber test, Rinne test), and balance (Romberg test). (See Cranial Nerve VIII in Table 14.9 in this chapter.
2. Assess the external ear.
   a. Auricle: Assess size, shape, position, angle of attachment, and symmetry.
      (1) Normal findings: 4 to 10 cm in length; all structures present (e.g., helix, antihelix, antitragus, tragus, and lobule) (Fig. 14.17); top of ears level with eyes; ears vertical with 10° posterior tilt and symmetrical.

Fig 14.17 External structures of the ear. (From Wilkinson and Treas [2016]. *Fundamentals of nursing,* Vol. 2, 3rd ed. Philadelphia: F. A. Davis Company, with permission.)

MAKING THE CONNECTION

Auditory Stimuli and Interpretation of Sound

An auditory stimulus (sound) occurs. The external ear, consisting of the auricle and external auditory canal, collects and transmits the sound to the middle ear. The middle ear consists of the tympanic membrane, connection between middle ear and nasopharynx (eustachian tube), and three auditory bones (malleus, incus, and stapes). The tympanic membrane transmits the sound to the three auditory bones, and they in turn transmit the sound to the inner ear (labyrinth). The labyrinth consists of the vestibule and semicircular canals (both of which are concerned with balance) and the cochlea (which is concerned with hearing). The organ of Corti within the cochlea has specialized microvilli that contain endings of the cochlear branch of cranial nerve VIII that transmits the sound impulses to the temporal lobes of the cerebral cortex of the brain, where the sound is interpreted (Fig. 14.18).

(2) Deviations: Size <3 cm or >10 cm, absent external structures, low-set ears, exaggerated posterior tilt, asymmetrical ears.

b. External auditory canal: Use an otoscope to visualize the walls of the canal and tympanic membrane. Pull the helix up and back to straighten the canal of an adult, and pull the lobule down and back to straighten the canal of a child younger than age 3 years.

(1) Normal findings: Walls of canal light in color, patent, with a small amount of earwax *(cerumen)*; no drainage. Tympanic membrane pearly gray, shiny, semitransparent, and mobile.

(2) Deviations: Excessive and/or dry cerumen, possibly obscuring the tympanic membrane; redness of walls, possibly indicating infection; bloody drainage, indicating trauma; purulent drainage, indicating infection; clear drainage, possibly indicating spinal fluid from a head injury; tympanic membrane that is pink, red, yellow, amber, white, or blue; is dull or somewhat opaque; has limited mobility; and appears bulging or retracted.

H. Assessment of the integumentary system

For a review of assessment of the integumentary system including the skin, mucous membranes, teeth, hair and nails, and factors influencing tissue integrity see Chapter 18, "Tissue Integrity, Hygiene, and Wound Care."

I. Assessment of the respiratory system

For a review of assessment of the respiratory system, including structures and functions of the respiratory system, factors that influence respirations, and the techniques of inspection (including breathing patterns), auscultation

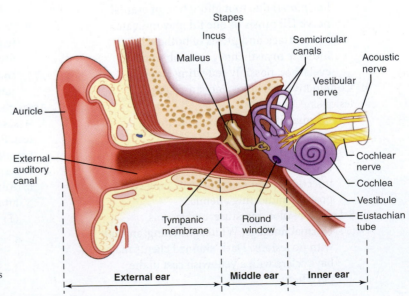

Fig 14.18 Cross section of the ear. (From Wilkinson and Treas [2016]. *Fundamentals of nursing,* Vol. 1, 3rd ed. Philadelphia: F. A. Davis Company, with permission.)

(including normal and abnormal breath sounds), percussion, and palpation, see Chapter 19, "Oxygenation."

J. Assessment of the gastrointestinal (GI) system
For a review of assessment of the GI system, including factors affecting bowel elimination, characteristics of stool, and common human responses associated with the GI system (e.g., diarrhea, constipation, fecal incontinence, hemorrhoids, and flatulence), see Chapter 23, "Bowel Elimination." For a nutritional assessment, including a health history, dietary history, factors that influence nutrition, and physical assessments focusing on nutritional status, see Chapter 20, "Nutrition."

K. Assessment of the musculoskeletal system
For a review of assessments of the musculoskeletal system, including anatomy and physiology of movement, balance, body alignment, coordination, gait, and range of motion of all joints of the body, see Chapter 17, Mobility.

L. Assessment of the urinary system
For a review of the urinary system, including structures and functions; factors affecting urinary function; assessments; diagnostic tests; urinary elimination problems, catheters, and diversions; and bladder irrigations see Chapter 22, "Urinary Elimination."

CASE STUDY: Putting It All Together

An older adult with a history of peripheral arterial disease and osteoarthritis is admitted to a hospital with a diagnosis of pneumonia. The nurse obtains the client's vital signs and performs a physical assessment, including the client's lungs, eyes, and ears. Some of the results of these assessments are as follows: temperature—102.4°F; apical pulse—96 beats/minute and regular; radial pulse—94 beats/minute and regular; respirations—26 breaths/minute, shallow, and use of accessory muscles of respiration; BP—146/88 mm Hg; oxygen saturation—88%; breath sounds—crackles in both lungs; eyes—glazed, limited red eye reflex; ears—difficulty hearing, excessive cerumen in both ears; abdomen—distended, hypoactive bowel sounds, tympany. The client reports feeling short of breath and having tingling in the feet.

Case Study Questions

A. What instruments did the nurse use to perform these assessments and what was the nurse assessing by using the instruments?

1. _____

2. _____

3. _____

4. _____

5. _____

6. _____

B. What techniques of physical assessment did the nurse use and what was the nurse assessing by using the techniques?

1. _____

2. _____

3. _____

4. _____

continued.

CASE STUDY: Putting It All Together   *cont'd*

Case Study Questions

C. The client has a history of peripheral arterial disease and reports feeling tingling in the feet. Describe the focused assessment the nurse should perform to collect additional information.

1. _____

2. _____

3. _____

4. _____

5. _____

6. _____

D. What is the priority commonality of assessment when auscultating a client's heart sounds, lung sounds, and bowel sounds and explain your answer?

1. _____

REVIEW QUESTIONS

Be sure to read the Introduction for valuable test-taking tips.

1. A nurse is obtaining a client's radial pulse and identifies that its rhythm is irregular. What should the nurse do **next**?
   1. Notify the client's primary health-care provider.
   2. Obtain the client's blood pressure.
   3. Take the pulse in the other arm.
   4. Assess the apical pulse.

2. Which client should the nurse perform a focused assessment on **first**?
   1. A client with obstructive pulmonary disease who is using pursed-lip breathing
   2. A client returning from a walk down the hall who is exhibiting nasal flaring
   3. A client with dyspnea who abruptly assumes the orthopneic position
   4. A client with asthma who is wheezing

3. A nurse is taking a client's temperature using the thermometer in the photograph. Which action is important when using this thermometer?

   1. Clean the probe before and after use.
   2. Use a new probe cover for each client.
   3. Slide the probe medially to laterally across the forehead to the temple.
   4. Pull the pinna of the ear upward when inserting the probe into the ear of an infant.

4. A nurse identifies that a client with cancer of the pancreas has an abdomen that is distended. What assessment should the nurse perform **next**?
   1. Weigh the client.
   2. Obtain the vital signs.
   3. Measure the girth of the abdomen.
   4. Inspect the characteristics of the next stool.

5. A client who is at high risk for breast cancer and who chooses to implement monthly self-breast examinations asks the nurse how to do a self-breast examination. Which techniques should the nurse teach the client to use when performing this examination? **Select all that apply.**
   1. Use the finger pads to palpate breast tissue.
   2. Assess the nipples before palpating the breasts.
   3. Palpate the breasts while in the supine position.
   4. Follow only a circular sequence of palpation of a breast from the nipples outward.
   5. Place a small pillow under the shoulder on the same side as the breast being palpated.

6. A nurse analyzes data collected about a client, including temperature, 101°F; apical pulse, 104 beats/minute; radial pulse, 72 beats/minute; respirations, 22 breaths/minute; pulse oximetry, 95%; and blood pressure, 138/72 mm Hg. What is the client's pulse deficit? **Record your answer using a whole number.**
   Answer: _____

7. Which client assessments documented by the nurse in the client's clinical record indicate a period of remission? **Select all that apply.**
   1. "Client continues to experience dull pain in the joints from osteoarthritis."
   2. "Client's response indicates a variation from the response that one would expect."
   3. "Client's readmission to the hospital was due to a return of signs and symptoms of leukemia."
   4. "Client's signs and symptoms of cancer have lessened in intensity since the last assessment a month ago."
   5. "Client continues to experience freedom from pain in the left foot after receiving a cortisone injection for plantar fasciitis."

8. A nurse is taking a tympanic temperature of an adult client who is in a right lateral position. Place the following steps in the order in which they should be implemented.
   1. Return the tympanic unit to its storage unit for recharging.
   2. Attach a disposable probe cover to the tympanic temperature unit.
   3. Use the left hand and gently pull the pinna of the right ear upward and backward.
   4. Remove the unit from the client's ear and discard the probe cover without contaminating the environment.
   5. Press the probe gently into the client's ear canal and hold the temperature button until a green light flashes and a temperature is displayed.
   Answer: _____

9. A nurse is caring for a client in the postanesthesia care unit who had surgery for a coronary artery bypass graft. The client has an intravenous catheter in the right forearm, a urinary retention catheter, and a nasogastric tube in place to low intermittent suction. Where should the nurse place the oxygen saturation sensor?
   1. Right nostril
   2. Left ear lobe
   3. Right great toe
   4. Left index finger

10. A nurse performs the following techniques when assessing a client. Which assessments use the technique of percussion? **Select all that apply.**
    1. Pressing down on the symphysis pubis to determine the presence of urinary retention
    2. Tapping on the abdomen to help identify the density of underlying structures
    3. Placing a stethoscope on the abdomen to assess the extent of bowel sounds
    4. Using a rubber-tipped hammer to elicit a deep tendon reflex
    5. Touching the skin over an artery to obtain a pulse rate

11. A nurse is caring for an older adult who was just transferred to the unit after being in the intensive care unit for the last 72 hours. The nurse is concerned about the client experiencing sensory overload. For which clinical manifestations of sensory overload should the nurse assess the client? **Select all that apply.**
    1. Pain
    2. Fatigue
    3. Confusion
    4. Restlessness
    5. Scattered attention
    6. Hearing impairment

12. When assessing a client's radial pulse, a nurse is unable to feel pulsations. What should the nurse do **first**?
    1. Release the pressure of the fingers slightly while compressing the artery.
    2. Apply more pressure when palpating the artery.
    3. Use a Doppler to assess the artery.
    4. Assess an artery in the other arm.

13. A nurse is completing an assessment of several newly admitted clients to a nursing home. For which clients should the nurse assess clinical indicators of sensory deprivation? **Select all that apply.**
    1. The client who was recently cared for in an intensive care unit
    2. The client who recently sustained an injury causing blindness
    3. The client who is experiencing quadriplegia
    4. The client who has a history of depression
    5. The client who is experiencing acute pain

14. A nurse is assessing a client's ability to focus on a cognitive skill. What questions are appropriate for the nurse to ask the client in relation to this assessment? **Select all that apply.**
    1. "What day of the week is it?"
    2. "What are you feeling right now?"
    3. "What did you have for lunch today?"
    4. "What is the result when you multiply 2 times 2?"
    5. "What city did you live in when you were 20 years old?"

15. A nurse is assessing a client's oculomotor nerve, cranial nerve III. How should the nurse assess the functioning of this nerve? **Select all that apply.**
    1. Instruct the client to smile.
    2. Inspect the location of the eyelids.
    3. Shine a light onto the client's pupil.
    4. Ask the client to raise the shoulders against resistance.
    5. Place a padded tongue blade gently against the client's posterior oropharynx.

16. A nurse analyzes data collected about a client, including temperature, 98.6°F; apical pulse, 90 beats/minute; radial pulse, 60 beats/minute; respirations, 24 breaths/minute; pulse oximetry, 98%; and blood pressure, 110/60 mm Hg. What is the client's pulse pressure? **Record your answer using a whole number.**
    Answer: _____

17. A nurse is collecting a past medical history of a newly admitted client with chest pain. Which information should the nurse include in this assessment? **Select all that apply.**
    1. Allergies
    2. Vital signs
    3. Prior surgeries
    4. Immunizations
    5. Childhood illnesses
    6. Present signs and symptoms

18. A nurse is assessing a female client's external genitalia. Which finding should be reported to the primary health-care provider?
    1. The vaginal introitus has a discharge that is clear and odorless.
    2. The pubic hair extends to the upper inner thighs.
    3. The urethra is midline below the clitoris.
    4. The clitoris is 4 cm long and 2 cm wide.

19. Which peripheral pulse sites are commonly accessed when performing cardiopulmonary resuscitation for infants and children? **Select all that apply.**
    1. Carotid
    2. Femoral
    3. Brachial
    4. Dorsalis pedis
    5. Posterior tibial

20. At which site should the nurse position a stethoscope when assessing the apical pulse rate for an adult?

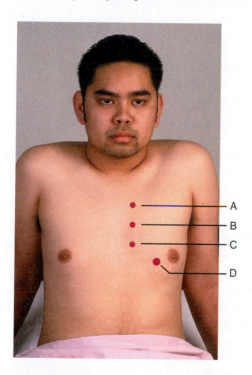

    1. A
    2. B
    3. C
    4. D

21. A nurse is obtaining a client's blood pressure. What is reflected by the diastolic blood pressure?
    1. Contraction of the left ventricle
    2. Volume of cardiac output
    3. Resting arterial pressure
    4. Pulse pressure

22. A primary health-care provider asks the nurse for a report on the quality of a client's pulse. Which information collected by the nurse will answer this question posed by the primary health-care provider?
    1. The pulse rate is 65 beats/minute.
    2. The pulse volume is full and bounding.
    3. The pulse rate is slower than the heart rate.
    4. The pulse has 2 beats that repeatedly occur close together.

23. A parent brings a 4-year-old child to the urgent care center stating, "I think she has a bad cold." The nurse takes the child's vital signs, performs an inspection, and interviews the parent. What assessment should the nurse perform **next**?
    1. Auscultate the lungs.
    2. Palpate the abdomen.
    3. Obtain the apical heart rate.
    4. Ask the child where it hurts.

Client's Clinical Record

Vital Signs

Temperature: 100.4°F, temporal scanner
Pulse: 94 beats/minute, regular rhythm, radial
Respirations: 30 breaths/minute

Inspection

Facial flushing, slight supraclavicular and intercostal retractions, nonproductive cough, restless, sitting in the tripod position on bed. Abdomen appears soft, no signs of guarding noted.

Parental Interview

Mother states, "She started coughing about 2 days ago, but the cough is getting worse. She is not bringing up phlegm, but she keeps coughing. I kept her home from school thinking that it was just a cold and she would get better, but she has gotten worse. She doesn't want to drink and her urine is very dark. When her face got so red, I got scared and brought her here."

---

24. Which site should the nurse use when monitoring the heart rate prior to administering a cardiac medication?
    1. Brachial
    2. Carotid
    3. Apical
    4. Radial

25. A client is experiencing the onset of a fever. Which nursing actions are appropriate during this phase? **Select all that apply.**
    1. Ensuring that there are no environmental drafts
    2. Applying cloth covered ice packs to the groin
    3. Using tepid water for a sponge bath
    4. Covering the client with a blanket
    5. Lowering the heat in the room
    6. Ensuring that bed linen is dry

26. A primary health-care provider prescribes a dose of a medication for a child at 2 mg/kg of body weight. The child weighs 64 pounds. Before determining the prescribed dose, the nurse must convert the child's weight from pounds to kilograms. How many kilograms does this child weigh? **Record your answer using a whole number.**
    Answer: _____ kilograms

27. A nurse is assisting several male clients with physical hygiene. While performing perineal hygiene the nurse assesses the external genitalia. Which assessments should be reported to a primary health-care provider? **Select all that apply.**
    1. The scrotum appears taut with few rugae.
    2. The urethral meatus has a white discharge.
    3. The foreskin can be retracted back from the glans.
    4. The scrotum is darker than the rest of the client's skin.
    5. The anus constricts when touched with a gloved finger.

28. A nurse is caring for a variety of clients. Place the clients in the order in which they should be attended to by the nurse. Begin first with the client who has the highest priority and progress to the client who has the lowest priority.
    1. A client who just returned from the operating room with a temperature of 100°F
    2. A client who returned from rigorous physical therapy who has a temperature of 99°F
    3. A client who had surgery three days ago and has developed a temperature of 100.2°F
    4. A client who received two intravenous antibiotic doses in the last 24 hours for a urinary tract infection and has a temperature of 100.6°F
    5. A client who was admitted to the hospital after receiving multiple bruises as a result of an automobile collision and has a temperature of 100.4°F
    Answer: _____

29. A nurse is performing a complete physical assessment of a 16-year-old child. What is an important approach to use with the client?
    1. Pull the curtain so that the parents are beyond the curtain during the examination.
    2. Limit questions from the adolescent to after the examination is completed.
    3. Allow the adolescent to keep underpants on during the examination.
    4. Have the parents remain outside the room during the examination.

30. A nurse is caring for an infant who has a core body temperature of 104.8°F. The infant has a prescription for acetaminophen 10 mg/kg PO every 6 hours prn for a temperature more than 102°F. Place the following nursing interventions in priority order from highest priority to lowest priority.
    1. Obtain all vital signs.
    2. Institute seizure precautions.
    3. Remove the blanket that is covering the infant.
    4. Administer acetaminophen as per the prescription.
    5. Inform the primary health-care provider of the infant's status.
    Answer: _____

31. A nurse is caring for a client who is presenting with diarrhea, abdominal cramps, diaphoresis, shortness of breath, and severe anxiety. Which thermometer should the nurse use to obtain this client's temperature?
    1. Tympanic thermometer
    2. Paper strip thermometer
    3. Plastic rectal thermometer
    4. Electronic oral thermometer

32. A nurse obtains a client's temperature using an oral thermometer indicated in the illustration. What is the client's temperature? **Record your answer using one decimal place.**
    Answer: _____ °F

33. A nurse assesses that an adult client's skin feels warm to touch. The nurse obtains a tympanic temperature of 97.2°F via the client's right ear. What should the nurse do?
    1. Take the client's temperature in the other ear while pulling the pinna upward and back.
    2. Retake the client's temperature in the same ear while pulling the pinna upward and back.
    3. Take the client's temperature in the other ear while pulling the pinna downward and back.
    4. Retake the client's temperature in the same ear while pulling the pinna downward and back.

34. A nurse in the emergency department is obtaining the temperatures of several clients using a temporal scanner thermometer. Which clients should the nurse identify as requiring an alternate route for the assessment of body temperature? **Select all that apply.**
    1. Client who is diaphoretic
    2. Client who is a mouth breather
    3. Client who is wearing a ski hat
    4. Client who is exhibiting male pattern baldness
    5. Client who is sleeping in the side-lying position with the head on a pillow

35. A nurse is assessing a client with a history of liver disease. Which part of the eye should the nurse assess for jaundice?

1. A
2. B
3. C
4. D

REVIEW ANSWERS AND RATIONALES

1. ANSWER: 4.

Rationales:

1. This is premature. The nurse should obtain additional data about the client's status.

2. Although obtaining the blood pressure may eventually be done, it is premature at this time.

3. Although assessing the radial pulse in the other arm may eventually be done, it is premature at this time.

4. The nurse should first assess the apical pulse and rhythm and then determine the pulse deficit. These assessments provide valuable information about the rate and rhythm of the client's apical and radial pulse rates.

TEST-TAKING TIP: Identify the word in the stem that sets a priority. The word *next* in the stem sets a priority. Identify options that contain a clang association. The word *pulse* in the stem and in options 3 and 4 are clang associations. Consider options 3 and 4 carefully.

Content Area: Physical Assessment
Integrated Processes: Nursing Process: Assessment
Client Need: Physiological Integrity; Reduction of Risk Potential
Cognitive Level: Application
Concept: Perfusion

2. ANSWER: 3.

Rationales:

1. Although this client should be assessed frequently, pursed-lip breathing is a technique that may be used constantly by clients with obstructive pulmonary disease. Pursed-lip breathing prolongs exhalation, preventing collapse of alveoli and small bronchial passages, which promotes gas exchange.

2. Although additional assessments may be performed to assess this client's response to physical exertion, this client is not the priority from among the client situations presented. Nasal flaring commonly is associated with physical effort because it reduces the friction of air entering and exiting the body.

3. A client who has difficulty breathing and assumes an upright leaning forward position is attempting to expand the thoracic cavity to promote respirations. This client should be assessed first because medical intervention may be necessary to relieve this client's respiratory distress.

4. Although this client should be monitored closely for an escalation of the wheezing, wheezing is associated with asthma because of constricted airways.

TEST-TAKING TIP: Identify the word in the stem that sets a priority. The word *first* in the stem sets a priority.

Content Area: Physical Assessment
Integrated Processes: Nursing Process: Assessment
Client Need: Safe and Effective Care Environment; Management of Care
Cognitive Level: Analysis
Concept: Patient-Centered Care; Oxygenation

3. ANSWER: 2.

Rationales:

1. The probe does not have to be cleaned before and after use unless it is touched by the client or is contaminated by touching something in the environment that is contaminated.

2. The use of a new probe sheath for each client is an infection control practice that prevents the transmission of microorganisms from one client to another. Each used probe sheath is ejected into a trash container or onto a paper towel, which is then discarded into a trash container.

3. This technique is used when using a temporal artery thermometer.

4. The pinna should be pulled upward and backward when using a tympanic thermometer to obtain the temperature of an adult. The pinna should be pulled downward and backward when using a tympanic thermometer to obtain the temperature of a child less than 3 years of age. These actions straighten the ear canal, which allows the probe to access the tympanic membrane.

Content Area: Physical Assessment
Integrated Processes: Nursing Process: Implementation
Client Need: Health Promotion and Maintenance
Cognitive Level: Analysis
Concept: Safety

4. ANSWER: 3.

Rationales:

1. Although this should be done, it is premature to weigh the client at this time.

2. Although this should be done, it is premature to obtain the vital signs at this time.

3. Measuring the abdominal girth with a tape measure around the body at the level of the umbilicus is an objective measurement of the circumference of the abdomen. Repeat assessments can be compared with the first assessment to determine progression of the distention.

4. This is unrealistic. It could take hours or days before the client has a bowel movement. Abdominal distension usually is related to gas in the intestine (flatus) or fluid in the abdominal cavity (ascites). Assessing bowel sounds may provide information related to flatus, and a fluid wave test may provide information related to ascites.

TEST-TAKING TIP: Identify the word in the stem that sets a priority. The word *next* in the stem sets a priority. Identify the clang association. The word *abdomen* in the stem and in option 3 is a clang association.

Content Area: Physical Assessment
Integrated Processes: Nursing Process: Assessment
Client Need: Physiological Integrity; Reduction of Risk Potential
Cognitive Level: Application
Concept: Cellular Regulation

5. ANSWER: 1, 3, 5.

Rationales:

1. Placing the pads of three fingers flat against the breast is the correct technique for palpation of the breast. There are

numerous nerve endings in the pads of the fingers that promote the sense of touch. Research does not demonstrate a clear benefit of physical breast exams done by a primary health-care provide or clients themselves for screening for breast cancer. However, clients should be aware of how their breasts look and feel normally and report any changes to their primary health-care provider. Clients who are at high risk for breast cancer and who choose to implement monthly self-breast examinations should be taught how to correctly implement a self-breast examination.

2. This sequence of assessment is not required.

3. **The client should be in the supine position when performing palpation of the breasts. The supine position allows breast tissue to spread out evenly over the chest wall. This permits lumps or thickening of tissue to become more evident during palpation.**

3. Any systematic method can be used: concentric circles, vertical strip, or pie wedge. The vertical strip method is the preferred method.

5. **Placing a small pillow under the shoulder raises the site that is being palpated accentuating the soft tissue in the area of the breast and the tail of Spence, which is the extension of breast tissue that extends into the axilla.**

TEST-TAKING TIP: Identify the option with a specific determiner. Option 4 contains the word *only*, which is a specific determiner; this option can be eliminated from consideration.

Content Area: Physical Assessment
Integrated Processes: Nursing Process: Assessment
Client Need: Health Promotion and Maintenance
Cognitive Level: Application
Concept: Patient-Centered Care; Cellular Regulation

6. **ANSWER: 32.**

The pulse deficit is calculated by subtracting the radial pulse rate from the apical pulse rate. Therefore, 104 – 72 = 32.
Content Area: Physical Assessment
Integrated Processes: Nursing Process: Analysis
Client Need: Physiological Integrity; Reduction of Risk Potential
Cognitive Level: Application
Concept: Perfusion

7. **ANSWER: 4, 5.**
Rationales:
1. The statement in option 1 indicates the concept of chronicity, not remission; Chronicity (chronic disease) refers to a disease of long duration or demonstrating progressive deterioration over a long period of time.
2. The statement in option 2 indicates the concept of deviation or deviance, not remission. Deviation or deviance refers to a departure from the norm.
3. The statement in option 3 indicates the concept of exacerbation, not remission. Exacerbation refers to a return of symptoms or increase in the severity of symptoms.
4. **A remission occurs when the clinical manifestations of a client's illness diminish or evidence of the disease no longer is demonstrated.**
5. **The statement in option 5 indicates the concept of remission, a period whereby signs and symptoms lessen in severity or abate.**

Content Area: Physical Assessment
Integrated Processes: Communication and Documentation; Nursing Process: Assessment
Client Need: Physiological Integrity; Physiological Adaptation
Cognitive Level: Application
Concept: Cellular Regulation

8. **ANSWER: 2, 3, 5, 4, 1.**
Rationales:
2. A disposable probe cover reduces the spread of microorganisms between clients.
3. Using the right hand to hold the unit when using the left ear and using the left hand to hold the unit when using the right ear helps to attain the best angle for a good seal when the probe is placed in the ear. Pulling the pinna upward and backward for an adult helps to straighten the ear canal and provide better access to the tympanic membrane. This helps to attain an accurate reading.
5. Pressing the probe gently into the client's ear canal facilitates a seal and helps to attain an accurate reading. A flashing green light and the display of a temperature reading indicate that the reading is complete.
4. Once the reading is established the unit is then removed from the client's ear and the probe cover discarded in an appropriate trash receptacle to prevent cross-contamination.
1. The unit should be returned to its base unit for recharging for future use.
Content Area: Physical Assessment
Integrated Processes: Nursing Process: Planning
Client Need: Health Promotion and Maintenance
Cognitive Level: Analysis
Concept: Thermo-regulation

9. **ANSWER: 2.**
Rationales:
1. This placement would be uncomfortable because the client already has a nasogastric tube in place.
2. **The ear lobes have many capillary beds that are appropriate for placement of an oxygen saturation sensor. The ear lobes are not distal appendages that may be affected by a decreased cardiac output.**
3. The client had cardiac surgery because of inadequate cardiac output. The capillary refill time in the toes may be prolonged, which will interfere with accurate oxygen saturation results.
4. The client had cardiac surgery because of inadequate cardiac output. The capillary refill time in the fingers may be prolonged, which will interfere with accurate oxygen saturation results.

TEST-TAKING TIP: Identify the equally plausible options. Options 3 and 4 are equally plausible because both are distal points on the extremities. One is no better than the other. Eliminate both from further consideration.
Content Area: Physical Assessment
Integrated Processes: Nursing Process: Assessment
Client Need: Health Promotion and Maintenance
Cognitive Level: Application
Concept: Oxygenation

10. **ANSWER: 2, 4.**
    Rationales:
    1. Using the fingers to assess for distention of the urinary bladder employs the technique of palpation.
    2. Percussion is the use of the fingers to strike a client's body part to elicit a sound or vibration. This provides information about the presence and density (e.g., solid or air filled) of underlying structures.
    3. Listening to sounds produced within the body by use of a stethoscope employs the assessment technique of auscultation.
    4. Striking a client's body part with the fingers or a rubber-tipped hammer to elicit a sound, vibration, or response involves the assessment technique of percussion.
    5. Measuring a pulse rate by using the fingers employs the assessment technique of palpation.
    Content Area: Physical Assessment
    Integrated Processes: Nursing Process: Assessment
    Client Need: Health Promotion and Maintenance
    Cognitive Level: Application
    Concept: Patient-Centered Care

11. **ANSWER: 2, 3, 4, 5.**
    Rationales:
    1. Pain is a contributing factor, not a clinical manifestation, of sensory overload.
    2. Fatigue is a common clinical manifestation of sensory overload. Sensory overload prevents the brain from ignoring environmental stimuli, interfering with the ability to sleep.
    3. Confusion occurs because many stimuli cause difficulty recognizing the environment in a way that makes sense.
    4. Constant stimuli attack both the physical and emotional domains of the client, contributing to restlessness.
    5. As a result of constant stimuli, a client's mind can race in many directions, contributing to scattered attention.
    6. Hearing impairment is a contributing factor, not a clinical manifestation, of sensory deficit, not sensory overload.
    Content Area: Physical Assessment
    Integrated Processes: Nursing Process: Assessment
    Client Need: Safe and Effective Care Environment; Safety and Infection Control
    Cognitive Level: Analysis
    Concept: Sensory Perception

12. **ANSWER: 1.**
    Rationales:
    1. Excessive compression of an artery sometimes will obliterate a pulse. Releasing pressure of the fingers slightly will allow the blood to flow through the artery.
    2. This will further compound the problem of obstructing blood flow through the artery, obliterating the pulse.
    3. Using a Doppler may eventually be done; however, the nurse's assessment technique should be adjusted first.
    4. Assessing an artery in the other arm may eventually be done; however, the nurse's assessment technique should be adjusted first.

TEST-TAKING TIP: Identify the word in the stem that sets a priority. The word *first* in the stem sets a priority. Identify options that are opposites. Options 1 and 2 are opposites. Examine options 1 and 2 carefully.
Content Area: Physical Assessment
Integrated Processes: Nursing Process: Assessment
Client Need: Health Promotion and Maintenance
Cognitive Level: Application
Concept: Perfusion

13. **ANSWER: 2, 3, 4.**
    Rationales:
    1. A person in an intensive care unit (ICU) may experience sensory overload, not deprivation. A client in an ICU is exposed to an increase in the quantity and/or intensity of internal and/or external stimuli and can become overwhelmed, resulting in ICU psychosis. The clinical manifestations of ICU psychosis include confusion, disorientation, fatigue, irritability, anxiety, restlessness, reduced ability to problem-solve, increased muscle tension, and scattered attention span.
    2. A person experiencing sudden blindness may require several months or more to develop compensatory coping behaviors to deal with the loss of vision. This person can no longer watch television, read a book, or recognize others by sight, resulting in sensory deprivation. Fear of new environments and depression may occur, maximizing the initial isolation caused by blindness.
    3. The person who is experiencing quadriplegia and other clients with impaired mobility may have less exposure to stimulating environments and activities because of the effort it takes to become involved or to leave the home.
    4. A client with a history of depression is at risk for sensory deprivation because of the emotional and physical withdrawal from others.
    5. The client with acute pain is more likely to experience sensory overload, not sensory deprivation. The client with chronic, not acute, pain is more likely to experience sensory deprivation because the client may not have the stamina or interest to engage in stimulating and socializing activities.
    Content Area: Physical Assessment
    Integrated Processes: Nursing Process: Assessment
    Client Need: Safe and Effective Care Environment; Safety and Infection Control
    Cognitive Level: Analysis
    Concept: Sensory Perception

14. **ANSWER: 1, 4.**
    Rationales:
    1. This question assesses the person's orientation to time. It is part of the assessment of time, place, and person, which is related to cognitive functioning.
    2. Assessing feelings is in the affective, not cognitive, domain.
    3. This question assesses short-term memory.
    4. This question requires the client to perform a mathematical calculation, which is a cognitive skill.
    5. This question assesses long-term memory.

Content Area: Physical Assessment
Integrated Processes: Communication and Documentation;
Nursing Process: Assessment
Client Need: Physiological Integrity; Reduction of Risk
Potential
Cognitive Level: Analysis
Concept: Cognition

15. **ANSWER: 2, 3.**
Rationales:
1. The facial nerve, cranial nerve VII, promotes facial expressions, facial muscle strength, and taste. The client should be instructed to smile, wrinkle the forehead, puff out the cheeks, purse the lips, squeeze the eyes shut, and bear the teeth. Deviations from expected responses indicate impairment of the facial nerve.
2. There should be no lid lag if the oculomotor nerve (cranial nerve III) is functioning properly. Cranial nerve III is impaired if there is drooping of an eyelid (ptosis).
3. Shining a light onto the client's pupil should cause the pupil to constrict. If it is slow to constrict or does not constrict then the oculomotor nerve, cranial nerve III, is impaired.
4. The accessory nerve, cranial nerve XI, is associated with raising the shoulders and turning the head from side to side. Asymmetrical movements, limited or absent movements, or pain indicate an impaired accessory nerve.
5. The glossopharyngeal nerve, cranial nerve IX, is involved with the gag reflex, swallowing, tongue movements, taste, and secretion of saliva. Absence of the gag reflex, dysphagia, impaired tongue movements, alterations in taste, and dry mouth all indicate malfunctioning of the glossopharyngeal nerve.
Content Area: Physical Assessment
Integrated Processes: Nursing Process: Assessment
Client Need: Physiological Integrity; Reduction of Risk
Potential
Cognitive Level: Analysis
Concept: Neurologic Regulation

16. **ANSWER: 50.**
Rationales:
Pulse pressure is calculated by subtracting the diastolic blood pressure from the systolic blood pressure. Therefore, 110 – 60 = 50.
Content Area: Physical Assessment
Integrated Processes: Nursing Process: Analysis
Client Need: Physiological Integrity; Reduction of Risk
Potential
Cognitive Level: Application
Concept: Perfusion

17. **ANSWER: 1, 3, 4, 5.**
Rationales:
1. Allergies are information that is associated with a past medical history.
2. Vital signs are associated with the current health problem; current vital signs are not part of a past medical history.
3. Prior surgeries are information that is associated with a past medical history.

4. Immunizations are information that is associated with a past medical history.
5. Childhood illnesses are information that is associated with a past medical history.
6. Present signs and symptoms are associated with the current health problem, not data related to a past medical history.
Content Area: Physical Assessment
Integrated Processes: Communication and Documentation;
Nursing Process: Assessment
Client Need: Physiological Integrity; Physiological Adaptation
Cognitive Level: Analysis
Concept: Patient-Centered Care

18. **ANSWER: 4.**
Rationales:
1. A clear discharge can occur because the vaginal canal is lined with mucous membranes.
2. Pubic hair is coarse, full, and symmetrical over the mons pubis and can extend to the inner upper thighs.
3. The normal location of the urethra is midline below the clitoris and above the vagina.
4. The expected size of the clitoris is 2 cm long and 0.5 cm wide. An enlarged clitoris may indicate excess androgens and therefore should be reported to the primary health-care provider.
TEST-TAKING TIP: Identify the words in the stem that indicate negative polarity. The words *should be reported* in the stem indicate negative polarity. The question is asking "What physical assessment is not within the expected range?" Identify the option that is unique. Option 4 is unique because it is the only option that contains numbers. Consider option 4 carefully.
Content Area: Physical Assessment
Integrated Processes: Communication and Documentation;
Nursing Process: Assessment
Client Need: Physiological Integrity; Reduction of Risk
Potential
Cognitive Level: Application
Concept: Sexuality

19. **ANSWER: 1, 3.**
Rationales:
1. The carotid arteries are closest to the heart and can be palpated to assess cardiac function in adults and children older than 1 year of age.
2. The femoral site is used to determine circulation to a lower extremity.
3. The brachial arteries are major arteries that can be assessed to determine cardiac function in infants from birth to 1 year of age.
4. The dorsalis pedis site is used to determine circulation to the foot.
5. The posterior tibial site is used to determine circulation to the foot.
Content Area: Physical Assessment
Integrated Processes: Nursing Process: Assessment
Client Need: Physiological Integrity; Physiological adaptation
Cognitive Level: Application
Concept: Perfusion

20. **ANSWER: 4.**

    Rationales:

    1. This is not the site for assessing an apical pulse rate in an adult. This is the site to assess heart sounds generated at the pulmonic valve. It is two or three finger-breadths below the clavicular notch at the second intercostal space.

    2. This is not the site for assessing an apical pulse rate in an adult. This is Erb's point. This is the left third intercostal space and is used to assess heart sounds generated at the mitral valve.

    3. This is not the site for assessing an apical pulse rate in an adult. This is the left-lateral sternal border. It is used to assess heart sounds generated at the tricuspid valve.

    4. This is the point of maximum impulse. It is the apex of the heart, where the heart contraction is the strongest, and is the site for assessing an apical pulse rate in an adult. It is located at the end of the left ventricle, which is near the fifth intercostal space and 3 to 4 inches to the left of the sternum at the midclavicular line.

    Content Area: *Physical Assessment*
    Integrated Processes: *Nursing Process: Assessment*
    Client Need: *Health Promotion and Maintenance*
    Cognitive Level: *Analysis*
    Concept: *Perfusion*

21. **ANSWER: 3.**

    Rationales:

    1. Contraction of the left ventricle is reflected by the systolic pressure.

    2. The volume of cardiac output is computed by multiplying the stroke volume by the number of heart beats per minute.

    3. Diastole is the period when the ventricles are relaxed and reflects the pressure in the arteries when the heart is at rest.

    4. Pulse pressure is the difference between the systolic and diastolic pressures.

    TEST-TAKING TIP: Identify options with a clang association. The word *pressure* in the stem and in options 3 and 4 are clang associations. Examine options 3 and 4 carefully.

    Content Area: *Physical Assessment*
    Integrated Processes: *Nursing Process: Assessment*
    Client Need: *Physiological Integrity; Reduction of Risk Potential*
    Cognitive Level: *Comprehension*
    Concept: *Perfusion*

22. **ANSWER: 2.**

    Rationales:

    1. The rate is not related to the quality of a pulse. It is related to the number of beats per minute.

    2. The amount of circulating blood volume will influence the quality of the pulse. An increased circulating blood volume will result in a bounding pulse. A decreased circulating blood volume will result in a weak, thready pulse.

    3. This is known as a pulse deficit. It is related to the rate of a pulse and reflects either a dysrhythmia or a decrease in the strength of ventricular contractions.

    4. Two beats repeatedly occurring close together (bigeminy) is related to a dysrhythmia, not quality of the pulse.

    Content Area: *Physical Assessment*
    Integrated Processes: *Communication and Documentation; Nursing Process: Assessment*
    Client Need: *Health Promotion and Maintenance*
    Cognitive Level: *Application*
    Concept: *Perfusion*

23. **ANSWER: 1.**

    Rationales:

    1. The nurse should perform a focused assessment. The child is in respiratory distress and the lungs should be auscultated to determine the presence of wheezes and/or crackles. The expected respiratory rate of a 6-year-old child is 21 breaths/minute. The child is exhibiting retractions when breathing and is assuming the tripod position, indicating dyspnea. Facial flushing is one of the clinical manifestations of asthma, along with the respiratory signs of dyspnea.

    2. Although abdominal palpation should be done eventually, the data collected via inspection and the parental interview do not indicate that the child is in pain or is experiencing urinary retention. Another assessment is the priority.

    3. Although the apical heart rate should be obtained eventually, the radial rate is sufficient initially. Another assessment is the priority.

    4. Although asking the child where it hurts may be done eventually, the data collected via inspection and the parental interview do not indicate that the child is in pain. Another assessment is the priority.

    TEST-TAKING TIP: Identify the word in the stem that sets a priority. The word *next* in the stem sets a priority.

    Content Area: *Physical Assessment*
    Integrated Processes: *Communication and Documentation; Nursing Process: Assessment*
    Client Need: *Physiological Integrity; Reduction of Risk Potential*
    Cognitive Level: *Analysis*
    Concept: *Patient-Centered Care; Oxygenation*

24. **ANSWER: 3.**

    Rationales:

    1. The brachial site generally is used when assessing the heart rate of an infant during cardiopulmonary resuscitation. It is also used when obtaining a blood pressure in an arm.

    2. The carotid site generally is used when preforming cardiopulmonary resuscitation and assessing circulation to the brain.

    3. The apical pulse is assessed at the apex of the heart. It is the most accurate because the pulse rate is generated by the contraction of the left ventricle of the heart as blood is pumped away from the heart.

    4. The radial pulse generally is used for routine assessment of the heart rate. However, due to various factors, there may be a difference between the heart rate and radial pulse rate (pulse deficit), and therefore it is not as accurate as another site.

    Content Area: *Physical Assessment*
    Integrated Processes: *Nursing Process: Assessment*
    Client Need: *Health Promotion and Maintenance*
    Cognitive Level: *Application*
    Concept: *Medication; Perfusion*

25. ANSWER: 1, 4.
    Rationales:
    1. During the onset (cold or chill) phase of a fever a client will feel cold, shiver, and have pilo erection ("gooseflesh"). Drafts will make the client feel colder and accentuate these clinical adaptations. Drafts should be avoided.
    2. Ice packs to the groin during the onset phase of a fever can cause excessive chilling and shivering, which will cause the temperature to increase, not decrease. Ice packs are never appropriate applications at any phase of a fever.
    3. A tepid sponge bath during the onset stage of a fever will cause vasoconstriction and shivering. Shivering should be avoided because it can increase body temperature. Also, a tepid sponge bath used to reduce a fever is a dependent function of a nurse and requires a prescription.
    4. When the temperature increases and the body has not yet reached the new set point, the client usually feels chilly and may shiver. A blanket helps prevent a client from shivering. Shivering should be avoided because it can increase body temperature.
    5. Decreasing the temperature in the room is associated with the second phase (course) of a fever when the temperature reaches the new set point and the client generally feels flushed and warm.
    6. Keeping bed linen dry is important when the client is experiencing diaphoresis that accompanies the third phase (defervescence or crisis phase) of a fever.
    Content Area: Physical Assessment
    Integrated Processes: Nursing Process: Implementation
    Client Need: Safe and Effective Care Environment; Reduction of Risk Potential
    Cognitive Level: Application
    Concept: Thermo-regulation

26. ANSWER: 29.
    Rationale:
    Recall that 1 kilogram equals 2.2 pounds. Divide the child's weight in pounds by 2.2 to determine the child's weight in kilograms. 64 ÷ 2.2 = 29 kilograms. The formula for ratio and proportion also can be used to solve this problem.

    $$\frac{\text{Desire 64 pounds}}{\text{Have 2.2 pounds}} = \frac{x \text{ kilograms}}{1 \text{ kilogram}}$$
    $$2.2x = 64 \times 1$$
    $$2.2x = 64$$
    $$x = 64 \div 2.2$$
    $$x = 29 \text{ kilograms}$$

    Content Area: Physical Assessment
    Integrated Processes: Nursing Process: Planning
    Client Need: Physiological Integrity; Pharmacological and Parenteral Therapies
    Cognitive Level: Application
    Concept: Medication; Safety

27. ANSWER: 1, 2.
    Rationales:
    1. Tautness of the scrotal skin with few rugae may indicate the presence of fluid, infection, torsion, or a mass. The primary health-care provider should be notified.
    2. There should be no discharge from the urethral meatus. A white, yellow, or green discharge may indicate the presence of a sexually transmitted infection.
    3. This is done when performing perineal care for an uncircumcised client. The primary health-care provider should be notified if the foreskin cannot be retracted.
    4. This is expected. The scrotum in most men is darker than the rest of their skin.
    5. This is an expected response and is called the anal reflex.
    TEST-TAKING TIP: Identify the words in the stem that indicate negative polarity. The words *should be reported* in the stem indicate negative polarity. The question is asking "What physical assessment is not within the range of normal?"
    Content Area: Physical Assessment
    Integrated Processes: Nursing Process: Assessment
    Client Need: Physiological Integrity; Reduction of Risk Potential
    Cognitive Level: Application
    Concept: Sexuality

28. ANSWER: 3, 5, 1, 2, 4.
    Rationales:
    3. An increased temperature three days after surgery indicates a potential postoperative infection. The nurse should assess this client immediately (e.g., vital signs, characteristics of the incision) and notify the primary health-care provider of the client's status.
    5. Having a temperature of 100.4°F is expected after receiving multiple bruises in an automobile collision. However, this patent should be monitored for other possible sequela of the event.
    1. Having a low-grade fever immediately after surgery is not unusual; it occurs as a result of an increased metabolic rate in response to the trauma of surgery.
    2. Having a low-grade fever after rigorous physical therapy is not uncommon because of the increased metabolic rate. The client should be assessed to ensure that the other vital signs have returned to the expected range.
    4. The client's urinary tract infection is being treated. The client's increased temperature may persist for several days until the antibiotics take full effect.
    Content Area: Physical Assessment
    Integrated Processes: Nursing Process: Planning
    Client Need: Safe and Effective Care Environment; Management of Care
    Cognitive Level: Analysis
    Concept: Patient-Centered Care

29. ANSWER: 4.
    Rationales:
    1. Although pulling the curtain provides some privacy, the parents will still be able to hear the conversation between the nurse and adolescent.

2. This is an authoritative and restrictive approach. The adolescent should be encouraged to ask a question whenever desired.

3. This is unrealistic. Physical assessment includes inspection of the genitalia because of the development of secondary sexual characteristics during adolescence.

4. An adolescent is more likely to give an honest answer to a sensitive question and is more apt to ask the nurse a sensitive question if the examination is conducted in private. Privacy also promotes a trusting relationship between the nurse and adolescent.

TEST-TAKING TIP: Identify the options that are opposites. Options 1 and 4 are opposites because in option 1 the parents are within hearing distance of the interaction between the adolescent and the primary health-care provider and in option 4 the parents are not in hearing distance. Consider options 1 and 4 carefully because more often than not one of the opposites is the correct answer.

Content Area: Physical Assessment
Integrated Processes: Caring; Nursing Process: Assessment
Client Need: Psychosocial Integrity
Cognitive Level: Application
Concept: Legal

30. **ANSWER: 2, 1, 3, 4, 5.**
    Rationales:
    2. An infant with a temperature of 104.8°F is at high risk for seizures and therefore should be placed on seizure precautions to prevent injury if a seizure does occur. Seizure precautions include padding raised bed rails, ensuring the bed is in the lowest position, and communicating the infant's status to other members of the health-care team providing direct client care.
    1. Obtaining a full set of vital signs is important to gain more data. The vital signs must be taken before administration of the acetaminophen because acetaminophen will lower the temperature, thus providing artificially low temperature readings. Before contacting the client's primary health-care provider, the nurse should always take the client's vital signs.
    3. Removing the infant's blanket will help slightly to reduce the child's temperature through radiation.
    4. Administering acetaminophen (Tylenol) will help reduce the temperature, although not immediately.
    5. Informing the infant's primary health-care provider should be done after the previous interventions. The client is the center of the health team, and the client's needs must be met first.

    Content Area: Physical Assessment
    Integrated Processes: Nursing Process: Planning
    Client Need: Safe and Effective Care Environment; Management of Care
    Cognitive Level: Analysis
    Concept: Thermo-regulation

31. **ANSWER: 1.**
    Rationales:
    1. A tympanic thermometer is the preferred thermometer to use in this scenario. It will not impose on the client's respiratory or gastrointestinal system and it

should not increase the client's anxiety because it is not invasive.

2. A paper strip thermometer is contraindicated for a client with diaphoresis because it will not adhere to the skin, resulting in an inaccurate result.

3. A rectal thermometer is contraindicated for a client with a potential intestinal problem. A rectal thermometer may irritate the mucous membranes of the anus and rectum.

4. Any type of oral thermometer is contraindicated for a client who is short of breath. People who are short of breath frequently become mouth breathers and will be unable to seal the lips around the thermometer to ensure an accurate result.

Content Area: Physical Assessment
Integrated Processes: Nursing Process: Implementation
Client Need: Health Promotion and Maintenance
Cognitive Level: Analysis
Concept: Thermo-regulation

32. **ANSWER: 98.6.**
    Each short line above 98 is equal to 2 tenths. The line of the temperature indicator is almost at the third short line after the line indicating 98. The result should be moved up to the next nearest line. Therefore, the client's temperature is 98.6°F.
    Content Area: Physical Assessment
    Integrated Processes: Nursing Process: Assessment
    Client Need: Health Promotion and Maintenance
    Cognitive Level: Analysis
    Concept: Thermo-regulation

33. **ANSWER: 1.**
    Rationales:
    1. The other ear should be used because the client may have excessive ear wax (cerumen) in the right ear that is causing an inaccurate low reading. Pulling the pinna upward and back in an adult straightens the ear canal so that the sensor can assess the tympanic membrane.
    2. Pulling the pinna upward and back is the appropriate technique for straightening the external ear canal in an adult. However, the same ear should not be used because the temperature was below the expected range, indicating that excessive cerumen may be interfering with an accurate assessment.
    3. Although it is appropriate to access the other ear, pulling the pinna downward and back will not straighten the external ear canal in an adult. This technique is appropriate for children less than 3 years of age.
    4. The other ear should be used because the client may have excessive cerumen in the right ear that is interfering with an accurate reading. Pulling the pinna downward and back is the appropriate technique to straighten the external ear canal of children less than 3 years of age, not an adult.

    TEST-TAKING TIP: Identify the options with duplicate facts. Four concepts are presented: taking the temperature in the same ear, taking the temperature in the other ear, pulling the pinna upward and back, and pulling the pinna downward and back. If you know just one of these concepts in relation to the question you can eliminate two options from consideration.

Content Area: Physical Assessment
Integrated Processes: Nursing Process: Assessment
Client Need: Physiological Integrity; Reduction of Risk
Potential
Cognitive Level: Application
Concept: Thermo-regulation

34. **ANSWER: 1, 3, 5.**

    Rationales:

    1. Excessive perspiration may interfere with contact between the skin and the temporal scanner probe, resulting in an inaccurate result.

    2. Being a mouth breather will not interfere with obtaining an accurate temperature with a temporal scanner probe.

    3. A hat helps retain surface body heat and may result in an inaccurate high result when using a temporal scanner probe.

    4. Obtaining an accurate temperature is not influenced by a client who has male pattern baldness. However, excessive hair that flows over the forehead may help retain surface body heat, producing an inaccurate high result when using a temporal scanner probe.

    5. Sleeping in the side-lying position with the head on a pillow may result in the retention of surface body heat that may result in an inaccurate high result when using a temporal scanner probe.

    TEST-TAKING TIP: Identify the words that indicate negative polarity. The words *requiring an alternate route* indicate

negative polarity. The question is asking, "Which clients are not candidates for the use of a temporal scanner?"
Content Area: Physical Assessment
Integrated Processes: Nursing Process: Assessment
Client Need: Health Promotion and Maintenance
Cognitive Level: Analysis
Concept: Thermo-regulation

35. **ANSWER: 2.**

    Rationales:

    1. The upper eyelid is not the site to assess for the presence of jaundice.

    2. The sclera of the eyes, mucous membranes of the oral cavity, and skin are the common sites to assess for the presence of jaundice. The yellow appearance of the sclera, mucous membranes, and skin is caused by deposition of bile pigments (jaundice, icterus).

    3. The pupil is not the site to assess for the presence of jaundice.

    4. The iris is not the site to assess for the presence of jaundice.

    Content Area: Physical Assessment
    Integrated Processes: Nursing Process: Assessment
    Client Need: Physiological Integrity; Physiological Adaptation
    Cognitive Level: Analysis
    Concept: Metabolism

Pain, Comfort, Rest, and Sleep

KEY TERMS

Bruxism—Repetitive cienching and grinding of teeth that last 4 to 5 seconds, usually occurring during stage 2 non–rapid eye movement sleep

Comfort—Exists when an individual experiences a feeling of well-being and a sense of being strengthened

Dyssomnias—Sleep disorders related to abnormal physiological mechanisms that regulate sleep and wakefulness

Insomnia—Inability to fall asleep, remain asleep, or go back to sleep, resulting in an inadequate quantity or quality of sleep

Narcolepsy—Sudden uncontrollable urge to sleep during the day, lasting seconds to 30 minutes

Nightmare disorder—Repeated episodes of frightening dreams that result in awakening

Nocturnal enuresis—Repeated episodes of involuntary urination when sleeping after toilet training is well established

Pain—An unpleasant emotional or sensory experience initiated by potential or actual tissue damage

Pain threshold—The smallest stimulus that is needed to establish a perception of pain within a person

Pain tolerance—The maximal amount of pain a person is willing to endure before seeking relief

Parasomnias—Disorders characterized by patterns of abnormal behaviors that intrude on sleep or occur at the threshold between waking and sleeping

Rest—State when the body's physical and emotional energy expenditure is limited

Restless leg syndrome—Uncontrollable movements of the legs when resting or just before onset of sleep

Sleep—Cyclical physiological process characterized by decreased perception and motor activity

Sleep apnea—Periodic interruption of breathing when sleeping that lasts from 10 seconds to 2 minutes and occurs 50 to 600 times a night

Sleep deprivation—Situation in which a person experiences extended periods of time without sustained, natural, recurring states of unconsciousness

Sleep terrors—Repeated episodes of abrupt awakening along with a panicky scream

Somnambulism (sleepwalking)—Episodic walking around while asleep with minimal awareness of surroundings

I. Concepts Related to Pain

Pain, which is commonly referred to as the "fifth vital sign," is an unpleasant emotional or sensory experience initiated by potential or actual tissue damage. It is a subjective experience, and therefore its presence and characteristics are whatever the client says they are. Nurses must understand the factors that influence pain, the proper method for performing a comprehensive assessment of pain, and independent and dependent nursing interventions that can help to relieve clients' pain.

A. Types
1. Nociceptive.
    a. Results from stimulation of pain receptors at the site of trauma, ischemia, or inflammation.
    b. Involves visceral pain (i.e., from internal organs) and somatic pain (i.e., from skin, connective tissue, muscles, and bones).
    c. Commonly described as aching, pounding, dull, or gnawing.
2. Neuropathic.
    a. Results from repeated transmission of pain signals from a site of injury that affected nerve cells.
    b. Associated with chronic problems, such as phantom limb sensation, brain attack, and diabetes.
    c. Commonly described as burning, numbness, or "pins and needles."

B. Pain threshold
1. **Pain threshold** is the smallest stimulus that is needed to establish a perception of pain within a person.
2. Varies from person to person but usually does not vary within a person.

C. Pain tolerance
1. **Pain tolerance** is the maximal amount of pain a person is willing to endure before seeking relief.
2. Varies from person to person and within a person, depending on the situation.

D. Factors that influence pain perception
1. Emotions.
    a. Influenced by previous pain experiences.
    b. Common emotions that may increase pain perception include anxiety, fear, anger, depression, helplessness, and hopelessness.
2. Fatigue: Decreases a person's coping abilities, which increases pain intensity.
3. Ethnic and cultural values.
    a. Behavior and beliefs related to pain are commonly learned through interaction with members of the family and social groups; however, people are individuals and may not reflect the values of their ethnic or cultural group.

MAKING THE CONNECTION

A Painful Stimulus and the Perception of Pain

Pain-sensitive nociceptors are found in the skin, subcutaneous tissue, walls of arteries, joints, and many internal organs. When a mechanical, thermal, or chemical stress damages tissues, the tissues release biochemical mediators (e.g., bradykinin, histamine, and prostaglandins) that activate nociceptors in adjacent tissue. This activation converts the noxious stimulus into an electrical stimulus (transduction). Peripheral nerves then carry the pain message to the dorsal horn of the spinal cord and then via the spinothalamic tracts of the spinal cord to the brain stem and thalamus (transmission). Finally, the pain message travels from the thalamus to the brain, where the pain message is perceived (perception). It involves the somatosensory cortex, where physical sensations are perceived and interpreted; the limbic system, which is involved in emotional reactions to the pain message; and the frontal cortex, which is involved with the affective expression of pain. These physiological processes involved in pain perception are known as *nociception.*

---

    b. May influence communication of pain (e.g., demonstrative or silent endurance), extent of family involvement, and intensity of pain willing to be tolerated before seeking relief.
4. Extent of physical and emotional support.
    a. Supportive family, friends, and health team members may help to decrease perception of and increase tolerance to pain.
    b. Lack of empathy may increase intensity of pain.
5. Environment.
    a. A strange environment, such as a hospital or long-term care facility, has noises, odors, lights, and activity that can increase anxiety, which may increase pain intensity.
    b. A familiar environment, such as one's home and bed, may decrease the intensity of pain.
6. Spirituality or religious beliefs.
    a. Pain and suffering may be perceived as penance for one's wrongdoings or an avenue to salvation.
    b. Prayers and religious rituals may offer comfort and hope.
7. Multiplicity of stressors: Intensity of pain increases as the number of issues impacting on an individual's ability to adapt increase.
8. Developmental level: Age and experiential background influence pain perception and physical and behavioral responses to pain (Table 15.1).

Table 15.1 Developmental Variations Associated With Pain and Related Nursing Care

Developmental Level	Perception of Pain and Pain-Related Behaviors	Nursing Interventions
Infants	• Preterm infants: May have a greater sensitivity to pain. • Newborns: Have the same sensitivity to pain as infants and older children. • Are unable to convey characteristics of pain, such as location, intensity, and description. • Respond by increased physical activity, pulling away, resisting stimuli, quivering chin, and crying.	• Encourage parents to hold the infant to provide comfort. • Encourage skin-to-skin contact against the chest of the parent (kangaroo care) for newborns. • Use a sucrose pacifier. • Play comforting auditory stimuli, such as soft music or heartbeat.
Toddlers and preschoolers	• Perceive pain as a threat to safety and security. • May consider pain as punishment. • Begin to have the ability to point to location of pain and describe intensity and characteristics. • Toddlers: Respond by crying, screaming, behavioral regression, and difficulty being comforted. • Preschoolers: Respond by a low frustration level, crying, struggling against restraint, and verbal and physical aggressiveness.	• Encourage the parents to remain with the child. • Be honest about the possibility of and acknowledge the presence of pain or discomfort. • Hold to provide comfort. • Use distractions. • Correct misconceptions about pain.
School-aged children	• Able to convey characteristics of pain, such as location, intensity, and description. • Understand simple explanations for pain. • May regress to an earlier stage of development as a coping mechanism.	• Provide emotional support. • Role-play what will happen when a therapeutic painful procedure is performed and what it will feel like.
Adolescents	• Desire to appear brave in front of others, especially peers. • May be slow to admit the presence of pain.	• Encourage expression of feelings. • Allay fears and anxiety. • Provide privacy during painful procedures.
Adults	• May ignore pain as a result of the desire to be strong, fear of the cause of the pain, or beliefs associated with analgesic use.	• Encourage expression of feelings. • Explore beliefs and correct myths. • Encourage independence as indicated. • Assess presence and characteristics of pain, especially intensity.
Older adults	• May accept pain as part of aging, which it is not; pain in older adults is related to health problems. • May have decreased sensitivity to painful stimuli. • May ignore pain because fear of treatment, lifestyle changes, or fear of becoming dependent.	• Same as Adults.

E. Nursing care for clients who are in pain

🛑 1. Accept the client's perception of pain because it is a subjective symptom that is what the client says it is; validate the presence of pain.

🛑 2. Be nonjudgmental; do not impose own attitudes, beliefs, or expectations onto a client.

3. Assess characteristics of pain.
   a. Onset.
      (1) Ask, "When did the pain start?"
      (2) Abrupt or gradual onset.
   b. Origin and location.
      (1) Ask, "Where do you feel the pain?"
   (2) Identify the origin and location of pain (Table 15.2 and Fig. 15.1).
   (3) Use anatomical landmarks.
   c. Quality.
      (1) Ask, "What does the pain feel like?" and "Is this pain different from the pain that you have been experiencing all along?"
      (2) Possible descriptions include burning, stabbing, throbbing, crushing, pressure, sharp, dull, and achy.
      (3) Allow the client to describe the pain without offering descriptive words.

Table 15.2 Origin of Pain

Type	Location	Examples
Superficial or cutaneous	• Skin or subcutaneous tissue.	• Superficial cut.
Visceral	• Deep internal pain receptors.	• Abdominal organ cancer. • Labor pain.
Somatic	• Ligaments, tendons, blood vessels, and bones.	• Arthritis. • Bone cancer.
Radiating	• Arises in one site and extends to another.	• Sciatic pain from lumbar vertebrae. • Pain with lymphatic streaking associated with infection.
Referred	• Arises in one site but is felt in a distant site (See Figure 15.1).	• Heart ischemia felt as pain in jaw. • Appendicitis causing pain at McBurney's point (halfway between the umbilicus and right anterior iliac crest).
Phantom	• Perceived as arising from a site that was surgically removed.	• Sensations or pain in a limb that was amputated.
Psychogenic	• Perception of pain without a physical cause.	• Any site perceived by the client.

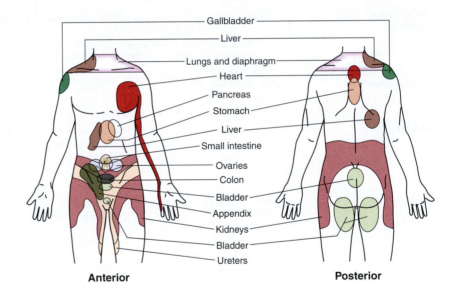

Fig 15.1 Sites of referred pain. (From Williams and Hopper [2015]. *Understanding medical surgical nursing*, 5th ed., Philadelphia: F. A. Davis Company, with permission.)

(4) Is helpful in diagnosing illness because there are commonalities in perceptions of pain, such as with myocardial infarction (crushing); intestinal infections (cramping); urinary tract infection (burning); and arthritis (aching).

d. Intensity.

(1) Ask, "How severe is the pain?"

(2) Use a quantitative pain scale to provide objectivity and consistency in assessments.

(a) For individuals aged 12 years and older, use a numerical pain scale (Fig. 15.2).

(b) For children of different ages, use the Wong-Baker FACES Pain Scale (Fig. 15.3).

(c) For infants and children from birth to 3 years, cognitively impaired clients, and those who are unable to use other scales, use the FLACC Pain Scale (Fig. 15.4).

No pain	Mild pain	Moderate pain	Severe pain	Worst pain

0   1   2   3   4   5   6   7   8   9   10

Fig 15.2 Numerical pain scale 0 to 10. (From Ward and Hisley [2009]. *Maternal-child nursing care, enhanced revised reprint.* Philadelphia: F. A. Davis Company, with permission.)

Wong-Baker FACES® Pain Rating Scale

0	2	4	6	8	10
No Hurt	Hurts Little Bit	Hurts Little More	Hurts Even More	Hurts Whole Lot	Hurts Worst

©1983 Wong-Baker FACES Foundation. www.WongBakerFACES.org
Used with permission. Originally published in *Whaley & Wong's Nursing Care of Infants and Children.* ©Elsevier Inc.

Fig 15.3 Wong-Baker FACES pain rating scale. (From Hockenberry and Wilson [2009]. *Wong's essentials of pediatric nursing,* ed. 8. St. Louis, MO: Mosby. Used with permission.)

FLACC Behavioral Scale

Categories	Scoring		
	0	1	2
Face	No particular expression or smile	Occasional grimace or frown, withdrawn, disinterested	Frequent to constant frown, clenched jaw, quivering chin
Legs	Normal position or relaxed	Uneasy, restless, tense	Kicking, or legs drawn up
Activity	Lying quietly, normal position, moves easily	Squirming, shifting back and forth, tense	Arched, rigid, or jerking
Cry	No cry (awake or asleep)	Moans or whimpers, occasional complaint	Crying steadily, screams or sobs, frequent complaints
Consolability	Content, relaxed	Reassured by occasional touching, hugging, or being talked to; distractible	Difficult to console or comfort

Each of the 5 categories—(F) Face; (L) Legs; (A) Activity; (C) Cry; (C) Consolability—is scored from 0–2, which results in a total score between 0 and 10.

Fig 15.4 FLACC behavioral scale. (© 2002 The Regents of the University of Michigan. All Rights Reserved.)

e. Duration.
  (1) Ask "How long does the pain last?"
  (2) Seconds, minutes, hours, or days.
  (3) Identify characteristic associated with acute versus chronic pain (Table 15.3.)
f. Pattern.
  (1) Ask, "Is there a pattern to the pain?"
  (2) Continuous or intermittent, frequency, predictable occurrences, and time of day it occurs.
g. Precipitating factors.
  (1) Ask, "What initiates or increases the pain?"

  (2) Can be helpful in diagnosing the cause and/or location of pain.
    (a) Bending, lifting, and coughing: Vertebral pain.
    (b) Lying flat: Heartburn.
    (c) Valsalva maneuver: Hemorrhoids.
    (d) Deep breaths: Pancreatitis, fractured ribs.
h. Relieving factors.
  (1) Ask, "What helps to diminish or eliminate the pain?"
  (2) Examples may include immobility, repositioning, eating or eliminating specific

Table 15.3 Comparison of Acute and Chronic Pain

	Acute Pain	Chronic Pain
Onset	• Rapid. • Related to potential or actual tissue damage.	• Gradual. • Related to a lingering or progressive illness. • May be related to no current tissue damage.
Duration	• Short length of time; usually 6 months or less. • Continuous, diminishes, and resolves.	• Long length of time; usually more than 6 months. • Continuous, recurring (exacerbations and remissions). • Relief difficult to achieve and never permanently resolves (intractable pain).
Client's physical responses	*Autonomic nervous system responses* • Tachycardia. • Hyperpnea. • Hypertension. • Diaphoresis. • Dilated pupils. • Pressured speech.	*Parasympathetic nervous system responses* • Decreased pulse rate and blood pressure. • Variable breathing patterns. • Constricted pupils. • Slow, monotonous speech.
Client's behavioral responses	• Restlessness. • Anxiety. • Guarding. • Groaning, wincing, or crying. • Grimacing. • Client usually reports presence of pain.	• Usual or apathetic facial expression. • Resting or sleeping. • Attempting to focus on distracting activities. • Client usually does not report presence of pain unless asked.
Psychological impact	• Briefly diminishes physical and emotional energy, but client usually is able to cope knowing it will eventually end.	• Depletes physical and emotional resources because of no anticipated end. • May be permanently disabling, resulting in interruption in activities of daily living, employment, interpersonal relationships, and so on.
Response to interventions	• Relief may occur in response to nursing interventions, such as repositioning, back rub, imagery, and distraction, if pain is mild. • Relief usually occurs due to primary healthcare provider prescriptions, such as medications and application of heat or cold.	• Often unresponsive to conventional interventions; relief may be difficult to achieve (intractable pain). • Requires multiple modalities. • Complementary and alternative modalities commonly used, such as acupuncture, therapeutic touch, imagery, yoga, hypnosis, and biofeedback.

foods, analgesics, application of heat or cold, and repetitive behaviors, such as rocking, rubbing, and pacing.

  i. Behavioral effects.

    (1) Identify what behavioral indicators of pain are being exhibited.

    (2) Vocalizations (e.g., moaning, grunting, and crying); body movements (e.g., restlessness, muscle tension, wringing the hands, guarding and holding or rubbing a part of the body); social interactions (e.g., withdrawal, avoiding conversation, and reduced attention span); facial expressions (e.g., wrinkled forehead, tightly closed eyes, grimacing, clenched teeth, and open mouth associated with crying).

4. Provide emotional support and answer questions the client has to relieve anxiety and fears.

5. Use distraction techniques, such as soft music, television, conversation, and play appropriate to the client's developmental level.

6. Alter irritating stimuli, such as by limiting noise in the environment, closing curtains or doors, dimming environmental lights, and adjusting room temperature.

7. Teach the client to use relaxation techniques, such as diaphragmatic breathing, guided imagery, and progressive muscle relaxation.

8. Provide cutaneous stimulation, such as back rubs, warm or cold applications, and transcutaneous electrical nerve stimulation (TENS), that uses the gate-control theory of pain to limit pain; with

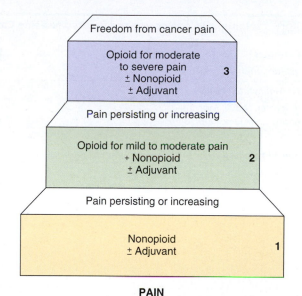

PAIN

Fig 15.5 The WHO's pain relief ladder. (Reprinted with permission from the World Health Organization [2016]. *WHO's pain relief ladder.* Retrieved June 27, 2016, from www.who.int/cancer/palliative/painladder/en/.)

MAKING THE CONNECTION

Gate-Control Theory of Pain and Effectiveness of Cutaneous Stimulation Therapy

The gate-control theory of pain claims that the transmission of pain impulses to the central nervous system is modulated by large A-delta fibers and small C fibers. These fibers terminate in the substantia gelatinosa of the dorsal horn cells of the spinal cord. Stimulation of the small C fibers opens the pain gate, enhancing the transmission and perception of pain. Stimulation of the large A-delta fibers through touch, vibration, and thermal stimuli cause the pain gate to close, diminishing the transmission and perception of pain. The large A-delta fibers are stimulated by cutaneous stimulation therapy, such as application of heat or cold, massage, and TENS.

---

the exception of a back rub, these interventions require a prescription.

F. Nursing care for clients receiving medications for pain
  1. Ensure that the five rights of medication administration are met.
      a. Right drug: The World Health Organization (WHO) three-step analgesic ladder (Fig. 15.5). Although the ladder focuses on pain associated with cancer, it can be applied to pain from any cause.
          (1) Nonopioids: acetaminophen (Tylenol); NSAIDs, such as aspirin and ibuprofen (Advil, Motrin, Aleve). (See Table 15.4.)
          (2) Opioids: codeine, hydrocodone (Hycodan), oxycodone (OxyContin), hydromorphone (Dilaudid), and fentanyl (Duragesic). (See Table 15.5.)
          (3) Adjuvant analgesics.
              (a) Medications given to manage mild pain or concurrently with nonopioid or opioid analgesics to limit escalating doses of the nonopioid or opioid medication.
              (b) Examples include anticonvulsants, antidepressants, psychostimulants, muscle relaxants, neuroleptics, and corticosteroids.
      b. Right dose.
          (1) Computed by weight for infants and children.
          (2) Lower doses given to older adults due to decreased metabolism and elimination.
          (3) Higher doses may be given for intractable pain.
      c. Right route: Although analgesics can be given by any route, the intravenous route provides

the most rapid relief from pain, and the transdermal route provides the most prolonged relief from pain.
      d. Right time.
          (1) Administer at time prescribed to maintain a continuous therapeutic blood level.
          🛑 (2) Administer prn medications before pain becomes too intense because doing so helps them to be more effective than when they are administered when the pain is at the high end of a pain scale.

  2. Maintain patient-controlled analgesia (PCA) to eliminate highs and lows in the intensity of pain and manage pain at a consistent level that is tolerable.
      a. Teach the client that the pump will deliver a basic dose (basal dose) of analgesic periodically and that compressing the trigger will deliver an extra dose as needed up to a certain point (lockout). A lockout prevents the delivery of excessive doses when the trigger is pushed prematurely.
      b. Ensure that the flow rate is set at the prescribed rate.
      c. Monitor the catheter insertion site, such as the peripheral vein or epidural space (Fig. 15.6), for integrity of the line; ensure that the catheter and tubing are not compressed or dislodged.
      d. Monitor the number of times the client uses the trigger in an attempt to relieve pain; excessive

Table 15.4 Nonopioid Analgesics and Related Nursing Care	
Examples	**Nontherapeutic Effects**
acetaminophen (Tylenol)	• *Hepatic toxicity.*
Nonsalicylate NSAID	
ibuprofen (Advil, Motrin) *naproxen (Aleve, Naprosyn)*	• *Rash.* • *Tinnitus.* • *Flu-like syndrome.*
Salicylate NSAID	
acetylsalicylic acid (aspirin, Ecotrin)	• *Agitation.* • *Hyperventilation.* • *Lethargy.* • *Confusion.* • *Diarrhea.* • *Bleeding.* **Toxicity** • *Diaphoresis.* • *Tinnitus (eighth cranial nerve damage).*

Nursing Care

• *Assess level of pain.*
• *Encourage the client to take the medication with 8 oz of water; sit up 15 to 30 minutes after ingestion, and take the medication with food, except for naproxen and ibuprofen.*
• *Monitor for nontherapeutic effects.*
• *Monitor for GI bleeding, such as anemia and melena.*
• *Encourage the client to avoid alcohol and OTC medications.*
• *Acetaminophen: Encourage the client not to exceed 4 g in 24 hours because an overdose may cause liver damage.*
• *Salicylates.*
  • *Monitor serum salicylate levels.*
  • *Warn the client to avoid toxicity by not exceeding the recommended 24-hour dose.*
  • *Withhold 1 week before invasive procedures to decrease the risk of bleeding.*
  • *Understand that salicylates are contraindicated in pregnant women, lactating women, and children younger than 2 years of age (associated with Reye's syndrome).*

Table 15.5 Opioid (Narcotic) Analgesics and Related Nursing Care	
Examples	**Nontherapeutic Effects**
codeine *fentanyl (Duragesic): 72-hour transdermal patch for chronic/intractable pain* *hydrocodone (Hycodan)* *hydromorphone (Dilaudid)* *methadone HCl (Dolophine)* *morphine sulfate (MS Contin, Roxanol): For intractable pain, myocardial infarction, pulmonary edema* *oxycodone (OxyContin)*	• *Decreased respiratory rate.* • *Drowsiness, sedation, confusion.* • *Hypotension.* • *Constipation.* • *Nausea and vomiting.* • *Pruritus.* • *Fentanyl: Dry mouth, diaphoresis, weakness.*
Opioid/nonopioid analgesic combinations	
propoxyphene napsylate and acetaminophen (Darvocet-N) *hydrocodone and acetaminophen (Vicodin)* *oxycodone and acetaminophen (Percocet)* *codeine phosphate and acetaminophen (Tylenol with codeine 1, 2, 3, or 4)*	

Nursing Care

• *Assess level of pain using a pain rating scale before and after administration (see Figs. 15.2, 15.3, and 15.4).*
• *Administer before pain is severe; regularly scheduled doses maintain therapeutic blood levels, which increase effectiveness.*
• *Administer combinations of analgesics cautiously; combined effect is greater than when each is given independently (synergistic).*
• *Administer additional prescribed medication for breakthrough pain; common with continuous infusion or sustained-release medications or intractable pain.*
• *Encourage coughing and deep breathing every 2 hours to prevent pooling of respiratory secretions.*
• *Encourage increased fluids, dietary fiber, and exercise to limit constipation; administer stool softeners or laxatives if prescribed.*

Table 15.5 Opioid (Narcotic) Analgesics and Related Nursing Care—cont'd

Nursing Care

- *Provide for safety, such as teaching the client to avoid hazardous activities and to change positions slowly.*
- *Teach the client how to self-administer medication via various routes.*
- *Monitor pain relief, vital signs, hypotension, drowsiness, confusion, constipation, nausea, and vomiting.*
- *Monitor for severe respiratory depression; if rate is less than 10 breaths/minute, withhold the next dose and notify the primary health-care provider.*
- *Assess for signs of a decreased physiological response (tolerance); usually requires an increase in dose to achieve effectiveness.*
- *Assess for signs of physical or emotional reliance on the medication to maintain its effect (dependence); formerly called habituation or addiction.*
- *Keep naloxone (Narcan) readily available for toxicity or overdose.*

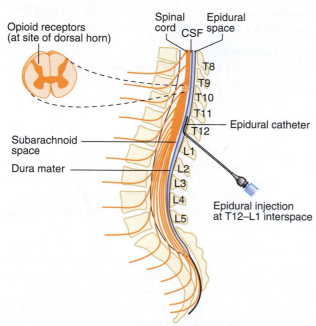

Fig 15.6 Placement of an epidural needle and catheter.
(From Wilkinson and Treas [2016]. *Fundamentals of nursing*, Vol. 1, 3rd ed. Philadelphia: F. A. Davis Company, with permission.)

attempts to administer a bolus dose may occur when the basal rate is inadequate.

3. Correct misconceptions regarding tolerance as well as physical and psychological dependence.
4. Consult with the primary health-care provider regarding measures to prevent constipation, such as adequate dietary fiber intake, intake of 2 to 3 L of fluid daily, out-of-bed activities, and a stool softener if the client is receiving an opioid.
5. Evaluate the client's response to interventions, such as the extent of pain relief; decrease in vital signs, particularly respirations; and presence of constipation if an opioid is given.
6. Notify the primary health-care provider if pain is not relieved or the respiratory rate is 10 or fewer breaths/minute; modify the plan as prescribed.

II. Concepts Related to Comfort

Comfort exists when an individual experiences a feeling of well-being and a sense of being strengthened. It involves being at ease, content, and rising above discomforts when they cannot be lessened. Comfort is more complex than just achieving a state of relief from discomfort or pain and requires a comprehensive plan of care to promote comfort. Although comfort measures are defined by and are unique to an individual, some common nursing interventions provide comfort related to physical, environment, sociocultural, and psychospiritual contexts. Clients expect nurses to help them achieve comfort and nurses should meet these expectations.

A. Dimensions of comfort—Kolcaba
   1. *Relief:* Discomfort or pain is lessened.
   2. *Ease:* Absence of discomforts and feeling content.
   3. *Transcendence:* Rising above discomforts when they cannot be lessened.
B. Contexts in which comfort needs occur and related nursing care
   1. Physical.
      a. Relates to homeostasis, bodily sensations, and basic physiological needs.
      b. Nursing care.
         (1) Administer prescribed medications.
         (2) Assist the client to maintain regular bowel functioning.
         (3) Assist the client to maintain regular urinary elimination.
         (4) Monitor and maintain fluid, electrolyte, and acid-base balance.
         (5) Ensure adequate oxygenation.
         (6) Provide hygiene, such as bathing, grooming, and oral care.
         (7) Ensure clean, smooth, dry linens.
         (8) Turn and position the client.
         (9) Maintain tissue integrity.
         (10) Manage physical discomforts such as pain, nausea, vomiting, and dyspnea.
         (11) Provide a back rub (See "Back Rub," later in this chapter).

2. Environmental.
   a. Relates to that which is outside the body, such as surroundings, location, and ambiance.
   b. Nursing care.
      (1) Limit noxious noise in the environment.
      (2) Adjust room temperature to the client's preference.
      (3) Modify light in room to the client's preference.
      (4) Arrange furniture so that the client has a window view if desired and possible.
      (5) Transport the client to other surroundings if desired and able, such as to a lounge on the unit, coffee shop, or outside patio.
      (6) Provide environmental stimuli desired by the client, such as music.
3. Sociocultural.
   a. Relates to family and societal interpersonal relationships, family traditions, rituals, and cultural customs.
   b. Nursing care.

   🛑 (1) Be nonjudgmental and provide an attitude of caring.

      (2) Ensure continuity of care, such as sharing a written plan of care, assigning consistent caregivers, and performing thorough change-of-shift reports.
      (3) Provide the client with information and teaching; include family members when appropriate.
      (4) Enhance support of family and friends by encouraging staying with the client, involving family in direct care if desired by the client, and ensuring liberal visiting hours if desired and beneficial to the client.
      (5) Support cultural customs, such as involving the person who is viewed as the decision maker in the family, supporting the ability to wear culturally appropriate clothing or head coverings, and assigning a specific gender nurse, depending on the client's culture.

DID YOU KNOW?

People often learn how to respond to pain based on interactions with family members and the culture in which they are raised. For example, in stoical cultures, people avoid demonstrating behavioral responses to or reports of pain because their culture values bravery. Cultural groups generally associated with a stoical response to pain include European American, Native American, Irish, and Filipino cultures. People of Japanese heritage often bear pain without outward expressions as a matter of family honor and may have taboos against use of opioids for relief of pain. People who respond to pain in an outspoken manner may have been raised in a culture where moaning, crying, and responding loudly to pain is common and acceptable. Cultural groups generally associated with an outspoken response to pain include Italian, Puerto Rican, and Jewish cultures. Although certain patterns of responses to pain are associated with certain cultural groups, the nurse must avoid expecting people of a particular heritage to respond in a manner related to their cultural group. Although nurses should strive to provide culturally competent care, the nurse must avoid stereotyping clients. Pain is a multidimensional experience, and each client should be cared for as a unique person with individual needs.

4. Psychospiritual.
   a. Relates to personal awareness of self, self-esteem, personal meanings in one's life, sexuality, and a relationship to a higher being or force.

   🛑 (1) View each client as a unique individual.

      (2) Use communication techniques, especially active listening.
      (3) Support self-esteem, such as by treating the client with respect, providing for privacy, ensuring confidentiality, and meeting client needs as they arise.
      (4) Promote independence, such as involving the client in planning and providing choices.
      (5) Increase relaxation to relieve anxiety, such as by encouraging activities, such as imagery, progressive muscle relaxation, and breathing techniques.
      (6) Provide emotional support and instill hope.
      (7) Accommodate the client's desired religious practices, such as by contacting a spiritual advisor and arranging for religious practices such as distribution of Holy Communion or religious sacraments.

III. Concepts Related to Rest and Sleep

Rest is a state when the body's physical and emotional energy expenditure is limited. **Sleep** is a cyclical physiological process characterized by decreased perception and motor activity.

Rest and sleep are universal needs of all humans and are essential for physiological and psychological health. The amount of rest and sleep required by healthy individuals may vary, but all individuals with health problems usually require an increased need for rest and sleep (restorative sleep). Nurses must understand the basic concepts related to rest and sleep, particularly sleep cycles, to provide appropriate nursing care to clients.

A. Rest
1. Is a state when the body's physical and emotional energy expenditure is limited.
2. While resting, the individual is calm, relaxed, alert, and at ease physically and emotionally.
3. Promotes relaxation, conserves energy, and reduces physical and emotional stress; after an episode, the individual should feel refreshed.
4. May involve activities viewed by the individual as relaxing, such as praying, listening to music, watching television, reading, and engaging in needlework.
5. Although beneficial, rest is not as restorative as sleep because it does not filter external stimuli by altering the level of consciousness.

B. Sleep
1. Is a cyclical physiological process characterized by decreased perception and motor activity.
2. While sleeping, the individual exhibits minimal physical activity; has varied levels of consciousness; lacks awareness of the environment but responds selectively to external stimuli; and has varied physiological responses, depending on the stage of sleep.
3. Conserves energy, prevents fatigue, allows physiological processes (e.g., such as metabolism, vital signs) to slow down, and promotes physiological functioning, such as by boosting the immune system, stimulating protein synthesis for tissue repair, and increasing red blood cell production; after an episode of sleep, an individual should feel refreshed, rejuvenated, and satisfied with the amount of sleep achieved.
4. Promotes emotional functioning, such as by restoring balance among parts of the nervous system and reducing brain activity in areas that control emotions, decision making, and interpersonal communication.
5. Amount needed varies by age and other individual factors, such as lifestyle, environment, and illness.
   a. Newborns: Need 16 to 20 hours a day.
   b. Adults: May need only 7 to 8 hours a day.
6. Sleep states/cycles.
   a. Sleep is preceded by a 10- to 30-minute period when an individual begins to feel sleepy.
   b. Sleep involves two stages: Non–rapid eye movement (NREM), which has four phases, and rapid eye movement (REM) (see Table 15.6 and Table 15.7).

Table 15.6 Comparison of NREM and REM Sleep

Characteristic	NREM Sleep	REM Sleep
Additional name	• *Slow-wave sleep* because of the presence of delta waves.	• *Paradoxical sleep* because of high brain activity with decreased muscle tension.
Physiological contribution	• *Contributes to body tissue restoration.* • *Biological functions slow, protein synthesis increases, and growth hormone is released, promoting cellular and functional repair.* • *Parasympathetic nervous system dominates.*	• *Contributes to cognitive and emotional restoration.* • *Cerebral blood flow changes, cortical activity increases, and epinephrine is released, promoting filtering of stored information about the day's activities, memory storage, and learning.* • *Less restful than NREM sleep.*
Eye movements	• *No eye movements or slow rolling movements.*	• *Periodic episodes of rapid eye movements.*
Vital signs	• *Temperature, pulse, respirations, and blood pressure progressively decrease during stages 1 through 4.*	• *Pulse, respirations, and blood pressure increase and fluctuate.*
Muscle tone	• *Muscles relax.* • *Occasionally, the whole body twitches.*	• *Skeletal muscles become immobile.*

Clinical manifestations of deprivation	• *Precipitate physiological deficiencies.*
	  • *Fatigue.*
	  • *Lethargy.*
	  • *Restlessness.*
	  • *Delayed wound healing.*
	  • *Immunosuppression.*
	  • *Increased sensitivity to pain.*
	  • *Tremors.*
		• *Precipitate cognitive, emotional, and behavioral changes.*
		  • *Anxiety.*
		  • *Irritability.*
		  • *Confusion.*
		  • *Apathy.*
		  • *Inability to concentrate.*
		  • *Combativeness.*
		  • *Disorientation.*
		  • *Delusions.*
		  • *Hallucinations.*
		  • *Paranoia.*

Table 15.7 Stages of Sleep

Stage	Characteristics
NREM Stage 1	
• Time between wakefulness and sleep. • 5 to 10 minutes long. • 5% of total sleep.	• Light sleep, easy to awaken. • Relaxed but aware of surroundings. • Regular, deep breathing. • Eyes may open and close slowly.
NREM Stage 2	
• 10 to 15 minutes long. • 50% of total sleep.	• Light sleep, easy to awaken. • Muscles are relaxed. • Vital signs slightly decreased. • Eyes closed with almost no movement.
NREM Stage 3	
• 5 to 15 minutes long. • 8% of total sleep.	• Deep sleep, difficult to awaken. • Muscles are more relaxed. • Vital signs decreased. • Snoring may occur. • Eyes closed with almost no movement.
NREM Stage 4	
• 20 to 50 minutes long. • 11% of total sleep.	• Deepest sleep, difficult to awaken. • Confused when awakened. • Muscles are very relaxed. • Eyes closed with almost no movement.
REM, also called Stage 5	
• 5 to 30 minutes long. • 25% of total sleep.	• Paradoxical sleep. • Reacts normally when awakened. • Large muscle inactivity; small muscles may twitch, deep-tendon reflexes are depressed. • Vital signs increase; pulse may be rapid and irregular, periods of apnea may occur. • Dreaming may occur.

c. Once asleep, an individual usually has four or five complete sleep cycles per night, lasting 90 to 100 minutes each; with successive cycles, NREM stage 1 is excluded, NREM stages 3 and 4 shorten, and the REM stage lengthens (Fig. 15.7).

d. Amount of time in each cycle varies over the life span; infants and children spend more time in stages 3 and 4 than do older adults.

C. Nursing care to promote effective rest and sleep

1. Teach client to engage in restful activities

   a. Encourage client to identify preferred restful activities.

   b. Encourage client to set a routine for restful activities (e.g., after work, after dinner).

   c. Teach client that engaging in restful activities releases "feel good" hormones (e.g., serotonin, prolactin, and oxytocin) and lowers stress hormones (e.g., cortisol).

   d. Provide a back rub to reduce muscle tension, heart rate, and blood pressure; human touch also releases serotonin.

2. Teach clients that sleep hygiene involves activities that control all behavioral and environmental factors that precede sleep or interfere with sleep.

   a. Identify personal activity and sleep patterns.

   b. Engage participation in activity and exercise during the day to reduce stress and deplete energy.

   c. Avoid daytime naps unless they are less than 30-minute naps (power naps) to prevent insomnia at night.

   d. Avoid physical exertion for 1 to 2 hours before bedtime to limit stimulation before attempting sleep.

   e. Avoid heavy and spicy meals for 2 to 3 hours before bedtime to reduce the risk of gastrointestinal (GI) distress and esophageal reflux.

   f. Avoid nicotine and caffeine-containing foods and beverages, such as coffee, tea, colas, and chocolate, for 4 hours before bedtime to limit the stimulating effects of these products (half-life of nicotine is 1 to 2 hours).

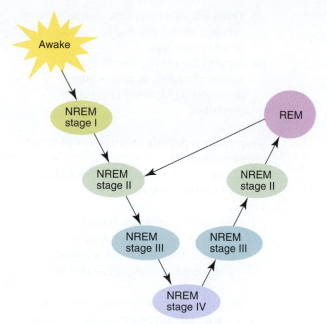

Fig 15.7 The normal adult sleep cycle. (From Wilkinson and Treas (2016). *Fundamentals of nursing,* Vol. 1, 3rd ed. Philadelphia: F. A. Davis Company, with permission.)

g. Avoid alcohol for 4 hours before bedtime to limit the need to void during the night because of alcohol's diuretic effect and to limit early awakening.

h. Consume products containing sleep-promoting constituents: Small snack of carbohydrates and protein, such as cheese and crackers; carbohydrates limit the sensation of hunger while protein reduces the sugar boost of the carbohydrate.

i. Establish a daily bedtime routine, such as reading, taking a warm bath, listening to music, performing specific hygiene practices, and choosing a consistent time to go to bed and arise.

j. Control the environment, such as by turning off lights, limiting environmental noise, setting a preferred environmental temperature, and using "white noise," such as sounds of raindrops or wind, to limit stimuli that may delay or interrupt sleep.

k. Perform relaxation techniques, such as imagery, diaphragmatic breathing, and progressive muscle relaxation, to reduce muscle tension and promote relaxation.

l. Get out of bed if not asleep within 30 minutes and return to bed when sleepy to establish an expectation that sleep should follow when in bed; use the bed only for sleeping and sexual activity.

🛑 m. Avoid consistent use of medication for sleep to prevent physical or emotional dependence.

IV. Sleep Deprivation

Sleep deprivation refers to a situation in which a person experiences extended periods of time without sustained, natural, recurring states of unconsciousness. It results from deprivation of REM sleep, NREM sleep, or both. Nurses should understand the problems associated with sleep deprivation, the clinical manifestations of sleep deprivation, and the nursing care that can promote sleep.

A. Factors that contribute to sleep deprivation
1. Conditions that interfere with the ability to go to sleep, remain asleep, or return to sleep, such as insomnia, restless leg syndrome, sleep apnea, and sensory overload.
2. Illnesses that interfere with sleeping, such as fever, pain, and dyspnea.
3. Situations impacting the sleep-wake cycle, such as rapid change in time zones (jet lag), rotating shift work, multiple interruptions by health-care providers during sleep, and environmental lights and noise that interfere with sleeping (e.g., intensive care unit [ICU] psychosis).

B. Assessment of clients for physiological manifestations of sleep deprivation
1. Drooping eyelids *(ptosis)*.
2. Slowed response time.
3. Depressed reflexes.
4. Decreased fine motor skills.
5. Slowed reasoning and judgment.
6. Decreased auditory and visual alertness.
7. Cardiac dysrhythmias.

C. Assessment of clients for psychological manifestations of sleep deprivation
1. Excessive sleepiness.
2. Irritability, agitation, and hyperactivity.
3. Decreased motivation, apathy, and withdrawal.
4. Increased sensitivity to pain.
5. Confusion and disorientation.

D. Nursing care for clients experiencing sleep deprivation
   See "Nursing care to promote effective rest and sleep" earlier in this chapter.

V. Sleep Disorders and Related Nursing Care

The most common disorders that impact sleep are classified as dyssomnias or parasomnias. **Dyssomnias** are sleep disorders related to abnormal physiological mechanisms that regulate sleep and wakefulness. **Parasomnias** are sleep disorders characterized by patterns of abnormal behaviors that intrude on sleep or occur at the threshold between waking and sleeping. There are commonalities of nursing care to promote sleep in clients with these sleep disorders. However, each sleep disorder has unique characteristics that require specific nursing interventions. Nurses should be knowledgeable about these sleep disorders and their specific treatments as well as have a comprehensive repertoire of strategies to assist clients to improve their ability to achieve restorative sleep.

A. Commonalities of nursing care for clients experiencing sleep disorders
1. Assess clients at risk for sleep disorders.
2. Validate the client's and significant other's frustration and anxiety regarding the problem and physical and emotional consequences.
3. Have the client keep a sleep/activity/dietary diary.
4. Teach sleep hygiene practices.
5. Encourage specific interventions appropriate for the disorder.
6. Document assessments, nursing interventions, and client responses.

B. Dyssomnias and specific nursing care
1. Insomnia.
   a. **Insomnia** is the inability to fall asleep, remain asleep, or go back to sleep, resulting in an insufficient quantity or quality of sleep.
   b. May be transient (lasting less than a month) or chronic (lasting longer than a month).
   c. Characterized by awakening without feeling refreshed and excessive daytime sleepiness.
   d. Specific nursing care.
      (1) Assess for risk factors, including female gender, advanced age, anxiety, substance misuse, caffeine intake, inadequate sleep hygiene, and use of medications, such as amphetamines, bronchodilators, decongestants, and beta-adrenergic blockers.
      (2) Support the use of short-term prescribed sedatives-hypnotics to help prevent chronic insomnia.
2. Restless leg syndrome.
   a. **Restless leg syndrome** is characterized by uncontrollable movements of the legs when resting or just before onset of sleep.
   b. Caused by a central nervous system (CNS) disorder.
   c. Characterized by unpleasant sensations in the legs, such as tingling, itching, creeping, and crawling.
   d. Specific nursing care.
      (1) Assess for risk factors, including a family member with the disorder, advanced age, low levels of iron, and use of certain antidepressants, such as sertraline (Zoloft), a selective serotonin reuptake inhibitor (SSRI).
      (2) Teach the client to avoid stimulants, such as caffeine.

(3) Teach self-care measures, such as walking, massage, stretching, and application of heat or cold to the legs.
(4) Support the use of prescribed neuroleptic agents, vibration, or acupressure; clonazepam (Klonopin) may be prescribed.

3. Sleep apnea.
   a. **Sleep apnea** is periodic interruption of breathing when sleeping.
   b. Lasts from 10 seconds to 2 minutes and may occur 50 to 600 times a night.
   c. Types.
      (1) *Obstructive sleep apnea* (OSA).
         (a) Caused by airway obstruction due to tongue, tonsils, adenoids, deviated septum, or collapse of soft palate.
         (b) Characterized by struggling to breathe with snoring, gasping, and snorting sounds; client usually is not aware of awakening.
         (c) Treatment directed at cause.
      (2) *Central sleep apnea* (CSA).
         (a) Caused by dysfunction of central respiratory control.
         (b) Attempts to breathe cease; client usually is aware of awakening.
         (c) Presently has no effective treatment.
   d. Characterized by excessive daytime sleepiness, fatigue, morning headache, irritability, and difficulty concentrating.
   e. Causes physiological problems if untreated, such as dysrhythmias, hypertension, heart failure, brain attack, and impotence.
   f. Causes emotional problems if untreated, such as mood swings, personality changes, and depression.
   g. Specific nursing care.
      (1) Assess for risk factors, including male gender, age older than 40, and overweight; enlarged tonsils; deviated septum; and associated physical and emotional conditions.
      (2) Obtain the sleeping partner's report about the client's behavior when sleeping, such as snoring, snorting, and gasps, alternating with periods of silence and flailing of the arms and legs during apneic episodes.
      (3) Encourage diagnostic testing while sleeping, such as electrocardiography, arterial oxygen saturation, electroencephalography, and oral and nasal air flow.

(4) Specific nursing care for clients with OSA.

🛑 (a) Encourage consistent nighttime use of continuous positive airway pressure (CPAP) to maintain an open airway if prescribed.

(b) Encourage weight loss and avoidance of alcohol and smoking, if applicable.

(c) Provide perioperative care for procedures, such as tonsillectomy, repair of deviated septum, or laser removal of excess tissue of the platelet and pharynx.

4. Narcolepsy.
   a. **Narcolepsy** is a sudden uncontrollable urge to sleep during the day, lasting seconds to 30 minutes.
   b. Thought to be caused by a genetic defect of the CNS in which REM sleep cannot be controlled.
   c. Characterized by slurred speech, abrupt bilateral loss of muscle tone *(cataplexy)*, and abruptly falling asleep *(sleep attack, sleep episode)*.
   d. Associated with client reports of sleeping well at night; weakness of the knees or inability to move during onset of sleep attack or when waking up *(sleep paralysis)*; vivid, bizarre dreams while falling asleep that last 1 to 15 minutes; and awakening from sleep episodes refreshed.
   e. Specific nursing care.
      (1) Assess for risk factors, including onset between 15 and 30 years of age and a family member with the disorder.
      (2) Determine whether the client sleeps well at night to distinguish between narcolepsy and sleep deprivation; sleep attacks caused by sleep deprivation resolve with sufficient sleep.
      (3) Teach avoidance of shift work, which usually is not tolerated, and passive activities, such as watching television or reading that precipitate sleep.
      (4) Encourage several naps a day at consistent times to decrease sleepiness.

🛑 (5) Recommend avoidance of activities that may result in injury during a sleep attack, such as driving a car and using machinery.

      (6) Encourage intake of prescribed medications, including CNS stimulants, such as amphetamines, methylphenidate (Ritalin), or modafinil (Provigil), and antidepressants, such as monoamine inhibitors and serotonergics.

C. Parasomnias and specific nursing care
   1. Bruxism.
      a. **Bruxism** is repetitive clenching and grinding of teeth; episode lasts 4 to 5 seconds.
      b. Occurs usually during stage 2 NREM sleep.
      c. May erode tooth enamel, loosen teeth, and cause jaw pain.
      d. May become a habit after the initial cause resolves.
      e. Specific nursing care.
         (1) Assess for risk factors, including increased stress, abnormal bite, and GI disturbances.
         (2) Encourage use of relaxation techniques as part of the bedtime routine.
         (3) Encourage the use of a prescribed mouth guard over the teeth when sleeping.

   2. Somnambulism (sleepwalking).
      a. **Somnambulism** is episodic walking around while asleep with minimal awareness of surroundings; episode lasts 3 minutes or longer.
      b. Occurs during stage 3 or 4 NREM sleep, 1 to 2 hours after falling asleep.
      c. Clients may have glassy eyes, look through other people as if they do not exist, or perform activities, such as making coffee or dusting furniture.
      d. Clients report no awareness or memory of the episode.
      e. Specific nursing care.
         (1) Assess for risk factors: More common in children but can occur in adults.

🛑 (2) Encourage the use of safety devices, such as bed and house alarms that alert others when the person exits the bed or leaves the house.

   3. Nightmare disorder.
      a. **Nightmare disorder** is characterized by repeated episodes of frightening dreams that result in awakening; clients commonly report that the dreams jeopardize their personal safety.
      b. Occurs during REM sleep and may occur every 90 to 110 minutes.
      c. Characterized by increased vital signs, diaphoresis, and difficulty falling back to sleep for fear of having another nightmare.
      d. Specific nursing care.
         (1) Assess for risk factors.
            (a) Occurs most commonly in children 3 to 5 years of age but can occur in older children and adults.
            (b) Is associated with stress; traumatic events; anxiety; guilt; insecurity; depression; fever; medication use, such as stimulants, antidepressants, and antihypertensives; and emotional problems, such as post-traumatic stress disorder, borderline personality, and dissociative disorder.

(2) Encourage the client to engage in activities to limit stress, such as daily exercise, relaxation techniques, yoga, and self-hypnosis.

(3) Support taking or discontinuing medications as prescribed.

(4) Teach significant others to provide emotional support.

4. Sleep terrors (night terrors).

a. **Sleep terrors** are repeated episodes of abrupt awakening along with a panicky scream.

b. Occurs during stage 4 NREM sleep and lasts from 10 to 30 minutes.

c. Characterized by crying or screaming in fear, thrashing about, and resisting attempts at consolation; appearing awake but not being awake; being difficult to awaken; and reporting no awareness or memory of the episode.

d. Specific nursing care.

(1) Assess for risk factors: Most common in children.

(2) Teach significant others that attempts to hold or comfort may be resisted.

🛑 (3) Remain physically close to provide emotional support and maintain safety.

5. Nocturnal enuresis (bed wetting).

a. **Nocturnal enuresis** is repeated episodes of involuntary urination when sleeping after toilet training is well established.

b. Occurs when arousing from stages 3 and 4 NREM sleep, 1 to 2 hours after falling asleep.

c. Client may or may not awaken during the episode.

d. Has multifactorial causes, including hormonal, bladder, and sleep problems; genetics; and medical conditions, such as small bladder, diabetes mellitus, and urinary tract infection.

e. May limit social activities, such as sleepovers and camp; precipitate social exclusion by peers; or cause anger and frustration in significant others.

f. Specific nursing care.

(1) Assess for clients at risk: More common in males than in females; clients with a family member who has or had the disorder; and clients with developmental delays or medical problems associated with the disorder.

(2) Teach the client to reduce the volume of urine in the bladder at night by limiting fluid intake after 6 p.m. and voiding before going to bed and to decrease bladder irritability by eliminating caffeine in the diet.

(3) Support the use of behavior modification strategies.

(a) Rewards for waking up dry.

(b) Positive imagery, such as thinking about waking up dry.

(c) Use of a bedwetting alarm if prescribed; an alarm is activated when the sleeper begins to wet the bed which awakens the sleeper who should attempt to stop the urinary stream and use a toilet to void; its use is controversial.

🛑 (4) Teach parents to be nonjudgmental when episodes occur and have a nonchalant demeanor when changing soiled linens and bedclothes.

🛑 (5) Teach the client about the disorder and provide emotional support to increase self-esteem and limit embarrassment, shame, and guilt.

VI. Medications That Promote Rest and Sleep and Related Nursing Care

Many independent and dependent nursing interventions may be inadequate to promote rest or achieve restorative sleep. Medications, such as anxiolytics, sedatives, and hypnotics, may be prescribed. Clients may self-prescribe over-the-counter medications, such as antihistamines, dietary supplements, and herbs, to promote sleep. Nurses should know the mechanisms of action, therapeutic and nontherapeutic effects, and nursing care related to the common medications that are specifically designed to address client needs in relation to rest, and sleep.

A. Anxiolytics, sedatives, and hypnotics: Reduce anxiety and promote rest and sleep (Table 15.8)

B. Over-the-counter (OTC) products used to promote sleep

1. Types of products.

a. Antihistamines: diphenhydramine (Benadryl).

b. Dietary supplements: melatonin.

c. Herbs: kava, valerian, chamomile, passion flower, and lemon balm.

2. Nursing care.

a. Advise the client that self-medicating with OTC products can be dangerous.

(1) Products may potentiate, diminish, or interact with other medications being taken. (See Table 9.1 "Common Herbal Supplements and Related Nursing Care" in Chapter 9, Medications).

(2) Products may be habit forming, promoting physical or emotional dependence.

(3) Products such as dietary supplements and herbs are not regulated by the U.S. Food and Drug Administration.

Table 15.8 Anxiolytics, Sedatives, and Hypnotics and Related Nursing Care

Types	Examples	Nontherapeutic Effects
Benzodiazepines		
• *Increase action of gamma-aminobutyric acid (GABA) inhibitory neurotransmitter.*	**Short acting** alprazolam (Xanax) midazolam (Versed) **Medium acting** lorazepam (Ativan) **Long acting** chlordiazepoxide (Librium) clonazepam (Klonopin) diazepam (Valium)	• *Decreased mental alertness.* • *Decreased blood pressure.* • *Drowsiness.* • *Dizziness.* • *Headache.* • *Nausea and vomiting.* • *Paradoxical reactions, such as euphoria and excitement.*
Nonbarbiturates		
• *All have CNS depressant effects but variable action depending on the medication.*	buspirone (BuSpar) hydroxyzine (Atarax, Vistaril) zaleplon (Sonata) zolpidem (Ambien)	

Nursing Care
- *Assess sleep patterns.*
- *Teach the client sleep hygiene practices to promote effectiveness of medication.*
- *Encourage avoidance of products that potentiate effects, such as alcohol, or diminish effects, such as caffeine.*
- *Teach the client to provide for personal safety because of decreased mental alertness.*
- *Discontinue the medication slowly as prescribed to prevent clinical manifestations associated with withdrawal; use longer than 2 weeks may lead to dependence.*
- *Assess therapeutic effectiveness and for signs of dependence.*

---

b. Encourage the client to discuss the desire to use these products with the primary health-care provider.

VII. Strategies to Decrease Pain and Promote Comfort, Rest, and Sleep

Specific interventions can be used to decrease mild to moderate pain and promote comfort, rest, and sleep by closing the gate for painful stimuli and using emotions and the conscious mind to interfere with the interpretation and perception of pain. The gate-control theory of pain is involved with relaxation techniques that stimulate cutaneous tissues (e.g., back rub). Positive thoughts and emotions (e.g., guided imagery) stimulate the release of endorphins that also are thought to have an effect on closing the gate to painful stimuli. In addition, techniques that require the mind to focus on issues other than the pain (e.g., distraction, progressive muscle relaxation, and breathing techniques) help to interfere with the interpretation and perception of pain because the brain can process only a certain amount of information at one time. These techniques are included within the role of the nurse and do not require a primary health-care provider's prescription.

A. Guided imagery
1. Use of auditory suggestions, from a nurse or from an internal dialog, that have the client picture in the mind places or situations that stimulate emotions that promote relaxation.
2. Nursing care.
   a. Have the client assume a position of comfort with the eyes closed; maintain a quiet environment.
   b. Speak in a soft, slow manner.
   c. Make suggestions that use a variety of senses in relation to the image selected by the client, such as, "Hear the waves lapping on the shore," "Smell the roses in the garden," "Savor the taste of the food you are eating," and "Feel the wind blowing through your hair."

B. Distraction
1. Focusing on something else other than the pain.
2. Nursing care.
   a. Carry on a conversation with the client.
   b. Suggest the use of distraction techniques.
      (1) Visual: Reading, watching television.
      (2) Tactile: Taking a warm bath, petting an animal, cuddling with a significant other.
      (3) Auditory: Listening to music or books on tape, an infant listening to a heartbeat or soothing whispering from a parent.
      (4) Intellectual: Completing crossword or Sudoku puzzles, playing card games alone, such as solitaire, or playing more complex games with another person.

C. Breathing techniques
1. Inhalation and exhalation of air to maximize lung expansion or require the mind to focus on the pattern of breathing rather than discomfort or pain.
2. May be as simple as diaphragmatic breathing, which utilizes the diaphragm, rather than thoracic muscles, to achieve maximal expansion of the lungs on inhalation and promote muscle relaxation.
3. May involve complex patterns that alternate depths and rates of breaths to distract a person from an uncomfortable or painful experience; can be used by a woman during labor and birth.
4. Nursing care.
   a. Have the client assume a position of comfort with the hands positioned over the upper abdomen; maintain a quiet environment.
   b. Instruction for the client.
      (1) Inhale slowly through the nose while counting to the number 4; the client should first feel the abdomen expand and then the chest.
      (2) Hold the breath at the height of inhalation while counting to the number 4.
      (3) Exhale gently and smoothly while counting to the number 8; the client should feel the abdomen move toward the middle of the body.
      (4) Repeat steps 1 through 4.

D. Progressive muscle relaxation
1. Tensing and relaxing muscles in the body in a sequential pattern to reduce muscle tension and engage the mind in an activity.
2. Nursing care.
   a. Have the client assume a position of comfort with the eyes closed; maintain a quiet environment.
   b. Encourage the client to engage in diaphragmatic breathing throughout the procedure.
   c. Begin the sequence of tensing and relaxing muscles with the facial muscles and progress toward the toes.
   d. Instruct the client to breathe in through the nose while tensing a group of muscles; hold the tension for 15 seconds and then relax the muscles while breathing out.
   e. Instruct the client to rest for several seconds and then progress to another group of muscles.

E. Back rub
1. Therapeutic effects.
   a. Relieves muscle tension.
   b. Promotes physical and emotional relaxation.
   c. Facilitates induction of sleep.
   d. Limits transmission of pain impulses via the gate-control theory of pain.
   e. Increases circulation to the skin (friction causes heat that promotes dilation of capillaries).
2. Contraindications.
   a. Personal preference not to receive a back rub; always ask a client's desire for and permission to perform a back rub.
   b. Rib fractures and vertebral disorders.
   c. Impaired tissue integrity, such as burns, pressure ulcers, and open wounds.
   d. Within 48 hours of an acute neurological (e.g., brain attack) or cardiac (e.g., myocardial infarction, cardiac surgery) problem; client may not tolerate the stimulation of a back rub.
3. Types of back rub strokes.
   a. *Effleurage:* Long, smooth strokes with gentle pressure that slide over the skin from the small of the back to the shoulders; promotes relaxation and circulation to the skin.
   b. *Friction:* Continuous, small, circular movements on either side of the vertebrae from the shoulders to the small of the back and then from the small of the back to the shoulders; promotes circulation to the skin.
   c. *Pétrissage:* Kneading of the skin and muscles; promotes circulation to the skin and reduces muscle stiffness and spasms.
   d. *Tapotement:* Gentle, rhythmic tapping over tense muscles; reduces muscle tension.
   e. *Feathering:* Long, soft, fingertip strokes from the shoulders to the small of the back; soothing stroke that signals the end of the back rub.
4. Nursing care.
   a. Identify whether the client has any contraindications to a back rub to prevent injury.
   b. Assess the client's desire for a back rub.
   c. Wash hands to limit the transfer of microorganisms.
   d. Raise the bed to a working height and lower the side rails to prevent reaching and straining of own back and legs.
   e. Close the door, pull the curtain, and drape the client, exposing just the back, to provide privacy and emotional comfort.
   f. Place the client in a side-lying or prone position.
   g. Warm the lotion to promote comfort and dilation of the capillaries.
   h. Place the lotion on own hands first to prevent startling the client.
   i. Massage using a variety of strokes for 3 to 5 minutes ending with feathering; variety provides several therapeutic effects.

j. Reposition the client and cover with bed linen.

k. Document the back rub and the client's response in the client's clinical record.

F. Aromatherapy

1. Use of natural essential oils extracted from parts of plants to enhance mood, cognition, psychological or physical well-being.

2. Effective via two mechanisms: Olfactory system influences the limbic system of the brain and the direct pharmacological effects of essential oils.

3. These oils are used through topical application, massage, inhalation or water immersion to promote a desired response; specific oils precipitate specific human responses.

4. Use is controversial. Risk of adverse effects versus benefit makes their use uncertain; some oils are highly toxic particularly if taken internally; can be hazardous to pregnant and lactating women.

G. Acupressure

1. Application of physical pressure to acupressure points along invisible lines of energy flow

(*meridian system*) in the body with the aim of cleaning blockages to restore health and balance in the body.

2. Has its roots in traditional Chinese medicine; vital energy flows along at least 14 meridians that connect organs with other parts of the body.

3. Thought to enhance or unblock energy flow thereby improving well-being; belief that blocked energy along a meridian can cause ailments that can precipitate disease.

4. Thought to decrease human responses such as nausea, vomiting, lower back pain, and tension headaches to name a few.

5. Should not be used instead of western medical care. Should be avoided: when pregnant because some pressure points stimulate uterine contraction; over areas with burns, infection, inflammation, contagious disease of the skin, and varicose veins; when client has active cancer or high or low blood pressure.

CASE STUDY: Putting It All Together

A nurse is caring for an older man who is being admitted to the hospital for pain management due to progressive metastatic disease. The nurse interviews the client, completes a pain assessment, and reviews the admitting primary health-care provider's prescriptions.

Client's Clinical Record

Client Interview

Client states that the pain was significantly reduced after surgery 1 year ago to remove as much of a malignant intestinal tumor as the surgeon was able to remove. The client said that the pain was initially manageable. However, for the last 7 months, the pain has progressively increased in intensity to where now it is "unbearable." Reports constant fatigue. Expressed that he "feels helpless" because nothing seems to help and stated, "I am so angry that this is happening to me. I was careful about what I ate and lived a healthy lifestyle. I can't take much more of this, and I am afraid of what is going to happen next. I lost my wife 4 months ago because she was hit by a drunk driver and I had to move into my daughter's house because I could no longer take care of myself." He said his family is great and they are always there for him but that he feels like a burden. He shared that his daughter has three small children and the house is always noisy and busy, so it is hard to rest. He went on to say, "Sometimes I think that this suffering is what has to happen because of the things that I did during the Vietnam War that I regret. It was a terrible time in my life."

Pain Assessment

• Pain level before coming to the hospital was "11" on a scale of 0 to 10, and now, 2 hours later, after the first dose of morphine 6 mg, is a level 6.

• The client stated, "The pain is sharp and piercing and is concentrated all around my belly," as he rubbed his hand in a circular motion over the surface of the abdomen.

• Guarding his abdomen with his hands.

• Makes facial grimaces, clenches the teeth, and tightly closes the eyes when making slight changes in position.

Vital Signs	
Temperature:	99.6°F
Pulse:	120 beats/minute
Respirations:	24 breaths/minute, shallow
Blood pressure:	165/92 mm Hg

Primary Health-Care Provider's Prescriptions

Morphine sulfate 6 mg Sub-Q every 4 hours prn for severe pain.

Percocet 2.5 mg oxycodone/325 mg acetaminophen: 1 tablet PO every 6 hours prn for mild pain and 2 tablets PO every 6 hours prn for moderate pain.

Tylenol 500 mg capsule: 1 capsule PO every 4 hours prn for temp over 101°F.

Colace 100 mg PO every 12 hours.

Senokot 2 tablets PO h.s. prn for constipation.

continued.

CASE STUDY: Putting It All Together

cont'd

OOB to chair with assistance.
Regular diet.
Vital signs every 8 hours.

Psychiatry consult for depression.
Oncology consult.
Palliative medicine consult.

Case Study Questions

A. What information collected by the nurse are factors that influence this client's pain experience?

1. _____
2. _____
3. _____
4. _____
5. _____
6. _____
7. _____
8. _____
9. _____

B. Identify at least five additional questions that the nurse should ask the client to arrive at a more complete pain assessment.

1. _____
2. _____
3. _____
4. _____
5. _____

C. Identify at least 15 independent nursing interventions that the nurse should implement to address this client's pain and comfort needs.

1. _____
2. _____
3. _____
4. _____
5. _____
6. _____
7. _____
8. _____
9. _____
10. _____
11. _____
12. _____
13. _____

CASE STUDY: Putting It All Together

cont'd

_____ **Case Study Questions** _____

14. _____

15. _____

D. Identify five dependent nursing interventions that the nurse should implement that address this client's pain and comfort needs.

1. _____

2. _____

3. _____

4. _____

5. _____

REVIEW QUESTIONS

Be sure to read the Introduction for valuable test-taking tips.

1. A nurse is caring for an overweight client who was diagnosed with obstructive sleep apnea. Which should the nurse encourage the client to do because they are effective in supporting restful sleep? **Select all that apply.**
   1. Teach the importance of weight loss.
   2. Maintain a side-lying position when going to bed.
   3. Employ breathing exercises for relaxation before bedtime.
   4. Use a prescribed positive pressure device when going to sleep.
   5. Position several pillows under the head when going to bed at night.

2. A client with a history of inflammation of the gallbladder (cholecystitis) comes to the urgent care center with acute pain in the upper right quadrant of the abdomen. The client states, "We went out for dinner last night and I ate spare ribs, macaroni and cheese, and ice cream. I really overdid it." Where should the nurse anticipate that the client will report referred pain associated with inflammation of the gallbladder?

   1. A
   2. B
   3. C
   4. D

3. A client on a medical unit tells a nurse, "My heart hurts." What is the nurse's **most** appropriate response?
   1. Say, "Your heart hurts."
   2. Alert the rapid response team.
   3. Obtain the client's vital signs.
   4. State, "Please be more specific about how it hurts."

4. A nurse is caring for a school-aged child who is to have a bone marrow biopsy. Although a local anesthetic will be used during the biopsy, it may be frightening and uncomfortable for the child. What should the nurse say that will **best** help the child tolerate the procedure?
   1. "Let's practice what will happen during the procedure."
   2. "Do you have any questions about the procedure that you would like to ask?"
   3. "You need to be strong during the procedure and before you know it will be over."
   4. "Would you like me to play a disk with your favorite songs during the procedure?"

5. A nurse is caring for a client who is reporting pain in the jaw as a result of cardiac ischemia. What word should the nurse use to describe this pain when writing progress notes?
   1. Cutaneous
   2. Radiating
   3. Referred
   4. Visceral

6. An older adult with rheumatoid arthritis comes to the clinic during an exacerbation of the disease. Which client responses are associated with chronic pain? **Select all that apply.**
   1. Pressured speech
   2. Constricted pupils
   3. Increased heart rate
   4. Decreased blood pressure
   5. Increased respiratory rate

7. A nurse is assessing the presence of pain in a variety of clients. Which client conditions may precipitate phantom pain? **Select all that apply.**
   1. Vertebral stenosis causing sciatica
   2. Above the knee amputation
   3. Myocardial infarction
   4. Acute appendicitis
   5. Loss of an arm

8. A nurse is caring for a postoperative client who is receiving patient-controlled analgesia to control postoperative pain. Which concept about controlling pain is **most** important for the nurse to convey to the client?
   1. A basal dose will deliver a basic dose of analgesic periodically.
   2. Excessive doses are locked out if a triggered dose is premature.
   3. Pain medication should be administered before pain becomes intense.
   4. An extra dose of medication is delivered whenever the trigger is compressed.

9. A nurse is caring for a client who reports feeling tense and "up tight." The nurse decides to administer a back rub. Which back rub stroke is **most** effective in producing both relaxation and circulation to the skin?
   1. Friction
   2. Pétrissage
   3. Effleurage
   4. Feathering

10. A toddler must undergo a painful dressing change. How can the nurse **best** provide emotional support for this child?
    1. Hold the child.
    2. Provide a sucrose pacifier.
    3. Encourage the child to cry.
    4. Obtain a prescription for an opioid.

11. A nurse is assessing a client with acute pain. What clinical indicators should the nurse expect the client to exhibit? **Select all that apply.**
    1. Anxiety about the pain
    2. Apathetic facial expression
    3. Relief after taking an analgesic
    4. Grimacing when the pain is intense
    5. Actual tissue damage that caused the pain

12. A nurse plans to administer a back rub to a client. What should the nurse do **first** before administering the back rub?
    1. Wash the hands.
    2. Warm the lotion.
    3. Pull the curtain for privacy.
    4. Identify any contraindications.

13. Which of the following is unique to sleep that does not occur with rest?
    1. Prevents fatigue
    2. Slows vital signs
    3. Conserves energy
    4. Reduces perception

14. A nurse identifies that a client has been awakening frequently during the night and comes to the conclusion that the client is experiencing REM sleep deprivation. Which clinical manifestations identified by the nurse support this conclusion? **Select all that apply.**
    1. Fatigue
    2. Tremors
    3. Disorientation
    4. Combativeness
    5. Delayed wound healing
    6. Increased sensitivity to pain

15. Which statements indicate that the client is experiencing narcolepsy? **Select all that apply.**
    1. "I grind my teeth at night to the point that my jaw is sore in the morning."
    2. "My family says that I snore so loud that I keep everyone awake at night."
    3. "I unexpectedly fall asleep for several minutes in the middle of the day at work."
    4. "Sometimes when I wake up in the morning I feel very weak and I am unable to move."
    5. "My mother says that I walk around in my sleep at night, but I don't remember anything."

16. A nurse has implemented interventions to promote rest and sleep in a postoperative client. What assessment **best** indicates that the client probably is sleeping rather than just resting?
    1. Eyes are closed.
    2. Appears physically at ease.
    3. Arms are resting at the side of the body.
    4. Lacks a response to environmental noises.

17. A nurse is caring for a client who has a prescription for a medication that will provide a palliative reaction. Which client response indicates that the medication is effective?
    1. The client has not become pregnant.
    2. The client's pain has subsided to a tolerable level.
    3. The client no longer has clinical manifestations of an infection.
    4. The client's blood glucose level has returned to the normal range.

18. A client is explaining the pain that is felt in the lower legs as a result of impairment of nervous tissue secondary to diabetes. What words generally expressed by clients to describe this type of neuropathic pain should the nurse expect the client to use? **Select all that apply.**
    1. Pins and needles
    2. Numbness
    3. Pounding
    4. Burning
    5. Aching

19. A nurse is caring for an adolescent who is scheduled for a painful dressing change after a burn injury caused by "cooking" an illicit medication. Which statement by the nurse is **most** helpful?
    1. "This may cause you some pain, so it is all right if you cry."
    2. "We are going to pull the curtain around your bed for privacy."
    3. "If you experience any pain, it is not because we are trying to punish you."
    4. "I know that you want to be brave, so we will do this as quickly as possible."

20. A nurse asks a client, "What does the pain feel like?" What characteristic of pain is the nurse assessing?
    1. Quality
    2. Intensity
    3. Behavioral effects
    4. Precipitating factors

21. Which nursing intervention is **most** important when providing nursing care to a client experiencing pain?
    1. Validate the presence of pain.
    2. Encourage breathing exercises.
    3. Employ a distraction technique.
    4. Teach muscle relaxation techniques.

22. A nurse is assessing a client with chronic pain. Which clinical indicators should the nurse expect the client to exhibit? **Select all that apply.**
    1. Gradual onset
    2. Dilated pupils
    3. Pressured speech
    4. Recurrent in nature
    5. Variable breathing patterns

23. A nurse is caring for a client who reports difficulty sleeping for several weeks. What should the nurse encourage the client to do that will facilitate sleeping? **Select all that apply.**
    1. Drink a small glass of alcohol to relax
    2. Take a warm bath prior to bedtime
    3. Avoid consuming milk at bedtime
    4. Read in bed to induce drowsiness
    5. Establish a daily bedtime routine

24. A nurse awakens a client who is sleeping to implement a required nursing intervention. The nurse identifies that the client is in the deepest stage of sleep and is difficult to awaken. Which stage of sleep is the client experiencing?
    1. REM sleep stage 5
    2. NREM sleep stage 1
    3. NREM sleep stage 2
    4. NREM sleep stage 4

25. A nurse is caring for a client who reports having difficulty going to sleep and staying asleep at night. What should the nurse encourage the client to do? **Select all that apply.**
    1. Limit naps to 1 hour at a time during the day.
    2. Avoid products with nicotine 2 hours before bedtime.
    3. Engage in vigorous exercise 1 to 2 hours before bedtime.
    4. Avoid caffeine-containing food and liquids 4 hours before bedtime.
    5. Eat a small snack of carbohydrates and protein, such as cheese and crackers, just before going to bed.

26. A nurse is caring for an older adult who just had alprazolam prescribed for anxiety that has been interrupting sleep. What nursing action is **most** important at this time when caring for this client?
    1. Institute fall precautions.
    2. Assess for elevated blood pressure.
    3. Monitor the client for clinical indicators of dependence.
    4. Discontinue immediately if the client experiences drowsiness.

27. A nurse is caring for a client who is receiving codeine for pain. Which is **most** important for the nurse to do before administering this medication?
    1. Encourage coughing and deep breathing.
    2. Assess for signs and symptoms of tolerance.
    3. Ensure that pain is 7 or higher on a 0 to 10 pain scale.
    4. Monitor for a respiratory rate fewer than 10 breaths/minute.

28. A nurse is caring for a client in the intensive care unit who has been exhibiting clinical indicators of sleep deprivation. Which interventions should the nurse implement to assist this client to remain asleep? **Select all that apply.**
    1. Group care into blocks of time.
    2. Encourage naps during the day.
    3. Implement the client's bedtime ritual.
    4. Avoid unnecessary environmental noise.
    5. Provide a back rub at the client's bedtime.

29. A nurse is caring for an older adult male who was admitted to the hospital with an exacerbation of rheumatoid arthritis. The nurse interviewed the client, performed a physical assessment, and reviewed the client's clinical record. Based on the data collected, what statement is **most** likely related to this client's situation?
    1. Lack of sleep because of noise made by a roommate has made him irritable.
    2. The multiplicity of stresses may have reduced the client's tolerance to pain.
    3. The dose of the client's pain medication should be increased to provide pain relief.
    4. He is experiencing respiratory depression due to excessive amounts of pain medication.

Client's Clinical Record

Client Interview

Client states that his wife of 52 years died 3 months ago after a sudden heart attack. He said that she took care of him and that he had to put his house up for sale and move to a nursing home because he could not take care of himself. He shared that finances are tight and that he could not afford to pay for a private room. He currently shares a room with another man who snores a lot at night, making it difficult for him to sleep. He said that he is able to take a few naps during the day. He is estranged from his son, an only child, because they quarrelled over the details of his wife's burial and the sale of the house.

Client Assessment

Client is rubbing his knees with the palms of his hands and says that they hurt on a level 3 all the time, even with pain medication. He said that when his wife was alive he was able to deal with the pain but since she passed away he has experienced more pain in his knees. The knees appear slightly swollen, erythema is present, and they are warm to the touch. Temperature is 100.2°F, pulse is 78 beats/minute, respirations are 14 breaths/minute, blood pressure is 110/60 mm Hg. IV fluids running as prescribed; IV site is clean, dry, and intact.

Primary Health-Care Provider's Prescriptions

Regular diet.
Activity as tolerated.
Physical therapy consult.
CBC with differential, basic metabolic panel, rheumatoid factor, antinuclear antibody, sedimentation rate, C-reactive protein.
Celecoxib (Celebrex) 200 mg PO daily.
Hydrocortisone (Solu-Cortef) 60 mg IVPB every 12 hours.
Oxycodone/acetaminophen (Percocet) 5 mg/325 mg, 1 tablet for moderate joint pain every 4 hours prn
Hydromorphone (Dilaudid) 2 mg Sub-Q every 4 hours, prn for severe joint pain.
Docusate sodium (Colace) 100 mg PO twice daily.

30. A nurse is caring for a client who reports restless leg syndrome. Which nursing intervention should help reduce unpleasant sensations related to this sleep disorder?
    1. Wrapping the client's legs with ace bandages snugly before sleeping
    2. Teaching the client how to perform stretching exercises of the legs
    3. Encouraging the client to drink warm tea before bedtime
    4. Assisting the client to implement a weight loss program

31. A client has a prescription for hydromorphone (Dilaudid) 1.5 mg Sub-Q every 4 hours prn for moderate pain. Hydromorphone is available in 1 mg per mL. How many mL should the nurse administer? **Record you answer using one decimal place.**
    Answer: _____ mL

32. A nurse is teaching a client about the acetaminophen prescribed to relieve mild pain. Which information is important to include in this discussion? **Select all that apply.**
    1. Avoid hazardous activities.
    2. Do not exceed the prescribed dose.
    3. Use a stool softener when taking this medication.
    4. Advise the client to avoid alcohol when taking this medication.
    5. Instruct the client to immediately report a rash and stop taking the medication.

33. A nurse is caring for an adult who is receiving an opioid Sub-Q every 6 hours prn for pain. Place the following statements in sequence according to the nursing process.
    1. Evaluate the effectiveness of the opioid.
    2. The client will report that the pain level is tolerable.
    3. Pain is a level 8 on a pain scale of 0 to 10, with 10 being the most severe pain.
    4. Administer the opioid according to the primary health-care provider's prescription.
    5. Acute pain related to tissue trauma and reflex muscle spasms secondary to surgery.
    Answer: _____

34. A nurse suspects that a client is experiencing bruxism. Which question should the nurse ask the client?
    1. "Do you walk in your sleep?"
    2. "Do you urinate in your sleep?"
    3. "Do you grind your teeth at night?"
    4. "Do you awaken from sleep with panicky screams?"

35. A client who is cachectic reports hip discomfort when attempting to sleep. What should the nurse do to limit this discomfort?
    1. Place trochanter rolls on the lateral side of each of the client's hips when in bed.
    2. Request that a mild analgesic be prescribed for the client prior to bedtime.
    3. Arrange for a pillow-top mattress to be placed on the client's bed.
    4. Manipulate environmental factors that will promote client rest.

REVIEW ANSWERS AND RATIONALES

1. **ANSWER: 1, 2, 4.**
   Rationales:
   1. Obesity is a risk factor for sleep apnea because of excessive tissue in the neck area and soft palate. In extreme cases a uvulopalatoplasty is performed; this surgery revises the soft palate to prevent tissue from blocking the airway.
   2. Positioning may help to keep the tongue, tonsils, adenoids, or soft palette from obstructing the airway, thereby providing for more restful sleep.
   3. Breathing exercises will not help to minimize airway obstruction when sleeping. The client does not need to be more relaxed to sleep. The client needs the airway to be patent.
   4. A continuous positive airway pressure (CPAP) machine has either a mask worn over the nose or prongs positioned in the nostrils. It increases the amount of air entering the respiratory tract through continuous positive airway pressure. CPAP also helps prevent airway collapse during exhalation.
   5. Several pillows under the head may cause flexion of the head, further obstructing the airway. Pillows placed under the shoulders and head may help to maintain an open airway.
   TEST-TAKING TIP: Identify the clang associations. The word *weight* in the stem and option 1 and the word *sleep* in the stem and in option 4 are clang association. Examine options 1 and 4 carefully.
   Content Area: Pain, Comfort, Rest, and Sleep
   Integrated Processes: Teaching/Learning; Nursing Process: Implementation
   Client Need: Physiological Integrity; Basic Care and Comfort
   Cognitive Level: Application
   Concept: Sleep and Rest

2. **ANSWER: 3.**
   Rationales:
   1. Pain that radiates to the sternal area of the chest usually originates in the stomach.
   2. Pain that radiates to the right groin area usually originates in the appendix, kidneys, or ureters.
   3. Sensory innervation of the gallbladder is provided by the right phrenic nerve (C3, 4, and 5). An inflamed gallbladder may irritate this nerve so that pain is referred to the right shoulder.
   4. Pain that radiates to the left arm usually originates in the heart.
   Content Area: Pain, Comfort, Rest, and Sleep
   Integrated Processes: Communication/Documentation; Nursing Process: Assessment
   Client Need: Physiological Integrity; Basic Care and Comfort
   Cognitive Level: Analysis
   Concept: Comfort

3. **ANSWER: 4.**
   Rationales:
   1. An open-ended question in a potential emergency situation may not gather pertinent information.
   2. Alerting the rapid response team is premature at this time.
   3. Although obtaining the client's vital signs is an appropriate intervention and should be done eventually, it is premature at this time.
   4. This response gathers more specific information from the client. The location, intensity, and characteristics of the pain should be assessed first.
   TEST-TAKING TIP: Identify the word in the stem that sets a priority. The word *most* in the stem sets a priority. Identify options with clang associations. The words *heart hurts* in the stem and in option 1 and the word *hurts* in the stem and in option 4 are clang associations. Consider options 1 and 4 carefully.
   Content Area: Pain, Comfort, Rest, and Sleep
   Integrated Processes: Communication/Documentation; Nursing Process: Assessment
   Client Need: Physiological Integrity; Basic Care and Comfort
   Cognitive Level: Application
   Concept: Comfort

4. **ANSWER: 1.**
   Rationales:
   1. Role-playing enables the child to learn what will happen; it provides an opportunity for the nurse to allay the child's fears and for the child to ask questions and receive answers in a nonthreatening environment. The procedure should be less frightening and threatening when a school-aged child knows what to expect.
   2. Asking if the child has any questions is not as good as a response presented in another option. The school-aged child may not know what to ask about the procedure.
   3. Stating that the child needs to be strong denies the child's feelings.
   4. Although playing a disk with the child's favorite songs during the procedure may be done, it is not the best intervention presented in the options.
   TEST-TAKING TIP: Identify the word in the stem that sets a priority. The word *best* in the stem sets a priority. Identify the statement that denies the child's feelings, needs, or concerns. Option 3 denies the feelings that a school-aged child would most likely have regarding an unfamiliar and potentially uncomfortable procedure.
   Content Area: Pain, Comfort, Rest, and Sleep
   Integrated Processes: Caring; Communication/Documentation; Nursing Process: Implementation
   Client Need: Physiological Integrity; Reduction of Risk Potential
   Cognitive Level: Application
   Concept: Patient-Centered Care

5. **ANSWER: 3.**
   Rationales:
   1. Cutaneous pain is associated with superficial cuts of the skin or subcutaneous tissue.
   2. Radiating pain is when pain arises in one site and extends to another site. For example, sciatic pain from the lumbar vertebrae or pain associated with lymphatic streaking.
   3. When heart ischemia is felt as pain in the jaw, it is identified as referred pain. Referred pain occurs when pain arises in one site but is felt in a distant site.

4. Visceral pain occurs when deep internal pain receptors are stimulated, such as during labor or in response to cancer of the abdominal organs.
Content Area: Pain, Comfort, Rest, and Sleep
Integrated Processes: Communication/Documentation; Nursing Process: Assessment
Client Need: Safe and Effective Care Environment; Management of Care
Cognitive Level: Knowledge
Concept: Comfort

6. **ANSWER: 2, 4.**
Rationales:
1. Pressured speech occurs with acute pain because it tends to accompany a crisis. A slow monotonous speech pattern is associated with chronic pain because chronic pain is debilitating, depleting physical and emotional resources; clients may become apathetic, stoical, or resigned to the pain.
2. **Constriction of the pupils occurs with chronic pain because of the action of the parasympathetic nervous system. Dilation of the pupils occurs with acute pain because of the action of the sympathetic nervous system.**
3. An increased heart rate occurs with acute pain because of the action of the sympathetic nervous system. A decreased heart rate occurs with chronic pain because of the action of the parasympathetic nervous system.
4. **A decreased blood pressure occurs with chronic pain because of the action of the parasympathetic nervous system. An increase in blood pressure is associated with acute pain because of the action of the sympathetic nervous system.**
5. An increase in the respiratory rate (tachypnea) occurs with acute pain because of the action of the sympathetic nervous system. The breathing rate may slow with chronic pain because of the action of the parasympathetic nervous system.
Content Area: Pain, Comfort, Rest, and Sleep
Integrated Processes: Nursing Process: Assessment
Client Need: Physiological Integrity; Basic Care and Comfort
Cognitive Level: Analysis
Concept: Comfort

7. **ANSWER: 2, 5.**
Rationales:
1. Direct extension of pain from one area (vertebrae) to another (sciatic nerve) is called radiating pain.
2. **Phantom sensation/pain is discomfort arising from a site that has been surgically removed. The discomfort is perceived as being in the part of the body that no longer exists.**
3. A myocardial infarction is associated with referred pain; it may feel as though the pain is originating in areas such as the jaw, left arm, or center of back.
4. Acute appendicitis may precipitate pain at McBurney's point, a site halfway between the umbilicus and the right anterior iliac crest. This is an example of referred pain.
5. **Phantom sensation/pain is discomfort arising from a site that has been traumatically or surgically removed. The discomfort is perceived as being in the part of the body that no longer exists.**

Content Area: Pain, Comfort, Rest, and Sleep
Integrated Processes: Nursing Process: Analysis
Client Need: Physiological Integrity; Basic Care and Comfort
Cognitive Level: Analysis
Concept: Comfort

8. **ANSWER: 3.**
Rationales:
1. Although this concept is important, it is not as important as the concept in another option.
2. Although this concept is important, it is not as important as the concept in another option.
3. **Receiving pain medication before the pain becomes intense is an important concept for the client to understand. Research demonstrates that medicating a client for pain before it becomes intense avoids the highs and lows of pain levels and maintains a tolerable consistent level, which is more effective in controlling pain, requiring less medication overall.**
4. An extra dose of medication is delivered only when the trigger is activated after the lockout time has expired and not before.
TEST-TAKING TIP: Identify the word in the stem that sets a priority. The word *most* in the stem sets a priority. Identify the unique option. Option 3 is unique because it is the only statement that does not directly relate to the functioning of the patient-controlled analgesia machine. Option 3 is a general principle about pain. Identify the option with a clang association. The word *pain* in the stem and in option 3 is a clang association. Examine option 3 carefully.
Content Area: Pain, Comfort, Rest, and Sleep
Integrated Processes: Teaching/Learning; Nursing Process: Implementation
Client Need: Physiological Integrity; Pharmacological and Parenteral Therapies
Cognitive Level: Application
Concept: Comfort

9. **ANSWER: 3.**
Rationales:
1. Friction, employing continuous, small, circular movements on either side of vertebrae from the shoulders to the small of the back and then from the small of the back to the shoulders, promotes circulation. It generally does not produce relaxation.
2. Pétrissage, kneading of skin and shoulder muscles, promotes circulation. It generally does not promote relaxation.
3. **Effleurage, long, smooth strokes with gentle pressure that slide over skin from the small of the back to the shoulders, promotes relaxation and circulation to the skin.**
4. Feathering, long, soft, fingertip strokes from shoulders to the small of the back, promotes relaxation. It generally does not increase circulation.
TEST-TAKING TIP: Identify the word in the stem that sets a priority. The word *most* in the stem sets a priority.
Content Area: Pain, Comfort, Rest, and Sleep
Integrated Processes: Nursing Process: Implementation
Client Need: Physiological Integrity; Basic Care and Comfort
Cognitive Level: Analysis
Concept: Sleep and Rest

10. **ANSWER: 1.**

Rationales:

1. Toddlers perceive pain as a threat to their safety and security. Holding the toddler provides comfort and emotional support.

2. The use of a sucrose pacifier is more appropriate for infants rather than toddlers.

3. Toddlers should be permitted to cope with discomfort in their own way. Although they may cry, they also may respond by struggling against the provider of care or use physical or verbal aggression.

4. Obtaining a prescription for an opioid may be unnecessary. Other nonprescription interventions should be attempted first. If a medication is prescribed, opioids should be used as a last resort after other analgesics.

TEST-TAKING TIP: Identify the word in the stem that sets a priority. The word *best* in the stem sets a priority. Identify the options with clang associations. Options 1 and 3 and the stem contain the word *child,* which are clang associations. Examine these two options carefully. More often than not, an option with a clang association is the correct answer.

Content Area: Pain, Comfort, Rest, and Sleep
Integrated Processes: Caring; Nursing Process: Implementation
Client Need: Physiological Integrity; Basic Care and Comfort
Cognitive Level: Application
Concept: Comfort

11. **ANSWER: 1, 3, 4, 5.**

Rationales:

1. Acute pain usually has an abrupt onset, may be severe, and requires a diagnostic workup to determine its cause; these factors increase anxiety.

2. An apathetic facial expression often is associated with chronic pain because chronic pain is debilitating, depleting physical and emotional resources; apathy and resignation are common responses to chronic pain.

3. Acute pain usually responds to the administration of analgesics, whereas chronic pain may not. Chronic pain may require multiple modalities to relieve pain.

4. Behavioral responses (e.g., grimacing, wincing, groaning, crying) often occur with acute pain because it is related to a new situation. People with chronic pain due to a lifelong condition reach a point where they become apathetic, resigned, or develop coping mechanisms other than overt signs of pain.

5. Acute pain is always related to body tissue changes. Chronic pain may not be related to tissue damage.

TEST-TAKING TIP: Identify the options that are opposites. Options 2 and 4 are opposites. One or the other should be eliminated; rarely are both opposite options correct answers in this type of question. Identify the clang associations. The word *pain* in the stem and in options 1, 4 and 5 are clang associations. Examine these options carefully.

Content Area: Pain, Comfort, Rest, and Sleep
Integrated Processes: Nursing Process: Assessment
Client Need: Physiological Integrity; Basic Care and Comfort
Cognitive Level: Analysis
Concept: Comfort

12. **ANSWER: 4.**

Rationales:

1. Washing the hands is not the first thing that the nurse should do before administering a back rub.

2. Warming the lotion is not the first thing that the nurse should do before administering a back rub.

3. Pulling the curtain for privacy is not the first thing that the nurse should do before administering a back rub.

4. The stimulation of a back rub may not be tolerated by some clients. A back rub is contraindicated when a client has certain conditions, such as impaired skin integrity (e.g., pressure ulcer, burn, or open wound), rib fractures, or a vertebral disorder or within 48 hours of experiencing the onset of an acute neurological or cardiac problem.

TEST-TAKING TIP: Identify the word in the stem that sets a priority. The word *first* in the stem sets a priority. Identify the option that is unique. Option 4 is unique. It is the only option that is not a physical action associated with providing direct care to the client.

Content Area: Pain, Comfort, Rest, and Sleep
Integrated Processes: Nursing Process: Planning
Client Need: Physiological Integrity; Basic Care and Comfort
Cognitive Level: Application
Concept: Comfort

13. **ANSWER: 4.**

Rationales:

1. Sleep and rest both prevent fatigue.

2. Sleep and rest both slow vital signs.

3. Sleep and rest both conserve energy.

4. Reduced perception occurs with sleep, but not with rest, because the client is unconscious.

TEST-TAKING TIP: Identify the equally plausible options. Options 1 and 3 are equally plausible. One is no better than the other. Eliminate both from further consideration.

Content Area: Pain, Comfort, Rest, and Sleep
Integrated Processes: Nursing Process: Evaluation
Client Need: Physiological Integrity; Basic Care and Comfort
Cognitive Level: Analysis
Concept: Sleep and Rest

14. **ANSWER: 3, 4.**

Rationales:

1. NREM sleep deficiency precipitates physiological deficiencies, such as fatigue and lethargy.

2. NREM sleep deficiency precipitates physiological deficiencies, such as tremors.

3. REM sleep deficiency precipitates cognitive, emotional, and behavioral changes that include disorientation. Also, the person may experience anxiety, apathy, an inability to concentrate, delusions, hallucinations, and/or paranoia.

4. REM sleep deficiency precipitates cognitive, emotional, and behavioral changes that include combativeness and irritability.

5. NREM sleep deficiency precipitates physiological deficiencies, such as immunosuppression and delayed wound healing.

6. NREM sleep deficiency precipitates physiological deficiencies, such as increased sensitivity to pain.

TEST-TAKING TIP: Identify the options that are unique. Options 2 and 3 are unique and relate to each other within the cognitive/behavioral domain. Options 1, 4, and 5 are unique and relate to each other within the physiological domain. If you know the effects of deficient REM or NREM sleep, you can narrow down the options to the correct answers.

Content Area: Pain, Comfort, Rest, and Sleep
Integrated Processes: Nursing Process: Assessment
Client Need: Physiological Integrity; Basic Care and Comfort
Cognitive Level: Analysis
Concept: Sleep and Rest

15. **ANSWER: 3, 4.**
    Rationales:
    1. Grinding the teeth while sleeping is bruxism. It may include repetitive clenching of teeth; it can erode tooth enamel, loosen teeth, and cause pain in the jaw.
    2. Snoring is a clinical indicator of obstructive sleep apnea, not narcolepsy.
    3. Abruptly falling asleep unexpectedly is a clinical indicator of narcolepsy. Additional clinical indicators include slurred speech and abrupt bilateral loss of muscle tone (cataplexy). The client may report weakness of the knees, an inability to move during the onset of a sleep attack (sleep paralysis), and vivid or bizarre dreams while falling asleep. These clinical indicators are the result of the sleep cycle beginning with the REM rather than the NREM stage of sleep for people with narcolepsy.
    4. An inability to move upon awakening is a common symptom of narcolepsy. It is called sleep paralysis. This clinical indicator is the result of the sleep cycle beginning with the REM rather than the NREM stage of sleep for people with narcolepsy.
    5. Episodic walking around while asleep with minimal awareness of the environment is sleepwalking (somnambulism), not narcolepsy.

    Content Area: Pain, Comfort, Rest, and Sleep
    Integrated Processes: Communication/Documentation; Nursing Process: Assessment
    Client Need: Physiological Integrity; Basic Care and Comfort
    Cognitive Level: Application
    Concept: Sleep and Rest

16. **ANSWER: 4.**
    Rationales:
    1. When the eyes are closed, the individual may be resting or sleeping. The client may have the eyes closed when engaged in such activities as praying and imagery.
    2. Appearing physically at ease with a reduction in muscle tension can occur with both rest and sleep.
    3. A client may keep the arms at the side of the body when either resting or sleeping.
    4. A client will experience altered levels of consciousness when sleeping, with a lack of response to insignificant environmental noises. A client at rest will be alert and have no altered level of consciousness.

    TEST-TAKING TIP: Identify the word in the stem that sets a priority. The word *best* in the stem sets a priority.

    Content Area: Pain, Comfort, Rest, and Sleep
    Integrated Processes: Nursing Process: Evaluation

Client Need: Physiological Integrity; Basic Care and Comfort
Cognitive Level: Application
Concept: Sleep and Rest

17. **ANSWER: 2.**
    Rationales:
    1. Not being pregnant is an outcome associated with contraceptive therapy, not palliative therapy. Contraceptive therapy prevents a pregnancy.
    2. Pain that has subsided to a tolerable level is an outcome that reflects palliative care, whereby the illness is not cured, but relief of signs and symptoms make the illness more tolerable.
    3. When a client has no clinical manifestations of an infection it reflects an outcome associated with curative care, not palliative care. Curative care completely resolves an illness.
    4. A blood glucose level returning to the normal range is an outcome associated with health maintenance or substitutive medication therapy, whereby a medication is administered to support normal body function (e.g., regular insulin for diabetes).

    Content Area: Pain, Comfort, Rest, and Sleep
    Integrated Processes: Nursing Process: Evaluation
    Client Need: Physiological Integrity; Pharmacological and Parenteral Therapies
    Cognitive Level: Application
    Concept: Medication; Comfort

18. **ANSWER: 1, 2, 4.**
    Rationales:
    1. The feeling of pins and needles generally is associated with neuropathic pain. Neuropathic pain is caused by nerve fibers that are damaged or dysfunctional, which can occur in either the peripheral or central nervous system.
    2. A lack of sensation (numbness) generally is associated with neuropathic pain due to dysfunctional nerve fibers.
    3. Pain described as pounding generally results from stimulation of pain receptors at the site of trauma, ischemia, or inflammation. Also, it is associated with pain from internal organs and pain from skin, connective tissue, muscles, and bones.
    4. A burning sensation generally is associated with neuropathic pain due to dysfunctional nerve fibers.
    5. An aching sensation generally results from stimulation of pain receptors at the site of trauma, ischemia, or inflammation. Also, it is associated with pain from internal organs and pain from skin, connective tissue, muscles, and bones.

    Content Area: Pain, Comfort, Rest, and Sleep
    Integrated Processes: Communication/Documentation; Nursing Process: Assessment
    Client Need: Physiological Integrity; Basic Care and Comfort
    Cognitive Level: Application
    Concept: Comfort

19. **ANSWER: 1.**
    Rationales:
    1. Adolescents generally want to appear brave in front of others, especially peers. Stating that it is OK to cry is

client centered because it gives the adolescent permission to cry when confronted with pain.
2. Although pulling the curtain addresses the privacy needs of an adolescent, it is not as important as a statement presented in another option.
3. Although stating "If you experience any pain, it is not because we are trying to punish you" may be verbalized, it is not as important as a statement presented in another option. Toddlers, not adolescents, may consider pain as punishment.
4. Stating "I know that you want to be brave, so we will do this as quickly as possible" is not a client-centered statement. This statement places the nurse's beliefs onto the client as well as presents an expected client response that may be unrealistic.

TEST-TAKING TIP: Identify the word in the stem that sets a priority. The word *most* in the stem sets a priority.
Content Area: Pain, Comfort, Rest, and Sleep
Integrated Processes: Caring, Communication/ Documentation; Nursing Process: Implementation
Client Need: Physiological Integrity; Basic Care and Comfort
Cognitive Level: Application
Concept: Stress

20. **ANSWER: 1.**
Rationales:
1. **Asking, "What does the pain feel like?" is a question that assesses the quality of the pain. Descriptions generally include such words as burning, stabbing, throbbing, crushing, pressure, sharp, dull, achy, and so on.**
2. A question that assesses intensity is "How severe is your pain on a scale of 0 to 10?" A numerical scale provides objective and consistent assessment of pain intensity.
3. The question in the stem does not assess behavioral responses to pain. Observing moaning, grunting, crying, increased muscle tension, hand wringing, guarding, holding or rubbing a part of the body, and so on are examples of observed behaviors associated with a painful experience.
4. A question that assesses precipitating factors is "What initiates or increases the pain?" Participating factors may include such actions as bending, lifting, coughing, eating, or breathing deeply.
Content Area: Pain, Comfort, Rest, and Sleep
Integrated Processes: Communication/Documentation; Nursing Process: Assessment
Client Need: Physiological Integrity; Basic Care and Comfort
Cognitive Level: Application
Concept: Comfort

21. **ANSWER: 1.**
Rationales:
1. **It is essential that clients know that nurses believe that they are experiencing pain and that the pain is real.**
2. Although breathing exercises may reduce the client's pain, they are not as important as another option.
3. Although a distraction technique may reduce the client's pain, it is not as important as another option.
4. Although muscle relaxation techniques may reduce the client's pain, they are not as important as another option.

TEST-TAKING TIP: Identify the word in the stem that sets a priority. The word *most* in the stem sets a priority. Identify the clang association. The word *pain* in the stem and in option 1 is a clang association. Identify equally plausible options. Options 2, 3, and 4 are strategies to manage pain. Option 1 is the only option that acknowledges the client's painful experience. Option 1 is unique and reflects nursing care that is client centered.
Content Area: Pain, Comfort, Rest, and Sleep
Integrated Processes: Caring; Communication/ Documentation; Nursing Process: Implementation
Client Need: Psychosocial Integrity
Cognitive Level: Application
Concept: Comfort

22. **ANSWER: 1, 4, 5.**
Rationales:
1. **A gradual onset is associated with chronic pain. A quick onset is associated with acute pain.**
2. Constricted, not dilated, pupils are related to stimulation of the parasympathetic nervous system associated with chronic pain. Dilated pupils are related to stimulation of the sympathetic nervous system associated with acute pain.
3. Pressured speech is related to stimulation of the sympathetic nervous system associated with acute pain. Slow, monotonous speech is associated with chronic pain in response to stimulation of the parasympathetic nervous system.
4. **Recurring pain is associated with remissions and exacerbations, which are related to chronic pain. Chronic pain is related to a time frame longer than 6 months.**
5. **Variable breathing patterns are associated with chronic pain in response to stimulation of the parasympathetic nervous system. Hyperpnea is related to acute pain in response to stimulation of the sympathetic nervous system.**
Content Area: Pain, Comfort, Rest, and Sleep
Integrated Processes: Nursing Process: Assessment
Client Need: Physiological Integrity; Basic Care and Comfort
Cognitive Level: Analysis
Concept: Comfort

23. **ANSWER: 2, 5.**
Rationales:
1. Alcohol should be avoided because it contributes to early awakening. Also, it has a diuretic effect, which may cause nocturia that will interrupt sleeping.
2. **A warm bath should be encouraged because it reduces muscle tension and facilitates relaxation.**
3. Milk at bedtime may be encouraged, not avoided. L-tryptophan in milk converts to melatonin, which maintains the body's circadian rhythms and promotes sleep.
4. The bed should only be used for sleeping and sexual activity. A person should get out of bed if not asleep within 30 minutes and return to bed when sleepy. This trains the body and mind to associate a bed with sleeping.
5. **Rituals and routines promote comfort and relaxation. Also, they precipitate the expectation that sleep will follow.**

Content Area: Pain, Comfort, Rest, and Sleep
Integrated Processes: Teaching/Learning; Nursing Process: Implementation
Client Need: Physiological Integrity; Basic Care and Comfort
Cognitive Level: Application
Concept: Patient-Centered Care; Sleep and Rest

24. **ANSWER: 4.**
    Rationales:
    1. Reacting normally when awakened and paradoxical sleep is associated with REM sleep stage 5.
    2. Light sleep and easy to awaken is associated with NREM sleep stage 1.
    3. Light sleep and easy to awaken is associated with NREM sleep stage 2.
    4. Deep sleep and difficulty awakening is associated with NREM sleep stage 4.
    Content Area: Pain, Comfort, Rest, and Sleep
    Integrated Processes: Nursing Process: Assessment
    Client Need: Physiological Integrity; Basic Care and Comfort
    Cognitive Level: Analysis
    Concept: Sleep and Rest

25. **ANSWER: 2, 4, 5.**
    Rationales:
    1. Daytime naps should be avoided unless they are less than 20 to 30 minutes. Excessive napping contributes to insomnia at night.
    2. Nicotine is stimulating. The half-life of nicotine is 1 to 2 hours.
    3. Physical exertion should be avoided 1 to 2 hours before bedtime because it is too stimulating.
    4. Caffeine is stimulating and should be avoided 4 hours before bedtime.
    5. Carbohydrates limit the sensation of hunger, which provides for comfort; protein reduces the sugar boost of the carbohydrates.
    Content Area: Pain, Comfort, Rest, and Sleep
    Integrated Processes: Teaching/Learning; Nursing Process: Implementation
    Client Need: Physiological Integrity; Basic Care and Comfort
    Cognitive Level: Application
    Concept: Patient-Centered Care; Sleep and Rest

26. **ANSWER: 1.**
    Rationales:
    1. An increase in falls is associated with older adults receiving alprazolam (Xanax). Alprazolam, a benzodiazepine, depresses the central nervous system, which may cause impaired coordination, drowsiness, fatigue, confusion, and tremors.
    2. The blood pressure decreases, not increases, in response to alprazolam (Xanax) because it may cause central nervous system depression.
    3. Monitoring for clinical indicators of dependence is not the priority at this time. Receiving alprazolam (Xanax) longer than 2 weeks may lead to dependence.

4. Alprazolam (Xanax) should be discontinued slowly, not immediately, to prevent signs and symptoms of withdrawal.
TEST-TAKING TIP: Identify the word in the stem that sets a priority. The word *most* in the stem sets a priority.
Content Area: Pain, Comfort, Rest, and Sleep
Integrated Processes: Nursing Process: Implementation
Client Need: Physiological Integrity; Pharmacological and Parenteral Therapies
Cognitive Level: Application
Concept: Medication; Safety

27. **ANSWER: 4.**
    Rationales:
    1. Although encouraging coughing and deep breathing should be done to prevent hypostatic pneumonia, it is not the priority.
    2. Although assessing for signs and symptoms of tolerance should be done because tolerance can occur with an opioid, it is not the priority.
    3. Codeine, a low-dose opioid, is prescribed for mild pain generally reported as 4 to 6 on a 0 to 10 pain rating scale. A client prescribed codeine for pain should be medicated when pain is rated as 4 before pain becomes more intense. Doing so helps codeine to be more effective than when pain is at the high end of a pain rating scale. Pain rated as 7 is considered severe pain and requires a high-dose opioid such as hydrocodone, methadone, morphine sulfate, or oxycodone.
    4. Codeine depresses respirations. If a client experiences a respiratory rate of less than 10 breaths per minute, withhold the next dose and notify the primary health-care provider about the status of the client. The dose of the codeine should be reduced or a prescription for a different medication may be necessary.
    TEST-TAKING TIP: Identify the word in the stem that sets a priority. The word *most* in the stem sets a priority.
    Content Area: Pain, Comfort, Rest, and Sleep
    Integrated Processes: Nursing Process: Evaluation
    Client Need: Physiological Integrity; Pharmacological and Parenteral Therapies
    Cognitive Level: Application
    Concept: Medication; Oxygenation

28. **ANSWER: 1, 4.**
    Rationales:
    1. Frequent awakenings to implement nursing care generally are the underlying cause of sleep deprivation in critical care environments. Clustering nursing care provides blocks of uninterrupted periods of time in which the client can attempt to sleep.
    2. Encouraging naps during the day will not help the client remain asleep.
    3. Although supporting a bedtime ritual may help a client fall asleep, it does not support uninterrupted sleep.
    4. Noise stimulates the mind. Therefore, it is important to maintain as quiet an environment as possible to calm the mind, which facilitates uninterrupted sleep.

5. Although a back rub may relax a client and facilitate falling asleep, this intervention will not facilitate uninterrupted sleep.
Content Area: Pain, Comfort, Rest, and Sleep
Integrated Processes: Nursing Process: Implementation
Client Need: Physiological Integrity; Basic Care and Comfort
Cognitive Level: Application
Concept: Sleep and Rest

29. ANSWER: 2.

Rationales:

1. There is no evidence in the client interview that indicates that the client is irritable.
2. Multiplicity of stress can overwhelm a client physically and emotionally, reducing a client's pain threshold.
3. A pain level of 3 is within the realm of pain that a person should be able to tolerate. The client's respirations are 14 breaths/minute. A larger or more frequent dose of an opioid will depress the central nervous system, causing respiratory depression, and should be avoided. In addition, opioids can precipitate constipation, hypotension, drowsiness, and confusion.
4. The expected range of respirations for an adult is 12 to 20 breaths/minute. The client's respiratory rate is 14 breaths per minute. If the respirations are less than 10 breaths/minute, the next dose of the opioid should be held and the primary health-care provider notified. The opioid dose may need to be adjusted or the medication changed. In extreme situations, the antidote naloxone (Narcan) may be required.
TEST-TAKING TIP: Identify the word in the stem that sets a priority. The word *most* in the stem sets a priority.
Content Area: Pain, Comfort, Rest, and Sleep
Integrated Processes: Communication/ Documentation; Nursing Process: Analysis
Client Need: Physiological Integrity; Pharmacological and Parenteral Therapies
Cognitive Level: Analysis
Concept: Patient-Centered Care; Stress

30. ANSWER: 2.

Rationales:

1. Wrapping the legs with ace bandages is not associated with reducing unpleasant sensations of restless leg syndrome.
2. Stretching exercises of the leg muscles often provide some relief of the unpleasant tingling, itching, creeping, and crawling sensations associated with restless leg syndrome.
3. Tea contains caffeine, which is a stimulant, and should be avoided in clients with restless leg syndrome.
4. Excessive weight is associated with sleep apnea, not restless leg syndrome.
TEST-TAKING TIP: Identify the clang associations. The word *leg* in the stem and the word *legs* in options 1 and 2 are clang associations. Examine options 1 and 2 carefully.
Content Area: Pain, Comfort, Rest, and Sleep
Integrated Processes: Teaching/Learning; Nursing Process: Implementation

Client Need: Physiological Integrity; Basic Care and Comfort
Cognitive Level: Application
Concept: Sleep and Rest

31. ANSWER: 1.5.
Rationale:
Solve the problem by using the formula for ratio and proportion.

$$\frac{\text{Desire 1.5 mg}}{\text{Have 1 mg}} = \frac{x \text{ mL}}{1 \text{ mL}}$$
$$1x = 1.5 \times 1$$
$$1x = 1.5$$
$$x = 1.5 \div 1$$
$$x = 1.5 \text{ mL}$$

Content Area: Pain, Comfort, Rest, and Sleep
Integrated Processes: Nursing Process: Planning
Client Need: Physiological Integrity; Pharmacological and Parenteral Therapies
Cognitive Level: Application
Concept: Medication; Comfort

32. ANSWER: 2, 4, 5.

Rationales:

1. Avoiding hazardous activities is unnecessary. Acetaminophen does not depress the central nervous system.
2. Intake of greater than 4 g of acetaminophen in 24 hours may cause liver damage.
3. Constipation is not related to the intake of acetaminophen.
4. Ingesting alcohol with acetaminophen can increase the risk of liver damage.
5. A rash when taking acetaminophen is associated with two of the most serious, rare skin conditions. Stevens-Johnson Syndrome (SJS) and toxic epidermal necrolysis (TEN) usually require hospitalization and can cause death.
Content Area: Pain, Comfort, Rest, and Sleep
Integrated Processes: Teaching/Learning; Nursing Process: Implementation
Client Need: Physiological Integrity; Pharmacological and Parenteral Therapies
Cognitive Level: Application
Concept: Medication; Safety

33. ANSWER: 3, 5, 2, 4, 1.

Rationales:

3. The first step in the nursing process is assessment. The client's pain is a level 8.
5. The second step in the nursing process is identifying the problem. The problem is that the client is experiencing acute pain related to tissue trauma and reflex muscle spasms secondary to surgery.
2. The third step in the nursing process is planning. Planning includes identifying the expected outcome and planned interventions.
4. The fourth step of the nursing process is implementation. Administering the opioid according to the primary health-care provider's prescription is an action that should achieve the expected outcome.

1. The fifth and last step of the nursing process is evaluation. Evaluating the effectiveness of the administered opioid requires the nurse to reassess the client's pain to ensure that the expected outcome was achieved.
Content Area: Pain, Comfort, Rest, and Sleep
Integrated Processes: Nursing Process: Planning
Client Need: Physiological Integrity; Pharmacological and Parenteral Therapies
Cognitive Level: Analysis
Concept: Patient-Centered Care; Medication

34. ANSWER: 3.

Rationales:

1. Episodic walking around while asleep with minimal awareness of surroundings is called somnambulism (sleep walking). It occurs during stage 3 or 4 NREM sleep and lasts 3 minutes or longer.

2. Repeated episodes of involuntary urination when sleeping after toilet training is well established is called nocturnal enuresis (bed wetting). It occurs when arousing from stages 3 and 4 NREM sleep, 1 to 2 hours after falling asleep.

3. Bruxism is the repetitive clenching and grinding of the teeth when sleeping. Episodes usually occur during stage 2 NREM sleep and last 4 to 5 seconds. It is associated with increased stress, abnormal bite, and gastrointestinal disorders.

4. Repeated episodes of abrupt awakening along with panicky screams is called sleep terrors (night terrors). It occurs during stage 4 NREM sleep and lasts from 10 to 30 minutes.

Content Area: Pain, Comfort, Rest, and Sleep
Integrated Processes: Communication and Documentation; Nursing Process: Assessment
Client Need: Physiological Integrity; Basic Care and Comfort
Cognitive Level: Application
Concept: Sleep and Rest

35. ANSWER: 3.

Rationales:

1. Trochanter rolls prevent external rotation of the hips, not discomfort related to cachexia.

2. Analgesics should be used as a last resort. Other interventions should be attempted first.

3. Clients who are cachectic have little body fat and subcutaneous tissue to pad bony prominences. A pillow-top mattress will provide padding to limit discomfort from lying on a flat surface.

4. Although manipulating environmental factors should be done (e.g., comfortable room temperature, dimmed lights, limited noise), these factors do not address the specific problem the client has reported.

Content Area: Pain, Comfort, Rest, and Sleep
Integrated Processes: Communication and Documentation; Nursing Process: Implementation
Client Need: Physiological Integrity; Basic Care and Comfort
Cognitive Level: Application
Concept: Comfort

Chapter 16

Inflammation, Infection, Immunity, and Wound Care

KEY TERMS

Active immunity—Antibodies are formed within the body

Bacterium (pl. bacteria)—Single-celled microorganism that replicates independently outside of cells with the appropriate environment

Carrier—Person who harbors a microorganism capable of causing disease while not exhibiting clinical manifestations of the disease

Fomite—Any substance (e.g., food, water, object) that conveys a microorganism to a portal of entry

Fungus (pl. fungi)—Microorganism that requires nutrients from decaying organic matter; includes yeasts and molds

Immune response—Body's reaction to and interaction with substances identified by the body as being foreign.

Extent of resistance to a pathogen—Degree and integration of the body's response (immune response) to foreign matter (antigen).

Immunizations (vaccines)—Administration of an antigen that precipitates the immune system to produce antibodies that protect the individual from a specific disease

Infection—Invasion and multiplication of a pathogenic organism within the body

Mode of transmission—Method by which a microorganism is transferred from an infectious agent to a host

Parasite—Organism living in or on another living being and feeding off its cells and tissues

Passive immunity—Antibodies acquired from a source other than the individual's body

Pathogenicity—Ability to produce pathophysiological changes and disease

Sterile—Absence of microorganisms

Sterile technique (surgical asepsis)—Interventions to prevent the introduction of microorganisms into an area (e.g., sterile field) or body part (e.g., skin).

Sterilization—Process by which microorganisms are destroyed

Vector—Animal or insect that transports microorganisms to a portal of entry

Virulence—Degree of pathogenicity possessed by a microorganism

Virus—Tiny microorganism that lives inside a host cell and takes over metabolism of the cell to replicate

Wound—Disruption in the integrity of the skin.

I. Body's Defenses Against Infection

The human body fights infection on three levels. Primary defenses involve body systems or parts of body systems that resist or confine invading pathogens. Secondary defenses are physiological responses to toxins produced by invading pathogens. Tertiary defenses are immune responses that react to the presence of an antigen and precipitate protective mechanisms or act directly against antigenic cells. Nurses must not only understand the way in which this three-level defense system helps to protect the body from infection but also the types of immunity, the role of immunizations (vaccines) that produce immunity to communicable diseases, and nursing care specific to these issues.

A. Primary defenses
1. Skin and mucous membranes.
   a. Sebum on skin protects the skin.
   b. Ongoing desquamation of skin cells removes microorganisms.
   c. Low pH limits microbial growth.
   d. Mucous membranes produce mucus that traps microorganisms.
   e. Macrophages and lysozymes destroy bacteria on mucous membranes.
2. Respiratory system.
   a. Cilia capture and move microorganisms out of the respiratory tract.
   b. Mucous membranes secrete lysozymes that destroy microorganisms.
3. Gastrointestinal (GI) system.
   a. Saliva contains microbial inhibitors, such as lysozymes, lactoferrin, and immunoglobulin A (IgA).
   b. Low pH (*acetic*) of stomach and high pH (*alkaline*) of small intestine create inhospitable environments for microorganisms.
   c. Goblet cells lining the GI system produce secretions that prevent penetration by microorganisms and destroy (*lyse*) the cell walls of microorganisms.
   d. Peristalsis moves microorganisms out of the anus.
4. Circulatory system.
   a. Blood carries components of the inflammatory response (e.g., fibrinogen; thromboplastin; platelets; and white blood cells, including neutrophils and monocytes).
   b. Blood carries components of the immune response (e.g., immunoglobulins, T cells, and antibodies).
5. Eyes.
   a. Tears and blinking flush microorganisms out of the eyes.
   b. Tears contain lysozymes that destroy microorganisms.
6. Genitourinary system.
   a. The vagina has a low pH that creates an inhospitable environment for microorganisms.
   b. The low pH of urine and flushing action of urination limits microbial growth.

B. Secondary defenses
1. Fever.
   a. Products of pathogenic microorganisms (*pyrogens*) stimulate production of prostaglandins that reset the body's temperature thermostat in the hypothalamus to a higher level.
   b. An elevated temperature facilitates some immune reactions and inhibits the action of pathogens (exact mechanisms are still being debated).
2. Complement cascade.
   a. Proteins in the blood trigger chemicals that destroy pathogens by rupturing their cell membranes.
   b. Proteins in the blood stimulate basophils, a type of white blood cell, to release histamine, which is involved in the inflammatory response.
3. Inflammatory response: Local adaptation syndrome (LAS)—Hans Selye.
   a. A cellular response to irritation, injury, or infection attempts to neutralize pathogens and repair body tissues.
   b. A similar response occurs regardless of the stressor.
      (1) Physical (external body factors): such as heat, cold, radiation, and pressure, result in ischemia.
      (2) Pathogens: such as bacteria and viruses.
      (3) Chemicals: such as acid or alkaline burns.
      (4) Physiological (internal body factors): such as enzymes leaking into the abdomen, antigen-antibody reactions, and autoimmune diseases.
   c. Nursing care can help to detect or disrupt the inflammatory response. (Table 16.1)

DID YOU KNOW?

Infection is always accompanied by the inflammatory response, but the inflammatory response can occur without the presence of infection.

C. Tertiary defenses
1. The **immune response** is the body's reaction to and interaction with substances identified by the body as being foreign.
   a. Humoral immunity.
      (1) The humoral immune response reacts to the presence of an antigen (e.g., toxins, foreign substances, or particulates, such as bacteria, viruses, and proteins originating from within the body).

Table 16.1 **Stages of the Inflammatory Response and Related Nursing Care**

Commonalities of Nursing Care for Clients Experiencing the Inflammatory Response

1. Collect information to identify the causative factor.
2. Use standard precautions.
3. Perform physical assessment to identify the stage of the inflammatory response.
4. Inspect the site and surrounding area to determine the presence of lymphatic streaking.
5. Obtain vital signs to identify potential progression to sepsis, such as hyperthermia, tachycardia, and tachypnea.

 6. Obtain specimens for culture and sensitivity tests, if necessary, before initiating antibiotics.

 7. Institute transmission-based precautions if the client has a known or suspected communicable infection or infestation.

8. Implement prescribed interventions, such as application of warm soaks and administration of antibiotics or other medications.

Stage	Physiological Response	Specific Nursing Care
Vascular response	• Initially, blood vessels briefly constrict (vasoconstriction) at the site of injury. • Histamine is released at the site of injury, causing blood vessel dilation (vasodilation) and increasing blood flow to the site. • Kinins released by destroyed cells make capillaries permeable, and fluid moves into the interstitial compartment at the site of injury.	• Assess the site for paleness when blood vessels are constricted. • Assess the site for redness (hyperemia) and heat when blood vessels are dilated. • Assess the site for swelling (edema), pain, and loss of function.
Cellular response	• Blood flow slows in dilated vessels. • White blood cells (WBCs), specifically neutrophils and monocytes, migrate to the site of injury and pass into tissues. • WBCs engulf foreign material, damaged cells, and microorganisms and destroy them (phagocytosis). • Bone marrow responds by increasing the number of WBCs in circulation (leukocytosis).	• Monitor continuation of signs of redness, heat, edema, pain, and loss of function. • Assess WBC count (expected level is 5,000 to 10,000/mm^3; rate may increase to 15,000 to 20,000/mm^3).
Exudate formation	• A fluid forms that contains protein and cellular debris (exudate) as a result of the inflammatory response. • Fibrinogen, thromboplastin, platelets, and WBCs may make a barrier around the site (abscess) to limit the injury. • Abscesses contain thick liquid made up of cellular debris, destroyed tissue, phagocytic cells, and microorganisms (pus); generally they are associated with infection. • The nature and amount of exudate depends on the type and extent of injury. **Serous:** Clear, watery liquid that is like plasma. **Sanguineous:** Fluid that is red like blood. **Serosanguineous:** Pink, watery fluid; a mixture of serous and sanguineous fluid. **Purulent:** Thick fluid that appears yellow, green, tan, or brown; may be free flowing or contained in an abscess.	• Assess the amount and characteristics of exudate. • Perform irrigations and dressing changes as prescribed.
Reparative phase	**Healing by primary intention** • Wounds with approximated edges and minimal tissue destruction heal with minimal scar formation. • Tissue is replaced by identical or similar cells to original tissue (regeneration). **Healing by secondary intention** • Wounds with extensive tissue damage that do not have approximated edges heal from the inner layer to the outer surface. • Initially fragile, gelatinous tissue made up of newly formed capillaries forms (granulation). • Eventually, capillaries constrict, the tissue shrinks, collagen fibers contract, and firmer fibrous tissue remains (scar). **Healing by tertiary intention** • Two surfaces of granulated tissue are brought together and sutured in the absence of edema, foreign matter, or infection.	• Assess for fragile, gelatinous tissue that appears pink or red at the base of the injury. • Assess for shrinkage of tissue because, as it occurs, bleeding may recur. • Perform irrigations and dressing changes as prescribed.

(2) Macrophages and helper T cells stimulate B lymphocytes to produce antibodies, also called immunoglobulins (e.g., IgM, IgG, IgA, IgD, and IgE).

(3) Antibodies target antigens and destroy them through a variety of processes, such as phagocytosis, neutralization, agglutination, and activation of the complement cascade.

  b. Cellular immunity.

    (1) T cells act directly against antigenic cells.

    (2) Cytotoxic (killer) T cells attack and destroy cells infected with pathogens.

    (3) Helper T cells stimulate B cells in humoral immune responses.

    (4) Memory T cells form in response to an antigen and increase the speed and extent of T cell responses to subsequent invasion by the same antigen.

    (5) Suppressor T cells interrupt the immune response when infection is contained, acting like a feedback loop.

2. Types of immunity.

  a. **Active immunity:** Antibodies are formed within the body.

    (1) *Natural active immunity.*

      (a) Antibodies are formed during the course of the disease.

      (b) Usually produces lifelong immunity, such as to measles, chickenpox, and smallpox.

    (2) *Acquired active immunity.*

      (a) Antigen (e.g., vaccine or toxoid) is administered to stimulate the formation of antibodies.

      (b) Usually produces lifelong immunity or requires revaccination to maintain titers.

  b. **Passive immunity:** Antibodies are acquired from a source other than the individual's body.

    (1) *Natural passive immunity.*

      (a) Passage of antibodies occurs from a mother to a fetus via the placenta or to a neonate via colostrum.

      (b) Provides immunity for 6 months to 1 year.

    (2) *Acquired passive immunity.*

      (a) Antibodies produced from another source (immune serum) are injected into a person.

      (b) Provides immunity for 2 to 3 weeks.

3. Immunizations (vaccines).

  a. An immunization is a specific substance that precipitates the immune system to produce antibodies that protect an individual from a specific disease.

  b. Administered at specific developmental timetables (Figs. 16.1 and 16.2).

II. Chain of Infection and Related Nursing Care

An **infection** is the invasion and multiplication of a pathogenic organism within the body. The transmission of an infection requires an uninterrupted cycle that consists of an infectious agent, a reservoir, a portal of exit, a mode of transmission, a portal of entry, and a susceptible host (Fig. 16.3). The transmission of microorganisms can be prevented if the chain is broken by practices performed by nurses, other health-care providers, and clients. Each link of the chain of infection necessitates specific interventions to prevent transmission of an infectious agent.

A. Infectious agent (microorganism)

1. Extent to which a microorganism can cause an infection.

  a. **Pathogenicity:** Ability to produce pathophysiological changes and disease.

  b. **Virulence:** Degree of pathogenicity possessed by a microorganism, including invasiveness, such as ability to survive in the environment, method of transfer to another host, ability to grow once attached to the new site, and ability to produce harmful substances.

  c. Amount of microorganisms present.

2. Type of microorganism.

  a. **Virus:** Tiny microorganism that lives inside a host cell and takes over metabolism of the cell to replicate.

  b. **Bacterium:** Single-celled microorganism that replicates independently outside of cells with the appropriate environment.

  c. **Fungus:** Microorganism with cell walls that contain chitin and cellulose that resist destruction; requires nutrients from decaying organic matter; includes yeasts and molds.

  d. **Parasite:** Organism living in or on another living being and feeding off cells and tissues, causing tissue destruction.

3. Nursing care.

  a. Use soap and water or disinfectant to decrease microorganisms on the skin.

  b. Teach clients to:

    (1) Avoid taking antibiotics unless absolutely necessary to prevent antibiotic-resistant mutations and superinfections.

    🛑 (2) Complete the full course of prescribed antibiotics to avoid resistance.

    (3) Not share antibiotics with others.

Fig 16.1 Recommended immunization schedule for persons aged 0 through 18 years—United States, 2016. (From Centers for Disease Control and Prevention [2016]. *Recommended immunization schedule for persons aged 0 through 18 years—United States, 2016.* Retrieved June 9, 2016, from www.cdc.gov/vaccines/schedules/download/child/0-18yrs-schedule.pdf.)

Fig 16.2 Recommended adult immunization schedule—United States, 2016. (From Centers for Disease Control and Prevention [2016]. *Recommended adult immunization schedule—United States, 2016.* Retrieved June 9, 2016, from www.cdc.gov/vaccines/schedules/downloads/adult/adult-schedule.pdf.)

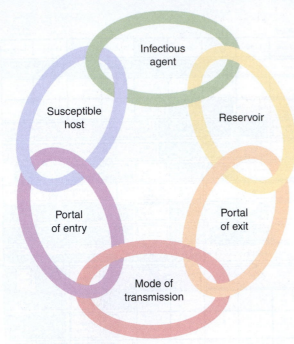

Fig 16.3 Chain of infection. (From Wilkinson and Treas [2016]. *Fundamentals of nursing*, Vol. 1, 3rd ed. Philadelphia: F. A. Davis Company, with permission.)

B. Reservoir (source)
1. Place where microorganism can survive and may or may not multiply.
2. Living reservoirs include humans, animals, and insects.
3. Nonliving reservoirs include contaminated water, garbage, sinks, toilets, bed rails, and linens.
4. Characteristics of environments that support microbial growth.
   a. Moist.
   b. Dark.
   c. Available nutrients.
   d. Temperature of 68°F to 109°F and pH of 5 to 8.
   e. Presence of oxygen (supports aerobic microorganisms) or absence of oxygen (supports anaerobic microorganisms), depending on type of microorganism.
5. **Carrier:** Person who harbors a microorganism capable of being transmitted and causing disease in another while not exhibiting clinical manifestations of the disease.
6. Nursing care.
   a. Ensure potentially contaminated surfaces, such as sinks, toilets, and overbed tables, are regularly cleaned.
   b. Change bed linens regularly or whenever contaminated.
   c. Use medical asepsis, such as fluid-impervious garbage bags and linen hampers, and avoid touching sinks and toilets in public restrooms.

d. Clean and change water in covered water jugs every 8 hours.
e. Empty suction and drainage bottles at regular intervals (e.g., every 8 hours, end of each shift).
f. Teach clients to:
   (1) Store food in a cool environment.
   (2) Clean surfaces where food is prepared regularly.
   (3) Perform hand hygiene regularly, particularly before and after handling food.

C. Portal of exit
1. Contaminated reservoir is a source of infection only when a microorganism exits the reservoir.
2. Human portals of exit.
   a. Respiratory tract (nose and mouth): Sneezing, coughing, talking, and breathing; includes oral, pharyngeal, or tracheal suctioning.
   b. Skin and mucous membranes: Breaks (e.g., tears, sores, fissures) in integrity of skin and mucous membranes; includes site of an IV catheter, injection, or blood drawn for laboratory tests.
   c. GI tract: Saliva, vomitus, and feces; includes discharges from GI tubes or ostomies.
   d. Reproductive tract: Vaginal secretions or discharge and semen.
   e. Urinary tract: Urine.
   f. Blood: Blood or plasma exiting from a wound or contained in a body fluid.
3. Nursing care.
   a. Maintain the integrity of closed systems, such as urinary catheters, portable wound drainage systems, and wound dressings.
   b. Limit talking when performing sterile procedures, such as dressing changes.
   c. Teach clients to:
      (1) Cough and sneeze into an elbow or upper arm.
      (2) Formula feed infants if mother is HIV positive because breast milk may contain the HIV.
      (3) Wash hands after toileting.

D. Mode of transmission
1. The **mode of transmission** is the method by which a microorganism is transferred from an infectious agent to a host.
2. Depends on characteristic of the microorganism and the disease it produces.
   a. *Direct:* Transfer of microorganism via contact between the infectious agent and host via touching, sexual intercourse, or kissing.
   b. *Droplet:* Transfer of large microorganisms in fluid droplets that can travel a maximum of 3 feet through activities such as sneezing, coughing, and talking.

c. *Airborne:* Transfer of small microorganisms suspended in air for extended periods of time and travel via air currents.

d. *Vehicle-borne:* Transfer via any substance that conveys a microorganism to a portal of entry, such as contaminated food or water; contaminated inanimate object that acts as a vehicle (**fomite**), such as tissues, toys, linens, clothing, and medical equipment.

e. Vector-borne: Animal or insect (**vector**) that transports microorganisms to a portal of entry; vectors may deposit feces on skin, inject salivary fluid during biting, or carry microorganisms on their legs.

3. Nursing care.

a. Maintain standard precautions. (See "Standard Precautions" in Chapter 1, Safety, and "Transmission-Based Precautions" in Table 16.2 in this chapter.)

b. Teach clients to:

(1) Dispose of used tissues into a fluid-impervious bag.

(2) Use a sharps container for used puncture devices associated with self-blood glucose monitoring or needles and syringes for injection of medication.

E. Portal of entry

1. Microorganisms can enter the body through the same routes as portals of exit from the body.

2. Human portals of entry include the respiratory, GI, reproductive, and urinary tracts and the skin and mucous membranes.

3. Protecting clients from infection involves maintaining protective tissues (e.g., mucous membranes of the mouth, nose, vagina, urethra, anus, and rectum) in the host.

4. Nursing care.

🛑 a. Use sterile technique when performing invasive procedures, such as injections, urinary catheterizations, dressing changes, and catheter irrigations.

b. Ensure all drainage tubes and drainage containers are kept below the insertion site.

c. Change dressings as soon as they become moist.

d. Provide perineal care with soap and water daily and when necessary, such as after toileting.

e. Teach clients to:

(1) Perform perineal care after toileting and to wash the genital area with soap and water daily.

(2) Maintain medical or surgical asepsis concerning tubes that enter the body (e.g., urinary catheter, portable wound

drainage systems) and procedures that must be performed (e.g., dressing changes, injections).

(3) Use insect repellent and wear long-sleeve shirts and long pants when in areas where insect-causing diseases are endemic.

F. Susceptible host

1. Person who is at risk for infection because of inadequate defenses against microorganisms, such as the very young, very old, or immunocompromised; those with multiple chronic illnesses, inadequate nutrition, tissue destruction related to trauma or medical or surgical interventions; and people who smoke cigarettes.

2. Susceptibility depends on the extent of resistance to a pathogen (immune response).

3. Defenses protect the body from infection. (See "Body's Defenses Against Infection" in this chapter.)

4. Nursing care.

a. Implement protective environmental precautions when the client is immunocompromised (see "Protective environmental precautions" in Table 16.2).

b. Ensure the client has received all age-appropriate immunizations (see Figs. 16.1 and 16.2).

c. Provide vaccine information, including the safety, benefits, and risks concerning immunizations; correct misconceptions regarding immunizations.

d. Teach the parents potential adverse effects and appropriate interventions (e.g., prescribed dose of acetaminophen to minimize discomfort).

🛑 e. Do not administer live virus vaccines (e.g., measles, mumps, and rubella [MMR] and varicella [chickenpox]) to a person who has a depressed immune system, had a temperature within the last 24 hours, received another vaccination within the last month, had an allergic reaction to the vaccination in the past, or who lives in a home with very young children.

f. Teach clients to follow a healthy lifestyle.

(1) Avoid tobacco-related habits.

(2) Eat a healthy diet.

(3) Drink adequate fluids daily (e.g., 2 to 3 L/day).

(4) Cough and deep breathe hourly when at an increased risk for stasis of respiratory secretions (e.g., when sedentary or on bedrest, after receiving anesthesia).

(5) Maintain the integrity of the skin and mucous membranes, such as by bathing, using moisturizing lotions, performing oral care, and alternating positions.

Table 16.2 Transmission-Based Precautions and Protective Environmental Precautions and Related Nursing Care

Commonalities of Nursing Care for Clients Receiving Transmission-Based and Protective Environmental Precautions

1. Institute specific precautions as indicated (e.g., with a primary health-care provider's prescription or when a client's condition meets the criteria identified in agency protocol).
2. Explain to the client the nature of the condition, the need for precautions, and the specifics of required interventions.
3. Involve the client in the plan of care and provide the client with choices to support independence.
4. Ensure that the client understands how to use the call bell to summon health team members.
5. Demonstrate a supportive, nonjudgmental attitude about the need for precautions; ensure that verbal and nonverbal communication does not convey negative feelings, such as disgust or revulsion.
6. Schedule time to converse with and provide nursing care to the client on a regular basis; use touch appropriately after donning personal protective equipment (PPE).
7. Assess the need for stimulation and encourage the client to engage in activities within abilities, such as watching television, reading a book, sitting in a chair, or walking around the room.
8. Assess for clinical manifestations of sensory deprivation, such as boredom, apathy, anxiety, increased sleeping, and disorganized thoughts.
9. Screen visitors to prevent entry of a person who may place clients or visitors at risk, such as a visitor with a respiratory tract infection or an unimmunized person.
10. Instruct visitors about specific precautions they must use.
11. Dedicate client-care equipment to prevent transmission of microorganisms to others.
12. Limit client movement outside of the room.
13. When wearing only a mask: Untie the mask, touching just the ties; discard the mask into an appropriate receptacle; and wash the hands.
14. When wearing a mask, gloves, and gown: Remove the gloves first; untie the mask, touching just the ties; discard the mask into an appropriate receptacle; untie the ties of the gown at the neck and the waist because these areas are considered clean; remove the gown, touching just the inside of the gown; and wash the hands.

Transmission-Based Precautions

Type	Description	Specific Nursing Care
Airborne precautions	• Used for clients suspected or known to be colonized or infected with an infectious agent that is transmitted via the air. • Based on the concept that droplet nuclei smaller than 5 mcg can remain suspended in the air and travel air currents. • Examples: Pulmonary tuberculosis, measles, chickenpox (varicella), and disseminated varicella zoster.	• Place in a private airborne infection isolation room (AIIR) with the door closed with negative pressure air flow of 6 to 12 air exchanges per hour via HEPA filtration or discharged to outside air. • Wear a mask or a particulate filter mask (N95 respirator) prior to entering the room depending on disease specific recommendations. • *Wear a gown, gloves, and face shield if splashing of body fluids is anticipated.* • Place a surgical mask on the client during transport. • Ensure nonimmune people do not enter rooms of clients with vaccine-preventable airborne diseases, such as measles, chickenpox, and smallpox.
Droplet precautions	• Based on the concept that microorganisms larger than 5 mcg within 3 feet of the client can be transmitted to others through direct contact with the client or via contaminated objects. • Examples: Rubella, influenza virus, adenovirus, rhinovirus, and group A streptococcus.	• Place the client in a private room or cohort with another client who has the same microorganism after consultation with infection control personnel. • Wear a mask when entering the room (respirator mask not necessary) when close contact with the client is anticipated. • *Wear gown, gloves, and goggles/face shield when client has substantial respiratory secretions or splashing of body fluids is anticipated.* • Place a surgical mask on the client during transport.
Contact precautions	• Based on the concept that microorganisms can be transmitted by direct contact with the client or indirect contact with contaminated objects in the client's environment. • Examples: Clostridium difficile, respiratory syncytial virus, methicillin-resistant Staphylococcus aureus (MRSA), vancomycin-resistant enterococci (VRE), scabies, and conditions in which excretions or secretions are difficult to contain, such as draining wounds and fecal incontinence.	• Place in a private room or cohort with another client who has the same microorganism after consultation with infection control personnel. • Wear gloves and gown when anticipating contact with the client or the client's environment. • Wear additional PPE if splashing of body fluids is anticipated (e.g., goggles, face shield).

Table 16.2	**Transmission-Based Precautions and Protective Environmental Precautions and Related Nursing Care—cont'd**	
Protective Environmental Precautions		
Reverse isolation, protective isolation, neutropenic precautions	• Based on the concept that immunocompromised individuals are at risk for contracting invasive environmental infections, such as aspergillosis. • Examples: Clients who have a neutrophil count ≤500 cells/mL; are receiving immunosuppressive therapy, such as chemotherapy, radiation, antirejection agents, or allogeneic hematopoietic stem cell transplant; and those with chronic illnesses.	• Use transmission-based precautions as prescribed. • Ensure air quality of the environment (e.g., HEPA filtration of incoming air, positive room air pressure relative to corridor, 12 air exchanges per hour, well-sealed room). • Ensure strategies to limit dust, such as wet dusting solid surfaces daily. • Ban dried and fresh flowers and potted plants from the client's room. • Place a face mask/N95 respirator on the client during transport for essential reasons (recommended but under-valued).

Siegel JD, Rhinehart E, Jackson M, Chiarello L, and the Healthcare Infection Control Practices Advisory Committee. (2007) *Guideline for isolation precautions: Preventing transmission of infectious agents in healthcare settings.* Retrieved December 2, 2016, from http://www.cdc.gov/ncidod/dhqp/pdf/isolation2007.pdf

MAKING THE CONNECTION

Chain of Infection and Nursing Care to Interrupt the Chain of Infection

To help prevent the spread of infection, nurses must make the connection between an organism's chain of infection and nursing actions that interrupt the chain at each point. For example, pulmonary tuberculosis is caused by the bacterium *Mycobacterium tuberculosis (infectious agent)*. It lives and multiplies in the body of an infected person *(reservoir)*. The infectious agent exits the respiratory tract via respiratory secretions from an infected person *(portal of exit)*. It is transmitted via respiratory secretions that are released into the air when an infected person exhales, coughs, sneezes, or talks. The secretions are aerosolized and carried by air currents (mode of transmission). Generally, the infectious agent is inhaled through the nose as aerosolized nuclei *(portal of entry)*. People with reduced immunity because of receiving chemotherapy for cancer, acquired immunodeficiency syndrome, chronic alcohol abuse, or advanced age *(susceptible host)* are at an increased risk for contracting the disease if exposed to the agent. To help prevent the spread of tuberculosis, nurses should be involved in activities that interrupt the chain of infection at each point along the chain. For example:

• *Infectious agent:* Obtain a sputum specimen to send to the laboratory to identify the presence of *M. tuberculosis.*

• *Reservoir:* Screen using purified protein derivative (PPD) to identify people who have been exposed to tuberculosis and may be harboring the *M. tuberculosis* bacterium. Verify the presence of *M. tuberculosis* via a sputum culture.

• *Portal of exit:* Place a mask on a client when transported outside a negative pressure room.

• *Mode of transmission:* Institute airborne transmission-based precautions. Maintain the client in a negative pressure room with multiple air exchanges per hour.

• *Portal of entry:* Wear a high-efficiency particulate air (HEPA) respirator when in the client's room.

• *Susceptible host:* Do not allow people with immature or inadequate immune systems to visit a client with active tuberculosis.

III. Sterile Technique (Surgical Asepsis)

Sterile technique *(surgical asepsis)* involves interventions that prevent the introduction of microorganisms into an area (e.g., sterile field) or body part (e.g., skin). The situations in which a nurse must use sterile technique are numerous. Regardless of the sterile procedure being performed, certain principles should be employed to maintain sterility. This section discusses these issues and relates nursing care associated with each principle.

A. Introduction
  1. **Sterile** means absence of microorganisms.
  2. **Sterilization** is a process that destroys microorganisms (e.g., moist heat, gas, boiling water, and radiation).
  3. Human skin harbors many microorganisms, is not sterile, and cannot be sterilized; however, techniques can be used to limit the number of microorganisms, such as the use of hand washing, alcohol-based antimicrobial gels, and surgical scrubs.
  4. Sterile technique involves using practices to prevent the introduction of microorganisms into an area.
  5. Sterile technique is used in a variety of instances, including:
    a. When intentionally piercing a client's skin, such as inserting an intravenous catheter into a vein or creating a surgical incision.

b. When a client's skin or membranes are breached or not intact, such as with burns, wounds, postoperative incisions, and childbirth.

c. When inserting catheters into body cavities, such as a urinary catheter or tracheobronchial suctioning.

d. When providing care in specialty environments, such as a birthing room, an operating room, and certain diagnostic procedure rooms, such as cardiac catheterization laboratories.

B. Principles of surgical asepsis (Table 16.3)

IV. Wounds and Wound Care

A **wound** is a disruption in the integrity of the skin. Wounds can be classified by duration of healing, amount of microorganisms present, depth of injury, and integrity of the skin. They heal by primary, secondary, or tertiary intention; however, many factors can delay wound healing.

Nurses must know how to assess wounds, collect a specimen of exudate, and provide care for all types of wounds. These topics are reviewed in this section.

A. Classification of wounds
  1. Duration of healing.
     a. *Acute.*
        (1) Healing occurs over a short duration, such as for a surgical incision.
        (2) Most commonly heals by primary intention.
     b. *Chronic.*
        (1) Healing occurs over a long duration.
        (2) Healing is delayed due to the presence of infection, ischemia, edema, impaired circulation, or another underlying disease process, such as diabetes.
        (3) Generally heals by secondary intention.
  2. Depth of the wound.
     a. *Superficial wound:* Involves loss of only the epidermal layer (e.g., a superficial excoriation

Table 16.3 Principles of Surgical Asepsis and Related Nursing Care

Principle	Nursing Care
• All objects placed on a sterile field must be sterile and be kept sterile.	• Keep sterile objects in a clean, dry storage area. • Check sterile packages for intactness, dryness, and expiration dates and discard torn, wet, or outdated packages. • Check sterile packages for indication of sterilization (e.g., the word STERILE is on a closure tape that changes color when sterilized). • Place sterile objects inside a 1-inch margin of all edges of a drape because this area is considered sterile; the 1-inch border around the entire edge of the drape is considered unsterile. • The flat surface of a sterile field is considered sterile; draping material falling over the side of the surface is considered unsterile.
• Sterile objects remain sterile when touched by something sterile.	• Manipulate objects on a sterile field with sterile forceps or hands wearing sterile gloves. • Change sterile gloves if they become contaminated. • Remember "sterile to sterile."
• Sterile objects become unsterile when touched by unsterile, clean, or contaminated objects or fluid.	• Discard sterile objects that come in contact with unsterile, clean, or contaminated objects; discard object when sterility is questionable. • Refrain from reaching over a sterile field with ungloved hands or moving unsterile objects over a sterile field. • Keep the lip of a bottle of liquid several inches above a sterile receptacle when pouring sterile liquid because the edge of the bottle is considered unsterile. • Use a moisture-proof barrier between the table and sterile objects. • Discard a sterile field that is pervious to liquid if it becomes wet by fluid from under or on the sterile field because capillary action will draw microorganisms onto the field. • Hold wet swabs with forceps held downward to keep fluid from flowing up toward the hands and becoming contaminated. • Hold hands above the elbows during a surgical hand scrub to prevent contaminated fluid from flowing onto the hands. • Wear surgical caps in operating rooms and birthing and burn units.
• Sterile objects become contaminated by exposure to air.	• Limit air currents in the room by closing the door, closing the bed curtain, and limiting unnecessary movement of people in the room. • Prepare the sterile field immediately before use. • Limit talking over the sterile field, and avoid laughing, sneezing, or coughing in the room. • Avoid walking between a sterile field and the client.
• Sterile objects are considered unsterile when out of the nurse's sight or below the nurse's waist.	• Prepare and hold sterile objects above the waist. • Keep sterile objects and sterile gloved hands in the line of vision; they are considered contaminated when they are outside the line of vision. • Never leave a sterile field unattended.

caused by friction); may take several days to a week to heal.

b. *Partial-thickness wound:* Involves loss of the epidermis and possibly partial loss of the dermis (e.g., a partial-thickness burn); may take 2 to 3 weeks to heal.

c. *Full-thickness wound:* Involves loss of the epidermis and dermis; may extend into deeper structures, such as subcutaneous tissue, muscle, joint, and bone, which are nonregenerative (e.g., a stage III or IV pressure ulcer); may take months or years to heal; some chronic full-thickness wounds may never heal because of underlying pathology, such as inadequate circulation secondary to a peripheral occlusive disorder or diabetes.

3. Presence and extent of microorganisms in the wound.

a. *Clean wound:* Uninfected wound.

b. *Clean-contaminated wound:* Surgical incision that penetrates the GI, respiratory, or genitourinary tract, and areas that commonly harbor pathogenic microorganisms.

c. *Contaminated wound:* Colonized with microorganisms but has not progressed to an infection; generally associated with traumatic breaks in the skin; usually less than 100,000 organisms per gram of tissue.

d. *Infected wound:* Colonized with bacteria causing erythema, swelling, and warmth around the wound; foul odor; drainage; and discomfort or pain; presence of greater than 100,000 organisms per gram of tissue; however, any number of beta-hemolytic streptococci present is considered an infection.

B. Types of healing (Fig. 16.4) (see "Reparative Phase" in Table 16.1 Stages of the Inflammatory Response and Related Nursing Care)

1. Primary intention.
2. Secondary intention.
3. Tertiary intention.

Primary intention

Clean wound   Sutured early   Results in hairline scar

Secondary intention

Wound gaping and irregular   Granulation occurring   Epithelium fills in scar

Tertiary intention

Wound not sutured   Granulation partially fills in wound   Granulating tissue sutured together

Fig 16.4 Types of healing. (From Wilkinson and Treas [2016]. *Fundamentals of nursing,* Vol. 1, 3rd ed. Philadelphia: F. A. Davis Company, with permission.)

C. Factors that delay wound healing
1. Increased age.
   a. Aging skin loses elasticity.
   b. Collagen replacement is diminished.
   c. Circulation, phagocytic, and immune responses are reduced.
   d. Wound contraction occurs slowly.
   e. Scars are less strong.
2. Chronic illness and impaired health.
   a. The essential factors needed to facilitate wound healing are absent.
   b. The immune system is depressed because of the illness or therapy (e.g., radiation, chemotherapy).
3. Edema.
   a. Fluid in the interstitial space increases the distance from the circulation to body cells.
   b. Edematous tissue reduces transport of nutrients to a wound and removal of debris from a wound.
4. Fever.
   a. Fever increases the metabolic rate and the demand for oxygen on a cellular level.
   b. Fever may precipitate dehydration, which limits the amount of circulating blood volume to the injured area.
5. Infection.
   a. Infection interferes with the inflammatory response and causes edema.
   b. Pathogenic organisms increase the extent of exudate in the wound.
6. Lifestyle.
   a. Personal behaviors, such as inadequate nutrition, do not provide the vitamins and proteins needed for adequate wound healing.
   b. Smoking (nicotine) constricts blood vessels, reducing the oxygen needed for healing.
7. Medications.
   a. Anti-inflammatory drugs, such as steroids and aspirin, impair the inflammatory process.
   b. Antineoplastics are cellular toxic and depress the bone marrow, resulting in decreased leukocyte production, which increases the risk of infection.
8. Multiple wounds.
   a. Multiple wounds compete for nutrients, such as enzymes and protein, needed for tissue repair.
   b. Multiplicity of stressors increases the demand on the sympathetic nervous system, precipitating hormonal and metabolic changes that interfere with the synthesis of inflammatory mediators.
9. Nutrition.
   a. Inadequate calories; protein; zinc; fluid; and vitamins C, A, and E impair healing.
   b. Vitamin C is needed for collagen synthesis, capillary growth, and fibroblast and immunologic function.
   c. Protein is needed for tissue growth, angiogenesis, collagen formation, immune function, and wound remodeling.
   d. Overeating results in obesity; excessive adipose tissue has fewer blood vessels, predisposing a person to wound complications.
10. Tissue perfusion.
    a. Impaired perfusion to a wound decreases the delivery of nutrients and oxygen to the area (e.g., lung and heart disease, anemia, peripheral edema, or peripheral artery disease).
    b. Impaired perfusion away from a wound decreases the removal of waste, carbon dioxide, and cellular debris (e.g., peripheral venous insufficiency or peripheral edema).
11. Radiation.
    a. The initial stages of the inflammatory response are severely inhibited.
    b. Radiation breaks down underlying connective tissue and bone marrow.
    c. Radiation slows the growth of granulation tissue and the reepithelialization process.
12. Wound tension.
    a. Vomiting, coughing, sneezing, and obesity strain wound edges, which may cause them to pull apart.
    b. Tension can lead to wound dehiscence or evisceration. (See "Dehiscence" and "Evisceration" in "Postoperative Wound Complications" in Chapter 24, Perioperative.)

D. Culture and sensitivity testing of wound exudate
1. Culture and sensitivity test.
   a. Identifies microorganisms present in a specimen.
   b. Identifies antibiotics that are most effective in destroying an identified microorganism.
   🛑 c. Requires the nurse to obtain a specimen before initiating antibiotic therapy.
2. Nursing care for obtaining a wound specimen.
   a. Wash hands.
   b. Collect the appropriate equipment (e.g., clean gloves, sterile culturette tube that contains a cotton-tipped swab).
   c. Confirm the client's identity.
   d. Explain the procedure.
   e. Provide for the client's privacy.
   f. Don personal protective equipment as indicated, such as a gown, a face shield, and clean gloves.
   g. Place the client in a position that provides easy access to the wound.
   h. Assess the characteristics of the wound and drainage.

i. Irrigate the wound surface with sterile normal saline solution to remove surface bacteria.

j. Rotate the tip of the sterile swab from a culturette tube in the wound bed, avoiding areas that have drainage or necrotic tissue and the wound edges (Fig. 16.5).

k. Place the sterile swab back into the culturette tube and then seal the tube.

l. Place identifying information on the culturette tube and the outside of the fluid-impervious bag before sending the specimen to the laboratory.

m. Document all assessments, interventions, and client responses.

E. Commonalities of nursing care for clients with all types of wounds

1. Support the client emotionally.

a. Encourage the client to express feelings about the wound and its implications.

b. Identify whether the client is anxious or fearful about the size, location, appearance, or odor of the wound; accept the client's feelings about the wound.

c. Avoid excessive exposure of the client to the wound until the client is ready to look at the wound or participate in wound care.

d. Avoid body language that may communicate a negative reaction to the wound.

🛑 e. Help the client to maintain a positive body image when the body is altered due to such events as mastectomy, colostomy, burns, or facial scarring.

2. Monitor the client's vital signs, including temperature, pulse, respirations, blood pressure, and pain.

3. Assess the characteristics of the wound.

a. Identify the location of the wound.

Fig 16.5 Obtaining a specimen from a wound for culture and sensitivity. (From Burton and Ludwig [2015]. *Fundamentals of nursing care: Concepts, connections & skills,* 2nd ed. Philadelphia: F. A. Davis Company, with permission.)

b. Measure the dimensions of the wound, including length, width, and depth and amount of undermining and tunneling, using an objective measuring device.

c. Describe the wound edges, such as approximation or nonapproximation of wound edges *(dehiscence).*

d. Assess the condition of the surrounding skin for clinical indicators of an infection such as swelling, warmth, and redness.

e. Identify type of exudate. (See "Exudate Formation" in Table 16.1 in this chapter.)

f. Document the number of saturated gauze or abdominal pads; document output from wound drains in milliliters (mL); and, if two or more drains are present, ensure that they are numbered.

g. Describe the status of the wound using the red, yellow, and black classification system.

(1) Red.

(a) Reflects newly granulating tissue.

(b) Care involves gentle cleaning and a moist dressing (transparent or hydrocolloid).

(2) Yellow.

(a) Reflects oozing exudate, which may be purulent.

(b) Care includes cleansing or irrigating the wound; using a wet-to-moist dressing, foam absorptive dressing, hydrogel, or alginate to debride the wound; and possibly seeking a prescription for a topical antimicrobial.

(3) Black.

(a) Indicates necrotic tissue *(eschar);* color variations of eschar include gray, tan, or brown.

(b) Care involves removal of eschar *(debridement)* (see "Wound debridement and related nursing care" in this chapter).

h. Identify the stage of the wound by indicating the tissue layers involved when assessing wounds healing by secondary or tertiary intention (see Table 17.4, "Pressure Ulcer Stages," in Chapter 17, Mobility).

i. Identify pain or discomfort associated with the wound using an objective rating scale, and administer an analgesic as prescribed 30 minutes before a dressing change if pain is anticipated.

4. Cleanse and dress a wound.

a. Wear clean gloves, remove the soiled dressing, discard the dressing and gloves in a trash container, and discard the dressing in a biohazard container if the dressing is saturated with blood or body fluids.

b. Wash hands, establish a sterile field with all needed equipment, and don sterile gloves.

c. Clean the wound using a systematic approach, moving from clean to dirty (Fig. 16.6).

d. Clean the pins of an external fixation device.

  (1) Swipe the base of each pin where it exits from the skin using a circular motion, making one complete revolution with a 4 × 4 gauze pad moistened with normal saline solution.

  (2) Repeat using a new wet 4 × 4 gauze pad for each revolution.

  (3) Apply a topical antibiotic ointment around each pin if prescribed.

DID YOU KNOW?

External fixation devices are used to stabilize a crushing or splintering bone injury with soft tissue damage. Pins are inserted into the bone and attached to an external metal framework that prevents bone movement. An external fixation device, rather than a cast, prevents pressure on traumatized, edematous soft tissue, permitting soft tissue to heal.

Fig 16.6 Cleaning a wound. Swipe along the line numbered 1 in either illustration A or B first with a 4 × 4 gauze pad moistened with normal saline solution. Use a new 4 × 4 gauze pad to swipe along each line numbered 2 through 5 or 2 through 8, depending on the cleansing method used. (From Nugent and Vitale [2014]. *Fundamentals of nursing: Content review PLUS practice questions.* Philadelphia: F. A. Davis Company, with permission.)

e. Apply a dressing.

  (1) Use the three-tape method because it uses less tape; protects skin from excessive adhesive, which may impair skin integrity; allows for flexibility of skin; and permits air to circulate under the gauze.

  (2) Use the window method of taping to secure the dressing on all sides and contain wound drainage within the gauze window; use for dressings with moist packing.

  (3) Use Montgomery straps to secure the dressing if indicated (Fig. 16.7).

F. Wound infection and related nursing care

1. Invasion of a wound by a pathogen that proliferates, resulting in inflammation and purulent drainage.

2. Clinical manifestations.

  a. Local erythema, edema, heat, and pain.

  b. Extent of approximation of wound edges.

  c. Amount and characteristics of purulent exudate, such as color and presence of foul odor.

  d. Increased vital signs.

  e. Increased white blood cell count.

3. Nursing care.

  a. Institute contact precautions.

  b. Obtain a wound specimen for a wound culture and sensitivity test.

  c. Notify the primary health-care provider of clinical indicators of infection.

  d. Irrigate and dress the wound as prescribed.

  e. Encourage foods high in protein and vitamin C to promote wound healing.

  f. Administer antibiotics and pain medication as prescribed.

  g. Monitor the incision for clinical indicators of dehiscence and evisceration. (See "Dehiscence" and "Evisceration" in Chapter 24, Perioperative.)

  h. Assist with debridement of a wound if prescribed.

Fig 16.7 Montgomery straps. (From Wilkinson and Treas [2016]. *Fundamentals of nursing*, Vol. 1, 3rd ed. Philadelphia: F. A. Davis Company, with permission.)

G. Wound debridement and related nursing care

1. Assist the primary health-care provider with surgically cutting away devitalized tissue with a scalpel or scissors (*surgical debridement*) at the bedside. Wear a gown, mask, face shield, and sterile gloves. If the wound is large, expect this procedure to be completed in an operating room.
2. Employ other prescribed debridement methods, such as scrubbing the wound with gauze (*mechanical debridement*), using collagenase enzyme products (*chemical debridement*), or using a dressing that promotes the body to generate enzymes to break down eschar (*autolytic debridement*).
3. Apply prescribed ointment or paste to the skin surrounding the wound to protect the skin from contact with debridement products and exudate, which can macerate tissue.
4. Apply the dressing prescribed by the primary health-care provider and according to the manufacturer's instructions (see Table 16.4).

H. Wound irrigation and related nursing care

1. Irrigate the wound with the prescribed solution.
2. Wear personal protective equipment (e.g., gloves, gown, and face shield) to protect from splashing of the client's blood or body fluid (Fig. 16.8).
3. Position the client so that the irrigating solution will flow into an emesis basin.
4. Hold a piston syringe with irrigating solution 2 inches from the wound surface, just inside the top edge of the wound.
5. Spray back and forth gently across the inside of the wound and progressively move down the surface of the wound so that the solution and debris move out of the wound via gravity without disrupting granulated tissue in the wound bed.
6. Refill the syringe and continue the procedure until the entire surface of the wound is cleansed.

I. Packing a wound and related nursing care

1. Obtain the prescribed solution to moisten the packing gauze.
2. Establish the sterile field and don sterile gloves.
3. Separate the wound edges gently to ensure that the entire wound is accessible so that granulation and healing can occur from the bottom of the wound bed outward.
4. Open and fluff moistened rolled gauze to increase the surface area for contact with the wound bed (Fig. 16.9A).
5. Fill the wound completely with the moistened gauze while avoiding the surrounding skin and cover with a dry abdominal pad (Fig. 16.9B).
6. Use Montgomery straps to secure a dressing that requires frequent changes due to excessive wound drainage; avoids trauma to the skin caused by constant application and removal of tape (Fig.16.7).

Table 16.4 Types of Wound Dressings and Related Nursing Care

- A dressing facilitates healing.
- Keeps the wound dry (dry sterile dressing) for an approximated incision or laceration.
- Keeps the wound bed continuously moist (wet-to-moist dressing) for wounds with unapproximated edges to promote granulation in the wound bed.
- Controls exudate without dehydrating or drying the wound bed.
- Fills the wound cavity and undermining areas to avoid dead space.
- Keeps surrounding intact skin dry because it prevents maceration and skin impairment.
- Nursing care provided for a client with a wound dressing varies by the type of dressing prescribed.

Type of Dressing	Related Nursing Care
Transparent Dressing	
- See-through, film-like, thin sheet that is semipermeable, allowing for an interchange of oxygen between the wound and the environment. - Self-adhesive. - Elastic and pliable, making it comfortable. - Used over intact skin to reduce shearing or to protect a small, superficial wound, such as a blister, stage I or II pressure ulcer, abrasion, skin tear, IV site, or minor burn. - Used for a wound that has minimal drainage. - Maintains a moist wound bed. - Protects the wound from contamination. - Examples: Op-Site, Tegaderm, Acu-derm, Bioclusive, and Polyskin.	- Clean the wound as prescribed and then thoroughly dry the skin around the wound. - Apply the dressing to a dry skin surface. - *Do not stretch or wrinkle the dressing when applying it to the area to prevent pulling on the skin and promote adherence.* - Remove and replace the dressing if its edges roll, its seal breaks, or after 24 to 72 hours, depending on manufacturer's instructions. - Assess the area daily for clinical indicators of a problem.

Continued

Table 16.4 **Types of Wound Dressings and Related Nursing Care—cont'd**

Type of Dressing	Related Nursing Care
Hydrocolloid Dressing	
• *Occlusive adhesive dressing that adheres to wet and dry sites.* • *Available in many sizes and shapes that contour to fit different body parts.* • *Also available as a paste, granules, or powder that can be applied to the wound cavity.* • *Becomes an absorbent gel on contact with drainage.* • *Protects the wound from contamination, serving as an excellent microbial barrier.* • *Is moisture retentive.* • *Cushions the wound.* • *Serves as a thermal insulator.* • *Used for wounds with light to moderate drainage; contraindicated with heavy drainage because this type of dressing absorbs drainage slowly.* • *Used for shallow to medium depth skin ulcers and donor sites and with packing for small cavity wounds.* • *Some can be used on intact skin and others in the presence of dry eschar, necrosis, or slough.* • *Facilitates autolytic debridement.* • *Does not permit visualization of the wound.* • *Contraindicated for infected wounds, wounds with exposed tendon or bone, and foot ulcers associated with diabetes mellitus.* • *Examples: DuoDERM, Intact, IntraSite, Ultec, Comfeel, Restore, and Tegasorb.*	• *Ensure a 1-inch margin of healthy skin around the wound when sizing the dressing.* • *Round off the edges to reduce the likelihood of the edges catching on gowns or linens.* • *Warm the dressing by rubbing it between the hands before application to improve adhesion if it is an adhesive product.* • *Apply to dry skin with a secondary dressing if indicated (a secondary dressing is unnecessary if it is an adhesive dressing).* • *Avoid applying the dressing by stretching the product or using too much tension to prevent a tourniquet effect; do not reinforce it with tape.* • *Remove and replace the dressing if the edges roll, the seal breaks, after 3 to 7 days according to the manufacturer's directions, or whenever necessary.* • *Assess for maceration of the skin around wound margins.*
Hydrogel Dressing	
• *Available in flexible sheets or as a powder, beads, or paste.* • *80% to 90% glycerin or water, adding moisture to a wound.* • *Devitalizes tissue to assist with autolytic debridement.* • *Forms a gelatinous mass when in contact with exudate to maintain a moist wound environment.* • *Does not adhere to the wound.* • *Pads the wound, increasing comfort and reducing shearing.* • *Softens eschar via autolytic debridement.* • *Used for partial-thickness and full-thickness wounds, necrotic wounds, and superficial burns.* • *Contraindicated with wounds that are infected, have excessive exudate, or are bleeding.* • *Examples: Aquasorb, Vigilon, IntraSite Gel, Nu-Gel, and Hypergel.*	• *Gently insert the flexible sheet to fill the contour of the wound; apply powder, beads, paste, or spray as indicated by the manufacturer's instructions to fill the wound cavity; avoid skin surrounding the wound.* • *Apply a secondary dressing over the hydrogel product.* • *Change the dressing every 8 to 48 hours as indicated by the manufacturer's instructions.* • *Irrigate the hydrogel residue from the wound; then reapply a new dressing.* • *Assess the skin around the wound for clinical indicators of maceration or infection; however, do not be confused with expected gel residue that looks like pus and is malodorous.*
Alginate Dressing	
• *Made of soft, nonwoven fibers developed from seaweed in the form of pads, ropes, or ribbons for application to various-shaped wounds.* • *Becomes a gel on contact with exudate and absorbs 20 times its weight.* • *Used for wounds with moderate to high amounts of drainage.* • *Used for partial-thickness and full-thickness wounds, venous status ulcers, pressure ulcers, diabetic ulcers, graft sites, traumatic and surgical wounds, and infected wounds.* • *Contraindicated in dry wounds and full-thickness wounds with exposed tendons or bone.* • *Examples: Sorbsan, AlgiDerm, Curasorb, Kaltostat, and Dermacea, SeaSorb, and Melgisorb.*	• *Cut or fold the dressing so that it fits the wound; do not overlap the wound margins.* • *Secure the dressing with a nonocclusive secondary dressing.* • *To change the dressing, gently remove the secondary dressing; if the area looks dry, saturate it with sterile normal saline solution, gently remove the alginate, and then discard it appropriately.* • *Irrigate the wound with a wound cleanser as prescribed before applying a new dressing.* • *Change the dressing as needed (possibly every 24 hours depending on the volume of exudate).*

Table 16.4 Types of Wound Dressings and Related Nursing Care—cont'd

Type of Dressing	Related Nursing Care
Foam Dressing	
• A highly absorbent dressing that wicks exudate off the wound, decreasing maceration of surrounding tissue. • Available in many shapes to fit the contours of the body. • Protects the wound. • Maintains wound moisture. • May have hemostatic, debriding, antimicrobial, and odor-controlling activities and inactivate proteolytic enzymes in chronic wounds. • May be adhesive. • Used for heavily exudating wounds, such as deep cavity wounds, weeping ulcers, and chronic wounds. • Used in wound vacuum-assisted closure systems. • Contraindicated for wounds with little drainage because of its drying effect. • Examples: Foam, Polyderm, Curafoam, Mepilex, and Allevyn.	• Clean the wound as prescribed. • Place the foam over the wound, extending over the wound margins or cut it to fit the wound cavity. • Secure the dressing in place with tape, elastic gauze, or tube gauze if the dressing is not adhesive; *avoid excessive tightness because, as foam absorbs moisture, it will place increased pressure on the wound bed.* • Leave the dressing in place for 2 to 7 days, per the manufacturer's directions or when evidence indicates that the foam is full of exudate (e.g., dressing becomes heavy). • For nursing care related to vacuum-assisted closure, see "Negative Pressure Wound Therapy" in this chapter.
Growth Factor–Impregnated Dressing	

• Growth factors are small protein hormones that enhance wound healing at various places along the healing cascade.
• Attract immune cells to fight infection, promote production of connective tissue, facilitate new blood vessel growth to nourish the area, and promote remodeling.
• May be impregnated into a dressing or applied topically and covered with a dressing.
• Most common growth factors.
  • Platelet-derived growth factor (PDGF).
  • Epidermal growth factor (TGF).
  • Transforming growth factor-beta (TGF-Beta).
  • Vascular endothelial growth factor (VEGF).
  • Insulin growth factor-1 (IGF-1).
• Each works differently; for example, PDGF recruits stem cells to the wound site, promotes angiogenesis, and initiates tissue regeneration and remodeling.
	• Apply a growth factor–impregnated dressing as prescribed.
	• Apply growth factor directly to a wound bed and cover with a dressing as prescribed.

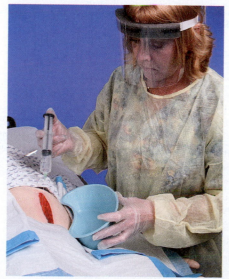

Fig 16.8 Irrigating a wound. (From Wilkinson and Treas [2016]. *Fundamentals of nursing*, Vol. 2, 3rd ed. Philadelphia: F. A. Davis Company, with permission.)

J. Negative pressure wound therapy and related nursing care
1. Vacuum-assisted closure (VAC); an occlusive dressing is attached via tubing to a negative pressure machine that removes exudate, thereby reducing edema and promoting granulation (Fig. 16.10).
2. Ensure that the device is appropriate for the client's wound—for example, the wound should not have necrotic tissue.
3. Cut the prescribed foam dressing to a size that fills just the wound cavity.
4. Apply a liquid product around the outside of the wound to protect the skin.
5. Apply a transparent film that extends 3 to 5 cm (1 to 2 inches) beyond the wound margins.
6. Cut a 2-cm round hole in the center of the transparent film and attach the suction device with tubing directly over the hole in the transparent film.

Fig 16.9 Packing a wound. (A) Fluffing moistened gauze. (B) Filling wound with moistened gauze. (From Wilkinson and Treas [2016]. *Fundamentals of nursing,* Vol. 2, 3rd ed. Philadelphia: F. A. Davis Company, with permission.)

7. Connect the tubing to negative pressure as prescribed (continuous or intermittent, 5 to 125 mm Hg).

8. Ensure that negative pressure is maintained.

   a. The film will collapse or wrinkle as pressure is applied.

Fig 16.10 Vacuum-assisted closure. (From Wilkinson and Treas [2016]. *Fundamentals of nursing,* Vol. 2, 3rd ed., Philadelphia: F. A. Davis Company, with permission.)

   b. Audible leaks can be heard if the film dressing is not secure.

9. Change the collection container when full or at least once a week.

10. Observe the site for signs of infection.

11. Document the amount of drainage, characteristics, and wound assessments.

V. Medications Associated With Infection or Infestation and Related Nursing Care

When a person is diagnosed with an infection caused by a bacteria, virus, or fungus or is diagnosed with an infestation of a parasite or helminthic, the primary health-care provider prescribes appropriate medication to cause death of the invading agent. Nurses need to know the mechanisms of action, therapeutic and nontherapeutic effects, and nursing care related to common antibiotics, anti-infectives, antivirals, antifungals, antiparasitics, and anthelminthics (Table 16.5).

Table 16.5 Medications Associated With Infection or Infestation and Related Nursing Care

Antibiotics and Anti-infectives

- *Decrease growth of or destroy susceptible microorganisms.*

Mechanism of Action	Examples	Nontherapeutic Effects
Anti-infectives • *Decrease protein and DNA synthesis, bacteriocidal, trichomonacidal, and amebicidal.*	metronidazole (Flagyl)	• *Nausea and vomiting.* • *Diarrhea.* • *Hypersensitivity reactions, such as skin rash and anaphylaxis.* • *Possibly, hepatotoxicity, nephrotoxicity, and bone marrow depression.*
Aminoglycosides • *Decrease protein synthesis.*	azithromycin (Zithromax) clarithromycin (Biaxin) gentamicin (Garamycin)	
Cephalosporins • *Bind to cell wall, causing cell death.*	cefazolin (Ancef) cephalexin (Keflex)	
Penicillins • *Bind to cell wall, causing cell death.*	amoxicillin (Amoxil) penicillin V (Veetids, V-cillin)	
Quinolones • *Decrease DNA synthesis.*	ciprofloxacin (Cipro) levofloxacin (Levaquin)	
Sulfonamides • *Decrease protein synthesis.*	doxycycline (Vibramycin)	

Table 16.5	**Medications Associated With Infection or Infestation and Related Nursing Care—cont'd**

Nursing Care

- Obtain a specimen for culture and sensitivity testing before administering the first dose of medication.
- Assess for and teach about clinical manifestations of infection.
- Administer evenly spaced doses to maintain therapeutic blood levels of the medication.
- Teach the client to complete the entire antibiotic regimen to prevent resistance.
- Teach the client not to chew or crush extended-release tablets.
- Assess for clinical manifestations of superinfection, such as furry overgrowth on the tongue, vaginal discharge, and foul-smelling stool.
- Obtain a blood specimen 1 to 3 hours after a dose to measure the peak level (depends on medication's half-life). A **peak level** is the highest blood concentration of a medication.
- Obtain a blood specimen 30 to 60 minutes before the next dose to measure the trough level. A **trough level** is the lowest blood concentration of a medication.

Antifungals

Decrease fungal growth.

Mechanism of Action	Examples	Nontherapeutic Effects
Systemic - Impair fungal plasma membrane.	clotrimazole (Mycelex) fluconazole (Diflucan) nystatin (Mycostatin)	- Nausea and vomiting. - Diarrhea. - Hypersensitivity reactions, such as rash and anaphylaxis. - Possible harm to fetus if woman being treated is pregnant (teratogenic). - Ototoxicity. - Hepatotoxicity. - Nephrotoxicity. - Burning and irritation at the site of application.
Topical - Disrupt fungal cell wall and cell metabolism.	clotrimazole (Lotrimin) ketoconazole (Nizoral) nystatin (Mycostatin) amphotericin B (Fungizone)	

Nursing Care

Systemic
- Teach the client to refrain from intercourse to prevent pregnancy during therapy.
- Teach the client to complete the entire regimen.
- Monitor for ototoxicity, nephrotoxicity, and hepatotoxicity.

Topical
- Clean the skin with tepid water before application.
- Monitor for skin or mucous membrane irritation.
- Teach the client how to insert a vaginal suppository or cream.
- Teach the client how to insert a rectal suppository.
- Teach the client difference between "swish and spit" and "swish and swallow."

Antiparasitics and anthelminthics

Cause death of a parasite or helminthic.

Mechanism of Action	Examples	Nontherapeutic Effects
Parasiticide - Absorbed into parasites and eggs. - Used for scabies and lice.	lindane (Kwell)	- Central nervous system toxicity. - Seizures.
	permethrin (Nix)	- Tingling. - Pruritus.
Antihelminthic - Prevents worm growth and reproduction. - Used for pinworms.	mebendazole (Vermox)	- Hypersensitivity, such as skin rash and anaphylaxis. - Abdominal pain.

Nursing Care

- Teach the client to wash linens and clothing in hot water and dry in a dryer.
- Teach the client to seal nonwashables in plastic bags for a minimum of 2 weeks.
- Teach the client to vacuum carpets and furniture daily.
- Ensure that all persons living within the household are treated.

Continued

Table 16.5 Medications Associated With Infection or Infestation and Related Nursing Care—cont'd

Nursing Care

For pinworms
- *Obtain a specimen via cellophane tape test in the morning before a bowel movement.*
- *Monitor for GI distress and for irritation of the perianal area.*

For head lice
- *Teach the client to wash hair for 5 minutes with an antiparasitic shampoo.*
- *Teach the client to comb hair with fine-tooth comb to remove eggs (nits).*
- *Teach the client to assess for the continued presence of nits at the base of hair shafts, particularly hair at the nape of the neck and behind the ears.*
- *Maintain contact precautions (e.g., gown and gloves; hair covering is recommended) when providing client care before treatment and for 24 hours after initiation of topical treatment.*

For scabies
- *Maintain contact precautions (e.g., gown and gloves; hair covering is recommended) when providing client care before treatment and for 24 hours after initiation of topical treatment.*
- *Teach the client to scrub the body with soap and water, dry, and apply antiparasitic medication, avoiding the face, eyes, mucous membranes, and open wounds.*

Antivirals

Decrease severity of infections (not curative).

Mechanism of Action	*Examples*	*Nontherapeutic Effects*
Anti-herpes agents • *Decrease viral DNA synthesis.*	acyclovir (Zovirax) famciclovir (Famvir) valacyclovir (Valtrex)	• *Anorexia.* • *Nausea and vomiting.* • *Diarrhea.* • *Headache.*
Anti-cytomegalovirus (CMV) agents • *Decrease viral DNA synthesis.*	cidofovir (Vistide) ganciclovir (Cytovene) valganciclovir (Valcyte)	• *Dizziness.* • *Insomnia.* • *Moniliasis or vaginitis.* • *Nephrotoxicity.*
Anti-hepatitis agents • *Depending on the drug, cause viral DNA death by inhibiting viral replication and phagocytizing cells.*	adefovir (Hepsera) interferon (Intron A) lamivudine (Epivir HBV)	**Anti-CMV agents** • *Hepatotoxicity.*
Anti-influenza agents • *Prevent penetration of virus into host cells or inhibit the neuramidase enzyme needed for viral replication.*	amantadine (Symmetrel) oseltamivir (Tamiflu) rimantadine (Flumadine) zanamivir (Relenza)	• *Central nervous system and bone marrow depression.* • *Teratogenicity.* **Anti-hepatitis agents (adefovir, interferon)** • *Clinical depression.* **Anti-influenza agents** • *Headache.* • *Dizziness.* • *Fatigue.*

Nursing Care

- *Obtain a specimen for culture and sensitivity testing before the first dose is administered.*
- *Teach the client to take the medication exactly as prescribed to maintain therapeutic blood levels.*
- *Teach the client to drink adequate fluids to prevent nephrotoxicity.*
- *Assess for and teach the client about clinical manifestations of nephrotoxicity, hepatotoxicity, and bone marrow and CNS depression.*
- *Employ safety interventions if the client is experiencing headache, dizziness, or fatigue.*
- *Teach the client to avoid pregnancy if the medication can harm a fetus (teratogenic).*

Anti-herpes agents
- *Teach the client to take the medication when pain or pruritus occurs because these precede eruptions.*
- *Teach the client to avoid sexual activity during exacerbations to prevent transmission of the virus.*
- *Teach the client the need for continued health-care supervision because of the increased risk of cervical cancer.*

CASE STUDY: Putting It All Together

An older adult female is admitted to a hospital with extensive weeping lesions over her scalp, neck, axillae, and groin and under her breasts. The client says that she has experienced many rashes over the years and generally uses home remedies that her mother had used when she was a child; however, this time nothing worked to eliminate the rash and itching. She went on to say that, when the lesions spread to her chest and looked like they were infected, she became frightened and short of breath and immediately went to the emergency department. The primary health-care provider admits the client with a diagnosis of atopic dermatitis R/O methicillin-resistant *Staphylococcus aureus* (MRSA) infection. The client's 45-year-old daughter is notified of her mother's admission to the hospital and plans to visit after work.

Primary Health-Care Provider Prescriptions

- Regular diet.
- OOB ad lib.
- Contact precautions.
- IV 0.9% sodium chloride, 100 mL/hour.
- C&S of lesion exudate.
- Wash scalp with fluocinolone acetonide 0.01% (Capex shampoo) daily. Massage into the scalp, allow to stay on for 5 minutes, and then rinse thoroughly.
- Apply a thin layer of desonide 0.05% (Desonate) topical gel to lesions on the neck, chest, axillae, and groin BID.
- Hydrocortisone (Solu-Cortef) 60 mg IVPB times 1 dose, then hydrocortisone 30 mg IVPB every 8 hours.
- Diphenhydramine (Benadryl) 50 mg IVPB times 1, then diphenhydramine 50 mg PO every 6 hours.
- Vancomycin 1g IVPB times 1 dose; then check vancomycin level and report results to primary health-care provider.

Case Study Questions

A. Which nursing action should the nurse implement first? Explain your answer.

_____

B. What nursing actions, including the use of personal protective equipment, should the nurse implement to maintain contact precautions?

1. _____
2. _____
3. _____
4. _____
5. _____
6. _____
7. _____

C. What teaching points should the nurse discuss with people who are visiting this client?

1. _____
2. _____
3. _____
4. _____
5. _____

D. Can alcohol-based and non–alcohol-based hand sanitizers be used to reduce the risk of transmission of MRSA when soap and water are not available? Explain your answer.

_____

REVIEW QUESTIONS

Be sure to read the Introduction for valuable test-taking tips.

1. A nurse is caring for an older adult who sustained a skin tear on the forearm. What type of dressing should the nurse anticipate might be prescribed for this injury?
   1. Hydrogel dressing
   2. Dry sterile dressing
   3. Wet-to-moist dressing
   4. Transparent film dressing

2. A nurse is assessing a client who has a wound on the leg as the result of a bicycle accident. Which clinical manifestations indicate a localized inflammatory response? **Select all that apply.**
   1. Surrounding area is warm.
   2. Body temperature is 101.4°F.
   3. Heart rate is 102 beats/minute.
   4. Area around the wound is swollen.
   5. Immediate vicinity adjoining the wound is painful.
   6. Exudate from the injury is greenish yellow in color.

3. A nurse is caring for a client with gastroenteritis who is receiving contact precautions. Which actions are required when caring for this client? **Select all that apply.**
   1. Keeping visitors 3 feet away from the client
   2. Wearing gloves when entering the client's room
   3. Wearing a gown when entering the client's room
   4. Wearing an eye-protective surgical mask if working within 3 feet of the client
   5. Placing the client in a private room or cohort with another client with the same organism

4. A nurse is assessing a client. Which information indicates that the client may be at risk for infection because a primary defense is impaired? **Select all that apply.**
   1. Oral mucous membranes are pink.
   2. Hair can be seen in the nostrils.
   3. Low white blood cell count.
   4. Eyes appear moist.
   5. Skin is dry.

5. Which actions are unique to maintaining airborne precautions for a client with a diagnosis of suspected pulmonary tuberculosis? **Select all that apply.**
   1. Keeping the door closed after entering and leaving the room
   2. Maintaining negative air pressure in the room
   3. Wearing a surgical mask when in the room
   4. Donning a gown when entering the room
   5. Wearing gloves when entering the room

6. A group of women who are positive for HIV are attending a program about how to prevent the transmission of the virus. Which activity should the nurse teach them to avoid? **Select all that apply.**
   1. Hugging
   2. Breastfeeding
   3. Shaking hands
   4. Using public toilet seats
   5. Washing personal laundry with family clothes

7. A nurse is administering an immunization to a female client. Which questions should the nurse ask the client before administering the immunization? **Select all that apply.**
   1. "Are you menstruating?"
   2. "Do you live in a home with very young children?"
   3. "Have you had a temperature within the last 24 hours?"
   4. "Have you received another vaccination within the last 30 days?"
   5. "Did you ever have an allergic reaction to a vaccination in the past?"

8. A nurse is assessing several clients with a variety of wounds. Which type of wounds should the nurse anticipate will heal by secondary intention? **Select all that apply.**
   1. Abrasion
   2. Paper cut
   3. Pressure ulcer
   4. Abdominal incision from surgery
   5. Superficial slash caused by a knife

9. A nurse is assessing a client who had numerous sutures several days ago for a traumatic injury to the base of the right index finger. Which assessments indicate that the inflammatory response has progressed to an infectious process? **Select all that apply.**
   1. Foul odor
   2. Yellow exudate
   3. Swelling around the site
   4. Inability to flex the finger
   5. Elevated body temperature
   6. Feeling of heat when touched

10. A nurse is counseling a sexually active male client about the ways HIV is transmitted. Which situations that increase the risk of acquiring HIV should the nurse discuss with this client? **Select all that apply.**
    1. Oral sex with another person
    2. Anal sex with another person
    3. Sex with a menstruating woman
    4. Sex when one person has a genital lesion
    5. Use of intravenous drug equipment used by another person

11. A nursing staff development educator is monitoring the sterile technique of a newly hired nurse in a simulation laboratory. What behavior by the newly hired nurse alerts the nurse educator that further teaching is necessary? **Select all that apply.**
1. Wears a mask because of a seasonal cold
2. Opens sterile gauze packages with ungloved hands
3. Uses a sterile bottle of normal saline that was opened by another nurse
4. Discards sterile gauze that may have touched the edge of the sterile field
5. Uses sterile wet swabs with forceps with the hand held higher than the wrist
6. Keeps sterile objectives inside a half inch boarder around the edge of the sterile field

12. A nurse is working in a long-term care facility. Which client should the nurse assess **first**?
1. The client who reports nausea after eating lunch
2. A newly admitted client who says that under her breasts are itchy
3. A client who just sustained an uncomfortable scratch on the forearm
4. The older adult client who reported feeling dizzy when moving from lying to sitting while in bed

13. A nurse is removing personal protective equipment when exiting an isolation room. Place the following steps in the order in which they should be implemented.
1. Untie the gown at the waist.
2. Release the ties of the mask and dispose of the mask in an appropriate trash container.
3. Place fingers of the dominant hand inside cuff of the other sleeve and pull gown sleeve over the nondominant hand.
4. Remove one glove by touching the outside of the glove with the other gloved hand and without contaminating oneself; dispose of it in an appropriate trash container.
5. With the ungloved hand, slip a finger inside the cuff of the other glove and remove it without contaminating oneself and dispose of it in an appropriate trash container.
6. With a gown covered hand, pull gown down over the dominant hand, folding the gown inward and gathering it together as it is pulled down; dispose of it in an appropriate container.
Answer: _____

14. A nurse is working on a medical unit in an acute care agency. For which clients should the nurse institute transmission-based droplet precautions? **Select all that apply.**
1. HIV infection
2. Influenza virus
3. MRSA infected wound
4. Pulmonary tuberculosis
5. *Streptococcal* pneumonia

15. A nurse's assessment of a client's wound that is healing by secondary intention indicates the presence of some raw-looking tissue with extensive necrosis. How should the nurse classify the wound using the color classification system?
1. Red
2. Black
3. Green
4. Yellow

16. A nurse in a home health-care agency is teaching a class about infection control to a group of nursing assistants. Which interventions did the nurse include that interrupts the chain of infection at the mode of transmission stage? **Select all that apply.**
1. Maintain a urinary collection bag below the level of the client's bladder.
2. Shut off the handles of water faucets with a clean, dry paper towel.
3. Clean bedside tables routinely with a disinfectant.
4. Reposition clients every two hours.
5. Keep your fingernails short.

17. A nurse is caring for a client with *Staphylococcus aureus* who is to receive an antibiotic. Which statement should the nurse include in a teaching session that explains the reason for the medication?
1. "This medication should eradicate the organism that is causing your symptoms."
2. "This medication will help to avoid a recurrence of your infection in the future."
3. "The intention of this medication is to support normal body function."
4. "The principle purpose of this medication is palliative."

18. DuoDERM, a hydrocolloid dressing, is prescribed for a client with a break in the skin that has a small amount of drainage. What should the nurse do when applying this dressing? **Select all that apply.**
    1. Stretch the dressing while placing it over the wound.
    2. Apply tape on all four sides of the dressing after its application.
    3. Round off the edges of the dressing when preparing the dressing.
    4. Warm the dressing between the hands before applying the dressing.
    5. Ensure a quarter-inch margin of healthy skin around the wound when sizing the dressing.

19. A nurse teaches a client about a health-related regimen associated with acquired active immunity. For which client is the nurse providing teaching?
    1. A child who has chickenpox
    2. A woman who is learning how to breastfeed
    3. An older adult who is to receive a vaccine to reduce the risk of pneumonia
    4. An adolescent with an inadequate history of immunization who stepped on a rusty nail

20. A nurse is assessing several clients with a variety of wounds. Which wounds should the nurse anticipate will heal by primary intention? **Select all that apply.**
    1. Infected abrasion as a result of a bicycle accident
    2. Ulcer on the greater trochanter as a result of pressure
    3. Sore on a toe as a result of impaired arterial perfusion
    4. Abdominal incision as a result of gastrointestinal surgery
    5. Surgical amputation of the tip of a finger due to a traumatic injury

21. Which actions are associated with droplet precautions? **Select all that apply.**
    1. Keeping the door of the client's room closed
    2. Keeping visitors three feet away from the client
    3. Wearing gloves when entering the client's room
    4. Wearing a surgical mask when working within three feet of the client
    5. Placing a surgical mask on the client when transporting for procedures

22. The nurse receives a prescription to mechanically debride a client's wound. Which action should the nurse expect to perform in relation to this prescription?
    1. Scrubbing the wound with gauze
    2. Placing a collagenase enzyme product into the wound
    3. Assisting with cutting away devitalized tissue from the wound with a scalpel
    4. Applying a dressing to the wound that promotes the body to generate enzymes

23. A nurse is providing teaching to a client who is taking an antibiotic for a bacterial infection. Which is important for the nurse to teach the client to do to help prevent resistance to this antibiotic in the future?
    1. "Eat some food when taking the medication."
    2. "Assess yourself for signs of a superinfection."
    3. "Take the pills evenly spaced around the clock."
    4. "Complete the entire regimen of medication prescribed."

24. During the initial assessment of a newly admitted client, the nurse observes several small red excoriated lines on the client's wrists. What is the nurse's **best** intervention at this time?
    1. Place the client on contact precautions.
    2. Place the client in a negative pressure room.
    3. The client should be oriented to the assigned bedroom.
    4. The client's condition should be communicated to the primary health-care provider.

25. A nurse is changing a client's sterile dressing and performing wound irrigation. Which actions by the nurse maintained sterile technique? **Select all that apply.**
    1. Wore an eye shield and a gown
    2. Used a new sterile piston syringe
    3. Started the flow of irrigating solution just inside the top edge of the wound
    4. Dried the skin on either side of the wound by using one gauze pad for each swipe
    5. Held sterile gloved hands below the waist as much as possible during the procedure
    6. Poured fluid from a previously opened bottle of normal saline sitting on the client's bedside table

26. An adult is diagnosed with an infection, and penicillin G 1,000,000 units via intermittent infusion every 6 hours is prescribed. The vial instructions state to add 1.8 mL of sterile water to yield 250 mg/mL. How many mL should the nurse prepare to add to the intravenous infusion? **Record your answer using a whole number.**
Answer: _____ mL

27. A nurse is collecting equipment for several procedures that need to be performed. For which procedures should the nurse wear sterile gloves? **Select all that apply.**
    1. Collecting a urine specimen from a closed drainage system for a culture and sensitivity test
    2. Instilling solution into a nasogastric tube to reestablish patency of the catheter
    3. Suctioning the oropharynx to maintain airway patency
    4. Obtaining a specimen for blood glucose monitoring
    5. Changing a dressing on a central venous catheter
    6. Inserting a urinary retention catheter

28. Protective isolation (neutropenic precautions) is prescribed for a client who is immunocompromised. What should the nurse do? **Select all that apply.**
    1. Wear gloves when entering the client's room.
    2. Remove fresh flowers from the client's room.
    3. Place a N95 respirator on the client during transport when outside the room.
    4. Ensure positive room air pressure of the client's room relative to the corridor.
    5. Have people with a respiratory infection wear a mask when in the client's room.
    6. Ensure that housekeeping staff use a dry mop when cleaning the floor of the client's room.

29. A client is to begin a regimen of cephalexin by mouth for a pneumococcal infection. What actions should the nurse take to help the client avoid complications from this regimen? **Select all that apply.**
    1. Suggest that the client eat an active culture yogurt while taking the medication.
    2. Tell the client to inform the clinic if the tongue develops a white coating.
    3. Inform the client to call the clinic if there is blood in the stool.
    4. Advise the client to take the medication with food.
    5. Encourage the client to drink more fluids.

30. A school nurse is planning a health class for seniors in high school about interrupting the chain of infection at the reservoir stage. What should the nurse include in the teaching plan? **Select all that apply.**
    1. Storing food in a cool environment
    2. Keeping a kitchen garbage can clean
    3. Obtaining age-appropriate immunizations
    4. Covering a cough by coughing into an elbow
    5. Eliminating stagnant water in the environment
    6. Wearing long pants in an area where ticks are endemic

31. A client has a wound that is healing by secondary intention. The nurse is using sterile technique to irrigate the wound before applying a wet to damp dressing. Which step of this procedure is an intervention associated with sterile technique?
    1. Wipe the outside of edges of the wound first.
    2. Wash the hands again after setting up the sterile field.
    3. Place the irrigating solution on the side of the field farthest from the client.
    4. Direct the flow of sterile irrigating solution to the inside top of the client's wound.

32. A nurse is caring for a client who is to have a midstream urine specimen collected. Which action interrupts the chain of infection at the mode of transmission?
    1. Giving the client a sterile container for the collection of urine
    2. Cleansing the urethral orifice with an antiseptic solution soaked cotton ball
    3. Instructing the client to collect the specimen after initiating the urine stream
    4. Placing the urine specimen container into a transport bag using aseptic technique

33. Place the photographs in the order in which the steps should be implemented when donning sterile gloves.

1.

2.

3.

4.

5.

Answer: _____

34. A client is diagnosed as having herpes simplex type 2, and acyclovir is prescribed for use during recurrent outbreaks. Which statement indicates that the client understands the nurse's instructions about this medication?
1. "I should discontinue the medication if I develop dizziness."
2. "I have to increase fiber in my diet because the medication may cause constipation."
3. "I must take my pulse before I take this medication because it can increase my heart rate."
4. "I need to take this medication as soon as I feel tingling in the area where I get the lesions."

35. A nurse is assessing the vaccines received by an infant. Which vaccine should have been received at least twice by 4 months of age? **Select all that apply.**
1. Tetanus vaccine
2. Varicella vaccine
3. Influenza vaccine
4. Diphtheria vaccine
5. Inactivated poliovirus vaccine
6. Measles, mumps, and rubella vaccine

36. Clindamycin palmitate hydrochloride (Cleocin) oral suspension 60 mg by mouth three times a day is prescribed for 10 days for a young child. The bottle of medication indicates that there are 75 mg per 5 mL of solution. How many milliliters of solution should the nurse plan to administer for each dose? **Record your answer using a whole number.**
Answer: _____ mL

37. A nurse is caring for a postoperative client who requires the use of the device that appears in the illustration. In what situation should the nurse use this type of device?

1. A wound that requires frequent dressing changes
2. A dressing that should dry out between changes
3. A wound that has a small amount of drainage
4. A dressing that the client will care for

38. A nurse is caring for a client who has a prescription for wound irrigation. Which should the nurse do when implementing this procedure? **Select all that apply.**
1. Use a 60 mL piston syringe to cleanse debris from the wound.
2. Use sterile gauze to dry the wound edges after completion of the procedure.
3. Spray around the wound, then spray the inside of the wound from top to bottom.
4. Hold a piston syringe 4 inches from the wound surface when applying the solution.
5. Position the client so that the irrigating solution will flow from the wound into an emesis basin.

39. A nurse is caring for a client who has a pressure ulcer with a vacuum-assisted closure device. Which should the nurse do when applying this device? **Select all that apply.**

1. Place the suction apparatus over a hole at the edge of the transparent film.
2. Cut the foam dressing so that it extends 1 inch beyond the wound cavity.
3. Make sure wrinkles are present in the film when pressure is applied.
4. Connect the tubing to the positive pressure machine as prescribed.
5. Apply the transparent film 2 inches beyond the wound margins.

40. A client is admitted to the hospital for multiple, extensive, severe abrasions and a concussion after being hit and dragged by an automobile. The nurse reviews the client's past medical history, interviews the client, and performs a physical assessment. Based on this information, what risk factors for delayed wound healing should the nurse identify? **Select all that apply.**

1. Advanced age
2. Chronic illnesses
3. Dependent edema
4. Inadequate nutrition
5. Presence of an infection
6. History of smoking cigarettes

Client's Clinical Record
Past Medical History
77 years old; developed type 2 diabetes 10 years ago; gave up smoking cigarettes 5 years ago when diagnosed with congestive heart failure; status stable receiving furosemide (Lasix) and enalapril (Vasotec).
Client Interview
Client states, "A car turned the corner, hit me while I was crossing the street, and dragged me for about a half a block. I live alone and it has been hard for me since my wife died." Client indicates that he has become a good cook and has meals on wheels delivered during the week.
Physical Assessment
Height: 5 feet, 10 inches Weight: 150 pounds Temp: 99°F, temporal route Pulse: 92 beats per minute, bounding Respirations: 18 breaths per minute, regular depth and rhythm Blood Pressure: 156/88 mm Hg 2+ edema in distal lower extremities Oriented to time, place, and person Pink-tinged serous oozing from abrasions on arms and legs

REVIEW ANSWERS AND RATIONALES

1. ANSWER: 4.
Rationales:
1. A hydrogel dressing helps to maintain a moist wound environment and should be covered with other dressing materials, which makes it too bulky for a superficial injury such as a skin tear. Hydrogel dressings are most often used on pressure ulcers with moderate drainage.
2. A dry sterile dressing is inappropriate for a skin tear because it will dry out the wound, interfering with wound healing.
3. A wet-to-moist dressing is inappropriate for a skin tear. It is more often used for a larger wound. Also, excess moisture will cause maceration of tissue around the wound, inhibiting wound healing.
4. Transparent film dressings have an adhesive side that adheres to dry tissue but not moist tissue. It provides a protective barrier and moist inner surface that facilitates epithelialization of a wound. They are not used for stage III and IV pressure ulcers; draining wounds; infected, puncture, or arterial wounds; or full-thickness burns.
Content Area: Inflammation, Infection, Immunity, and Wound Care
Integrated Processes: Nursing Process: Planning
Client Need: Physiological Integrity; Physiological Adaptation
Cognitive Level: Analysis
Concept: Tissue Integrity

2. ANSWER: 1, 4, 5.
Rationales:
1. Because of an increase in blood flow to a wound on the leg, the area will feel warm to the touch.
2. An increased body temperature is a systemic, not local, response that is associated with infection, not inflammation.
3. An elevated heart rate is a systemic, not localized, response that is associated with infection, not inflammation.
4. A localized swelling around a wound indicates the presence of edema. Vasodilation and increased permeability of the capillaries promote the shift of fluid from the intravascular compartment to the interstitial compartment.
5. Localized swelling around a wound due to vasodilation and increased permeability of the capillaries promote a shift of fluid from the intravascular compartment to the interstitial compartment causing pressure on pain receptors resulting in pain.
6. Greenish-yellow exudate from a wound indicates infection, not inflammation. A clear, watery (serous) discharge is associated with the inflammatory response.
TEST-TAKING TIP: Identify the clang associations. The word *wound* in the stem and in options 4 and 5 are clang associations. Examine these options carefully.
Content Area: Inflammation, Infection, Immunity, and Wound Care
Integrated Processes: Nursing Process: Assessment
Client Need: Physiological Integrity; Reduction of Risk Potential
Cognitive Level: Analysis
Concept: Inflammation

3. ANSWER: 2, 3, 5.
Rationales:
1. As long as the visitor wears gloves and a gown and wears a mask if splashing with blood or body fluids is likely, the visitor may enter the client's room as well as move within 3 feet of the client. The need to keep a visitor, without a surgical mask, farther than 3 feet from the client refers to droplet precautions, not contact precautions.
2. Gloves always must be worn when entering a room when a client is on contact precautions. Gloves protect the hands from exposure to the client's pathogens.
3. A gown must be worn when entering the room of a client who is on contact precautions who has diarrhea, has a colostomy, is incontinent, has a wound not contained by a dressing, or when giving direct client care. A gown protects a person's clothing from being exposed to the client's pathogens.
4. A mask with eye protection is necessary in a room when a client is on contact precautions only if there is a likelihood of the caregiver being splashed with a client's body fluids.
5. A client on contact precautions must either be in a private room or have a roommate with the same pathogenic microorganism; this contains pathogens within a controlled environment, protecting noninfected clients.
Content Area: Inflammation, Infection, Immunity, and Wound Care
Integrated Processes: Nursing Process: Implementation
Client Need: Safe and Effective Care Environment; Safety and Infection Control
Cognitive Level: Application
Concept: Safety

4. ANSWER: 3, 5.
Rationales:
1. The mucous membranes have an abundant capillary network that carries blood to the area; as a result, the mucous membranes appear pink. Also, the mucous membranes produce mucus that traps microorganisms.
2. Hair in the nostrils and cilia and mucus in the respiratory tract capture and move microorganisms out of the respiratory tract.
3. White blood cells are a primary defense against infection. If a white blood cell count is lower than the expected range, the ability to fight an infection may be impaired.
4. Tears contain lysosomes that destroy microorganisms. Tears and blinking flush microorganisms out of the eyes.
5. Sebum, a secretion of the sebaceous glands of the skin, is an oily substance that softens and lubricates the skin; it also has a bactericidal effect that protects the skin from microorganisms.
TEST-TAKING TIP: Identify the words in the stem that indicate negative polarity. The words *defense is impaired* indicate that the stem has negative polarity.
Content Area: Inflammation, Infection, Immunity, and Wound Care
Integrated Processes: Nursing Process: Assessment
Client Need: Physiological Integrity; Safety and Infection Control
Cognitive Level: Application
Concept: Infection

5. **ANSWER: 1, 2.**
   Rationales:
   1. To maintain negative air pressure in a room required for airborne precautions, the door to the room must be kept closed except when entering or exiting the room.
   2. A private room that has negative air pressure (6 to 12 exchanges of air per hour, or discharge of air to the outside, or a filtration system for the air in the room) is required for airborne precautions.
   3. A respiratory device (N95 respirator), not a surgical mask, is necessary to protect a caregiver from the *M. tuberculosis* or *M. bovis* emanating from the client's respiratory tract.
   4. Donning a gown is necessary only when the caregiver is at risk for coming into contact with the client's body fluids, contaminated items, or nonintact skin.
   5. Gloves are only necessary when it is likely that the nurse will come into contact with the client's body fluids, contaminated items, nonintact skin, or mucous membranes.
   Content Area: Inflammation, Infection, Immunity, Wound Care
   Integrated Processes: Nursing Process: Implementation
   Client Need: Safe and Effective Care Environment; Safety and Infection Control
   Cognitive Level: Application
   Concept: Safety

6. **ANSWER: 2, 5.**
   Rationales:
   1. HIV is not spread casually through hugging.
   2. **Breast milk can transmit HIV to a newborn.**
   3. HIV is not spread casually through hand shaking.
   4. HIV is not spread through the use of public toilet seats.
   5. **Personal clothing or linen may be contaminated with blood or body fluids. Personal soiled clothing and linen should be contained in a plastic bag until it is washed. These items should be washed with hot water and laundry detergent as well as a cup of bleach in each load.**
   TEST-TAKING TIP: Identify the word in the stem that indicates negative polarity. The word *avoid* indicates a stem with negative polarity. The test-taker is being asked, "What behavior *should not* be performed to help prevent the transmission of HIV?"
   Content Area: Inflammation, Infection, Immunity, and Wound Care
   Integrated Processes: Teaching/Learning; Nursing Process: Implementation
   Client Need: Safe and Effective Care Environment; Safety and Infection Control
   Cognitive Level: Application
   Concept: Patient-Centered Care; Immunity

7. **ANSWERS: 2, 3, 4, 5.**
   Rationales:
   1. Menstruation has no effect on the administration of vaccinations.
   2. **If the person has very young children, the primary health-care provider should be consulted because the vaccine may contain a live virus or bacterium that has the potential for causing an infection in young children.**
   3. **A temperature is a contraindication for receiving a vaccination because the body is fighting an infection.**

Vaccines are stressors that challenge the immune system.
4. **If a client had another vaccination within the last month, the client should be referred to the primary health-care provider to ensure that the two vaccines will not interact.**
5. **If a client had an allergic reaction to a vaccine or any of its ingredients (e.g., eggs), the client should not receive the vaccine again without consultation with the primary health-care provider.**
TEST-TAKING TIP: Identify the options with a clang association. The word *immunization* in the stem and the word *vaccination* in options 4 and 5 are obscure clang associations. Examine these options carefully.
Content Area: Inflammation, Infection, Immunity, and Wound Care
Integrated Processes: Communication and Documentation; Nursing Process: Assessment
Client Need: Physiological Integrity; Pharmacological and Parenteral Therapies
Cognitive Level: Analysis
Concept: Immunity

8. **ANSWER: 1, 3.**
   Rationales:
   1. **An abrasion is a scraping away of skin or mucous membrane due to traumatic injury or mechanical means. This type of wound involves tissue loss that prevents approximated wound edges, thereby necessitating healing from inner skin layers to the surface of the skin (secondary intention).**
   2. A paper cut will heal by primary intention because the injury is superficial and the wound edges are approximated. Primary intention healing involves minimal formation of granulated tissue and scarring.
   3. **A pressure ulcer does not have approximated wound edges. Pressure ulcers usually involve the epidermis and dermis that require healing by secondary intention. Secondary intention healing occurs from inner skin layers to outer skin layers. Fragile granulated tissue fills in the wound and eventually the capillaries constrict, tissue shrinks, collagen fibers contract, and firmer fibrous tissue remains (scar).**
   4. Surgery is conducted using sterile technique and the abdominal incision has approximated wound edges. An abdominal incision usually heals by primary intention.
   5. A superficial slash will heal by primary intention because it has minimal tissue destruction and approximated wound edges.
   Content Area: Inflammation, Infection, Immunity, and Wound Care
   Integrated Processes: Nursing Process: Analysis
   Client Need: Physiological Integrity; Safety and Infection Control
   Cognitive Level: Analysis
   Concept: Tissue Integrity

9. **ANSWER: 1, 2, 5.**
   Rationales:
   1. **A foul odor to a wound indicates infection. The odor is the result of purulent drainage consisting of pyogenic**

bacteria, protein-rich fluid filled with white blood cells, and cellular debris.

2. **Purulent drainage, which may be yellow, green, tan, or brown, indicates the presence of an infectious process. The discharge contains cellular debris, destroyed tissue, phagocytic cells, and microorganisms (pus). The discharge associated with the inflammatory response usually is clear (serous) and contains cellular debris proteins and plasma fluid; it also may contain blood (e.g., serosanguineous, sanguineous).**

3. Swelling around the site is part of the local inflammatory response. Histamine released at the site of the trauma causes vasodilation, and kinins released by destroyed cells increase capillary permeability; both allow fluid to move from the intravascular compartment into the interstitial compartment, resulting in an accumulation of fluid (edema).

4. Edema and pain associated with the local inflammatory response interfere with the ability to flex the finger.

5. **An increased body temperature is a systemic response to an infection. The body is creating a hostile environment that can interfere with the replication of bacterial cells.**

6. Local heat is part of the local inflammatory response. Dilation of blood vessels brings more warm blood to the site and there is an increase in metabolic processes at the site; both increase heat at the site of the injury.

Content Area: Inflammation, Infection, Immunity, and Wound Care
Integrated Processes: Nursing Process: Evaluation
Client Need: Physiological Integrity; Safety and Infection Control
Cognitive Level: Analysis
Concept: Infection

10. **ANSWER: 1, 2, 3, 4, 5.**
Rationales:

1. **Engaging in unprotected oral sex increases the risk of HIV transmission because of mucous membrane contact with potentially infected body fluids.**

2. **Trauma to mucous membranes that may result in bleeding increase the risk of transmission of the HIV during unprotected anal sex.**

3. **Unprotected sex with a menstruating woman increases the risk of HIV transmission because the virus resides in blood.**

4. **The risk of contracting the HIV from unprotected sex with an infected person is greater when the uninfected person has a genital lesion because the skin or mucous membranes are not intact.**

5. **Sharing intravenous equipment exposes the second person using the equipment to the blood of a potentially HIV-infected individual.**

Content Area: Inflammation, Infection, Immunity, and Wound Care
Integrated Processes: Teaching/Learning; Nursing Process: Implementation
Client Need: Safe and Effective Care Environment; Safety and Infection Control
Cognitive Level: Application
Concept: Patient-Centered Care; Infection

11. **ANSWER: 1, 3, 5, 6.**
Rationales:

1. **Wearing a mask because of a seasonal cold was not an appropriate decision on the part of the nurse. A nurse who has an upper respiratory infection should not be caring for any client, especially a client with a wound. Although this was just a simulation, the nurse should have said to the educator, "I cannot put clients at risk by caring for them when I have a cold. I will proceed as if I did not have a cold for the purpose of this simulation."**

2. The outside of sterile gauze packages are not sterile; they can be touched with the hands.

3. **The nurse cannot vouch for the sterility of the bottle of saline. A new bottle of saline should be used.**

4. If a sterile item is believed to have touched a nonsterile surface or item, the sterile item must be discarded as contaminated. The outer one inch of a sterile field is always considered contaminated.

5. **Sterile wet swabs held with forceps must be held downward, not upward, to keep fluid from flowing up toward the hands and becoming contaminated.**

6. **The nurse must keep all sterile objects within a 1-, not half-, inch border around the entire sterile field because only objects within the 1-inch border are considered sterile.**

TEST-TAKING TIP: Identify the words in the stem that indicate negative polarity. The words *further teaching is necessary* in the stem indicate negative polarity. The question is asking, "What is unacceptable technique when changing a sterile dressing?" Identify the unique option. Option 1 is unique because it is the only option that does not contain the word *sterile*. Examine option 1 carefully. Identify the clang associations. The word *sterile* in the stem and in options 2, 3, 4, 5, and 6 are clang associations. Unfortunately, identifying clang associations will not help you explore potential correct options in this question.

Content Area: Inflammation, Infection, Immunity, and Wound Care
Integrated Processes: Teaching/Learning; Nursing Process: Evaluation
Client Need: Safe and Effective Care Environment; Management of Care
Cognitive Level: Application
Concept: Patient-Centered Care; Infection

12. **ANSWER: 2.**
Rationales:

1. Although it is important to assess a client experiencing nausea, this situation is not the priority.

2. **The newly admitted client may have scabies. This is a condition where a mite burrows under the skin; it generally involves the wrists, auxiliary area, and/or under the breasts. Scabies are contagious, and contact precautions should be instituted until the client is assessed. If scabies is diagnosed, contact precautions should be maintained for 24 hours after the client receives treatment.**

3. Although it is important to address this client's needs because the scratch may become a portal of entry for microorganisms, this situation is not the priority.

4. It is not uncommon for an older person to experience orthostatic hypotension when moving from a lying to a sitting position. Although it is important to assess this client, this situation is not the priority.

TEST-TAKING TIP: Identify the word in the stem that sets a priority. The word *first* in the stem sets a priority.

Content Area: Inflammation, Infection, Immunity, and Wound Care
Integrated Processes: Nursing Process: Planning
Client Need: Safe and Effective Care Environment; Safety and Infection Control
Cognitive Level: Analysis
Concept: Patient-Centered Care; Safety

13. **ANSWER: 1, 4, 5, 2, 3, 6.**
Rationales:
1. The tie at the waist is released first while still wearing gloves. The tie at the waist is considered contaminated because it is at or below the level of the waist, which is always considered contaminated.
4. The gloves are removed next so as not to contaminate the hands or the environment. The first glove is removed by touching only the outside of the gloves.
5. After the first glove is removed, the second glove is removed by touching only the inside of the contaminated glove.
2. The ties of the mask can be untied with the hands because the ties are considered clean.
3. The gown is removed by touching only the inside of the gown. A hand can be used by placing the fingers of one hand up the inside of the other sleeve and pulling the sleeve down over the hand.
6. With the other hand inside the gown, the gown should be folded downward and gathered inward to itself. The gown acts as a barrier and protects the nurse from contact with the contaminated outer surface of the gown. Gathering the soiled gown together as it is pulled down contains the contaminated surface of the gown. A paper gown is then placed in an appropriate trash container while a material gown is placed in a designated linen hamper. Before leaving the client's room, the hands are washed.

Content Area: Inflammation, Infection, Immunity, and Wound Care
Integrated Processes: Nursing Process: Planning
Client Need: Safe and Effective Care Environment; Safety and Infection Control
Cognitive Level: Analysis
Concept: Safety

14. **ANSWER: 2, 5.**
Rationales:
1. HIV is transmitted via blood, semen, vaginal secretions, and breast milk. Standard precautions, which are instituted for all clients, should be followed.
2. The influenza virus is transmitted by large-particle respiratory droplets. Droplet precautions should be instituted.

3. Methicillin-resistant *Staphylococcus aureus* (MRSA) in a wound is transmitted by contact with the infected individual or a MRSA-contaminated surface or object. Contact precautions should be instituted.
4. *Mycobacterium tuberculosis* microorganisms are transmitted via airborne nuclei. Airborne precautions should be instituted.
5. *Streptococcal* pneumonia is transmitted by large-particle respiratory droplets. Droplet precautions should be instituted.

TEST-TAKING TIP: Identify the unique option. Option 5 is unique. It is the only option that contains an italicized word.

Content Area: Inflammation, Infection, Immunity, and Wound Care
Integrated Processes: Nursing Process: Implementation
Client Need: Safe and Effective Care Environment; Safety and Infection Control
Cognitive Level: Analysis
Concept: Safety

15. **ANSWER: 2.**
Rationales:
1. A wound with newly granulating tissue is classified as red. This is a sign of the reparative stage of wound healing.
2. Necrotic tissue indicates cell death caused by the progressive degradative action of enzymes. Wounds exhibiting necrotic tissue are classified as black.
3. The color green is not part of the color classification system of wounds.
4. A wound with purulent exudate is classified as yellow. It usually indicates the presence of infection.

Content Area: Inflammation, Infection, Immunity, and Wound Care
Integrated Processes: Nursing Process: Assessment
Client Need: Physiological Integrity; Safety and Infection Control
Cognitive Level: Analysis
Concept: Tissue Integrity

16. **ANSWER: 2, 3, 5.**
Rationales:
1. Keeping a urinary collection bag below the level of the client's bladder will prevent the backflow of urine into the urinary bladder. This will prevent microorganisms from entering the bladder. Portals of entry in humans include the respiratory, gastrointestinal, reproductive, and urinary tracts and the skin and mucous membranes.
2. Shutting off the handle of a water faucet with a clean, dry paper towel is an action that interrupts the chain of infection at the mode of transmission stage. Microorganisms thrive on the handles of water faucets and are transmitted to others when touched.
3. The mode of transmission stage of the chain of infection is related to how a microorganism is transferred from an infectious agent to the portal of entry of a host. Microorganisms can thrive on surfaces that the client uses and be transmitted to a portal of entry in the client.

4. Repositioning a client every 2 hours maintains tissue integrity. This interrupts the chain of infection at the susceptible host stage.

5. Microorganisms thrive under fingernails because the area is warm, dark, and moist. Therefore, they should be kept short to prevent the harboring of microorganisms. Also, artificial nails and nail polish should be avoided.

Content Area: *Inflammation, Infection, Immunity, and Wound Care*
Integrated Processes: *Teaching/Learning; Nursing Process: Implementation*
Client Need: *Safe and Effective Care Environment; Safety and Infection Control*
Cognitive Level: *Analysis*
Concept: *Infection*

17. ANSWER: 1.

Rationales:

1. Antibiotics are used to destroy disease-producing pathogens. Antibiotics are curative in nature.

2. Antibiotics will not prevent a recurrence of the infection.

3. Antibiotics are not classified as health maintenance drugs. Drugs that support normal body function are called "substitutive" medications or provide for "health maintenance" (e.g., levothyroxine [Synthroid] for an underactive thyroid gland).

4. Antibiotics are not drugs that are palliative in nature. A palliative drug is used to relieve signs or symptoms of disease, not cure the disease (e.g., acetaminophen to relieve a fever).

Content Area: *Inflammation, Infection, Immunity, and Wound Care*
Integrated Processes: *Communication and Documentation; Teaching/Learning; Nursing Process: Implementation*
Client Need: *Physiological Integrity; Pharmacological and Parenteral Therapies*
Cognitive Level: *Application*
Concept: *Medication; Infection*

18. ANSWER: 3, 4.

Rationales:

1. Avoid applying the dressing by stretching the product or using too much tension to prevent a tourniquet effect.

2. Applying tape around all four sides of the dressing after its application is unnecessary; it is a self-adhesive dressing.

3. Rounding off the edges of the dressing reduces the likelihood of the edges catching on gowns or linens causing a rolling of the edges of the dressing.

4. Warming the dressing between the hands before application improves adhesion of the dressing to the client's skin.

5. The nurse should ensure that there is a 1-inch margin of healthy skin around the wound when sizing the dressing.

TEST-TAKING TIP: Identify the option with a specific determiner. Option 2 contains the word *all* which is a specific determiner.

Content Area: *Inflammation, Infection, Immunity, and Wound Care*
Integrated Processes: *Nursing Process: Implementation*
Client Need: *Physiological Integrity; Safety and Infection Control*
Cognitive Level: *Application*
Concept: *Tissue Integrity*

19. ANSWER: 3.

Rationales:

1. A person with a disease develops immunity to the disease in the future because the body produced antibodies in response to the original antigen. This is known as natural active immunity.

2. A breastfeeding mother transmits antibodies to her infant through colostrum in breast milk. This is known as natural passive immunity.

3. A medication that stimulates the production of antibodies that limit or prevent future infection is called an immunization or vaccine. This is known as acquired active immunity.

4. An adolescent who stepped on a rusty nail and has an inadequate immunization history will be treated with an antitoxin that contains antibodies (human tetanus immune globulin—TIG). This is known as acquired passive immunity.

Content Area: *Inflammation, Infection, Immunity, and Wound Care*
Integrated Processes: *Teaching/Learning; Nursing Process: Implementation*
Client Need: *Health Promotion and Maintenance*
Cognitive Level: *Analysis*
Concept: *Patient-Centered Care; Immunity*

20. ANSWER: 4, 5.

Rationales:

1. An abrasion is an area of skin that is denuded by a mechanical process, such as friction. An abrasion does not have wound edges that are approximated and therefore heals by secondary intention.

2. A pressure ulcer usually involves the epidermis and dermis resulting in a crater that does not have approximated wound edges. It heals by secondary intention. In addition, a pressure ulcer results from impaired capillary perfusion due to pressure, which also delays wound healing.

3. An ulcer on a toe as a result of impaired arterial circulation can injure the epidermis, dermis, and underlying structures, such as muscle and bone. Wounds with impaired circulation can become chronic, are difficult to heal, and usually heal by secondary intention.

4. An abdominal incision is created under sterile conditions, and the wound edges are approximated and sutured in place. Surgical incisions usually heal by primary intention.

5. A surgical amputation is created under sterile conditions, and the wound edges are approximated and sutured in place. Surgical incisions usually heal by primary intention.

Content Area: *Inflammation, Infection, Immunity, and Wound Care*
Integrated Processes: *Nursing Process: Analysis*

Client Need: Physiological Integrity; Reduction of Risk Potential
Cognitive Level: Analysis
Concept: Tissue Integrity

21. **ANSWER: 2, 4, 5.**
    Rationales:
    1. The door to a client's room must be kept closed with airborne, not droplet, precautions.
    2. Keeping visitors 3 feet away from the client is required with droplet precautions to protect visitors from large-particle droplets emanating from the client's respiratory tract.
    3. Gloves are necessary only when coming into contact with body fluids, such as excretions and secretions, mucous membranes, or nonintact skin.
    4. Wearing a mask within 3 feet when working with the client is required with droplet precautions to protect the caregiver from large-droplet particles emanating from the client's respiratory tract.
    5. Placing a surgical mask on the client when transporting the client is required with droplet precautions to protect others and the environment from contamination with large-droplet particles emanating from the client's respiratory tract.
    Content Area: Inflammation, Infection, Immunity, and Wound Care
    Integrated Processes: Nursing Process: Implementation
    Client Need: Safe and Effective Care Environment; Safety and Infection Control
    Cognitive Level: Application
    Concept: Safety

22. **ANSWER: 1.**
    Rationales:
    1. Scrubbing a wound with gauze uses friction to remove devitalized, necrotic tissue. This type of debridement is known as mechanical debridement. A nurse can implement this procedure at the direction of a primary health-care provider.
    2. The use of a collagenase enzyme product to remove devitalized, necrotic tissue is known as chemical debridement. A nurse can implement this procedure after receiving a prescription from a primary health-care provider.
    3. Removal of devitalized, necrotic tissue with a scalpel or scissors is known as surgical debridement. A nurse does not perform this intervention independently but assists a primary health-care provider.
    4. The application of a dressing that promotes the body to generate enzymes to break down necrotic tissue is known as autolytic debridement. A nurse can apply this dressing after receiving a prescription from a primary health-care provider.
    TEST-TAKING TIP: Identify the options that are equally plausible. Options 2 and 4 both involve enzymes to debride the wound. More often than not, equally plausible options are distractors and can be eliminated from consideration.
    Content Area: Inflammation, Infection, Immunity, and Wound Care
    Integrated Processes: Nursing Process: Implementation

Client Need: Physiological Integrity; Physiological Adaptation
Cognitive Level: Application
Concept: Tissue Integrity

23. **ANSWER: 4.**
    Rationales:
    1. Taking an antibiotic with food prevents gastric irritation, not resistant bacteria. Not all antibiotics should be administered with food because some are absorbed more efficiently on an empty stomach.
    2. A superinfection is an infection occurring in a person who already is experiencing an infection. These signs generally include furry overgrowth on the tongue, vaginal discharge, and foul-smelling stool. A pathogen causing a superinfection usually is resistant to the medication being administered.
    3. Evenly spacing doses of antibiotic medication maintains a therapeutic blood level of the drug; it does not prevent bacterial resistance.
    4. Taking the entire regimen of antibiotic eradicates the pathogens that have invaded the body. Stopping the medication early promotes the development of resistant bacteria.
    Content Area: Inflammation, Infection, Immunity, and Wound Care
    Integrated Processes: Teaching/Learning; Nursing Process: Implementation
    Client Need: Physiological Integrity; Pharmacological and Parenteral Therapies
    Cognitive Level: Analysis
    Concept: Medication; Infection

24. **ANSWER: 1.**
    Rationales:
    1. These lines can be an indication of scabies, which are highly contagious; therefore, the client should be placed on contact precautions.
    2. Excoriated lines on a client do not indicate tuberculosis or any other disease requiring a negative pressure room.
    3. The nurse should orient the client to the room after another intervention is performed.
    4. The nurse should inform the client's primary health-care provider of the assessment findings after another intervention is performed.
    TEST-TAKING TIP: Identify the word in the stem that sets a priority. The word *best* in the stem sets a priority.
    Content Area: Inflammation, Infection, Immunity, and Wound Care
    Integrated Processes: Nursing Process: Implementation
    Client Need: Safe and Effective Care Environment; Safety and Infection Control
    Cognitive Level: Application
    Concept: Safety

25. **ANSWER: 2, 3, 4.**
    Rationales:
    1. Wearing personnel protective equipment does not maintain sterile technique during wound irrigation. Wearing an eye shield and gown protects the nurse from the client's blood and body fluids.

2. **A new sterile piston syringe should be used each time the wound is irrigated to avoid introducing a pathogenic microorganism.**

3. **The flow of irrigating solution should start at the top inner edge of the wound so that the solution flows down the wound and is collected as it flows out of the wound by gravity. Starting at the inner edge of the wound and not outside the edge of the wound reduces the risk of contaminating the wound with pathogenic microorganisms on the skin.**

4. **Drying the skin on either side of the wound by using one gauze pad for each swipe maintains sterile technique. One gauze pad should be used for each swipe because it prevents cross contamination. Dry skin will allow adherence of the tape used to secure the dressing.**

5. Holding sterile gloves below the waist violates sterile technique. Sterile gloved hands should be held above the waist and within the line of site at all times to ensure that they do not touch an unsterile surface or object.

6. Using fluid from a previously opened bottle of normal saline sitting on the client's bedside table violates sterile technique. The nurse has no knowledge about the sterility of the bottle of normal saline.

TEST-TAKING TIP: Identify the clang associations. The word *wound* in the stem and in options 3 and 4 are clang associations. Examine these options carefully.

Content Area: Inflammation, Infection, Immunity, and Wound Care
Integrated Processes: Nursing Process: Evaluation
Client Need: Safe and Effective Care Environment; Safety and Infection Control
Cognitive Level: Application
Concept: Infection

26. **ANSWER: 4.**
Rationale:
Solve the problem by using ratio and proportion.

$$\frac{\text{Desire } 1{,}000{,}000 \text{ units}}{\text{Have } 250{,}000 \text{ units}} = \frac{\text{x mL}}{1 \text{ mL}}$$

$$250{,}000\text{x} = 1{,}000{,}000 \times 1$$
$$250{,}000\text{x} = 1{,}000{,}000$$
$$\text{x} = 1{,}000{,}000 \div 250{,}000$$
$$\text{x} = 4 \text{ mL}$$

Content Area: Inflammation, Infection, Immunity, and Wound Care
Integrated Processes: Nursing Process: Planning
Client Need: Physiological Integrity; Pharmacological and Parenteral Therapies
Cognitive Level: Application
Concept: Medication; Infection

27. **ANSWER: 3, 5, 6.**
Rationales:
1. Sterile equipment (e.g., sterile syringe and sterile specimen container) and clean gloves should be used by the nurse to collect a urine specimen from a closed urinary drainage system for a culture and sensitivity test.
2. Instilling solution into a nasogastric tube to reestablish patency of the catheter is not a sterile procedure. Clean

gloves should be worn by the nurse while performing this procedure.

3. **Suctioning the oropharynx to maintain airway patency is a sterile procedure. A foreign object is being placed into the oropharynx, which makes the client vulnerable to being exposed to microorganisms.**

4. Obtaining a specimen for blood glucose monitoring is not a sterile procedure. Clean gloves should be worn by the provider of care during this procedure.

5. **A central venous catheter causes a break in the skin, and the catheter enters a large vein of the body. These factors place the client at risk for a systemic infection, and therefore the nurse must wear sterile gloves and maintain sterile technique when changing this dressing.**

6. **Inserting a urinary retention catheter requires the nurse to wear sterile gloves and maintain sterile technique because the catheter is entering a sterile body cavity.**

Content Area: Inflammation, Infection, Immunity, and Wound Care
Integrated Processes: Nursing Process: Planning
Client Need: Safe and Effective Care Environment; Safety and Infection Control
Cognitive Level: Analysis
Concept: Infection

28. **ANSWER: 2, 3, 4**
Rationales:
1. Wearing gloves is unnecessary. The nurse does not have to be protected from the client.
2. **Fresh flowers and potted plants harbor molds. They should be removed from the client's room to limit exposure to microorganisms that could harm the client.**
3. **Wearing an N95 respirator protects the client from airborne pathogens when outside the room.**
4. **Filtration of air coming into the client's room, 12 air exchanges per hour, a well-sealed room, and maintaining positive room air pressure relative to the corridor reduces the risk of the presence of airborne pathogens entering the room and placing the client at risk for infection.**
5. People with respiratory infections should not be permitted in the client's room with or without a mask.
6. Although the floor should be cleaned, it should be wet mopped, not dry mopped. Wet mopping will limit dust and help prevent microorganisms from becoming aerosolized.

Content Area: Inflammation, Infection, Immunity, and Wound Care
Integrated Processes: Nursing Process: Implementation
Client Need: Safe and Effective Care Environment; Safety and Infection Control
Cognitive Level: Application
Concept: Safety

29. **ANSWERS: 1, 2, 3, 4.**
Rationales:
1. **Oral antibiotics can interfere with the normal gastrointestinal (GI) flora. An active culture yogurt will help maintain proper GI flora.**
2. **A white tongue may indicate a super infection, and appropriate medical intervention is warranted.**
3. **Blood in the stool may indicate pseudomembranous colitis requiring medical intervention.**

4. Taking cephalexin (Keflex) with food will limit GI irritation.
5. An increased fluid intake will not alter the potential side effects of this medication.
Content Area: Inflammation, Infection, Immunity, and Wound Care
Integrated Processes: Nursing Process: Implementation
Client Need: Physiological Integrity; Pharmacological and Parenteral Therapies
Cognitive Level: Application
Concept: Medication; Infection

30. **ANSWER: 1, 2, 5.**
Rationales:
1. The reservoir stage of the chain of infection is where microorganisms survive (e.g., people, animals, insects, food, and surfaces). Cool environmental temperatures help to minimize microbial growth. Microorganisms survive best in environments with a temperature between 68°F and 109°F.
2. A soiled kitchen garbage can generally contains remnants of food matter, and it is a dark and moist environment. These factors support the growth of microorganisms. Keeping the inner and outer surface of a garbage can clean and then lining it with a plastic bag that contains garbage will help to break the chain of infection at the reservoir (source) stage of the chain of infection.
3. Immunizations protect an individual by stimulating the production of antibodies. This interrupts the chain of infection at the susceptible host stage.
4. Covering a cough will interrupt the chain of infection at the portal of exit stage.
5. Stagnant (nonflowing) water is a breeding ground for mosquitoes that transmit disease. Also, stagnant water often is contaminated with human and animal feces and is an incubator for the growth of bacteria and parasites. Eliminating stagnant water interrupts the chain of infection at the reservoir (source) stage of the chain of infection.
6. Wearing long pants in areas where ticks are endemic interrupts the chain of infection at the mode of transmission stage.
Content Area: Inflammation, Infection, Immunity, and Wound Care
Integrated Processes: Teaching/Learning; Nursing Process: Planning
Client Need: Safe and Effective Care Environment; Safety and Infection Control
Cognitive Level: Application
Concept: Patient-Centered Care; Infection

31. **ANSWER: 4.**
Rationales:
1. Wiping the outside edges of the wound first will bring microorganisms on the skin toward the wound opening; the opposite should be done. In addition, the center of a wound healing by secondary intention should not be wiped to prevent dislodging granulated tissue.
2. Washing the hands again after setting up the sterile field is unnecessary. The nurse should perform hand hygiene before collecting the equipment for the procedure and

positioning the client and then again just before beginning the procedure.
3. Placing the irrigating solution on the side of the field farthest from the client violates a principle of sterile technique. If the solution is farthest from the client, the irrigating solution may drip on and contaminate the sterile field when it is time to irrigate the wound.
4. Directing the flow of sterile irrigating solution to the inside top of the client's wound is appropriate sterile technique because it prevents microorganisms on the skin from being carried into the wound.
TEST-TAKING TIP: Identify the options with clang associations. The word *sterile* in the stem and in options 2 and 4 are clang associations. The word *wound* in the stem and in options 1 and 4 are clang associations. The word *irrigate* in the stem and *irrigating* in options 3 and 4 are clang associations. Examine option 4 carefully because it contains all three clang associations.
Content Area: Inflammation, Infection, Immunity, and Wound Care
Integrated Processes: Nursing Process: Implementation
Client Need: Safe and Effective Care Environment; Safety and Infection Control
Cognitive Level: Application
Concept: Infection

32. **ANSWER: 4.**
Rationales:
1. A sterile container will help prevent the contamination of the urine specimen, but it will not interrupt the chain of infection at the mode of transmission, thereby protecting others from infection.
2. Cleansing the urethral orifice with an antiseptic solution–soaked cotton ball will interrupt the portal of entry step in the chain of infection. In addition, it will help prevent the contamination of the specimen from microorganisms that are on the skin and mucous membranes. It will not prevent transmission of microorganisms to others.
3. Instructing the client to collect the specimen midstream prevents contamination of the specimen by flushing microorganisms from the urethra first, but it does not prevent the transmission of microorganisms to others.
4. Placing the urine specimen container into a transport bag using aseptic technique will interrupt the chain of infection at the mode of transmission step. Containing the specimen container in a bag prevents transmission of microorganisms that may be on the outside of the specimen container. This action protects others from the transmission of microorganisms.
TEST-TAKING TIP: Identify the clang association. The words *urine specimen* in the stem and in option 4 is a clang association. Examine option 4 carefully.
Content Area: Inflammation, Infection, Immunity, and Wound Care
Integrated Processes: Nursing Process: Implementation
Client Need: Safe and Effective Care Environment; Safety and Infection Control
Cognitive Level: Analysis
Concept: Infection

33. ANSWER: 2, 4, 3, 5, 1.
Rationales:
2. Picking up the first sterile glove, touching only the inside of the folded cuff edge, and inserting the dominant hand into the sterile glove is the first step in donning sterile gloves.
4. After the dominant hand is inside the sterile glove, the nurse uses the ungloved hand to pull the glove on until it fits snuggly, touching only the inside cuff of the sterile glove.
3. The sterile gloved hand is then slipped underneath the cuff of the second sterile glove. The second sterile glove touches only the sterile surface of the first glove. The nondominant hand is inserted into the second glove.
5. The nurse then pulls the second glove on until it fits snuggly, touching only sterile surface to sterile surface.
1. Last, the nurse uses the nondominant hand to pull up the cuff of the first glove, touching only sterile surface to sterile surface.
Content Area: Inflammation, Infection, Immunity, and Wound Care
Integrated Processes: Nursing Process: Planning
Client Need: Safe and Effective Care Environment; Safety and Infection Control
Cognitive Level: Analysis
Concept: Infection

34. ANSWER: 4.
Rationales:
1. A medication should not be discontinued without collaboration with the primary health-care provider. Safety precautions should be taken if the client develops dizziness or fatigue.
2. Acyclovir (Zovirax) will not precipitate constipation; it may cause anorexia, nausea, vomiting, and diarrhea.
3. Taking the pulse before the administration of acyclovir (Zovirax) is unnecessary; it does not influence the heart rate.
4. Acyclovir (Zovirax) should be taken at the first indication of an outbreak, such as tingling, itching (pruritus), or pain at the site where lesions develop (usually the perineal area).
Content Area: Inflammation, Infection, Immunity, and Wound Care
Integrated Processes: Teaching/Learning; Communication and Documentation; Nursing Process: Evaluation
Client Need: Physiological Integrity; Pharmacological and Parenteral Therapy
Cognitive Level: Application
Concept: Medication; Infection

35. ANSWER: 1, 4, 5.
Rationales:
1. Two doses of the tetanus vaccine should have been administered by 4 months of age.
2. The varicella vaccine should be administered at the minimum age of 12 months and is known as the VAR vaccine. The second dose may be administered before 4 years of age, provided that at least 3 months have elapsed since the first dose.
3. The influenza vaccine is not administered until an infant is at least 6 months of age and then yearly.

4. The diphtheria vaccine should have been administered twice by 4 months of age.
5. The inactivated poliovirus should have been administered at least twice by 4 months of age. Four or more doses should be administered before age 4 years and an additional dose should be administered at age 4 through 6 years of age.
6. The MMR vaccine consists of the measles, mumps, and rubella vaccines and should be administered at the minimum age of 12 months.
Content Area: Inflammation, Infection, Immunity, and Wound Care
Integrated Processes: Nursing Process: Evaluation
Client Need: Health Promotion and Maintenance
Cognitive Level: Application
Concept: Immunity

36. ANSWER: 4.
Rationale:
Solve the problem by using ratio and proportion.

$$\frac{\text{Desire } 60 \text{ mg}}{\text{Have } 75 \text{ mg}} = \frac{x \text{ mL}}{5 \text{ mL}}$$

$$75x = 300$$

$$\frac{75x}{75} = \frac{300}{75}$$

$$x = 300 \div 75$$

$$x = 4 \text{ mL}$$

Content Area: Inflammation, Infection, Immunity, and Wound Care
Integrated Processes: Nursing Process: Planning
Client Need: Physiological Integrity; Pharmacological and Parenteral Therapies
Cognitive Level: Application
Concept: Medication; Safety

37. ANSWER: 1.
Rationales:
1. Montgomery straps are used when frequent dressing changes are required because of a draining wound. This protects the skin from excessive removal and reapplication of tape that can injure skin. Montgomery straps attach with adhesive to the skin on either side of the wound and the portion that is nonadhesive lays over the dressing and is laced up with gauze strips that hold abdominal pads in place.
2. Moist to dry dressings are not advisable because the dry dressing will disrupt new granulated tissue when it is removed. Research demonstrates that a moist wound bed supports the growth of granulated tissue and wound healing.
3. The dressing in the illustration is not used for wounds with a small amount of drainage. A wound with a small amount of drainage generally is changed only once a day.
4. Although clients can be taught to change their own dressings, this is not the purpose of this type of dressing.
TEST-TAKING TIP: Identify the options that are opposites. Option 1, which indicates a wound that requires frequent dressing changes generally because of copious amounts of drainage, and option 3, which indicates a wound that has a

small amount of drainage, are opposites. Examine options 1 and 3 carefully. More often than not, an option that is an opposite is the correct answer.
Content Area: Tissue Integrity, Hygiene, and Wound Care
Integrated Processes: Nursing Process: Planning
Client Need: Physiological Integrity; Physiological Adaptation
Cognitive Level: Analysis
Concept: Tissue Integrity

38. **ANSWER: 1, 2, 5.**
    Rationales:
    1. **A wound should be gently cleansed using a piston syringe so that all surfaces of the wound are cleansed. A piston syringe provides more control than a bulb syringe when discharging the saline into the wound.**
    2. **Drying the skin will allow the tape used to secure the dressing to adhere to the skin.**
    3. The nurse should spray back and forth across the inside of the wound and progressively move down the surface of the wound. This prevents the introduction of microorganisms surrounding the wound from contaminating the wound.
    4. A piston syringe should be held 2, not 4, inches from the surface of the wound. Holding the piston syringe 2 inches away from the wound helps minimize splashing and prevents irrigating solution from contaminating the environment.
    5. **Positioning the client so that the irrigating solution flows into an emesis basin uses the principle of gravity to direct the flow of solution and debris away from the wound. Collecting the irrigating solution and debris in an emesis basin protects the environment from contamination.**
    TEST-TAKING TIP: Identify the clang association. The word *irrigation* in the stem and the word *irrigating* in option 5 is a clang association. Examine option 5 carefully.
    Content Area: Tissue Integrity, Hygiene, and Wound Care
    Integrated Processes: Nursing Process: Implementation
    Client Need: Physiological Integrity; Physiological Adaptation
    Cognitive Level: Application
    Concept: Tissue Integrity

39. **ANSWER: 3, 5.**
    Rationales:
    1. The suction device and tubing is positioned over a hole at the center, not edge, of the transparent film. This allows for the suction to be maintained over the entire wound, not just one edge.
    2. The foam dressing should be contained within the wound, not extended 1 inch over the edge of the wound cavity. This protects the tissue surrounding the wound from becoming macerated.
    3. **This is expected. In the absence of audible leaks, wrinkles indicate that the closure is secure when negative pressure is applied.**
    4. The tubing is connected to negative, not positive, pressure as prescribed. Suction can be continuous or intermittent and between 5 to 125 mm Hg.

5. **Applying the transparent film 2 inches beyond the wound margins is the correct way to apply the transparent film of a vacuum-assisted closure device. This ensures that the transparent film has a firm seal around the wound.**
TEST-TAKING TIP: Identify the clang associations. The word *wound* in the stem and in options 2 and 5 are clang associations. Examine options 2 and 5 carefully.
Content Area: Tissue Integrity, Hygiene, and Wound Care
Integrated Processes: Nursing Process: Implementation
Client Need: Physiological Integrity; Physiological Adaptation
Cognitive Level: Application
Concept: Tissue Integrity

40. **ANSWER: 1, 2, 3.**
    Rationales:
    1. **The client is 77 years old. As one ages, skin loses collagen and elasticity. In addition, circulation, phagocytic, and immune responses are reduced. All of these factors delay wound healing.**
    2. **Chronic illnesses can delay wound healing. With heart failure, circulation to the distal extremities is impaired, interfering with the bringing of oxygen and nutrients to tissues attempting to heal. Clients with type 2 diabetes have an increased amount of glucose in the tissues that promotes infection. In addition, the disruption in the metabolism of protein, carbohydrates, and fats can interfere with an adequate supply of nutrients needed for tissue repair.**
    3. **Fluid in the interstitial compartment increases the distance from the circulation to body cells. Edematous tissue reduces the transport of nutrients to wounds and removal of debris from a wound.**
    4. There are no data that indicate that the client has inadequate nutrition. The client receives meals on wheels and cooks for himself. In addition, his weight is appropriate for his height; the average weight of a person who is 5 feet 10 inches tall is 162 pounds, with a range of 144 to 180 pounds.
    5. There are no signs of an infection. The client's pulse and respirations are stable, and the drainage from the abrasions is a pink watery-like discharge. If an infection is present, then the drainage would be yellow, yellowish-green, green, or greenish-blue.
    6. The client's history of smoking cigarettes is not a current problem. If the client continued to smoke cigarettes, nicotine would constrict blood vessels, decreasing the amount of oxygen reaching the area for wound healing.
    Content Area: Inflammation, Infection, Immunity, and Wound Care
    Integrated Processes: Nursing Process: Assessment
    Client Need: Physiological Integrity; Physiological Adaptation
    Cognitive Level: Analysis
    Concept: Patient-Centered Care; Tissue Integrity

Chapter 17

Mobility

NURSING CONCEPTS

Elimination
Health Promotion
Metabolism
Mobility
Neurologic Regulation
Nutrition

Oxygenation
Patient-Centered Care
Perfusion
Safety
Tissue Integrity

KEY TERMS

Base of support—Points of the body that are touching the ground

Center of gravity—Point within the body where the greatest mass of the body exists

Contracture—Rigidity of a joint due to permanent shortening of a muscle, tendons, and ligaments

Embolus—When a clot or tissue debris moves via the circulation from its place of origin to a smaller vessel causing an occlusion.

Gait—Manner in which a person walks

Joints—Connections between bones

Line of gravity—Line that is drawn from the top of the head through the individual's center of greatest mass

Metabolic rate—Minimal energy expended to maintain the body's physical and chemical processes

Negative nitrogen balance—State caused by inadequate intake of protein to meet body needs, resulting in muscle breakdown that releases nitrogen from muscle cells

Orthostatic hypotension—Decrease in blood pressure when moving from a recumbent to a sitting or standing position resulting in dizziness

Range of motion (ROM)—Maximum extent of movement by a joint through sagittal, frontal, and transverse planes

Thrombus—Formation of a blood clot within the vascular system

Valsalva maneuver—Forceful exhalation against a closed glottis, resulting in increased intrathoracic and venous pressures, bradycardia, and decreased blood return to the heart

I. Foundations of Mobility

Movement involves a change in one's position, posture, or physical location. It requires the interaction of the muscles, skeletal system, and nervous system.. The way in which the body moves *(body mechanics)* involves balance, body alignment, coordination, joint mobility, and gait. Effective body mechanics facilitate the use of muscle groups to limit the amount of stress on body structures, reduce the amount of energy required for an activity, and decrease the risk of injury to both the client and nurse. Nurses should integrate principles of body mechanics when performing nursing activities to care for clients effectively and safely as well as to reduce the risk of occupational injuries.

A. Anatomy related to movement
   1. Skeletal system.
      a. Bones are rigid connective tissue composed mostly of calcium salts.
         (1) Skeletal system consists of 206 bones (Fig. 17.1).
         (2) Provides shape and support for the body; protects internal organs.

Fig 17.1 Skeletal system. (From Scanlon [2015]. *Essentials of anatomy and physiology,* 7th ed. Philadelphia: F. A. Davis Company, with permission.)

(3) Produces constituents of the blood (e.g., RBCs, WBCs, platelets) and stores calcium and phosphorus.

b. **Joints** are connections between bones.

(1) *Ball and socket:* Rounded head of one bone fits into a cuplike structure of another bone; moves in all planes of range of motion (ROM) as well as rotation. Examples include the joints of the shoulders (scapula and humerus) and hips (pelvic bone and femur).

(2) *Condyloid:* One oval-shaped bone fits into an elliptical cavity of another bone; moves

in one plane with some lateral movement. Examples include the wrists (radius and carpal bones).

(3) *Gliding:* Flat plane of the surface of one bone moves past the flat plane of another bone; moves from side to side. Examples include small bones of the wrists and ankles.

(4) *Hinge:* Convex surface of one bone fits into the cavity of another bone; moves in one plane, flexion and extension. Examples include elbow (humerus, ulna, and radius) and knee (femur, patella, and tibia).

(5) *Pivot:* Projection of one bone articulates with a ring or notch of another bone; moves by rotating around a single point. An example is the neck (atlas and axis).

(6) *Saddle:* Concave surface of one bone fits into the convex surface of another bone; moves in several planes. Examples include the thumbs (thumb's metacarpal bone and wrist's carpal bone).

c. Cartilage: Supportive connective tissue.

d. Ligaments: Bind joints together and connect bones and cartilages.

e. Tendons: Connect muscle to bone.

f. Bones serve as levers, and joints serve as fulcrums; a *lever* is a fixed bar that moves about a fixed point known as a *fulcrum.*

2. Nervous system.

   a. Autonomic nervous system: Innervates involuntary muscles, such as the heart, blood vessels, and glands.

   b. Somatic nervous system: Part of the peripheral nervous system that innervates voluntary skeletal muscles.

   c. The motor areas of the frontal lobes of the cerebrum generate the electrochemical impulses that initiate voluntary skeletal muscle contraction.

   d. The cerebellum coordinates the muscles involved in voluntary movement.

3. Muscles.

   a. Skeletal muscles consist of muscle fibers that can contract (shorten) or extend (stretch), thus moving a joint.

   b. Muscle attaches to bone at two points.
      (1) Origin: More stationary bone.
      (2) Insertion: More movable bone.

   c. Muscle pairs act antagonistically to each other—when one contracts, the other relaxes.

   d. A **contracture** is rigidity of a joint due to permanent shortening of a muscle, tendons, and ligaments; it decreases the angle of the joint. (Fig. 17.2)

MAKING THE CONNECTION

Anatomical Structures and Body Movement

Electrochemical impulses that initiate voluntary motor activity originate in the motor areas of the cerebrum. The cerebellum modifies these impulses, which progress to skeletal muscles, stimulating them to respond. The skeletal muscles respond to these modified impulses by contracting (shorten), which pulls on bones, producing body movement. Skeletal muscles also can extend (lengthen), which allows the muscle to return to its resting length after contraction. For movement to be exact, coordinated, smooth, and efficient, the nervous and skeletal systems and muscles must work together to produce a result not independently obtainable.

B. Assessment of client mobility

1. Assess bones for length, shape, and symmetry.

   a. Normal findings.
      (1) Length between arms and length between legs less than 1 cm.
      (2) Expected skeletal configuration reflected in shape of all bones.
      (3) Absence of sound on movement.

   b. Deviations.
      (1) Asymmetrical lengths.
      (2) Grating sound *(crepitus)* on movement.
      (3) Deformities of shape:
         (a) Rheumatoid arthritis: *Boutonnière deformity*—proximal interphalangeal joint flexion and distal interphalangeal joint hyperextension of the fingers; *swan-neck deformity*—proximal interphalangeal joint hyperextension and distal interphalangeal joint flexion of the fingers; *ulnar drift*—long axis of fingers deviates toward the ulnar side of the hand.
         (b) Osteoarthritis: *Heberden nodes*—enlarged distal interphalangeal joints of fingers; *Bouchard nodes*—enlarged proximal interphalangeal joints of fingers.

A. *Extension*

B. *Flexion*

Fig 17.2 Antagonistic muscles. (From Scanlon [2015]. *Essentials of anatomy and physiology,* 7th ed. Philadelphia: F. A. Davis Company, with permission.)

(c) Gouty arthritis: *Tophi*—sodium urate deposits in tissues of outer ear, hands, feet, elbows, or knees.

2. Assess muscles for tone while muscles are at rest; muscles firm when contracted; hand grip; leg strength via foot push/leg rise against resistance; and movement.
  a. Normal findings.
    (1) Muscles soft and pliable at rest.
    (2) Muscles firm when contracted.
    (3) Hand grip and foot push/leg rise strong and equal.
    (4) No involuntary movements.
  b. Deviations.
    (1) Strength in arm and legs weak, unequal, or absent.
    (2) Deviations in muscle tone.
      (a) Atony: Lack of muscle tone.
      (b) Hypotony: Decreased muscle tone.
      (c) Hypertony: Excessive tone.

3. Assess motor function for coordination; movement is initiated in the cerebral cortex and coordinated by the cerebellum because of an awareness of posture, movement, and position sense *(proprioception)*.
  a. Normal findings: All movements should be smooth and rhythmical.
  b. Deviations in movement.
    (1) *Ataxia:* Uncoordinated movements.
    (2) *Spasticity:* Uncontrolled contractions of skeletal muscles.
    (3) *Hemiparesis:* Weakness in arm and leg on same side of body.
    (4) *Hemiplegia:* Paralysis in arm and leg on same side of body.
    (5) *Paraplegia:* Paralysis of both legs.
    (6) *Quadriplegia:* Paralysis of both arms and both legs.
    (7) *Tremors:* Rhythmic, purposeless movements.
    (8) *Intention tremor:* Tremors occurring when attempting voluntary movement.
    (9) *Nonintention tremor (resting tremor):* Tremors occurring when muscles are at rest.
    (10) *Fasciculations:* Localized, uncontrollable twitching of a single muscle group innervated by a single motor nerve fiber.

4. Assess body alignment, including posture; symmetry of shoulders, scapula, and iliac crests; and cervical, thoracic, lumbar, and sacral curves.
  a. Normal findings.
    (1) Spine in a neutral position where the line of gravity passes through the center of gravity.

(2) Shoulders, scapula, and iliac crests are symmetrical, and the spinal curves are cervical, concave; thoracic, convex; lumbar, concave; and sacral, convex (Fig. 17.3).
  b. Deviations (Fig. 17.4)
    (1) Kyphosis: Accentuated thoracic curve
    (2) Lordosis: Accentuated lumbar curve
    (3) Scoliosis: Lateral "S" spinal deviation

5. Assess gait; **gait** is the manner in which a person walks such as posture, steadiness or unsteadiness, arm swing, cadence, width of feet apart, stride length, and toe position.
  a. Normal findings.
    (1) Posture erect with head midline.
    (2) Smooth, rhythmic movements with arms swinging in opposition.

Cervical (concave)
Thoracic (convex)
Lumbar (concave)
Sacral (convex)

Fig 17.3 Normal spine curves. (From Wilkinson and Treas [2016]. *Fundamentals of nursing,* Vol. 2, 3rd ed. Philadelphia: F. A. Davis Company, with permission.)

Scoliosis   Kyphosis

Fig 17.4 Scoliosis and kyphosis. (From Wilkinson and Treas [2016]. *Fundamentals of nursing,* Vol. 2, 3rd ed. Philadelphia: F. A. Davis Company, with permission.)

(3) Width of feet apart is 2 to 4 inches and toes point forward.

(4) Length of stride is 12 to 14 inches.

b. Deviations.

(1) Posture slumped with head not in midline.

(2) Uncoordinated movements.

(3) Lack of arm swing (associated with Parkinson disease).

(4) Wide base of support and shortened stride associated with muscle weakness, joint stiffness, CNS dysfunction (usually cerebellum), and problems with balance.

(5) Abnormal gaits.

(a) *Waddling:* Rolling motion in which the opposite hip drops when taking a stride, such as with developmental dysplasia of the hip and pregnancy.

(b) *Propulsive (cogwheel):* Small, shuffling steps with involuntary accelerations, such as with Parkinson disease.

(c) *Spastic:* Stiff, foot-dragging walk, such as with cerebral palsy.

(d) *Steppage:* Exaggerated lifting of the leg to avoid dragging the toes, such as with footdrop and Guillain-Barré syndrome.

6. Assess balance including Romberg test. (See Cranial Nerve VIII in Table 14.9 in Chapter 14, Physical Assessment.)

a. **Center of gravity** is the point within the body where the greatest mass of the body exists; usually is below the umbilicus to the top of the pelvis (Fig. 17.5).

b. **Line of gravity** is the line that is drawn from the top of the head through the individual's center of greatest mass.

c. **Base of support** is the points of the body that are touching the ground.

(1) The wider the base of support the more stable the body.

(2) Examples: A walker or cane increases the base of support.

d. Normal findings: Coordinated; ability to maintain balance with minimal swaying.

e. Deviations.

(1) Extending arms to the side with a wide base of support and shortened stride.

(2) Swaying or loss of balance related to cerebellar disorder or dorsal column problem.

7. Assess extent of joint mobility.

a. **Range of motion (ROM)** is the maximum extent of movement by a joint through the sagittal, frontal, and transverse planes.

b. See Movement of Joints, Table 17.1.

A   **B**

Fig 17.5 Center of gravity. (A) With a wide stance, the center of gravity (X) is closer to the base of support. (B) With a narrow stance, the body is less stable. (From Wilkinson and Treas [2016]. *Fundamentals of nursing,* Vol. 1, 3rd ed. Philadelphia: F. A. Davis Company, with permission.)

C. Nursing care related to body mechanics

1. *Body mechanics* is the efficient, coordinated, and safe use of the body to carry and move objects as well as perform the activities of daily living safely.

2. Raise the bed and overbed table to waist level when providing care to a client in bed to prevent stress and strain on the nurse's anatomical structures.

3. Use a wide base of support by spreading the feet apart or placing one in front of the other. The wider the base of support, the more stable the person or object.

DID YOU KNOW?

The risk of falls and musculoskeletal injuries increases when the center of gravity is outside the base of support.

4. Push, pull, or roll heavy objects when possible rather than lift to minimize strain because pulling is less strenuous than pushing.

5. Use gravity to facilitate movements. Doing so allows the client's weight to promote movement by moving from a higher to a lower plane and reduces stress and strain on the nurse and client.

6. Contract gluteal, abdominal, leg, and arm muscles before the actual move to prepare muscles for action.

7. Keep the neck, back, pelvis, and feet in alignment to avoid twisting to reduce stress and strain on the nurse's anatomical structures.

(Text continued on page 502)

Table 17.1 Movement of Joints (Range of Motion)

Range of Motion	Illustration
Neck: Pivotal joint	
Flexion: Move head from upright midline position forward, ending with chin on chest. *Extension:* Move head from flexed position to upright midline position. *Hyperextension:* Move head from upright midline position backward.	
Lateral flexion: Tilt head to side from midline position toward each shoulder.	
Rotation: Move head in circular motion as far to right or left as possible.	
Elbow: Hinge joint	
Flexion: Bend elbow to move forearm toward shoulder. *Extension:* Straighten arm to bring forearm forward and down.	
Supination: With elbow flexed at 90°, rotate hand and forearm so that palm is facing toward the ceiling. *Pronation:* With elbow flexed at 90°, rotate hand and forearm so that palm is facing toward the floor.	
Knee: Hinge joint	
Flexion: Bend knee to bring heel toward buttocks. *Extension:* Straighten knee to move heel away from buttocks.	

Table 17.1 **Movement of Joints (Range of Motion)—cont'd**

Range of Motion	Illustration
Hands and fingers: Condyloid joints and hinge joints (interphalangeal joints)	
Flexion: Form a fist with fingers. *Extension:* Straighten fingers. *Hyperextension:* Bend fingers back toward outer aspect of forearm.	
Abduction: Spread fingers apart. *Adduction:* Move fingers together.	
Thumb: Saddle joint	
Flexion: Move thumb across palm toward fifth finger. *Extension:* Move thumb laterally away from fingers.	
Opposition: Move thumb to tip of each finger.	
Abduction: Move thumb away from hand. *Adduction:* Move thumb toward hand.	(See illustration of abduction and adduction under Hands and Fingers above.)
Wrist: Condyloid joint	
Flexion: Bend hand toward inner aspect of forearm. *Extension:* Straighten wrist in same plane as forearm.	
Hyperextension: Bend hand toward outer aspect of forearm.	

Continued

Table 17.1 Movement of Joints (Range of Motion)—cont'd

Range of Motion	Illustration
Abduction (radial flexion): Bend hand toward thumb side. *Adduction (ulnar flexion):* Bend hand toward fifth finger side.	
Ankle: Hinge joint	
Flexion (dorsiflexion): Move toes and foot upward toward abdomen. *Extension (plantar flexion):* Move toes and foot downward away from abdomen.	
Foot: Gliding joint	
Eversion: Turn sole of foot outward, laterally. *Inversion:* Turn sole of foot inward, medially.	
Toes: Hinge joints; intertarsal joints are gliding joints	
Flexion: Curl toes downward. *Extension:* Straighten toes.	
Abduction: Spread toes apart. *Adduction:* Bring toes together.	
Shoulder: Ball-and-socket joint	
Flexion: Beginning with arm at side of body, raise arm forward and upward to alongside head. *Extension:* Move arm to side of body. *Hyperextension:* Beginning with arm at side of body, move arm straight backward.	

Table 17.1 **Movement of Joints (Range of Motion)—cont'd**

Range of Motion	Illustration
Abduction: Raise arm laterally with elbow straight to side of head with palm facing outward. *Adduction:* Move straight arm from side of body to across front midline of body.	
External rotation: Begin with upper arm out to side at shoulder level and elbow bent with fingers pointing downward; then move arm upward until fingers are higher than shoulder. *Internal rotation:* Move arm forward and downward until fingers are again pointing down below shoulder.	
Circumduction: Make a circle with the arm from the shoulder.	
Hip: Ball-and-socket joint	
Flexion: Move leg up and forward. *Extension:* Move leg down and back beside the other. *Hyperextension:* Move leg back behind body.	
Abduction: Move leg laterally away from body. *Adduction:* Move leg inward across front midline of body.	

Continued

Table 17.1 Movement of Joints (Range of Motion)—cont'd	
Range of Motion	**Illustration**
External rotation: Turn leg and foot so they point outward away from other leg. *Internal rotation:* Turn leg and foot so they point inward toward other leg.	
Circumduction: Make a circle with the leg from the hip.	

Figure credits: Wilkinson and Treas (2016). *Fundamentals of nursing,* Vol. 2, 3rd ed. Philadelphia: F. A. Davis Company, with permission.

8. Squat to lift objects off the floor. The lower the center of gravity, the more stable the body.

9. Use leg muscles and flex the knees, hips, and ankles when lifting. Doing so permits larger muscles of the body to provide the power and decreases strain on back muscles.

10. Use both hands and arms with elbows flexed when lifting objects because elbows act as fulcrums while the arms act as levers.

11. Keep an object close to the body when lifting or carrying it. The closer an object is to the center of gravity, the more stable the body and less strain on the muscles of the back.

II.   Exercise

Exercise is an activity that is planned and structured to promote muscle strength, maintain joint flexibility, and/or improve respiratory and cardiovascular status. Exercise often requires a client to perform repetitive actions that actively contract and relax muscles. Nurses must understand the types of exercises, their advantages, and examples of activities associated with each type to assist clients with the performance of exercises. ROM exercises are designed to prevent contractures and can be performed independently or with assistance or can be received passively when a caregiver puts a client's joints through their full planes of movement. Nurses must understand the principles associated with the provision of ROM exercises to administer these interventions effectively and safely.

A. Types of exercise
Exercises are classified based on the type of muscle contraction (e.g., isotonic, isometric, or isokinetic) and the source of energy (e.g., aerobic) (Table 17.2).

B. Range-of-motion (ROM) exercises
1. Movements to maintain joint mobility and function.
2. Help prevent permanent shortening of muscles, tendons, and ligaments that ultimately limits joint mobility *(contracture).*
3. Types of ROM exercise.
   a. Active ROM.
      (1) ROM performed by a client.
      (2) Requires muscle contraction that improves muscle strength.
   b. Active-assistive ROM.
      (1) ROM initiated by a client that is completed by a caregiver.
      (2) Requires some muscle contraction that eventually improves muscle strength.
   c. Passive ROM.
      (1) ROM performed for a client by a caregiver.
      (2) Passive ROM does not contract muscles and, therefore, does not improve muscle strength.
   d. Continuous-passive ROM.
      (1) ROM achieved for a client by a machine to improve extent of joint movement and prevent a contracture.

Table 17.2 **Types of Exercises**		
Type	**Advantages**	**Examples**
Isotonic • *Muscle shortens to produce muscle contraction and movement.*	• *Increases muscle tone, mass, and strength.* • *Promotes joint mobility.* • *Increases heart rate and circulation.*	• *Walking.* • *Swimming.* • *Calisthenics.* • *Lifting self with a trapeze.* • *Performing active ROM and activities of daily living.*
Isometric • *Change in muscle tension occurs without change in muscle length or joint movement.*	• *Strengthens muscles.* • *Increases heart rate and cardiac output slightly but not circulation.*	• *Tensing muscles, such as muscles of an extremity within a cast.* • *Exerting pressure against an immovable object.*
Aerobic • *Repetitive or continuous activity that increases the demand for oxygen at the cellular level.*	• *Strengthens skeletal muscles.* • *Increases heart and respiratory rates.*	• *Rapid, intense exercise, such as brisk walking, jogging, and cycling.*
Isokinetic • *Activity that includes a variable resistance to movement.*	• *Combines the best features of isotonic and isometric exercise.*	• *Activities with specialized machines that provide resistance at a constant, preset rate while muscle moves through full ROM.*

(2) An extremity is placed in a mechanical device that supports the limb from distal to proximal and sequentially flexes and extends a joint at a prescribed speed and degree of joint flexion (e.g., a machine placed under the upper thigh to the foot flexes the knee and hip). (See "Continuous Passive Motion Machine," Fig. 24.7, in Chapter 24, Perioperative.)

4. Nursing care when providing ROM exercises.
 a. Review the primary health-care provider's prescription for the type and extent of ROM exercises and restrictions to ensure that the exercises are permitted and not contraindicated.
 b. Schedule ROM exercises to permit adequate time to complete the planned routine or complete during another activity, such as a bed bath. Doing so ensures that ROM exercises are performed and do not physically tax the client.
 c. Wash your hands, identify the client, introduce yourself, explain the procedure to the client, and provide privacy.
 d. Assess the client's status, such as presence of joint stiffness, swelling, or pain; physical ability to perform or assist with exercises; level of motivation; and cognitive ability to follow instructions. Doing so provides data that influence the extent to which ROM exercises should be performed.
 e. Apply heat before ROM to relax muscles and increase contractility; however, be aware that the application of heat requires a prescription from a primary health-care provider.

 f. Encourage the client to perform active ROM exercises to the extent that the client's health and mobility permit; assist the client with those exercises that cannot be performed independently. This promotes independence, and assistance ensures that the exercises are performed.
 🛑 g. Begin each movement with the extremity in functional alignment to prevent strain and injury to the client's body structures.
 ⚠ h. Assess the client's response to ensure that ROM exercises do not cause pain. Doing so prevents the joint from being moved beyond its ability to be moved.

 i. Put each joint through ROM, moving the body part to the point of resistance and applying slow, gentle pressure if rigidity or a contracture is present. Doing so ensures that the joint is put through the fullest range possible and stretches muscle fibers (Table 17.1).
 j. Place hands distal and proximal to the joint (Fig. 17.6) or support the joint with one hand

Fig 17.6 Supporting a limb during ROM. (From Nugent and Vitale [2014]. *Fundamentals of nursing: Content review PLUS practice questions.* F. A. Davis Company, with permission.)

while cradling the distal portion of the extremity with the forearm to support the joint while it is being put through ROM.

k. Implement ROM slowly, smoothly, and rhythmically to limit stress on the client's anatomical structures; repeat each movement three to five times to stretch muscle fibers.

l. Monitor the client's physical, verbal, and nonverbal responses to interventions to provide data that influence continuation of or future implementation of ROM.

m. Use the opportunity to perform other assessments, such as the condition of the skin.

n. Document interventions, extent of mobility of joints, and client's responses. Doing so documents that the nursing care was provided and communicates information to other members of the health team.

III. Positioning Clients

A position is the physical arrangement the human body can assume. Various positions are used to maintain clients in functional body alignment with the goal of placing the least stress and strain on the body. Clients generally reposition themselves regularly and move to positions of comfort. However, clients who are physically compromised (e.g., paralyzed, unconscious, or frail), experiencing pain, or cognitively impaired require assistance to change positions. Frequent change in position (every 1 to 2 hours) helps maintain muscle tone and stimulates postural reflexes; it also helps prevent muscle discomfort, compression of blood vessels, damage to superficial nerves, and contractures.

A. Positions and specific nursing care
   Each position has its advantages and requires the nurse to place the client's body, head, and extremities in specific arrangements to maintain body alignment (Table 17.3).

Table 17.3 Positions and Specific Nursing Care

Position	Specific Nursing Care
Supine *Advantages:* • *Promotes comfort.* • *Facilitates assessment of the abdomen, breasts, extremities, and pulses.* • *Prevents headache after spinal anesthesia.*	• *Keep the head of the bed flat.* • *Position the client in the flat, back-lying position with the legs extended.* • *Place a pillow behind the head and shoulders to prevent hyperextension of the neck.* • *Keep the arms at the client's sides.* Note: Supported supine position • *Elevate the forearms on pillows.* • *Position a small pillow under the lumbar curvature to limit lordosis.* • *Place a pillow under the legs from below the knees to above the ankles to keep the heels off the bed.* • *Place a trochanter roll lateral to each thigh to prevent external rotation.* • *Use high-top sneakers to support dorsiflexion if prescribed.*
Dorsal recumbent *Advantages:* • *Reduces tension on abdominal muscles.* • *Facilitates assessment of the abdomen, breasts, extremities, pulses, and pelvis.*	• *Keep the head of the bed flat.* • *Position the client in the flat, back-lying position.* • *Place a pillow behind the head and shoulders to prevent hyperextension of the neck.* • *Position the client with the hips and knees slightly flexed and the feet flat on the bed.* • *Place a pillow under the thighs to support flexion of the knees if necessary.* • *Place the arms over the head or at the side of the body.*
Prone *Advantages:* • *Allows full extension of the hips and knees.* • *Promotes drainage of secretions from the mouth, which helps prevent aspiration.* • *Relieves pressure on the sacrum and greater trochanter.*	• *Position the client on the abdomen.* • *Turn head to the side on a small pillow to prevent lateral flexion of the neck.* • *Flex one or both arms.* • *Change the position in 1 hour or less because the weight of the body on the chest impedes breathing and exerts pressure on the breasts and male genitalia.* Note: Supported prone position • *Place a small pillow under the abdomen to prevent hyperextension of the lumbar curvature.* • *Place a small pillow under the lower legs to limit plantar flexion.*

Table 17.3 Positions and Specific Nursing Care—cont'd

Position	Specific Nursing Care
Lateral (Side Lying) **Advantages:** • Relieves pressure on the sacrum and heels. • Facilitates assessment of the back and perianal areas. • Permits access to the anus to provide perineal care, obtain a rectal temperature, permit insertion of a suppository, or perform an enema. • Promotes rest and sleep.	• Position the client on a side with a small pillow under the head to prevent lateral flexion of the neck. • Keep lower hip and knee extended to promote functional alignment. • Flex upper hip and knee in front of the body on a pillow to prevent adduction and lordosis, promote back alignment, and provide a wider triangular base of support. • Place a pillow behind the back to maintain the lateral position.
Sims' (Semiprone) **Advantages:** • Facilitates drainage of secretions from the mouth, which helps prevent aspiration. • Relieves pressure on the sacrum, greater trochanter, and heels. • Allows access for perineal assessment or suppository insertion.	• Position the client halfway between the lateral and prone positions. • Place a small pillow under the head to prevent lateral flexion of the neck. • Keep the lower arm extended behind the body with the palm facing the ceiling and the upper arm in front of the body with the shoulder and elbow flexed on a pillow to prevent internal rotation. • Keep the lower hip and knee extended and the upper hip and knee flexed in front of the body on a pillow to prevent adduction and keep the foot off the mattress.
Fowler **Advantages:** • Promotes lung expansion. • Limits risk of aspiration associated with gastric feedings and nasotracheal suctioning. • Facilitates intake of oral feedings.	• Position the client in the back-lying position with the head elevated. Low-Fowler: Head and trunk raised to 15°. Semi-Fowler: Head and trunk raised 16° to 45°. High-Fowler: Head and trunk raised 46° to 90°. • Place a pillow under the head and shoulders to prevent neck flexion and under both arms to limit tension on the shoulders if indicated. • Use high-top sneakers to support dorsiflexion if prescribed.
Orthopneic **Advantages:** • Permits maximum lung expansion. • Facilitates exhalation.	• Raise the head of the bed to the high-Fowler position. • Place the client in the sitting position with a pillow behind the back and leaning on a pillow on an overbed table. • Raise the side rails that do not interfere with placement of the overbed table. • Place client in a chair leaning forward on a pillow on an overbed table if permitted.

Continued

Table 17.3 Positions and Specific Nursing Care—cont'd

Position	Specific Nursing Care
Lithotomy **Advantages:** • Permits access to female perineal area for visual inspection, pelvic examination, perineal hygiene, and vaginal birth. • Facilitates insertion of vaginal suppositories or administration of a douche.	• Position the client in the back-lying position with the head of the bed flat. • Assist client with lifting both legs at the same time while placing them in stirrups to limit strain on pelvic structures or place the feet flat on the bed close to the buttocks with the knees flexed and spread apart. • Drape the client as much as possible to provide for privacy. • Support the legs during the procedure to help a frail client to maintain the position.
Sitting **Advantages:** • Permits assessment of anterior and posterior chest. • Permits assessment of heart and lung sounds. • Promotes function of body systems, especially cardiopulmonary and urinary systems.	• Assist the client to move from the lying to the sitting position on the side of the bed. • Stand in front of the client with one foot placed forward between the client's feet and the other foot placed backward to provide a wide base of support. • Ask whether the client feels light-headed or dizzy and, if so, return the client to the lying position if the sensation does not resolve within 1 to 2 minutes. • Ensure that client's hips and knees are at a 90° angle and that the feet are flat on the floor with foot coverings. • Client may be assisted to stand and transferred to a chair or wheelchair.

Figure credits: Wilkinson and Treas (2016). *Fundamentals of nursing,* Vol. 1, 3rd ed. Philadelphia: F. A. Davis Company, with permission.

B. Commonalities of nursing care when moving or positioning clients

1. Review the primary health-care provider's activity prescription and implement it accordingly (e.g., bedrest, out of bed in a chair for 2 hours twice a day, out of bed). The client's level of activity requires a prescription and is a dependent function of the nurse.

2. Assess factors that may influence mobility, such as age, weight, pain, stiffness, contractures, hemiparesis, paraplegia, and mental status. Assessment ensures that nursing care is individualized according to the client's status and needs.

3. Assess the task to be performed and the client's status to determine the need for environmental alterations, assistive devices, and additional staff members.

4. Use appropriate assistive devices to move or transfer clients (e.g., pull sheet, gait belt, transfer roller sheet, sit-to-stand lift, and mechanical lift); ensure that all devices are in working order and that wheels on all devices and the client's bed are locked. Doing so ensures safety of the client and health team members.

5. Encourage the client to assist within the limits of his or her physical status to promote independence and limit muscle atrophy. For example, encourage use of the side rails and trapeze bar to facilitate movement.

6. Follow the principles of body mechanics.

   🛑 a. **Ensure that a client is in functional alignment before changing the client's position to prevent strain or injury to the client's body structures.**

   b. Use a wide base of support. For example, place one foot 8 inches to 10 inches to the side and in front of the other; open the lower support bars of a mechanical lift. Doing so provides a wider base that supports stability.

   c. Push, pull, or roll heavy objects when possible rather than lifting to limit the energy and stress required to accomplish the task.

   d. Use gravity to facilitate movements because doing so uses the client's weight and gravity to accomplish the movement and requires less energy to perform the activity. For example, position a bed higher than a chair when getting a client out of bed and lower the head of the bed before moving a client up in bed.

e. Use a client's body mass to help turn the client. For example, place the client's arm and leg across the body in the direction the client is going to turn.

f. Use own body mass and move in the direction the client is being moved to enhance the power of muscles. For example, rock your body forward when moving clients away from you or backward when moving clients toward you.

g. Allow the person with the heaviest load to coordinate movements when two or more health team members are involved in moving a client. Doing so ensures coordination of the actions of all health team members involved. Synchronized, smooth movements reduce client and occupational injuries. For example, direct the movement to begin on the count of three.

h. Turn a client as a unit *(log roll)* using two to three caregivers to maintain spinal alignment following trauma or neuro/orthopedic procedures.

7. Assess the client's reaction to the activity and record it in the client's clinical record. Doing so documents that the activity was performed and communicates the reaction to team members.

IV. Negative Effects of Immobility and Related Nursing Care

Immobility is a decrease in the amount and control of movement. It can have major negative effects on many body systems. The longer the inactivity, the greater the risk of the development of a complication of immobility. Nurses can implement a variety of dependent and independent interventions to prevent the negative consequences of immobility. Some of these nursing interventions are general in nature and affect several body systems (Box 17.1), and others are related to specific body systems.

A. Musculoskeletal system
   1. Disuse atrophy.
      a. Muscles that are not used decrease in size and physiological ability *(atrophy)*.
      b. Muscle begins to lose contractile strength after 24 to 36 hours of inactivity.
      c. Inactivity or bedrest can lead to 7% to 10% loss of muscle strength in 1 week.
   2. Contractures.
      a. When a muscle does not contract and relax, it eventually permanently shortens *(contracture)*.
      b. Contractures limit joint mobility.
   3. Joint stiffness and pain.
      a. Inactive muscles cause connective tissue at joints to become permanently immobile *(ankylosis)*.

Box 17.1 Commonalities of Nursing Care for Clients With Limited Mobility

- *Encourage the client to be as independent as possible.*
- *Ensure that immobility is not maintained beyond that which is necessary.*
- *Encourage the client to change position or change a client's position every 1 to 2 hours, particularly from horizontal to vertical, such as high-Fowler position and out of bed in a chair.*
- *Encourage fluid intake (2 to 3 L daily), if not restricted, to help prevent responses such as dehydration, hypercoagulability, thickened respiratory secretions, and constipation.*
- *Maintain client safety at all times, such as by using side rails on the bed, positioning the bed in the lowest position, locking wheels on movable objects, assisting with ambulation, and encouraging the use of the bathroom and corridor hand rails.*
- *Coordinate and support activities performed by other health team members, such as physical, respiratory, and occupational therapists.*

---

   b. Demineralization of bone *(osteoporosis)* occurs because of lack of weight bearing.
   c. As bones demineralize, calcium deposits in joints contribute to stiffness and pain.
   d. Demineralized bones may become deformed or fracture easily.
   4. Nursing care.
      a. Encourage active ROM or perform passive ROM exercises to maintain joint mobility.
      b. Encourage weight-bearing exercise, such as lifting small handheld weights or using a tilt table, if permitted.
      c. Support joints and limbs when moving clients.
      d. Use assistive devices to maintain body alignment (e.g., trochanter roll, sand bag) or prescribed position (e.g., pillow between the legs after hip surgery to keep the legs apart [abduction]).
      e. Apply splints or braces as prescribed to maintain functional alignment and prevent contracture formation.
      f. Encourage and assist with ambulation if the client has a prescription for out of bed.

B. Cardiovascular system
   1. Orthostatic hypotension.
      a. **Orthostatic hypotension** occurs when the autonomic nervous system results in an inability to equalize blood pressure when moving from a recumbent to a sitting or standing position, causing syncope.
      b. Venous blood pools in the lower extremities because of a decrease in the vasopressor mechanism that normally causes muscle contractions that exert pressure on the veins, promoting venous return.

c. Orthostatic neurovascular reflex control of blood vessels decreases because of habituation to the lower pressure, higher flow, and increased diameter of vessels in the recumbent position.

2. Increased workload of the heart.
   a. The heart works harder when a person is in the supine position than in an erect position.
   b. Decreased gravity pressure redistributes blood from the legs to other parts of the body, resulting in an increased heart rate, stroke volume, and cardiac output.
   c. Release of the breath pressed forcibly against a closed glottis (*Valsalva maneuver*) causes a surge of blood to enter the heart, which can cause a dysrhythmia and cardiac arrest.

3. Thrombus formation.
   a. A **thrombus** is the formation of a blood clot within the vascular system. Circulatory stasis, activation of clotting, and vessel injury can lead to clot formation (*Virchow's triad*).
   b. Venous stasis results from a lack of muscle contraction that promotes venous return.
   c. Hypercoagulability results from an increased concentration of formed elements in blood, a decreased blood volume related to dehydration that often accompanies immobility, and an increased blood calcium level.
   d. Pressure on blood vessels from bed-bound or sitting positions causes intima damage that begins the cascade of clot formation.
   e. An **embolus** occurs when a clot or tissue debris moves from its place of origin to a smaller vessel causing an occlusion. A pulmonary embolus occurs when this happens in the lungs.

4. Nursing care.
   a. Assess vital signs routinely.
   b. Assess the lower extremities for clinical manifestations of a thrombus, such as localized pain, heat, swelling, and redness.
   c. Teach the client to avoid the Valsalva maneuver, such as by exhaling when having a bowel movement or changing positions. The Valsalva maneuver causes a surge of blood flow when the held breath is released, which can dislodge a thrombus.
   d. Maintain safety due to the potential for orthostatic hypotension.
   e. Apply prescribed venous compression devices (e.g., sequential compression devices, antiembolism stockings) that apply pressure to the legs to promote venous return. (See "Lower Extremity Compression Devices" in Fig. 24.5 in Chapter 24, Perioperative.)

🛑 f. Avoid massaging the legs because doing so can cause a thrombus to become a pulmonary embolus.

🛑 g. Encourage intake of 2 to 3 L of fluid daily to prevent dehydration and hypercoagulability.

C. Respiratory system
1. Decreased respiratory movement.
   a. Counterresistance of a bed or chair limits chest movements.
   b. Recumbent positions permit abdominal organs to compress the diaphragm, limiting its usual descent on inspiration.
   c. Muscle disuse or decreased innervation limits the effectiveness of the accessory muscles of respiration.
   d. Central nervous system depressants, such as opioids and sedatives, may decrease mobility and the rate and depth of respirations.
   e. Decreased lung expansion limits gas exchange.

2. Stasis of respiratory secretions.
   a. Gravity permits secretions to pool in the lungs.
   b. The ability to cough is reduced by a loss of muscle tone and medications that depress the cough reflex.
   c. Clients with mobility problems may have inadequate fluid intake, be dehydrated, or be taking anticholinergic medications that increase the viscosity of secretions.
   d. Secretions may impede exchange of gases between the atmosphere and the lungs and jeopardize a patent airway.
   e. Retained secretions provide a medium for pathogenic microorganisms, resulting in hypostatic pneumonia.

3. Oxygen–carbon dioxide imbalance.
   a. Decreased respiratory movement and stasis of secretions result in deficient ventilation.
   b. Deficient ventilation with a decrease in surfactant results in collapse of alveoli (*atelectasis*).
   c. Respiratory acidosis occurs as blood oxygen concentration decreases and carbon dioxide (as hydrogen ions and carbonic acid) increases.

4. Nursing care.
   a. Assess respiratory status, such as rate, regularity, depth (shallow or deep), thoracic or abdominal, easy or labored, length of inhalation and exhalation, productive or nonproductive cough, and oxygen saturation level.
   b. Identify the use of accessory muscles of respiration (e.g., intercostal and sternocleidomastoid).
   c. Assess breath sounds regularly, particularly for crackles and diminished breath sounds.
   d. Assess for central nervous system manifestations of hypoxia, such as restlessness, confusion, forgetfulness, and anxiety.

⊘ e. Monitor for clinical manifestations of a pulmonary embolus, such as unilateral chest pain, shortness of breath, dyspnea, tachycardia, tachypnea, and decreased breath sounds on auscultation. Initiate the rapid response team and report the client's status to the primary health-care provider immediately.

f. Maintain semi-Fowler or high-Fowler position if permitted to allow abdominal organs to drop by gravity and promote contraction of the diaphragm.

g. Encourage the client to change positions, use an incentive spirometer, and cough every hour to expand the lungs and raise sputum.

h. Teach the client to use abdominal muscles to increase the depth of inhalation and prolong exhalation.

i. Administer oxygen as prescribed.

j. Coordinate activities of the respiratory therapist (e.g., cupping, clapping, postural drainage, nebulizer treatment) if prescribed to facilitate mobilization of respiratory secretions.

D. Integumentary system

1. Reduced skin turgor.

a. Atrophy of skin can occur.

b. Skin elasticity may decrease because the health of the dermis is affected by fluid shifts between fluid compartments.

2. Skin breakdown.

a. Decreased circulation as a result of decreased muscle contraction limits the delivery of oxygen and nutrients to cells.

b. When pressure on a capillary exceeds 15 to 32 mm Hg, its lumen is occluded, resulting in deprivation of oxygen to tissues (*tissue ischemia*) and accumulation of metabolic wastes.

3. Nursing care

a. Use predictive measures, such as the Norton Scale (Fig. 17.7), to assess each client's risk of pressure ulcer development.

b. Reposition the client every 1 to 2 hours to relieve pressure over bony prominences that can lead to pressure ulcers (Fig. 17.8).

c. Employ actions to avoid shearing, such as using a pull sheet or transfer board and placing the client in the low-Fowler position.

d. Use assistive devices to limit the development of pressure ulcers, such as gel pads, synthetic sheepskin, and an air mattress.

e. Keep skin clean and dry; use a moisture barrier in the perineal area and implement incontinence management.

f. Encourage adequate nutritional and fluid intake, especially foods high in protein and vitamin C.

g. Massage dependent areas, except calves of the legs, to promote circulation.

h. Use dressings as prescribed (e.g., DuoDERM, transparent adhesives, or films) to protect skin from frictional forces.

i. Assess for the first signs of pressure ulcer development; assess the stage of a pressure ulcer if present (Table 17.4).

Norton Scale for Assessing Risk of Pressure Ulcers

	Physical Condition		Mental Condition		Activity		Mobility		Incontinent		
	Good	4	Alert	4	Ambulant	4	Full	4	Not	4	Total Score
	Fair	3	Apathetic	3	Walk/help	3	Slightly limited	3	Occasional	3	
	Poor	2	Confused	2	Chair-bound	2	Very limited	2	Usually/urine	2	
	Very bad	1	Stupor	1	Bed	1	Immobile	1	Doubly	1	
Name/Date											

The Norton scale uses five criteria to assess patients' risk for pressure ulcers. Scores of 14 or less indicate liability to ulcers; scores of less than 12 indicate very high risk.

Fig. 17.7 Norton scale for assessing risk of pressure ulcers. (From Norton, D., McLaren, R., & Exton-Smith, A. N. [1975]. *An investigation of geriatric nursing problems in hospital.* Edinburgh: Churchill Livingstone, with permission.)

Sitting Position

Lateral Position

Vertebrae
(spinal processes)

Sacrum   Pelvis
(ischial tuberosity)

Heels
(calcaneus)

Ear   Ilium   Knee (medial
and lateral
condyles)

Side of head
(parietal and
temporal bones)

Shoulder
(acromial
process)

Greater
trochanter

Malleolus
(medial
and
lateral)

Supine Position

Prone Position

Back of head
(occipital bone)

Scapulae   Elbows
(olecranon
process)

Sacrum   Heels
(calcaneus)

Cheek and
ear (zygomatic
bone)

Shoulder
(acromial
process)

Breasts
(women)

Genitalia
(men)

Knees
(patellas)

Toes
(phalanges)

Fig 17.8 Common sites for pressure ulcer development. (From Wilkinson and Treas [2016]. *Fundamentals of nursing*, Vol. 1, 3rd ed. Philadelphia: F. A. Davis Company, with permission.)

Table 17.4 Pressure Ulcer Stages

Illustration	Clinical Manifestations	Photograph
Stage I: Involves only the epidermis. Epidermis / Dermis / Fat / Muscle / Bone	• *Erythema that remains for 15 to 30 minutes after release of pressure* (reactive hyperemia). • *Skin that may appear darker than adjacent skin in dark-skinned people.* • *Lack of blanching when touched with a finger.* • *Skin that may feel firm, soft, or boggy and warmer or cooler than adjacent tissue.* • *Tingling or burning at the site.*	
Stage II: Involves the epidermis and partial-thickness loss of the dermis.	• *Serum-filled blister(s) that has ruptured.* • *Shallow crater that may be pink or red and shiny or dry.* • *Erythema surrounding skin breakdown that may feel warm to touch.*	
Stage III: Involves the epidermis, full-thickness loss of the dermis, and damage to subcutaneous tissue.	• *Deep crater extending down to but not through the fascia.* • *Damage under outer margins of the ulcer (undermining).* • *Possible presence of exudate.*	

Table 17.4	**Pressure Ulcer Stages—cont'd**	
Illustration	**Clinical Manifestations**	**Photograph**
Stage IV: Involves full-thickness skin loss with damage or destruction to muscle, supportive structures, and bone.	• *Deep full-thickness crater.* • *Possible visible or palpable bone or tendon.* • *Possible undermining.* • *Possible development of a sinus tract under the epidermis* (tunneling). • *Tan, yellow, green, gray, or brown necrotic tissue that does not obscure the wound bed* (slough). • *Tan, black, or brown leather-like necrotic tissue that does not obscure the wound bed* (eschar).	
Unstageable: Involves full-thickness skin loss and the base of the wound is obscured by necrotic tissue.	• *Base of the wound obscured by slough or eschar.*	

Figure credits: From Dillon (2016). *Nursing health assessment: The foundation of clinical practice,* 3rd ed. Philadelphia: F. A. Davis Company, with permission; Wilkinson and Treas (2016). *Fundamentals of nursing,* Vol. 1, 3rd ed. Philadelphia: F. A. Davis Company, with permission; and Burton and Ludwig (2015). *Fundamentals of nursing care: Concepts, connections & skills,* 2nd ed. Philadelphia: F. A. Davis Company, with permission.

E. Gastrointestinal system
1. Constipation.
   a. A slowed metabolic rate decreases gastrointestinal motility and delays gastric emptying.
   b. Dehydration, often associated with immobility, results in decreased fluid content in stool.
   c. Ignoring the urge to have a bowel movement may occur due to need to use a bedpan, embarrassment, or inadequate privacy; this weakens the defecation reflex.
   d. Dry, hard stool is more difficult to expel, which may lead to the client excessively using the Valsalva maneuver.
2. Decreased appetite *(anorexia).*
   a. Appetite diminishes when peristalsis slows, resulting in decreased caloric intake.
   b. Decreased caloric intake results in an inability to meet the body's nutritional needs.
3. Nursing care.
   a. Assess the characteristics of stool, such as frequency, color, and consistency.
   b. Assess for the presence and extent of bowel sounds.
   c. Identify the client's food preferences and incorporate them into the client's prescribed diet when possible.
   d. Encourage the intake of dietary fiber if permitted, such as from whole grains, fruits, and vegetables.
   e. Encourage the client to assume the sitting position if possible when eating to facilitate the passage of food from the esophagus to the stomach and eventually the intestine.
   f. Teach the client to respond to the urge to defecate. Toilet a client immediately when the client indicates the need to have a bowel movement.
   g. Provide privacy when the client is attempting to have a bowel movement.
   h. Encourage the client to use the sitting position for bowel movements, if permitted, to promote gravitational forces and to allow the client to lean forward to increase intra-abdominal pressure without using the Valsalva maneuver.

F. Metabolism
1. Decreased metabolic rate.
   a. **Metabolic rate** is the minimal energy expended to maintain physical and chemical processes, decreases.
   b. Decreased metabolic rate results in a negative nitrogen balance and fatigue.
2. Negative nitrogen balance.
   a. **Negative nitrogen balance** is the state caused by an inadequate intake of protein to meet body needs, resulting in muscle breakdown that releases nitrogen from muscle cells.
   b. Protein synthesis decreases and protein breakdown increases.

c. Catabolized muscles release nitrogen, which is excreted over time, impeding tissue building and wound healing.

3. Nursing care.

a. Obtain weekly body weights.

b. Monitor laboratory values, such as serum albumin and total protein.

c. Provide preferred foods that are high in protein, such as meat, poultry, fish, eggs, dairy products, and legumes.

d. Provide small, frequent feedings.

e. Encourage intake of nutritional supplements (e.g., Boost, Ensure) between meals as prescribed.

G. Urinary system

1. Urinary stasis.

a. When in a horizontal position, urinary stasis occurs due to incomplete emptying of the urinary bladder.

b. Bladder functioning is further compromised by a decrease in muscle tone.

2. Urinary retention or incontinence.

a. Urine accumulates in the bladder and is unable to be excreted (retention) because of decreased muscle tone or altered innervation.

b. An inability to relax perineal muscles sufficiently occurs due to unnatural positioning for urination, inadequate privacy, and embarrassment about using a bedpan.

c. Excessive bladder distention results in involuntary urination (incontinence) or involuntary dribbling of urine indicating urinary retention with overflow.

3. Urinary tract infection (UTI).

a. Demineralization of bone causes hypercalcemia, resulting in urine becoming more alkaline, which supports bacterial growth.

b. The urinary tract may become contaminated by Escherichia coli from inadequate perineal hygiene.

c. Contaminated urine may back up into the renal pelvis distending the kidneys.

4. Renal calculi.

a. Demineralization of bone causes hypercalcemia, resulting in calcium salts in urine.

b. These salts precipitate out as crystals to form renal stones (calculi).

5. Nursing care.

a. Assess the characteristics of the client's urine, such as color, clarity, and odor.

b. Assess intake and output.

c. Encourage the intake of 2 to 3 L of fluid daily if not contraindicated to help flush the kidneys and bladder.

d. Provide privacy when the client is urinating.

e. Encourage assumption of as normal a position as possible when urinating to allow gravity to assist, such as standing for men and sitting for women.

f. Use techniques to help stimulate urination, such as a warm cloth over the symphysis pubis, hands in a basin of warm water, sound of flowing water from a faucet, and pressure against the suprapubic area with the hands (Credé's maneuver).

g. Assess for clinical manifestations of renal calculi, such as blood in the urine (hematuria) and flank pain radiating to the pubic area (renal colic).

h. Assess for clinical manifestations of UTI, such as frequency, urgency, hematuria, pus in urine (pyuria), and painful urination (dysuria).

i. Strain urine if calculi are suspected.

j. Administer prescribed urinary tract analgesics and antibiotics for UTIs.

H. Psychoneurological system

1. Psychosocial changes.

a. An inability to fulfill one's role and dependence on others may lower self-esteem and precipitate changes in mood, such as sadness, hostility, and depression.

b. Narrowed opportunities for socialization may precipitate apathy and withdrawal.

2. Mental changes.

a. A decrease in a variety of stimuli may precipitate a decreased ability to perceive time accurately, concentrate, problem-solve, and recall sequential events.

b. A decrease in endorphins, generally released with activity, causes a negative effect on mood.

3. Nursing care.

a. Assess for clinical indicators of emotional responses associated with limitations in mobility and alterations in body image, such as anxiety, depression, frustration, and anger.

b. Involve the client in planning care.

c. Offer choices whenever possible.

d. Ensure safety if the client is cognitively impaired.

V. Assistive Devices to Increase Client Mobility and Related Nursing Care

Assistive devices are types of equipment that promote independence and safety in clients with varying limitations in mobility because of musculoskeletal, neurological, or cardiovascular problems. The nurse should assess each client to determine the most appropriate device to use because each device serves a purpose and requires specific client abilities. A major responsibility of the nurse is to assist clients to use these devices safely.

A. Cane
1. A cane is a device that has a shaft with a handle at one end and one or more points (prongs) that touch the floor.
2. Purposes.
   a. Provides independent mobility.
   b. Limits pressure on weight-bearing joints.
   c. Provides a wide base of support to promote stability.
   d. Promotes walking on flat surfaces as well as using stairs.
3. Nursing care.
   a. Ensure that the client has the ability to use a cane.
      (1) Ability to bear some weight on both lower extremities.
      (2) Ability to use upper extremity opposite to affected lower extremity.
   b. Ensure appropriate cane length.
      (1) Handle should be level with the greater trochanter.
      (2) Elbow flexed 30° with the wrist extended when holding the handle.
   c. Ensure that the rubber tips on prongs of the cane are intact.
   d. Teach the client how to use the cane.
      (1) Hold the cane in the hand opposite to the affected lower extremity.
      (2) Distribute weight evenly between the cane and feet.
      (3) Walk erect without leaning forward or toward the cane.
      (4) Advance the cane and the affected lower extremity at the same time and then the other leg.
      (5) Maintain the same length of stride with both lower extremities.
      (6) Climb stairs by advancing the unaffected lower extremity and then placing the cane and affected lower extremity on the same step; reverse the procedure when descending the stairs.

B. Walker
1. A walker is a U-shaped device with four points that touch the floor; some have two or four wheels and some have a seat.
2. Purposes.
   a. Provides independent mobility.
   b. Limits pressure on weight-bearing joints.
   c. Promotes greater stability by providing a wider base of support than a cane.
   d. Promotes walking on flat surfaces.
   e. Cannot be used on stairs.

3. Nursing care.
   a. Ensure that the client has the ability to use a walker.
      (1) Ability to bear some weight on both lower extremities.
      (2) Adequate strength in elbow extensors, shoulder depressors, and hand and wrist muscles of both upper extremities to lift or move the walker.
   b. Ensure appropriate walker height.
      (1) Handle should be level with the greater trochanter.
      (2) Elbow flexed 30° with the wrist extended when holding the handle.
   c. Teach the client how to use the walker.
      (1) Stand between the back legs of the walker.
      (2) Move the walker forward a short distance.
         (a) Four-prong walker: Lift the walker off floor, place all four prongs flat on the floor, and then step between the walker.
         (b) Two-wheeled walker: Lift the back prongs off the floor, roll the walker forward, place the back prongs flat on the floor, and then step between the walker.
         (c) Four-wheeled walker: Push the walker forward and then step between the walker.

C. Crutches
1. A crutch is a device that has a shaft with an axillary bar at the top, a bar for the hands to hold about halfway down the length of the shaft, and one point at the end of the shaft that rests on the floor.
2. Purposes.
   a. Promotes independent ambulation.
   b. Limits or eliminates weight bearing on a lower extremity.
   c. Promotes walking on flat surfaces as well as using stairs.
3. Nursing care.
   a. Ensure that the client has the ability to use crutches.
      (1) Ability to bear full weight on one leg or partial weight on both legs.
      (2) Adequate strength in the triceps, finger flexors, and wrist and elbow extensors.
      (3) Ability to coordinate sequence of upper and lower extremity movements.
   b. Ensure appropriate crutch height.
      (1) Measure the distance from the anterior axillary fold to 6 inches (15 cm) outside of the heel of the foot.

(2) Allow 2 inches (5 cm) between the axilla and the axillary bar of the crutch.

(3) Ensure that the hand bar allows extension of the arm with the elbows flexed 30° when weight is placed on the hand.

c. Ensure that padding on the axillary bars is adequate and the rubber tips on the ends of the crutches are intact.

d. Teach the client how to use crutches.

(1) Use the proper sequence of advancing the crutches and the lower extremities (Table 17.5).

🛑 (2) Bear weight on the hands, not on the axillae, because bearing weight on the axillae compresses the nerves under the arm, resulting in nerve damage that affects the arms and hands.

(3) Look forward, not down, when walking to maintain a correct center of gravity; looking down moves the center of gravity forward, jeopardizing stability.

(4) Maintain balance when using just one lower extremity by keeping the affected lower extremity slightly forward rather than with the knee flexed; flexing the knee on the affected extremity moves the center of gravity backward, jeopardizing stability.

(5) Climb stairs by advancing the unaffected lower extremity and then placing the crutches and affected lower extremity on the same step; reverse the procedure when descending the stairs.

D. Wheelchair

1. A wheelchair is a device that consists of a seat with a back, sides to support the arms, foot rests to support the lower extremities, and wheels that allow propulsion by the client, another person, or a motor.

2. Purposes.

a. Promotes independent mobility.

b. Provides mobility for clients who cannot ambulate.

c. Provides mobility for clients who are too unsteady or frail to use an alternate device.

d. Eliminates the need to ambulate, thereby decreasing the workload on the heart and oxygen demands of the body.

3. Nursing care.

a. Maintain safety.

(1) Ensure that all parts of the wheelchair are in correct working order.

🛑 (2) Lock the wheels when not moving the wheelchair.

(3) Keep the wheelchair in close proximity to the bed or chair during a transfer.

(4) Initiate the transfer by leading from the client's stronger side.

(5) Raise the foot rests before transferring the client to the wheelchair, and place the client's feet on lowered foot plates after the transfer to the wheelchair.

Table 17.5 Crutch-Walking Gaits	
Type of Gait	**Client Teaching**
Two-point gait • *Both lower extremities must be capable of partial weight bearing.* • *Requires more balance and strength than the four-point gait.* • *Maintains two points on the floor at all times.*	• *Move the right crutch and left lower extremity forward simultaneously.* • *Then move the left crutch and right lower extremity forward simultaneously.*
Three-point gait • *One lower extremity must be able to support body weight.* • *Requires more balance and strength in the arms than the two-point and four-point gaits.*	• *Move both crutches and the affected lower extremity forward simultaneously.* • *Then move the stronger lower extremity forward.*
Four-point gait • *Both legs must be able to support partial body weight.* • *Requires coordination to alternate movements among extremities.* • *Maintains three points on the floor at all times.*	• *Move the right crutch forward.* • *Then move the left lower extremity forward.* • *Then move the left crutch forward.* • *Then move the right lower extremity forward.*
Swing crutch gaits • *Both lower extremities must be able to support partial body weight.* • *Requires more strength in both upper extremities than other gaits.* • *Maintains two points on the floor at all times.*	*Swing-to gait* • *Move both crutches forward simultaneously.* • *Swing both lower extremities to the level of the crutches.* *Swing-through gait* • *Move both crutches forward simultaneously.* • *Then swing both lower extremities slightly past the level of the crutches.*

(6) Position the client so that the client is sitting well back in the wheelchair, with the back of the knees at the edge of but not touching the seat.

🛑 (7) Enter or exit an elevator, maneuver over irregularities in sidewalks, and go down curbs with the large wheels first.

🛑 (8) Place your body between the wheelchair and the lower side of an incline (e.g., push a wheelchair up an incline and back a wheelchair down an incline).

b. Teach the client about self-care when using a wheelchair.
   (1) Prevent the development of pressure ulcers over the ischial tuberosities.
      (a) Use a padded cushion or gel pad on the seat to provide a soft surface and distribute body weight more evenly.
      (b) Perform push-ups using the arms of the wheelchair or shift weight side to side several times every hour to relieve compression of the capillary beds.

(2) Prevent hip and knee flexion contractures.
   (a) Avoid sitting in the wheelchair for prolonged periods of time.
   (b) Extend the knees or stand in place if possible every 2 hours to extend the knee and hip joints.
   (c) Assume the prone position when in bed for 20 minutes twice a day to extend the hips and knees.
(3) Perform assessments to identify early signs of complications.
   (a) Assess the body or have a significant other assess the body routinely to identify early signs of impaired tissue integrity.
   (b) Identify stiffening of joints that may indicate beginning contractures.
   (c) Notify the primary health-care provider if early signs or symptoms of complications of immobility are identified.
(4) Inform the client of the availability of wheelchair accessories (e.g., lap boards, seat-belts, removable arms, extended leg panels, motor propulsion).

CASE STUDY: Putting It All Together

An older male client is admitted to the hospital with a diagnosis of pneumonia and an 8-year history of Parkinson disease. When transferring the client from a wheelchair to the bed, a nurse identifies that the client has stiff joints and is walking with small, shuffling steps with involuntary accelerations. The client states, "I'm afraid to leave the house because I have difficulty maintaining my balance and I fell twice recently. I hold on to furniture and walls as I walk around my house. Occasionally, I get a little light-headed when I stand up. I really just sit around the house all day because I get too tired and out of breath when I'm more active." When completing a skin assessment, the nurse identifies in the sacral area several small (1 cm) shallow, red, shiny breaks in the client's skin that are surrounded by erythema. The nurse also notes rhonchi in the left and right lung fields; moist cough; occasional expectoration of thick yellow secretions; delayed capillary refill in the toes; respiratory rate of 28 breaths/minute and shallow respirations at rest; and dyspnea on exertion. The client's oxygen saturation is 88% on room air and 95% with nasal oxygen at 2 L/minute. The primary health-care provider prescribes passive ROM exercises. Just before leaving the client's room, the nurse decides to move the client up in bed.

Case Study Questions

A. Place in order of priority the following concerns identified by the nurse and explain the reasoning behind the sequence identified.

Risk for injury:

_____

_____

continued.

CASE STUDY: Putting It All Together
cont'd

Case Study Questions

Impaired walking:

_____

_____

Ineffective airway clearance:

_____

_____

B. What word(s) should the nurse use when describing the small, shuffling steps with involuntary accelerations?

_____

C. What stage pressure ulcer is associated with several small (1 cm) shallow, red, and shiny breaks in the skin surrounded by erythema?

_____

D. Identify two complications of immobility that affect the cardiovascular system other than orthostatic hypotension, which is already identified in the scenario, and explain why they occur.

1. _____

2. _____

E. Identify six nursing interventions that the nurse should implement to reduce the risk of thrombus formation.

1. _____

2. _____

3. _____

4. _____

5. _____

6. _____

F. Identify seven nursing interventions that the nurse should implement when assisting with or providing ROM exercises.

1. _____

2. _____

3. _____

4. _____

5. _____

6. _____

7. _____

CASE STUDY: Putting It All Together

cont'd

Case Study Questions

G. Identify 10 principles of body mechanics that the nurse should follow when moving a client up in bed and explain their purposes.

1. _____
2. _____
3. _____
4. _____
5. _____
6. _____
7. _____
8. _____
9. _____
10. _____

12. A nurse is teaching a client with weakness in the left leg how to use a cane. The nurse first positions the client in a standing position with the cane in the hand opposite the affected leg. Place the following steps in the order in which they should be implemented.
    1. Position the tip of the cane 6 inches in front of the strong foot.
    2. Move the affected leg forward opposite to the cane.
    3. Move the cane forward 4 to 6 inches.
    4. Move the unaffected leg forward.
    5. Put weight on the affected leg.
    6. Repeat the sequence of steps.
    Answer: _____

13. A nurse is planning to assist a client with active-assistive range-of-motion exercises. What should the nurse do **first?**
    1. Encourage the client to be as independent as possible when doing range-of-motion exercises.
    2. Identify any restrictions regarding the type and extent of range-of-motion exercises.
    3. Explain what range-of-motion exercises are and why they are being done.
    4. Schedule range-of-motion exercise to occur during the client's bath.

14. A nurse is completing a head-to-toe assessment of a newly admitted client. The nurse identifies a lesion that looks like a broken blister over a bony prominence on the client's foot. Which condition should the nurse conclude the client is exhibiting?
    1. Pressure ulcer
    2. Plantar wart
    3. Callus
    4. Corn

15. A nurse is positioning a client in the supported prone position. What actions should the nurse implement when positioning this client? **Select all that apply.**
    1. Change the client's position hourly.
    2. Put pillows under the client's thighs.
    3. Align pillows alongside the client's hips.
    4. Place a small pillow under the client's head.
    5. Put a small pillow under the client's abdomen.

16. For which of the following consequences associated with the muscular system should the nurse assess a client who has been on prolonged bedrest?
    1. Atrophy
    2. Osteoporosis
    3. Pressure ulcers
    4. Skin breakdown

17. Which position is least likely to be used to position a client with a stage III pressure ulcer of the right greater trochanter?

18. A nurse is caring for a bed-bound client. In which position should the nurse place the client to prevent a hip flexion contracture?
    1. Prone
    2. Supine
    3. Fowler
    4. Lateral

19. A nurse must transfer a client from a bed to a wheelchair. Place the following nursing actions in the order that they should be performed.
    1. Lock the brakes on the wheelchair.
    2. Place the wheelchair parallel to the client's bed.
    3. Stand up and pivot the client toward the wheelchair.
    4. Inform the client how the transfer will be performed.
    5. Bend your knees and place your arms under the client's axillae.
    6. Allow the client to sit on the side of the bed for several minutes.
    Answer: _____

20. What should the nurse do **first** before moving a client?
    1. Consider all of the principles of body mechanics that should be followed.
    2. Select assistive devices to support the client's functional alignment.
    3. Assess for all the factors that may influence the client's mobility.
    4. Verify the primary health-care provider's activity prescription.

21. A nurse receives the following prescription: "Teach the client to engage in aerobic exercise." Which exercise should the nurse discuss with the client? **Select all that apply.**
    1. Bicycle riding
    2. Tensing and relaxing muscles
    3. Using a machine for resistance while moving a joint
    4. Jogging while progressively increasing the distance over time
    5. Walking around the neighborhood in a gentle but steady pace

22. A nurse is caring for a client who is comatose and determines that the client has a stage IV pressure ulcer. Which observations support this conclusion? **Select all that apply.**
    1. Wound obscured with sloughing tissue
    2. Soft tissue over a bony prominence
    3. Deep crater with an intact fascia
    4. Tunneling under the epidermis
    5. Full-thickness skin loss

23. A nurse is positioning a client in the semi-Fowler position. Which actions should be implemented by the nurse when positioning this client? **Select all that apply.**
    1. Place 2 pillows under the client's head.
    2. Raise the head of the client's bed 45 degrees.
    3. Place hand rolls in the palms of both the hands.
    4. Apply foam boots to maintain dorsiflexion of the feet.
    5. Put trochanter rolls alongside the client's knees to the ankles.

24. A nurse receives a prescription to institute active range-of-motion exercises with a client. What nursing action is unique to providing active range-of-motion exercises?
    1. Assisting the client who is unable to complete the exercises through all planes of movement
    2. Encouraging the client to perform the exercises independently
    3. Providing a warm bath before the exercises
    4. Demonstrating how to do the exercises

25. Which principles of body mechanics should the nurse implement when providing nursing care? **Select all that apply.**
    1. Hold an object away from the body.
    2. Extend the arms when lifting objects.
    3. Squat when lifting objects off the floor.
    4. Keep feet together when moving an object.
    5. Put weight on the balls of the feet, one foot ahead of the other to pivot.

26. A nurse is caring for a client with a pressure ulcer on the right trochanter. In which position should the nurse place this client? **Select all that apply.**
    1. Semi-Fowler
    2. Right lateral
    3. Left Sims'
    4. Supine
    5. Prone

27. A nurse is caring for a client who is at risk for thrombus formation due to decreased mobility. For which clinical manifestation that is the **most** serious should the nurse monitor the client?
    1. Faint pedal pulse
    2. Edema of the calf
    3. Pain in the lower leg
    4. Unilateral chest pain

28. A nurse is providing passive range-of-motion exercises. Which principle is important?
    1. Increase the speed of the exercises progressively and according to the client's activity tolerance.
    2. Assist the client to complete all planes of movement when the client is unable to do so.
    3. Support above and below the joint being exercised.
    4. Repeat each movement a dozen times twice a day.

29. Which position requires that the client be repositioned after only 1 hour, rather than after 2 hours, which is generally the norm?
    1. Sims'
    2. Prone
    3. Lateral
    4. Orthopneic

30. A nurse is caring for a client who has a prescription for bedrest. The nurse is concerned about the client's increased risk for hypostatic pneumonia. Which nursing actions should be implemented by the nurse to minimize this risk? **Select all that apply.**
    1. Assess lung sounds for crackles.
    2. Position the client in a chair for meals.
    3. Turn the client from side to side every 2 hours.
    4. Apply sequential compression devices to the lower legs as prescribed.
    5. Encourage the use of an incentive spirometer 5 times an hour when awake.

31. A nurse is caring for a newly admitted client who has a urinary tract infection and is recovering from a brain attack (cerebrovascular accident, stroke) that left her with mild hemiparesis of the right side. She uses a cane and a lower right leg brace to enable her to walk more normally without having to lift her leg and have her foot slap down on the ground due to a slight footdrop. The primary health-care provider prescribes an IV antibiotic, out of bed to a chair twice a day, and a regular diet. The nurse reviewed the client's clinical record, interviewed the client, and completed a brief physical assessment. What should the nurse do **first** based on the collected data?
    1. Apply a protective skin ointment to the perineal area.
    2. Teach the client to limit fluid intake after 6:00 p.m.
    3. Take the client's vital signs every 4 hours.
    4. Administer the antibiotic.

Client's Clinical Record

Laboratory Results: Urinalysis

Cloudy, concentrated.
RBCs greater than 3 (per high-power field).
WBCs greater than 6 (per high-power field).
Specific gravity: 1.023.
pH: 8.5.
Presence of casts.
Culture positive for Pseudomonas.

Client Interview

States that she spends most of her time lying on the couch. She said that she is limiting her fluid intake starting in the early afternoon so that she does not have to get up so much. However, she said, "Lately I feel as though I have to get up all the time to pass my water. I know that it sounds childish, but I have been wearing an adult incontinence pad so that I don't have to get up so much. The doctor prescribed an antibiotic because he said that I have a urinary tract infection."

Physical Assessment

Temperature: 102.4°F, oral.
Pulse: 100 beats/minute, occasional missed beat at irregular intervals.
Respirations: 24 breaths/minute, no dyspnea.
Blood pressure: 138/84 mm Hg.
Voiding small amounts of urine frequently, concentrated, cloudy.
Abdomen does not feel distended.
Client states that it burns when she urinates.
Perineal area appears red and inflamed, but skin is intact.
IVF running at 125 mL per hour as prescribed, site dry and intact with no S&S of infection or infiltration.

32. A nurse identifies that a client is walking with a propulsive cogwheel gait. Which client behaviors observed by the nurse supports this conclusion? **Select all that apply.**
    1. Rolling motion in which the opposite hip drops when taking a stride
    2. Exaggerated lifting of the leg to avoid dragging the toes
    3. Involuntary acceleration when walking
    4. Stiff, foot dragging when ambulating
    5. Small, shuffling steps

33. A nurse is caring for a client with a diagnosis of thrombophlebitis of the lower left leg. Which independent nursing action is important for the nurse to implement?
    1. Elevate the left leg on a pillow.
    2. Apply a warm soak to the left leg twice a day.
    3. Massage the legs gently from distal to proximal.
    4. Maintain venous compression devices to both legs.

34. A nurse is caring for a client who recently sustained a brain attack (cerebrovascular accident, stroke), which caused right-sided hemiparesis. The nurse is concerned about the client developing contractures related to immobility. Which action is **most** important for the nurse to implement?
    1. Providing active and passive range-of-motion exercises
    2. Turning the client from side to side every 2 hours
    3. Placing the client on a tilt table 2 times a day
    4. Encouraging coughing and deep breathing

35. Which nursing actions are effective in minimizing tissue ischemia due to shearing forces? **Select all that apply.**
    1. Massaging gently around the client's bony prominences every two hours
    2. Using a transfer board to move a client from a bed to a stretcher
    3. Placing an air mattress on the bed under the client
    4. Positioning the client in a semi-Fowler position
    5. Using a pull sheet to move the client up in bed

36. A client who has been immobile because of a spinal cord injury develops hypercalcemia. Hydrochlorothiazide 50 mg twice a day by mouth is prescribed. The medication is supplied in capsules of 12.5 mg. How many capsules should the nurse administer for each dose? **Record your answer using a whole number.**
    Answer: _____ capsules

37. A nurse is caring for a client who is prescribed OOB in a chair for 1 hour twice a day. The nurse is concerned about the complication of orthostatic hypotension. What nursing action employed by the nurse will help to minimize the risk of orthostatic hypotension?
    1. Encourage use of an incentive spirometer every 2 hours.
    2. Massage the client's legs gently before moving to a sitting position.
    3. Teach ways to avoid the Valsalva maneuver when changing position.
    4. Dangle the client on the side of the bed for 1 minute before standing.

38. A nurse is repositioning a client who is on bedrest to the orthopneic position. What actions should the nurse implement when repositioning this client? **Select all that apply.**
    1. Position trochanter rolls alongside the hips to the knees of both legs.
    2. Position an overbed table with a pillow on it across the lap.
    3. Elevate the head of the bed to a high-Fowler position.
    4. Lift both legs into the stirrups at the same time.
    5. Help the client to stand from a sitting position.

39. A nurse is caring for a client who is on bedrest and is concerned about the risk of urinary stasis. Which nursing action is effective in reducing the risk of complications associated with urinary stasis?
    1. Strain urine if calculi are suspected.
    2. Pour warm water over the symphysis pubis.
    3. Assist the client to a normal position when voiding.
    4. Encourage the intake of three liters of fluid daily if permitted.

40. A nurse is caring for a client with the potential for developing a pressure (decubitus) ulcer. Which are the reasons why the nurse places a synthetic sheepskin under the client? **Select all that apply.**
    1. Absorbs urine
    2. Minimizes friction
    3. Keeps the skin warm
    4. Distributes weight more evenly
    5. Allows air to circulate under the client

REVIEW ANSWERS AND RATIONALES

1. ANSWER: 3.
Rationales:
1. Extension is straightening the finger joints.
2. Adduction is bringing the fingers in alignment next to one another.
3. Opposition is the correct term to describe touching the thumb to the tip of each finger of the same hand.
4. Circumduction is a circular motion of the hip or shoulder joint.
Content Area: Mobility
Integrated Processes: Nursing Process: Implementation
Client Need: Physiological Integrity; Basic Care and Comfort
Cognitive Level: Knowledge
Cognitive Level: Mobility

2. ANSWER: 1.
Rationales:
1. Pressure ulcers occur when the pressure in the capillaries exceeds that of the arterioles (15 to 32 mm Hg). Pathologic changes begin within 1 to 2 hours when tissues are deprived of oxygen and nutrients. If pressure is not relieved, tissue breakdown and cellular death (necrosis) occur.
2. Desquamation (shedding of the epidermis) is seen in postmature infants. It is not a cause of pressure ulcers.
3. Skin breakdown is the response to pressure, not the cause of a pressure ulcer; also, skin breakdown may be caused by stressors other than pressure.
4. Cellular necrosis is the death of tissues in response to prolonged pressure and oxygen deprivation; cellular necrosis is the response to pressure, not the cause of a pressure ulcer.
TEST-TAKING TIP: Identify the option that is unique. Option 1 is unique because it is not an example of tissue breakdown but rather the cause of deprivation of oxygen to tissue, which can cause death to cells. Identify equally plausible options. Options 2, 3, and 4 are equally plausible. They all are examples of tissue breakdown.
Content Area: Mobility
Integrated Processes: Nursing Process: Analysis
Client Need: Physiological Integrity; Reduction of Risk Potential
Cognitive Level: Comprehension
Concept: Tissue Integrity

3. ANSWER: 3.
Rationales:
1. Turning the client's arm so that the palm is facing the floor results in pronation, not supination, of the forearm and hand.
2. Bending the fingers of a hand back as far as possible so that the nails of the fingers are facing the forearm results in hyperextension of the wrist, not supination of the arm.
3. Turning the client's arm so that the palm is facing toward the ceiling results in supination of the forearm and hand.
4. Moving the arm so that it is 90 degrees away from the side of the body results in abduction of the shoulder, not supination of the arm.
TEST-TAKING TIP: Identify the options that are opposites. Options 1 and 3 are opposites. In option 1, the arm is positioned so that the palm is facing downward toward the

floor. In option 3, the arm is positioned so that the palm is facing upward toward the ceiling. More often than not, the correct answer is one of the options that is an opposite. Examine options 1 and 3 carefully.
Content Area: Mobility
Integrated Processes: Nursing Process: Implementation
Client Need: Physiological Integrity; Basic Care and Comfort
Cognitive Level: Analysis
Concept: Mobility

4. ANSWER: 3, 5.
Rationales:
1. The lower hip and knee should be extended, not flexed.
2. The right arm should be positioned behind the body in extension with the palm facing toward the ceiling.
3. The left arm should be positioned in front of the body when implementing the right Sims' position.
4. Both legs should be slightly flexed in front of the body with the left leg in front of the right leg.
5. Turning the body halfway between the lateral and prone position is the correct position of the body when a client is placed in the Sims' position.
Content Area: Mobility
Integrated Processes: Nursing Process: Implementation
Client Need: Physiological Integrity; Basic Care and Comfort
Cognitive Level: Application
Concept: Mobility

5. ANSWER: 1, 4, 5.
Rationales:
1. Entering an elevator with the wheelchair's big wheels first result in the client's head facing the door after entering; this is an acceptable practice. The client should be facing out toward the door as other people in the elevator tend to face. Also, when exiting an elevator the wheelchair's big wheels should exit first. Doing so will allow the wheelchair's big wheels to navigate the space between the floor and the elevator with less interference and promote client safety.
2. It is unsafe to move a wheelchair down a ramp leading with the small wheels. Having the wheelchair in front when going down a steep ramp will not prevent it from rolling down the hill in the event the person pushing the wheelchair loses control.
3. It is unsafe to use the footrests of the wheelchair to push a swinging door open. The pressure of the door may injure the client's feet or break the footrests of the wheelchair.
4. Pushing a wheelchair up a hill leading with the small wheels is a safe practice. Having the wheelchair in front when going up a hill will help prevent the wheelchair from rolling backward in the event the person pushing the wheelchair loses control. The body of the person pushing the wheelchair will prevent the wheelchair from rolling backward.
5. Locking the brakes when a wheelchair is not being moved is a safe practice. It is important to lock the brakes when a wheelchair is not in motion to prevent it from moving.
Content Area: Mobility
Integrated Processes: Teaching/Learning; Communication and Documentation; Nursing Process: Evaluation

Client Need: Safe and Effective Care Environment; Safety and Infection Control
Cognitive Level: Application
Concept: Patient-Centered Care; Mobility

6. ANSWER: 1.
Rationales:
1. The focus of the abduction pillow is to prevent adduction of the right leg, which can cause dislocation of the prosthesis. However, the other joints in the body should be maintained in functional alignment. Either a trochanter roll should be aligned along the side of the left leg from the hip to the knee or the left leg should be more securely positioned to the abduction pillow to prevent external rotation of the left hip.
2. The left forearm and hand are positioned across the abdomen, which is acceptable. This position helps prevent dependent edema in the left hand via the principle of gravity.
3. The trapeze is the correct distance from the client. If it is too close to the client, the client will not have room to lift the upper body off the bed.
4. The low-Fowler position is acceptable. However, a high-Fowler position is contraindicated. The hip flexion angle should not exceed 90 degrees because this can cause the prosthetic hip to dislocate.
TEST-TAKING TIP: Identify the word in the stem that indicates negative polarity. The word *wrong* in the stem indicates negative polarity. Identify the clang association. The word *hip* in the stem and in option 1 is a clang association.
Content Area: Mobility
Integrated Processes: Nursing Process: Evaluation
Client Need: Physiological Integrity; Basic Care and Comfort
Cognitive Level: Analysis
Concept: Mobility

7. ANSWER: 3.
Rationales:
1. Assessing vital signs routinely is an independent, not dependent, action of the nurse. Although taking vital signs routinely will help identify the client's cardiovascular status, it will not prevent a complication such as thrombophlebitis due to venous stasis.
2. Encouraging a client to do ankle-pumping exercises is an independent, not dependent, action of the nurse that will help minimize venous stasis due to immobility.
3. Applying sequential compression devices prescribed by a primary health-care provider will help minimize the risk of complications associated with venous stasis because it promotes venous return. This is a dependent function of the nurse because it must be prescribed by the primary health-care provider.
4. This action is unsafe and may injure the client. The supine, not semi-Fowler, position was prescribed for this client.
Content Area: Mobility
Integrated Processes: Nursing Process: Implementation
Client Need: Physiological Integrity; Basic Care and Comfort
Cognitive Level: Application
Concept: Perfusion

8. ANSWER: 1, 2.
Rationales:
1. Resting the head on one pillow prevents right lateral flexion of the neck and positions the client's head in functional alignment.
2. Flexing the left arm on a pillow is the correct position when in the right lateral position.
3. A trochanter roll is unnecessary. The right hip and leg are positioned against the mattress. A trochanter roll is used to prevent external rotation of the hip when the client is in a supine position.
4. The left hip and knee should be flexed slightly in front of the right leg and positioned on enough pillows to maintain functional alignment of the left hip, knee, and ankle.
5. This is the position of the right arm when in the right Sims', not lateral, position.
Content Area: Mobility
Integrated Processes: Nursing Process: Implementation
Client Need: Physiological Integrity; Basic Care and Comfort
Cognitive Level: Application
Concept: Mobility

9. ANSWER: 1.
Rationales:
1. Exerting pressure against an immovable object is an example of isometric exercise. It requires muscle tension with no change in muscle length or movement.
2. Performing active range-of-motion exercises is an example of isotonic, not isometric, exercise. Isotonic exercise involves a shortening and then lengthening of muscles to produce movement.
3. Walking briskly is associated with aerobic, not isometric, exercise. Aerobic exercise involves sustained periods of exertion whereby oxygen is metabolized to support energy.
4. Lifting the body using a trapeze is an example of isotonic, not isometric, exercise. Isotonic exercise involves a shortening and then lengthening of muscles to produce movement.
Content Area: Mobility
Integrated Processes: Teaching/Learning; Nursing Process: Evaluation
Client Need: Physiological Integrity; Basic Care and Comfort
Cognitive Level: Application
Concept: Patient-Centered Care; Mobility

10. ANSWER: 1, 2, 4.
Rationales:
1. An ischial tuberosity is a bony prominence located at the base of each ischium bone at the base of the pelvic girdle. No weight is placed on these bony prominences when in the Sims' position.
2. An ischial tuberosity is a bony prominence located at the base of each ischium bone at the base of the pelvic girdle. No weight is placed on these bony prominences when in the prone position.
3. The orthopneic position should be avoided. An ischial tuberosity is a bony prominence located at the base of each ischium bone at the base of the pelvic girdle. Body weight rests on these bony prominences when the body is in the sitting position.

4. An ischial tuberosity is a bony prominence located at the base of each ischium bone at the base of the pelvic girdle. No weight is placed on these bony prominences when in the right lateral position.

5. The high-Fowler position should be avoided. An ischial tuberosity is located at the base of each ischium bone at the base of the pelvic girdle. Body weight rests on these bones when the body is in the high-Fowler position.

Content Area: Mobility
Integrated Processes: Nursing Process: Implementation
Client Need: Physiological Integrity; Basic Care and Comfort
Cognitive Level: Application
Concept: Tissue Integrity

11. **ANSWER: 2.**
    Rationales:
    1. Keeping the back as straight as possible prevents injuries to the back and is an acceptable practice. Keeping the back as straight as possible prevents twisting (torsion). Twisting the back puts strain on the vertebrae, muscles, and tendons.
    2. Holding the object away from the body is improper body mechanics. It does not keep the weight close to the body's center of gravity, which minimizes stress on the back's vertebrae, muscles, and tendons. Objects should be held as close to the body as possible without touching the nurse's uniform; this prevents contamination of the nurse's uniform or the object being carried.
    3. Placing the feet wide apart is proper body mechanics because it promotes stability by increasing the base of support.
    4. Bending the knees while lifting an object demonstrates proper body mechanics. It allows the larger muscles of the legs to assist with the lift rather than the weaker muscles of the back. If the legs are not bent, the individual will have to bend at the waist and lean over to pick up the object, putting undue strain on the back.
    TEST-TAKING TIP: Identify the word in the stem that indicates negative polarity. The word *inappropriate* in the stem indicates negative polarity. The question is asking, "What action by the nursing assistant is wrong and violates the principles of body mechanics?" Identify the option that contains a clang association. The word *object* in the stem and in option 2 is a clang association.
    Content Area: Mobility
    Integrated Processes: Nursing Process: Evaluation
    Client Need: Safe and Effective Care Environment; Management of Care
    Cognitive Level: Application
    Concept: Mobility

12. **ANSWER: 1, 3, 2, 5, 4, 6.**
    Rationales:
    1. When a client is in the standing position, a cane should be placed 6 inches from the front of the unaffected foot. This distance supports balance in the erect position.
    3. The cane is moved forward only 4 to 6 inches because this distance keeps the cane within a tolerable distance from the client's center of gravity.

2. The affected leg is then moved an equal distance forward opposite to the cane. While the affected leg is being moved, the unaffected leg is bearing the weight of the body.
5. When weight is put on the affected leg, the cane shares the body's weight.
4. When the unaffected leg is moved forward, the affected leg and cane share the body's weight.
6. This sequence is repeated as the client moves forward.

Content Area: Mobility
Integrated Processes: Nursing Process: Planning
Client Need: Physiological Integrity; Basic Care and Comfort
Cognitive Level: Analysis
Concept: Mobility

13. **ANSWER: 2.**
    Rationales:
    1. Although encouraging the client to be as independent as possible should be done, it is not the first nursing action implemented by the nurse.
    2. Assessment is the first step of the nursing process. Before a client engages in range-of-motion exercises, the nurse should identify any factors that should be taken into consideration before teaching or providing range-of-motion exercises, such as the presence of contractures, pain, weakness, or impaired cognition.
    3. Although explaining what range-of-motion exercisers are and why they are being done should be implemented, it is not the first thing that the nurse should do.
    4. Although scheduling range-of-motion exercises during a bath may be arranged, it is not the first thing that the nurse should do.
    TEST-TAKING TIP: Identify the word in the stem that sets a priority. The word *first* in the stem sets a priority.
    Content Area: Mobility
    Integrated Processes: Nursing Process: Assessment
    Client Need: Physiological Integrity; Basic Care and Comfort
    Cognitive Level: Application
    Concept: Mobility

14. **ANSWER: 1.**
    Rationales:
    1. A blister over a bony prominence is a stage II pressure ulcer.
    2. A plantar wart is a painful growth caused by a virus; generally, it occurs on the sole of a foot, not over a bony prominence.
    3. Although a callus may be found over a bony prominence, it is hardened skin, not a blister-like lesion. It is similar to a corn but generally covers a larger surface area and clients report that they are not painful.
    4. Although a corn may be found over a bony prominence, it is a thickening of the skin caused by pressure or friction; usually it is due to ill-fitting shoes, and clients report that corns are painful.
    Content Area: Mobility
    Integrated Processes: Nursing Process: Analysis
    Client Need: Physiological Integrity; Basic Care and Comfort
    Cognitive Level: Analysis
    Concept: Tissue Integrity

15. ANSWER: 1, 4, 5.

Rationales:

1. The client's position should be changed every hour, not every 2 hours which generally is the rule, because the weight of the body impedes breathing and exerts pressure on the breasts and male genitalia.

2. Pillows should not be positioned under the thighs. This will result in lordosis, which puts stress on the vertebrae and muscles of the back. A pillow should be placed under the lower legs; this will keep the feet off the bed, minimizing planter flexion (extension of the ankle).

3. Pillows alongside the hips are unnecessary to maintain functional alignment in this position.

4. A small pillow should be positioned under the client's head to maintain the head in functional alignment. A large pillow under the head causes lateral flexion of the neck, which may cause stress and strain on the muscles of the neck and should be avoided.

5. A small pillow under the client's abdomen supports functional alignment because it prevents hyperextension of the lumbar curvature. In addition, it minimizes pressure on the genitalia of male clients and pressure on the breasts of female clients.

TEST-TAKING TIP: Identify the unique option. Option 1 is unique. It is the only option that does not contain the word *pillow*. Examine option 1 carefully.

Content Area: Mobility
Integrated Processes: Nursing Process: Implementation
Client Need: Physiological Integrity; Basic Care and Comfort
Cognitive Level: Application
Concept: Mobility

16. ANSWER: 1.

Rationales:

1. Lack of contraction of muscles that occurs with immobility results in a decrease in the size of muscles (atrophy). Muscle strength begins to decline within 48 hours of the initiation of bedrest or immobility.

2. Osteoporosis is the loss of bone mass and is associated with the skeletal system, not muscles. Immobility contributes to bone loss. Weight-bearing exercises, such as walking, are associated with bone buildup.

3. A pressure ulcer is a lesion caused by tissue compression when capillary occlusion pressure exceeds 15 to 32 mm Hg, causing tissue ischemia and eventual cell death. Pressure ulcers most often are associated with the skin (integumentary system).

4. Skin breakdown is associated with pressure ulcers and is associated with the skin (integumentary system).

TEST-TAKING TIP: Identify the options that are equally plausible. Options 3 and 4 are equally plausible. Pressure ulcers are examples of skin breakdown. Option 3 is no better than option 4. Eliminate both options from further consideration because they are distractors.

Content Area: Mobility
Integrated Processes: Nursing Process: Assessment
Client Need: Physiological Integrity; Basic Care and Comfort
Cognitive Level: Application
Concept: Mobility

17. ANSWER: 2.

Rationales:

1. The high-Fowler position does not put pressure on the right greater trochanter. It places pressure on the vertebrae, sacrum, pelvis (ischial tuberosities), and heels (calcaneus).

Vertebrae (spinal processes)

Sacrum   Pelvis (ischial tuberosity)   Heels (calcaneus)

2. The right side-lying position (right lateral position) places pressure on the right greater trochanter and should be avoided when a client has a pressure ulcer in this area. Additional pressure areas associated with the right side-lying position include the side of the head (parietal and temporal bones), ear, shoulder (acromial process), ilium, knee (medial and lateral condyles), and ankle (medial and lateral malleolus).

Ear   Ilium   Knee (medial and lateral condyles)

Side of head (parietal and temporal bones)   Shoulder (acromial process)   Greater trochanter   Malleolus (medial and lateral)

3. The supine position does not put pressure on the right greater trochanter. It places pressure on the back of the head (occipital bone), scapulae, elbows (olecranon process), sacrum, and heels (calcaneus).

Back of head (occipital bone)   Scapulae   Elbows (olecranon process)   Sacrum   Heels (calcaneus)

4. The prone position does not put pressure on the right greater trochanter. It places pressure on the cheek and ear (zygomatic bone), shoulder (acromion process), breasts in women, genitalia in men, and toes (phalanges).

Cheek and ear (zygomatic bone)   Shoulder (acromial process)   Breasts (women)   Genitalia (men)   Knees (patellas)   Toes (phalanges)

TEST-TAKING TIP: Identify the word in the stem that indicates negative polarity. The word *least* in the stem indicates negative polarity.
Content Area: Mobility
Integrated Processes: Nursing Process: Implementation
Client Need: Physiological Integrity; Basic Care and Comfort
Cognitive Level: Analysis
Concept: Mobility

18. **ANSWER: 1.**
Rationales:
1. **Placing the client in the prone position (lying face down on the abdomen) will prevent a hip flexion contracture because the mattress will push against and prevent the hip muscles from contracting. This position should be assumed twice a day for approximately 30 to 60 minutes as long as the client's respiratory status is adequate.**
2. The supine position will not fully prevent hip flexion contracture because there will be no force to resist hip muscle flexion.
3. The Fowler position may accelerate hip flexion contractures because the hips will be partially flexed and there will be no counterresistance to prevent contractures.
4. The lateral position will not prevent hip flexion contractures because it will not offer any counterresistance to natural muscle contraction.
Content Area: Mobility
Integrated Processes: Nursing Process: Implementation
Client Need: Physiological Integrity; Basic Care and Comfort
Cognitive Level: Application
Concept: Mobility

19. **ANSWER: 4, 2, 1, 6, 5, 3.**
Rationales:
4. **Informing the client about the procedure should be done first to decrease the client's anxiety and promote teamwork during the transfer.**
2. **Placing the wheelchair parallel to the client's bed minimizes the distance the client has to transfer and keeps it in the client's and nurse's line of vision.**
1. **Locking the brakes of the wheelchair prevents it from moving after it has been placed next to the client's bed.**
6. **Prior to transferring the client, the nurse should let the client sit on the side of the bed with shoes on and the feet on the floor. This decreases the risk of orthostatic hypotension when the client stands.**

5. **Bending the knees and placing arms under the client's axillae with the hands supporting the back allows the nurse to control the client's movement.**
3. **Standing up assists the client to an upright position and pivoting, rather than twisting, prevents injury to the client's and nurse's backs.**
Content Area: Mobility
Integrated Processes: Nursing Process: Planning
Client Need: Physiological Integrity; Basic Care and Comfort
Cognitive Level: Planning
Concept: Mobility

20. **ANSWER: 4.**
Rationales:
1. Although considering the principles of body mechanics is important, it is not the first thing that the nurse should do before moving a client.
2. Although selecting assistive devices to support the client's functional alignment is important, it is not the first thing that the nurse should do before moving a client.
3. Although identifying factors that may influence a client's activity, such as age, weight, pain level, presence of contractures, weakness, and mental status is important, it is not the first action by the nurse.
4. **Verifying the activity prescription is the first nursing action before moving a client. Maintaining a client's activity is a dependent nursing action and requires a prescription by the primary health-care provider.**
TEST-TAKING TIP: Identify the word in the stem that sets a priority. The word *first* in the stem sets a priority. Identify the options with specific determiners. The word *all* in options 1 and 3 are specific determiners. Rarely is an option with a specific determiner the correct answer. Delete options 1 and 3 from further consideration.
Content Area: Mobility
Integrated Processes: Nursing Process: Implementation
Client Need: Safe and Effective Care Environment; Safety and Infection Control
Cognitive Level: Application
Concept: Mobility

21. **ANSWER: 1, 3.**
Rationales:
1. **Bicycle riding is an aerobic activity that increases the heart rate and promotes increased use of oxygen to improve overall body functioning.**
2. Tensing and relaxing muscles is an example of isometric, not aerobic, exercise. It requires muscle tension with no change in muscle length or movement.
3. Using a machine for resistance while moving a joint is an example of isokinetic, not aerobic, exercise.
3. **Jogging is an example of aerobic exercise. It is an intense exercise that metabolizes oxygen to support energy.**
4. Walking at a gentle, steady pace is an example of isotonic, not aerobic, exercise. It involves shortening and lengthening of muscles to produce movement. When done gently at a steady pace, it does not fall into the realm of aerobic exercise.

Content Area: Mobility
Integrated Processes: Teaching/Learning; Nursing Process: Implementation
Client Need: Physiological Integrity; Basic Care and Comfort
Cognitive Level: Analysis
Concept: Patient-Centered Care; Mobility

22. **ANSWER: 4, 5.**
    Rationales:
    1. A wound obscured with sloughing tissue describes an unstageable pressure ulcer, not a stage IV pressure ulcer. An unstageable pressure ulcer involves full-thickness skin loss with the base obscured by necrotic tissue. Slough is necrotic tissue that is tan, yellow, green, gray, or brown in color.
    2. Soft, boggy tissue over a bony prominence indicates a stage I, not stage IV, pressure ulcer.
    3. A deep crater with an intact fascia indicates a stage III, not stage IV, pressure ulcer. Stage III ulcers extend down to, but not through, the fascia. Undermining and exudate may be present.
    4. Tunneling under the epidermis (sinus tract) occurs because of the deep tissue injury and is associated with a stage IV pressure ulcer.
    5. Full-thickness skin loss describes a stage IV pressure ulcer. The pressure ulcer may also have tunneling, undermining, and necrotic tissue that is tan, yellow, green, gray, or brown that does not obscure the wound bed. In addition, a stage IV pressure ulcer may have eschar (tan, black, or brown leathery necrotic tissue) that does not obscure the wound bed.
    Content Area: Mobility
    Integrated Processes: Nursing Process: Analysis
    Client Need: Physiological Integrity; Basic Care and Comfort
    Cognitive Level: Analysis
    Concept: Tissue Integrity

23. **ANSWER: 2, 4.**
    Rationales:
    1. One pillow is sufficient to maintain functional alignment of the head and neck. Two pillows will cause unnecessary flexion of the head, which should be avoided.
    2. Raising the head of the bed between 16 to 45 degrees is associated with the semi-Fowler position.
    3. Hand rolls are used to prevent flexion contractures of the hands, not to provide support of a client in the semi-Fowler position.
    4. Foam boots or foot/ankle splints support dorsiflexion, which helps prevent footdrop (planter flexion).
    5. Trochanter rolls generally are used to prevent external rotation of the hips when the client is in the supine position. Trochanter rolls are positioned alongside the hips to the knees, not the knees to the ankles.
    Content Area: Mobility
    Integrated Processes: Nursing Process: Implementation
    Client Need: Physiological Integrity; Basic Care and Comfort
    Cognitive Level: Application
    Concept: Mobility

24. **ANSWER: 2.**
    Rationales:
    1. When a client needs assistance to complete these exercises, it is called active-assistive range-of-motion exercises, not active range-of-motion exercises.
    2. Active range-of-motion exercises require the client to complete the exercises independently. Active range-of-motion exercises require muscle contraction that eventually improves muscle strength.
    3. Although a warm bath may relax the client, reducing stiffness, it is not a required or unique action associated with implementing range-of-motion exercises.
    4. Demonstrating how to do the exercises is not unique to instituting active range-of-motion exercises. Explaining what is to be done and why should be implemented before providing all nursing care.
    TEST-TAKING TIP: Identify the option that contains a specific determiner. Option 1 contains the word *all* which is a specific determiner. Identify the options that are opposites. Options 1 and 2 are opposites. Option 1 has the nurse assisting the client and option 2 encourages the client to perform the exercises independently. Examine option 1 and 2 carefully. More often than not, an option that is an opposite is the correct answer.
    Content Area: Mobility
    Integrated Processes: Teaching/Learning; Nursing Process: Implementation
    Client Need: Physiological Integrity; Basic Care and Comfort
    Cognitive Level: Application
    Concept: Mobility

25. **ANSWER: 3, 5.**
    Rationales:
    1. Objects should be held close to the body when lifting or carrying an object. The closer the object is to the center of gravity, the more stable the body and less strain on the muscles of the back.
    2. Elbows should be flexed when lifting objects; elbows act as fulcrums (the point on which a lever moves).
    3. Squatting uses the stronger muscles of the legs to provide the power when lifting an object, rather than the smaller and weaker muscles of the arms and back. This decreases strain on the weaker muscles.
    4. Feet should be spread wide apart when lifting an object. This provides a wide base of support. The wider the base of support, the more stable the object or person.
    5. Putting weight on the balls of the feet, one foot ahead of the other, when pivoting reduces frictional surface with the floor and knees are not twisted when turning.
    Content Area: Mobility
    Integrated Processes: Nursing Process: Implementation
    Client Need: Physiological Integrity; Basic Care and Comfort
    Cognitive Level: Application
    Concept: Mobility

26. **ANSWER: 1, 3, 4, 5.**
    Rationales:
    1. There is no pressure on the right trochanter when the client is positioned in the semi-Fowler position.
    2. The right lateral position should be avoided because it places direct body pressure on the right trochanter.
    3. There is no pressure on the right trochanter when the client is positioned in the left Sims' position.
    4. There is no pressure on the right trochanter when the client is positioned in the supine position.
    5. There is no pressure on the right trochanter when the client is positioned in the prone position.
    Content Area: Mobility
    Integrated Processes: Nursing Process: Implementation
    Client Need: Physiological Integrity; Basic Care and Comfort
    Cognitive Level: Application
    Concept: Mobility

27. **ANSWER: 4.**
    Rationales:
    1. A faint pedal pulse indicates impaired circulation to the foot. Although this is serious, another clinical indicator is life threatening and takes priority.
    2. Although edema of the calf indicates the presence of a thrombus in a vein in the calf, it is a localized problem that has not yet become life threatening. Another option is more serious because it is a clinical indicator of a life-threatening event.
    3. Although pain in the lower leg may indicate the presence of a thrombus in a vein in the calf, it is a localized problem that has not yet become life threatening. Another option is more serious because it is a clinical indicator of a life-threatening event.
    4. Unilateral chest pain that occurs in the presence of a thrombophlebitis indicates that a part of the thrombus has become an embolus that has lodged in the lung. When this occurs, it has the potential to be life threatening.
    TEST-TAKING TIP: Identify the word in the stem that sets a priority. The word *most* in the stem sets a priority. Identify the option that is unique. Options 1, 2, and 3 all refer to a lower extremity. Option 4 is unique because it relates to the chest.
    Content Area: Mobility
    Integrated Processes: Nursing Process: Assessment
    Client Need: Safe and Effective Care Environment; Reduction of Risk Potential
    Cognitive Level: Application
    Concept: Perfusion

28. **ANSWER: 3.**
    Rationales:
    1. Each movement should be implemented slowly, smoothly, and rhythmically. This minimizes undue stress and strain on the structures of the joint and adjoining muscles.
    2. With passive range-of-motion exercises, the caregiver moves the client's joints through their full range to the point of resistance without active participation on the part of the client.

    3. Supporting above and below the joint being moved is most important because it prevents undue stress, strain, or injury to the muscles, joints, and ligaments that can occur when a joint is unsupported.
    4. Three to five repetitions twice a day is sufficient to maintain full range of motion. Twelve repetitions twice a day are unnecessary.
    TEST-TAKING TIP: Identify the option with a specific determiner. Option 2 contains the word *all* which is a specific determiner. Identify the options that contain a clang association. The stem contains the word *exercises* and options 1 and 3 contain the words *exercises* and *exercised*, respectively. Consider options 1 and 3 carefully because they each contain a clang association.
    Content Area: Mobility
    Integrated Processes: Nursing Process: Implementation
    Client Need: Physiological Integrity; Basic Care and Comfort
    Cognitive Level: Application
    Concept: Mobility

29. **ANSWER: 2.**
    Rationales:
    1. The client can remain in the Sims' position for 2 hours unless circumstances require more frequent repositioning.
    2. Because respiratory exertion is reduced in the prone position due to the pressure of body weight on the chest and because of pressure on the breasts in women and genitalia in men, clients should be repositioned after 1 hour.
    3. The client can remain in the lateral position for 2 hours, unless circumstances require more frequent repositioning.
    4. The client can remain in the orthopneic position for 2 hours, unless circumstances require more frequent repositioning.
    Content Area: Mobility
    Integrated Processes: Nursing Process: Implementation
    Client Need: Physiological Integrity; Basic Care and Comfort
    Cognitive Level: Application
    Concept: Mobility

30. **ANSWER: 3, 5.**
    Rationales:
    1. Assessing a client for clinical indicators of a hypostatic pneumonia does not lower the risk of hypostatic pneumonia. It only reflects the presence of adventitious breath sounds.
    2. The client has a prescription for bedrest. The client should not be sitting in a chair for meals.
    3. Inactivity allows secretions to pool by gravity, thereby providing an excellent media for the growth of microorganisms. Moving the client from side to side every 2 hours helps to mobilize secretions, better enabling the client to cough up and expel secretions.
    4. Sequential compression devices will not reduce the risk of hypostatic pneumonia; they increase peripheral venous return in the legs.
    5. An incentive spirometer helps the client increase the depth of inhalations, which aerates the lower lobes of the lung; also, it facilitates movement of secretions into

upper areas of the lungs whereby coughing may enable expectoration of the secretions. Aeration of the lower lobes of the lungs and expectoration of secretions help reduce stasis of secretions, which can precipitate hypostatic pneumonia.
Content Area: Mobility
Integrated Processes: Nursing Process: Assessment
Client Need: Safe and Effective Care Environment; Reduction of Risk Potential
Cognitive Level: Application
Concept: Oxygenation

31. **ANSWER: 4.**
Rationales:
1. Although a protective skin ointment should be applied to the perineal area, it is not the priority.
2. The client should drink 2 to 3 L of fluid daily to flush the urinary system of invading pathogens; however, it is not the priority.
3. Although the client's vital signs should be monitored every 4 hours because the client has a urinary tract infection, it is not the priority.
4. A urinary tract infection is a complication associated with urinary stasis as a result of impaired mobility. Administering the antibiotic is the priority as long as the urine specimen has been collected and sent to the laboratory; this is the case in this situation because the laboratory section of the medical record indicates results of a urinalysis and urine culture.
TEST-TAKING TIP: Identify the word in the stem that sets a priority. The word *first* in the stem sets a priority.
Content Area: Mobility
Integrated Processes: Communication and Documentation; Nursing Process: Implementation
Client Need: Safe and Effective Care Environment; Management of Care
Cognitive Level: Analysis
Concept: Patient-Centered Care; Medication

32. **ANSWER: 3, 5.**
Rationales:
1. A rolling motion in which the opposite hip drops when taking a stride is a waddling gait associated with developmental dysphagia of the hip or due to the enlarged abdomen associated with pregnancy.
2. Exaggerated lifting of the leg to avoid dragging the toes is a steppage gait. It is associated with footdrop and Guillain-Barré syndrome.
3. Involuntary acceleration is a component of the propulsive cogwheel gait associated with Parkinson's disease.
4. Stiff, foot dragging when ambulating is a spastic gait. It is associated with cerebral palsy.
5. Small shuffling steps are a component of the propulsive cogwheel gait associated with Parkinson's disease.
TEST-TAKING TIP: Identify the option with a clang association. The word *walking* in the stem and in option 3 is a clang association.
Content Area: Mobility
Integrated Processes: Nursing Process: Analysis

Client Need: Physiological Integrity; Basic Care and Comfort
Cognitive Level: Comprehension
Concept: Mobility

33. **ANSWER: 1.**
Rationales:
1. Elevating the left leg on a pillow is an independent function of the nurse and does not require a prescription from the primary health-care provider. This action uses the principle of gravity to facilitate venous return and reduce edema in interstitial tissue.
2. Applying heat is a dependent function of the nurse and cannot be implemented without a prescription from the primary health-care provider. If prescribed, the nurse can apply a warm soak to the area. This action causes vasodilation, which increases blood flow to the area.
3. Massaging the legs is contraindicated because it can cause a thrombosis to become an embolus, which can travel to a lung, causing a life-threatening situation.
4. Applying a venous compression device to the left leg is contraindicated. This may cause a thrombosis to become an embolus, which can travel to a lung. This is a life-threatening event. In addition, applying venous compression devices requires a prescription by a primary health-care provider; it is a dependent function of the nurse.
TEST-TAKING TIP: Identify options with a clang association. The words *left leg* in the stem and in options 1 and 2 are clang associations. Examine options 1 and 2 carefully. More often than not, an option with a clang association is the correct answer. Identify equally plausible options. Options 3 and 4 are equally plausible. They both apply external pressure to the legs. Option 3 is no better than option 4. Eliminate options 3 and 4 from further consideration.
Content Area: Mobility
Integrated Processes: Nursing Process: Implementation
Client Need: Physiological Integrity; Physiological Adaptation
Cognitive Level: Application
Concept: Perfusion

34. **ANSWER: 1.**
Rationales:
1. Range-of-motion exercises minimize the formation of contractures. Putting joints through their full range several times daily averts shortening of muscles, which causes contractures.
2. The main purpose of repositioning a client is to prevent tissue ischemia over bony prominences, which causes pressure ulcers, not to prevent contractures. Also, repositioning can minimize stasis of respiratory secretions, thereby reducing the risk of hypostatic pneumonia.
3. The use of a tilt table will not prevent contractures. A tilt table is used to place weight on the long bones of the body, helping to reduce bone demineralization. Also, it is used to help the body adapt to changes in circulation when moved from a lying to a standing position.
4. Coughing and deep breathing will not prevent contractures associated with right-sided hemiparesis. Coughing and deep breathing helps to mobilize respiratory secretions, thereby reducing the risk of hypostatic pneumonia.

TEST-TAKING TIP: Identify the word in the stem that sets a priority. The word *most* in the stem sets a priority.
Content Area: Mobility
Integrated Processes: Nursing Process: Implementation
Client Need: Physiological Integrity; Basic Care and Comfort
Cognitive Level: Application
Concept: Mobility

35. **ANSWER: 2, 5.**
Rationales:
1. Although massaging around bony prominences every 2 hours increases circulation in an effort to minimize the risk of a pressure ulcer, it does not prevent shearing.
2. A transfer board helps to prevent shearing forces when moving a client from a bed to a stretcher. Shearing occurs when the epidermal layer slides over the dermis, causing injury to the vascular bed; in addition, when shearing occurs, it reduces the amount of pressure needed to occlude vessels by half. In addition, shearing often occurs when a client slides down in bed when the head of the bed is elevated higher than the low-Fowler position and when a client is dragged across the surface of a mattress when being moved up in bed without the use of a pull sheet.
3. An air mattress helps to distribute body weight over a larger surface area, thereby minimizing the risk of tissue ischemia due to pressure; it does not prevent shearing.
4. A low-Fowler, not semi-Fowler, position reduces the risk of shearing forces. Shearing forces occur when the epidermal layer slides over the dermis, causing injury to the vascular bed. Shearing forces occur when the head of a client's bed is elevated to a semi- or high-Fowler position and the client slides lower in the bed in response to gravity.
5. A pull sheet helps to prevent shearing forces when moving a client up in bed. Shearing occurs when the epidermal layer slides over the dermis, causing injury to the vascular bed. When a pull sheet is used, the sliding of the epidermal layer over the dermis does not occur.
Content Area: Mobility
Integrated Processes: Nursing Process: Implementation
Client Need: Safe and Effective Care Environment; Reduction of Risk Potential
Cognitive Level: Application
Concept: Tissue Integrity

36. **ANSWER: 4.**
Rationale:
Solve the problem by using the formula for ratio and proportion.

$$\frac{\text{Desire 50 mg}}{\text{Have 12.5 mg}} \times \frac{x \text{ capsules}}{1 \text{ capsule}}$$
$$12.5x = 50 \times 1$$
$$12.5x = 50$$
$$x = 50 \div 12.5$$
$$x = 4 \text{ capsules}$$

Content Area: Mobility
Integrated Processes: Nursing Process: Planning

Client Need: Physiological Integrity; Pharmacological and Parenteral Therapies
Cognitive Level: Application
Concept: Medication; Fluid and Electrolyte Balance

37. **ANSWER: 4.**
Rationales:
1. An incentive spirometer helps minimize the risk of stasis of respiratory secretions, not orthostatic hypotension.
2. The nurse should never massage a client's legs because doing so could cause a thrombus to become an embolus, which could cause a pulmonary embolus or other life-threatening vascular occlusion.
3. Avoiding the Valsalva maneuver (exhalation pressed forcibly against a closed glottis) causes a surge of blood to enter the heart, which can cause tachycardia and cardiac arrest, not orthostatic hypotension.
4. When moving from a sitting and then to a standing position after being on bedrest, venous blood pools in the lower extremities because of a decrease in the vasopressor mechanism (muscle contraction causing pressure on veins promotes venous return). Having a client sit for a minute after raising the head of the bed and then having the client sit on the side of the bed with the legs resting on the floor (dangle) for a minute allows time for the blood pressure to equalize, which minimizes the risk of orthostatic hypotension and a fall.
Content Area: Mobility
Integrated Processes: Nursing Process: Implementation
Client Need: Physiological Integrity; Basic Care and Comfort
Cognitive Level: Application
Concept: Perfusion

38. **ANSWER: 2, 3.**
Rationales:
1. Trochanter rolls are used to prevent external rotation of the hips when a client is in the supine, not orthopneic, position.
2. Positioning an overbed table with a pillow on it provides a comfortable surface upon which the client can rest when sitting upright to breathe.
3. This is the correct position of the head of the bed when that client is in the orthopneic position. Once in the high-Fowler position, a pillow should be placed behind the client to maintain the client in a forward leaning position. The orthopneic position allows gravity to move abdominal organs downward away from the thoracic cavity permitting fuller lung expansion.
4. Lifting both legs into the stirrups at the same time is associated with the lithotomy, not orthopneic, position.
5. This client is on bedrest and should not be standing.
Content Area: Mobility
Integrated Processes: Nursing Process: Implementation
Client Need: Physiological Integrity; Basic Care and Comfort
Cognitive Level: Application
Concept: Oxygenation

39. ANSWER: 4.

Rationales:

1. Straining urine if calculi are suspected will not prevent them from forming.

2. Although pouring warm water over the symphysis pubis may be implemented to stimulate voiding, there is no information in the question that indicates that the client is having difficulty voiding. This will not reduce the risk of complications associated with urinary stasis.

3. Although a sitting position for women and a standing position for men will facilitate voiding, it is not as effective as another option to prevent complications associated with urinary stasis.

4. An increase in fluid intake will help to flush the urinary system of pathogens that invade the urinary tract via the urethra.

Content Area: Mobility
Integrated Processes: Nursing Process: Implementation
Client Need: Health Promotion and Maintenance
Cognitive Level: Application
Concept: Elimination

40. ANSWER: 2, 4, 5.

Rationales:

1. Synthetic sheepskin is not designed to absorb urine; wet sheepskin will contribute to skin breakdown.

2. Soft tuffs of synthetic sheepskin reduce friction under the client.

3. Synthetic sheepskin helps to keep skin cool, not warm, by allowing air to circulate through the tuffs of synthetic sheepskin.

4. The tuffs in synthetic sheepskin distribute weight more evenly so that body weight is not concentrated in one area predisposing the client to skin breakdown.

5. Synthetic sheepskin allows air to circulate through the tuffs of synthetic sheepskin which prevents accumulation of moisture.

Content Area: Mobility
Integrated Processes: Nursing Process: Analysis
Client Need: Physiological Integrity; Basic Care and Comfort
Cognitive Level: Comprehension
Concept: Tissue Integrity

Chapter 18

Tissue Integrity and Hygiene

NURSING CONCEPTS

Culture
Growth and Development
Inflammation
Nutrition
Patient-Centered Care

Perfusion
Safety
Sensory Perception
Tissue Integrity

KEY TERMS

Cyanosis—Bluish-gray color of the skin

Ecchymosis—Blue-purple area that progresses to green-yellow caused by shallow bleeding under the skin or mucous membrane

Erythema—Redness of the skin due to congestion of the capillaries

Flushed—Redness of the skin due to dilated capillaries

Jaundice—Yellow-orange cast to the skin, mucous membranes, and sclerae caused by deposition of bile salts

Keloid—Raised, irregular scar due to excess collagen formation (hypertrophic scar)

Pallor—Decrease in skin color or ashen gray appearance in dark-skinned people

Petechiae—Small, red-purple spots caused by intradermal or submucosal hemorrhaging

Prepuce (foreskin)—Loose skin covering the end of the penis

Scar—Formation of replacement connective tissue and fibrotic changes following healing of a wound

Shearing force—When gravity pulls down on deep body structures and frictional resistance occurs between the skin and a firm surface

Smegma—Thick, cheesy, odoriferous secretion from sebaceous glands found under the labia minor and around the clitoris in the female and under the foreskin in the male

Sordes—Collection of bacteria, debris, and thick, sticky secretions on the tongue, teeth, and lips

Ulcer—Irregularly shaped loss of skin, extending into or through the dermis

I. Integumentary System

The integumentary system is the largest organ in the body. It includes not only the skin but mucous membranes, hair, and nails. Nurses must know the anatomy and functions of the components of the integumentary system to provide knowledgeable nursing care to clients.

A. Structures of the integumentary system
  1. Epidermis (outer layer).
     a. In addition to skin, includes mucous membranes and lips.

b. Contains melanocytes that produce melanin, which gives skin its color.

2. Dermis.
   a. Consists of vascular fabric of collagen and elastic fibers that produce flexibility and strength.
   b. Contains touch receptors.

3. Glands.
   a. *Eccrine:* Sweat glands; secrete clear fluid through pores.
   b. *Apocrine:* Scent glands; found in axillary, mammary, and genital areas.
   c. *Sebaceous:* Sebum-secreting gland at base of hairs and open into upper portion of hair follicles.
   d. *Mammary:* Milk-secreting glands; discharges milk through nipples during lactation.

4. Mucous membranes.
   a. Lining of passages and cavities opening directly to the exterior of the body (e.g., oral cavity, rectum, nose, urethra, gastrointestinal tract).
   b. Consist of epithelial surface layer, basement membrane, and underlying layer of connective tissue.
   c. Secrete mucus, a thick, slippery material that keeps the membranes moist and protected.
   d. Condition of the mucous membranes is influenced by changes in oxygenation, circulation, nutrition, and hydration.

5. Hair.
   a. Keratinized, threadlike outgrowth from epidermal structures called follicles.
   b. Routinely shed and replaced; replacement may not keep pace of hair loss due to genetic predisposition, alopecia, radiation, chemotherapy.
   c. Distribution affected by gender, genetics, and age.

6. Nails.
   a. Hardened, horny cutaneous plates overlying the dorsal surface of the ends of fingers and toes.
   b. Consist of nail body, root, cuticle, and nailbed; grows about 0.5 mm a week; fingernails faster than toenails; growth faster in summer than winter.
   c. Contain abundant blood vessels and appear pink and translucent; easily monitored for signs of cyanosis.
   d. Condition influenced by local problems, systemic problems, and aging.

B. Functions of the integumentary system
   1. Largest organ of the body, the condition of which reflects the effects of the body's metabolism and nutritional status.
   2. Protects the body.
      a. Acts as a barrier between the internal and external environments.
      b. Prevents injury to underlying structures; nails protect distal appendages from mechanical injury.
      c. Provides protection from microorganisms; "acid mantle" (pH between 4 and 5.5).
      d. Cilia in nostrils filter and warm air entering the nasal cavities.
      e. Eyelashes and eyebrows keep sweat and debris out of eyes.
   3. Regulates body temperature.
      a. Dilates blood vessels and activates sweat glands to cool the body via processes of perspiration, evaporation, conduction, and radiation.
      b. Constricts blood vessels and inactivates sweat glands to conserve heat.
      c. Hair on head, arms, legs, and torso provides thermal insulation.
   4. Receives sensations of heat, cold, touch, pressure, and pain via nerve receptors.
   5. Produces vitamin D when skin is exposed to ultraviolet light from the sun.
   6. Secretes sebum from sebaceous glands, which lubricates skin and hair; reduces heat loss from skin because of its oily nature; and reduces bacterial growth.
   7. Excretes water, sodium chloride, and nitrogenous waste via perspiration.

II. Assessment of the Integumentary System

When assessing the integumentary system, the nurse should know the normal and abnormal characteristics of skin, such as variations in color, temperature, moisture, texture, and presence of lesions that impair skin integrity. In addition, the nurse should know the normal and abnormal characteristics of the mucous membranes, hair, and nails, which are components of the integumentary system. This foundation of knowledge is necessary before the nurse can implement a comprehensive assessment, identify problems, and plan and implement nursing interventions associated with the integumentary system.

A. Principles of assessment of the skin
   1. Obtain the client's permission for assessment because it invades the client's personal space.
   2. Ensure adequate lighting and that the color of curtains and wall paint does not influence assessments.
   3. Use inspection before palpation; rub hands to warm them before placing them on the client's skin.
   4. Consider the mucous membranes, hair, and nails as extensions of the skin.

B. Assessment of skin color
   1. Recognize that skin color varies according to age and race and that exposed areas are darker than

unexposed areas; palms of the hands, soles of the feet, and nailbeds are the lightest areas.

2. Note variations in skin color.
   a. **Cyanosis:** Bluish-gray color of the skin; may appear ashen gray in dark-skinned people; more obvious in the conjunctivae, tongue, buccal mucosa, palms of the hands, and soles of the feet; associated with hypoxia or exposure to extreme cold.
   b. **Ecchymosis:** Blue-purple area larger than petechiae that progresses to green-yellow; commonly called a bruise; due to shallow bleeding under the skin or mucous membrane; associated with blunt trauma.
   c. **Erythema:** Redness of the skin due to congestion of the capillaries; associated with inflammation, vasodilation, prolonged pressure, and application of heat or cold.
   d. **Flushed:** Redness of the skin due to dilated capillaries; most commonly associated with increased body temperature.
   e. **Jaundice:** Yellow-orange cast to the skin caused by deposition of bile salts; most obvious in sclerae of the eyes, mucous membranes, palms of the hands, and soles of the feet; associated with liver or biliary impairment.
   f. **Pallor:** Pale skin or ashen gray appearance in dark-skinned people; more obvious in oral mucous membranes, conjunctivae, nailbeds, palms of the hands, and soles of the feet; associated with anemia and malnutrition.
   g. **Petechiae:** Small, red-purple spots caused by intradermal or submucosal hemorrhaging; associated with thrombocytopenia and some febrile illnesses.

C. Assessment of skin temperature
   1. Use the back of the hand or fingers to assess skin temperature (see Fig. 14.8 in Chapter 14, Physical Assessment); skin should feel warm to touch.
   2. Assess extremities bilaterally and compare for symmetry.
   3. Assess a client with excessively warm skin further because this finding may indicate a fever; obtain body temperature to verify.
   4. Assess a client with excessively cool skin further because it may indicate conditions such as impaired circulation, shock, or hypothyroidism.

D. Assessment of skin moisture
   1. Use inspection and palpation; skin usually is warm and dry.
   2. Assess a client with excessively moist skin *(profuse diaphoresis)* further because this finding may indicate conditions such as hyperthermia, anxiety, exposure to hot environment, or hyperthyroidism.

3. Assess a client with excessively dry skin further because this finding may indicate conditions such as dehydration, excessive exposure to the sun, overzealous bathing, or hypothyroidism.
4. Assess a client with oily skin further because this finding may be due to excessive sebaceous gland secretion or sebaceous gland inflammation *(acne)*, commonly associated with adolescence.
5. Assess skin turgor to determine elasticity of the skin, which reflects hydration status; pinch skin on anterior chest below the clavicle, sternum, forehead, or inner thigh and note how long it takes to return to its original position (see Fig. 21.7 in Chapter 21, Fluids, Electrolyte, and Acid-Base Balance).
   a. Prolonged tenting (longer than 2 to 3 seconds) is associated with dehydration and aging.
   b. Resistance to pinching is associated with edema; client may report that the skin "feels tight" or that rings and shoes do not fit.

E. Assessment of skin texture
   1. Recognize that skin texture varies according to age and the area being assessed.
      a. Exposed areas and elbows and knees tend to be drier and coarser than unexposed areas.
      b. Skin of infants and children is softer and smoother than that of adults because of lack of exposure to the environment and extent of hydration of tissues.
   2. Identify changes in skin texture related to impaired circulation to the lower extremities.
      a. Peripheral arterial insufficiency is associated with pale-colored skin when the legs are elevated and reddish-blue colored skin when dependent. Additional clinical manifestations include dry, scaling skin; yellowed, brittle nails; loss of hair; ulcerations near the toes; and pain with activity *(intermittent claudication)*.
      b. Peripheral venous insufficiency is associated with thick, rough skin that frequently is hyperpigmented; edematous; superficial vein dilation; and ulcerations around the ankle. Red blood cells exit ruptured vessels and then degenerate, leaving a brownish discoloration of the tissues.

F. Assessment of skin lesions
   1. Use standard precautions when assessing skin lesions.
      a. Wash hands before and after.
      b. Wear gloves.
   2. Identify the type of lesion.
      a. Primary lesions occur in response to a change in the internal or external environment of the skin due to a disease process (Table 18.1).
      b. Secondary lesions occur as a result of changes in a primary lesion due to trauma, scratching, or infection (Table 18.2).

Table 18.1 **Primary Skin Lesions**

Type of Lesion	Depiction of Lesion	
Bulla • *Elevated, fluid-filled vesicle more than 1 cm in size (A)* • *Examples include blister (B), deep partial-thickness burn, and contact dermatitis*	A	B
Cyst • *Mass of fluid-filled tissue that extends to the subcutaneous tissues or dermis and is more than 1 cm in size (A)* • *Examples include epidermoid cysts (B) and sebaceous cyst*	A	B
Macule • *Flat, circumscribed area from 1 to several centimeters in size (A)* • *Examples include cherry angioma (B); freckles; flat, pigmented moles; and measles*	A	B
Nodule • *Raised solid mass that extends into the dermis and is 1 to 2 cm in size (A)* • *Examples include pigmented nevus (B) and fibroma*	A	B
Papule • *Raised, circumscribed area less than 1 cm in size due to superficial thickening in the epidermis (A)* • *Examples include raised mole (B), ringworm, and wart*	A	B
Pustule • *Vesicle or bulla filled with pus that is more than 1 cm in size (A)* • *Examples include acne vulgaris (B) and impetigo*	A	B

Table 18.1	**Primary Skin Lesions—cont'd**

Type of Lesion	Depiction of Lesion
Vesicle • *Raised collection of fluid less than 1 cm in size (A)* • *Examples include herpes simplex (B), chickenpox, and poison ivy*	
Wheal • *Round, raised superficial collection of fluid due to dermal edema and surrounding capillary dilation, extending 1 mm to several cm in size (A)* • *Examples include hives, also known as urticaria (B), and mosquito bites*	

Figures from Dillon (2007). *Nursing health assessment,* 2nd ed. Philadelphia: F. A. Davis Company, with permission.

Table 18.2	**Secondary Skin Lesions**

Type of Lesions	Depiction of Lesion
Crust • *Dried residue from serum, blood, or pus (A)* • *Examples include dried herpes simplex (B) and impetigo*	
Erosion • *Nonbleeding loss of superficial epidermis (A)* • *Examples include candidiasis (B) and chickenpox rupture*	
Fissure • *Linear crack in the skin (A)* • *Examples include cheilitis (B) and athlete's foot*	

Continued

Table 18.2 Secondary Skin Lesions—cont'd	
Type of Lesions	**Depiction of Lesion**
Keloid • *Raised, irregular scar due to excess collagen formation (hypertrophic scar) (A)* • *Examples of common sites include surgical incisions (B), ear piercings, and tattoos*	
Scale • *Exfoliation (shedding) of dead skin cells. May be dry or oily, loose or adherent, and vary in color (A)* • *Examples include psoriasis (B) and dandruff*	
Scar • *Formation of replacement connective tissue and fibrotic changes following healing of a wound (A)* • *Examples of common sites include surgical incisions (B) and cuts*	
Ulcer • *Irregularly shaped loss of skin, extending into or through the dermis* • *Surface may bleed, may become necrotic (A)* • *Examples include stasis ulcer (B) and pressure ulcer*	

Figures not supplied by the authors are from Dillon (2016). *Nursing health assessment,* 3rd ed. Philadelphia: F. A. Davis Company, with permission.

3. Identify the size and shape of the lesion.
    a. Note size in millimeters.
    b. Identify whether the lesion is circumscribed or diffuse, round or oval.
    c. Identify the depth of the lesion.
4. Identify the texture of the lesion: Depressed, flat, or elevated; hard, solid, or soft; rough or thickened; fluid filled or flakey.
5. Identify the presence and characteristics (e.g., color, odor) of exudate.
6. Identify the color of lesion: May have no color, one discrete color, or several colors; color may be red, brown, black, blue, purple, or yellow.
7. Identify the distribution of lesions: Document the location of the lesion(s); symmetry or asymmetry of lesions.
8. Identify the pattern (configuration) of lesions: Arrangement of lesions in relation to each other, such as circular, linear, clustered, arcing, merged together, or following the course of cutaneous nerves.

G. Assessment of mucous membranes

1. Inspect oral cavity, rectum, nares, and urinary meatus; mucous membranes should be pink, moist, and intact.
2. Assess the mouth and oropharynx via inspection.
   a. Lips.
      (1) Should be pink or color of the person's skin, smooth, moist, intact, and free from lesions.
      (2) Deviations include dryness, fissures, pallor, cyanosis, involuntary movement, and drooping.
   b. Inner surface of mouth, buccal mucosa, roof of mouth, and floor of mouth.
      (1) Same assessment results as lips.
      (2) Deviations include inflammation of the oral mucosa *(stomatitis)*.
   c. Tongue.
      (1) Should be shiny, pink, and moist, with an even distribution of papillae organized in an inverted "V."
      (2) Deviations include dryness, fissures, or inflammation of the tongue *(glossitis)*.
   d. Uvula and tonsils.
      (1) Uvula should be in midline and rise when client says "ah."
      (2) Tonsils should be pink, smooth, with no discharge and should be behind the tonsillar pillars; deviations include inflammation of the tonsils *(tonsillitis)*.
   e. Teeth and gums.
      (1) Teeth should be free from tartar, hardened deposits of debris from bacteria, saliva, epithelial cells, and leukocytes *(plaque)*.
      (2) Gums should be pink, moist, and firm; deviations include receding from teeth and swollen, inflamed gums *(gingivitis)*.

H. Assessment of hair

1. Color of hair.
   a. Black, brown, blond, red, gray, or white.
   b. Loss of pigment as one ages results in gray or white hair.
2. Quantity of hair.
   a. Thick, thin, sparse; none *(alopecia)*; abnormal hairiness *(hirsutism)*.
   b. Amount of hair may decrease on the lower extremities, pubic and axillary areas, and head as one ages, as the result of chemotherapy, or because of thyroid disease.
3. Distribution of hair.
   a. Symmetrical; hair in expected or unexpected areas; multiple bald spots; male pattern baldness.
   b. Male pattern of hair distribution in women is associated with endocrine disorders and steroid medications; lack of hair on distal extremities may indicate inadequate peripheral circulation.
4. Texture of hair.
   a. Coarse or fine; straight, wavy, or curly; oily or dry.
   b. Dry hair is associated with malnutrition, aging, and hypothyroidism; fine, silky hair is associated with hyperthyroidism; hair return after chemotherapy may have a different color and/or texture.
5. General condition of hair: Clean and combed; dirty, unkempt, and matted.
6. Condition of scalp: Should be shiny, smooth, mobile, and nontender.
7. Presence of infection or infestations.
   a. Wash hands before and after wearing clean gloves.
   b. Systematically part hair in multiple sections, particularly behind the ears and at the nape of the neck, to assess for sores, lice eggs *(nits)*, ringworm *(tinea capitis)*, dry flakes *(dandruff)*, or oily scales *(seborrhea)*.

I. Assessment of nails

1. Color of nails.
   a. Usually pink or light brown.
   b. Yellow nails are related to cigarette smoking, fungal infections, or psoriasis.
   c. Blue nails are related to peripheral disease or hypoxia.
   d. White nails are related to trauma and liver or renal disease.
   e. Black nails are related to trauma; color due to accumulation of blood under the nail.
2. Shape and nail plate angle.
   a. Convex curve expected with an angle of 160 degrees between the fingernail and nailbed (Fig. 18.1A).
   b. Angle equal to or greater than 180 degrees *(clubbing)* is related to long-term lack of oxygen (Fig. 18.1B).
   c. Spoon-shaped nail is related to iron-deficiency anemia.
3. Texture of nails.
   a. Smooth surface expected.
   b. Excessively thick nails are related to impaired circulation, chronic fungal infection, and aging.
   c. Excessively thin nails or the presence of grooves or furrows are related to iron-deficiency anemia.
   d. Brittle nails are related to malnutrition, calcium, and iron deficiency.
   e. Longitudinal ridges are related to arterial insufficiency.
4. Cuticle and surrounding tissue.
   a. Smooth intact epidermis expected.
   b. Edema, erythema, or exudate indicates inflammation or infection; assess for ingrown nails.

Normal angle
160°

A

Finger clubbing
>180°

B

Fig 18.1 Nail plate angle (normal, clubbing). (From Dillon [2016]. *Nursing health assessment,* 3rd ed. Philadelphia: F. A. Davis Company, with permission.)

5. Capillary refill.
   a. Compression of the nail produces blanching and color returns in <3 seconds after pressure is released *(blanch test).*
   b. Return of circulation >3 seconds (>5 seconds in older adults) indicates cardiopulmonary problems or anemia.

III. Risk Factors for Impaired Tissue Integrity and Related Nursing Care

The integrity of the skin must be maintained to preserve one of the first protective lines of defense of the body. Factors such as moisture, excessive or inadequate hydration of the skin, inadequate nutrition, prolonged pressure, and shearing forces can compromise tissue integrity. Nurses must have a thorough understanding of these factors as they relate to skin breakdown because many of them can be prevented or minimized by nurses when caring for clients.

A. Moisture
   1. Incontinence and perspiration because of fever in response to disease or illness can cause prolonged dampness, which softens skin *(maceration).*
   2. Feces and gastric tube drainage that contain digestive enzymes and urine that contains urea can cause loss of superficial layers of the skin *(excoriation, denuded skin).*
   3. Abdominal and perineal skin folds and under the breasts are particularly at risk because these touching skin surfaces confine moisture and are warm, dark, moist places that facilitate growth of bacteria and fungi.
   4. Nursing care.
      a. Keep the client clean and dry, especially skinfolds for a client who is obese, perspiring,

incontinent of urine or stool, or has a gastric or urinary tube.

🛑 b. **Assess the skin and mucous membranes of clients who are incontinent regularly.**

🛑 c. **Change wet clothing and linens immediately.**

   d. Provide a skin barrier to the perineal area or around the entry of a gastrostomy or urostomy tube as prescribed; many facilities have standing protocols that permit the nurse to use professional judgment concerning the application of products such as A&D ointment.
   e. Engage in a bowel or bladder training program if the client is a candidate and it is prescribed.
   f. Implement a toileting schedule to reduce episodes of incontinence; assist with toileting before and after meals to take advantage of the gastrocolic reflex (food/fluid entering an empty stomach stimulates peristalsis), when awakening in the morning and when going to bed at night, and every 2 hours when awake.

B. Dehydration and edema
   1. Fluid loss due to fever, diarrhea, or vomiting or inadequate fluid intake contributes to dry, cracking skin and mucous membranes.
   2. Excessive fluid in interstitial tissue *(edema)* decreases elasticity and flexibility of skin and interferes with oxygenation and clearing of waste from cells, increasing the risk of tissue breakdown.
   3. Nursing care.

🛑 a. **Ensure that the client has adequate fluid intake (2 to 3 liters daily) to maintain body function.**

      (1) Administer IV fluids as prescribed.
      (2) Provide fresh water and preferred fluids and assist a client who is unable to acquire fluid, such as by offering sips of water whenever passing the client's room.
   b. Maintain fluid restriction as prescribed.
   c. Provide pressure relief devices to protect skin surfaces.
   d. Elevate the legs of a client with dependent edema as long as the client has no acute cardiac insufficiency. (See "Alterations in Fluid Balance" in Chapter 21.)

C. Inadequate nutrition
   1. Insufficient protein, carbohydrates, and vitamin C contribute to muscle wasting, insufficient subcutaneous tissue, and weight loss.
   2. Insufficient protective cushioning of bony prominences by adequate tissue layers increases the risk of skin breakdown due to pressure.
   3. Nursing care.
      a. Assess self-feeding ability; condition of oral cavity, such as lesions, stomatitis, and problems

with dentures; current weight; and weight history.

  b. Ensure that the client receives adequate nutrition; evaluate and document the percentage of each meal ingested; avoid using relative terms such as "good" and "poor" to describe intake.

🛑 c. Assist a client with meals as needed and encourage intake of foods high in calories, protein, and vitamin C to maintain weight and facilitate wound healing.

  d. Conduct a calorie count when prescribed to evaluate the client's nutritional intake.

D. Prolonged immobility

1. When pressure exceeds 15 to 32 mm Hg (capillary occlusion pressure) due to tissue compression between a bony prominence and a hard surface, such as a bed or chair, tissue ischemia occurs, contributing to cell death.
2. Three factors are a concern:
   a. Intensity of pressure.
   b. Duration of pressure.
   c. Degree of tissue tolerance to the pressure due to a concurrent problem.
3. Concurrent problems that contribute to prolonged pressure and skin breakdown include presence of edema, inadequate nutrition, moisture, dehydration, reduced sensation, and impaired cognition that influences the ability to move.
4. Nursing care.
   a. Encourage independence but assist with activities that the client cannot complete or care for areas that the client cannot reach.

🛑 b. Turn and reposition the client every 2 hours and document on a turning and positioning flow sheet; may be done hourly for clients at risk for skin breakdown.

  c. Teach the client how to shift weight frequently to reduce the duration of pressure.
  d. Use pressure-relief devices, such as gel cushions, an air mattress, pillows, and elbow and heel pads to distribute weight over a greater area, thereby decreasing the intensity of pressure.
  e. Provide massage, skin care, and range of motion every time a client's position is changed to increase local circulation and prevent contractures.

E. Shearing force

1. **Shearing force** occurs when gravity pulls down on deep body structures and frictional resistance occurs between the skin and a firm surface.
2. The epidermal layer slides over the dermis and underlying tissue layers.
3. Shearing and frictional forces damage the vascular bed of skin and superficial tissue.
4. Capillary occlusion pressure is significantly reduced when shearing occurs; the combination of

pressure and shearing dramatically increases the risk of skin breakdown.
5. Nursing care.
   a. Use a pull sheet to move a client up in bed.
   b. Avoid using a high- or semi-Fowler position or limit the use of this position to alternating 2-hour intervals.
   c. Use a sliding board when transferring a client from a bed to a stretcher and back.
   d. Use a mechanical lift to transfer a client from a bed to a chair and back if the client is unable to move independently.

IV. Factors Affecting Hygiene Practices and Related Nursing Care

Personal hygiene consists of activities that maintain body cleanliness, promoting physical and psychological well-being. It is highly individualized and determined by numerous personal, cultural, religious, socioeconomic, environmental, and physical factors. Nurses must have a comprehensive understanding of these factors to aid in the assessment of clients and in the planning of nursing interventions that are specific for each client.

A. Personal preferences

1. Some people prefer to take a shower versus a bath, bathe in the morning versus the evening, and have specific opinions about the type of products they desire.
2. Personal habits develop on the basis of factors such as culture, home environment, family patterns, and economic circumstances.
3. Nursing care.
   a. Ask about preferences regarding hygiene and grooming activities.
   b. Accept hygiene practices nonjudgmentally.
   c. Support hygiene routines whenever possible using products preferred by the client.

B. Culture and religion

1. Maintaining personal cleanliness is not as important in some cultures as in others; North Americans commonly bathe daily, and those in other cultures may bathe only once a week.
2. Some cultures expect a person to use deodorant, and others believe that it is unnecessary.
3. Different cultures have different beliefs about nudity and privacy; North Americans generally bathe in private, and people in other cultures may bathe communally (Box 18.1).
4. Nursing care.
   a. Identify and meet specific preferences based on cultural and religious customs.

🛑 b. Provide privacy for hygiene and grooming activities; expose only the area of the body being washed.

Box 18.1 **Examples of Cultural and Religious Bathing Preferences**

- *Orthodox Jewish women engage in a ritual bath after each menstruation and after childbirth.*
- *In some cultures, family members provide hygiene and grooming care for ill relatives.*
- *Women who practice the Islam or Hindu religion can receive personal care only from another woman.*
- *Muslims use the left hand for cleaning and the right hand for eating and praying.*
- *In some cultures, family members may perform religious ceremonial washing when a client dies.*

🛑 c. Assign a gender-specific caregiver to a client when touching between unrelated males and females is forbidden in the client's culture.

   d. Include a family member in meeting hygiene needs if it is the client's preference.

   e. Support ceremonial washing of a client by family members when requested.

C. Developmental level

1. Common nursing care.
   a. Encourage clients to provide for their own hygiene needs as independently as possible within developmental, physical, emotional, and mental abilities.
   b. Provide a bath or assist with bathing activities when a client is unable to reach body parts or when cognitively immature or impaired.
   c. Use hygiene products that are the client's preference and/or that are designed for a specific developmental age, such as gentle soaps or soap substitutes for infants and older adults.
   d. Use protective skin barrier ointments in the perineal area when a client is not toilet trained or is incontinent.

🛑 e. Test the temperature of bath water before use, including water in a shower.

2. Infants and children.
   a. Have fragile, easily injured skin.
   b. Are incontinent of urine and feces that promote skin breakdown.
   c. Have hygiene activities provided for by parents and caregivers.
   d. Progressively assume more self-care activities as they grow older.
   e. Eventually provide self-care independently.
   f. Specific nursing care.
      (1) Change diaper as soon as soiled.
      (2) Allow children to engage in self-care as gross and fine motor skills develop.
      (3) Teach parents to never leave a child unattended in a bath tub.
      (4) Teach parents to bathe an infant in a plastic tub or bath tub rather than the kitchen sink; accidental turning on of the faucet may cause a thermal injury.

3. Adolescents.
   a. Have increased sebaceous gland growth and secretion, which makes the skin more oily and susceptible to acne.
   b. May shower several times a day as they become more concerned about personal appearance.
   c. Specific nursing care.
      (1) Support adolescents nonjudgmentally as they engage in meeting hygiene needs to enhance their self-esteem.
      (2) Support use of prescribed acne medications.

4. Older adults.
   a. Have many integumentary changes that result in fragile, easily injured skin (Fig. 18.2).
   b. May need assistance with hygiene because of problems such as physical or physiological limitations and reduced sensation, resulting in an inability to sense pressure, heat, cold, and friction or chemical irritants.

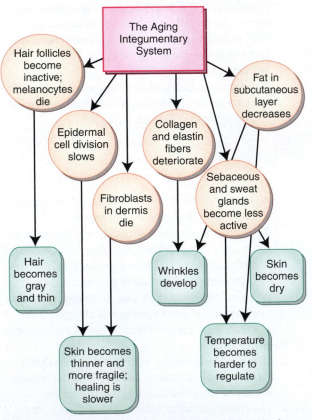

Fig 18.2 The aging integumentary system. Note: Circles indicate physiologic changes; squares indicate observable results of physiologic changes. (From Williams and Hopper [2015]. *Understanding medical surgical nursing,* 5th ed. Philadelphia: F. A. Davis Company, with permission.)

c. May be reluctant to seek assistance because of fear that they will be viewed as unable to cope.

d. Specific nursing care.

(1) Bathe less frequently according to a client's preference to avoid drying the skin.

(2) Use mild cleansing products to maintain pH balance of skin and prevent removal of natural moisturizers and lipids that protect the skin.

(3) Use a soft cloth and pat skin surfaces dry to avoid damage by abrasion.

(4) Allow client to progress at own pace because of developmental decline in mobility; doing so reduces stress, conserves energy, and prevents activity intolerance.

(5) Apply a moisturizer/emollient after bathing and at least twice a day to make skin supple and less dry; ensure safety precautions because these products can be slippery.

(6) Teach the client to assess all body surfaces, especially bony prominences, daily using a mirror, if needed, to identify tissue trauma.

D. Knowledge, values, beliefs, and motivation

1. Knowledge alone may not precipitate healthful behaviors.

2. An opinion about the worth of something (value) and thoughts that a person considers to be true, which may or may not be based on fact (belief) influence personal hygiene behaviors.

3. Changes in behavior related to health beliefs are based on the client's perception of these factors:

(1) Seriousness of the illness.

(2) Personal risk of developing the illness.

(3) Personal benefit of the actions to be taken.

4. The desire or incentive to learn (motivation) influences whether a behavior is instituted and/or sustained. (See "Motivation Facilitates Learning" in Chapter 8, Teaching and Learning.)

5. Nursing care.

a. Identify the client's values and beliefs in relation to hygiene.

b. Identify the client's understanding of actions and inactions that impact personal hygiene and bodily functions.

c. Teach principles associated with hygiene and that are within the client's values and beliefs.

d. Help the client to set goals and outcomes and assist clients to meet these goals and outcomes.

E. Socioeconomic status and personal environment

1. Inadequate income influences the environment in which one lives and the ability to afford hygiene products.

2. A person renting a room or living in a rooming house may not have easy access to bathing facilities.

3. Homeless people carry all belongings with them and may bathe in a sink in a public bathroom.

4. Attaining food, clothing, and shelter may be more important than bathing to people who live in poverty.

5. Nursing care.

a. Be sensitive to an inability to provide for personal cleanliness due to poverty or homelessness.

b. Advocate for the client and initiate contact with an appropriate social service agency that can address the multiple physical and emotional needs of the client.

c. Direct the client to a food bank that provides hygiene products or a shelter that provides facilities in which to bathe.

d. Direct the client to community agencies that help acquire funding for people living in poverty.

F. Health status and energy level

1. Clients challenged with physical, physiological, emotional, mental, or cognitive problems may not have the physical strength, dexterity, endurance, or psychic energy to provide for their own hygiene needs safely.

2. Common health issues that impact the self-performance of hygiene.

a. Pain due to problems such as surgery, trauma, and acute or chronic health problems.

b. Impaired mobility due to problems such as Parkinson disease, multiple sclerosis, spinal cord injury, or brain attack.

c. Sensory deficits, such as impaired vision or hearing and neuropathies.

d. Cognitive deficits, such as delirium, dementia, traumatic brain injury, or lowered level of consciousness.

e. Emotional, mental, or cognitive issues, such as an altered reality state, severe anxiety, or depression.

3. Assess the level of client assistance needed to meet hygiene needs.

a. Independent: Client is able to provide total self-care without assistance.

b. Set-up with partial assistance: Client can physically and mentally bathe most body parts when equipment is positioned in easy reach; caregiver assists with body parts that the client is unable to reach, such as lower legs and feet, back, and buttocks.

c. Supervision: Client can physically provide self-care but, because of a mental or emotional impairment, needs coaching to stay focused or complete the steps in a task.

d. Complete assistance: Client is physically, emotionally, or mentally incapable of providing self-care; all hygiene and grooming tasks are implemented by the caregiver.

4. Nursing care.
   a. Complete a nursing history and physical and identify factors that may interfere with a client's ability to provide self-care.
   b. Identify the client's level of ability to participate in self-care.
   c. Plan and implement a plan of care that addresses hygiene and grooming needs.
   d. For nursing care for clients with specific needs associated with an impaired ability to meet personal hygiene and grooming needs, see "Providing Hygiene for Clients With Special Needs" in this chapter.

V. Nursing Care to Support Hygiene

Activities of daily living related to personal care generally include bathing, perineal care, foot care, oral care, hair care, nail care, and shaving. They also include insertion, removal, and storage of hearing aids and dentures. Each of these activities includes specific nursing interventions that incorporate the principles of medical asepsis and client safety. Nurses must understand not only what should be done but also the rationale for each of these interventions.

A. Purposes of hygiene
   1. Cleanses the skin by minimizing microorganisms and removing secretions, excretions, and debris from the skin; removes and inhibits unpleasant body odors.
   2. Increases circulation by bringing oxygen and nutrients to the cells of the skin and removing cellular waste.
   3. Promotes a sense of well-being and fosters relaxation and comfort.

B. Scheduled hygiene
   1. Hourly.
      a. Rounding hourly is also known as "comfort or safety rounds."
      b. Ensures client's comfort, positioning, and toileting needs are met in a timely manner.
   2. Upon awakening.
      a. Also known as "early morning care."
      b. Client is toileted upon awakening, hands and face are washed, and oral care and comfort interventions (e.g., positioning, medications) are performed in preparation for breakfast and diagnostic testing.
   3. Morning care.
      a. Also known as "a.m. care."
      b. After breakfast, clients are assisted with hygiene and grooming activities, such as toileting, bathing, oral care, skin care, shaving if desired, dressing, and positioning in a chair. At this time, linens generally are changed and the room is organized and cleaned.

   4. Afternoon care.
      a. Sometime after lunch, clients may be assisted with toileting and returned to bed for rest.
      b. Care also may include performing hand hygiene, providing oral care, repositioning, straightening linens, and providing comfort measures, such as medication for pain.
   5. Hour of sleep care.
      a. Also known as "p.m. care."
      b. Includes the same care as afternoon care; in addition, a back rub may be performed to promote relaxation.
      c. The television and lights should be turned off and the door closed, per the client's preferences.

C. Bathing
   1. Commonalities of nursing care for all types of bathing methods.
      a. Explain what is going to be done and why to meet the client's right to know and promote motivation and participation.
      b. Ask the client about his or her usual routine and provide for preferences.
      c. Complete hand hygiene to minimize cross-contamination, and collect all equipment to avoid interrupting the bath.
      d. Close the door, pull the curtain, and close all windows to provide privacy and reduce heat loss via convection.
      e. Offer to toilet the client. Doing so addresses the urge to void that might be stimulated by bathing.
      f. Position a bath blanket over the client, and remove the top linen from under the bath blanket. Expose only those areas being washed, rinsed, or dried. Doing so provides privacy, comfort, and warmth.
      g. Encourage independence but assist the client as needed. Self-care supports self-esteem and increases circulation and range of motion.
      h. Use warm (105°F to 115°F), not hot, water to promote vasodilation and prevent dry skin caused by hot water, which excessively removes sebum.
      i. Change water when cool, soiled, or soapy. Doing so promotes vasodilation, supports comfort, and minimizes contamination.
      j. Make a bath mitt with a washcloth by laying a hand on the washcloth, folding one side over the hand then the other, folding the top down across the hand, and tucking it under the folded edge at the wrist. Doing so retains water and heat and prevents the ends from being tossed about, contaminating the environment.
      k. Wash (softens dirt and debris), rinse (removes debris and soap), and dry (removes moisture

Box 18.2 Safety Measures Implemented After Hygiene Care

- *Leave the bed in the lowest position.*
- *Position the call bell within the client's reach.*
- *Place the overbed table within easy reach with fresh water, tissues, and other desired items.*
- *Provide additional blankets if desired by the client.*

that supports microbial growth) each part of the body.

l. Reposition the client in functional alignment to support comfort and reduce stress and strain on bones, joints, muscles, ligaments, and tendons.

m. Implement safety measures before leaving the client's bedside (Box 18.2).

n. Discard soiled towels and washcloths in soiled linen hamper; discard bath water into the toilet; clean the basin and return it to the client's bedside table. Doing so maintains medical aseptic technique and prepares equipment for future use.

o. Evaluate and document the client's outcomes and tolerance of the activity. Doing so ensures that the client's status is evaluated and information is communicated to other health-care team members.

MAKING THE CONNECTION

Providing Hygiene Care and Making Nursing Assessments

There is no better time to assess body systems than during the administration of a bath. During this activity, the nurse not only has an opportunity to assess the client's skin, mucous membranes, hair, and nails but also may be directed to a more focused assessment in response to an unexpected observation. For example, the nurse may identify an impairment in cognition (e.g., altered level of consciousness, impaired problem-solving ability, inability to follow directions), mobility impairment (e.g., inability to turn and move as expected, presence of fatigue, or weakness), or altered respiratory status (e.g., shortness of breath on exertion, activity intolerance). After identifying an unexpected response, the nurse should make a more detailed assessment of the related system. In addition to the opportunity to make focused assessments, the time spent performing personal care also affords clients the opportunity to share emotions and concerns that they might not have expressed otherwise. Lastly, it is an ideal time to establish a professional rapport with the client and support the development of trust in the caregiver.

2. Bathing methods and related nursing care.

a. *Complete bed bath:* Involves washing, rinsing, and drying a client's entire body; may be performed independently or with some or total assistance from a caregiver (who addresses areas that the client cannot reach, such as the back and feet).

(1) Start at the head and work down the body; moves from clean to dirty.

(2) Cleanse the far side of the body first, then the near side; prevents contamination of the clean side of the body by a dripping washcloth.

(3) Wash the face with plain water, beginning with the eyes from inner to outer canthus; avoid soap, which has a drying effect and can irritate the eyes, and minimizes secretions entering lacrimal duct by moving from inner to outer canthus.

(4) Use a different side of the washcloth for each eye to reduce the risk of transferring microorganisms from one eye to the other.

(5) Wash, rinse, and dry the face, ears, and neck.

(6) Place a towel under one upper extremity and wash, rinse, and dry the arm, axillae, and hand; stroke from distal to proximal. Repeat for the other arm. Use of a towel keeps the bed dry, and stroking from distal to proximal promotes venous blood return.

(7) Rest the client's hand in the washbasin if hand or nails are excessively soiled to loosen dirt.

(8) Apply deodorant or antiperspirant per client preference to reduce the risk of body odor.

(9) Wash, rinse, and dry the chest and then abdomen while exposing only the area being washed.

(10) Clean and dry under the breasts of women or men with enlarged breasts due to obesity or gynecomastia to minimize risk of odor and skin irritation.

(11) Place a towel under a lower extremity and wash, rinse, and dry, stroking from distal to proximal. Repeat for the other leg and foot.

(12) Rest the client's foot in the washbasin if foot or toenails are excessively soiled to loosen dirt.

(13) Change the water and provide perineal care. See "Perineal Care" later in this chapter.

(14) Change the water before moving to the client's back. Doing so ensures clean, warm water and prevents contamination.

(15) Turn the client on the side and place a towel on the bed along back and buttocks.

(16) Wash, rinse, and dry the back and then the buttocks; moves from clean to dirty.

(17) Provide a backrub if not contraindicated. Doing so increases local circulation, promotes relaxation, and supports comfort. (See "Back Rub" in Chapter 15, Pain, Comfort, Rest, and Sleep.)

(18) Assist the client with grooming (e.g., oral care, shaving, hair care).

(19) Put a clean gown on the client, and make the bed with clean linens; remove the bath blanket from under the clean top sheet.

b. *Partial bed bath:* Generally includes body areas that have secretions or excretions, cause an odor, are at risk for skin breakdown and infection, or need to be freshened for the day.

(1) Wash the client's face, hands, axillae, back, perineal area, and under the breasts (for women and men with enlarged breasts). Doing so cleanses essential areas of the body while conserving the client's energy.

(2) Follow the progression indicated in a complete bed bath to adhere to the principle of clean to dirty.

c. *Bath-in-a-bag:* Includes a package of 8 to 10 disposable washcloths premoistened with a no-rinse surfactant, diluent substance to trap moisture (humectant), and an emollient; proven to reduce overall skin dryness, skin flaking, and scaling; preferred in critical care and long-term care settings because it is less physically stressful for clients.

(1) Use a microwave or warming unit to warm washcloths to 105°F, following the manufacturer directions.

🛑 **(2) Ensure that washcloths are not too hot before use to prevent unintentional burns.**

(3) Use one washcloth for each area of the body to follow the concept of clean to dirty, which prevents cross-contamination.

(4) Do not rinse to prevent removal of the emollient.

(5) Allow each area to air dry to ensure that the emollient and skin protectant remain on the skin surface.

d. *Blanket/towel bath:* Involves placing a bath blanket, towel, and washcloth in a plastic bag and saturating them with a commercially prepared solution of disinfectant, nonrinse cleaning agent, moisturizer, and water and then warming according to manufacturer's directions; proven to provide client satisfaction and takes less time than a traditional bath; commonly a method of choice for clients with mild to moderate impaired skin integrity, activity intolerance, or cognitive impairment.

(1) Follow agency procedure or manufacturer's directions for the amount of water and products to add to the bag with the bath blanket, towel, and washcloth and warm according to the directions. Doing so ensures that appropriate products and equipment are added, avoids excessive suds, and ensures that the temperature is not too warm.

(2) Place a dry bath blanket over the client to provide for privacy and protect the client from drafts.

(3) Replace the dry blanket with the fan-folded wet blanket. Starting at the neck, move the dry blanket down while unfolding the fan-folded wet blanket until the client is completely covered from the neck to the feet with the wet blanket.

(4) Wash the client with the wet blanket, fan-folding up the wet blanket as you move and replacing it with a fan-folded dry blanket as you work. Doing so ensures that the principle of clean to dirty is maintained because different parts of the wet blanket are used for each body part and the wet blanket is folded and replaced with the dry blanket as the bath progresses.

(5) Wash the face with plain water, beginning with the eyes from inner to outer canthus. This avoids soap, which has a drying effect and can irritate the eyes; minimizes secretions from entering lacrimal duct by moving from inner to outer canthus.

(6) Use a different side of the washcloth for each eye to reduce the risk of transferring microorganisms from one eye to the other.

(7) Wash, rinse, and dry the face, ears, and neck.

(8) Don gloves to protect self from the client's blood or body fluids.

(9) Turn the client on his or her side, unfold the wet bath towel over the client's back and buttocks, and wash the back and buttocks.

(10) Remove gloves, wash hands, don clean gloves, reposition the client, and then provide perineal care. For more information, see "Perineal care (female and male)" in this chapter.

e. *Shower and tub baths:* Require a prescription because the extent of exposure to warm water causes vasodilation and requires more client effort and energy than other bathing methods; may be prescribed as therapeutic baths, such as oatmeal baths, for clients with skin conditions or hydrotherapy-type baths after a burn injury.

(1) Shower: Client stands or sits on a shower chair under a continuous flow of water.

(2) Tub bath: Involves immersion in a tub of water; provides more thorough washing and rinsing than other types of baths; generally requires a transfer in a chair lift or bathing stretcher to the tub.

(3) Nursing care.

(a) Ensure that the shower or tub is clean before and after use to prevent cross-contamination.

(b) Ensure a nonskid area around the tub or shower, such as by not using a towel on the floor, to promote safety and prevent a fall.

(c) Hang an "in-use" sign outside the tub or shower room to support privacy.

(d) Explain to the client the steps in the transfer procedure to reduce anxiety and support a sense of control.

(e) Use a shower chair if the client has activity intolerance. Secure the client in a transfer chair or stretcher to ensure a safe transfer.

(f) Assist the client in entering and exiting the shower or tub. Doing so widens the base of support to help prevent a fall.

(g) Encourage the use of handrails and grab bars to facilitate movement and help prevent a fall.

(h) Ensure that the water temperature is no higher than 115°F to avoid unintentional burns.

🛑 (i) **Stay with the client or wait on the other side of a curtain throughout the shower or bath, depending on the client's ability to be independent and safe.**

(j) Limit a bath to 20 minutes to prevent prolonged exposure to warm water, which can cause vasodilation and dizziness, precipitating a fall.

D. Perineal care (female and male)

1. Involves washing the area from the symphysis pubis to the anus.

2. Performed a minimum of once daily, usually as part of a complete or partial bed bath.

3. Performed as often as necessary because of incontinence of urine or feces, profuse diaphoresis, or urethral, vaginal, or rectal discharge.

4. Requires use of a firm but gentle touch to minimize stimulation.

5. Nursing care.

a. Gather clean, warm water; a towel; and a washcloth to prevent having to interrupt the procedure later to gather additional equipment.

b. Explain what is to be done and close the door and curtain around the client's bed. Doing so provides information and maintains the client's privacy.

🛑 c. **Don clean gloves to protect self from the client's body fluids.**

d. Position the client for the procedure to access the site that requires hygiene care.

(1) Female: Place the client in the supine position with the knees bent and the feet flat on the bed.

(2) Male: Place the client in the supine position with the hips and knees extended.

e. Drape the client for the procedure to provide for warmth, comfort, and privacy.

(1) Female: Arrange a bath blanket over the client in a diamond position with one point at the head, one at the feet, and one point at each side; wrap a side point of the bath blanket around each leg and foot; then drape the point at the feet over the perineal area, where it can be lifted up and folded back (Fig. 18.3).

(2) Male: Position the bath blanket above the client's waist and the bed linens over the legs from the thighs to the feet.

f. Cleanse the perineal area with soap and water using a different side of the wash cloth for each stroke and cleaning the area of the urinary

Fig 18.3 Draping a female client for perineal care. (From Wilkinson and Treas [2016]. *Fundamentals of nursing*, Vol. 2, 3rd ed. Philadelphia: F. A. Davis Company, with permission.)

meatus first and then progressing to more soiled perineal areas. Doing so prevents contamination of clean areas with a soiled part of the washcloth and adheres to the principle of clean to dirty. Soap and water removes thick, cheesy odoriferous secretion of sebaceous glands, desquamated epithelial cells, and mucus (**smegma**), under the loose skin at the end of the penis (**foreskin, prepuce**) of a male or under the labia minora and around the clitoris of the female and minimizes bacterial growth.

(1) Female.
    (a) Spread the labia with one hand and wash the far side, near side, and then down the middle of the vulva from the urinary meatus to the anus, using a separate part of the wash cloth for each stroke (Fig. 18.4); repeat until clean.
    (b) Rinse the vulva using the same principles of clean to dirty.
    (c) Pat dry with a clean towel.

(2) Male.
    (a) Begin with the penile head; retract the foreskin (if uncircumcised) and wash in a circular motion around the tip of the penis and glans and then working down the shaft toward the suprapubic area (Fig. 18.5); repeat until clean.
    (b) Rinse the penis using the same principles of clean to dirty.
    (c) Pat dry with a clean towel.
    🛑 (d) Return the foreskin to its natural position over the glans penis if the client is uncircumcised to prevent constriction of blood flow that may precipitate edema, pain, and even necrosis of the glans penis.
    (e) Spread the client's legs and gently wash, rinse, and pat dry the scrotum.

Fig 18.4 Cleansing the labia. (From Wilkinson and Treas [2016]. *Fundamentals of nursing*, Vol. 2, 3rd ed. Philadelphia: F. A. Davis Company, with permission.)

Fig 18.5 Male perineal care. (From Wilkinson and Treas [2016]. *Fundamentals of nursing*, Vol. 2, 3rd ed. Philadelphia: F. A. Davis Company, with permission.).

g. Turn the client on the side and wash, rinse, and dry the buttocks and then the anus; work from the urinary meatus toward the anus; this follows the principle of clean to dirty.
h. Assess the area for skin breakdown due to contact with urine and feces.
i. Clean a urinary retention catheter if present.
    (1) Hold the catheter with one hand close to the urinary meatus and wash with soap and water down the tubing in a circular motion away from the meatus toward the distal end of the catheter; repeat with a different area of the washcloth until clean. Doing so avoids traction on the catheter, preventing trauma to the urethra, and follows the principle of clean to dirty.
    (2) Rinse and dry tubing to remove moisture minimizes the growth of microorganisms.
j. Continue with the rest of the bath if perineal care is part of a complete bed bath.

E. Foot care
1. Involves cleaning the feet from the ankles to the toes.
2. Performed as part of a complete bed bath.
3. The feet should be assessed before and reassessed after care; compare assessments for symmetry.
    a. Bilateral dorsalis pedis pulses.
    b. Temperature and color of skin and toenails.
    c. Capillary refill.
    d. Movement and sensation.
4. Nursing care.
    a. Maintain standard precautions because of the potential to be exposed to impaired skin, particularly if the client has health problems such as peripheral vascular disease or diabetes.
    b. Position the client in a sitting position in bed or a chair; soak each foot for 5 to 10 minutes at a time in a basin of warm water (105°F to 115°F) that is positioned on a waterproof pad. Do not soak the feet of a client with peripheral vascular disease or diabetes. Warm water softens dirt

and promotes circulation and relaxation. However, it also removes natural oils, promoting drying and cracking of the skin.

c. Wash, rinse, and dry each foot gently and thoroughly, especially between the toes, and then place feet on a clean pad or towel. Doing so cleanses the skin, removes irritating soap, and prevents skin maceration. A clean surface provides a safe place on which to provide additional foot care.

d. Apply lotion to the feet but avoid areas between the toes and excessive amounts of lotion. Doing so lubricates the skin, but excessive amounts can cause skin maceration, especially if applied between the toes.

e. Provide a bed cradle if the client has a foot problem to raise linens off the legs and feet, relieving pressure and supporting comfort.

f. Teach the client precautions to protect the feet.

(1) Assess the feet daily using a mirror, visit a podiatrist routinely, and notify a primary health-care provider if a problem is identified.

(2) Wear well-supporting shoes when out of bed, and ensure that linings and surfaces of shoes are smooth and intact.

(3) Wear socks without seams.

(4) Avoid excessively soaking the feet and dry between the toes well.

(5) Have toenails cut by a podiatrist to ensure professional assessment and care.

(6) Avoid self-treatment of corns, calluses, and other problems with over-the-counter remedies.

F. Oral care

1. Involves maintaining the integrity of a client's oral mucous membranes, teeth, gums, tongue, and lips. Includes caring for dentures if present.

2. Performed as part of a partial or complete bed bath, before and after meals, and in the morning and evening.

3. Provided more frequently for clients who are on nothing-by-mouth (NPO) status, mouth breathing, receiving oxygen, or have a nasogastric tube because these situations contribute to dry mucous membranes and collection of bacteria and thick, sticky secretions on the tongue, teeth, and lips (**sordes**).

4. The oral mucosa, teeth, gums, and lips should be assessed for color, extent of tissue hydration (moist), and presence of lesions (absence of lesions).

5. Products based on the client's preference should be used (e.g., toothbrush, toothpaste, mouthwash, and floss).

6. Oral care for a conscious client.

a. Wash hands, and then don clean gloves. Doing so minimizes microorganisms on the hands and protects the caregiver from the client's body fluids.

b. Place the client in the Fowler's position to minimize the risk of aspiration.

c. Place a towel under the chin and across the client's chest.

d. Apply a small amount of toothpaste on a moistened toothbrush to avoid excessive foaming, and have the client brush his or her own teeth if able; if unable, complete the procedure for the client.

e. Instruct the client to hold the brush at a 45-degree angle and brush the base of the teeth at the gum line with short, vibrating, circular motions; repeat for all surfaces where teeth contact gums. This dislodges plaque that adheres at the base of the tooth.

f. Instruct the client to brush back and forth over biting surfaces as well as the tongue to dislodge food debris, plaque, and sordes from crevices of teeth and on the tongue.

g. Instruct the client to rinse the mouth with water or mouthwash and spit (*expectorate*) it into an emesis basin.

h. Floss the teeth by stretching the floss between the fingers and sliding the floss between two teeth down to the gum line; then move the floss with an up and down motion several times. Use a systematic progression to include all teeth. Doing so loosens and removes debris between teeth.

i. Wipe the client's mouth with a towel; clean the equipment and return it to the client's bedside table.

j. Remove gloves and dispose in an appropriate trash container; wash hands.

7. Oral care for an unconscious client.

a. Position the client in the side-lying position with the head turned to the side to facilitate drainage of secretions and fluids used in oral care via gravity, which minimizes the risk of aspiration.

b. Place a towel under the client's chin and across the pillow and mattress; position an emesis basin slightly under the client's chin.

c. Wear gloves and a gown and face shield if splashing is likely to protect self from contact with the client's body fluids.

d. Dip a gauze-covered tongue blade or sponge swab in half water and half mouthwash; swab the tongue, teeth, hard palate, and inside of the cheeks and the lips (Fig. 18.6). Gentle friction helps to loosen debris.

Fig 18.6 Oral care for an unconscious client. (From Wilkinson and Treas [2016]. *Fundamentals of nursing*, Vol. 2, 3rd ed. Philadelphia: F. A. Davis Company, with permission.)

🛑 e. Avoid swabbing the last third of the back of the tongue to prevent stimulation of the gag reflex.

   f. Rinse the oral cavity using a clean, wet gauze-covered tongue blade or sponge swab.

🛑 g. Do not leave the client until all cleaning solution has drained from the client's mouth to prevent aspiration.

🛑 h. Stop the procedure and suction the client if the client coughs or demonstrates signs of choking; do not leave the client until the client's respirations return to the client's normal rate and rhythm. Doing so minimizes aspiration of solution into breathing passages and provides for client safety.

8. Care of a client with dentures.
   a. Dentures should be removed and cleaned according to the client's usual routine; usually removed, cleaned, and stored when sleeping and reinserted in the beginning of the day.
   b. Dentures should be inspected for integrity and not be used if cracks or rough edges are present.
   c. The mouth, especially the gums under dentures, should be assessed for redness, irritation, lesions, or signs of infection. Ensure that dentures are not loose or tight. Seek a referral for a dental consult if there is a concern.
   d. Removal of dentures.
     (1) Encourage the client to remove the dentures or remove the dentures for the client if necessary.
     (2) Remove the top denture before the bottom denture to ease removal of the larger top denture.
     (3) With a gauze pad, grasp the upper denture with a thumb and forefinger and move the denture up and down to release suction.
     (4) Use your thumbs to push up gently on the bottom denture at the gum line to release suction.

     (5) Tilt the dentures vertically slightly when removing them from the mouth to avoid stretching the client's lips.
   e. Cleaning of dentures.
     (1) Transport dentures in an emesis basin or denture cup and wash them in a sink padded with a towel. Doing so minimizes risk of breaking the dentures if dropped.
     (2) Use denture cleaner, a soft toothbrush, and warm, not hot, water to clean dentures. Regular toothpaste and a firm toothbrush may be too abrasive. Denture material can warp or become sticky when exposed to hot water.
     (3) Brush gums and tongue with a soft toothbrush; assist to rinse mouth with water or dilute mouthwash.
   f. Storage of dentures.
     (1) Soak dentures overnight in a labeled (client's name and other identifying information) denture cup with dental cleanser and cool water per the client's preference. This keeps dentures clean and white and prevents warping when stored in cool water.
     (2) Place the denture cup in the bedside table to help prevent loss.
   g. Insertion of dentures.
     (1) Apply denture adhesive to the underside of the top denture if preferred by the client to securely seal the denture to the hard palate and upper gum.
     (2) Tilt the top denture at a slight angle to ease insertion and press into place with a thumb on the palate to promote adherence.
     (3) Repeat with the bottom denture; press gently downward into place. This securely seals the bottom denture to the bottom gum.

G. Hair care
1. Condition of hair can be a measure of physical and emotional health. See "Assessment of Hair" in this chapter.
2. The scalp perspires and secretes oils, and hair is a perfect environment for the collection of secretions and dirt.
3. Hair care should include brushing/combing daily and shampooing weekly.
4. Nursing care.
   a. Brushing or combing hair.
     (1) Place a towel over the client's shoulders.
     (2) Position the client in the sitting position if able or, if not, the side-lying position.
     (3) Brush or comb hair beginning from distal ends in small sections moving up toward the scalp every 2 to 3 inches as tangles are

removed. This removes tangles and stimulates scalp circulation. Attending to small sections and lengths at a time avoids scalp trauma and pain.

(4) Style hair according to client's preference; use hair clips or braid long hair per the client's preference. Avoid inappropriate styles, such as pigtails for older adults. Hair clips or braiding helps prevent matting and facilitates movement in bed when a client has long hair. Instituting client preferences supports self-esteem, dignity, and a sense of control.

(5) Provide additional interventions for hair that is dry, coarse, curly, or kinky in texture.

    (a) Apply mineral oil or a moisturizing hair cream before combing to lubricate hair and scalp, which limits tangles and matting.

    (b) Use a wide-tooth comb when combing hair to minimize breakage of hair.

(6) Clean the brush or comb and store it in the bedside table; fold the towel into itself and place it in a linen hamper.

b. Shampooing hair.

  (1) Comb or brush the hair to remove tangles before shampooing.

  (2) Place the client in the supine position.

  (3) Place a waterproof pad or plastic garbage bag on the bed, position a shampoo cradle under the client's head, and place a towel around the client's neck.

  (4) Position a trough over the side of the bed to a collection receptacle to direct water off the bed and contain it in a collection receptacle.

  (5) Have the client protect the eyes by holding a towel over the eyes if able and wet the hair with warm water using a water pitcher.

  (6) Apply shampoo and then wash the hair, using products per the client's preference.

  (7) Cover hair styled in cornrows or braids with a stocking cap and shampoo through the cap. This technique cleans the hair while preserving the hair style.

  (8) Massage the scalp with the fingertips to stimulate scalp circulation and promote relaxation.

  (9) Double-rinse with warm water, and then apply a cream rinse per the client's preference. Doing so removes shampoo, which may irritate and dry the scalp, causing itching.

  (10) Dry hair well using a hairdryer if available.

(11) Comb hair and style according to the client's preference to support self-esteem, a sense of control, and dignity.

(12) Replace soiled linens with clean linens; dispose of soiled linens in a soiled linen hamper.

(13) Clean equipment and return to storage areas.

H. Shaving

1. Total or partial removal of hair from the face of a man is a personal preference.

  a. Some men consider it an important daily grooming measure.

  b. Some men do not shave because it is forbidden in their culture.

2. Grooming the hair on the face involves its removal or washing, combing, and trimming a beard or mustache.

3. The face and neck should be assessed for skin lesions, eczema, or ingrown hairs because these areas should be avoided during shaving or may be a contraindication for shaving.

4. Nursing care.

  a. Identify the type of razor to use; when possible, defer to the client's preference.

  🛑 b. **Use an electric shaver if the client is receiving an anticoagulant or has a low platelet count. Doing so prevents breaks in the skin that can result in excessive bleeding.**

  c. Don gloves to protect self from the client's blood if shaving breaks the client's skin.

  d. Use a disposable safety razor.

    (1) Position a warm washcloth on the beard for a few minutes to soften and lift whiskers.

    (2) Spread shaving cream over the beard and mustache area liberally to reduce skin irritation.

    (3) Hold the skin taut and shave in the direction that hair grows (Fig. 18.7). Doing

Fig 18.7 Shaving a client. (From Wilkinson and Treas [2016]. *Fundamentals of nursing*, Vol. 2, 3rd ed. Philadelphia: F. A. Davis Company, with permission.)

so helps maintain the 45-degree angle of a safety razor blade to the skin, thereby preventing the blade from irritating the skin or causing ingrown hairs.
  (a) Shave cheeks down toward the ridge of the chin.
  (b) Instruct the client to position the upper lip over the teeth to increase access to the skin under the nose.
  (c) Shave down from nose to upper lip.
  (d) Shave down from lower lip to chin.
  (e) Shave neck upward to chin.
  (4) Shave the ridge of the chin carefully to minimize the potential for a cut because of its contour.
  (5) Place the disposable razor in a sharps container to reduce the risk of injury.
  (6) Wash the face with a wet washcloth to remove shaving cream and debris, and then pat dry.
  (7) Apply aftershave lotion per the client's preference to soothe irritated skin.
e. Use an electric razor.
  (1) Apply preshave lotion to the beard and mustache area to soften and raise whiskers.
  (2) Hold skin taut and shave in the direction that hair grows to prevent ingrown hairs and skin irritation.
    (a) Use a circular motion to shave the cheeks.
    (b) Shave the mustache area in a downward motion.
    (c) Shave the neck in an upward circular motion.
  (3) Apply aftershave lotion per the client's preference to soothe irritated skin.
  (4) Clean the razor: Remove the head, brush out debris with the small brush provided with the razor, replace the head, and return it to its storage container in the middle draw of the bedside table. Doing so minimizes growth of microorganisms and protects the razor from damage or loss.
f. Care of a mustache and/or beard.
  (1) Ask the client's permission to trim a beard or mustache and identify the extent of trimming according to the client's preference. Doing so supports the client's preference and avoids removing too much of the mustache or beard.
  (2) Secure signed consent if the client wants a mustache or beard removed. This protects the caregiver if the client should regret the change and blame the caregiver.

  (3) Use a scissor or razor (disposable or electric) to trim a beard.
    (a) Comb a mustache straight down, and trim the length just above the upper lip.
    (b) Trim the line of a beard so that it is clearly defined.
I. Nail care
  1. Nails grow continuously and should be groomed during a complete bed bath.
  2. Seek a referral for a podiatrist for care of toenails, especially for people who have diabetes or vascular occlusive disease. Doing so avoids causing a break in the skin or an ingrown toenail if toenails are clipped too short, which could precipitate an injury or foot ulcer.
  3. Nursing care.
    a. Soak the client's hands or feet in a basin of warm water for 5 minutes to soften nails and cuticles.
    b. Dry hands and feet well, especially between digits to prevent skin maceration and infection.
    c. Use a washcloth or the flat end of an orange stick to gently push back the cuticle; use the pointed end to gently clean under the nails.
    d. Use an emery board to gently file nail edges if permitted by agency policy and procedure. Doing so removes sharp edges, which prevents scratches.
    e. Apply moisturizing lotion to the hands and feet but not between toes. Lotion makes skin soft and supple and avoiding between toes prevents skin maceration and infection.

VI. Providing Hygiene for Clients With Special Needs

Nurses should provide hygiene to or assist all clients with hygiene-related activities every day and whenever needed. The challenges of these activities increase when clients have issues that interfere with understanding what is being done, are unable to participate with the activities, or have unique physical or physiological needs.
A. Clients with impaired cognition
  1. May be unaware of the need for hygiene care, unable to remember how to bathe and groom oneself, or unable able to follow directions.
  2. Includes unconscious clients.
  3. Nursing care.
    a. Assess the client's ability to comprehend what is to be done and the ability to participate in care.
    b. Teach the benefits and risks of hygiene and grooming activities if the client is receptive to teaching.
    c. Administer prescribed analgesic or anxiolytics to promote relaxation.

d. Postpone bathing if the client is agitated to prevent escalation of the agitation.

e. Use a bath-in-bag product if available. Doing so limits the perception that interventions are threatening and is quicker to implement than a traditional bath.

f. Use simple commands in short phrases, and avoid multiple or complicated directions to support understanding.

g. Avoid using mouthwash to prevent it from being swallowed.

🛑 h. Avoid putting hands in the client's mouth to reduce the risk of caregiver injury.

🛑 i. Apply an eye lubricant and tape the eyes closed or apply an humidified eye shield as prescribed for an unconscious client or for a client who has an absent blink reflex when preparing for sleep. Eye care should be provided every 2 to 4 hours and when necessary. Doing so protects the cornea and delicate mucous membranes of the eye from becoming dry.

B. Clients with physiological impairments
1. Causes of impairments:
   a. Physiological problems that affect the neuro-musculoskeletal system, such as immobility due to a brain attack or multiple sclerosis.
   b. Lack of energy due to anemia or a chronic debilitating disease, such as chronic obstructive pulmonary disease.
   c. Pain from surgery or disease processes that impairs ability to move.
2. Nursing care.
   a. Assess the client's overall strength, hand grasp strength, balance, flexibility, coordination, ability to sit unsupported, range of motion, dexterity, and activity tolerance. This assessment helps to determine which aspects of care can be implemented independently and which require assistance.
   b. Encourage independence but provide assistance to complete tasks the client is unable to complete; provide assistive devices, such as a padded handle on a brush, as indicated to promote independence and support self-esteem.
   c. Provide prescribed pain medication if indicated to reduce pain, which will enable the client to participate in the activities.

🛑 d. Pace care and provide rest periods to conserve energy and prevent activity intolerance.

C. Clients with physical limitations
1. Physical limitations, such as casts; traction; nasogastric, gastrostomy, or urinary retention catheters; surgical drains; and restraints may interfere with a client's ability to provide self-care.

2. Nursing care.
   a. Identify the presence of equipment and how it interferes with independence. This assessment determines what activities may require adjustments to meet the client's hygiene needs without interrupting a therapeutic modality.
   b. Identify the number of caregivers necessary to provide required care to ensure that the safety of the client and caregivers is maintained.
   c. Provide specific interventions depending on the physical limitation.
      (1) Casts: Protect cast edges with plastic wrap to keep it from getting wet during a bath.
      (2) Traction.

🛑 (a) Do not release weights because weights maintain the pull of traction and therefore alignment of the bone.

      (b) Instruct the client to sit forward to provide access to the client's back for administering care.
      (c) Instruct the client to use the trapeze to lift the body off the mattress to provide access to the client's buttocks for administering care.
      (3) Restraints: Remove only one wrist or mitt restraint at a time while providing care to prevent the client from injuring self or caregiver.

D. Clients with impaired vision
1. A visually impaired client may be challenged when managing the environment and providing for self-care safely.
2. Nursing care.
   a. Determine the extent of the client's visual impairment and how it impacts self-care. Assessment allows for appropriate planning of care.
   b. Describe the location of items in the environment, especially the bedside call bell and nurse alert cord in the bathroom, to reduce anxiety and support safety.
   c. Describe the location of items on the overbed table using the numbers on a clock to support independence, which promotes self-esteem.
   d. Remain nearby when the client is providing self-care to support safety.
   e. Assist with activities that the client is unable to complete.

E. Clients with impaired mental health
1. Clients with mental illness may be unaware of the need for hygiene; lack the energy to engage in hygiene activities (e.g., with depression); or not take the time to engage in hygiene activities (e.g., with bipolar disorder, manic episode).

2. A person with a mental illness may experience an altered state of reality, such as delusions or hallucinations, paranoia, inability to make decisions, or moderate or severe anxiety that interferes with the ability to provide for one's own hygiene and grooming.

3. Nursing care.
   a. Assess the client's feelings, mood, and behavior and how they may impact on the performance of hygiene activities.
   b. Administer prescribed anxiolytics before starting care to minimize the client's anxiety when indicated.
   c. Speak calmly using a soft tone; use unhurried, slow motions to limit the perception that actions are threatening.
   d. Provide a bath-in-a-bag or towel bath. Doing so minimizes stress of the procedure, is less threatening, and is quicker to use than a traditional bath.
   e. Postpone activities if the client is agitated to prevent escalation of the agitation.
   f. Avoid touching an angry, hostile, or paranoid client to provide hygiene care. Doing so prevents an escalation of the client's feelings or behavior because touching the client may be perceived as a threat.

F. Clients with body piercings
   1. Body piercing is the insertion of barbells, rings, or precious stones in a setting into skin or mucous membranes.
   2. Piercings can be found in such areas as around the eyebrow, external ear, nose, lip, umbilicus, tongue, and genitalia.
   3. Nursing care.
      a. Assess the sites of piercings for clinical manifestations of inflammation or infection, such as redness, discomfort, swelling, and drainage. Assessment provides for early identification of a problem.
      b. Identify the way in which the client usually provides self-care; refer to the agency's procedure manual for details (generally, soap and water or alcohol is used to cleanse sites). Doing so limits microorganisms at the site of piercing, preventing infection.

DID YOU KNOW?

Piercings have to be removed because they can interfere with magnetic resonance imaging (MRI) and surgery (e.g., a tongue barbell may interfere with the insertion of an endotracheal tube). Most piercings have at least one end that can be unscrewed to allow removal. These sites close in a few days; therefore, piercings must be reinserted as soon as possible.

G. Clients with a hearing aid
   1. A hearing aid is a device that is placed in the external auditory canal; it magnifies sound to improve hearing.
   2. Nursing care.
      a. Identify the type of hearing aid used by a client (Fig. 18.8).
      b. Inspect for cracks, broken cords, or torn ear molds; a device should not be inserted if it is not intact.
      c. Remove a hearing aid.
         (1) Turn off the hearing aid and remove it from the client's ear.
         (2) Wipe the hearing aid and ear mold with a damp cloth and dry well.
         (3) Remove earwax that may be in the small opening in the ear piece using the cleaning instrument provided by the manufacturer. If the device has a screen or filter to block earwax, gently tap the aid against a clean cloth on a table to remove earwax.

Behind the ear   **A**   In the ear canal   **B**

In the ear   **C**

Fig 18.8 Types of hearing aids. (A) Behind the ear. (B) In the ear canal. (C) In the ear. (From Wilkinson and Treas [2016]. *Fundamentals of nursing*, Vol. 1, 3rd ed. Philadelphia: F. A. Davis Company, with permission.)

(4) Clean the external auditory canal with a washcloth wrapped around a finger; rinse and dry well.

(5) Inspect the ear for any signs or symptoms of irritation, infection, sores, or drainage; notify the primary health-care provider if any are present and do not reinsert the ear mold or hearing aid until the client is assessed by the primary health-care provider.

d. Store a hearing aid.

(1) Remove the battery and store the hearing aid in its case, which generally is a labeled, moisture-control container. This prolongs battery life.

(2) Place the case in the client's bedside drawer to protect it from moisture, damage, or loss.

e. Insert a hearing aid.

(1) Identify whether the hearing aid or mold is labeled right or left to ensure that the correct hearing aid or ear mold is inserted into the correct ear.

(2) Check the battery by turning on the device, turning the volume to its highest capacity, and listening for a whistle. If no whistle occurs, check the battery and replace it if necessary.

(3) Turn down the volume and turn off the hearing aid.

(4) Insert the hearing aid into the correct ear; turn it on, and adjust the volume according to the client's preference.

VII. Bedmaking

A bed is the client's most immediate environment. The linens on the bed usually are changed daily as part of morning care or as needed if they become wet or soiled. The pillow and draw sheet should be changed daily, even if the other linens are not because they are a reservoir for microorganisms. Linens include flat sheets or fitted sheets. Flat sheets require specific techniques to secure them to the mattress and limit wrinkles and are discussed in this section.

A. Making an unoccupied bed

1. Wear gloves if the risk of exposure to blood or body fluids is present.

2. Loosen tucked-in linen and fold it into itself; carry it positioned away from the body, and place it in a soiled linen hamper. These actions contain soiled linen while avoiding contaminating the caregiver's uniform.

3. Place a clean bottom sheet on the bed and unfold it lengthwise so the center crease is along the center of the bed to ensure that enough clean linen will be available to cover the sides of the bed.

4. Avoid shaking or fluffing linens to avoid raising microorganisms into air currents unnecessarily.

5. Secure a flat sheet to the mattress.

a. Line up the edge of the bottom sheet at the edge of the mattress at the foot of the bed to allow more linen to be tucked in at the head of the bed.

b. Tuck the bottom sheet at the top of the bed under the mattress. This secures the sheet, making it less likely to be displaced when the head of the bed is raised.

c. Make mitered corners on the bottom sheet at the head of the bed. Securing the bottom sheet helps to eliminate wrinkles, which can cause pressure injuring skin and be uncomfortable.

(1) Pick up the top edge of the sheet or spread about 12 to 18 inches from the end of the bed; lift it on top of the mattress (Fig. 18.9A).

(2) Tuck the sheet hanging below the mattress under the mattress (Fig. 18.9B).

(3) Lift the sheet off the top of the mattress and let it hang free on the side of the bed if it is a top sheet or spread (Fig. 18.9C); tuck in

A

B

C

Fig 18.9 Mitered corner. (From Wilkinson and Treas [2016]. *Fundamentals of nursing*, Vol. 2, 3rd ed. Philadelphia: F. A. Davis Company, with permission.)

under the mattress along the entire side of the bed if it is a bottom sheet.

6. Secure a fitted sheet to the mattress.
   a. Tuck the edge of the top corner of the sheet under the mattress followed by the bottom corner.
   b. Move to the other side of the bed and tuck the edge of the top corner of the sheet under the mattress followed by the bottom corner.

7. Spread a draw sheet across the center of the bed and secure it tightly under the mattress on both sides of the bed. A draw sheet helps secure the bottom sheet in place, protects the bottom sheet from minor soiling, and can be used to lift and turn a client. Often times a draw sheet is no longer used, particularly with fitted sheets, because it increases the risk of wrinkles that promote pressure against the client's skin.

8. Unfold the top sheet 4 inches down from the head of the bed with the center fold in the center of the bed; open up the sheet and let it hang free over the sides and bottom of the bed. This ensures that there is enough linen on each side and bottom of the bed.

9. Unfold a spread with the center fold in the center of the bed; position it 8 inches from the top of the top sheet; open up the spread and let it hang free over the sides and bottom of the bed; fold the top sheet over the top edge of the spread.

10. Tuck both the top sheet and spread under the mattress at the foot of the bed on each side of the bed. Make a mitered corner with the top sheet and blanket or spread on both sides at the bottom of the bed; do not tuck it in as with the bottom sheet, but let it hang free.

11. Make a toe pleat by raising the top linen and making a 2-inch fold down by the feet (Fig. 18.10). Doing so allows for movement of the client's feet and prevents tight fitting linens from causing footdrop or pressure sores on the toes or heels.

12. Put on a pillowcase.
    a. Grasp the closed end of the pillowcase and turn the pillowcase inside out over the same hand holding it; with the same hand gasp the pillow in the middle of one end and slide the pillowcase down over the pillow with the other hand.
    b. Change the pillowcase daily or more frequently if necessary; pillowcases generally harbor the most microorganisms because of the secretions of the nose and mouth.
    c. Position the pillow at the head of the bed.

B. Making an occupied bed
1. Raise the side rail on the nonworking side of the bed to prevent the client from rolling off the bed.
2. Turn the client toward the nonworking side of the bed.
3. Position the pillow under the client's head to support functional alignment and prevent unnecessary strain on neck muscles.
4. Unfold a bath blanket over the client and remove the top linens from under the bath blanket. Doing so provides for privacy and supports comfort and warmth.
5. Loosen the soiled bottom linen and fanfold it toward the client, tucking it just under the legs, buttocks, back, and shoulders (Fig. 18.11).

🛑 6. Fanfold the clean linen up to just short of the edge of the soiled linen; it may be necessary to position a towel or pad between the soiled linen and clean linen (Fig. 18.12).

7. Raise the side rail and assist the client to turn to the other side of the bed; explain that it may feel like rolling over a "hump"; position the pillow under the client's head. This informs the client about what to expect and maintains the client's head in functional alignment.

Fig 18.10 Toe pleat. (From Wilkinson and Treas [2016]. *Fundamentals of nursing*, Vol. 2, 3rd ed. Philadelphia: F. A. Davis Company, with permission.)

Fig 18.11 Fanfolding dirty linen. (From Wilkinson and Treas [2016]. *Fundamentals of nursing*, Vol. 2, 3rd ed. Philadelphia: F. A. Davis Company, with permission.)

Fig 18.12 Fanfolding clean linen. (From Wilkinson and Treas [2016]. *Fundamentals of nursing*, Vol. 2, 3rd ed. Philadelphia: F. A. Davis Company, with permission.)

8. Go to the other side of the bed, lower the rail and remove the soiled linen by rolling it up into itself, hold it away from the body, and dispose of it in a soiled linen hamper or laundry bag; doing so contains soiled linen and avoids contaminating the caregiver or the environment. Do not put it on the floor or a chair.

Fig 18.13 Pulling through clean linen. (From Wilkinson and Treas [2016]. *Fundamentals of nursing*, Vol. 2, 3rd ed. Philadelphia: F. A. Davis Company, with permission.)

9. Pull through the clean linen from under the client and finish making the bed (Fig. 18.13).
10. Assist the client to the supine position in the middle of the bed and then reposition the pillow under the client's head.
11. Position the top sheet and spread over the bath blanket and remove the bath blanket from underneath.
12. Make the top of the bed and change the pillowcase as indicated in the procedure for an unoccupied bed.

CASE STUDY: Putting It All Together

A nurse is admitting a 70-year-old woman, who practices the Islam faith, from a nursing home to a medical unit at the local hospital. The client states that she has chronic back pain as a result of an automobile accident 6 months ago and is unable to care for herself. She spends a lot of time in bed or in a wheelchair and says, "If I don't move much, the pain is tolerable, but if I move even just a little bit, the pain becomes unbearable." The client was admitted for treatment of a large lesion at the base of the sacrum with exudate that has a foul odor and for pain management. The client states, "I avoid using a bedpan because it is so uncomfortable to use so I wet myself. I am embarrassed to call for help, so I just stay wet."

Case Study Questions

A. Considering that the client follows the Islam faith, what information is important when assigning caregivers to this client?

_____

B. List four components of a thorough assessment of the client's sacral lesion.

1. _____

2. _____

3. _____

4. _____

C. List at least three concerns the nurse may have because of the client's age and data.

1. _____

2. _____

3. _____

D. Identify at least four actions the nurse should implement when providing for this client's hygiene needs.

1. _____

2. _____

3. _____

4. _____

E. A principle related to hygiene is that bathing strokes should follow a specific directional progression based on the body part being washed. In which direction should the nurse wash the following areas of the body and explain your answer.

1. Eye: _____

_____

_____

2. Arms and legs: _____

_____

3. Female genitalia: _____

_____

4. Male genitalia: _____

_____

_____

REVIEW QUESTIONS

Be sure to read the Introduction for valuable test-taking tips.

1. A nurse teaches a new nursing assistant to give a partial bed bath. The nurse identifies that the teaching is understood when the nursing assistant makes which of the following statements?
   1. "I should help the client to wash the face, hands, underarms, back, and perineal area."
   2. "I must direct the client to wash as much as possible and assist with the rest."
   3. "I need to assist the client to wash only one part of the body at a time."
   4. "I will instruct the client to wash the face, hands, and perineal area."

2. A nurse educator is teaching a class about client hygiene and grooming to nursing assistants. What problem can be prevented by daily brushing of the client's hair that the nurse needs to include in the teaching?
   1. Pediculosis
   2. Dandruff
   3. Alopecia
   4. Tangles

3. A nurse is assessing a client's ability to perform activities of daily living. Place the following classifications of self-care abilities in order from the most independent to the most dependent.
   1. Requires help from another person for assistance or supervision
   2. Requires help from another person and equipment or device
   3. Totally dependent; does not participate in activity
   4. Requires use of equipment or device
   5. Completely independent
   Answer: _____

4. A nurse finishes assisting a client with a complete bed bath. What is **most** important for the nurse to do before leaving the client's room, besides moving the bed to its lowest position?
   1. Secure the call bell within easy reach.
   2. Place the overbed table next to the bed.
   3. Leave the door to the client's room open.
   4. Pull all the side rails up on both sides of the client's bed.

5. A nurse is caring for a client whose hair is dry and has a coarse texture with tight little curls. Which hair care implement should the nurse use when grooming this client's hair?

   1. A
   2. B
   3. C
   4. D

6. An adolescent with the diagnosis of severe nodular acne vulgaris is unresponsive to conventional therapy. The client is registered in the government-regulated iPledge program, and isotretinoin (Claravis) 0.5 mg/kg PO daily divided into two doses is prescribed. The adolescent weighs 132 lb. How many milligrams should the nurse administer for each dose?
   Answer: _____ mg

7. What action should the nurse include in the plan of care that is a common hygiene need of all older adults?
   1. Remove the bottom denture first.
   2. Assist with daily bathing.
   3. Apply a skin moisturizer.
   4. Use deodorant soap.

8. Which actions should be implemented when bathing a client? **Select all that apply.**
   1. Bathe from head to toe.
   2. Use contact precautions.
   3. Bathe from clean to dirty.
   4. Use warm water for bathing.
   5. Wash from proximal to distal for extremities.
   6. Change the water after perineal care, not before.

9. Which is the **most** important nursing action when making an occupied bed?
   1. Change all of the linens on the bed.
   2. Make just one side of the bed at a time.
   3. Put the side rail up on the nonworking side of the bed.
   4. Lower the head of the bed until the client is in the supine position.

10. How can a nurse **best** prevent footdrop in a client when making an occupied bed?
   1. Tuck the top sheet in loosely.
   2. Make a toe pleat in the top linens.
   3. Place the pillow under the client's ankles.
   4. Make a square corner when securing the client's bottom sheet.

11. A nurse is providing oral care for a client who is wearing full dentures. Which actions should the nurse implement when providing care for this client? **Select all that apply.**
   1. Clean dentures with cool water using a firm toothbrush and toothpaste.
   2. Use thumbs to push up gently on the bottom denture at the gum line to release the suction.
   3. Soak dentures overnight in a commercial dental cleanser if this is the preference of the client.
   4. Store dentures in a labeled dry denture cup in the bedside drawer if the client does not want to wear them.
   5. With a gauze pad, grasp the upper denture with the thumb and forefinger and move the denture up and down to release the suction.

12. Which should the nurse do **first** before initiating a.m. care with a client?
   1. Ask the client about preferences.
   2. Raise the bed to working height.
   3. Change the linens on the bed.
   4. Feed the client breakfast.

13. An unconscious client's mouth is dry and coated with sticky mucous from mouth breathing. Which actions are essential to prevent aspiration when providing oral care? **Select all that apply.**
   1. Insert 10 mL of diluted mouthwash with a syringe into the side of the mouth to remove toothpaste.
   2. Brush inner and outer teeth surfaces and the gum line with short circular motions.
   3. Use a moderate amount of toothpaste to cleanse the teeth and gums.
   4. Use a padded tongue blade to access various sections of the mouth.
   5. Use an unpadded tongue blade to scrap debris from the tongue.

14. A nurse washes a bed-bound client's entire body without assistance from the client. The nurse uses a washcloth, several basins of warm water, gentle soap, and a towel to dry the skin. What type of bath should the nurse record in the progress notes of the client's clinical record?
   1. Complete bath
   2. Partial bath
   3. Towel bath
   4. Bag bath

15. A nurse is providing care for a client with a hearing aid. Which should the nurse do when caring for this client? **Select all that apply.**
   1. Wipe the ear mold with a damp cloth and dry well.
   2. Ensure the client's hearing aid is turned off before insertion.
   3. Immerse the aid in warm soapy water and wash thoroughly weekly.
   4. Inspect the ear before insertion and after removal of the hearing aid.
   5. Remove earwax from the opening in the ear piece with the tool provided by the manufacturer.

16. A nurse, caring for a client with type I diabetes, includes foot care in the client's plan of care. What actions should be included in the plan? **Select all that apply.**
   1. Assess bilateral dorsalis pedis pulses daily.
   2. Use an antifungal powder liberally between the toes.
   3. Apply moisturizing lotion sparingly to the feet, avoiding between the toes.
   4. Trim the toenails straight across and smooth the edges with an emery board.
   5. Teach the client to inspect feet daily and use a mirror to see the soles of the feet.
   6. Soak the feet in a basin of warm water for half an hour before trimming toenails if they appear brittle.

17. A nurse performs a physical assessment of an older adult. Which observations does the nurse conclude are related to the aging process? **Select all that apply.**
   1. Dry, thin skin
   2. Thick toenails
   3. Fine, silky hair
   4. Translucent skin
   5. Sparse pubic hair

18. A nurse identifies the condition below when assessing a client. Which should the nurse document on the client's physical assessment form?

1. Macule
2. Fissure
3. Keloid
4. Scar

19. A nurse identifies that an older adult has long, torturous, yellow toenails. What should the nurse do?
1. File the client's toenails with an emery board.
2. Get a referral to a podiatrist to trim the toenails.
3. Cut the toenails straight across with a nail clipper.
4. Soak the client's feet in hot water to soften the toenails.

20. A nurse is preparing a class for adolescents about the common causes of problems with the teeth. Which problems should the nurse include? **Select all that apply.**
1. Periodontal disease
2. Dental caries
3. Stomatitis
4. Cheilosis
5. Halitosis

21. A nurse is caring for a comatose client. Which intervention is **essential** when providing eye care for this client?
1. Apply eye shields to protect the eyes.
2. Place a folded washcloth over the eyes to block the light.
3. Administer antibiotic eye drops daily to lubricate the eyes.
4. Wash the eyes from the inner to outer canthus every eight hours.

22. Which is **most** important to do, as evident in the photograph, when cleaning a client's dentures?

1. Place a washcloth in the bottom of the sink.
2. Ensure a continuous flow of water.
3. Brush the upper appliance first.
4. Wear sterile gloves.

23. What should the nurse do if a client with a urinary retention catheter experiences a urethral discharge? **Select all that apply.**
1. Increase oral fluid intake.
2. Provide more frequent catheter care.
3. Replace the catheter with a larger size.
4. Apply an antibiotic ointment to the perineal area.
5. Report the observation to the primary health-care provider.

24. A nurse is caring for several clients. Which client is at **greatest** risk for skin breakdown?
    1. Client who is dehydrated
    2. Client who has diaphoresis
    3. Client who is incontinent of feces
    4. Client who has difficulty moving up in bed

25. Which outcomes associated with physical hygiene are appropriate and should be included in a client's plan of care? **Select all that apply.**
    1. Will comb hair unassisted
    2. Offer pain medication before providing a bath
    3. Mouth is clean and free of debris after oral hygiene
    4. Provide clothing with Velcro fasteners instead of buttons
    5. Expresses satisfaction with body cleanliness after morning care

26. A nurse is planning nursing care for an older adult who was admitted to the hospital with a diagnosis of brain attack (cerebrovascular accident, stroke). After reviewing the client's clinical record, which of the following should the nurse identify as **most** important when providing for this client's hygiene and grooming needs?
    1. Providing a complete bed bath daily
    2. Pacing care to avoid activity intolerance
    3. Asking the client to choose personal bath products
    4. Implementing range-of-motion exercises during the bath

Client's Clinical Record

Vital Signs

Temperature: 97.8°F orally
Pulse: 98 beats/min
Respirations: 23 breaths/min, shallow
Blood pressure: 160/86 mm Hg
Oxygen saturation: 95% on room air while resting

Nurse's Progress Note

Client admitted 9 days ago with a diagnosis of brain attack. The client has half strength of the right upper and lower extremities. Client occasionally is incontinent of stool. States that the perineal area is tender; slight perianal erythema identified; skin barrier applied as per standing protocol. Able to turn on right side unassisted but needs assistance to turn on left side. High-top sneakers to prevent foot drop utilized at all times except when bathing and providing for range-of-motion exercises. Measured for hand/wrist and leg splint. Social worker visit to discuss posthospital rehabilitation plan of care.

27. Clients with which conditions should the nurse anticipate will need assistance in making decisions regarding hygiene care? **Select all that apply.**
    1. Moderate pain
    2. Altered reality
    3. Sensory deficit
    4. Limited mobility
    5. Developmental delay
    6. Short-term memory loss

28. A client with diabetes is admitted to the hospital with the concurrent diagnosis of peripheral vascular insufficiency. Which client assessments indicate that the vascular impairment is arterial rather than venous? **Select all that apply.**
    1. Skin of the lower extremities is pale when the legs are elevated.
    2. Distal capillary refill is less than 3 seconds.
    3. There is a lack of hair on the lower extremities.
    4. Toenails on both feet are translucent.
    5. Pain occurs in the legs with activity.
    6. Skin of the feet is warm to touch.

29. A child is diagnosed with a head lice infestation, and permethrin (Nix) is prescribed. What should the nurse recommend that the parents do to help control this infestation? **Select all that apply.**
    1. Soak bed linens in cold water daily.
    2. Brush the hair vigorously twice a day.
    3. Ensure that everyone in the family is treated.
    4. Comb hair with a fine-tooth comb to remove nits.
    5. Wash hair for 5 minutes with the prescribed shampoo.
    6. Seal nonwashable items in plastic bags for a minimum of 2 weeks.

30. Which actions should nurses take to reduce the risk of transmitting microbes in a hospital setting? **Select all that apply.**
    1. Wash the hands when entering a client's room.
    2. Bring the linen hamper into a client's room.
    3. Use alcohol-based hand cleaners.
    4. Avoid wearing dangling apparel.
    5. Keep fingernails short.

REVIEW ANSWERS AND RATIONALES

1. ANSWER: 1.

Rationales:

1. The face, hands, underarms, back, and perineal area should be washed daily because they harbor the most microorganisms.

2. Directing the client to wash as much as possible and assist with the rest is considered a complete bed bath with assistance, not a partial bed bath.

3. Assisting the client to wash only one part of the body at a time is considered a complete bed bath with assistance.

4. The axillary areas and the back must also be washed along with the areas presented in option 3 in a partial bed bath.

TEST-TAKING TIP: Identify the option with a specific determiner. Option 3 contains the word *only*, which is a specific determiner.

Content Area: *Tissue Integrity and Hygiene*
Integrated Processes: *Teaching/Learning; Communication and Documentation; Nursing Process: Evaluation*
Client Need: *Physiological Integrity; Basic Care and Comfort*
Cognitive Level: *Application*
Concept: *Patient-Centered Care; Tissue Integrity*

2. ANSWER: 4.

Rationales:

1. Pediculosis is caused by direct contact with lice or their eggs (nits); brushing the hair will not prevent head lice.

2. Shampooing the hair and rubbing the scalp help to limit dandruff.

3. Loss of hair (alopecia) may be caused by nutritional, emotional, iatrogenic, and genetic factors; it is not prevented by brushing.

4. Brushing separates tangles and evenly distributes secretions and oils down the hair shafts.

Content Area: *Tissue Integrity and Hygiene*
Integrated Processes: *Teaching/Learning; Nursing Process: Planning*
Client Need: *Physiological Integrity; Basic Care and Comfort*
Cognitive Level: *Application*
Concept: *Patient-Centered Care; Tissue Integrity*

3. ANSWER: 5, 4, 1, 2, 3.

Rationales:

5. A person who is able to provide complete self-care is the most independent.

4. A person who is completely independent but uses equipment or a device to provide self-care is the second-most independent person of the options offered.

1. A person who requires some assistance or supervision from another person is the third-most independent person of the options offered.

2. A person who needs help from another person and equipment is more in need of help than a person who only needs assistance or supervision from another person.

3. A person who is totally dependent and is unable to participate in activities is the most dependent person of the options offered.

Content Area: *Tissue Integrity and Hygiene*
Integrated Processes: *Nursing Process: Analysis*
Client Need: *Safe and Effective Care Environment; Management of Care*
Cognitive Level: *Analysis*
Concept: *Patient-Centered Care; Safety*

4. ANSWER: 1.

Rationales:

1. It is most important that a client have the ability to call for help when needed. It is a major safety issue.

2. Although moving the overbed table next to the client's bed is helpful, it is not essential.

3. The client may prefer to have the door closed. The nurse should determine the client's preference.

4. Pulling up all of the side rails of a bed without the client's consent is considered a restraint. A nurse can engage all of the side rails of a bed if it is necessary to maintain the safety of the client, but the need for their use must be documented by the nurse and prescribed by the primary health-care provider.

TEST-TAKING TIP: Identify the word in the stem that sets a priority. The word *most* in the stem sets a priority. Identify the option with a specific determiner. Option 4 contains the word *all*, which is a specific determiner.

Content Area: *Tissue Integrity and Hygiene*
Integrated Processes: *Nursing Process: Implementation*
Client Need: *Safe and Effective Care Environment; Safety and Infection Control*
Cognitive Level: *Application*
Concept: *Safety*

5. ANSWER: 3.

Rationales:

1. This is a regular-tooth comb for hair that is straight, relaxed, or slightly curly and has a regular or fine texture. A regular-tooth comb can be used on curly hair if used gently.

2. This is a brush that helps to remove tangles; massage the scalp, which increases circulation; and move oil down the hair shafts proximal to distal. It is used for hair that is straight or curly and has a regular or fine texture.

3. A wide-tooth comb is used for hair that is dry and has a coarse texture to limit hair breakage. Applying mineral oil or moisturizing hair cream before combing also helps to minimize hair breakage.

4. This is a fine-tooth comb mainly used to remove head lice eggs (nits) after the scalp and hair are treated with an antiparasitic agent.

Content Area: *Tissue Integrity and Hygiene*
Integrated Processes: *Nursing Process: Implementation*
Client Need: *Physiological Integrity; Basic Care and Comfort*
Cognitive Level: *Analysis*
Concept: *Tissue Integrity*

with this type of bath, and it takes less time than a traditional bath. Often, it is a method of choice for clients with mild to moderate impaired skin integrity, activity intolerance, or cognitive impairment.

4. A bag bath refers to bathing a client with premoistened, disposable washcloths. This product generally contains a no-rinse surfactant, a diluent substance to trap moisture (humectant), and an emollient. Research demonstrates that this type of bathing system reduces overall skin dryness, skin flaking, and scaling. It is preferred in critical care and long-term care settings for clients who are unable to bathe themselves. The package of 8 to 10 disposable washcloths is warmed in a microwave in preparation for use.

TEST-TAKING TIP: Identify the obscure clang association. The word *entire* in the stem and the word *complete* in option 1 is an obscure clang association.

Content Area: Tissue Integrity and Hygiene
Integrated Processes: Communication and Documentation; Nursing Process: Implementation
Client Need: Physiological Integrity; Basic Care and Comfort
Cognitive Level: Analysis
Concept: Tissue Integrity

15. **ANSWER: 1, 2, 4, 5.**
    Rationales:
    1. **A damp cloth will remove dirt and debris from the ear mold and drying well will prevent moisture from damaging the mechanism of the hearing aid.**
    2. **A hearing aid should be off during insertion. Once inserted, the hearing aid should be turned on and the volume adjusted from the lowest setting to the setting of the client's preference. This provides for client comfort.**
    3. Immersing a hearing aid in warm soapy water will destroy the mechanism of the hearing aid.
    4. **An ear should be inspected before insertion and after removal of a hearing aid; ear wax and debris may collect in the external auditory canal, and pressure of the ear mold may irritate the tissues of the ear.**
    5. **Ear wax can collect in the opening of the ear mold. An instrument provided with the hearing aid allows for removal of the ear wax so that sound can be transmitted unobstructed from the environment to the tympanic membrane of the ear.**

    TEST-TAKING TIP: Identify the options with clang associations. The words *hearing aid* in the stem and in options 2 and 4 are clang associations. Examine options 2 and 4 carefully.

    Content Area: Tissue Integrity and Hygiene
    Integrated Processes: Nursing Process: Implementation
    Client Need: Physiological Integrity; Basic Care and Comfort
    Cognitive Level: Application
    Concept: Sensory Perception

16. **ANSWER: 1, 3, 5.**
    Rationales:
    1. **Decreased circulation to the feet is a complication of diabetes because the basement membrane of capillaries**

becomes impaired. Assessing the dorsalis pedis pulses daily monitors the quality of peripheral circulation and is considered part of care of the feet.
    2. Antifungal powder should be applied only if prescribed by a primary health-care provider for athlete's foot; if prescribed, it should be used sparingly, not liberally. An excessive amount of a powdered substance, when moistened, becomes sandpaper-like, which can contribute to further skin breakdown.
    3. **Applying moisturizing lotion sparingly to the feet, avoiding between the toes is an appropriate nursing action. Excessive moisturizing lotion, especially between the toes, may cause skin maceration or a fungal infection.**
    4. A podiatrist, not a nurse, should trim the toenails of a client who has diabetes. An emery board should be avoided because, if not used properly, it can cause an abrasion and foot-related complications. Breaks in the skin of the feet of a client who has diabetes may not heal and may become gangrenous, leading to an amputation.
    5. **It is important that a client who has diabetes inspect the feet thoroughly every day. Early recognition and treatment of a problem may prevent a more serious complication.**
    6. Soaking the feet of a client who has diabetes should be avoided because it removes natural oils, causing skin cracks. Also, the appropriate temperature for foot soaks (e.g., 105° to 115°F) may cause burns in a client who has diabetes. Foot soaks for individuals without foot problems should last only 5 to 10 minutes because it removes natural oils, causing skin cracks.

    TEST-TAKING TIP: Identify the slightly obscure clang associations. The word *foot* in the stem and the word *feet* in options 3, 5, and 6 are clang associations. Examine these options carefully. Options 3 and 5 are correct answers. Option 6 is a distractor.

    Content Area: Tissue Integrity and Hygiene
    Integrated Processes: Communication and Documentation; Nursing Process: Planning
    Client Need: Physiological Integrity; Reduction of Risk Potential
    Cognitive Level: Application
    Concept: Tissue Integrity

17. **ANSWER: 1, 2, 4, 5.**
    Rationales:
    1. **Dry, thin skin is associated with aging. The skin is dry because sebaceous and sweat glands are less active. The skin appears thinner because of the loss of dermis and subcutaneous fat.**
    2. **Thick toenails are associated with slow nail growth related to aging.**
    3. Fine, silky hair is not a result of aging. Fine, silky hair is associated with hyperthyroidism. Thin, dry, graying hair is associated with aging. Graying hair occurs as the number of pigment cells in hair bulbs (melanocytes) decrease, causing darker hair to be replaced with nonpigmented hair. A reduction in thyroid hormone production can cause the hair to have a coarse texture and slower rate of

growth as well as increased hair loss. Thyroid hormone affects cell division at the hair follicle.

4. The skin of older adults is translucent due to loss of dermis and subcutaneous fat associated with aging.

5. Sparse pubic hair is associated with hormone decline that occurs with aging. Overall hair loss is specifically linked with a decrease in testosterone and thyroid hormone levels.

Content Area: Tissue Integrity and Hygiene
Integrated Processes: Nursing Process: Analysis
Client Need: Physiological Integrity; Basic Care and Comfort
Cognitive Level: Application
Concept: Tissue Integrity

18. **ANSWER: 3.**
Rationales:
1. A macule is a flat, circumscribed area from 1 to several centimeters in size. Examples include cherry angioma, freckles, flat pigmented moles, and measles.
2. A fissure is a linear crack in the skin. Examples include cheilitis and athlete's foot.
3. A keloid is a raised, irregular scar due to excess collagen formation (hypertrophic scar). Examples of common sites include surgical incisions, body piercings, and tattoos.
4. A scar is the formation of replacement connective tissue and fibrotic changes following healing of a wound. Examples of common sites include surgical incisions and cuts.
Content Area: Tissue Integrity and Hygiene
Integrated Processes: Communication and Documentation; Nursing Process: Analysis
Client Need: Physiological Integrity; Physiological Adaptation
Cognitive Level: Analysis
Concept: Tissue Integrity

19. **ANSWER: 2.**
Rationales:
1. Filing the toenails with an emery board is unsafe and may injure already impaired tissues.
2. Long, torturous, yellow toenails often are associated with problems such as impaired arterial circulation to the feet or a fungal infection. The nails usually are thick, brittle, and difficult to trim. These toenails should be cut by an appropriate practitioner.
3. Cutting the toenails straight across with a nail clipper is unsafe and may injure already impaired tissues. Clients with normal nails may provide self-care in the home by cutting the toenails straight across. This technique prevents ingrown toenails.
4. Yellow toenails indicate that the client may have inadequate perfusion to the distal extremities. Often, this is accompanied by altered sensation in the extremities. Warm, not hot, water should be used to wash the feet to prevent injury to impaired tissues. A podiatrist may prescribe that the feet be soaked for a short period of time just prior to clipping because it can soften the toenails.

TEST-TAKING TIP: Identify the option that is unique. Option 2 is unique. It is the only option that does not provide direct care to the client's feet or toenails.
Content Area: Tissue Integrity and Hygiene
Integrated Processes: Nursing Process: Implementation
Client Need: Safe and Effective Care Environment; Management of Care
Cognitive Level: Application
Concept: Tissue Integrity

20. **ANSWER: 1, 2.**
Rationales:
1. Periodontal disease (pyorrhea) is one of the most common causes of tooth loss. Bleeding and receding gums and destruction of adjacent bone structures lead to infected gums and loosening of teeth that may require their removal.
2. Dental caries (cavities) generally are caused by failure to remove an invisible, destructive bacterial coating that builds up on teeth and destroys the enamel. The nurse should teach people to avoid refined sugars, to floss and brush the teeth at least three times during the day, and to consult a dentist at least two times a year for an oral assessment and appropriate intervention, including plaque removal.
3. Stomatitis, an inflammation of the oral mucosa, is not one of the most common causes of problems with the teeth. Stomatitis is caused by mechanical trauma, irritants, nutritional deficiencies, and systemic infection. This is not a problem with teeth.
4. Cheilosis is a cracking and ulceration seen as reddened fissures at the angles of the mouth, generally caused by vitamin B–complex deficiencies. This is not a problem with teeth.
5. Halitosis, or bad breath, is not a cause of problems with the teeth. It is a sign of inadequate oral hygiene; dental caries; infection of the mouth; tobacco use; systemic disease, such as liver disease or diabetes; and the eating of such foods as garlic and onions.
Content Area: Tissue Integrity and Hygiene
Integrated Processes: Teaching/Learning; Nursing Process: Planning
Client Need: Health Promotion and Maintenance
Cognitive Level: Application
Concept: Health Promotion; Tissue Integrity

21. **ANSWER: 1.**
Rationales:
1. Eye shields protect the eyes of a comatose client; they prevent debris from entering the eyes and trauma from linens; they limit drying of ocular structures, particularly if they are a humidified eye shield.
2. A folded washcloth over the eyes may damage the client's corneas.
3. Antibiotic eye drops treat an eye infection; they are not used to lubricate the eyes of a comatose client. Saline eye drops or artificial tears may be used to lubricate the eyes. Also, the primary health-care provider may prescribe a lubricating ointment to protect the eyes from becoming dry.
4. Eight hours is too long a time period between cleansing the eyes of a comatose client. The client should have eye

care every 2 to 4 hours and whenever necessary. It is correct technique to wash the eyes from the inner to outer canthus to minimize contamination of the lacrimal duct with debris from the eye.

TEST-TAKING TIP: Identify the word in the stem that sets a priority. The word *essential* in the stem sets a priority.
Content Area: Tissue Integrity and Hygiene
Integrated Processes: Nursing Process: Implementation
Client Need: Physiological Integrity; Reduction of Risk Potential
Cognitive Level: Application
Concept: Tissue Integrity

22. **ANSWER: 1.**
Rationales:
1. **Of the four options presented, the placement of a washcloth in the bottom of the sink is the most important action. This minimizes the risk of damaging the denture if the nurse should accidentally drop the denture in the sink.**
2. The flow of water does not have to be continuous; it has to flow only when rinsing the denture cleanser off the denture after being cleaned.
3. It does not matter which denture is cleansed first.
4. Clean, not sterile, gloves are necessary to protect the nurse from the client's oral secretions when cleaning a client's dentures.

TEST-TAKING TIP: Identify the word in the stem that sets a priority. The word *most* in the stem sets a priority.
Content Area: Tissue Integrity and Hygiene
Integrated Processes: Nursing Process: Implementation
Client Need: Physiological Integrity; Basic Care and Comfort
Cognitive Level: Analysis
Concept: Safety

23. **ANSWER: 2, 5.**
Rationales:
1. Increasing oral fluids will not decrease the urethral discharge.
2. **More frequent catheter care will remove secretions, reducing the risk of skin breakdown and infection. The nurse should notify the primary health-care provider of the urethral discharge. It may be due to irritation from the catheter, but it could also be a sign of an infectious process requiring medical intervention.**
3. A larger catheter is indicated if urine leakage occurs around a catheter, not by the presence of a urethral discharge.
4. Application of an antibiotic ointment is a dependent function of the nurse and requires a prescription by a primary health-care provider.
5. **A urethral discharge may be due to irritation from the catheter, but it could also be a sign of an infectious process requiring medical intervention.**

TEST-TAKING TIP: Identify the options with a clang association. The stem and options 2 and 3 contain the word *catheter,* which are clang associations. Carefully consider options 2 and 3. Option 2 is a correct answer and option 3 is a distractor. An option with a clang association is often, but *not always,* a correct answer.

Content Area: Tissue Integrity and Hygiene
Integrated Processes: Nursing Process: Implementation
Client Need: Physiological Integrity; Reduction of Risk Potential
Cognitive Level: Application
Concept: Tissue Integrity

24. **ANSWER: 3.**
Rationales:
1. Although a decrease in interstitial fluid is a risk factor for skin breakdown, it is not as great a risk factor as that which is presented in another option.
2. Although the secretions of sweat glands (perspiration) increase moisture on the skin causing maceration of skin, perspiration is not as destructive as that which is presented in another option.
3. **Feces contain fluid and digestive enzymes that injure the skin if not removed immediately. In addition, urine contains urea and is acidic. Urine and feces can cause loss of superficial layers of the skin (excoriation, denuded skin).**
4. Although people who have difficulty moving up in bed may slide up in bed, exerting a frictional resistance between the skin and the bed (shearing force), they can be taught to use an overbed trapeze that eliminates this problem.

TEST-TAKING TIP: Identify the word in the stem that sets a priority. The word *greatest* in the stem sets a priority.
Content Area: Tissue Integrity and Hygiene
Integrated Processes: Nursing Process: Analysis
Client Need: Physiological Integrity; Basic Care and Comfort
Cognitive Level: Analysis
Concept: Tissue Integrity

25. **ANSWER: 3, 5.**
Rationales:
1. "Will comb hair unassisted" is an incomplete outcome statement because it does not establish a time frame when it should be achieved.
2. "Offer pain medication before providing a bath" is a nursing intervention, not a client-centered goal.
3. **"Mouth is clean and free of debris after oral hygiene" is an acceptable outcome statement. It objectively establishes the criteria for achievement, *mouth is clean and free of debris,* and it establishes a time frame in which it should be achieved, *after oral hygiene.***
4. "Provide clothing with Velcro fasteners instead of buttons" is a nursing intervention, not a client-centered goal.
5. **"Expresses satisfaction with body cleanliness after morning care" is an appropriate outcome. It objectively establishes the criteria for achievement, *expresses satisfaction with body cleanliness,* and it establishes a time frame in which it should be achieved, *after morning care.***

Content Area: Tissue Integrity and Hygiene
Integrated Processes: Communication and Documentation; Nursing Process: Planning
Client Need: Safe and Effective Care Environment; Management of Care
Cognitive Level: Application
Concept: Patient-Centered Care; Tissue Integrity

26. ANSWER: 2.

Rationales:

1. A complete bath generally is unnecessary for a client who is an older adult because of decreased sebaceous gland activity and increased drying of skin associated with aging. A complete bath twice a week and partial baths and perineal care provided when necessary is most appropriate when meeting the hygiene needs of an older adult.

2. Providing for the client's hygiene needs without causing activity intolerance is the most important action presented. Older adults experience a decrease in lung expansion and reduced vital capacity due to weakened thoracic muscles and calcification of costal cartilage associated with aging. Also, older adults have a decreased ability to deliver and diffuse oxygen to cells due to changes in respiratory and vascular tissues secondary to the aging process. This client's respiratory status (increased respiratory rate, shallow respirations, and oxygen saturation at the lower range of normal) indicates impaired respiratory functioning. The nurse should avoid unnecessarily straining the client physically.

3. Although it is important to provide the client with the opportunity to participate in care by making choices because choices support a sense of control, it is not the most important action of the options presented.

4. Although range-of-motion exercises should be implemented when providing care to this client, it is not the most important action of the options presented.

TEST-TAKING TIP: Identify the word in the stem that sets a priority. The word *most* in the stem sets a priority. Identify the option that is unique. Option 2 is the only option that contains a rationale. Examine option 2 carefully. Use Maslow's hierarchy of needs and Airway, Breathing, and Circulation (ABCs) to help establish the priority. Meeting a client's need for oxygen is a first-level need, according to Maslow, and breathing, according to the ABCs, is essential for life. Preventing activity intolerance is the most important option of the options presented.

Content Area: Tissue Integrity and Hygiene
Integrated Processes: Communication and Documentation; Nursing Process: Planning
Client Need: Physiological Integrity; Basic Care and Comfort
Cognitive Level: Analysis
Concept: Patient-Centered Care; Oxygenation

27. ANSWER: 2, 5, 6.

Rationales:

1. Pain may limit a person's ability to participate in hygiene care but should not impair one's ability to make independent decisions regarding care.

2. Altered reality related to delusions, hallucinations, or impaired cognition may impair a person's ability to make personal care decisions.

3. Sensory deficits may interfere with a client's ability to perform hygiene care independently; however, it should not interfere with the person's ability to make independent decisions regarding care.

4. Limited mobility may interfere with a client's ability to perform hygiene care independently; however, it should not interfere with the person's ability to make independent decisions regarding care.

5. A developmental delay is a maturational lag whereby an individual matures at a slower rate than an individual of the same age who consistently meets developmental milestones. An individual with a developmental delay may not be cognitively capable of making decisions about their own hygiene care.

6. An individual with short-term memory loss has a decreased ability to register, retain, and retrieve information and may not be capable of making decisions about his or her hygiene care. In addition, impaired attention span and possible perceptual distortions of incoming stimuli occur with loss of short-term memory, which will affect whether or not a person can make decisions about his or her hygiene care.

Content Area: Tissue Integrity and Hygiene
Integrated Processes: Caring; Nursing Process: Planning
Client Need: Physiological Integrity; Basic Care and Comfort
Cognitive Level: Application
Concept: Cognition

28. ANSWER: 1, 3, 5.

Rationales:

1. Inadequate circulation to the legs and feet causes the skin to appear pale when the legs and feet are elevated. When the legs are dependent, they may develop a dusky red color known as *dependent rubor*.

2. When blanching returns to pink after release of compression of peripheral tissues it indicates that cardiac output and circulation to the feet are adequate. Capillary refill that takes longer than 3 seconds, or longer than 5 seconds in an older adult, indicates impaired cardiac or peripheral vascular functioning.

3. Prolonged lack of oxygen to hair follicles results in lack of hair on the legs. Hair loss begins distally and progressively moves upward. The abrupt demarcation between where there is hair and a lack of hair gives it the appearance of a sock where there is no hair (sock effect).

4. Healthy toenails are translucent (i.e., not transparent but allows for slight penetration by light rays) or have variations of pink. Arterial insufficiency will cause the toenails to be yellow, thick, and brittle.

5. With arterial insufficiency, not enough oxygen is able to reach the muscles during activity, resulting in pain. The pain resolves once the activity is stopped.

6. The skin of the feet should feel warm to touch with adequate arterial circulation because warm blood reaches the capillary beds of the feet. The feet will feel cool to touch when there is impaired peripheral arterial circulation to the feet.

Content Area: Tissue Integrity and Hygiene
Integrated Processes: Nursing Process: Assessment
Client Need: Physiological Integrity; Reduction of Risk Potential
Cognitive Level: Analysis
Concept: Perfusion

29. **ANSWER: 3, 4, 6.**

Rationales:

1. Bed linens should be washed in hot, not cold, water and dried in a dryer to kill lice and their eggs (nits).

2. The hair should be treated with the prescribed medication and then combed with a fine-tooth comb to remove dead lice and nits.

3. **Head lice are an easily transmitted infestation. All members of the household must be treated to prevent repeated cross contamination.**

4. **Combing the hair with a fine-tooth comb after use of the antiparasitic shampoo is the most effective way to remove dead lice and lice eggs (nits).**

5. The hair must be washed and then treated for 10 minutes with Nix, which contains permethrin, the active ingredient that kills head lice.

6. **Head lice can live for 24 hours, and nits can survive for 7 to 12 days away from a client's head. Therefore, containing nonwashable items in a sealed plastic bag for 14 days will decontaminate nonwashable items.**

Content Area: Tissue Integrity and Hygiene
Integrated Processes: Teaching/Learning; Nursing Process: Implementation
Client Need: Physiological Integrity; Pharmacological and Parenteral Therapies
Cognitive Level: Application
Concept: Medication; Infection

30. **ANSWER: 1, 3, 4, 5.**

Rationales:

1. **Hand washing is the single most important way to prevent the transmission of microbes. Soap, water, friction, and rinsing the hands limit the amount of microorganisms on the hands.**

2. The linen hamper should not be brought into a client's room because it is a vector that can transmit microorganisms. The linen hamper should be left in the hall just outside a client's room.

3. **Although not as effective as washing with soap and water, alcohol-based hand cleaners are effective in limiting the amount of most microorganisms on the hands.**

4. **Dangling apparel has the potential of touching a client's clothing or bed linens. Contaminated apparel can act as a vector when the health-care provider visits another client.**

5. **Keeping fingernails short can help prevent the spread of microbes by eliminating areas where they can collect and multiply.**

Content Area: Tissue Integrity and Hygiene
Integrated Processes: Nursing Process: Implementation
Client Need: Physiological Integrity; Safety and Infection Control
Cognitive Level: Application
Concept: Safety

Chapter 19

Oxygenation

NURSING CONCEPTS

Acid/Base Balance
Collaboration
Communication
Growth and Development
Medication

Neurologic Regulation
Oxygenation
Patient-Centered Care
Perfusion
Sleep and Rest

KEY TERMS

Accessory muscles of respiration—Use of intercostal, abdominal, and trapezius muscles to help expand the chest cavity

Aspiration—Breathing foreign matter into the lungs

Atelectasis—Incomplete expansion of the lung

Barrel chest—Increase in anteroposterior diameter of the thoracic cavity

Clubbing—Bulbous swelling of the soft tissue of the end of the phalanx of fingers, causing the nail plates to be equal to or greater than 180 degrees

Cor pulmonale—Right-sided heart failure

Diaphragmatic (abdominal) breathing—Expansion of the abdomen on deep inhalation and tightening of the abdominal muscles on exhalation, increasing the amount of air entering and exiting the lungs

Dyspnea—Difficulty breathing

Exertional dyspnea—Difficulty breathing with activity

Expectoration—Coughing up and spitting out of sputum

External respiration—Gas exchange at the alveolar-capillary junction

Expiratory grunting—When a grunt or moan occurs at the beginning of exhalation as the glottis opens; it is caused by the sound of air expelled through the larynx.

Hypercarbia (hypercapnia)—Increased level of carbon dioxide in the blood

Hypocarbia (hypocapnia)—Decreased level of carbon dioxide in the blood

Hypoxemia—Decreased level of oxygen in the blood

Hypoxia—Inadequate oxygen in organs and tissues

Incentive spirometer—Device that provides a visual goal to increase the volume of breaths

Internal respiration—Gas exchange at the capillary-tissue junction

Nasal flaring—Widening of nares during inhalation that reduces resistance to airflow

Nebulizer—Device with a mouthpiece or mask placed over the nose that produces a medicated aerosol spray that is inhaled

Orthopnea—Difficulty breathing in the supine position, necessitating an upright position to breathe

Orthopneic (tripod) position—Forward-leaning position utilized while sitting to facilitate breathing

Oximetry—Identification of the oxygen saturation of arterial blood

Paroxysmal nocturnal dyspnea—Extreme shortness of breath during sleep that causes an abrupt awakening and immediate need to assume the upright position for relief

Pneumothorax—Air or gas in the pleural cavity

Postural drainage—Sequential positioning of a client in a variety of positions that use gravity to drain secretions from lobes of the lungs

Pursed-lip breathing—Exhalation through the mouth with lips creating a small opening to prolong exhalation, which keeps alveoli open longer for gas exchange

Continued

I. The Respiratory System

The exchange of oxygen and carbon dioxide in the body is essential for life. This exchange takes place in the lungs and at the cellular level. The mechanisms of respiration are complex and require an integration of factors involving the nervous system, chemoreceptors in the cardiovascular system, as well as the respiratory system. Knowledge of the anatomy and physiology that influences breathing is the basis for understanding how to best care for clients with oxygenation problems.

A. Structures of the respiratory system (Fig. 19.1)
 1. Airways.
    a. Consist of *upper airways* (located above the larynx; include nasal passages, oral cavity, and pharynx) and *lower airways* (located below the larynx; include trachea, bronchi, and bronchioles).
    b. Humidify the air: Moist mucous membranes add water to the inhaled air.
    c. Warm the air: Heat is transferred from the blood circulating in the capillary beds of the airways to the inhaled air.
    d. Filter the air: Sticky mucus traps debris, and tiny hairlike projections from the walls of the airway *(cilia)* move debris up and out of the airway.
 2. Lungs.
    a. Soft, spongy, cone-shaped organs.
    b. Right lung has three lobes, and left lung has two lobes.
    c. Each lung extends from its top portion (apex), which is just above the clavicle, to its bottom portion (base), which rests on the diaphragm.
    d. Composed of tiny, thin-walled air sacks *(alveoli)* surrounded by an extensive network of capillaries.
    e. Alveoli consist of type I cells that are involved with gas exchange and type II cells that produce a lipoprotein that lowers the surface tension to facilitate alveoli inflation.

B. Functions of the respiratory system
 1. Ventilation.
    a. Movement of air into and out of the lungs through the process of breathing.
    b. Involves inhalation and exhalation.
       (1) *Inhalation:* Expansion of the chest cavity and lungs resulting from contraction of the diaphragm that pulls the chest cavity downward and contraction of the intercostal muscles that pulls the ribs outward; lung expansion causes negative pressure that draws air into the respiratory system.
       (2) *Exhalation:* Chest cavity and lungs return to their original size and position when the diaphragm and intercostal muscles relax; this is a passive response that requires no effort.
    c. Factors that affect adequacy of ventilation.
       (1) Respiratory rate and depth: Fast, deep respirations result in hyperventilation; slow, shallow respirations result in hypoventilation.
       (2) Lung compliance: Extent of effort to inflate the lungs; conditions such as pulmonary edema and inadequate surfactant cause reduced lung compliance.
       (3) Airway resistance: Impairment of airflow within the airways; conditions that reduce the diameter of the airways, such as excess respiratory secretions and bronchospasms, cause increased airway resistance.
       (4) Lung elasticity: Ability of elastin fibers to return to their original position during exhalation; conditions that overstretch the alveoli, such as emphysema, result in a reduction of elastic recoil, leaving excess air trapped in the alveoli at the end of exhalation.
 2. Respiration.
    a. Exchange of gases that provides oxygenation of blood and body tissues and elimination of carbon dioxide from the lungs.
    b. Occurs at two levels, known as external and internal respiration (Fig. 19.2).
       (1) External respiration.
          (a) **External respiration** involves alveolar-capillary gas exchange.
          (b) Oxygen diffuses from the alveoli, through the alveolar capillaries, and into the blood.

Fig 19.1 Anterior view of the respiratory system. The upper airway lies above the larynx. The lower airway, located below the larynx, is considered sterile. (From Scanlon [2015]. *Essentials of anatomy and physiology*, 7th ed. Philadelphia: F. A. Davis Company, with permission.)

(c) Carbon dioxide diffuses out of the blood, through the alveolar capillaries, and into the alveoli.

(d) Rate of diffusion depends on the thickness of the membranes and extent of lung tissue.

(e) Conditions that impair external respiration include pleural effusion, bronchospasm, excessive secretions, and air or gas in the pleural cavity **(pneumothorax).**

(2) Internal respiration.

(a) **Internal respiration** involves capillary-tissue gas exchange.

(b) Oxygen diffuses from the blood, through the peripheral capillaries, and into tissue cells; oxygen is used for cellular metabolism.

(c) Carbon dioxide, which is a waste product of cellular metabolism, diffuses from tissue cells, through the peripheral

capillaries, and is transported via the blood to the lungs for exhalation.

(d) The effectiveness of internal respiration depends on adequate peripheral circulation and external respiration.

(e) Conditions that impair internal respiration include peripheral arterial and venous occlusive diseases; decreased cardiac output; impaired oxygen-carrying capacity of the blood, such as in anemia; and conditions that increase metabolism, such as fever, cancer, and hyperthyroidism.

c. Regulated by various mechanisms.

(1) The respiratory center, located in the medulla oblongata in the brain stem, sends impulses to the phrenic nerve, which precipitate contraction of the diaphragm and intercostal muscles.

(2) Chemoreceptors in the medulla, carotid arteries, and aorta identify changes in the

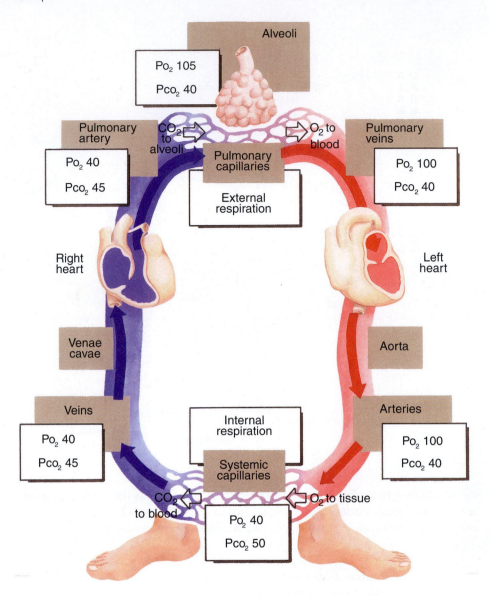

Fig 19.2 External and internal respiration. (From Scanlon [2015]. *Essentials of anatomy and physiology*, 7th ed. Philadelphia: F. A. Davis Company, with permission.)

level of circulating carbon dioxide, pH, and oxygen and send a message to the medulla to increase or decrease respirations accordingly.

(a) When the carbon dioxide level increases and the pH and oxygen levels decrease, the rate and depth of respirations increase.

(b) When the carbon dioxide level decreases and the oxygen and pH levels increase, the rate and depth of respirations return to normal.

(3) The system involves a feedback loop to return to usual respirations when circulating gases and pH are within expected levels.

(4) Regulation of respirations is usually under involuntary control; however, voluntary control via messages from the cerebral cortex can override involuntary control by the medulla for activities

such as swimming, talking, swallowing, and whistling.

d. Internal respirations can be disturbed by problems that affect gas exchange.

(1) **Hypoxemia** is a decreased level of oxygen in the blood.

(2) **Hypoxia** is inadequate oxygen in organs and tissues due to hypoxemia or circulatory disorders.

(a) Early clinical indicators: Restlessness, irritability, anxiety, tachypnea, tachycardia, headache, disorientation, and decreased level of consciousness.

(b) Late clinical indicators: Retractions, bradypnea, bradycardia, cardiac dysrhythmias, and cyanosis.

(3) **Hypercarbia (hypercapnia)** is increased level of carbon dioxide in the blood; may be due to an acute problem,

such as airway obstruction or drug overdose, or associated with chronic lung diseases.

(4) **Hypocarbia (hypocapnia)** is decreased level of carbon dioxide in the blood due to hyperventilation.

(5) Infections: Conditions include upper respiratory infections, such as colds; conditions that affect the lower respiratory tract, such as bronchitis, pneumonia, and tuberculosis; and conditions that can involve both the upper and lower respiratory tracts, such as influenza.

(6) Conditions that impede inhalation: Includes such conditions as fractured ribs, kyphosis, laryngospasm, and food/foreign body obstruction.

(7) Alveolar-capillary membrane problems: Includes conditions that interfere with the exchange of gases within the alveoli, such as pulmonary edema, emphysema, and pulmonary fibrosis.

(8) Inadequate lung surface for gas exchange: Includes such conditions as alveolar collapse, incomplete expansion of the lung (**atelectasis**), pleural effusion, and pneumothorax.

(9) Pulmonary circulation problems: Includes conditions that interfere with circulation to the alveolar capillary beds; thrombus entry into pulmonary artery (*pulmonary embolus*); and increased pressure within the pulmonary arterial system causing right-sided heart failure (**cor pulmonale**).

II. Factors That Affect Respiratory Function

The respiratory system does not function within an enclosed vacuum. It interacts with other physiological processes within the body and with issues external to the body. Factors that influence respiratory functioning include a person's age, multiple environmental stressors, various lifestyle behaviors, and pregnancy. Understanding these factors provides a basis for future nursing assessments and nursing interventions in relation to a client's respiratory status.

A. Developmental level
1. Infants (particularly premature infants).
   a. Airways are narrow, small, and immature.
   b. Central nervous system is immature, leading to impaired breathing patterns and periods of apnea.
   c. Small structures and immature immune systems increase the risk of respiratory infections.
   d. Putting small objects in mouth may lead to mechanical obstruction of the airway.
   e. Respiratory distress and sudden infant death syndrome are associated with this age group.
2. Toddlers and preschoolers.
   a. Tonsils and adenoids are large, increasing the risk of tonsillitis.
   b. Putting small objects in the mouth may lead to mechanical obstruction of the airway.
   c. Exposure to children in preschool and transmission of infection via toys increase the risk of upper respiratory infections.
   d. Viral infections, croup, and pneumonia are associated with this age group.
3. School-aged children.
   a. Although the lungs are developed, they are still vulnerable to infections and exercise-induced asthma.
   b. Exposure to children in school and after-school activities increases the risk of acquiring a respiratory infection.
4. Adolescents.
   a. Lungs develop adult characteristics.
   b. Vulnerability to peer pressure leads this age group to engage in habits that can impair the lungs, such as smoking and inhaling drugs or toxins.
   c. Although lung diseases generally are uncommon, exercise-precipitated asthma continues to be evident.
5. Young and middle-aged adults.
   a. Prior habits that impair the lungs may continue into adulthood.
   b. Subtle progressive respiratory system changes begin in middle adulthood.
   c. Issues such as anesthesia, infections, and diseases may stress the respiratory system, which is becoming less efficient.
6. Older adults.
   a. Reduced lung compliance, increased airway resistance, and decreased lung elasticity impair ventilation.
   b. Drier mucus, fewer cilia, a less effective cough, air trapping in the alveoli, and declining immunity increase the risk of respiratory tract infections.
   c. Problems such as gastroesophageal reflux disease and brain attack may result in inhalation of foreign matter (**aspiration**), which also can precipitate a respiratory tract infection.

B. Environmental factors
1. Air quality: Air pollution, such as cigarette smoke, automobile emissions, mold spores, and radon, can precipitate disease in vulnerable people (e.g., infants, toddlers, older adults, people with heart or lung disease).

2. Pulmonary allergens: Allergens, such as dust, animal dander, cockroach particles, environmental grasses, and foods such as peanuts and gluten, can precipitate respiratory hypersensitivity responses and allergies.

3. Altitude: Low oxygen levels place strain on the cardiopulmonary system and lead to increased ventilation, production of red blood cells and hemoglobin, and vascularity of lungs and body tissues.

C. Lifestyle factors

1. Smoking tobacco and inhaling second-hand smoke.

   a. Tobacco smoke contains tars, toxins, and nicotine; tars and toxins are known to precipitate cancer and nicotine constricts bronchioles.

   b. Smoke also causes mucous membrane inflammation, increases respiratory secretions, breaks down elastin, and decreases the numbers and efficiency of cilia.

   c. Prolonged use results in chronic bronchitis, smaller diameter of airways, and loss of alveolar elasticity, leading to emphysema.

2. Improper nutrition: Inappropriate balance of proteins, carbohydrates, and fats may reduce the immune system, impair cellular functioning, impede tissue repair, and cause obesity.

3. Lack of exercise: Sedentary lifestyle results in a depressed metabolic rate and an inability of the cardiopulmonary system to respond when any situation causes an increased metabolic rate; regular exercise increases the heart and respiratory rates, which helps condition the body so that the body can better adapt to physical or emotional stressors.

4. Obesity.

   a. A body mass index more than 30 increases the risk of respiratory infections because excess abdominal adipose tissue limits chest expansion and gas exchange in the alveoli.

   b. Sleep apnea occurs due to increased neck girth and fat deposits in the upper airway that obstruct the pharynx.

5. Occupational hazards.

   a. Toxic agents include chemical fumes from cleaning products; carbon monoxide from automobile or machine combustion; particles from construction debris, such as asbestos; and coal dust from coal mines.

   b. Toxic agents can cause chronic inflammation of the mucous membranes of the respiratory system and lung cancer.

6. Substance use or misuse.

   a. Alcohol and medications that depress the respiratory center in the medulla (e.g., opioids, sedatives, anxiolytics, and hypnotics) can cause hypoventilation, aspiration, apnea, and death.

   b. Stimulants, such as amphetamines and cocaine, hallucinogens, and marijuana, also adversely affect lung tissue, increase the risk of aspiration, and depress respirations.

D. Pregnancy

1. Body metabolism increases by 15% and oxygen consumption increases by 15% to 25%.

2. The enlarging uterus rises into the abdominal cavity, limiting enlargement of the chest cavity and downward movement of the diaphragm.

3. Maternal respiratory rate increases, and the mother may experience shortness of breath with activity.

III. Assessment of Respiratory Function

A respiratory assessment can be performed as part of a comprehensive health assessment or as a focused assessment. It begins with obtaining a health history to identify risk factors for potential respiratory problems. The physical examination includes assessing breathing patterns and breath sounds; determining whether the results of inspection, palpation, and percussion of the thoracic cavity are significant; exploring the characteristics of a cough if present; and examining the characteristics of sputum. Data collected from these assessments help determine whether the client's respiratory status is functioning adequately or further definitive action is required.

A. Obtain a health history

1. Identify age and assess for developmental stressors and changes.

2. Identify environmental and occupational stressors.

3. Identify lifestyle behaviors that impact the cardiopulmonary system.

4. Obtain list of prescribed, over-the-counter, and "recreational" medications taken by the client.

5. Assess overall physical and emotional health status and determine whether the client has any problems that impact the respiratory status.

B. Assess breathing pattern

1. Perform assessment of breathing patterns unobtrusively; involuntary breathing efforts are more desirable to assess than voluntary breathing efforts.

2. Note the client's position.

   a. Sitting allows the chest to expand and the diaphragm to move downward with inspirations.

   b. **Orthopnea** is difficulty breathing in the supine position; may occur because the abdominal organs press against the diaphragm and impede chest expansion.

   c. **Orthopneic (tripod) position** is leaning forward while sitting; it increases the thoracic area, allowing for greater chest expansion.

3. **Paroxysmal nocturnal dyspnea** is extreme short-ness of breath during sleep that causes an abrupt awakening and immediate need to assume the upright position for relief.
4. Observe the rate, depth, and rhythm of respirations. (Table 19.1; see also "Measurement of Respirations" in Chapter 14, Physical Assessment)
5. Identify the degree of respiratory effort.
   a. Breathing should be effortless.
   b. **Dyspnea** is difficulty breathing; occurs with inadequate oxygenation.
   c. **Exertional dyspnea** is difficulty breathing with activity; occurs with inadequate oxygenation.
   d. Shortness of breath and fatigue are subjective symptoms that can be reported only by the client.
   e. Physical signs of increased respiratory effort usually accompany difficulty breathing.
6. Identify signs of increased respiratory effort.
   a. Use of **accessory muscles of respiration** is the use of intercostal, abdominal, and trapezius muscles to help expand the chest cavity.
   b. **Retractions** occur when intercostal, supracla-vicular, and subcostal tissues recede during inspiration as a result of excessive negative pressure required to increase the depth of respirations.
   c. **Nasal flaring** occurs when nares widen during inhalation to reduce resistance to airflow; more common in infants and young children.
   d. **Expiratory grunting** is when a grunt or moan occurs at the beginning of exhalation as the glottis opens; it is caused by the sound of air expelled through the larynx; closure of the glottis at the height of inhalation keeps alveoli open to enhance gas exchange.
   e. **Pursed-lip breathing** is exhalation through the mouth with lips positioned to create a small opening to prolong exhalation; keeps alveoli open longer for gas exchange and more efficiently expels trapped air.

C. Perform inspection
1. Determine whether the chest expands and recoils with inhalation and exhalation, respectively.
   a. Movement should be symmetrical.
   b. Asymmetrical expansion may indicate a pneumothorax.

Table 19.1 Breathing Patterns

Pattern	Explanation
Eupnea (normal)	• *12 to 20 breaths/min* • *Not too deep or too shallow* • *Unlabored* • *Regular rhythm*
Bradypnea	• *Less than 12 breaths/min* • *Regular rhythm* • *Associated with neuromuscular disorders, electrolyte imbalances, and opioid medications*
Tachypnea	• *More than 20 breaths/min* • *Regular rhythm* • *Associated with physical exertion, anxiety, pain, and central nervous system and metabolic disorders*
Kussmaul	• *Increased rate and depth of respirations* • *Regular rhythm* • *Associated with metabolic acidosis, fear, and panic*
Biot	• *Varying depths of respirations (usually shallow), alternating with periods of apnea* • *Irregular rhythm* • *Associated with severe, persistent increased intracranial pressure and damage to the respiratory center in the medulla*
Cheyne-Stokes (periodic breathing)	• *Gradual increase in depth of respirations, followed by a gradual decrease and then a period of apnea* • *Regular rhythm* • *Associated with increased intracranial pressure, drug toxicity, and damage to the respiratory center in the medulla*
Apnea	• *Absence of breathing* • *Respiratory arrest* • *Requires mechanical ventilation or cardiopulmonary resuscitation*

Figures adapted from Dillon (2016). *Nursing health assessment: The foundation of clinical practice*, 3rd ed. F. A. Davis Company, with permission.

2. Measure the chest's anteroposterior-to-lateral ratio.
   a. The expected ratio should be 1:2.
   b. An increase in the anteroposterior diameter (**barrel chest**) is associated with chronic retention of carbon dioxide, which occurs with chronic obstructive pulmonary disease (COPD) (Fig. 19.3).
3. Assess the mucous membranes, which should be pink, moist, and intact.
   a. Dry mucous membranes indicate dehydration or a side effect of such medications as anticholinergics.
   b. Pale or bluish color indicates inadequate oxygenation.
4. Assess the lips, which should be slightly lighter or darker than skin color.
   a. Pale lips may indicate anemia or hypoxia.
   b. Cherry-red lips may indicate carbon monoxide poisoning or acidosis.
   c. Pallor around the lips (*circumoral pallor*) may indicate inadequate oxygenation.
5. Assess the fingers and nail plate angles for signs of bulbous swelling of the soft tissue of the end of the phalanx of fingers, causing the nail plates to be equal to or greater than 180 degrees (**clubbing**), which indicates prolonged inadequate oxygenation. (See Fig. 18.1 in Chapter 18, Tissue Integrity and Hygiene.)
6. Assess the color of fingers and nails.
   a. Yellow or brown color indicates nicotine stains from a prolonged history of smoking.
   b. Pallor or cyanosis indicates impaired oxygenation.
D. Perform palpation
   1. Assess the extent of respiratory excursion: Place your thumbs on either side of the client's vertebrae with the fingers flaring outward away from the vertebrae; the hands will move apart when the client inhales; provides a gross measurement of chest expansion on inspiration.
      a. Lack of movement on one side is associated with pneumothorax and lobectomy.
      b. Limited excursion is associated with obstructive airway diseases.
   2. Assess *tactile fremitus:* Place the palmar surface of your hands on either side of the client's sternum while keeping the fingers raised off of the chest wall; vibrations should be detected when the client vocalizes "99" repeatedly.
      a. Increased tactile fremitus is associated with pulmonary edema.
      b. Decreased tactile fremitus is associated with decreased air movement related to obstructive airway diseases.
   3. Assess for tenderness, masses, and crackling; air in subcutaneous tissue when compressed by palpation exhibits a crackling sensation (**subcutaneous emphysema**); air leaking into subcutaneous tissue usually is due to a pneumothorax or associated with a chest tube site.
E. Perform percussion
   1. Percuss over the intercostal spaces rather than over the ribs or scapulae.
   2. Note whether sounds are drumlike (tympanic), hollow (resonant), hyperresonant (echoing), quiet and thudding (dull, flat) to determine whether underlying structures are solid or hollow and contain fluid or air.
   3. Assess diaphragmatic excursion: Percuss the base of the lung at the posterior chest while the client holds a deep breath and then while the client holds a breath after exhalation; mark each point with a pen on the posterior chest wall and measure the difference in centimeters to determine diaphragmatic excursion.

Fig 19.3 Anteroposterior diameter of chest: Normal adult chest, barrel chest. (From Wilkinson and Treas [2016]. *Fundamentals of nursing,* Vol. 1, 3rd ed. Philadelphia: F. A. Davis Company, with permission.)

Normal adult chest

Posterior

Barrel chest

Posterior

F. Assess for presence of coughing and sputum

1. Recognize that coughing and sputum are protective mechanisms that remove mucus and debris from the respiratory airways.
2. Coughing and sputum can be caused by irritants such as smoke, dust, and chemical fumes; food, fluid, or a foreign object that gets lodged in the respiratory airways; and inflammation associated with respiratory tract infections or tumors.
3. Identify whether mucus is being produced by the mucous membranes of the trachea, bronchi, and lungs (**sputum**).
4. Identify whether coughing is not bringing up sputum (*nonproductive cough*) or is bringing up sputum (*productive cough*).
5. Identify the characteristics of sputum.
   a. Amount: From slight to copious.
   b. When produced: From once to continuous; in the morning; when lying down; after behaviors such as smoking.
   c. Color.
      (1) Clear/white: Associated with viral infections.
      (2) Yellow/green: Associated with bacterial infection.
      (3) Black: Associated with inhalation of smoke, soot, or coal dust.
      (4) Red/rust colored: Associated with the presence of blood (*hemoptysis*), tuberculosis, and pneumococcal pneumonia.
      (5) Pink/frothy: Associated with pulmonary edema.
   d. Odor: Foul smelling, associated with bacterial infections such as pneumonia and abscesses of the lung.
6. Obtain a sputum specimen for culture and sensitivity (see "Culture and sensitivity of sputum" under "Diagnostic Tests to Assess Respiratory Function and Related Nursing Care" in this chapter).

G. Auscultate breath sounds

🛑 1. **Clean the ear pieces and diaphragm of the stethoscope before and after use; have a dedicated stethoscope for a client receiving transmission-based precautions.**

2. Place the client in a sitting position to provide access to the client's anterior, posterior, and lateral chest; warm the diaphragm of the stethoscope with your hands before use to promote client comfort.
3. Place the diaphragm directly on the client's skin and follow a systematic sequence to ensure all lung fields are assessed (Fig. 19.4).
4. Instruct the client to breathe deeply through the mouth; provide for a period of regular breathing when necessary to prevent hyperventilation and respiratory alkalosis.

A

B

C

Fig 19.4 Sequence of auscultation of breath sounds. (A) Sequence of anterior auscultation sites. (B) Sequence of lateral auscultation sites for both sides. (C) Sequence of posterior auscultation sites. (From Dillon [2016]. *Nursing health assessment: The foundation of clinical practice*, 3rd ed. F. A. Davis Company, with permission.)

5. Note the duration of inspiration and expiration; inspiration should be longer than expiration.

6. Note the pitch, intensity, and other characteristics of sounds; if you hear air moving through fluid, have the client cough and reassess breath sounds to help distinguish between crackles and rhonchi (coughing will eliminate rhonchi but will not eliminate crackles).

7. Identify expected breath sounds: Bronchial, bronchovesicular, and vesicular (Fig. 19.5 and Table 19.2).

8. Identify abnormal breath sounds: Crackles (rales), rhonchi (sonorous wheezes), stridor, wheezes (sibilant wheezes), and pleural friction rub (Fig. 19.6 and Table 19.3).

IV. Diagnostic Tests to Assess Respiratory Function and Related Nursing Care

Physical examination alone may be inadequate to provide comprehensive information concerning a client's respiratory status. Additional diagnostic tests may be prescribed by the primary health-care provider. Some are essential to arrive at a medical diagnosis (e.g., tuberculin skin testing, sputum culture and sensitivity), whereas others are employed to identify specific information about a client's oxygenation status or the extent of functioning of a client's respiratory system (e.g., peek expiratory flow rate). Nurses must understand these tests because some of them are performed by the nurse and all of them require client teaching.

A. Pulse oximetry

Oximetry identifies the percentage of arterial oxygen saturation by assessing the percentage of hemoglobin molecules carrying oxygen. (See "Measurement of Arterial Oxygen Saturation" in Chapter 14, Physical Assessment.)

B. Peak expiratory flow rate (PEFR)

1. Identifies the amount of air that can be exhaled with forcible effort, expressed in liters per minute (Fig. 19.7).

2. Compared to the individual's "personal best" baseline result to determine dosage and effectiveness of respiratory medications.

   a. Green: Peak flow is within 80% to 100% of personal best baseline; continue prescriptions as prescribed.

   b. Yellow: Peak flow is within 50% to 80% of personal best baseline; reflects onset of airway

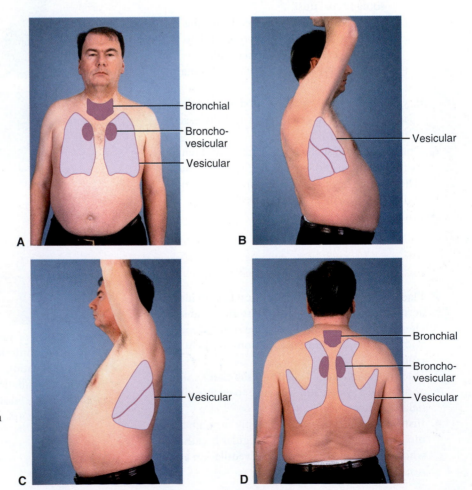

Fig 19.5 Locations of normal breath sounds. (From Dillon [2016]. *Nursing health assessment: The foundation of clinical practice*, 3rd ed. F. A. Davis Company, with permission.)

Table 19.2 Normal Breath Sounds

Breath Sound	Description	Location
Bronchial Inspiration / Expiration *(graph: inverted-V, inspiration line shorter rising, expiration line descending longer)*	• Caused by air moving through the trachea • Loud, high-pitched, hollow, blowing sound • Inspiration shorter than expiration	• Over the trachea anteriorly • Nape of the neck posteriorly
Bronchovesicular Inspiration / Expiration *(graph: tall symmetric inverted-V)*	• Caused by air moving through large bronchi • Medium-pitched, medium intensity, blowing sounds • Inspiration and expiration equal in length	• Over the first and second intercostal space on either side of the sternum anteriorly • Between the scapulae posteriorly
Vesicular Expiration / Inspiration *(graph: long rising inspiration line, short descending expiration)*	• Caused by air moving through smaller airways of the respiratory tract • Soft, low-pitched, breezy sounds • Inspiration is louder, higher pitched, and longer than expiration	• Over the periphery of the lung

Figures adapted from Dillon (2016). *Nursing health assessment: The foundation of clinical practice*, 3rd ed. F. A. Davis Company, with permission.

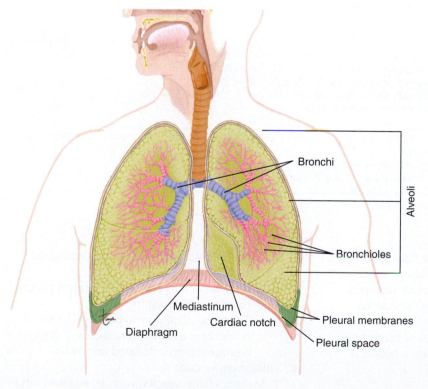

Fig 19.6 Location of abnormal breath sounds: Crackles—yellow; rhonchi—orange and blue; wheeze—pink; pleural friction rub—green. (Adapted from Scanlon [2015]. *Essentials of anatomy and physiology*, 7th ed. Philadelphia: F. A. Davis Company, with permission.)

Table 19.3 Abnormal Breath Sounds

Breath Sound	Description and Location	Etiology

Crackles (rales)
 	
 Crackles diagram (I–E)
	• Air bubbling through moisture in the alveoli
	 • Not cleared by coughing
	 • Heard in periphery of lung
	 • Classified as:
	   • *Fine:* Soft, high-pitched crackling sound heard at height of inspiration
	   • *Medium:* Lower-pitched, popping sound heard during the middle of inspiration
	   • *Coarse:* Loud, bubbling sound heard throughout inspiration
		• Inflammation due to pneumonia or bronchitis
		 • Hypervolemia due to congestive heart failure or fluid overload
		 • Alteration in structure or function, such as in emphysema

Rhonchi (sonorous wheeze) *Rhonchi* diagram (I–E)	• Mucus accumulated in large bronchi • Loud, coarse, low-pitched sound heard during inspiration and/or expiration • May be cleared by coughing • Heard over larger bronchi	• Inflammation due to bronchitis • Narrowed airways • Alteration in structure or function, such as in emphysema or fibrotic lungs
Wheeze (sibilant wheeze) *Mild wheeze* diagram (I–E) *Moderate wheeze* diagram (I–E) *Severe wheeze* diagram (I–E)	• Air moving through narrowed airways • High-pitched, musical sound that may be heard throughout inspiration and expiration; more prominent during expiration • Heard over bronchi • May be audible without a stethoscope	• Narrowing of small airways by spasms, inflammatory process, mucus accumulation, or tumors
Pleural friction rub *Friction rub* diagram (I–E)	• Inflamed pleural surfaces rubbing together • Low-pitched, grating sound during inspiration and/or expiration; more prominent at height of inspiration • Disappears when the breath is held (versus pericardial friction rub, which continues when the breath is held) • Heard at lateral, anterior, base of lung	• Inflammation of the pleural membranes (pleurisy)
Stridor	• High-pitched crowing sound; more prominent during inspiration • Heard over larynx and trachea • May be audible without a stethoscope	• Tracheal or laryngeal spasm • Partial airway obstruction

Figures adapted from Dillon (2016). *Nursing health assessment: The foundation of clinical practice*, 3rd ed. F. A. Davis Company, with permission.

changes that are reducing peak flow by 20% to 50%; may require increase in dosage of maintenance medications or use of rescue therapies.

  c. Red: Peak flow is less than 50% of personal best baseline; reflects severe reduction in peak flow rate; immediate use of rescue therapies is indicated; emergency intervention needed if condition does not improve.

3. Nursing care.

  a. Instruct the client to take a maximal deep breath and to forcefully exhale fully with lips sealed around the mouthpiece.

  b. Obtain three readings, and document the highest reading.

  c. Implement the prescribed treatment protocol based on PEFR results.

  d. Teach the client how to perform the test at home, keep a record of results, and determine treatment protocols based on results.

C. Pulmonary function tests

1. Identifies lung capacity, volume, and flow rates (Fig. 19.8).

  a. *Tidal volume:* Amount of air moving in and out of the lungs with a normal breath (e.g., 500 mL);

Fig 19.7 Peak expiratory flow rate (PEFR). (From Williams and Hopper [2015]. *Understanding medical surgical nursing*, 5th ed. Philadelphia: F. A. Davis Company, with permission.)

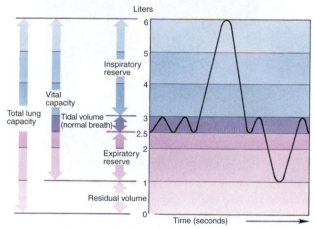

Fig 19.8 Pulmonary function test. (From Scanlon [2015]. *Essentials of anatomy and physiology*, 7th ed. Philadelphia: F. A. Davis Company, with permission.)

normally increases when oxygen demand increases and decreases with conditions such as obstructive lung diseases, muscular weakness, and paralysis of the diaphragm.

b. *Inspiratory reserve volume:* Maximum amount of air that can be inhaled beyond the tidal volume (e.g., 2,000 to 3,000 mL); reflects the extent to which tidal volume can increase when oxygen demand increases.

c. *Expiratory reserve volume:* Maximum amount of air that can be exhaled after exhalation of the tidal volume (e.g., 1,000 to 1,500 mL); decreases with conditions that collapse the alveoli and airways, thus trapping air in the lungs.

d. *Residual volume:* Amount of air remaining in the lungs after forceful exhalation (e.g., 1,000 mL); increases with conditions that trap air in the lungs.

e. *Vital capacity:* Amount of air that is forcefully exhaled after forcefully inhaling with the deepest inspiratory effort possible (e.g., 3,000 to 5,000 mL); reflects a combination of the inspiratory reserve volume, tidal volume, and the expiratory reserve volume.

f. *Total lung capacity:* A combination of the inspiratory reserve volume, tidal volume, expiratory reserve volume, and the residual volume.

2. Nursing care.

a. Identify clients who may not be capable of participating in the test, such as those who have pain on inspiration or expiration, are cognitively impaired, or have a lowered level of consciousness.

b. Teach the client to avoid smoking, bronchodilators, metered-dose inhalers, and aerosol therapies for 6 hours before the test unless otherwise indicated by the primary health-care provider.

c. Obtain current weight and height measurements, and record the results on the client's clinical record.

d. List all prescribed medications on the laboratory form.

e. Explain that deep breathing may precipitate lightheadedness, and instruct the client to report this occurrence to the test administrator.

f. Encourage rest after the test because it commonly causes fatigue in clients with respiratory problems.

DID YOU KNOW?

Inhalation studies may precipitate an asthmatic episode. Therefore, some medications may be permitted before a diagnostic test of the respiratory system.

D. Tuberculin skin testing

1. Identifies past or present exposure to tubercle bacilli but does not diagnose that the client has tuberculosis (TB); clients with positive purified protein derivative (PPD) results require a chest x-ray and sputum culture for a definitive diagnosis.

2. PPD of the tubercle bacillus is inserted via an intradermal injection.

3. Annual testing is recommended for health-care workers, immigrants from countries with an increased incidence of tuberculosis, and people residing in congregate living environments, such as prisons, low-income housing, and dormitories.

4. Nursing care.

a. Determine whether the client has a contraindication for the test (e.g., had tuberculosis, had a previous positive test, has a history of hypersensitivity to skin tests, has eczema, is receiving chemotherapy, or is pregnant).

b. Determine whether the client is taking steroids or immunosuppressants because these substances can cause a false-negative result.

c. Explain that the test results must be evaluated
48 to 72 hours after PPD injection; otherwise
results may be inaccurate.

d. Perform intradermal injection on the forearm
and encircle the area with an indelible pen.
(See "Intradermal (ID) Injections" in
Chapter 9, Medication.)

e. Measure the diameter of a raised, thickened
area (induration) if it occurs, not redness;
≤5 mm is a negative reaction; ≥5 mm, ≥10 mm,
or ≥15 mm associated with subgroups of the
population indicates a positive response.

f. Refer clients with a positive result to their
primary health-care provider for additional
testing.

E. Culture and sensitivity of sputum

1. The culture result identifies organisms in the
sputum.

2. The sensitivity result suggests appropriate
antimicrobial agents for treatment.

3. Nursing care.

🛑 a. Obtain the sputum specimen before initiation of
antibiotic therapy; otherwise the result of the test
may be inaccurate.

b. Place the client in the semi-Fowler or Fowler
position.

c. Obtain the specimen.

(1) Via expectoration: Have the client breathe
deeply several times, cough deeply, and
expel sputum directly into the sterile
specimen container.

(2) Via suction.

(a) Use a sterile inline sputum specimen
container.

(b) Administer oxygen before the procedure for 2 minutes (*preoxygenate*)
to increase the serum oxygen level
because suctioning will interfere
with the intake of oxygen during the
procedure.

🛑 (c) Don protective eyewear and sterile
gloves. Keep one hand sterile and one
hand clean.

(d) Hold the catheter with the sterile
gloved hand while attaching it to
the suction source tubing and lubricate the tip of the suction catheter
with sterile normal saline solution
(Fig. 19.9A).

(e) Use the sterile gloved hand to insert
the catheter through the nasopharynx,
endotracheal tube, or tracheostomy
tube and advance it to the trachea.

Fig 19.9 Obtaining a sputum specimen via suction. (From
Wilkinson and Treas [2016]. *Fundamentals of nursing*, Vol. 2, 3rd ed.
Philadelphia: F. A. Davis Company, with permission.)

(f) Apply suction with the clean gloved
hand for 5 to 10 seconds when the
client coughs.

(g) Remove the suction tubing and
connect the tubing on the specimen
container to the attached adapter
(Fig. 19.9B).

d. Label the container with the client's name,
identification number, test, and collection
date and time.

e. Place the specimen in a biohazard bag and
immediately send it to the laboratory.

V. Nursing Care for Clients With Respiratory Problems

Nursing interventions related to the respiratory system
focus on the promotion of efficient respiratory functioning, the prevention of respiratory difficulties, and the treatment of respiratory problems. Many of these interventions
are independent functions of the nurse, but some require
a primary health-care provider's prescription or a standing
protocol. Nurses must have a thorough understanding of

when and how to implement these interventions. Some support comfort and rest, but other actions maintain life.

A. Promote coughing out or spitting out of sputum (**expectoration**)

1. Prevent dehydration.
   a. Encourage intake of a minimum of 2 to 3 L of fluid by mouth per day if permitted.
   b. Provide prescribed intravenous fluids.
2. Encourage activity, such as walking, and alternating side-lying positions to mobilize secretions.
3. Encourage coughing and deep breathing; instruct the client to exhale deeply and take a deep breath and then exhale using abdominal muscles while keeping the glottis open (huff technique); repeat this technique several times and then take a deep breath and cough deeply to raise sputum.
4. Administer prescribed expectorants.
5. Ensure that supplemental oxygen is humidified.
6. Perform chest physiotherapy for clients too weak to cough or at risk for retained secretions; perform between meals to prevent nausea and vomiting or an unpleasant taste that may limit eating; administer a prescribed nebulizer treatment before the procedure to dilate airways and provide humidification; perform oral care after the procedure to limit an unpleasant taste. Chest physiotherapy may be implemented by a respiratory therapist. For more information about a **nebulizer,** see nonpressurized aerosol (handheld nebulizer), nursing intervention specific to administering medication via an aerosol handheld nebulizer, and Fig 9.5A in Chapter 9, Medication.
   a. **Postural drainage** involves placing the client sequentially in a variety of positions so that gravity drains secretions from all lobes of the lungs.
   b. *Percussion:* Strike the chest wall using cupped hands to generate sounds and slight negative pressure that loosen secretions (Fig. 19.10).
   c. *Vibration:* Apply vibrations to the chest wall with the hands (Fig. 19.11) or an inflatable

Fig 19.11 Chest wall vibration. (From Wilkinson and Treas [2016]. *Fundamentals of nursing,* Vol. 2, 3rd ed. Philadelphia: F. A. Davis Company, with permission.)

high-frequency chest wall oscillation vest can be worn that generates pulses of air into the vest that vibrate the client's chest wall, loosening secretions.

7. Teach the client how to use a vibratory positive expiratory pressure device to vibrate the airways (which loosens mucus from the walls), intermittently increase endobronchial pressure (which helps maintain airway patency during exhalation), and maximize expiratory airflow (which moves mucus toward the mouth) (Fig. 19.12).
   a. Sit in a chair with the head tilted slightly upward.
   b. Hold the stem of the device horizontal to the floor; this angle may be raised or lowered to achieve the maximum fluttering effect; vibrations during exhalation can be felt internally by the client or by the nurse by placing one hand on the client's back and one hand on the chest.
   c. Slowly inhale 75% of a usual breath and hold for 2 to 3 seconds and suppress coughing.

Fig 19.10 Chest wall percussion. (From Wilkinson and Treas [2016]. *Fundamentals of nursing,* Vol. 2, 3rd ed. Philadelphia: F. A. Davis Company, with permission.)

Perforated cover

Stainless steel ball

Mouthpiece

Fig 19.12 Flutter mucus clearance device. When the client blows into the mouthpiece, the stainless steel ball bounces up and down, causing airways to vibrate. (Courtesy of Axcan Scandipharm, Birmingham, AL.)

d. Place the mouthpiece in the mouth with the lips firmly around the stem.

e. Exhale through the device at a somewhat fast but not forceful speed while keeping cheeks stiff (stiff cheeks allow airways to vibrate rather than the cheeks).

f. Repeat steps c through e 5 to 10 times.

g. Perform two additional breaths through the device, but this time inhale fully and exhale forcefully with each breath.

h. Cough to raise mucus to the mouth, and then expectorate the mucus.

i. Perform the technique as prescribed because it is goal based rather than time based; usually, it is performed in the morning and late afternoon or evening.

j. Disassemble the device, rinse all components with tap water, dry with a clean towel, reassemble, and store in a dry place; clean with a mild soap or detergent every 2 days and then rinse, dry, reassemble, and store the device.

B. Promote lung expansion

1. Have the client assume a position that allows the diaphragm to contract without pressure from abdominal organs and permits thoracic excursion, such as semi-Fowler, high-Fowler, or orthopneic (tripod) position.

2. Encourage **diaphragmatic (abdominal) breathing** which is an intake of air that expands the abdomen on deep inhalation and abdominal muscles tighten on exhalation to increase the amount of air entering and exiting the lungs.

3. Encourage **pursed-lip breathing** which is exhaling through the mouth with the lips positioned to create a small opening to prolong exhalation. Doing so keeps alveoli open longer for gas exchange and

more efficiently expels trapped air. This breathing technique is beneficial for clients with obstructive airway diseases, such as emphysema, asthma, and chronic bronchitis.

4. Encourage use of an **incentive spirometer** which is a device that promotes deep breaths by providing a visual goal to progressively increase the volume of breaths; it should be performed 10 times every hour to help prevent atelectasis and reexpand collapsed alveoli (Fig. 19.13).

5. Administer prescribed bronchodilators and nebulizer treatments. (See Figures 9.5 and 9.7 and related information in Chapter 9, Medication.)

C. Maintain a balance between rest and activity

1. Organize care so that the client has uninterrupted periods of rest.

2. Anticipate the client's needs and assist with care.

3. Pace activities so that the client does not experience dyspnea.

4. Encourage use of a shower stool rather than standing when showering.

5. Teach the client to place several chairs throughout the home so that the client can rest when walking from one place to another.

6. Encourage the client to schedule rest periods or short naps several times a day.

7. Refer the client to a social service agency to arrange for a motorized chair.

D. Maintain a patent airway

1. Keep suction apparatus at the bedside.

🛑 2. Maintain aspiration precautions for a client who has a decreased level of consciousness, difficulty swallowing, or a diminished or absent gag or cough reflex.

a. Maintain the client in a side-lying position to promote drainage of secretions from the mouth.

Fig 19.13 Incentive spirometers. (A) Voldyne volumetric deep-breathing exerciser. (B) Triflow II incentive breathing exerciser. (From Williams and Hopper [2015]. *Understanding medical surgical nursing,* 5th ed. Philadelphia: F. A. Davis Company, with permission.)

b. Request medications in liquid form or crush medications (if not enteric coated or sustained release) and place them in a teaspoon of applesauce to promote swallowing.

c. Provide thick liquids, such as nectars, or use a thickening agent.

d. Place the client in the high-Fowler position for meals; have a nursing team member assist with the entire meal and ensure that client's mouth is empty of food after each mouthful and after the meal.

e. Offer small, frequent meals; alter the consistency of food as indicated, such as mechanical soft, soft, chopped, and pureed; feed slowly.

f. Keep the client in the semi- or high-Fowler position for at least 30 minutes after meals.

3. Maintain aspiration precautions for clients receiving enteral feedings.

a. Maintain the head of the bed at 30 degrees if the client is receiving continuous tube feedings.

b. Raise the head of the bed to 45 degrees before the client receives an intermittent tube feeding; intermittent tube feedings have a larger volume than continuous tube feedings, which increases the risk of aspiration; maintain head elevation for at least 30 minutes after the feeding.

c. Aspirate stomach contents to ensure that the nasogastric tube is in the stomach and to measure residual volume; withhold the next feeding if the residual volume exceeds the parameter indicated by the primary health-care provider or facility policy (depends on amount and frequency of feedings); re-instill the residual to prevent electrolyte imbalances.

4. Assess for signs of excessive secretions in the airways, such as rattling sounds in the throat, shortness of breath, ineffective cough, and rhonchi or crackles on auscultation.

🛑 5. Suction the client if respiratory secretions compromise the airway.

a. Commonalities of nursing care related to suctioning.
(1) Wash your hands.
(2) Provide for the client's privacy.
(3) Assess breath sounds, vital signs, and pulse oximetry before the procedure.
(4) Place the client in the semi- or high-Fowler position.
(5) Set the wall suction at an appropriate pressure (e.g., 100 to 150 mm Hg for adults, 100 to 120 mm Hg for children, and 50 to 95 mm Hg for infants).
(6) Don a face shield and appropriate gloves.
(7) Begin suctioning.

(8) Reposition the client and reinstitute the prescribed oxygen therapy after suctioning is completed.
(9) Assess breath sounds, vital signs, pulse oximetry, and the client's response to the procedure and document these results in the client's clinical record.
(10) Discard used equipment in appropriate disposal containers.

b. Oropharyngeal suctioning.
(1) Don sterile gloves; some references state that clean gloves are adequate.
(2) Obtain equipment.
(a) Yankauer (tonsil-tip) suction tube (Fig. 19.14) to remove secretions from the oral cavity.
(b) Suction catheter (e.g., 12 to 18 French for adults, 8 to 10 French for children, and 5 to 8 French for infants) to remove secretions from the oropharyngeal or nasopharyngeal area.
(3) Lubricate the tip of the tube or catheter with sterile normal saline solution.

🛑 (4) Advance the tube or catheter (3 to 4 inches) along the inside of the cheek to the pharyngeal area; avoiding the center of the tongue limits gagging.

🛑 (5) Apply negative pressure for only 10 to 15 seconds to remove secretions and prevent hypoxia.

(6) Suction the cheek pouches and under the tongue to remove pocketed secretions.

c. Nasopharyngeal suctioning.
(1) Don sterile gloves; some references state that clean gloves are adequate.
(2) Measure from the tip of the client's nose to the tip of the client's earlobe to determine the extent the catheter should be inserted (Fig. 19.15A).

Fig 19.14 Yankauer suction tube. (From Wilkinson and Treas [2016]. Fundamentals of nursing, Vol. 1, 3rd ed. Philadelphia: F. A. Davis Company, with permission.)

Fig 19.15 Nasopharyngeal suctioning. (A) Measure from the tip of nose to tip of ear lobe. (B) Insert lubricated catheter into naris. (From Wilkinson and Treas [2016]. *Fundamentals of nursing,* Vol. 2, 3rd ed. Philadelphia: F. A. Davis Company, with permission.)

    (3) Lubricate the tip of the catheter with water-soluble jelly.

    (4) Extend the client's head and advance the catheter into a naris the predetermined length, usually 5 to 6 inches (Fig. 19.15B).

    🛑 (5) Apply intermittent negative pressure for 10 to 15 seconds only when rotating and withdrawing the catheter.

    (6) Suction sterile normal saline solution to clear the catheter of secretions.

    (7) Repeat previous steps alternating nares and waiting 30 seconds between each pass of the catheter to allow the client time to breathe.

  d. Endotracheal and tracheal suctioning.

    (1) Preoxygenate the client by using a resuscitation bag connected to an oxygen source; compress the bag three to five times.

    🛑 (2) Do not preoxygenate if the client has copious secretions because doing so can force secretions deeper into the lung and delay their removal.

    (3) Don sterile gloves.

    (4) Lubricate the tip of the catheter with sterile normal saline solution.

    (5) Advance the catheter without applying negative pressure until resistance is felt (usually just above the bifurcation of the mainstream bronchi; endotracheal tube—usually 5 to 6 inches for an adult; tracheostomy tube—usually 2 to 3 inches for an adult).

    🛑 (6) Apply intermittent negative pressure for 10 to 15 seconds only when rotating and withdrawing the catheter (Fig. 19.16).

E. Institute basic life support (cardiopulmonary resuscitation [CPR]) (Table 19.4)

  1. Perform external cardiac compression and ventilation to increase blood flow to the heart and brain, following the sequence of Circulation, Airway, Breathing (CAB).

  2. Assess breathing and pulse simultaneously. If no breathing, only gasping, and no pulse within 5 to 10 seconds then proceed with CPR procedure. Palpate carotid pulse for adults and children older than 1 year of age and brachial pulse for infants.

  3. If no response: If alone, for an adult, activate emergency system and get an automated external defibrillator (AED) before CPR; for child or infant, follow steps for adult if collapse is witnessed; if unwitnessed, give 2 minutes of CPR, then activate the emergency system, get an AED, and then resume CPR.

  4. Ensure that victim is on hard surface before starting compressions.

  5. Assess and establish an airway; open the airway (head tilt–chin lift maneuver or jaw thrust without neck hyperextension if cervical injury is suspected).

Fig 19.16 Tracheal suctioning. (From Wilkinson and Treas [2016]. *Fundamentals of nursing,* Vol. 2, 3rd ed. Philadelphia: F. A. Davis Company, with permission.)

Table 19.4 Performing CPR			
CPR	**Infant (<1 year)**	**Child (>1 year–adolescent)**	**Adult**
Rate of compressions	• *Administer at least 100 to 120 compressions per minute.* • *Rotate health-care providers every 2 minutes.* • *Keep interruptions to less than 10 seconds.*		
Compression landmark	• *Two fingers in center of chest just below nipple line (one rescuer).* • *Two thumbs with hands encircling center of chest just below nipple line (two rescuers).*	• *One hand for small child and two hands for larger child on lower half of sternum.*	• *Heel of one hand with fingers interlocked with the other on lower half of sternum.*
Depth of compressions (allow full recoil after each compression)	• *Compress the chest about 1.5 inches.*	• *Compress the chest about 1.5 to 2 inches, depending on the child's size.*	• *Compress the chest at least 2 inches but no more than 2.4 inches.*
Ratio of compressions to ventilations	• *Compress the chest 30 to 2 (one rescuer).* • *Compress the chest 15 to 2 (two rescuers).*		• *Compress the chest 30 to 2 regardless of whether there are one or two rescuers.*

6. If the client is not breathing, institute rescue breaths and compressions at the ratio indicated in Table 19.4 in the section "Ratio of compressions to ventilations."
7. Maintain the ratio of compressions to ventilations for five cycles and then reassess the pulse.
8. If successful, discontinue CPR and position the victim in a side-lying (recovery) position.
9. If unsuccessful, attempt defibrillation; minimize length of interruptions to less than 10 seconds.
10. If unsuccessful, resume compressions and then ventilations according to appropriate age and number of rescuers ratio; terminate CPR when directed by the primary health-care provider or when rescuer exhaustion occurs.

F. Prevent and manage partial and total airway obstructions
1. Education for family members with small children.
   a. Ensure toys are as large as a clenched fist and inspect toys for small removable parts.
   b. Store plastic bags where they cannot be reached by small children.
   c. Cut food into very small pieces, and avoid foods such as olives, grapes, and frankfurters.
   d. Do not give small children hard candy, nuts, popcorn, marshmallows, peanut butter, chewing gum, or balloons.
   e. Discuss how and when to perform the universal choking sign (Fig. 19.17).
2. Assess for the presence of partial or total airway obstruction and intervene accordingly (Table 19.5).

Fig 19.17 Universal sign for choking. (From Wilkinson and Treas [2016]. *Fundamentals of nursing*, Vol. 2, 3rd ed. Philadelphia: F. A. Davis Company, with permission.)

VI. Administration of Oxygen

A. Commonalities of nursing care for clients receiving oxygen
1. Perform all preliminary nursing interventions, such as verifying the prescription, washing your hands, collecting appropriate equipment, identifying the client, providing privacy, and explaining the procedure to the client.
2. Obtain vital signs, measure the client's pulse oximetry level (may not be a reliable indicator for clients with COPD or impaired peripheral circulation), and perform a focused respiratory assessment, including auscultation of breath sounds, before initiation of therapy to have baseline data.
3. Initiate oxygen flow according to the manufacturer's directions, and place the device on the client.

Table 19.5 **Airway Obstructions**

	Infant (<1 year)	Child/Adolescent (>1 year)	Adult
Assess extent of obstruction	*Partial Obstruction* • *Can cough and make sounds.* *Total Obstruction* • *Cannot cough, make sounds, or speak; has difficulty breathing, pallor, and cyanosis.* • *In addition, a child or adult may encircle the throat with the hands (universal choking sign). Nurse should ask the victim, "Are you choking?"*		
Victim is conscious	*Partial Obstruction* • *Continue to monitor; allow the victim's efforts to dislodge the object.*		
	Total Obstruction in an Infant • *Sit with infant face down on your forearm, head angled down.* • *Deliver 5 back blows, turn infant face upward and deliver 5 chest thrusts.* • *Repeat until object is expelled or victim is unresponsive.*	*Total Obstruction in a Child or an Adult* • *Initiate abdominal thrust maneuver: Encircle victim's waist and with intertwined clenched fists, thrust upward and inward against diaphragm.* • *Perform abdominal thrust maneuver until the object is expelled or victim is unresponsive.*	
Victim is unconscious	• *Head tilt–chin lift maneuver to open airway; inspect the mouth; remove the object if present in the pharynx.* • *Implement cardiopulmonary resuscitation, but inspect the mouth before each two rescue breaths.*		

4. Hang an "oxygen in use" sign near the client's bed, use cotton gowns and linens to prevent static electricity, and prohibit smoking and open flames near the client because oxygen supports combustion.

5. Routinely monitor delivery of oxygen, ensuring that all connections are secure.

6. Assess the client's skin where elastic straps, the mask, or oxygen tubing may produce pressure or friction that could cause skin trauma (e.g., nares and top of ears with a nasal cannula, ears, bridge of the nose, and zygomatic bones with masks).

7. Routinely assess the client's vital signs, pulse oximetry, breath sounds, and other client responses, and evaluate data in relation to expected outcomes of interventions.

8. Document the procedure and the client's response in the client's clinical record.

B. Nursing care for clients receiving oxygen via specific oxygen delivery systems: See Table 19.6.

C. Nursing care for clients with an artificial airway

1. Device used to permit air to enter and exit the lungs, thereby maintaining an open airway.

2. Used for clients who are unconscious, at risk for airway obstruction, or require mechanical ventilation.

3. Should be suctioned only when necessary to maintain an open airway and limit trauma to mucous membranes of the respiratory tract.

4. Nursing care varies by type of device (Table 19.7).

MAKING THE CONNECTION

Avoidance of High Levels of Oxygen Therapy for Clients With Obstructive Respiratory Diseases

The carbon dioxide level in the body is the primary regulator of breathing because increased or decreased levels affect the pH of the blood. Changes in the oxygen level in the blood do not change the blood's pH. Normally, when the carbon dioxide level in the body increases and pH and oxygen levels decrease, the chemoreceptors in the carotid arteries, aorta, and medulla identify these changes and send a message to the medulla to increase respirations accordingly. However, people with obstructive airway disease become accustomed to increased carbon dioxide levels, and their stimulus to breathe is no longer increased levels of carbon dioxide but rather low oxygen levels. Therefore, when administering oxygen to people with obstructive airway diseases, the delivery of oxygen should not exceed 2 L/min. Excessive exogenous oxygen decreases the respiratory drive, resulting in decreased breathing and increased carbon dioxide retention. In addition, the Haldane effect suggests that the adverse effects of increased oxygen are caused by the inability of oxygen-saturated hemoglobin molecules to transport carbon dioxide. Both issues relate to excessive levels of carbon dioxide in the body associated with excessive exogenous oxygen *(CO$_2$ narcosis)*. Clients with obstructive airway diseases who are receiving oxygen should be assessed for the clinical manifestation of CO$_2$ narcosis, which include decreased rate and depth of respirations, confusion, decreased level of consciousness, tremors, convulsions, and even death.

Table 19.6 Oxygen Delivery Systems and Related Nursing Care

Type	Description	Advantages and Disadvantages	Related Nursing Care
Simple face mask	• Delivers oxygen to the nose and mouth via a clear, flexible mask. • Liter flow: 5 to 10 L/min. • Fraction of inspired oxygen (FIO$_2$): 40% to 60%, depending on liter flow.	*Advantages* • Client may breathe through the nose or mouth. *Disadvantages* • Some clients feel claustrophobic. • Some clients feel hot because the mask retains body heat. • The mask must be removed for eating and drinking. • Speech is muffled.	• Place the mask securely over the nose and mouth with the elastic straps above the ears. • Ensure the flow rate is ≥5 L/min to prevent carbon dioxide accumulation in the mask. • *Switch to a nasal cannula when eating.*
Nasal cannula	• Delivers oxygen to the nares via clear, flexible prongs. • Liter flow: 1 to 6 L/min. • FIO$_2$: 24% to 44%, depending on liter flow.	*Advantages* • The device is comparatively comfortable. • The client may eat, drink, and talk unimpeded. *Disadvantages* • It may dry the nasal mucosa and irritate the nares. • Device's effectiveness decreases if the client breaths through the mouth.	• Place the nasal prongs curved downward into the nares with the elastic straps wrapped around the ears and the slider under the chin. • Assess for dryness of the nasal mucosa. • *Humidify oxygen if the flow rate is >3 L/min.*
Partial rebreather mask	• Delivers oxygen to the nose and mouth via a clear, flexible mask with an attached bag (reservoir). • Some exhaled air is rebreathed; most exhaled air is discharged through ports on the side of the mask. • Liter flow: 6 to 15 L/min. • FIO$_2$: 50% to 90%, depending on liter flow.	*Advantages* • Rebreathing some exhaled carbon dioxide lowers the pH of the gas, which stimulates breathing and helps prevent carbon dioxide narcosis. *Disadvantages* • Some clients feel claustrophobic.	• Flood the reservoir with oxygen before attaching the mask to the client. • *Ensure that the reservoir does not collapse during inhalation; a higher flow rate is required if this occurs.*
Nonrebreather mask	• Delivers oxygen to the nose and mouth via a clear, flexible mask with an attached bag (reservoir). • All exhaled air is discharged through ports on the side of the mask. • Liter flow: 6 to 15 L/min. • FIO$_2$: 70% to 100%, depending on liter flow.	*Advantages* • This is the only oxygen delivery system that can deliver 100% oxygen when liter flow is 15 L/min. It allows higher FIO$_2$ levels because the reservoir fills with oxygen; one-third of the air in the reservoir is depleted when the client inhales; the reservoir is then refilled by the oxygen flow. *Disadvantages* • Some clients feel claustrophobic.	• Flood the reservoir with oxygen before attaching the mask to the client. • *Ensure that the reservoir remains half full during inhalation; if not, a higher flow rate is required.*

Continued

Table 19.6 Oxygen Delivery Systems and Related Nursing Care—cont'd

Type	Description	Advantages and Disadvantages	Related Nursing Care
Venturi mask	• Delivers oxygen to the nose and mouth via a clear, flexible mask with a valve and tubing attached between the mask and the oxygen tubing. • Interchangeable color-coded valves permit a specific mix of room air and oxygen to deliver a precise percentage of oxygen. • Exhaled air is discharged through ports on the side of the mask to keep carbon dioxide build-up to a minimum. • Liter flow: Depends on valve being used. • FIO_2: 24% to 60%, depending on color-coded valve used.	*Advantages* • Precise percentages of oxygen can be delivered to individualize therapy to meet specific client's needs, particularly those with an obstructive respiratory disease. *Disadvantages* • Some clients feel claustrophobic. • Color codes of valves may differ among manufacturers.	• Connect the color-coded valve consistent with the FIO_2 prescribed by the primary health-care provider. • *Set the oxygen flow rate indicated on the color-coded plastic valve.*
Face tent	• Delivers oxygen to the nose and mouth via a clear mask that fits under the chin and is open on the top. • Liter flow: 8 to 12 L/min. • FIO_2: 30% to 55%.	*Advantages* • Most clients do not feel claustrophobic. • High levels of humidity can be used. *Disadvantages* • Exact levels of oxygen cannot be delivered.	• *Monitor pulse oximetry routinely because the percentage of oxygen delivered is not precise.*

Figures adapted from Wilkinson and Treas (2016). *Fundamentals of nursing*, Vol. 2, 3rd ed. Philadelphia: F. A. Davis, with permission.

Table 19.7 Types of Artificial Airways and Related Nursing Care

Type of Tube	Nursing Care	Illustration
Oropharyngeal • Hard plastic tube that extends from the front of the teeth to the pharynx. • Holds the tongue away from the back of the pharynx. • Used only for clients who are unconscious (often postoperative clients immediately after surgery) because it can precipitate gagging, vomiting, and laryngospasm in conscious clients.	• Begin insertion with the inner curve of the device facing the nose (A). • Rotate the device 180 degrees when the airway reaches the posterior wall of the pharynx (B). • Do not tape the airway in place. • *Remove the device as soon as the client's gag reflex returns.*	

Table 19.7 **Types of Artificial Airways and Related Nursing Care—cont'd**

Type of Tube	Nursing Care	Illustration
Nasopharyngeal • *Flexible tube that extends from the nares to the pharynx.* • *Provides an avenue for air to enter and exit the lungs.* • *Used for clients who are semiconscious and at risk for airway obstruction.* • *Does not stimulate gagging.*	• *Advance the airway along the floor of the nostril to the posterior pharynx; the outer flange should rest just outside the nostril and the distal tip of the tube in the posterior pharynx, which can be visualized by depressing the client's tongue with a tongue blade and inspecting the posterior pharynx.* • *Feel for the passage of air at the outer flange.* • *Auscultate for bilateral breath sounds.* • *Remove the tube every 8 hours to assess for mucous membrane irritation and to clean the tube.*	
Tracheostomy • *Insertion of a tube into the trachea through an incision in the neck.* • *Provides an avenue for air to enter and exit the lungs bypassing the upper airway.* • *May be temporary or permanent.* • *Has three parts: Outer cannula (with or without an inflatable cuff); obturator that fills the blunt end of the outer cannula to promote ease of insertion into the tracheotomy; and inner cannula (disposable or can be cleaned).* • *Cuff on an outer cannula is inflated to prevent aspiration of fluids or prevent an air leak if the client is receiving mechanical ventilation; "pillow" expands when cuff is inflated.*	• *Document the type and size of the tracheostomy tube.* • *Maintain the outer cannula in place with twill ties or Velcro tracheostomy tube holders.* ***Tracheostomy Care*** • *Provide tracheostomy care routinely, at least every 8 hours.* • *Don clean gloves and remove the dressing under tracheostomy tube and the inner cannula.* • *Don sterile gloves and replace the inner cannula with a new inner cannula if disposable or remove the inner cannula and clean with a solution of half hydrogen peroxide and half normal saline, rinse with normal saline, and dry the internal lumen with pipe cleaners.* • *Clean around the stoma with normal saline solution using a cotton-tipped applicator; clean the faceplate of the tracheostomy tube with 4 × 4 gauze dampened with sterile normal saline solution.* • *Replace twill ties or collar every 24 hours; inspect under ties or collar routinely for signs of pressure or excoriation.* • *Follow manufacturer's instructions for protocol for replacing the collar.* • *Teach client self-care if the tracheal stoma is permanent; teach the client to wear a stoma bib to warm air and protect the tracheal opening from debris, to avoid water-related activities, and to wear a tracheal shield when showering.*	 Outer tube with cuff and inflating tube Cuff Inner cannula Obturator

Continued

Table 19.7 Types of Artificial Airways and Related Nursing Care—cont'd

Type of Tube	Nursing Care	Illustration
Endotracheal • *Insertion of tube into the trachea through the mouth or nose (intubation).* • *Provides airway for mechanical ventilation.* • *Has an inflatable cuff to provide a seal to prevent an air leak when the client is receiving mechanical ventilation.*	• *Maintain cuff inflation with minimal occlusive volume to prevent necrosis of the mucous membranes.* • *Inflate the cuff with the volume of air recommended by the manufacturer; cuff pressure usually is 20 mm Hg.* • *Place the stethoscope over the trachea.* • *Remove a small amount of air from the cuff at a time until a slight air leak is identified at the height of inhalation.* • *Assess placement of the tube.* • *Assess for symmetrical chest movements.* • *Auscultate the bilateral lung fields to ensure the tube has not slipped into the right main bronchus.*	

Figures adapted from Wilkinson and Treas (2016). *Fundamentals of nursing*, Vol. 2, 3rd ed. Philadelphia: F. A. Davis Company, with permission; Burton and Ludwig (2015). *Fundamentals of nursing care: Concepts, connections & skill*, 2nd ed. Philadelphia: F. A. Davis Company, with permission; and Williams and Hopper (2015). *Understanding medical surgical nursing*, 5th ed. Philadelphia: F. A. Davis Company, with permission.

VII. Medications That Affect the Respiratory System

When a person is diagnosed with a respiratory problem, the primary health-care provider can prescribe appropriate medications to dilate the respiratory airways, decrease the viscosity of respiratory secretions, and limit coughing. Nurses should know the mechanisms of action and therapeutic and nontherapeutic effects related to the common bronchodilators, expectorants, and antitussives (Table 19.8).

Table 19.8 Medications That Affect the Respiratory System

Mechanism of Action	Examples	Nontherapeutic Effects
Bronchodilators (Inlarge the lumina of air passages)		
Sympathomimetics (beta-adrenergic agonists) • *Stimulate beta receptors to dilate bronchioles*	• *albuterol (Proventil)* • *metaproterenol*	• *Tachycardia* • *Tremors* • *Anxiety*
Xanthines • *Relax bronchial smooth muscle*	• *aminophylline* • *theophylline*	• *Tachycardia* • *Tremors* • *Anxiety* • *Nausea and vomiting*
Anticholinergics • *Decrease action of acetylcholine receptors in bronchial smooth muscle*	• *ipratropium (Atrovent)* • *tiotropium (Spiriva)*	• *Dizziness* • *Headache* • *Palpitations* • *Nervousness* • *Dry mouth* • *Blurred vision* • *Urinary retention*
Leukotriene receptor antagonists • *Inhibit leukotriene synthesis or activity* • *Minimize inflammation and edema*	• *montelukast (Singulair)* • *zafirlukast (Accolate)* • *zileuton (Zyflo)*	• *Headache* • *Weakness* • *Nausea and vomiting*

Table 19.8 Medications That Affect the Respiratory System—cont'd

Mechanism of Action	Examples	Nontherapeutic Effects
Inhaled and nasal-route steroids • *Decrease inflammatory response and edema*	• *budesonide (Pulmicort)* • *fluticasone (Flovent)* • *mometasone (Asmanex Twisthaler)* • *triamcinolone (Aristocort)*	• *Headache* • *Oropharyngeal fungal infections* • *Dysphonia* • *Hoarseness* • *Flulike syndrome (budesonide)*
Mast cell stabilizers • *Stabilize mast cells to decrease histamine release*	• *cromolyn (Intal)* • *nedocromil (Tilade)*	Uncommon but may include: • *Hoarseness* • *Nausea* • *Dry, irritated throat* • *Coughing* • *Bad taste in mouth*
Combination agents • *Depends on individual action of agents*	• *albuterol and ipratropium (Combivent)* • *budesonide and formoterol (Symbicort)* • *fluticasone and salmeterol (Advair)*	• *Headache* • *Sore throat* • *Upper respiratory infection* • *Additional effects depending on individual agents*
Expectorants (Decrease viscosity of respiratory secretions in trachea and bronchi, promoting mobilization and expulsion of mucus)		
• *Increases respiratory tract fluid*	• *guaifenesin (Mucinex, Robitussin)*	Uncommon but may include: • *Nausea and vomiting* • *Headache* • *Dizziness* • *Serious allergic reaction (rare): Itching/swelling of face, throat, and tongue; rash; severe dizziness; and difficulty breathing*
Antitussives (Suppress cough reflex)		
• *Suppression of the cough reflex in the central nervous system*	• *codeine* • *dextromethorphan (DM suffix in cough preparations)*	• *Sedation at high doses*

CASE STUDY: Putting It All Together

A nurse is admitting a 72-year-old obese woman to a medical unit after the client was stabilized in and transferred from the emergency department. The client has a history of obstructive airway disease. In addition, she was a smoker (two packs a day for 30 years) but stopped at age 48, had asthma as a child, and was diagnosed with emphysema at age 68. Last month, the client had an episode of bronchitis. Today, she was exposed to environmental smoke as a result of a house fire in her neighborhood. She tells the admitting nurse, "After breathing the smoke from the fire, I started wheezing, my voice became hoarse, my chest felt tight, and I could barely catch my breath. I used my rescue inhaler several times, but it didn't help, so I came to the hospital. I feel better since they gave me oxygen, a nebulizer treatment, and medications in the emergency department." The nurse reviews the client's clinical record from the emergency department.

Vital Signs

Temperature:	99.6°F orally
Respirations:	32 breaths/min, shallow, labored
Pulse:	115 beats/min
Blood pressure:	170/84 mm Hg

Primary Health-Care Provider's Prescriptions

High-flow humidified oxygen 100% nonrebreather mask
Chest x-ray
Complete blood count
Basic metabolic panel
ECG
Carboxyhemoglobin level (carbon monoxide level in the blood)
Support orthopneic/tripod position

continued.

CASE STUDY: Putting It All Together *cont'd*

Dexamethasone (Decadron) 10 mg, IVPB, every 8 hours

IVF: 0.9% sodium chloride 100 mL/hr

Albuterol/Atrovent nebulized solution 1-unit dose each via nebulizer mask every 4 hours

Albuterol nebulized solution 1-unit dose via nebulizer mask every 2 hours, prn for breakthrough wheezing or respiratory distress

Assessments on Admission to the Emergency Department

Oxygen saturation 86%

Client is restless

Sitting on the side of the bed, leaning forward, and resting arms on a pillow on the overbed table

Circumoral pallor; capillary refill of toenails is 4 seconds

Reports shortness of breath and fatigue

Subclavicular retractions noted on inspiration

Stridor on inspiration

Case Study Questions

A. Which assessment noted on the client's clinical record from the emergency department should cause the nurse the most concern? Explain your conclusion.

_____

B. Identify nine signs and symptoms of impaired respiratory function for which the nurse should assess the client.

1. _____
2. _____
3. _____
4. _____
5. _____
6. _____
7. _____
8. _____
9. _____

C. Identify five factors that placed this client at risk for a problem with pulmonary function, and explain why.

1. _____
2. _____
3. _____
4. _____
5. _____

D. Identify at least 10 independent nursing actions the nurse should implement when caring for this client.

1. _____
2. _____
3. _____
4. _____

CASE STUDY: Putting It All Together *cont'd*

_____ **Case Study Questions** _____

5. _____

6. _____

7. _____

8. _____

9. _____

10. _____

REVIEW QUESTIONS

Be sure to read the Introduction for valuable test-taking tips.

1. An unconscious client has excessive oral secretions. In which position should the nurse place the client to help prevent aspiration?
   1. Sims'
   2. Supine
   3. Fowler
   4. Contour

2. A nurse is to perform a purified protein derivative (PPD) test on a client who was exposed to a person with the diagnosis of tuberculosis. What are essential nursing interventions related to this test? **Select all that apply.**
   1. Encircle the injection site with an indelible pen.
   2. Identify whether the client is taking an immunosuppressant.
   3. Determine whether the client had a previous positive reaction.
   4. Inject the purified protein derivative via an intradermal injection.
   5. Explain that the results must be evaluated within twenty-four hours.

3. A client is scheduled to have pulmonary function tests. What should the nurse instruct the client to do before the test?
   1. Avoid smoking for 6 hours before the test.
   2. Take a bronchodilator 1 hour before the test.
   3. Abstain from food for 2 hours before the test.
   4. Drink 8 oz of water immediately before the test.

4. A nurse documents that a client is experiencing Kussmaul respirations. What observations about the client's respirations did the nurse make to come to this conclusion?
   1. More than twenty breaths/min
   2. Increased rate and depth of respirations
   3. Varying depths of respirations, generally shallow, alternating with periods of apnea
   4. Gradual increase in depth of inhalations, followed by a gradual decrease, and then a period of apnea

5. An older adult client asks a nurse, "Why am I experiencing more frequent respiratory tract infections now that I am older?" Which information about the aging process should the nurse include in a response to the client's question? **Select all that apply.**
   1. Thoracic and expiratory muscles are weaker.
   2. There is an increase in the cough and laryngeal reflexes.
   3. Vital capacity increases as the residual volume decreases.
   4. The ribcage becomes more rigid due to calcification of costal cartilage.
   5. Decreased mobility associated with aging causes less effective gas exchange.

6. A nurse is caring for a client with a bacterial infection of the lungs. What type of sputum should the nurse anticipate the client to expectorate?
   1. Yellow-green
   2. Clear white
   3. Pink frothy
   4. Red rust

7. A nurse is monitoring a client's respiratory status. What should the nurse instruct the client to do when teaching about the use of the device in the photograph?

   1. "Inhale and exhale normally."
   2. "Hold the inhalation for several seconds."
   3. "First fully inflate your lungs before you exhale fully."
   4. "Inhale slowly and as deeply as possible through the mouthpiece."

8. A nurse is caring for a client who is experiencing a laryngeal spasm. For which clinical indicator should the nurse assess the client?
   1. Stridor
   2. Wheeze
   3. Crackles
   4. Rhonchi

9. Which independent nursing actions are associated with caring for a client who is experiencing hypoxemia? **Select all that apply.**
   1. Elevate the head of the bed.
   2. Attach a pulse oximeter to the client's finger.
   3. Remain calm and speak in a normal tone of voice.
   4. Encourage the client to cough when the client has secretions.
   5. Administer oxygen at four liters/min via a nonrebreather mask.

10. A nurse is caring for a client requiring continuous pulse oximetry. What should the nurse do when using this monitoring device? **Select all that apply.**
    1. Compare the pulse rate on the oximeter with the client's radial rate occasionally.
    2. Clean the site for the sensor with an alcohol wipe before applying the sensor.
    3. Explain that the test is noninvasive but may cause discomfort.
    4. Dampen the site slightly before applying the sensor.
    5. Ensure that capillary refill is more than 4 seconds.
    6. Change the site of the device every 2 hours.

11. An older adult comes to the clinic reporting shortness of breath and yellow mucus. What factors in the client's history may have contributed to this situation? **Select all that apply.**
    1. Has a body mass index of 35
    2. Smokes 1 pack of cigarettes a day
    3. Drinks 1 glass of wine with dinner
    4. Takes a 2-mile walk every morning
    5. Reports eating a vegetarian diet for the last 3 years

12. A nurse identifies that a client is experiencing exertional dyspnea. Difficulty breathing in relation to what behavior led the nurse to this conclusion?
    1. Eating
    2. Exercise
    3. Lying down
    4. Leaning forward while sitting

13. A nurse is teaching a client how to use a vibratory positive expiratory pressure device to facilitate expectoration of respiratory secretions. What should the nurse teach the client to do to ensure an expected outcome?
    1. Sit in a chair with the chin tilted slightly toward the chest.
    2. Forcefully inhale 50% of a usual breath and hold it for 4 seconds.
    3. Place the mouthpiece in the mouth with the lips firmly around the stem while keeping the cheeks relaxed.
    4. Complete the procedure with 2 additional breaths using the device, but inhale fully and exhale forcefully with each breath.

14. When a nurse is performing a physical assessment, the client reports feeling short of breath. For what signs of dyspnea should the nurse assess the client? **Select all that apply.**
    1. Pursed-lips on exhalation
    2. Supraclavicular retractions
    3. Grunting just before exhaling
    4. Oxygen saturation level of 96%
    5. Respiratory rate of 20 inhalations per minute

15. A client who had been in a house fire is experiencing a productive cough. What color should the nurse expect the client's sputum to exhibit?
    1. Yellow
    2. White
    3. Black
    4. Red

16. A nurse must obtain a sputum specimen from a client with an endotracheal tube. Place the following steps in the order in which they should be performed.
    1. Verify the prescription and wash the hands.
    2. Don a protective eye shield and sterile gloves.
    3. Apply suction when the client coughs or when meeting resistance.
    4. Lubricate the catheter tip with normal saline and advance it into the endotracheal tube.
    5. Remove the catheter and attach the tubing on the specimen container to the attached adapter.
    Answer: _____

17. A nurse is auscultating a client's breath sounds. What actions should the nurse employ to achieve the most accurate results? **Select all that apply.**
    1. Examine lung bases first.
    2. Place the client in the supine position.
    3. Instruct the client to inhale through the nose.
    4. Keep the stethoscope at each site for at least one minute.
    5. Compare results in the left and right lungs at the same site.
    6. Identify the breath sound heard before moving to the next site.

18. When auscultating breath sounds, the nurse identifies the presence of stridor. What should the nurse do?
    1. Notify the rapid response team immediately.
    2. Plan to reassess the client in one hour.
    3. Implement oropharyngeal suctioning.
    4. Arrange for an x-ray examination.

19. A client arrives in the emergency department with portable oxygen at 3 liters per minute via nasal cannula. The nurse in the emergency department obtains the client's health history and vital signs and performs a focused physical assessment. What should the nurse do **first** based on this information?
    1. Walk the client from the triage area to a bed.
    2. Reduce the oxygen flow rate to 2 liters per minute.
    3. Increase the oxygen flow rate to 6 liters per minute.
    4. Encourage the client to perform pursed-lip breathing.

Client's Clinical Record

Health History From Spouse

68-year-old man, lives with wife.
60-year history of asthma, 10-year history of emphysema.
Gave up smoking 3 years ago because of progressive shortness of breath.
For years he has been using oxygen 2 L/min via nasal cannula whenever the shortness of breath intensifies.
Client has had a cold for 5 days and has been using the oxygen without relief.
Wife increased the oxygen to 3 L/min 6 hours ago.
Client has been lethargic all day; when he had profuse sweating, the wife brought him to the emergency department.

Vital Signs

Temperature: 100.2°F orally
Pulse: 92 beats/min, regular
Respirations: 10 breaths/min, shallow, regular
Blood Pressure: 150/88 mm Hg

Focused Physical Assessment

Reports feeling drowsy and dizzy
Confused and unable to report recent facts concerning his condition
Exhibiting fine muscle twitching
Auscultation reveals bilateral rhonchi and wheezes
Oxygen saturation: 84%

20. A nurse receives a prescription for an oropharyngeal tube for a client who is unconscious. Which nursing actions are associated with this tube? **Select all that apply.**
    1. Administer mouth care every 2 to 4 hours.
    2. Secure the tube in position by taping it in place.
    3. Remove the tube occasionally to assess for irritation of the nose.
    4. Begin the tube's insertion with the inner curve facing the tongue.
    5. Rotate the tube 180 degrees when it reaches the end wall of the pharynx.

21. A client with chronic obstructive pulmonary disease (COPD) who is receiving 2 L/min of oxygen via nasal cannula has dyspnea, is using accessory muscles of respiration to breathe, and is responsive. The client's oxygen saturation is 89%. Place the following actions in the order that they should be performed beginning with what the nurse should do **first**.
    1. Obtain the client's vital signs.
    2. Teach the client pursed-lip breathing.
    3. Place the client in the high-Fowler position.
    4. Inform the client's primary health-care provider.
    5. Monitor the client's pulse oximetry level continuously.
    Answer: _____

22. A client is admitted to the emergency department after sustaining injuries in an automobile collision. The client is semiconscious and the nurse is concerned about maintaining the client's airway while diagnostic tests are completed. Which should the nurse anticipate will be prescribed by the primary health-care provider?
    1. Endotracheal tube
    2. Tracheostomy tube
    3. Oropharyngeal tube
    4. Nasopharyngeal tube

23. Sixty percent oxygen is prescribed for a client. Which oxygen delivery equipment should the nurse use to administer the oxygen to this client?
    1. Nonrebreather mask
    2. Nasal cannula
    3. Venturi mask
    4. Face tent

24. A nurse must perform nasopharyngeal suctioning. Place the following actions in the order in which they should be performed.
    1. Don sterile gloves.
    2. Open the suction kit.
    3. Lubricate the suction catheter tip.
    4. Place the client in the high-Fowler position.
    5. Insert suction catheter into the client's nasopharynx.
    6. Determine the distance between the client's nose and earlobe with the catheter.
    Answer: _____

25. Oxygen 4 L/min via nasal cannula is prescribed for a client who is cachectic. What nursing actions should be implemented when caring for this client? **Select all that apply.**
    1. Position the prongs in the client's nares so that they curve upward.
    2. Position padding between the zygomatic bones and the tubing.
    3. Secure elastic straps around the client's head.
    4. Ensure that the oxygen is humidified.
    5. Provide oral hygiene every shift.

26. A nurse is caring for a client receiving intermittent enteral feedings. Which nursing intervention should the nurse implement to reduce the risk of aspiration?
    1. Place the client in the left Sim's position after the instillation.
    2. Elevate the head of the bed 45 degrees during the feeding.
    3. Thicken the formula with a thickening solution.
    4. Suction the client before initiating the feeding.

27. A nurse is planning a class for parents about how they can reduce the risk of their toddlers experiencing an airway obstruction. Which information should the nurse include in the program? **Select all that apply.**
    1. Cut hot dogs into small pieces.
    2. Do not give toddlers marshmallows.
    3. Teach a toddler the universal sign for choking.
    4. Ensure that toys are larger than a clenched fist.
    5. Store plastic bags where they cannot be reached by toddlers.

28. A nurse is caring for an adult client with excessive respiratory secretions. What should the nurse do when suctioning this client? **Select all that apply.**
    1. Set the wall pressure at approximately 60 mm Hg.
    2. Evaluate breath sounds after the procedure.
    3. Wear personal protective equipment.
    4. Place the client in a lateral position.
    5. Use a sterile 8 French catheter.

29. A nurse is caring for a client with a history of chronic obstructive pulmonary disease. Which is the **most** important nursing action when administering oxygen via a nasal cannula to this client?
    1. Assess the ears for irritation as a result of the oxygen tubing.
    2. Post a sign that says oxygen in use near the client's bed.
    3. Monitor the client's oxygen saturation routinely.
    4. Limit oxygen flow rate to 2 L/min.

30. One hundred percent oxygen is prescribed for a client experiencing respiratory difficulty. Which type of oxygen mask should the nurse use when implementing this prescription?
    1.

    2.

    3.

    4.

31. A client has a respiratory rate of 24 breaths per minute and is having shortness of breath. What should the nurse do **first**?
    1. Administer 100% oxygen.
    2. Obtain an oxygen saturation level.
    3. Elevate the head of the client's bed to a 60-degree angle.
    4. Inform the primary health-care provider of the client's status.

32. A nurse is admitting a client to a unit from the emergency department. The nurse reviews the client's clinical record and assesses the client. What concern should be the priority?
    1. Urinary retention
    2. Respiratory status
    3. Increased temperature
    4. Potential for dehydration

Client's Clinical Record

Vital Signs

Temperature: 104°F rectally
Pulse: 100 beats/min and regular
Respirations: 17 breaths/min and shallow
Blood pressure: 138/88 mm Hg

Transfer Nurse's Note 10-9-2013 1330

Client transferred to room via stretcher from the emergency department with side rails raised. Client in semi-Fowler position, skin appears flushed, and client is diaphoretic. Client reports: feels warm, has no pain, and is very sleepy. IV in right hand set at prescribed rate of 125 mL/hr. IV in left hand is an intravenous lock. Both catheter sites are dry and intact, no clinical indicators of infiltration or inflammation noted. Client attempted to void but was unsuccessful. Has not voided since 1030. Oxygen running at 2 L/min via nasal cannula. Tylenol 650 mg administered at 1300.

Primary Health-Care Provider's Prescriptions 10-9-2013

1. Bedrest
2. Regular diet
3. Vital signs every 4 hours
4. I&O
5. Tylenol 650 mg PO every 4 hours prn for temperature 101.2°F
6. IVF 1000 mL 0.45% NaCl with 20 mEq KCl at 125 mL/hr
7. Oxygen 2 L via nasal cannula

---

33. A client has a respiratory rate of 24 breaths per minute with mild labored breathing. The nurse raises the head of the client's bed, but the client's breathing does not improve. What should be the nurse's **next** action?
    1. Perform cupping and clapping on the client's back.
    2. Call the client's primary health-care provider.
    3. Obtain a pulse oximetry level and vital signs.
    4. Administer 100% oxygen.

34. A nurse is caring for a client receiving a steroidal nasal spray. For which nontherapeutic effects should the nurse assess the client? **Select all that apply.**
    1. Dry mouth
    2. Swollen lips
    3. Blurred vision
    4. Urinary retention
    5. Difficulty breathing
    6. Oral fungal infection

35. A client has a respiratory infection and ciprofloxacin (Cipro) 750 mg PO every 12 hours is prescribed. A unit-dose package indicates that the dose is 250 mg/tablet. How many tablets should the nurse administer every 12 hours? **Record your answer using a whole number.**
    Answer: _____ mL

36. A nurse receives a prescription for a culture and sensitivity of a nasal specimen. Place the following steps in the order in which they should be implemented.
    1. Check the nasal passage with a flashlight.
    2. Offer the client a tissue to clean or blow the nose.
    3. Gently rotate culture swab at site of purulent/inflamed tissue.
    4. Position the client in a semi-Fowler position with head hyperextended.
    5. Insert culture swab into nasal passage without touching nasal structures.
    6. Remove swab without touching nasal structures and insert into culture tube.
    Answer: _____

37. A nurse identifies clubbing when assessing a client's hands. Which conclusion can the nurse make concerning this observation?
    1. The client has liver disease.
    2. The client has diabetes mellitus.
    3. The client has a nutritional deficiency.
    4. The client has a long-term oxygen deficit.

38. A nurse is auscultating a client's chest. The heart rate is irregular. The nurse proceeds to auscultate the base of the client's right lung. The nurse identifies the presence of crackles (rales). What should the nurse do **next**?
    1. Palpate the radial pulse to identify if there is a pulse deficit.
    2. Auscultate the base of the left lung to detect if there are crackles.
    3. Perform chest physiotherapy to loosen the retained respiratory secretions.
    4. Obtain a blood pressure measurement to determine the presence of hypervolemia.

39. A nurse is preparing to perform oropharyngeal suctioning using a Yankauer suction device. Which step of this procedure is different from performing nasopharyngeal suctioning?

1. Use sterile normal saline to clear the catheter of secretions between reinsertions of the device.
2. Wear clean gloves throughout the entire procedure using the device.
3. Apply negative pressure only when withdrawing the device.
4. Use sterile normal saline to lubricate the tip of the device.

40. Which should a nurse do when obtaining a client's peek expiratory flow rate (PEFR)?

1. Obtain three readings and document the highest reading.
2. Inform the primary health-care provider if the result is within the green range.
3. Have the client always use a rescue medication before performing the procedure.
4. Instruct the client to keep the lips sealed around the mouthpiece while forcefully inhaling.

REVIEW ANSWERS AND RATIONALES

1. ANSWER: 1.
Rationales:
1. The Sims' position is the most effective position to prevent aspiration, particularly in an unconscious client because excessive oral secretions will drain out of the side of the mouth. In addition, this position will be easy to maintain in a client who is unconscious.
2. The supine position will not aid in the prevention of aspiration because lying on the back will promote the flow of secretions to the back of the oropharynx and trachea.
3. The Fowler position may assist in the prevention of aspiration but will not be as effective as another position. In addition, an unconscious client may have difficulty maintaining the Fowler position.
4. The contour position will have minimal effect in preventing aspiration because the head will not be elevated enough. In addition, an unconscious client may have difficulty maintaining this position.
TEST-TAKING TIP: Identify the equally plausible options. Options 3 and 4 are equally plausible because both positions elevate the head of the bed and position the body in a sitting position.
Content Area: Oxygenation
Integrated Processes: Nursing Process: Implementation
Client Need: Physiological Integrity; Physiological Adaptation
Cognitive Level: Application
Concept: Oxygenation

2. ANSWER: 1, 2, 3, 4.
Rationales:
1. Encircling the injection site with an indelible pen ensures that the appropriate site is evaluated.
2. Immunosuppressants can cause a false-positive result.
3. A severe reaction may occur when the PPD is injected into a client who had a previous positive reaction; the client has been immunosensitized.
4. The intradermal route is used for this test. The allergen is injected just below the epidermis where a reaction can be observed.
5. The site of the intradermal injection of PPD should be evaluated within 48 to 72, not within 24, hours after the PPD is injected.
TEST-TAKING TIP: Identify the clang association. The words *purified protein derivative* in the stem and in option 4 is a clang association. Examine option 4 carefully because, more often than not, an option with a clang association is a correct answer.
Content Area: Oxygenation
Integrated Processes: Nursing Process: Implementation
Client Need: Physiological Integrity; Reduction of Risk Potential
Cognitive Level: Analysis
Concept: Oxygenation

3. ANSWER: 1.
Rationales:
1. Smoking constricts the bronchi and bronchioles, which will cause inaccurate test results; therefore, the client
should be instructed to avoid smoking for 6 hours before the test.
2. Taking a bronchodilator 1 hour before the test should be done only when advised to do so by the primary health-care provider. Medications that influence the respiratory tract may invalidate test results.
3. It is not necessary to abstain from food for any length of time before the test.
4. It is not necessary to drink fluid before the test.
Content Area: Oxygenation
Integrated Processes: Teaching/Learning; Nursing Process: Implementation
Client Need: Physiological Integrity; Reduction of Risk Potential
Cognitive Level: Application
Concept: Oxygenation

4. ANSWER: 2.
Rationales:
1. More than 20 breaths/min is tachypnea. Respirations should be between 12 to 20 breaths/min, have a regular rhythm, and be unlabored.
2. Increased rate and depth of respirations is Kussmaul respirations. They occur as hydrogen ions in the body increase as a result of acidosis. The body is attempting to blow off carbon dioxide.
3. Varying depths of respirations, generally shallow, alternating with periods of apnea is Biot respirations.
4. A gradual increase in depth of inhalations, followed by a gradual decrease, and then a period of apnea is Cheyne-Stokes respirations.
TEST-TAKING TIP: Identify the clang associations. The word *respirations* in the stem and in options 2 and 3 are clang associations. Examine these options carefully.
Content Area: Oxygenation
Integrated Processes: Communication and Documentation; Nursing Process: Assessment
Client Need: Physiological Integrity; Reduction of Risk Potential
Cognitive Level: Analysis
Concept: Oxygenation

5. ANSWER: 1, 4, 5.
Rationales:
1. Thoracic and expiratory muscles are weaker as one ages. There is a loss of muscle tone due to a more sedentary lifestyle and an increase in thoracic rigidity as one ages.
2. There is a decrease, not increase, in the cough and laryngeal reflexes as one ages. As one ages, there is an increase in airway resistance, a loss of muscle tone, and a reduced elastic recoil in the lungs and thoracic muscles, which all contribute to a decrease in the cough and laryngeal reflexes.
3. Vital capacity decreases, not increases, as the residual volume increases with aging. The amount of air left in the lung after expiration increases as a result of loss of muscle tone and reduced elastic recoil in the lungs and thoracic muscles.
4. The ribcage becomes more rigid due to calcification of costal cartilage as one ages. With less lung expansion, the

risk of respiratory infection increases because of insufficient lung inflation and decreased ability to expel foreign or accumulated material.

5. A more sedentary lifestyle associated with aging causes less effective gas exchange and decreased lung inflation, increasing the risk of respiratory infection.

Content Area: Oxygenation
Integrated Processes: Communication and Documentation; Nursing Process: Planning
Client Need: Health Promotion and Maintenance
Cognitive Level: Application
Concept: Growth and Development

6. **ANSWER: 1.**
Rationales:

1. **Yellow-green-colored sputum is associated with bacterial infections. It consists of cellular debris, phagocytic cells, and microorganisms.**
2. Clear-white-colored sputum is associated with viral infections.
3. Pink frothy sputum is associated with fluid in the lung due to pulmonary edema. The pink color is related to blood in the sputum.
4. Red-rust-colored sputum is associated with the presence of blood (hemoptysis).

Content Area: Oxygenation
Integrated Processes: Nursing Process: Analysis
Client Need: Physiological Integrity; Reduction of Risk Potential
Cognitive Level: Application
Concept: Infection

7. **ANSWER: 3.**
Rationales:

1. Inhaling and exhaling normally is not the correct way to use this device.
2. Holding an inhalation for several seconds is associated with a nebulizer treatment, not the device in the photograph. Holding the inhalation for several seconds when using a nebulizer facilitates longer contact of the fine mist of a nebulized drug to be in contact with the alveoli.
3. **This device is used to monitor peak expiratory flow rates. The client should exhale fully into the peak flow-meter after fully inflating the lungs with a deep breath. It measures in liters per minute the volume of air a person can exhale after fully inflating the lungs.**
4. Inhaling slowly and as deeply as possible through the mouthpiece is associated with an incentive spirometer, not the device in the photograph. An incentive spirometer promotes deep breathing, stimulates coughing to help remove mucus from the respiratory system, and prevents atelectasis.

TEST-TAKING TIP: Identify the options that are opposites. Options 1 and 3 are opposites. More often than not, an option that is an opposite is the correct answer. Examine these options carefully.

Content Area: Oxygenation
Integrated Processes: Teaching/Learning; Nursing Process: Implementation
Client Need: Physiological Integrity; Physiological Adaptation
Cognitive Level: Analysis
Concept: Patient-Centered Care; Oxygenation

8. **ANSWER: 1.**
Rationales:

1. **Laryngeal spasm is characterized by stridor, which is a high-pitched crowning sound more prominent during expiration; it is caused by constriction of the larynx.**
2. A wheeze is a high-pitched, musical sound that may be heard more prominently during expiration. It is associated with narrowing of small airways by spasms, inflammatory processes, mucus accumulation, or tumors.
3. Crackles, also known as rales, are fine, medium, or coarse sounds caused by air bubbling through moisture in the alveoli. It is associated with inflammation due to such conditions as pneumonia, bronchitis, hypervolemia due to congestive heart failure, or emphysema.
4. Rhonchi, also known as a sonorous wheeze, is a loud, coarse, low-pitched sound heard during inspiration and/or expiration. It may be cleared by coughing. It is associated with inflammation due to bronchitis, narrowed airways, alterations in structure or function associated with emphysema, and fibrotic lungs.

Content Area: Oxygenation
Integrated Processes: Nursing Process: Assessment
Client Need: Physiological Integrity; Reduction of Risk Potential
Cognitive Level: Analysis
Concept: Oxygenation

9. **ANSWER: 1, 2, 3, 4.**
Rationales:

1. **Elevating the head of the bed is an independent nursing action. It does not require a prescription from a primary health-care provider. Raising the head of the bed uses gravity to move abdominal organs away from the diaphragm, facilitating respirations.**
2. **Attaching a pulse oximeter to the client's finger is an independent function of the nurse. The nurse does not need a prescription from a primary health-care provider to monitor a client's oxygen saturation level. Nurses are permitted to assess clients.**
3. **Remaining calm and speaking in a normal tone of voice are independent functions of the nurse. Impaired oxygenation is a frightening experience. It is important for the nurse to remain calm and not contribute to the client's fear and/or anxiety.**
4. **Encouraging the client to cough when the client has secretions is an independent function of the nurse. Coughing facilitates expulsion of secretions from the respiratory tract. When secretions are cleared from the respiratory tract, more air can be inhaled into the alveoli and carbon dioxide exhaled.**
5. The nurse can administer 2 L/min of oxygen by nasal cannula in an emergency without a prescription from a primary health-care provider. Other oxygen delivery systems, such as a nonrebreather mask or elevating the oxygen level higher than 2 L/min, require a prescription from a primary health-care provider.

Content Area: Oxygenation
Integrated Processes: Nursing Process: Implementation
Client Need: Physiological Integrity; Physiological Adaptation
Cognitive Level: Application
Concept: Oxygenation

10. **ANSWER: 1, 2, 6.**
    Rationales:
    1. A significant difference between the oximeter pulse rate and the client's radial rate indicates a malfunction of the sensor.
    2. Cleaning the site ensures a more accurate reading because dirt and debris may interfere with accurate measurement.
    3. A pulse oximetry sensor does not cause discomfort.
    4. The skin should be dry before applying the sensor.
    5. Capillary refill should be less than 3 seconds; otherwise test results will not be accurate. Circulation to the area must be adequate for accurate test results.
    6. The sensor site should be changed every 2 hours to prevent tissue necrosis from pressure if monitoring is continuous.
    TEST-TAKING TIP: Identify the clang associations. The word *device* in the stem and in option 6 and the word *pulse* in the stem and in option 1 are clang associations. The word *oximetry* in the stem and the word *oximeter* in option 1 is a clang association. Examine options 1 and 6 carefully.
    Content Area: Oxygenation
    Integrated Processes: Nursing Process: Implementation
    Client Need: Physiological Integrity; Reduction of Risk Potential
    Cognitive Level: Application
    Concept: Oxygenation

11. **ANSWER: 1, 2.**
    Rationales:
    1. A body mass index more than 30 increases the risk for respiratory problems because abdominal adipose tissue limits chest expansion and gas exchange in the alveoli.
    2. Tobacco smoke contains tars, toxins, and nicotine. Tars and toxins irritate the mucous membranes of the respiratory system, making them more vulnerable to disease processes. Nicotine constricts blood vessels, which impairs oxygenation of body tissues.
    3. One glass of wine has been reported to promote cardiopulmonary functioning. However, excessive intake of alcohol may depress the respiratory center, resulting in hypoventilation and aspiration.
    4. Exercise increases the metabolic rate and functioning of the heart and lungs; these responses condition the body, which promotes adaptation to physical stressors.
    5. A vegetarian diet provides all the basic nutrients required for a healthy diet. An imbalance of proteins, carbohydrates, and fats may reduce the immune system and impair cellular functioning.
    Content Area: Oxygenation
    Integrated Processes: Communication and Documentation; Nursing Process: Assessment
    Client Need: Health Promotion and Maintenance
    Cognitive Level: Analysis
    Concept: Oxygenation

12. **ANSWER: 2.**
    Rationales:
    1. Although a full stomach impedes contraction of the diaphragm and expansion of the thoracic cavity, its relationship to dyspnea is not known as exertional dyspnea.
    2. Exercise increases the metabolic rate, causing an increase in the heart and respiratory rates. Exertion increases the demand for oxygen; when the body cannot meet the demand for oxygen, difficulty breathing results and is known as exertional dyspnea.
    3. Difficulty breathing when lying down necessitating having to sit up to breathe is known as orthopnea.
    4. Leaning forward when sitting in an effort to expand the thoracic cavity is a sign of difficulty breathing but is not known as exertional dyspnea; it is known as using the orthopneic or tripod position to facilitate breathing.
    TEST-TAKING TIP: Identify the word in the stem that is a clang association. The words *exertional* in the stem and *exercise* in option 2 are associated and is an obscure clang association.
    Content Area: Oxygenation
    Integrated Processes: Nursing Process: Analysis
    Client Need: Physiological Integrity; Reduction of Risk Potential
    Cognitive Level: Application
    Concept: Oxygenation

13. **ANSWER: 4.**
    Rationales:
    1. The client should sit in a chair with the head slightly tilted upward. This position facilitates movement of gases in and out of the upper airway and pharynx.
    2. The client should slowly, not forcefully, inhale 75%, not 50%, of a usual breath and then hold the breath for 2 to 3, not 4, seconds. This depth and rhythm of inhalations and the length of time for holding the breath provide for the most effective expectoration of respiratory secretions when using this device.
    3. Although the lips should be firmly around the stem, the cheeks should be kept stiff because this allows the airways rather than the cheeks to vibrate during the procedure.
    4. Taking two additional breaths using the device and inhaling fully and exhaling forcefully with each breath is the correct way to end the procedure. This helps to clear the lower airways once the upper airways are treated.
    TEST-TAKING TIP: Identify the clang association. The word *device* in the stem and in option 4 is a clang association. Examine option 4 carefully.
    Content Area: Oxygenation
    Integrated Processes: Teaching/Learning; Nursing Process: Implementation
    Client Need: Physiological Integrity; Reduction of Risk Potential
    Cognitive Level: Application
    Concept: Patient-Centered Care; Oxygenation

14. **ANSWER: 1, 2, 3.**
    Rationales:
    1. Making the opening to the mouth smaller during exhalation slows the flow of air out of the respiratory tract, which keeps the alveoli open longer for gas exchange and limits the collapse of small air passages that trap air in the respiratory tract.

2. Supraclavicular retractions reflect the use of accessory muscles of respiration, indicating the need for an increased effort to bring air into the respiratory tract.

3. Closing the glottis at the height of inspiration keeps air in the alveoli slightly longer, which promotes gas exchange in the alveolar capillary beds. A grunt results when the glottis opens during exhalation, as air passes through the vocal cords.

4. An oxygen saturation level of 96% is within the expected limits of 95% to 100%.

5. The expected respiratory rate is 12 to 20 breaths/min; in addition, it should have a regular rhythm and be unlabored.

Content Area: Oxygenation
Integrated Processes: Nursing Process: Assessment
Client Need: Physiological Integrity; Reduction of Risk Potential
Cognitive Level: Application
Concept: Oxygenation

15. ANSWER: 3.
Rationales:

1. Yellow and yellowish-green sputum are associated with bacterial infections.

2. White sputum most often is associated with viral infections.

3. **Black sputum is associated with exposure to a fire because of the inhalation of smoke.**

4. Red sputum reflects blood in the sputum (hemoptysis), which is associated with conditions such as pneumococcal pneumonia and pulmonary edema.

Content Area: Oxygenation
Integrated Processes: Nursing Process: Analysis
Client Need: Physiological Integrity; Reduction of Risk Potential
Cognitive Level: Application
Concept: Oxygenation

16. ANSWER: 1, 2, 4, 3, 5.
Rationales:

1. **Dependent functions of the nurse require a prescription from an individual with a prescriptive license. Washing the hands limits the transmission of microorganisms.**

2. **A protective eye shield protects the nurse in the event the splashing of body fluids occurs during the procedure. Wearing sterile gloves maintains the sterility of the catheter that is inserted into the client's endotracheal tube and the sterility of the specimen.**

4. **Lubricating the tip of the catheter with normal saline limits friction and trauma to the mucous membranes of the respiratory tract. Inserting the catheter into the endotracheal tube accesses the trachea where sputum can be obtained.**

3. **The catheter must be advanced to where sputum can be obtained. Coughing mobilizes sputum, facilitating its removal, and resistance indicates that it has reached the carina of the trachea.**

5. **The catheter should be removed slowly and the tubing secured to seal the specimen in the collection receptacle.**

Content Area: Oxygenation
Integrated Processes: Nursing Process: Planning
Client Need: Physiological Integrity; Reduction of Risk Potential
Cognitive Level: Analysis
Concept: Oxygenation

17. ANSWER: 1, 5, 6.
Rationales:

1. **Because most pathology occurs in the base of the lungs, the bases should be auscultated first before the client becomes fatigued.**

2. The client should be placed in a sitting, not supine, position so that the anterior and posterior aspects of the chest are accessible for auscultation.

3. The client should be instructed to breathe in through the mouth, not the nose; this reduces the friction associated with air passing through the nasal passages and allows a larger volume of air to enter the lungs.

4. It is not necessary to listen at each site for a full minute. This would prolong the assessment and could result in hyperventilation and fatigue.

5. **Auscultating each lung at the same position allows for a comparison of the sounds heard.**

6. **Each site should be assessed long enough to detect the presence of expected and abnormal breath sounds. The characteristics of the sounds, such as pitch and presence of fluid, length of inhalation and exhalation, and appropriateness of the sounds heard at the site, should be assessed.**

TEST-TAKING TIP: Identify the clang association. The words *breath sounds* in the stem and *breath sound* in option 6 is a clang association.

Content Area: Oxygenation
Integrated Processes: Nursing Process: Implementation
Client Need: Health Promotion and Maintenance
Cognitive Level: Application
Concept: Oxygenation

18. ANSWER: 1.
Rationales:

1. **Stridor is caused by narrowing of the larynx and/or trachea, which may be life threatening. The client needs immediate medical supervision and medical interventions.**

2. Reassessing the client in 1 hour will allow the client's condition to get progressively worse; this intervention does not meet the needs of the client.

3. Suctioning the client experiencing laryngospasm is contraindicated. The problem is not excessive secretions. Suctioning a client experiencing stridor may exacerbate the laryngospasm, precipitating total obstruction of the airway.

4. Arranging for an x-ray examination will delay medical attention, and the delay may compromise the client's physical status. Stridor involves narrowing of the larynx, while an x-ray examination focuses on lung tissue.

TEST-TAKING TIP: Identify the options that are opposites. Options 1 and 2 are opposites because option 2 delays doing something for 1 hour and option 1 does something immediately. Look at these options carefully; more often

than not, one of the opposite options is the correct answer.
Content Area: Oxygenation
Integrated Processes: Communication and Documentation; Nursing Process: Implementation
Client Need: Safe and Effective Care Environment; Management of Care
Cognitive Level: Application
Concept: Oxygenation

19. **ANSWER: 2.**
Rationales:
1. Activity will increase the metabolic rate and the demand for oxygen. The client should be transferred via a wheelchair. Sitting in a wheelchair promotes thoracic expansion because the diaphragm can expand downward without the abdominal organs compressing against the diaphragm. When transferred to a bed, the client should be maintained in the high-Fowler position.
2. The client probably is experiencing carbon dioxide narcosis (CO_2 narcosis). Because a person with emphysema has chronically increased carbon dioxide levels (the usual stimulus to breathe in a healthy person), a person with emphysema responds to decreased oxygen levels as the stimulus to breathe. Therefore, the stimulus to breathe decreases when excessive oxygen is administered to a person with emphysema. In addition, with an increase in exogenous oxygen, there is an increase in the degree to which diseased alveoli are perfused with blood relative to other less-diseased alveoli, resulting in a larger fraction of blood passing through parts of the lung that are poorly ventilated, which results in retained carbon dioxide. The primary health-care provider should be notified immediately because arterial blood gases may be drawn and the oxygen level lowered even more until the problem is corrected.
3. Administering additional oxygen is contraindicated. This will further complicate this client's problem. Also, this action requires a prescription because the flow rate is more than 2 L/minute.
4. Although encouraging the client to perform pursed-lip breathing should eventually be done, it is not the primary nursing intervention. Exhaling through the mouth with the lips positioned to create a small opening to prolong exhalation (pursed-lip breathing) keeps the alveoli open longer for gas exchange and more efficient exhalation of trapped air.
TEST-TAKING TIP: Identify the word in the stem that sets a priority. The word *first* in the stem sets a priority. Identify the options with a clang association. The word *liters* in the stem and in options 2 and 3 are clang associations. Identify the options that are opposites. Options 2 and 3 are opposites. Consider these options carefully. Often, one of the opposite options is the correct answer.
Content Area: Oxygenation
Integrated Processes: Communication and Documentation; Nursing Process: Implementation
Client Need: Physiological Integrity; Physiological Adaptation
Cognitive Level: Analysis
Concept: Patient-Centered Care; Oxygenation

20. **ANSWER: 1, 5.**
Rationales:
1. Administering mouth care every 2 to 4 hours is appropriate because the oral mucous membranes become dry and irritated with a foreign object in the mouth; keep suction equipment readily available at the bedside.
2. An oropharyngeal tube should not be taped in place. As the gag reflex returns, the client will attempt to spit out the tube. If it is taped in place and the gag reflex returns, it may cause retching, laryngospasm, vomiting, and aspiration.
3. An oropharyngeal tube is positioned in the mouth, not the nose. A nasopharyngeal tube is inserted in the nose and extends from the nares to the pharynx. A nasopharyngeal tube is used for clients who are semiconscious and are at risk for airway obstruction because it does not stimulate gagging and vomiting.
4. The tube should initially be inserted with the inner curve of the device facing the nose, not the tongue. This avoids potential occlusion of the airway. If the curve is facing the tongue, it could push the tongue to the rear of the mouth, occluding the airway.
5. The tube should be rotated from the curve facing the nose 180 degrees into place with the curve facing the tongue.
TEST-TAKING TIP: Identify the unique option. Option 1 is unique. It is the only option that does not contain the words *the tube*.
Content Area: Oxygenation
Integrated Processes: Nursing Process: Implementation
Client Need: Physiological Integrity; Physiological Adaptation
Cognitive Level: Application
Concept: Oxygenation

21. **ANSWER: 3, 1, 2, 4, 5.**
Rationales:
3. Placing a client in the high-Fowler position will lower the abdominal viscera, thus allowing the lungs to expand more effectively. Relieving distress is the priority.
1. Obtaining the client's vital signs is important but should be performed after implementing an intervention that may relieve the client's current distress.
2. Teaching the client pursed-lip breathing will help the client exhale more slowly, which will keep the alveoli expanded and prevent collapse of the bronchioles. This is done after an initial intervention to relieve the distress and collect more data. Teaching the client pursed-lip breathing may take a little time.
4. The client is the priority. Informing the client's primary health-care provider about the client's status will be necessary after attempts to alleviate the client's distress are instituted first.
5. The nurse already knows that the client's oxygen saturation is 89%. After performing essential nursing interventions to improve the client's physical status, the nurse should continue to monitor the client's oxygen saturation level. This will provide data about the client's response to care or identify a progressive deterioration

of the client's respiratory status. If the client's oxygenation status continues to decline, the rapid response team should be notified.

Content Area: Oxygenation
Integrated Processes: Nursing Process: Planning
Client Need: Physiological Integrity; Physiological Adaptation
Cognitive Level: Application
Concept: Oxygenation

22. ANSWER: 4.

Rationales:

1. An endotracheal tube is inappropriate in this situation. An endotracheal tube has an inflatable cuff to provide a seal, preventing an air leak when a client is receiving mechanical ventilation.

2. A tracheostomy tube is inappropriate in this situation. A tracheostomy tube is used for a client with an upper airway obstruction. This tube is surgically inserted and circumvents an obstruction. It can be temporary or permanent.

3. An oropharyngeal tube is contraindicated for a semiconscious client because it may stimulate gagging, laryngospasm, vomiting, and aspiration.

4. A nasopharyngeal tube is the most appropriate tube for the client in this situation. It maintains the airway without stimulating the gag reflex.

Content Area: Oxygenation
Integrated Processes: Nursing Process: Planning
Client Need: Physiological Integrity; Physiological Adaptation
Cognitive Level: Application
Concept: Oxygenation

23. ANSWER: 3.

Rationales:

1. A nonrebreather mask is not the appropriate oxygen delivery system to deliver 60% oxygen to the client. A nonrebreather mask delivers 70% to 100% oxygen, depending on the oxygen liter flow rate.

2. A nasal cannula is not the appropriate oxygen delivery system to deliver 60% oxygen to the client. A nasal cannula delivers 24% to 44% oxygen, depending on the oxygen liter flow rate.

3. A Venturi mask is the appropriate mask to deliver 60% oxygen to a client. A Venturi mask delivers 24% to 60% oxygen, depending on the oxygen liter flow rate and plastic valve used.

4. A face tent is not the appropriate oxygen delivery system to deliver 60% oxygen to the client. A face tent delivers 30% to 55% oxygen, depending on the oxygen liter flow rate.

Content Area: Oxygenation
Integrated Processes: Nursing Process: Implementation
Client Need: Physiological Integrity; Physiological Adaptation
Cognitive Level: Analysis
Concept: Oxygenation

24. ANSWER: 4, 2, 1, 6, 3, 5.

Rationales:

4. Placing the client in the high-Fowler position will facilitate nasal cannula insertion and allow for thoracic

expansion during suctioning. This should be done before donning sterile gloves.

2. Opening the suction kit should be done before donning sterile gloves because the outside of the kit is not sterile.

1. Donning sterile gloves should be done after opening the suction kit to allow the nurse to handle the kit's contents, which are sterile.

6. Determining the distance between the client's ear and nose with the catheter should be done before lubricating the catheter tip to avoid having the lubricant drip on the client or the catheter becoming contaminated. This measurement ensures that the catheter will reach the client's nasopharyngeal area to aspirate secretions.

3. Lubricating the catheter tip must be done to facilitate insertion of the catheter into the client's nares; it reduces friction and trauma to the mucous membranes.

5. Inserting the suction catheter should be done after the above steps have been completed.

Content Area: Oxygenation
Integrated Processes: Nursing Process: Planning
Client Need: Physiological Integrity; Physiological Adaptation
Cognitive Level: Analysis
Concept: Oxygenation

25. ANSWER: 2, 4.

Rationales:

1. The curved prongs should be positioned in the nose with the curve facing downward, not upward. This follows the natural curve of the internal pathway of the nose.

2. Padding between the zygomatic bones and the cannula tubing minimizes pressure, thereby maintaining tissue integrity.

3. A nasal cannula oxygen delivery system does not include elastic straps. The tubing of a nasal cannula is wrapped around the ears and the slider is positioned under the chin.

4. An oxygen flow rate higher than 3 L/min can dry the mucous membranes. Humidification of oxygen helps minimize drying of the mucous membranes.

5. Oral care should be provided every 4 hours or whenever necessary because oxygen therapy can dry mucous membranes.

TEST-TAKING TIP: Identify the clang association. The word *oxygen* in the stem and in option 4 is a clang association.

Content Area: Oxygenation
Integrated Processes: Nursing Process: Implementation
Client Need: Physiological Integrity; Physiological Adaptation
Cognitive Level: Application
Concept: Oxygenation

26. ANSWER: 2.

Rationales:

1. This position is unsafe after an enteral feeding. It will promote, not prevent, aspiration.

2. The head of the bed should be raised to 45 degrees during the feeding and for at least 1 hour after the feeding. This uses the principle of gravity to help keep the solution in the stomach, thereby minimizing the risk of regurgitation and aspiration.

3. Enteral feeding formulas should not be thickened because they may clog the feeding tube.

4. Suctioning should be implemented only when a client is unable to clear respiratory secretions that are threatening the airway.

TEST-TAKING TIP: Identify the clang associations. The word *feeding* in the stem and in options 2 and 4 are clang associations. Examine these options carefully.

Content Area: Oxygenation
Integrated Processes: Nursing Process: Implementation
Client Need: Physiological Integrity; Basic Care and Comfort
Cognitive Level: Application
Concept: Safety

27. ANSWER: 2, 4, 5.

Rationales:

1. Hot dogs should be avoided, not just cut into small pieces, because the casing is difficult to chew and swallow.

2. Toddlers should not be given marshmallows because they are sticky and difficult for toddlers to chew and swallow. Marshmallows can obstruct the airway.

3. Teaching a toddler the universal sign for choking is not an age-appropriate instruction; this is unrealistic for a toddler to understand.

4. Toys should be larger than a clenched fist and have no removable parts; these criteria prevent aspiration and an airway obstruction.

5. Plastic bags and plastic wrap should be stored out of the reach of young children. A plastic bag or plastic wrap can impair a child's ability to breathe by occluding the airway, causing hypoxia and death. Also, if a plastic bag is placed over the head, it can cause suffocation (asphyxiation).

TEST-TAKING TIP: Identify options with clang associations. The word *toddler* in the stem and in options 2, 3, and 5 are clang associations. Examine these options carefully. Options 2 and 5 are correct answers. Option 3 is a distractor.

Content Area: Oxygenation
Integrated Processes: Teaching/Learning; Nursing Process: Planning
Client Need: Health Promotion and Maintenance
Cognitive Level: Application
Concept: Health Promotion; Oxygenation

28. ANSWER: 2, 3.

Rationales:

1. Wall suction pressure should be set between 100 and 150 mm Hg for adults, 100 and 120 mm Hg for children, and 50 and 95 mm Hg for infants.

2. The nurse should assess breath sounds after suctioning to ensure that the client's airway is patent. In addition, pulse oximetry should be assessed before and after suctioning because it is objective data that reflects arterial blood oxygen saturation. After suctioning, a client's oxygen saturation level should increase.

3. Personal protective equipment protects the nurse from contamination with secretions that may be splashed during suctioning.

4. A client should be positioned in a semi- or high-Fowler position when being suctioned. These positions use gravity to move abdominal organs away from the thoracic cavity, facilitating lung expansion.

5. A 12 to 18 French catheter is used when suctioning an adult, an 8 to 10 French catheter is used when suctioning a child, and a 5 to 8 French catheter is used when suctioning an infant. The higher the catheter gauge, the larger the lumen.

Content Area: Oxygenation
Integrated Processes: Nursing Process: Implementation
Client Need: Physiological Integrity; Physiological Adaptation
Cognitive Level: Application
Concept: Oxygenation

29. ANSWER: 4.

Rationales:

1. Although assessing the ears for irritation due to the oxygen tubing should be done, it is not the priority.

2. Although hanging an "oxygen in use" sign is important, it is not the priority.

3. Although monitoring the client's oxygen saturation routinely may be done, it is not a reliable indicator for clients with chronic obstruction pulmonary disease or impaired peripheral circulation.

4. Do not exceed 2 L/min for clients with chronic obstructive lung disease because their bodies have become accustomed to increased carbon dioxide levels and their stimulus to breathe is a low oxygen level; assess for signs of carbon dioxide narcosis, such as mental confusion and lethargy.

TEST-TAKING TIP: Identify the word in the stem that sets a priority. The word *most* in the stem sets a priority. Identify the option that is unique. Option 4 is unique because it is the only option with a number.

Content Area: Oxygenation
Integrated Processes: Nursing Process: Implementation
Client Need: Physiological Integrity; Physiological Adaptation
Cognitive Level: Application
Concept: Oxygenation

30. ANSWER: 2.

Rationales:

1. This is a simple face mask and will not deliver 100% oxygen. A simple face mask usually is set at 5 to 10 L of oxygen and delivers 40% to 60% oxygen.

2. This is a nonrebreather mask that is used to deliver 100% oxygen. It has one or two side vents that open only when the client exhales and remains closed on inspiration. This mask prevents mixing of room air with oxygen and does not allow entry of exhaled air. It can deliver 70% to 100% oxygen.

3. This is a Venturi mask, and it will not deliver 100% oxygen. This mask allows for an exact mixing of room air and oxygen so that a specific amount of oxygen is delivered. Valves and oxygen flow rates are used to control the specific percentage of oxygen to be delivered.

4. This is a face tent and will not deliver 100% oxygen. It does not deliver an exact amount of oxygen because the

top is open; however, it does allow for delivery of high amounts of humidity. Because a face tent does not deliver precise amounts of oxygen, it is essential that the client's oxygen saturation be assessed.
Content Area: Oxygenation
Integrated Processes: Nursing Process: Implementation
Client Need: Physiological Integrity; Physiological Adaptation
Cognitive Level: Analysis
Concept: Oxygenation

31. **ANSWER: 3.**
Rationales:
1. Although oxygen may be needed, it is premature to administer oxygen without obtaining more data. In addition, administering oxygen will need a primary health-care provider's prescription unless it is an emergency situation.
2. Obtaining a pulse oximetry level will provide useful data, but it will not assist in alleviating the client's symptoms.
3. Elevating the head of the bed should be the first intervention because it is the least invasive, does not require a primary health-care provider's prescription, and may alleviate the problem. Raising the head of the bed allows the abdominal organs to drop by gravity, facilitating expansion of the thoracic cavity during inhalation.
4. Notifying the client's primary health-care provider may be necessary, but it is premature if done before additional data are collected and other interventions are attempted to alleviate the problem.
TEST-TAKING TIP: Identify the word in the stem that sets a priority. The word *first* in the stem sets a priority.
Content Area: Oxygenation
Integrated Processes: Nursing Process: Implementation
Client Need: Physiological Integrity; Physiological Adaptation
Cognitive Level: Application
Concept: Oxygenation

32. **ANSWER: 2.**
Rationales:
1. Although the client has not voided in 4 hours and 15 minutes and should be encouraged to void, it is not as serious a concern as another option at this time. If the client has not voided in 8 hours, the client's primary health-care provider should be informed.
2. Respirations of 17 shallow breaths per minute are a concern. One would expect the respiratory rate to be higher in light of the elevated temperature and concurrent increase in the basal metabolic rate. Also, the client currently is receiving 2 L/min of oxygen that obviously is ineffective in improving the client's respiratory status.
3. Although the temperature is high, the client was administered Tylenol 650 mg at 1300. Also, the client may be in the defervescence phase of fever abatement, as indicated by the clinical indicators of flushed appearance, diaphoresis, and reports of feeling warm.
4. Although the client may have been dehydrated on admission to the emergency department, the client has

been receiving 125 mL per hour of fluid for the past several hours and will continue to receive IV fluid until discontinued by the primary health-care provider.
TEST-TAKING TIP: Identify the word in the stem that sets a priority. The word *priority* in the stem sets a priority.
Content Area: Oxygenation
Integrated Processes: Communication and Documentation; Nursing Process: Analysis
Client Need: Physiological Integrity; Reduction of Risk Potential
Cognitive Level: Analysis
Concept: Patient-Centered Care; Oxygenation

33. **ANSWER: 3.**
Rationales:
1. Cupping and clapping are unnecessary. There is no indication that the client is having difficulty mobilizing respiratory secretions.
2. Calling the client's primary health-care provider at this time is premature. More information is needed regarding the client's status.
3. Vital signs, including oxygen saturation, are essential data that should be obtained to provide a better understanding of the client's cardiorespiratory status. This information will direct future interventions.
4. Administering oxygen may be necessary, but it is premature without gathering more information about the client's status.
TEST-TAKING TIP: Identify the word in the stem that sets a priority. The word *next* in the stem sets a priority.
Content Area: Oxygenation
Integrated Processes: Nursing Process: Implementation
Client Need: Physiological Integrity; Physiological Adaptation
Cognitive Level: Application
Concept: Oxygenation

34. **ANSWER: 2, 5, 6.**
Rationales:
1. Dry mouth is associated with an anticholinergic bronchodilator.
2. Swollen lips are an early sign of anaphylaxis; the medication should be discontinued and the rapid response team notified immediately.
3. Blurred vision is associated with an anticholinergic bronchodilator.
4. Urinary retention is associated with an anticholinergic bronchodilator.
5. Difficulty breathing is a sign of anaphylaxis; the medication should be discontinued and the rapid response team notified immediately.
6. Steroidal nasal sprays can depress the immune system, which can lead to an oropharyngeal fungal infection.
Content Area: Oxygenation
Integrated Processes: Nursing Process: Implementation
Client Need: Physiological Integrity; Pharmacological and Parenteral Therapies
Cognitive Level: Application
Concept: Medication; Oxygenation

Chapter 20

Nutrition

NURSING CONCEPTS

Collaboration
Communication
Fluid and Electrolyte Balance
Medication

Metabolism
Nutrition
Patient-Centered Care
Safety

KEY TERMS

Anorexia—Loss of appetite

Cachexia—Extreme loss of lean body mass, marked weakness, muscle wasting, and malnutrition

Carbohydrate—Organic compound that contains carbon, hydrogen, and oxygen

Cheilosis—Cracks or lesions at corners of the mouth

Complete protein—Nutrient that includes all of the essential amino acids required for protein synthesis

Dumping syndrome—Concentrated gastric contents rapidly enters the intestine, moving water from the bowel wall into the intestinal lumen causing osmotic diarrhea

Electrolytes—Chemical elements that when in solution dissociates as ions carrying either a positive or negative charge

Enteral nutrition—Administration of a liquid formula via tubing directly into the gastrointestinal tract

Essential amino acids—Amino acids that cannot be manufactured in the body and must be obtained from food or supplements

Gingivitis—Inflamed, swollen, spongy gums

Glossitis—Beefy, red, swollen, sore tongue, indicating inflammation

Incomplete protein—Nutrient that does not include all of the essential amino acids required for protein synthesis

Lipid (fat)—Organic compound that contains a carbon chain to which hydrogen, oxygen, and other elements are attached

Minerals—Inorganic simple elements that have varied roles related to the body's structure and function

Negative nitrogen balance—State caused by inadequate intake of protein to meet body needs, resulting in muscle breakdown that releases nitrogen from muscle cells

Nonessential amino acids—Amino acids that can be synthesized by the body and do not need to be obtained from food or supplements

Obese—Body mass index more than 30

Overweight (preobesity)—Body mass index more than 25 but less than 30

Parenteral nutrition—Administration of nutrients via a catheter directly into the bloodstream

Protein—Organic compound that contains amino acids linked by peptide bonds

Stomatitis—Sores on the lips or in the mouth, indicating inflammation

Underweight—Body mass index less than 18.5

Vitamins—Organic compounds necessary to catalyze metabolic processes in the body

I. Structures and Functions of the Gastrointestinal System

The structures and functions of the gastrointestinal (GI) system are associated with the ingestion of food and elimination of the waste products of digestion in the form of feces. Nurses must know the basic anatomy and physiology of the GI system when providing care to clients with alterations in nutrition. The anatomy and physiology of the GI system provides the foundation for understanding how essential nutrients are utilized in the body, assessing a client's nutritional status, implementing nursing care to support a client's nutritional status, and administering enteral and parenteral nutrition. (See Chapter 23, Bowel Elimination, for details concerning the structures and functions of the GI system and see Fig. 23.1, which illustrates the digestive organs.)

II. Essential Nutrients

Food contains chemical compounds and elements that provide the nutrients the body requires for the maintenance of life. The essential nutrients include macronutrients (e.g., carbohydrates, proteins, and lipids) and micronutrients (e.g., vitamins and minerals). Each nutrient has several types and specific functions and is digested via a process specific to the nutrient. This information is the foundation for understanding the role of nutrition in the promotion of health, prevention of disease, and recovery from illness.

A. Carbohydrates
1. Provides 4 kilocalories per gram.
2. Functions.
   a. Primary source of energy for muscle and organ function.
   b. Facilitates insulin secretion.
   c. Supports a feeling of fullness.
   d. Enhances absorption of sodium and excretion of calcium.
3. Types of carbohydrates.
   a. Simple carbohydrates.
      (1) Contain saccharide units (sugar); for example, monosaccharides (contain one saccharide unit) and disaccharides (contain two saccharide units).
      (2) Found in honey, table sugar, milk, sugar cane, molasses, sugar beets, corn syrup, and fruits.
   b. Complex carbohydrates.
      (1) Contain multiple chains of saccharide units, for example, polysaccharides.
      (2) Fiber: Consists of complex carbohydrates found in plants, such as grains, vegetables, and legumes; provides bulk to the diet,

which facilitates elimination of waste and fulfills the appetite.
      (3) Starches: Consist of insoluble, nonsweet forms of complex carbohydrates; exist in plants (e.g., grains, potatoes, legumes) and are in processed foods (e.g., bread, flour, and cereal).
4. Digestion.
   a. Starts in the mouth with salivary amylase.
   b. Continues in the small intestine with pancreatic amylase and intestinal sucrase, maltase, and lactase.
   c. Leads to excess carbohydrate compounds being converted to glycogen and stored in the liver or converted to adipose tissue.

B. Protein
1. Provides 4 kilocalories per gram.
2. Composed of amino acids.
   a. An **essential amino acid** is an organic compound that cannot be manufactured in the body and must be obtained from food or supplements.
   b. A **nonessential amino acid** is an organic compound that can be synthesized by the body and does not need to be obtained from food or supplements.
3. Functions.
   a. Necessary for tissue growth, maintenance, and repair.
   b. Necessary for production of digestive enzymes, hormones, lymphocytes, and antibodies.
   c. Facilitates fluid and acid-base balance.
   d. Serves as an energy source when carbohydrates and fats are insufficient to meet energy needs.
4. Types of protein.
   a. A **complete protein** is a nutrient that includes all of the essential amino acids required for protein synthesis, for example, eggs, cheese, and milk.
   b. An **incomplete protein** is a nutrient that does not include all of the essential amino acids required for protein synthesis, for example, nuts, corn, wheat, beans, seeds, and brown rice.
   c. A complete protein can be made by combining two incomplete proteins, such as red beans and brown rice or peanut butter and whole-grain bread.
5. Digestion.
   a. Starts in the mouth with pepsin.
   b. Continues in the small intestine by the pancreatic enzymes trypsin, chymotrypsin, and carboxypeptidase and the enzymes aminopeptidase and dipeptidase, which are secreted by glands in the intestinal wall.

6. Nitrogen balance.
   a. Reflects the extent of protein anabolism and catabolism in the body.
   b. **Negative nitrogen balance** is a state caused by inadequate intake of protein to meet body needs, resulting in muscle breakdown that releases nitrogen from muscle cells; nitrogen loss is greater than intake; occurs with conditions such as burns and malnutrition.

C. **Lipids** (Fats)
   1. Provides 9 kilocalories per gram.
   2. Functions.
      a. Main source of fuel for the body.
      b. Assist in the absorption of the fat-soluble vitamins A, D, E, and K.
      c. Provide satiety.
      d. Enhance the flavor of food.
      e. Contribute to the formation of adipose tissue, which cushions vital organs and aids thermoregulation by protecting the body from temperature extremes.
      f. Lubricates the skin via secretion of oil from sebaceous glands.
      g. Is an essential constituent of cell membranes and cellular function.
   3. Types of lipids.
      a. Glycerides.
         (1) Consist of one molecule of glycerol attached to various length fatty acid chains.
         (2) Types: Monoglyceride, diglyceride, and triglyceride.
      b. Sterols.
         (1) Necessary for the development of cell membranes, vitamin D, testosterone, and estrogen.
         (2) Cholesterol: Most important sterol; liver synthesizes 75% of body cholesterol, and 25% is provided from dietary sources, such as beef and pork (particularly the liver and heart), fish, poultry, dairy products, and egg yolk.
      c. Phospholipids.
         (1) Important element of lipoproteins that transport lipids throughout the body.
         (2) *Low-density lipoproteins (LDLs):* "Bad cholesterol"; saturated fats in the diet increase LDLs in the bloodstream, causing fatty deposits on vessel walls and contributing to cardiovascular disease.
         (3) *High-density lipoproteins (HDLs):* "Good cholesterol"; moves cholesterol from the bloodstream to the liver where it is used in bile or excreted.

4. Types of dietary lipids.
   a. Saturated fat.
      (1) Foods high in saturated fats raise the levels of LDL cholesterol, which increases the risk for cardiovascular disease and stroke.
      (2) Found in whole milk, butter, cheese, ice cream, red meat, coconut products, lard, chocolate, palm oil, and cocoa butter.
   b. Monounsaturated fat.
      (1) Contributes vitamin E to the diet, an antioxidant vitamin.
      (2) When substituted for saturated fats and trans fats it reduces LDL, which lowers the risk of heart disease and stroke.
      (3) Found in olive, canola, and peanut oils; nuts, such as cashews, almonds, and peanuts; and avocados.
   c. Polyunsaturated fat.
      (1) Provides omega-6 and omega-3 fatty acids, important for many bodily functions.
      (2) When substituted for saturated fats and trans fats it reduces LDL, which lowers the risk of heart disease and stroke.
      (3) Found in corn, safflower, soybean, sesame, and cottonseed oils; nuts and seeds; and fatty fish such as salmon, mackerel, herring, and trout.
   d. Trans fat.
      (1) Saturated fat produced when a manufacturer adds hydrogen to polyunsaturated plant oils (hydrogenation) to extend shelf life.
      (2) Foods high in trans fats raise the levels of LDL, which increases the risk for cardiovascular disease and stroke.
      (3) Found in vegetable shortening, most commercial baked goods, deep-fried chips, fast foods, and most margarines.
5. Digestion.
   a. Occurs in the small intestine by a variety of actions.
      (1) Lipids in the duodenum stimulate the release of cholecystokinin by glands in the wall of the intestine, which stimulates the contraction of the gallbladder.
      (2) Contraction of the gallbladder releases bile into the duodenum where bile emulsifies lipids and prepares them for further digestion.
      (3) Pancreatic enzymes act in the small intestine.
         (a) Lipase breaks down lipids, releasing the final products to be absorbed (e.g., fatty acids, diglycerides, monoglycerides, and glycerol).
         (b) Cholesterol esterase combines free cholesterol and fatty acids to form

cholesterol esters in preparation for absorption.

(4) Lecithinase, an intestinal enzyme, acts on lecithin, a phospholipid, to prepare it for absorption.

D. Vitamins

1. Organic compounds necessary to catalyze metabolic processes.
2. Essential for growth and development and act as coenzymes in enzymatic systems.
3. Supplied by the ingestion of plants and animals because they are not made by the body.

4. Fat-soluble vitamins.
   a. Include vitamins A, D, E, and K (Table 20.1).
   b. Are absorbed from the intestines like fats and primarily stored in the liver and adipose tissue.
   c. Excessive intake can cause toxicity.
   d. Deficiency occurs with inadequate intake or diseases that inhibit fat digestion and absorption.
5. Water-soluble vitamins.
   a. Include vitamin C, thiamin, riboflavin, niacin, vitamin B_6, folic acid, vitamin B_{12}, pantothenic acid, and biotin (Table 20.2).
   b. Are required daily because the body eliminates excesses in urine, which may result in deficiencies.

Table 20.1 Fat-Soluble Vitamins

Functions	Sources	Deficiency	Excess
Vitamin A			
• Important for night vision. • Promotes cellular growth and maturity. • Supports growth of bone and teeth. • Maintains healthy skin and mucous membranes. • Regulates energy. • Can be converted from beta carotene, a yellow-red pigment in some foods, in the gastric mucosa and act as an antioxidant.	• Pumpkin, sweet potatoes, carrots, spinach, collards, broccoli, cabbage, squash. • Apricots, cantaloupe. • Liver. • Fortified milk, butter, cream, egg yolk.	**Mild:** Night blindness, diarrhea, impaired vision, skin lesions, sore throat, mouth lesions, intestinal infections. **Severe:** Thickening and drying of the outer surface of the eyes, leading to blindness and inflammation of the eyes.	**Mild:** Gastrointestinal disturbances, blurred vision, impaired muscle coordination, fetal defects, yellow skin (carotenemia). **Severe:** Bone pain, reports of increased pressure in the skull, other signs and symptoms similar to a brain tumor.
Vitamin D			
• Essential for growth of bone and teeth. • Promotes absorption of calcium.	• Fortified dairy products and egg yolk. • Fatty fish and fish oils. • Synthesized by sunlight.	**Severe:** *Adults:* Osteomalacia (soft, fragile bones of the pelvis, spine, and legs). *Children:* Rickets (impaired growth plates, soft and fragile bones, growth retardation, bowlegs, and knock-knees).	**Mild:** Anorexia, nausea and vomiting, polyuria, weakness, and constipation. **Severe:** Calcium deposits in heart, brain, and kidneys; mental and physical growth retardation.
Vitamin E			
• Functions as an antioxidant. • Protects vitamin A and unsaturated fatty acids from oxidation.	• Wheat and rice germ. • Milk, butter, margarine, vegetable oils, shortening. • Nuts. • Eggs and fish. • Dark-green, leafy vegetables.	• Uncommon. • Myopathy, hyporeflexia, and ataxia. • Anemia in premature infants.	• Generally nontoxic. • Large supplemental doses for a year can cause excessive bleeding, impaired healing, depression, nausea, and impaired digestion.
Vitamin K			
• Important for blood clotting factors. • Necessary for bone development.	• Green leafy vegetables (e.g., kale, turnip greens, spinach, and collards). • Liver. • Made by bacteria in the intestine.	• Related to drug therapy, such as antibiotics that eliminate bacteria in the intestine or diseases that impair fat metabolism, which impedes vitamin K absorption.	*Adults:* No clinical indicators of toxicity reported. *Infants:* May cause hemolytic anemia or hyperbilirubinemia, leading to brain damage.

Table 20.2 **Water-Soluble Vitamins**

Functions	Sources	Deficiency	Excess
Thiamin (B$_1$)			
• Coenzyme for carbohydrate metabolism. • Needed to convert tryptophan to niacin. • Promotes nervous system functioning.	• Cooked dry beans. • Soy milk. • Whole-grain enriched bread and cereal. • Beef, liver, pork. • Nuts and peas.	**Beriberi** *Mild:* Anorexia, indigestion, constipation. *Severe:* Peripheral paralysis, fatigue, apathy, muscle weakness, cardiovascular problems, and alcoholism-related Wernicke-Korsakoff syndrome.	• No clinical indicators of toxicity reported.
Riboflavin (B$_2$)			
• Important in energy metabolism. • Assists in red blood cell production.	• Enriched breads and cereals. • Pork, liver, beef. • Eggs, milk, soft cheeses, such as ricotta and cottage cheese. • Mushrooms, soybeans, and spinach.	• Uncommon. • Lesions in the mouth and on the lips; swollen tongue; sore throat. • Facial dermatitis. • Vulval and scrotal skin changes. • Normocytic anemia.	• No clinical indicators of toxicity reported.
Niacin (B$_3$)			
• Needed for synthesis of fatty acids. • Important in maintaining muscle tone and function of the nervous system. • Coenzyme in creating energy from glucose.	• Enriched bread and cereal. • Chicken breast, liver. • Pickled herring, tuna. • Dairy products, peanuts, and coffee.	**Pellagra** Diarrhea, dermatitis, dementia, weakness, anorexia, and indigestion.	• Itching, facial flushing. • Nausea and vomiting, gastric ulcers, and liver damage.
Pantothenic Acid (B$_5$)			
• Important in metabolism of fat, carbohydrates, and protein. • Needed in synthesis of acetylcholine, a neurotransmitter.	• In most foods. • Best sources: Meats, liver, kidney, whole-grain cereals and bread, sweet potatoes, egg yolks, tomatoes, and legumes.	• No known deficiency.	• No clinical indicators of toxicity.
Pyridoxine (B$_6$)			
• Needed for amino acid synthesis and catabolism. • Related to metabolism of 60+ enzymes. • Coenzyme for dopamine and serotonin. • Role in production of antibodies. • Aids in amino acid transport.	• Meats, poultry, fish. • Nuts and seeds. • Milk and dairy products. • Whole grains and enriched cereals, wheat germ. • Bananas. • Potatoes and legumes.	• Uncommon. • Dermatitis. • Glossitis and stomatitis. • Depression and confusion. • Linked to 2- to 3-year use of oral contraceptives; infants of mothers who received oral contraceptives for greater than 30 months before pregnancy.	• Due to self-prescribed megadoses. • Neuropathy, such as sensory loss in hands and feet, causing ataxia and problems with walking.
Cyanocobalamin (B$_{12}$)			
• Necessary for hemoglobin synthesis. • Helps maintain myelin sheath. • Essential in metabolic reactions.	• Meat, poultry, fish, shellfish. • Milk, dairy products, and eggs.	• Numbness and tingling of hands and feet. • Impaired red blood cells. • Depression, confusion, dementia, delusions. • Unrestorable nerve damage and death. **Pernicious anemia** Inadequate intrinsic factor, a protein-binding factor secreted by gastric mucosal cells, causing inadequate absorption of vitamin B$_{12}$.	• No clinical indicators of toxicity.

Continued

Table 20.2 Water-Soluble Vitamins—cont'd

Functions	Sources	Deficiency	Excess
Vitamin C			
• *Promotes collagen synthesis.* • *Promotes healing of wounds and fractures.* • *Is an antioxidant.* • *Needed for adrenal gland function.* • *Facilitates iron absorption.* • *Converts folic acid to active form.* • *Plays a role in immune function.*	• *Citrus fruits, such as oranges, grapefruits, and lemons.* • *Apricot nectar and strawberries.* • *Green peppers, broccoli, and tomatoes.*	**Scurvy** *Mild:* Tender, sore gums; weak blood vessels, causing small skin hemorrhages. *Severe:* Skin changes, impaired wound healing, softening of ends of bones, tooth loss, hemorrhage in joints and around heart and stomach.	• *Gastrointestinal disturbances, such as abdominal cramping, diarrhea, and nausea.*
Folic Acid			
• *Needed for deoxyribonucleic acid (DNA).* • *Role in cellular metabolism and cell renewal.* • *Needed for hemoglobin formation.*	• *Liver.* • *Spinach, asparagus, broccoli, beans, turnip greens.* • *Oranges and cantaloupe.* • *Eggs.* • *Enriched cereals, yeast.*	• *Megaloblastic anemia.* • *Link between deficiency and neural tube defect in neonates.* • *Related to malabsorption, gastrointestinal problems, and illnesses that increase metabolic rate, such as infections, hyperthyroidism, cancer, serious burns, and hemorrhage.* • *Reduced cell division and protein synthesis, causing red, swollen tongue; heartburn; diarrhea; fatigue; and hypotension.*	• *Toxicity is rare.* • *Hives, rashes, pruritus.* • *Respiratory problems.* • *Seizures.*

E. Minerals and electrolytes
  1. **Minerals** are inorganic simple elements that have varied roles related to structure (e.g., calcium and phosphorous give strength to bones) and function (e.g., sodium and potassium help regulate fluid balance) in the body.
  2. **Electrolytes** are chemical elements that, when in solution, dissociate as ions carrying either a positive or negative charge.
  3. Some minerals are electrolytes and others are not; the major minerals in the body that are electrolytes are calcium, sodium, potassium, magnesium, chloride, and phosphorus. (For more information about these electrolytes, see "Electrolytes" in Chapter 21, Fluid, Electrolyte, and Acid-Base Balance.)

III. Factors That Affect Nutrition and Related Nursing Care

Although food choices should be made based on their essential nutrients, usually these choices are dramatically influenced by nonnutritional factors. Physical, developmental, psychosociocultural, individual issues, and medical therapies all impact a person's nutritional intake. Understanding these factors can aid nurses in assessing clients, maintaining a nonjudgmental attitude when working with diverse individuals and populations, and planning individualized approaches to nursing care.

A. Advertising
  1. Television commercials have a significant impact on the choices people make regarding food and beverages. Fast food establishments and advertisements for new food products, herbs, and supplements present information in a manner that communicates that these products are safe and fun to eat or drink.
  2. Nursing care.
    a. Encourage people to be cautious and examine the facts associated with products being advertised.
    b. Encourage clients to review caloric and nutritive value of meals when eating in restaurants.

B. Alcohol intake
  1. Excessive alcohol intake contributes to inadequate nutrition in various ways; for example, alcohol is high in calories leading to weight gain, it substitutes food in the diet, decreases appetite, and increases the demand for vitamin B because this vitamin is used to metabolize alcohol.
  2. Nursing care.
    a. Encourage judicious intake of alcohol.
    b. Refer clients to Alcoholics Anonymous for help with cessation if alcohol intake is a problem.

C. Beliefs about food
  1. If a person learns that foods high in animal fat are unhealthy and increase the risk of heart disease

and brain attack, the person may be motivated to eat foods that have less animal fat.

2. Some people consume certain foods or fluids because they are believed to be aphrodisiacs, impede aging, or prevent urinary tract infection.
3. Nursing care.
   a. Determine a person's beliefs regarding nutrition and food.
   b. Identify and correct misconceptions.

D. Culture and ethnicity
   1. Most cultures have certain foods that are traditional, such as Italian people prefer pasta, Asian people prefer rice, Latino people prefer rice and beans, and Indian people prefer food spiced with curry.
   2. Events are commonly accompanied by traditional meals or feasts. For example, when the Amish build a barn, the men build and the women provide a communal meal to celebrate the accomplishment.
   3. Nursing care.
      a. Identify cultural and ethnic influenced food preferences.
      b. Customize food choices when a person receives a therapeutic diet to best address nutritional needs within the client's cultural and ethnic food preferences. (See Table 20.3 for common food preferences of selected cultural groups.)

Table 20.3 Common Food Preferences of Selected Cultural Groups and Related Nursing Care

Group and Preferences	Related Nursing Care
Asians Rice, noodles, bread, dumplings, Chinese greens, bean sprouts, mushrooms, bamboo, bok choy, beef, poultry, pork, seafood, eggs, tofu, soybeans, soy sauce, and all fruits	• Encourage steamed rather than fried dumplings, fish, vegetables, and rice. • Discourage fried noodles, rice, eggrolls, tempura battered and fried foods, and spareribs to decrease fat intake.
Cubans Rice, onions, tomatoes, green peppers, black beans, pork, and chorizo (sausage)	• Encourage meals with chicken or beans with rice to reduce fat intake. • Encourage use of salsa to add spice to food.
Mexicans Tortillas; corn and corn products; chili peppers; tomatoes; onions; beets; cabbage; meat; poultry; eggs; pinto, calico, and garbanzo beans; and cheese	• Encourage substitution of low-fat cheese for cheese high in fat. • Discourage intake of refried beans, fried tortillas, and deep-fried foods. • Discourage intake of high-fat cheese and sour cream.
Puerto Ricans Red kidney beans, eggs, pork, chicken, fish, garbanzo beans, plantains, Puerto Rican bread, rice and starchy vegetables, and guava and other fruits	
Italians Pasta; pasta sauce with meat; pasta dishes made with cheese, butter, and cream; cheese; bread; salad with olive oil and vinegar dressing; vegetables high in starch; breaded and fried vegetables and meats; numerous types of sausage and seafood; green peppers; onions; and tomatoes	• Encourage grilled meats and seafood, nonfat salad dressing, pasta sauce without meat (substitute with clams). • Discourage fried foods; use of cream, butter, and cheese in pasta dishes; and sausage and fatty meats to decrease fat intake.
African Americans (particularly southern U.S.) Biscuits; grits; cornbread; white bread; rice; corn; sweet potatoes; yams; collard greens; okra; tomatoes; squash; cabbage; fried meat, pork, chicken, and catfish; black-eyed peas; beans; buttermilk; ice cream; melons; peaches; and bananas	• Encourage substitution of grilled or steamed foods rather than fried foods. • Discourage use of lard and bacon grease when cooking; encourage use of fat-free cooking sprays and various spices for flavoring food to decrease fat intake.
Middle Eastern Europeans Rice, pita bread, couscous, feta cheese, yogurt, figs, dates, peaches, grape leaves, tomatoes, onions, peppers, squash, okra, peas, legumes, fennel, lamb, goat, chicken, and fish	• Encourage the intake of grilled or baked meats, vegetables, legumes, dates, figs, citrus fruits, and yogurt for salad dressings to decrease fat intake. • Discourage fried foods, casseroles, sour cream, and excessive butter when making a recipe with filo (flakey pastry dough).
Native Americans Corn, wild rice and oats, Indian biscuits, choke-cherries, black cherries, crab apples, wild mushrooms, root vegetables, wild game, seafood, and nuts	• Encourage the removal of fat from game meats; broil, bake, or grill meats. • Discourage fried foods and use of lard in cooking.
Northern Europeans Dark breads, potatoes, beef, pork, poultry, fish, shellfish, sausage, eggs, all cheeses, milk and milk products, fruits, and vegetables	• Encourage use of poached, baked, or steamed lean meats, tomato-based sauces, and consommé. • Discourage use of sausage, fried potatoes, creamed soups and sauces, sour cream, whole milk, and whole-milk products.

E. Economics
1. People living in poverty have fewer food choices because meat and fresh vegetables generally are more expensive than food items such as pasta, rice, and beans.
2. People with adequate financial income generally eat more protein and fats.
3. People who are homeless have a limited ability to purchase, prepare, or store food and, therefore, generally eat an inadequate diet.
4. Nursing care.
   a. Suggest substituting beans and rice for meat.
   b. Encourage buying seasonal foods because they usually are less expensive.
   c. Teach the client to avoid prepared convenience foods because they are more expensive.

F. Lifestyle
1. Families often do not share meals because children are engaged in multiple sports and social activities, requiring a reliance on fast foods or eating "on the run"; fast food is high in carbohydrates and salt and usually does not contain the essential nutrients of a balanced diet.
2. Single-parent families and families in which both parents work commonly rely on convenience foods and processed and prepared foods that are quick to make; the majority of these foods are high in carbohydrates and salt.
3. A family may more likely be exposed to a greater variety of food experiences if a parent enjoys cooking.
4. Nursing care.
   a. Encourage making several healthy meals that can be frozen for use in the future when time is limited.
   b. Encourage parents to establish a mealtime that all or most members of the family can attend.

G. Medications and therapy
1. Antineoplastics can cause such problems as stomatitis, anorexia, nausea, vomiting, and diarrhea and diminish energy, which negatively affects nutritional intake.
2. Drug and food interactions may require a person to avoid certain foods; for example, clients taking warfarin should avoid foods high in vitamin K (e.g., leafy green vegetables) because it decreases the effectiveness of the drug.
3. Certain medications (e.g., aspirin) should be taken with food because they are irritating to the stomach lining; levothyroxine should be taken on an empty stomach because doing so helps the drug to be absorbed better than it would be if it were taken with food.
4. Some medications can damage the liver *(hepatotoxicity)* or kidney *(nephrotoxicity)* if intake exceeds the recommended daily dose; for example, exceeding the adult dose of 4 g of acetaminophen daily can cause nephrotoxicity.
5. Radiation therapy can affect nutrition; for example, radiation for head and neck cancers can cause dysphagia, altered taste, and decreased salivation; anorexia and fatigue are common side effects of radiation therapy that can significantly interfere with a person's ability to maintain an adequate diet.
6. Nursing care.
   a. Identify the medications and therapies that the client is receiving and the ways in which they affect the client's nutrition.
   b. Teach the client ways to improve nutritional intake in relation to the medications and therapies the client is receiving.

H. Personal preferences
1. Food has different meanings to people; some people live to eat and others eat to live.
2. Food preferences commonly are related to childhood experiences. For example, a person may like a certain food because it is associated with happy visits to a loved grandparent or dislike a food that is associated with an unhappy experience.
3. Foods have different tastes, smells, and flavors that affect what a person likes or dislikes. Color, texture, and spices have a significant impact on what people prefer to eat; for example, some people like crisp vegetables and others prefer them to be cooked until soft. Some people do not like the texture of mussels and clams or the flavor of garlic, spices (e.g., curry), or herbs (e.g., cilantro).
4. Some people are willing to try new foods and some prefer to eat the same foods with little variety.
5. Some people prefer a vegetarian diet that includes grains, nuts, vegetables, and fruit and eliminates meat or animal flesh and their by-products; some vegetarian diets are even more selective.

DID YOU KNOW?

The various types of vegetarians are classified according to the variety of foods they are willing to eat or eliminate from the diet. For example,

- Ovolactovegetarians: Ingest eggs and dairy products but avoid meat, fish, and poultry.
- Ovovegetarians: Ingest eggs but avoid dairy products, meat, fish, and poultry.
- Lactovegetarians: Ingest dairy products but avoid eggs, meat, fish, and poultry.
- Vegans: Generally ingest brown rice, other grains, and herbal teas and avoid all food of animal origin.
- Fruitarians: Ingest only fruits, nuts, honey, and vegetable oils.

6. Nursing care.
   a. Identify a client's food preferences and collaborate with the client and dietician so that preferences are provided in the prescribed diet when possible; this is essential for vegetarians.
   b. Encourage people to try different foods to expand their palate; teach parents to encourage their children to try different foods appropriate for their developmental level.
   c. Teach the client who is a vegetarian to follow healthy practices.
      (1) Select foods and plan meals carefully so that adequate nutrition is achieved.
      (2) Combine grains and legumes to provide different amino acids that will form proteins in the body.
      (3) Understand that processed soybeans, soy milk, processed protein products, and tofu enrich the nutritive value of a vegetarian diet and have protein value equal to animal-derived protein; this instruction is not recommended for fruitarians.
      (4) Consider taking vitamin and mineral supplements, such as vitamin B_{12}, vitamin D, calcium, iron, and zinc, and protein under the care of a dietician or primary health-care provider to ensure an adequate intake of essential elements.
      🛑 (5) Understand that children who follow a vegetarian diet are at risk for protein and vitamin deficiencies, such as vitamin B_{12} deficiency, if these needs are not adequately addressed.

I. Physical health
   1. Lack of teeth; lack of appetite (**anorexia**); difficulty or pain on swallowing; inability to adequately digest food; lack of energy for eating; and presence of nausea, vomiting, and diarrhea can interfere with nutrition.
   2. Some people have food allergies or are gluten or lactose intolerant, which limits the foods that a person can ingest and/or digest.
   3. Factors that increase the basal metabolic rate (BMR) increase the demand for calories and fluids—for example, fever, growth periods, cold environment, prolonged physical exertion, and disease processes, such as hyperthyroidism, cancer, cardiac failure, severe burns, and trauma.
   4. Traumatic injuries and large draining wounds increase the demand for protein and vitamin C needed for healing.
   5. Illnesses, such as diabetes, cancer, heart disease, and GI disorders, affect nutritional health by interfering with digestion, absorption, metabolism, transport, and utilization of nutrients and excretion of the by-products of nutrition.

6. Nursing care.
   a. Identify a client's risk factors or health problems that may interfere with nutritional status.
   b. Collaborate with the primary health-care provider, dietician, and client to ensure that the diet meets the client's physical needs and preferences.
J. Religious observances
   1. Nutritional practices are closely associated with religious customs and traditions; for example, Catholic people do not eat meat on Fridays during Lent and fast on Good Friday; some Jewish people follow many dietary laws, such as animals must be killed in a certain way, all blood must be drained from meat, pork is forbidden, and dairy products and meat cannot be eaten at the same meal; Native American ceremonies are celebrated with specific foods.
   2. For additional information about religious beliefs related to food see Table 11.2 in Chapter 11, Diversity and Spirituality/Religion.
K. Developmental level
   1. Nutritional needs vary across the life span.
   2. Nursing care: Care should be based on a client's developmental level (Table 20.4).

IV. Nutritional Assessment

A nutritional assessment collects objective and subjective data about a client's nutritional status. It includes personal factors that influence food choices, a health and dietary history, and a physical assessment. The data collected provides baseline information, identifies clients who are at risk for or are experiencing a form of malnutrition, and forms the foundation for the development of an individualized nutritional regimen.
A. Assess for factors that affect nutrition. (See previous section III in this chapter.)
B. Obtain a health history
   1. Ask about acute or chronic illnesses, such as allergies; infection; diabetes; cancer; gastroesophageal reflux disease (GERD); and cardiac, renal, GI, or liver disease.
   2. Ask about pathology associated with the tongue, gums and teeth, hard or soft palate, and nasopharynx.
   3. Ask about oral problems, such as difficulty chewing, ill-fitting dentures, and stomatitis.
   4. Ask about the use of medications, such as steroids, antineoplastics, antihypertensives, diuretics, antacids, proton pump inhibitors, laxatives, antidepressants, and potassium chloride.
   5. Ask about a history of such therapies as radiation, total parenteral nutrition, and enteral feedings.
   6. Ask about drug misuse, excessive alcohol intake, and smoking history.

Table 20.4 Nutritional Variations Across the Life Span and Related Nursing Care

Age Group	Developmental Considerations	Related Nursing Care
Birth to 1 year	• Most rapid growth period; weight doubles in 6 months and triples by 1 year. • Breastfeeding reduces food allergies and intolerances; is easier to digest than formula; is convenient and economical. • Breastfeeding and formula feeding are recommended until age 1 year. • Eruption of baby teeth begins. • Begin to eat solid food at age 6 months. • Begin to self-feed table food by age 1 year.	• Explain the value of breastfeeding or support the need to provide formula to meet growth needs. • Explain that cow's milk increases the risk of an allergic reaction; it is too concentrated for an infant's kidneys to manage, is a poor source of iron and vitamins C and E; and may cause gastrointestinal bleeding. *Teach the parents to:* • Provide finger foods, such as bananas and crackers, and to avoid foods that are choking hazards, such as hot dogs and fruit with edible skins.
Toddlers and preschoolers	• They strive for autonomy. • Coordination increases, improving the ability to self-feed and use a spoon and fork effectively. • Appetite may be irregular and variable. • They begin to develop likes and dislikes and varied attitudes toward food. • They may use food to manipulate parents. • Milk anemia (iron deficiency anemia) can occur if toddlers consume 24 or more ounces of milk daily because milk is an inadequate source of iron.	*Teach the parents to:* • Encourage self-feeding and to avoid feeding a child because it is faster and less messy. • Provide opportunities to explore foods with different tastes and textures. • Avoid the use of food to motivate, bribe, or punish the child because doing so may cause inappropriate food attitudes. • Cut food into small pieces. • Avoid foods that can cause an airway obstruction, such as peanuts, gum, popcorn, nuts, peanut butter, hard candy, and grapes.
School-aged children (6 to 12 years)	• They have an uneven growth pattern. • Permanent teeth replace baby teeth. • Activity increases energy requirements. • They socialize more and become more independent. • Obesity is increasing in this age group.	*Teach the parents to:* • Educate their children about a healthy diet, foods that are important, and foods that should be avoided to prevent obesity. • Provide foods with a high-nutritive value; provide nutritious snacks. • Encourage physical activity, such as participation in active sports.
Adolescents	• Experience an increase in physical, psychosocial, and sexual development. • The need for calories, protein, calcium, vitamins D and B, and iron increases to sustain growth. • Males increase in muscle, bone, and lean body tissue; females increase in fat deposition and begin menstruating. • Peer pressure influences food choices and eating habits. • Eat more calorie-dense foods, such as fast foods, donuts, chips, soda, and ice cream. • Eat more meals outside the home because of sports and social activities. • Deficient food intake, extreme weight loss, muscle wasting, and arrested sexual development is a serious eating disorder (anorexia nervosa) of adolescence; more common in females. • Gorging followed by self-induced vomiting and the use of diuretics and laxatives to purge is another serious eating disorder (bulimia nervosa) of adolescence. • Depression may develop if an adolescent has a negative body image related to being underweight or overweight.	*Teach parents and adolescents to:* • Learn about foods that support increased caloric requirements related to physical growth and development and involvement in sports. • Learn strategies to maintain a healthy weight, especially when concerned about gaining weight. • Avoid fad diets that are detrimental to health. • Avoid negative statements or self-talk about being over- or under-weight because this decreases self-esteem. • Consume healthy snacks, such as fruits and raw vegetables, instead of junk food that is high in carbohydrates and contains little nutritive value. • Avoid keeping unhealthy foods in the home. • Make a determined effort to schedule meals so that family members eat together; this fosters more regular eating habits. • Avoid conflicts that relate to food because adolescents need to develop responsibility for a healthy diet. • Seek professional help if exhibiting clinical indicators of depression, anorexia nervosa, or bulimia nervosa.

Table 20.4 **Nutritional Variations Across the Life Span and Related Nursing Care—cont'd**

Age Group	Developmental Considerations	Related Nursing Care
Adults	• Growth and development ceases. • BMR decreases with each decade; weight gain and obesity may become a problem. • Activity generally decreases due to stress of work and family responsibilities, which can lead to weight gain. • Postmenopausal women have an increased need for calcium because of the increased risk of osteoporosis.	Teach adults to: • Decrease caloric intake and increase exercise to avoid weight gain associated with a decrease in the metabolic rate. • Recognize that obesity contributes to chronic illnesses, such as diabetes, hypertension, and mobility problems. • Increase calcium and vitamin D intake to reduce the risk of osteoporosis in postmenopausal women.
Pregnant women	• Nutrition needs increase due to the growth of maternal tissue, placenta, and fetus, especially in the second and third trimesters. • Essential nutrients needed are protein, iron, folic acid, calcium, and iodine. • Inadequate nutrition can cause impaired growth and development of the fetus. • An enlarging uterus places pressure on the gastrointestinal tract and may cause nausea, vomiting, heartburn, and constipation, which influence nutrition. • Alcohol intake can cause fetal alcohol syndrome. • Fish commonly contains mercury and other toxic substances that should be avoided.	Teach the woman to: • Receive ongoing prenatal care. • Take prescribed vitamins and supplements. • Ingest 400 mcg of folic acid daily when trying to conceive and throughout pregnancy to reduce the risk of neural tube defect in the fetus. • Follow a prescribed diet for total weight gain based on prepregnancy body mass index. • Ingest small frequent meals and avoid spicy foods or other foods that contribute to heartburn and other gastrointestinal disturbances. • Avoid alcohol. • Avoid fish such as swordfish, shark, king mackerel, and tile fish; limit fish to 6 ounces of well-cooked fish weekly.
Lactating women	• Lactating women require 500 additional calories daily. • Inadequate nutrition affects breast milk; it is maintained at the expense of the woman's nutrition. • Alcohol, caffeine, and medications are transferred into breast milk. • Tobacco use decreases milk production.	Teach the woman to: • Ingest healthy foods to meet an increase in caloric intake of 500 calories daily and a balanced diet to meet nutritional needs of both mother and baby. • Avoid alcohol, caffeine, and tobacco while breastfeeding. • Avoid over-the-counter medications unless receiving medical supervision.
Older adults	• Energy output decreases, contributing to weight gain and obesity. • Periodontal disease, loss of teeth, and poorly fitted dentures may cause difficulty chewing. • Decline in taste and smell reduce appetite. • Reduced thirst sensation causes decreased fluid intake, precipitating dehydration and constipation. • Decrease in digestion, absorption, metabolism, and transport of nutrients causes a decline in nutritional status. • Acute and chronic illnesses may impair the ability to ingest, digest, absorb, metabolize, and/or transport nutrients to meet cellular needs and excrete by-products of nutrition. • May have limited financial income, which affects the ability to purchase food. • May be physically unable to procure food and prepare meals. • May be isolated at home due to illness or living alone, contributing to depression that decreases the interest in eating.	Teach the older adult to: • Seek regular dental care and keep dentures in good condition. • Chop food to facilitate eating. • Use spices other than salt to make food more palatable. • Eat calorie-dense foods high in nutritive value first to ensure adequate nutritional intake. • Eat high-fiber foods and drink 2 L of fluid daily to avoid constipation and dehydration. • Follow a prescribed therapeutic diet to treat medical conditions. • Use money-saving strategies, such as clipping coupons, buying foods on sale or store brands, substituting dairy products and beans for meat, avoiding convenience foods that generally cost more, and seeking assistance, such as food stamps or help from a food bank or Meals-on-Wheels–type program. • Become involved in senior citizen organizations to increase one's social life. • Seek medical intervention for depression.

C. Obtain a dietary history
1. Have the client complete a food diary for 3 to 5 days including all food and fluids consumed.
2. Identify foods that the client states are tolerated and those that cause problems.
3. Identify how many meals a day the client ingests and at what time they are ingested.
4. Identify food habits, such as preferences, types of snacks, and times meals are eaten.
5. Identify whether the client has been following a fad diet or taking supplements or health foods.
6. Identify clinical indicators of an eating disorder, such as excessive amount of food intake in a short period of time, induced vomiting after meals, multiple dental caries and eroded tooth enamel (associated with frequent vomiting), and excessive use of laxatives, diuretics, or weight loss medication.

D. Perform a physical assessment
1. Weight.
   a. **Underweight:** Body mass index (BMI) less than 18.5.
   b. *Cachexia:* Extreme loss of lean body mass, marked weakness, muscle wasting, and malnutrition.
   c. **Overweight (preobesity):** BMI more than 25 but less than 30.
   d. **Obese** *(obesity):* BMI of 30 or more.
   e. *Onset of change in weight:* Sudden or gradual.
   f. *Duration of change in weight:* Weight history, such as a 3-month, 6-month, or 1-year pattern of losing or gaining weight.
   g. Actions taken to promote weight loss or weight gain.
2. Skin.
   a. Dry, flaky: Aging, dehydration.
   b. Scaly: Vitamin A excess or deficiency, zinc deficiency, essential fatty acid deficiency.
   c. Petechiae or bruises: Vitamin C deficiency.
   d. Transparent: Protein deficiency.
   e. Purpura: Vitamin C deficiency, vitamin K deficiency.
   f. Edema: Protein deficiency, thiamin deficiency.
   g. Nonhealing wounds or lesions: Vitamin C deficiency, zinc deficiency, protein deficiency.
   h. Decreased skin turgor (tenting): Dehydration.
3. Hair.
   a. Dry, dull, brittle hair: Protein deficiency.
   b. Hair loss: Protein deficiency.
4. Eyes.
   a. Red or pale conjunctivae; dry, soft, dull corneas; dark skin under the eyes: Malnutrition, dehydration.
   b. Night blindness: Vitamin A deficiency.
5. Nails.
   a. Pale, brittle, ridged: Protein deficiency.
   b. Spoon shaped: Iron deficiency.
6. Mucous membranes. (See "Assessment of the Mucous Membranes" in Chapter 18, Tissue Integrity and Hygiene.)
   a. Lips.
      (1) Cracks or lesions at the corners of the mouth (**cheilosis**): Riboflavin or niacin deficiency.
      (2) Sores on the lips or in the mouth (**stomatitis**): Chemotherapy, Herpes simplex infection.
   b. Tongue.
      (1) Inflamed, beefy, red, swollen, sore tongue (**glossitis**): Vitamin B deficiency.
      (2) Atrophy: Riboflavin, niacin, vitamin B_{12}, folic acid, protein, or iron deficiency.
   c. Gums.
      (1) Inflamed, swollen, spongy gums that recede and bleed easily (**gingivitis**).
      (2) Problems due to vitamin C deficiency.
7. Teeth.
   a. Cavities or missing teeth, mottled teeth, or pain.
   b. Problems due to malnutrition and deficiencies in vitamin D and calcium.
8. Muscles.
   a. Flaccidity; poor tone; wasted, soft, underdeveloped muscles; weakness; and fatigue.
   b. Problems due to malnutrition and protein deficiency.
9. Nervous system.
   a. Neuropathy, paresthesia of the hands and feet, ataxia, decreased deep tendon reflexes and positional sense: Niacin, pyridoxine, and cyanocobalamin deficiencies.
   b. Tetany and increased deep tendon reflexes: Calcium and magnesium deficiencies.
   c. Confusion and irritability: Dehydration.
   d. Disorientation: Thiamin deficiency.
   e. Drowsiness, lethargy, apathy: Vitamins A and D excess.
10. Bones.
    a. Observed skeletal malformations and altered posture.
    b. Problems due to vitamin D deficiency.
11. Cardiovascular system.
    a. Tachycardia: Iron deficiency anemia.
    b. Increased blood pressure: Excessive salt intake, cardiovascular disease.
    c. Heart failure: Thiamin, phosphorus, and iron deficiencies.
12. Altered sensation.
    a. Decreased sense of taste or bad taste in mouth: Infection, medication side effect.
    b. Deficit in smell: Zinc deficiency.

13. Decreased ability to chew and swallow: Impaired dentition; weakness; fatigue; problems with the mouth, nasopharynx, and esophagus; dysphagia; impaired movement of the tongue; local inflammation or infection of the oral cavity.

14. GI system clinical manifestations such as anorexia, nausea and vomiting, diarrhea, constipation, epigastric discomfort, and distended abdomen: Related to specific illness or disease.
    a. Onset of GI distress: Sudden or gradual.
    b. Duration of GI distress: Short-term or long-term.
    c. Pattern of GI distress: Continuous or related to factors such as food intake or response to radiation, antineoplastic drugs, or activity.
    d. Actions taken to relieve the problem.

V. Diagnostic Tests Related to Nutritional Status

Diagnostic procedures are performed to obtain additional information about a client's nutritional status beyond just a history and physical. Noninvasive measures, such as anthropometry measurements, invasive measures, such as a gastrostomy, and blood tests performed either in the laboratory by technicians or at the client's bedside by nurses can provide valuable data. Because clinical manifestations of malnutrition take time to become evident, the results of laboratory tests may be the first indicator of a nutritional problem. The results of diagnostic tests related to a client's nutritional status are not evaluated in isolation but rather in conjunction with each other.

A. Anthropometry measurements
   1. Measurement of size, weight, and proportion of makeup of the body.
   2. Obtain height and weight and compare findings to the standard for height and weight relationships; provides a quick estimate of ideal body weight.
   3. Calculate BMI by dividing weight in kilograms by height in meters squared.
   4. Perform a skinfold measurement using special calipers to measure the thickness of the skinfolds, which indicates the amount of body fat; note that the calipers measure only the subcutaneous tissue, not underlying muscle.
   5. Mid-upper arm circumference measures muscle mass and protein reserve; client flexes the forearm and the circumference of the upper arm is measured at the midpoint.
   6. Abdominal girth measurement objectively measures abdominal distention; measure abdominal circumference with a measuring tape at a place indicated by an X made with an indelible pen or over the umbilicus; measure at the same site and time each day.

B. Gastrostomy
   1. Tube with fiber-optic capability is inserted into the mouth and advanced through the pharynx, esophagus, and stomach and sometimes into the duodenum to observe anatomical structures and check for the presence of polyps, lesions, tumors, and bleeding (Fig. 20.1).
   2. Using this procedure, polyps can be removed, bleeding sites cauterized, and biopsies obtained for diagnostic study.
   3. Teach the client about the procedure.
      a. Withhold food and fluid for 6 to 8 hours before the procedure.
      b. Remove dental appliances and eyewear.
      c. Explain that mild bloating, belching, or flatulence may occur after the procedure.
      d. Drinking and eating is permitted after the gag reflex and ability to swallow return.
      e. Notify the primary health-care provider immediately if any of the following occur: Difficulty swallowing; epigastric, substernal, or shoulder pain; black, tarry stools; vomiting of blood; or fever; these clinical manifestations may indicate a perforation of a structure of the GI tract.

C. Upper GI series
   1. Radiologic examination in which the client drinks contrast medium and films are taken every 20 minutes until the medium reaches the terminal ileum.
   2. Teach the client about the procedure.
      a. Maintain dietary restrictions, such as providing a low-residue diet for 48 hours before the test and withholding of food for 8 hours and fluid for 4 hours before the test.

Fig 20.1 Gastroscopy. (From Williams & Hopper [2015]. *Understanding medical surgical nursing,* 5th ed. Philadelphia: F. A. Davis Company, with permission.)

b. Implement bowel prep, such as tap water enema and/or cathartic the evening before the test.

c. Will be instructed to drink barium during the test; multiple x-rays will be obtained during the test.

d. Monitor stool, which will be chalky white for 72 hours or until the barium is completely evacuated; a cathartic may be prescribed to help evacuate the barium.

D. Laboratory tests

1. Laboratory tests are used to assess a client's nutritional status; no one test is used alone; some tests reflect changes within days, and some reflect a client's status over weeks.

2. They assess factors such as fluid balance, hydration, hemorrhage, presence of disease, liver and kidney function, and status of protein and nitrogen balance.

3. See Table 20.5 for a description of laboratory tests commonly used to assess nutritional status.

4. Blood glucose monitoring.

   a. Clients who have diabetes or who are receiving tube feedings or parenteral nutrition require blood glucose monitoring to ensure that blood glucose levels are maintained within the expected range of 70 to 110 mg/dL to avoid complications of hypoglycemia and hyperglycemia.

   b. Blood specimens may be sent to the laboratory for analysis of glucose (e.g., glucose tolerance, 2-hour postprandial, fasting glucose, random glucose) or performed by a nurse at regular and STAT intervals.

   c. Procedure for obtaining a fingerstick (capillary) blood specimen and measuring glucose level.

      (1) Verify the timing of the test, such as before a meal or at bedtime.

      (2) Wash your hands.

      (3) Calibrate the glucometer following the manufacturer's directions; ensure that the test strip has not expired.

      (4) Alternate sites to avoid overuse of one site, which may cause a problem with healing.

      (5) Wash the client's hands with soap and warm water to clean the skin and promote blood flow to the area; dry them well.

      (6) Don clean gloves.

      (7) Hold the finger in a dependent position to facilitate blood flow to the intended puncture site; do not milk blood toward the end of the finger to prevent an inaccurate test result.

      (8) Puncture the side of the middle or ring finger with a lancet because this area has fewer nerve endings than the fingertip (Fig. 20.2A).

      (9) Wipe away the first droplet with sterile gauze.

      (10) Position the test strip so that it makes contact with the second blood droplet (Fig. 20.2B).

      (11) Follow the manufacturer's instructions regarding the amount of time to leave the strip in the glucometer.

      (12) Apply gentle pressure with a gauze pad over the puncture site.

      (13) Dispose of the lancet in a sharps disposal container.

      (14) Read the result once it is displayed on the glucometer.

      (15) Discard your gloves appropriately and perform hand hygiene.

      (16) Document the results in the client's clinical record.

      (17) Administer insulin based on the guidelines prescribed by the primary healthcare provider if the client's blood glucose level is elevated.

DID YOU KNOW?

Soap and warm water are sufficient to clean the intended puncture site. If soap and water are unavailable, swipe the site with an alcohol swab but allow the alcohol to dry completely before puncturing the site. Doing so will prevent the alcohol from destroying the substance on the test strip that measures glucose levels. Squeezing or milking the finger of the intended puncture site, particularly after the finger has been punctured, can cause hemolysis and dilution of the blood specimen with fluid from local tissue. Both actions result in false low test results and should be avoided.

VI. Therapeutic Diets and Related Nursing Care

Although most everyone should follow the recommendations of the food guidance system called MyPlate that demonstrates the five food groups that are the foundation of a healthy diet, these guidelines may be inadequate or inappropriate for clients with health problems. The consistency of food, quantity of food, and constituents within foods may have to be altered to maintain health in the presence of physiological problems or to promote recovery from an illness. The provision of a diet to a client is a dependent function of the nurse and requires a prescription from a primary health-care provider.

Table 20.5 **Laboratory Tests to Assess Nutritional Status**

Factor	Increased Level	Decreased Level
Albumin *Normal value: 3.5–5 g/dL.* • *Synthesized by the liver from amino acids.* • *Important in fluid and electrolyte balance.* • *Half-life of 21 days.* • *Not an ideal indicator of acute protein depletion.*	• *>5 g/dL.* • *Dehydration.*	• *<3.5 g/dL indicates some extent of malnutrition or malabsorption.* • *Increased loss, such as through a fistula or burns.*
Blood glucose *Normal value: 70–110 mg/dL.* • *Primary energy source for cellular function.* • *Excess glucose is stored in the liver and muscles.* • *Lower than expected glucose levels stimulate metabolism of fat stores.*	**Hyperglycemia** • *>110 mg/dL fasting blood sample.* • *>126 mg/dL random blood sample.*	**Hypoglycemia** • *<50 mg/dL.*
Blood urea nitrogen *Normal value: 8–21 mg/dL.* • *End product of protein metabolism.* • *Reflects serum protein status.* • *Reflects balance of urea production and excretion.*	• *>21 mg/dL.* • *Acute renal failure.* • *Excessive protein intake.* • *Muscle wasting from starvation.* • *Total parenteral nutrition.*	• *<8 mg/dL.* • *Inadequate dietary protein.* • *Malabsorption.* • *Pregnancy.* • *Low-protein diet.* • *Severe liver disease.*
Creatinine *Normal value: 0.5–1.2 mg/dL.* • *Released during skeletal muscle metabolism.* • *Proportion to total body mass.*	• *>1.2 mg/dL.* • *Dehydration.*	• *<0.5 mg/dL.* • *Reduced total muscle mass.* • *Severe malnutrition.*
Hemoglobin *Normal value:* *Females: 12–16 g/dL.* *Males: 14–18 g/dL.* • *Measures oxygen and iron carrying capacity of blood.*	• *>16 or 18 g/dL for females and males respectively.* • *Dehydration.* • *Burns.* • *Congestive heart failure.*	• *<12 or 14 g/dL for females and males respectively.* • *Anemia.* • *Blood loss.* • *IV overload.* • *Fluid retention.*
Prealbumin *Normal value:* *15–40 mg/dL.* • *Protein produced by the liver.* • *Transports thyroxine and triiodothyronine.* • *Needed to transport vitamin A.* • *Half-life of 2 to 3 days.*	• *>40 mg/dL.* • *Alcoholism.* • *Steroid therapy.* • *Chronic renal failure.*	• *Mild protein depletion: <15 mg/dL.* • *Severe protein depletion: <11 mg/dL.* • *Malnutrition.* • *Acute-phase inflammatory response.* • *Liver disease.* • *Tissue necrosis.*
Total lymphocyte count *Normal values:* *1,000–4,800/mm^3 or 20%–40%.* • *Lymphocytes decrease as protein decreases.* • *Important in the immune response.*	• *>4,800/mm^3 or >40%.* • *Pathological conditions, such as appendicitis, inflammatory disorders, bone marrow disorders.*	• *<1,000/mm^3 or <20%.* • *Decreased nutritional intake.* • *Anemias.* • *Malnutrition.* • *Severe debilitating disease.* • *Antineoplastic drugs.*
Transferrin *Normal value:* *215–380 mg/dL.* • *Formed in the liver.* • *Transports up to 70% of the body's iron.* • *Half-life of 8 days.* • *Reacts quickly to changes in protein intake.*	• *>380 mg/dL.* • *Iron deficiency anemia.* • *Pregnancy.*	• *Moderate protein depletion: <200 mg/dL.* • *Severe protein depletion: <100 mg/dL.* • *Acute or chronic infection.* • *Excessive protein loss from renal disease.* • *Malnutrition from cancer.*
Lipid profile *Normal values:* LDL: <100 mg/dL. HDL: ≥60 mg/dL. Triglycerides: <150 mg/dL. Total cholesterol: ≤200 mg/dL. • *Used to assess risk of cardiovascular disease.*	Blood levels indicating increased risk for cardiovascular disease • *LDL: 160 to 189 mg/dL is high; ≥190 mg/dL is very high.* • *HDL: <40 mg/dL.* • *Triglycerides: 150 to 199 mg/dL is borderline; 200 to 499 mg/dL is high; ≥500 mg/dL is very high.* • *Total cholesterol: 201 to 240 mg/dL is borderline; >240 mg/dL is high.*	

Fig 20.2 Blood glucose monitoring: (A) using a lancet; (B) applying blood to a reagent strip test patch. (From Wilkinson and Treas [2016]. *Fundamentals of nursing*, Vol. 2, 3rd ed. Philadelphia: F. A. Davis Company, with permission.)

Details of therapeutic diets can be found in a health-care agency's dietary manual.

A. Commonalities of diet-related nursing care
1. Verify the diet prescribed by the primary health-care provider.
2. Arrange for a consult with a dietitian to ensure an individualized assessment and plan.
3. Provide for a client's personal food preferences as much as possible.
4. Encourage intake of nutrient-dense foods first from the meal tray when the client is anorexic.
5. Assist the client with eating as necessary.
6. Document the client's intake and tolerance objectively in the clinical record.

DID YOU KNOW?

Calorie-dense foods and nutrient-dense foods often are used interchangeably. However, they have very different meanings. Calorie-dense foods provide energy from calories but often have insignificant nutritive value. These foods are appropriate for people who have a high metabolic rate (e.g., clients with cancer or hyperthyroidism, athletes) or are underweight. Calorie-dense foods include foods such as potatoes, rice, beans, fruit juices, snack foods, and fast foods. Nutrient-dense foods provide more nutrients (e.g., protein, carbohydrates, vitamin B, iron, and potassium) than calories. Nutrient-dense foods are appropriate for people who have an inadequate oral

intake (e.g., clients with nausea or anorexia) or have increased nutritional needs (e.g., clients who are pregnant or lactating). Nutrient-dense foods include foods such as berries, melons, dark-green vegetables, lean meats, nuts, cheese, fish, and whole grains.

B. Nothing by mouth (*non per os* [NPO])
1. Restricted oral food and fluid intake.
2. Generally prescribed before surgery, procedures, or tests to minimize the risk of aspiration.
3. May be prescribed for a client with a problem, such as undiagnosed abdominal pain or vomiting, until the problem is diagnosed or the nausea and vomiting subside.
4. Nursing care.
   a. Explain to the client and family what "NPO" means and why it is prescribed; if NPO is violated, it may require postponement of an intervention or aggravate a medical condition.
   b. Remove the client's water pitcher from the bedside.
   c. Ensure that all members of the health-care team are informed of the client's NPO status; place an "NPO" sign in the client's room if permitted by policy.
   d. Provide frequent mouth care and instruct the client not to swallow water or mouthwash during mouth care.
   e. Administer intravenous (IV) fluids as prescribed.

C. Clear liquid diet
1. Provides for hydration and simple carbohydrates to meet a portion of a client's energy requirement.
2. Prevents dehydration.
3. Generally prescribed after surgery or when a client is recovering from a GI problem, such as vomiting and diarrhea because it reduces stimulation of the GI mucosa.
4. Allows intake of liquids that are transparent enough to see through, including frozen ice popsicles and gelatin, because they are clear when liquid.
5. Should be used only for a few days because it does not provide adequate protein, calories, or other nutrients necessary for a balanced diet.
6. Once tolerated, a client is progressed to a full liquid diet.
7. Nursing care.
   a. Teach the client the liquids that are permitted on a clear liquid diet, such as water; clear, fat-free soup (e.g., broth/bouillon); tea; coffee; clear juice (e.g., grape, cranberry, and apple); gelatin; popsicles; clear drinks with electrolytes (e.g., Gatorade, Pedialyte), and carbonated drinks (e.g., nondiet soda).
   b. Assess the client's tolerance, such as free from nausea, vomiting, and epigastric distress.

D. Full liquid diet
1. Includes all fluids on a clear fluid diet, fluids that are opaque, or food that becomes liquid at room temperature.
2. Generally prescribed as part of a progressive diet from clear to regular.
3. Prescribed when a client is unable to tolerate semisolid or solid food.
4. Is low in calories, protein, and iron.
5. Must be enhanced with a balanced oral supplement (e.g., Ensure, Boost) if the client is receiving it for more than a few days.
6. Nursing care.
   a. Teach the client that the liquids on a clear liquid diet also are included on a full liquid diet.
   b. Teach that additional fluids and foods include milk and milk drinks (e.g., milkshakes); puddings and custards; cream soups; yogurt; ice cream and sherbet; vegetable and fruit juices that are free from pulp; smooth peanut butter; refined cooked cereals (e.g., Cream of Wheat, Cream of Rice); and liquid supplements.
   c. Assess the client's tolerance, such as free from nausea, vomiting, and epigastric distress.

E. Soft diet
1. Easily chewed, swallowed, and digested foods; promotes the mechanical digestion of food.
2. Includes all foods on a full liquid diet plus soft, chopped, and shredded foods.
3. Prescribed for clients with difficulty chewing because of problems with the teeth, gums, jaw, or improperly fitted dentures and those who are weak.
4. Prescribed for clients with conditions such as Crohn's disease and ulcerative colitis to reduce stimulation of the GI mucosa.
5. Provides a balanced diet but is low in fiber and may increase the risk of constipation.
6. Nursing care.
   a. Teach the client that the diet includes all clear and full liquids; all soups; chopped or ground meats; well cooked, soft vegetables; cooked or canned fruit without membranes; applesauce; scrambled eggs; bananas; cottage cheese and other soft cheeses; rice; mashed or riced potatoes; pasta; cooked cereal and grits; pancakes; soft bread; bread pudding; and pastry.
   b. Encourage the intake of fluid, oatmeal, and cooked and canned fruit to minimize the risk of constipation.
   🛑 c. Teach the client to avoid nuts; foods with seeds, such as tomatoes and berries; raw fruits and vegetables; and whole grains because they are more irritating to the GI mucosa and are high in fiber.

d. Teach the client at risk for constipation to avoid rice, bananas, and other constipating foods.
e. Assess for clinical indicators of constipation.
f. Assess the client's tolerance, such as free from nausea, vomiting, epigastric distress, constipation, and diarrhea.

F. Pureed diet
1. Consists of foods that are processed in a blender or food processor so that the consistency is thicker than full liquids but can be served in scooped mounds on a plate.
2. Nursing care.
   a. Teach that all food can be included on this diet as long as it is blended to a semisolid consistency.
   b. Add a small amount of liquid to food if it is too thick to make it a semisolid consistency that is easy to swallow.

G. Regular diet
1. Provides a balanced diet of 2,000 calories daily.
2. Prescribed for clients with no unique or special nutritional needs.
3. Can be modified to meet specific needs or preferences, such as a kosher or vegetarian diet.
4. Generally avoids fatty, gas-forming, fried, and unpopular foods to appeal to a greater percentage of clients and to promote tolerance.
5. Nursing care.
   a. Teach clients which foods are most important to ingest first from the meal tray.
   🛑 b. Teach clients who have undergone surgery to ingest foods and fluids high in protein and vitamin C to facilitate wound healing.

H. Antigen-avoidance diet
1. Prescribed for a client who is allergic to or has intolerance to a food. The following are examples.
   a. Gluten-free diet: Essential for a person who cannot tolerate gluten because of celiac disease; diet free from grains such as wheat, bran, barley, rye, farina, and semolina.
   b. Lactose-free diet: Essential for a person who cannot tolerate lactose; diet is free from milk and dairy products.
   c. Peanut-free diet: Essential for a person who cannot tolerate peanuts and their products; diet free from peanuts and foods cooked with peanut oil.

DID YOU KNOW?
A client who cannot eat gluten should avoid foods that contain grains such as pasta, bread, bakery products, cereal, and fillers in processed foods. A client with lactose intolerance must avoid milk and milk products, such as cheese, bread, cereal, rice, or pasta prepared with milk; vegetables or salad dressings prepared with

milk or cheese; cream soups; dessert made with cream or milk products, such as sherbet, ice cream, pudding, and cake; anything made with milk solids, curds and whey, or skim milk solids. The nurse should suggest that the client try, with the primary health-care provider's permission, a nondairy creamer and reduced-lactose milk and cheese products because they may be tolerated. A client who is allergic to peanuts should avoid foods that contain peanuts or are cooked with peanut oil.

2. Nursing care.
   a. Teach the client foods to avoid that are high in the offending nutrient.
   b. Teach the client to investigate ingredients when buying food products or when dining in a restaurant to ensure that the offending nutrient is not used in the recipe.
   c. Identify restaurants that provide menus that address the needs of people with food intolerances and allergies (e.g., the Outback restaurant has extensive choices on a gluten-free menu).
   d. Ensure that a child's school has policies in place that protect children with food allergies or intolerances; some schools do not permit any child to bring food into the school that has peanuts or peanut oil in the food.
   🛑 e. Encourage a client who has a prescription for epinephrine (e.g., Epi-E-Pen, EpiPen Auto-Injector) to keep the device available at all times; teach the client how to self-administer an epinephrine injection.

I. Calorie-restricted diet
   1. Allows a reduced number of calories, such as 1,800; 1,200; or 1,000 calories as prescribed.
   2. Prescribed to facilitate weight loss.
   3. Nursing care.
      a. Encourage the client to participate in a program that provides counseling and support, such as individual counseling, Weight Watchers, or Overeaters Anonymous.
      b. Teach the client to limit foods that are high in fat and carbohydrates and to substitute foods that are low in calories and carbohydrates.
      c. Use positive, supportive statements to point out success in weight loss.
      d. Avoid negative statements because they can demoralize the client and negatively affect the nurse-client relationship.

J. American Diabetes Association (ADA) diet
   1. Maintains acceptable serum glucose levels (premeal level of 70 to 130 mg/dL and postmeal level of less than 180 mg/dL) and reduces lipid levels.
   2. Maintaining acceptable serum glucose levels may help minimize the risk of long-term complications

of diabetes, such as atherosclerosis, arteriosclerosis, retinopathy, nephropathy, neuropathy, infection, and foot ulcers.
   3. Nursing care.
      a. Encourage the client to seek guidance from a nurse who is a diabetes educator and a dietitian to help design and identify strategies to maintain a nutrition therapy plan.
      b. Encourage the client to become involved in efforts to reduce the intake of fats and calories to decrease weight and increase exercise because doing so will help reduce blood glucose levels.
      c. Teach the client high-glycemic foods to avoid because they are high in sugar and carbohydrates, such as pasta, rice, and bread.

K. High-calorie, high-protein diet
   1. Increases amount of calories and protein in the diet to promote wound healing and prevent catabolism.
   2. Prescribed for clients with conditions such as serious burns, developmental growth, increased metabolism associated with hyperthyroidism, and increased catabolism and wasting related to cancer.
   3. Nursing care.
      a. Teach the client foods that are high in calories and high in protein.
      b. Teach the client to augment the diet with high-calorie and high-protein supplements.
      c. Add protein powder supplements to soups and liquids as prescribed.

L. High-fiber diet
   1. Increases the movement of indigestible waste through the large intestine.
   2. Minimizes the risk of constipation and is a treatment regimen for diverticulosis.
   3. Nursing care.
      a. Teach the client foods that are high in fiber, such as raw vegetables, whole grains, and raw fruits, such as apples and oranges.
      b. Assess for clinical indicators of constipation and diarrhea.

M. Low-fat or fat-restricted diet
   1. Reduces the total fat ingested and substitutes monounsaturated fats for saturated and polyunsaturated fats.
   2. Prescribed to promote weight loss or lower cholesterol or triglyceride levels.
   3. Prescribed for people with atherosclerosis; coronary artery disease; and problems with fat malabsorption related to diseases of the liver, gallbladder, pancreas, lymphatic system, or intestines.

4. Nursing care.
   a. Teach the client to avoid foods that are high in fat, such as whole-milk products, fried foods, animal fat, gravies, sauces, and chocolate.
   b. Teach the client to limit use of butter, margarine, mayonnaise, oil, shortening, bacon, cream, and creamed cheese to 1 tablespoon a day or 1 teaspoon per meal.
   c. Encourage intake of fresh fruits and vegetables and fat-free milk and milk products.
   d. Encourage the client to substitute yogurt for sour cream in recipes.
   e. Teach the client to limit lean meats to no more than 18 oz weekly.
   f. Teach the client to limit the intake of foods high in cholesterol; U.S. dietary guidelines removed the limits on cholesterol intake. Others suggest that cholesterol intake should not exceed 300 mg/day in healthy people and 200 mg/day in those with elevated cholesterol levels.

N. Low-residue diet
  1. Contains foods with reduced fiber and cellulose.
  2. Decreases GI mucosal irritation.
  3. Used for clients with exacerbations of Crohn's disease, ulcerative colitis, and diverticulitis to reduce stimulation of the intestinal mucosa.
  4. May be prescribed before intestinal surgery.
  5. Nursing care.
     a. Teach the client to avoid foods high in fiber and cellulose, such as raw and dried fruits and vegetables and whole grains.
     b. Teach the client to reduce dairy products to two servings daily.
     c. Teach the client to avoid nuts and foods with seeds, such as tomatoes and berries (efficacy is controversial).

O. Protein-restricted diet
  1. Prescribed for clients with liver disease to decrease stress on the liver, which metabolizes protein.
  2. Prescribed for clients with kidney disease because of the need to limit levels of nitrogen, a by-product of protein metabolism.
  3. May be accompanied by fluid and sodium restriction.
  4. Nursing care.
     a. Teach the client to limit protein intake to the amount prescribed by the primary health-care provider (e.g., 20 g, 40 g, or 60 g daily).
     b. Teach the client to limit foods high in protein, such as meat and dairy products.

P. Sodium-restricted diet
  1. May be restricted to 2,000 mg (mild), 1,000 mg (moderate), 500 mg (strict), or 250 mg (severe).
  2. Prescribed because salt retains fluid in the body, which contributes to fluid retention.
  3. Prescribed for clients with hypertension, excess fluid volume, heart failure, and renal failure.
  4. Nursing care.
     a. Teach the client foods to avoid that are high in sodium (Box 20.1).
     b. Teach the client to substitute foods high in salt with fresh fruit; breads and pasta without salt; low-salt baked goods; low-sodium cheese; and spices, herbs, and vegetables that do not contain salt, such as allspice, almond extract, basil, bay leaves, chili powder, garlic, marjoram, onion powder, onions, oregano, parsley, pepper, rosemary, sage, tarragon, and thyme.
     c. Teach the client about the Dietary Approaches to Stop Hypertension (DASH) diet. It is a highly successful diet that emphasizes fruits, vegetables, whole grains, poultry, fish, low-fat dairy products, protein, and nuts and reduces red meat, sweets, and high-sodium foods. Also, it is rich in potassium, calcium, and magnesium.

VII. Nutrition Facts Labels

In May 2016 the U.S. Food and Drug Administration finalized the new nutrition facts label for packaged foods to reflect new scientific information. Manufacturers must implement the new label by July 26, 2018 (small manufacturers have an additional year). A nutrition facts label provides descriptive information about the food in the package.

A. Purpose of a nutrition facts label
  1. Provides information about the amount and nutrient content of the product in addition to other important information.

Box 20.1 Foods High in Sodium

- Condiments, such as catsup, mustard, barbecue sauce, and commercial salad dressing.
- Prepared stuffing, cake mixes, and baked goods with baking soda and baking powder.
- Milk from animals; yogurt; and regular cheese and cheese products.
- Treats such as salted pretzels, popcorn, crackers, and chips.
- Instant and prepared rice, pasta, and quick-cooking cereals.
- Bouillon cubes, tenderizers, gravy enhancers, and mixers.
- Canned soups and vegetables, especially sauerkraut.
- Oysters, clams, shrimp, and other shellfish.
- Soy, teriyaki, and Worcestershire sauce.
- Bacon, luncheon meat, and corned beef.
- Salted butter and margarine.
- Olives and pickles.
- Sugar substitutes.
- Egg substitutes.
- Peanut butter.
- Diet soda.

2. Assists people to make informed choices when purchasing food.

3. Assists people to adhere to a prescribed diet.

B. Sections of a nutrition facts label (Fig. 20.3)

1. Serving size: Identifies the volume of a serving size in household and metric measurements; identifies how many servings are in each package or can.

2. Calories: Identifies how many calories are contained in one serving.

3. Percentage of daily values: Includes nutrient information in the product (e.g., total fat, saturated fat, trans fat, cholesterol, sodium, total carbohydrates, dietary fiber, protein, total sugars and added sugars) within the context of a total daily diet; total sugars, including added sugars, was added to this section.

4. Vitamins and minerals: Includes nutrient information in the product (e.g., vitamin D, calcium, potassium, and iron) within the context of a total daily diet. Vitamins A and C were deleted because deficiencies in these vitamins are rare in the American diet and potassium and vitamin D were added.

5. The bottom section of the nutrition facts label explains that the % Daily Value reflects how much a nutrient in a serving of food contributes to a daily 2,000 calorie diet.

MAKING THE CONNECTION

Quantitative Value of Nutrients in a Product and Serving Size

Nurses must teach clients to read nutrition facts labels carefully to determine the total number of nutrients in a package. Many products contain more than one serving per package. For example, a nutrition facts label may indicate that a serving contains 100 calories; however, if the package/can contains three servings and the client eats the entire package, the total intake of calories is 300. This information is important to teach clients who must limit food intake to the number of calories prescribed for a specific diet, such as a 1,200- or 1,800-calorie diet. This concept also applies to the nutrients itemized on the nutrition facts label. A label may identify that a serving contains 200 mg of sodium; if the package/can contains three servings and the client eats two servings, the total intake of sodium by the client is 400 mg. This information is important to teach clients who are on sodium-restricted diets.

VIII. MyPlate

The Center for Nutrition Policy and Promotion, an organization of the U.S. Department of Agriculture, issued new dietary guidelines for Americans, 2015 to 2020, 8th edition. The food guidance system, MyPlate, introduced June 2011, reflects previous and present dietary guidelines and provides an easily understood icon to guide people regarding food categories and food choices for a healthier life. MyPlate demonstrates the five food groups that are the foundation of a healthy diet. It uses a plate divided into four sections—two of the groups fruits and vegetables together should be 50% of the plate, grains 30% of the plate, and protein 20% of the plate—and the fifth group, dairy, is represented by a circle that signifies a glass or cup. The plate design is based on the concept that a person should consider what is being put on a plate or in a bowl or cup when selecting foods and fluids in a daily diet (Fig. 20.4).

A. Fruits

1. Should include 2 cups of fruit daily.

2. Includes any fruit that is fresh, canned, or frozen and is whole, cut up, pureed, or 100% juice; however, whole fruits are preferable.

3. Examples: Apples, bananas, grapefruit, grapes, oranges, peaches, berries, melons, apricots, kiwi, lemons, limes, mangoes, pears, and papaya.

B. Vegetables

1. Should include 2.5 cups of vegetables daily.

2. Includes any vegetable that is raw, cooked, fresh, frozen, canned, dried, or dehydrated and can be cut up, mashed, or juiced (100%).

3. Examples arranged into five categories based on nutritive value.

a. Dark-green vegetables: Broccoli; collard greens; dark-green, leafy lettuce (e.g., romaine lettuce, spinach).

b. Legumes: Beans, such as black, kidney, pinto, white, navy, and soy beans; peas, such as split peas, chickpeas, black-eyed peas; and lentils. Note: Beans and peas also are counted as a subcategory of the protein food group.

c. Starchy vegetables: Such as corn, potatoes, green peas, green lima beans, water chestnuts, and plantains.

d. Red and orange vegetables: Such as carrots, sweet potatoes, tomatoes, pumpkin, red peppers, and butternut and acorn squash.

e. Other vegetables: Such as cauliflower, green beans, iceberg lettuce, mushrooms, onions, zucchini, artichokes, asparagus, avocado, beets, bean sprouts, cabbage, celery, cucumbers, eggplant, turnips, and wax beans.

C. Grains

1. Should be 30% of the plate daily; half should be whole-grain products.

2. Divided into whole grains and refined grains.

a. Whole grains.

(1) Food products made from the entire grain kernel, such as whole-wheat and

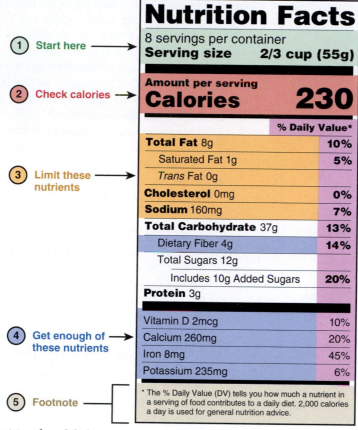

① Start here

② Check calories

③ Limit these nutrients

④ Get enough of these nutrients

⑤ Footnote

Nutrition Facts

8 servings per container
Serving size   2/3 cup (55g)

Amount per serving
Calories   230

	% Daily Value*
Total Fat 8g	**10%**
Saturated Fat 1g	**5%**
Trans Fat 0g	
Cholesterol 0mg	**0%**
Sodium 160mg	**7%**
Total Carbohydrate 37g	**13%**
Dietary Fiber 4g	**14%**
Total Sugars 12g	
Includes 10g Added Sugars	**20%**
Protein 3g	
Vitamin D 2mcg	10%
Calcium 260mg	20%
Iron 8mg	45%
Potassium 235mg	6%

* The % Daily Value (DV) tells you how much a nutrient in a serving of food contributes to a daily diet. 2,000 calories a day is used for general nutrition advice.

⑥ Calories from fat help people to keep fat intake to less than 30% of total calories

⑦ Quick guide to % DV

Shows how the food fits into the overall daily diet

• 5% or less is low

• 20% or more is high

% is based on a 2,000 calorie diet

Fig 20.3 Nutrition facts label. (From U.S. Food and Drug Administration, 2016.)

Fig 20.4 MyPlate. (USDA, www.ChooseMyPlate.gov, 2011.)

cracked-wheat flour, oatmeal, whole cornmeal, whole rye, whole-grain barley, millet, buckwheat, and brown rice.
  (2) Examples: Whole-wheat bread, crackers, pasta, and cereals; popcorn; wild rice; muesli; and rolled oats.

  b. Refined grains.
    (1) Food products using grains that are milled, which eliminates the bran and germ to make it a finer texture; it also removes fiber, iron, and many B vitamins.
    (2) Examples: White bread; white rice; corn bread; flour tortillas; grits; couscous; noodles; pretzels; spaghetti and other macaroni products; corn flakes; and crackers and pitas.
    (3) Some products made with refined grains are enriched with B vitamins, such as thiamin, riboflavin, and niacin; folic acid; iron; and fiber.
  3. Products made with grains must be reviewed to identify whether they used whole grains, refined grains, or are a mixture of whole and refined grains.
D. Protein
  1. Should be 20% of the plate daily.
  2. Includes foods in the following categories: meat, poultry, seafood, beans and peas, eggs, processed soy, nuts, and seeds.
  3. Lean cuts of meat and poultry should be substituted for fatty cuts of meat and poultry, with all visible fat and skin removed.

4. Two servings of seafood rich in omega-fatty acids should be included weekly.

5. Avoid meats, nuts, and seeds with added salt because excessive sodium intake is associated with fluid retention, high blood pressure, and brain attack.

6. Examples of protein.
   a. Meat such as beef, pork, ham, lamb, veal, bison, rabbit, and venison.
   b. Poultry such as chicken, duck, goose, and turkey.
   c. Beans, peas, lentils, and eggs.
   d. Nuts, such as almonds, cashews, mixed nuts, peanuts and peanut butter, walnuts, filberts, pecans, and pistachios; seeds, such as pumpkin, sesame, and sunflower.
   e. Soy products, such as tofu, tempeh, and texturized vegetable protein.
   f. Fish, such as salmon, catfish, cod, flounder, haddock, halibut, mackerel, porgy, sea bass, snapper, swordfish, trout, and tuna; canned fish, such as anchovies, tuna, and sardines.
   g. Shellfish, such as clams, crab, crayfish, lobster, mussels, octopus, oysters, scallops, squid, and shrimp.

E. Dairy
   1. Represented by the circle in the MyPlate icon.
   2. Includes not just milk, calcium-fortified soymilk, and reduced-lactose and lactose-free milk, but milk products, such as cheese and yogurt.
   3. Contributes approximately 18% of the protein ingested daily in the America diet, which is 3% to 4% of MyPlate; should include two or three fat-free or low-fat dairy products daily.
   4. Examples of dairy products.
      a. Fat-free (skim) milk, low-fat milk (1%), and products made with them; fat-free and low-fat milk should replace whole milk and products made with whole milk.
      b. Hard cheeses, such as cheddar, mozzarella, Swiss, and parmesan; soft cheeses, such as ricotta and cottage cheese; and processed cheeses, such as American cheese.
      c. Yogurt made with whole, reduced-fat, low-fat, or fat-free milk.
      d. Desserts made with low-fat milk, such as pudding, ice milk, frozen yogurt, and ice cream.
      e. Does not include cream cheese, cream, and butter because these foods contain little calcium.

IX. Nursing Care to Support Nutrition

Nursing responsibilities related to helping clients meet their dietary needs include teaching all clients basic concepts related to making healthy dietary choices, assisting clients who need help with feeding themselves, and providing specific nursing interventions related to health problems that interfere with one's nutritional status. Problems related to variations in ideal body weight, issues that impede the ability to eat, eating disorders, GI difficulties, and fluid and electrolyte imbalances all require nurses to further individualize nursing care to meet the client's needs related to the specific problem.

A. Client teaching to support healthy dietary choices
   1. Balance calories among food groups; eat a variety of foods in each group.
   2. Ensure that half of grains eaten are whole grains.
   3. Make sure half of each plate is fruits and vegetables.
   4. Choose foods that have the most nutritive value for the calories.
   🛑 5. Avoid exceeding the recommended daily calorie intake.
   🛑 6. Use a small plate, portion food before you eat, eat slowly, and recognize when you have had enough and stop eating to avoid overeating.
   7. Replace whole milk and whole-milk products with low-fat milk and low-fat milk products.
   8. Reduce the intake of foods high in solid fats, added sugars, and salt, such as ice cream, cake, cookies, candy, sweetened drinks, fried foods, and chips as well as fatty meats, such as sausage, bacon, and hot dogs. Include them once in a while as a treat.

DID YOU KNOW?
Fried foods, such as potato chips and french fries, are unhealthy because they are high in calories, unhealthy fats, and added salt. These foods contain "bad" fat (saturated fat) and increase "bad" cholesterol (LDLs), which stay in the body longer, raising circulating blood triglycerides that decrease "good" cholesterol (HDLs). Foods high in fat and salt are associated with heart disease and stroke (brain attack, cerebrovascular accident) and should be avoided or ingested only occasionally.

   9. Reduce sodium intake by comparing nutrition facts labels and selecting low-sodium products, such as those labeled as "no added salt" or "low sodium."
   10. Drink 8 glasses of water a day; avoid high-calorie beverages, such as nondiet soda.
   11. Balance food intake and physical activity.

B. Commonalities of nursing care
   1. Before a meal.
      a. Offer to toilet the client and provide oral care and hand hygiene before meals; if offered by your agency, provide prepackaged wet towels to wash hands before and after meals.
      b. Allow the client time to engage in religious rituals before a meal, such as saying a prayer.

c. Ask whether the client would like to listen to music during the meal to provide a pleasant mealtime environment.

d. Encourage family members to share meal-times when able; in residential settings, assist clients to the dining room to support socialization.

e. Provide a clean and pleasant eating environment.
   (1) Ensure that the client's room is free from unpleasant odors.
   (2) Remove offensive items from site, such as urinal, toilet paper, emesis basin, and soiled tissues and washcloths.
   (3) Clean the overbed table so that it is ready to receive the client's meal tray.

f. Provide privacy during meals if a client has difficulty eating and is embarrassed.

🛑 g. If the client wears dentures, ensure that they are in the client's mouth; if the client prefers not to wear dentures during meals, secure them in a labeled container stored in the client's bedside table rather than on the client's tray where they can be accidentally discarded.

🛑 h. Verify the diet prescribed against the menu form on the client's meal tray. Check the meal tray to ensure that the food on the tray is consistent with the prescribed diet.

2. During a meal.
   a. Position the client in an upright sitting position when possible. Have the client sit in a chair for meals if the client is able to get out of bed; if the client is in bed, raise the head of the bed to a comfortable position and place the overbed table over the client's legs so that the food tray is in easy reach. An upright position uses gravity to facilitate movement of food to the stomach once swallowed.
   b. Encourage self-feeding to support independence.
   c. Use a napkin, not a bib, over clothes to protect them from soiling to support dignity.
   d. Prepare the meal tray: Open food and fluid containers; position utensils in easy reach; cut meat; and season food and butter bread, as per the client's instructions.
   e. Locate food on the tray based on the face of a clock if the client is visually impaired.
   f. Explain and demonstrate use of assistive devices for eating and drinking when needed to facilitate intake.
   g. Feed a client who is unable to self-feed.
      (1) Sit at the client's eye level.
      (2) Ask the client the select foods to be presented and whether fluids should be provided after each mouthful.

🛑 (3) Serve small amounts of food at a time because too much food is difficult to manage and may cause aspiration.

🛑 (4) Provide ample time for the client to chew and swallow food; do not rush the client; ensure that food in the mouth is swallowed before offering the next bite.

(5) Provide finger foods that the client might be able to manage to self-feed, such as bread, to support independence.

(6) Provide one food at a time; avoid mixing several foods together, such as mashed potatoes and peas, unless this is the client's preference. Clients have a right to taste different textures and flavors and serving items individually may be more appetizing to the eye.

(7) Serve hot foods hot and cold foods cold.

(8) Have an informal conversation with the client to create a relaxed mealtime experience, but do not ask the client a question while the client has food or liquid in the mouth to minimize the risk of aspiration.

3. After a meal.
   a. Check the tray for dentures that may have been removed during the meal and wrapped in a napkin; they can be easily lost and are time consuming and expensive to replace.
   b. Assist the client to wash the hands or to toilet after the meal is completed.
   c. Encourage the client to remain upright for 40 to 45 minutes after the meal; gravity facilitates movement of food along the GI tract and helps to minimize the risk of aspiration.
   d. Identify and document feeding behaviors and tolerance, such as whether the client experienced coughing, difficulty swallowing.

🛑 e. Record the intake of food as a percentage and fluid in milliliters because these are objective measurements of the client's intake; avoid using words that are subjective, such as "good," "well," and "poor" to describe the client's intake.

C. Nursing care for clients with difficulty swallowing *(dysphagia)*
   1. Swallowing requires synchronized timing of sensory and motor systems to transport a bolus from the mouth, through the pharynx, and to the esophagus.
   2. Conditions that increase the risk of aspiration.
      a. Neuromuscular problems, such as brain attack, facial paralysis (Bell's palsy), cerebral palsy, Parkinson disease, multiple sclerosis, and myasthenia gravis.

b. Problems that influence the head, neck, and upper GI tract, such as cancer of the tongue, esophagus, or stomach.

3. Specific nursing care.

a. Assess for clinical indicators of dysphagia, such as statements by the client about pain, an inability to swallow, or food caught in the back of the mouth; drooling or leaking of liquid or food; pocketing of food; and gagging or coughing when eating food or drinking fluid.

b. Assess for the presence of cough and gag reflexes, level of consciousness, and swallowing ability.

c. Inform the primary health-care provider if clinical indicators of a swallowing problem are identified; suggest a referral for a swallowing consult by a speech-language pathologist to assess the client's swallowing ability.

d. Learn about the National Dysphagia Diet, which provides guidelines about the use of altering food textures and thickening liquids to facilitate safe swallowing.

🛑 e. **Institute aspiration precautions and communicate this action to all health-care team members in the plan of care and via a notice attached to the front of the client's clinical record.**

(1) Place the client in an upright position; instruct the client to flex the head slightly when swallowing to direct food toward the esophagus rather than the trachea.

(2) Provide the prescribed diet, such as pureed, ground, chopped, and soft food, to facilitate swallowing.

(3) Introduce food toward the back of the strong side of the mouth because doing so makes it easier to manage and control when swallowing.

🛑 (4) **Ensure that all food in the mouth is swallowed before offering the next bite; check the mouth as needed to ensure that food is not still between the gums or teeth and cheek (pocketed).**

(5) Avoid using a straw because fluid is more difficult to control when it enters the middle of the mouth versus directly from a glass or cup.

(6) Thicken fluids because they are easier to control and swallow than thin fluids. Thickness of fluids progresses from thin, nectar-like, honey-like to pudding-like thickness.

(7) Teach the client not to use liquids to promote the swallowing of food unless instructed to do so by the speech-language therapist.

(8) Avoid serving sticky foods, such as peanut butter and dry mashed potatoes.

(9) Encourage the client to dry swallow several times between bites.

(10) Ensure that a suction machine is accessible if needed to maintain a patent airway.

f. Collaborate with the primary health-care provider about the potential need for tube feedings if the client is not ingesting an adequate intake of calories daily.

D. Nursing care for clients who are overweight or obese

1. Overweight and obesity are a national epidemic in the United States; more than 68% of the population in the United States are overweight or obese (33.97% are obese, and 34.4% are overweight). Nearly 18% of children aged 6 to 11 years and 21% of adolescents 12 to 19 years are obese.

2. People who are overweight or obese have a greater incidence of chronic illnesses than individuals who are not overweight or obese.

3. Factors that place a client at risk.

a. Calorie intake greater than height, weight, activity, and energy requirements; may be due to high-fat diet and inappropriate food choices.

b. Reduced activity level without concurrent reduction in calorie intake; may be due to impaired mobility.

c. Cultural influences that support excess weight, such as frequent intake of fried foods or pasta.

d. Physiological situations, such as an underactive thyroid gland causing a low BMR and subsequent increase in weight.

e. Psychological factors, such as anxiety, that contribute to inappropriate food choices.

4. Specific nursing care.

a. Identify factors that place a client at risk for becoming overweight or obese.

b. Encourage the client to use a food diary to help develop insight into eating habits.

c. Help the client to identify realistic goals and to review them weekly.

d. Help the client understand that healthy eating needs to be an enduring lifestyle change.

e. Explain how to read a nutrition facts label to identify foods that are high in calories, fat, and carbohydrates that should be avoided in a low-fat, low-calorie diet; this knowledge will empower the client to have control over food choices.

f. Teach the client to avoid shopping for food when hungry to reduce the temptation to buy inappropriate comfort foods.

g. Identify foods to avoid that are high in fat, such as whole-milk products, fried foods, animal fat, gravies, sauces, nondiet soda, chocolate, and other treats that are high in carbohydrates and sugar.

h. Teach the client to limit the use of butter, margarine, mayonnaise, oil, shortening, bacon, cream, cream cheese, and other cheeses to 1 tablespoon a day or 1 teaspoon per meal.

i. Encourage the client to eat fresh fruits and vegetables; use fat-free milk and milk products; and substitute yogurt for sour cream in recipes.

j. Incorporate nutritious morning and afternoon snacks into the meal plan to minimize the desire to graze throughout the day.

k. Teach client to limit the intake of food containing cholesterol.

l. Encourage the client to serve food on small plates, eat small meals, take small bites, chew food well, eat slowly, and put the eating utensil down between bites.

m. Encourage the client to remain in a sitting position for 30 to 45 minutes after meals to use gravity to keep food in the stomach and minimize the risk of reflux and aspiration, which are associated with obesity.

n. Encourage the client to participate in counseling and/or a support group, such as Weight Watchers or Overeaters Anonymous.

o. Encourage the client to participate in an exercise program to burn calories and increase the BMR; clients should begin with less strenuous exercise at first and build to 40 minutes of exercise 6 days a week.

p. Encourage adequate sleep because sleep deprivation negatively affects the hormones leptin and ghrelin, which regulate appetite.

q. Use supportive statements to point out successes in efforts to lose weight; avoid negative statements because they can demoralize the client and negatively affect the nurse-client relationship.

r. Weigh the client weekly to evaluate progress; a sensible weight loss is approximately 2 lb a week; for a weight loss more than 2 lb a week, the client should be on a therapeutic weight loss diet and monitored by a primary health-care provider.

E. Nursing care for clients who have nausea and vomiting

1. Factors that place a client at risk.
   a. Electrolyte imbalances.
   b. Constipation or diarrhea.
   c. Anxiety.
   d. Pain.
   e. Pathological conditions, such as gastric ulcer, pancreatitis, and biliary disease.
   f. Radiation, medications, and/or anesthesia.

2. Specific nursing care.
   a. Monitor intake and output, fluid balance, and electrolyte levels.
   b. Avoid unpleasant procedures before and after meals.
   c. Provide frequent mouth care.
   d. Encourage the wearing of loose clothing to prevent pressure against the epigastric area.
   e. Teach the client to avoid the use of perfumes and scented hygiene products, such as soaps, aftershave, hairspray, and perfume, that may precipitate nausea.
   f. Provide food that the client likes, and identify and provide foods that the client tolerates; dry foods, such as crackers, breads, potatoes, pasta, and rice, may be better tolerated.
   g. Provide small, frequent meals; avoid odorous, high-fat, spicy, and hot food; some clients find that cold food is better tolerated than warm food.
   h. Teach the client to avoid food preparation areas; uncover food plates away from the client to allow food odors to dissipate somewhat before bringing the tray to the bedside.
   i. Remove the meal tray immediately when the client finishes eating or when the client is unable to eat because the sight and odor of food can precipitate nausea and vomiting.
   j. Encourage the client to eat slowly, chew food thoroughly, and rest after meals.

   🛑 k. Encourage intake of potassium-rich foods, such as orange juice, potatoes, and spinach, if low potassium is a concern with persistent vomiting.

   l. Seek a consult by a registered dietitian to address the client's nutritional needs if nausea or vomiting continues for more than a few days.

F. Nursing care for clients who are underweight, anorexic, or at risk for weight loss

1. Factors that place a client at risk.
   a. Chemotherapy or radiation therapy.
   b. Weakness or fatigue.
   c. Impaired dentition.
   d. Pain.
   e. Stomatitis or gingivitis.
   f. Impaired swallowing.
   g. Eating disorders, such as anorexia nervosa and bulimia nervosa.
   h. Conditions that increase the metabolic rate, such as hyperthyroidism, cancer, and serious burns.
   i. Conditions that interfere with absorption of nutrients, such as malabsorption syndromes, Crohn's disease, and colitis.
   j. Inadequate income to purchase food.
   k. Inability to shop and prepare meals.

2. Specific nursing care.
   a. Assess for factors that may place a client at risk for weight loss and for clinical indicators of being underweight or experiencing inadequate nutrition. Complete a 3-day calorie count if prescribed.
   b. Employ actions identified in "Nursing Care for Clients Who Have Nausea and Vomiting" previously presented in this chapter.
   c. Administer pain medication before meals to facilitate comfort during meals when appropriate.
   d. Encourage the client to eat protein and nutrient-dense foods on the meal tray first; offer milkshakes and other calorie-dense foods and liquids between meals.
   e. Provide five or six small meals daily because, over the course of the day, the total calorie intake should be higher than three meals a day and smaller portions are not as overwhelming as three large meals.
   f. Secure to modify the consistency of food, such as soft, chopped, or pureed, so that it is easier to swallow if swallowing or weakness is a concern.
   g. Limit the intake of fluids at meals because they may cause a feeling of fullness, which interferes with food intake.
   h. Avoid spicy, acidic, rough, hot, and salty foods for a client with stomatitis.
   🛑 i. Arrange for community services to assist a client who is unable to procure and prepare meals, such as Meals-on-Wheels, delivery of food from a food bank, application for food stamps, and a home-health aide to cook simple nutritious meals and to assist the client with eating.

G. Nursing care for clients with cognitive/mental impairments
   1. Diminished cognitive ability commonly interferes with a person's ability to comprehend the environment, communicate effectively, and eat independently.
   2. Factors that place a client at risk.
      a. Delirium and dementia.
      b. Intellectual or developmental impairment.
      c. Mental illness, such as major depression and bipolar disorder manic episode.
   3. Specific nursing care.
      a. Assess the client's ability to communicate, problem-solve, respond appropriately to stimuli, and self-feed and have an awareness of the need to eat.
      b. Reduce environmental stimuli, such as by turning off the radio or television and discouraging activity around the client during mealtimes.

   🛑 c. Remove unnecessary utensils and items that should not be eaten, such as packages of salt and pepper and container covers, from the food tray; position warm beverages out of reach to avoid a spill that could injure the client.
   d. Use simple phrases to cue the client, such as "open your mouth," "chew," and "swallow," when feeding the client.
   e. Help the client to self-feed as appropriate.
      (1) Position a hand over the client's hand and guide the client in feeding activities to initiate self-feeding.
      (2) Use hand gestures that the client may recognize and imitate.
      (3) Avoid feeding the client before the client has had time to self-feed.
      (4) Do not rush the client in self-feeding activities.
   f. Provide finger foods for a physically active client who is unable to sit through a meal.
   g. Provide positive reinforcement (e.g., say, "Good job") for efforts at self-feeding.
   h. Assist several people positioned at a feeding table (semicircular table generally used in long-term care facilities) for clients who need supervision, prompting to stay focused, or occasional assistance with eating; ensures client safety, supports socialization, and maximizes the use of a caregiver's time.
   🛑 i. Check the client's mouth for pocketed food after the meal to prevent aspiration.

H. Nursing care for clients with eating disorders (anorexia nervosa, bulimia nervosa)
   1. Eating disorders are characterized by an impaired relationship with food and body image.
   2. Clients perceive that they are overweight, fear obesity, and generally resist treatment.
   3. Clients do not see their eating patterns, lack of eating, and/or binging and purging as a problem because of impaired perception.
   4. Females are at greater risk for eating disorders, which occur most frequently during adolescence and young adulthood.
   5. Eating disorders can be life threatening if intervention is not provided before it is too late to reverse the damage to the body; mortality is as high as 20%.
   6. Persistent self-induced vomiting (*purging*) can precipitate clinical manifestations such as hypoglycemia, electrolyte imbalances (especially potassium and sodium); sore throat; excessive dental caries; enamel erosion and staining of the teeth due to contact with gastric acid; and swelling of the salivary glands.

7. *Anorexia nervosa.*
   a. Refusal to maintain body weight equal to or greater than expected weight for age and height; excessive fear of gaining weight or becoming obese even though underweight; disruption in the way one's body weight or contour is experienced; and denial of the gravity of the low body weight.
   b. Common physiological indicators include weight loss; muscle wasting; weakness; fatigue; lethargy; brittle hair and nails; lanugo on face; dry, pale, pasty skin; anemia; and amenorrhea. It can lead to severe fluid and electrolyte imbalances, dehydration, impaired sexual development, and death.
   c. Common behavioral clinical indicators include avoiding meals; reducing the amount and types of food ingested; compulsively arranging food; cutting food into small pieces; dieting and exercising excessively; denying hunger; wearing baggy clothes; vomiting after ingestion of food, which is common; and using diuretics and laxatives to reduce weight.
   d. Common emotions associated with anorexia nervosa include believing one is fat when really very thin; unhappiness with appearance; irritable; argumentative; overly sensitive to criticism; periods of depression; need for perfection; and low self-esteem.
8. *Bulimia nervosa.*
   a. Characterized by binge eating followed by purging which rids the body of excessive calories and other actions to prevent weight gain; and dissatisfaction with body contour and weight.
   b. Common physiological indicators associated with binging include dramatic variability in weight; abdominal swelling and pain; edema of the hands, feet and legs; fatigue; nausea; dizziness; and diarrhea from excessive laxative use, leading to dehydration.
   c. Common behavioral clinical indicators include behavior such as avoiding meals; vomiting after meals; evidence of binging, such as large volumes of food missing; hidden food wrappers; laxative, diuretic, and emetic use; stealing food or money to buy food; and night owl behavior so that binging occurs after others have gone to bed.
   d. Common emotions associated with bulimia include dissatisfaction with appearance; disinterest in social activities and work; moodiness; depression; irritability; overly sensitive to criticism; and low self-esteem.

9. Specific nursing care.
   a. Assess for clinical indicators of the eating disorder; identify verbal and nonverbal responses associated with the client's perceptions regarding body image.
   b. Maintain a consistent, nonjudgmental, non-argumentative, client-centered approach to support trust and a therapeutic relationship.
   c. Maintain a matter-of-fact approach; focus on emotional issues, not food.
   d. Assist with designing a contract for a behavior modification program.
   e. Monitor weight regularly.
   f. Monitor laboratory tests to identify electrolyte imbalances.
   g. Support and praise the client's efforts to control negative behaviors.
   h. Provide six small meals that are nutrient dense and several nutritious snacks daily.
   ⓘ i. Measure oral intake; monitor the client's behavior for 1 hour after meals to minimize the risk of self-induced vomiting.
   j. Support participation in individual, group, and/or family therapy.
   k. Assist the client in identifying and discussing concerns regarding low self-esteem, impaired identity, and family dysfunction.
   l. Provide prescribed IV therapy to restore electrolyte balance; administer enteral feedings when prescribed as a last resort.
I. Nursing care for clients with gastroesophageal reflux disease (GERD)
   1. Occurs when gastric contents flow up the esophagus.
   2. Factors that place a client at risk.
      a. Conditions that impair the ability of the lower esophageal sphincter to close firmly, such as protrusion of the stomach upward through the esophageal hiatus of the diaphragm *(hiatal hernia)*.
      b. Conditions that increase intra-abdominal pressure, such as obesity and pregnancy.
   3. Clinical indicators include epigastric discomfort or pain *(heartburn)*, dysphagia, regurgitation, aspiration, sore throat, and hoarse voice.
   4. Complications include respiratory system problems, such as wheezing, bronchitis, and pneumonia; chronic inflammation of the esophageal mucosa, leading to esophagitis; and epithelial changes known as Barrett's esophagus, a precancerous situation that in turn can lead to esophageal cancer.
   5. Specific nursing care.
      a. Encourage the client to lose weight if overweight or obese.

b. Teach the client practices to limit gastroesophageal reflux.

  (1) Use relaxation techniques before and after eating.

  (2) Eat six small meals a day.

  (3) Avoid foods that relax the lower esophageal sphincter, such as those high in fat, chocolate, peppermint, and spearmint; foods that stimulate gastric secretion, such as coffee and pepper; and foods that are irritating to the GI mucosa, such as alcohol, spicy foods, citrus fruits and juice, tomatoes, and tomato juice.

  (4) Avoid fluids for a half hour before meals; limit fluids to a half cup with meals; and avoid fluids for 1.5 hours after meals.

  (5) Maintain a sitting position for 2 hours after meals to allow gravity to keep gastric contents from ascending into the esophagus.

  (6) Limit food intake several hours before retiring to minimize the risk of reflux and aspiration.

  (7) Sleep with the head of the bed raised on 6- to 8-inch blocks to minimize gastroesophageal reflux at night.

  (8) Avoid clothing with tight belts to decrease pressure against the epigastric area.

  (9) Take over-the-counter antacids for mild reflux and proton pump inhibitors or histamine-2 receptor blockers as prescribed.

J. Nursing care for clients who have or are at risk for osteoporosis

1. Osteoporosis is a condition characterized by inadequate bone mass that causes fractures in response to mild trauma.

2. Caused by inadequate development of bone mass due to such factors as genetics; inadequate intake of calcium and vitamin D; excessive intake of protein, sodium, and caffeine that impairs calcium retention; insufficient exercise; and increased rate of bone loss later in life, especially in response to decreased estrogen in menopausal women.

3. Additional risk factors include reduced mobility, aging process, hyperthyroidism, use of corticosteroids and some antiseizure medications, being small and thin, family history, and intake of alcohol and tobacco.

4. Postmenopausal women are at risk due to the decrease in the protective effects of estrogen on bone; 80% of people with osteoporosis are women; 50% of women over the age of 50 experience a fracture related to osteoporosis.

5. The incidence of osteopenia and osteoporosis is increasing because of the aging of the U.S. population. Life expectancy for women is 81.2 years and for men is 75.9 years.

6. Clinical indicators include abnormal increased convexity of the curvature of the thoracic spine (kyphosis) and loss of height due to vertebral compression fractures; acute or chronic back pain, indicating vertebral fracture; pain that limits activities of daily living; and psychological problems, such as impaired body image, fear of falling or fractures, anxiety, and depression.

7. Bone density testing identifies the level of bone density and, when repeated every 1 or 2 years, can identify whether bones are losing density or staying the same; this is helpful in identifying a person's risk for a fracture and can assist in determining a person's treatment regimen.

8. Specific nursing care.

  a. Encourage intake of foods high in calcium, such as milk; cheese; yogurt; salmon; sardines; rainbow trout; oysters; cauliflower; tofu; and green, leafy vegetables, such as spinach, turnip greens, okra, and Chinese cabbage.

  b. Encourage exposure to sunlight because the sun's rays stimulate production of vitamin D, which promotes the absorption of calcium.

  c. Encourage intake of foods high in vitamin D, such as shiitake and button mushrooms, mackerel, salmon, herring, sardines, catfish, tuna fish, cod liver oil, eggs, and fortified cereals and soy products.

  d. Encourage a daily program of weight-bearing exercise, such as walking.

  e. Teach the client about prescribed medications.

    (1) Calcium supplements: 1,000 mg daily for clients 18 to 49 years of age and 1,200 mg daily for clients older than 50 years of age.

    (2) Vitamin D: 1,000 to 5,000 IU daily.

    (3) Bone forming drugs, such as teriparatide (Forteo).

    (4) Antiresorptive medications, such as alendronate (Fosamax) and ibandronate (Boniva).

X. Enteral Nutrition

Enteral nutrition is the delivery of liquid formula into the GI tract via a tube that bypasses the mouth, esophagus and, depending on the type of tube, sometimes the stomach. Enteral feedings are designed for clients who have a functioning GI system but have an inability to chew and swallow food, have a high metabolic need, or lack the stamina to eat. Nurses must be proficient in caring for clients with enteral feedings because of the risks associated with this type of therapy.

A. Enteral feeding tubes

1. Nasogastric tube.

  a. Tube inserted via a nostril (naris) through the nasopharynx and esophagus into the stomach.

b. Permits administration of a nutritional formula that enters the stomach *(gavage)*, bypassing the mouth and esophagus.

c. Used when a client is unable to swallow.

d. Usually used for less than 4 weeks.

e. Types.

   (1) Levin: Tube with one unvented lumen.

   (2) Salem sump: Double-lumen tube in which one lumen is used for gavage and the second, smaller lumen provides an air vent (blue pigtail) that permits inflow of air that keeps the tube from adhering to the stomach mucosa (Fig. 20.5).

   (3) Flexible, small-bore, weighted feeding tube.

      (a) Soft, flexible, small lumen tube inserted through a naris by the use of a wire within the lumen (stylet); stylet is removed when placement is verified.

      (b) Has less risk of mucosal trauma due to having a smaller diameter than other nasogastric tubes.

      (c) Can be used for a longer period of time than other nasogastric tubes.

2. Nasoenteric tube.

a. Long tube inserted via a naris and advanced further along the GI tract into the intestine.

b. Permits administration of a nutritional formula directly into the small intestine by bypassing the mouth, esophagus, and stomach.

c. Decreases the risk of aspiration in clients who have decreased level of consciousness, decreased or absent cough or gag reflex, endotracheal intubation, agitation, GERD, or gastric paresis.

d. Types.

   (1) Nasoduodenal tube: Inserted via a naris through the nasopharynx, esophagus, and stomach into the duodenum.

   (2) Jejunostomy tube (J-tube): Inserted via a naris through the nasopharynx, esophagus, stomach, duodenum, and into the jejunum.

3. Surgically implanted GI tubes.

a. Tube surgically or laparoscopically inserted through the abdominal wall into the stomach or intestine.

b. Generally used when nutritional support is required for longer than 4 weeks; however, now also used for short-term nutritional support because of new insertion techniques.

c. Types.

   (1) Percutaneous endoscopic gastrostomy (PEG) tube: Tube inserted through the abdomen into the stomach; can be converted to a gastrostomy button (G-button) after the insertion site heals; it can be capped between feedings and does not protrude from the abdomen (Fig. 20.6).

   (2) Percutaneous endoscopic jejunostomy (PEJ) tube: Tube inserted through the abdomen into the jejunum.

d. Advantages.

   (1) Provide reliable access to the GI tract.

   (2) Considered to be the most comfortable feeding tubes.

e. Disadvantages.

   (1) Require surgical or laparoscopic insertion through skin and abdominal wall into

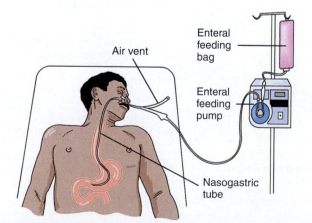

Fig 20.5 Salem sump tube attached to an enteral feeding pump. (From Williams & Hopper [2015]. *Understanding medical surgical nursing,* 5th ed. Philadelphia: F. A. Davis Company, with permission.)

Fig 20.6 Gastrostomy button (G-Button) for gavage. (From Wilkinson and Treas [2016]. *Fundamentals of nursing,* Vol. 1, 3rd ed. Philadelphia: F. A. Davis Company, with permission.)

stomach or intestine, which increases the risk of infection.

   (2) Insertion site requires surgical asepsis until healed (about 1 month) and then ongoing nursing assessment and meticulous skin care around site.

B. Enteral feeding formulas

1. Formulas include a variety of constituents and caloric values (Table 20.6).
2. Standard formulas require the client to have adequate digestion and absorption.
3. Special formulas contain constituents to meet a client's nutritional needs in relation to a specific health problem.

C. Nursing care for clients receiving enteral nutrition

1. Ensure accurate placement of the tube using several methods.
   a. Obtain x-ray confirmation of placement at the time of insertion per manufacturer or agency policy.
   b. Measure pH of the aspirate; low pH (1 to 5; acidic) indicates the tube is probably in the stomach; high pH (>6; alkaline) indicates the tube is probably in the intestine or respiratory tract.
   c. Inspect the aspirate for amount, color, and consistency.
      (1) Stomach: Greenish/yellow, clear with tan mucus, or brown (digested blood).
      (2) Esophagus: Scant amount, color unreliable.
      (3) Intestine: Yellow to brownish/green.
      (4) Lung: Off-white or tan.
   d. Ensure that the mark made on the tube during placement is just outside the naris.
   e. Instill 5 to 30 mL of air through the tube while auscultating over the epigastric area; "whoosh" sound with gurgling can be heard as air enters the stomach; most unreliable method.

🛑 f. Notify the primary health-care provider when in doubt to obtain a prescription for x-ray confirmation of placement.

2. Secure and monitor the tube in the naris.
   a. Secure the tube to the naris if specific placement is to be maintained; use a product

---

Table 20.6 Enteral Nutrition Formulas

Formula	Description	Indication for Use
Standard formula (isotonic–osmolality near that of body fluids)		
For example: Nutren, Osmolite.	• *Generally provides 1 kcal/mL.* • *Proportionally balanced among protein, fat, and carbohydrates depending on product.* • *Common minerals and vitamins.* • *Usually lactose free.*	• *Clients who are not ingesting adequate nutrients to meet daily energy requirements.* • *Clients with an inability to chew and swallow, but who have no problems with digestion or absorption.*
High-protein formula		
For example: Boost High-Protein.	• *Additional protein is added to normal nutrients needed daily.*	• *Clients with large draining wounds, serious burns, or malnutrition.*
Hydrolyzed formula (elemental formula)		
For example: Vital, Peptomen, Vivonex.	• *Contains partially or fully broken down nutritive elements that necessitate minimal digestion.* • *Fiber free.* • *Highly osmotic.*	• *Clients with a disorder that compromises digestion or absorption of nutrients.* • *Use is controversial.*
Renal formula		
For example: Nepro, Suplena.	• *Contains reduced amounts of protein, sodium, potassium, and nitrogen.*	• *Clients with renal insufficiency or failure who require enteral feedings.*
Pulmonary formula		
For example: Pulmocare, NutriVent.	• *High in calories and modified in carbohydrates and fats.* • *As oxygen is consumed, less carbon dioxide is produced.*	• *Clients with chronic emphysema, asthma, cancer of the lung, and pulmonary fibrosis who require enteral feedings.*
High-fiber formula		
For example: Jevity, Fibersource HN.	• *Contains more fiber than a standard formula to support digestive health and normal bowel function.* • *High in calories and protein.*	• *Clients with reduced physical activity.* • *Commonly prescribed for clients requiring prolonged enteral feedings.*

designed for this purpose or use tape (Fig. 20.7).

b. Inspect the site every 2 hours for signs of irritation because pressure and/or friction can cause skin breakdown (Fig. 20.8).

3. Provide PEG or PEJ tube site care; change sterile dressing every 8 hours until healed and then provide meticulous skin care with soap and water.

4. Maintain the head of the bed at a 30-degree to 45-degree angle to prevent regurgitation and aspiration.

5. Keep suction equipment at the bedside.

6. Provide frequent oral hygiene to keep mucous membranes moist.

Fig 20.7 Securing a nasogastric tube with ½-inch tape. (From Wilkinson and Treas [2016]. *Fundamentals of nursing*, Vol. 2, 3rd ed. Philadelphia: F. A. Davis Company, with permission.)

Fig 20.8 Pressure ulcer of a naris: Identified when a nasogastric tube was removed 18 hours after insertion.

7. Record accurate intake and output; include amount of formula and instillations used to flush the tubing in the intake.

8. Verify tube placement in the stomach before each intermittent feeding and every 4 hours with continuous or cyclic feedings.

9. Maintain tube patency.

a. Ensure that there are no dependent loops and that nothing is compressing the tube.

b. Flush the tube routinely according to agency policy, usually with 30 mL of water every 4 hours.

c. Ensure that liquid, powdered, and crushable medications are adequately diluted to prevent clogging the tube; flush the tube before and after instillation of medication.

10. Provide specific nursing care when administering an enteral feeding.

a. Verify the prescription for the formula, amount, rate of infusion, and type (continuous, intermittent [bolus], or cyclic [continuous feeding administered for less than 24 hours a day]).

b. Wash your hands.

c. Verify the expiration date on the formula and discard the formula if it is expired.

d. Label the feeding bag with the date, time, formula type, and rate of administration.

e. Flush the tubing with the formula to remove air before connecting the tubing to the client's access device and the enteric feeding pump; some pumps automatically purge the tubing.

f. Don clean gloves.

g. Verify placement and measure aspirate before each intermittent or cyclic feeding and every 4 hours with continuous or cyclic feedings; note that measurement of aspirate is not necessary with a PEJ tube because the jejunum is not a reservoir.

(1) Withhold the next feeding if the aspirate exceeds the amount specified by the primary health-care provider or agency protocol (e.g., more than the flow rate for 1 hour).

(2) Reinstill the aspirate to prevent fluid and electrolyte imbalances.

(3) Do not reinstill more than the flow rate for 1 hour; notify the primary health-care provider if the aspirate is excessive.

h. Flush the enteric tube with 30 mL of tap water before the administration of the formula.

i. Administer the feeding as prescribed.

(1) Continuous: Formula is administered continuously over 24 hours.

(2) Cyclic: Formula is administered in less than 24 hours; usually given at night when the client is sleeping.

(3) Intermittent: Formula is administered several times a day via a syringe by gravity (Fig. 20.9). Hold the syringe less than 18 inches above the insertion site to allow the solution to flow slowly and pinch the tubing as the formula reaches the bottom of the syringe to prevent air from entering the tube and eventually the stomach.

j. Flush the enteric tubing with 30 mL of water after completion of an intermittent feeding; flush the tubing of continuous or cyclic feedings with 30 mL of water every 4 hours as prescribed; some primary health-care practitioners prescribe a larger volume (e.g., 100 mL) of free water at routine intervals.

k. Assess the client's tolerance of feedings: Assess for clinical indicators of dumping syndrome, which indicates that the client is not tolerating the administration of a high-carbohydrate formula. (See the section "Dumping Syndrome" later in this chapter.)

l. Document the feeding and the client's response in the client's clinical record.

Fig 20.9 Feeding via a syringe by gravity. (From Wilkinson and Treas [2011]. *Fundamentals of nursing,* Vol. 2, 2nd ed. Philadelphia: F. A. Davis Company, with permission.).

m. Notify the primary health-care provider if intolerance or complications occur.

D. Complications of enteral nutrition and related nursing care

1. *Aspiration.*

   a. Occurs when gastric contents enter the respiratory tract due to gastric reflux or vomiting.

   b. Nursing care.

   (1) Monitor the client for clinical indicators of aspiration, such as coughing, shortness of breath, dyspnea, restlessness, tachycardia, tachypnea, and decreased oxygen saturation.

   (2) Ensure that suction equipment is readily available.

   (3) Ensure that tube placement is radiographically confirmed before use.

   (4) Keep the head of the bed (HOB) elevated 30 to 45 degrees throughout feedings; have a client with an intermittent feeding remain seated or elevate the HOB for 30 to 60 minutes after feedings.

   (5) Check for tube placement to ensure that it is in the stomach every 4 hours for continuous feedings and before an intermittent feeding.

   (6) Assess for residual volume to ensure that the feeding is being absorbed; every hour initially and then every 4 hours or when administering medication or adding more formula.

   (7) Withhold a feeding for 30 minutes to 1 hour if gastric residual is higher than the volume indicated by the primary health-care provider or based on protocol; usual protocol is to recheck the residual in 1 hour, and if it is within the prescribed volume, administer the feeding.

   (8) Place a continuous feeding pump on hold when administering care that requires the HOB to be lowered; after care is delivered, raise the HOB and reinstitute the feeding. When a client is receiving an intermittent feeding, provide care that requires the client's HOB to be lowered before a feeding when possible.

   (9) Do not overly sedate a client because doing so prolongs gastric emptying.

   (10) Administer medications that increase gastric motility, such as metoclopramide, as prescribed.

2. *Diarrhea.*

   a. Caused by situations such as a hyperosmolar formula, antibiotic therapy, bacterial contamination, and/or malabsorption.

b. Nursing care.

(1) Initiate the flow rate slowly and increase the flow rate after tolerance is determined. Continuous and cyclic feedings are preferred over bolus feedings because they are delivered over a longer period of time and, therefore, their volumes do not overwhelm the GI system.

(2) Prevent contamination of the system.

(a) Change the feeding set every 12 to 24 hours according to agency protocol and product recommendations.

(b) Discard a hanging formula after 8 hours if using an open system or after 24 to 48 hours depending on product recommendations if using a closed system.

(3) Administer prescribed medications, such as diphenoxylate/atropine (Lomotil) for diarrhea and Lactinex, a probiotic mixed culture of *Lactobacillus acidophilus* and *L. bulgaricus,* to restore and maintain normal bacterial balance of the GI tract.

(4) Consult with the primary health-care provider to prescribe a formula that is less hypertonic, fat-free, and/or lactose-free.

3. *Electrolyte imbalances.*

a. Occur with conditions such as cirrhosis, heart failure, diabetes, renal insufficiency, and excessive GI losses of electrolytes.

b. Nursing care.

(1) Monitor electrolyte levels regularly.

(2) Reinstill an aspirate when measuring residual volume to prevent fluid and electrolyte imbalances; do not reinstill more than the flow rate for 1 hour.

(3) Administer prescribed medications, such as potassium.

4. *Dumping syndrome.*

a. **Dumping syndrome** occurs when a concentrated formula rapidly enters the intestine, moving water from the bowel wall into the intestinal lumen, causing osmotic diarrhea.

(1) Mainly occurs 5 to 30 minutes after a bolus enteral feeding.

(2) Clinical indicators include: cramping, abdominal pain; hyperactive bowel sounds; vomiting; dizziness; weakness; heart palpitations; increased pulse rate; and sweating.

b. Concentrated formula causes blood glucose to rise and excessive insulin is released in response.

(1) Mainly occurs approximately 1 to 2 hours after a bolus enteral feeding.

(2) Clinical indicators include weakness, shakiness, anxiety, confusion, sweating, and tachycardia.

c. Nursing care.

(1) Assess for the clinical indicators of dumping syndrome and hyperglycemia.

(2) Initiate the flow rate slowly, and increase the flow rate after tolerance is determined.

(3) Encourage the client to rest in the semi-Fowler position for 1 hour after receiving a bolus enteral feeding to delay emptying of the stomach.

(4) Collaborate with the primary health-care provider to consider changing bolus feedings to a cyclical regimen.

5. *Impaired tissue integrity.*

a. Caused by gastric secretions leaking around a transabdominal tube site or by unrelieved pressure of an enteral tube taped too tightly to the nose (Fig. 20.8).

b. Nursing care.

(1) Tubes inserted via the nares.

(a) Monitor the naris every 2 hours for clinical indicators of skin breakdown.

(b) Use a tube fixation device to secure the tube to the client's nose, making sure to avoid excessive pressure against the naris (Fig. 20.7).

(c) Change fixation device/tape daily to allow for assessment of the naris.

(d) Clean the nares with a moistened cotton-tipped applicator, dry, and apply a water-soluble lubricant.

(e) Consult with the primary health-care provider regarding using a flexible, small-bore feeding tube or converting to a surgically implanted tube, such as a PEG tube.

(2) Transabdominal tubes.

(a) Monitor for clinical indicators of skin breakdown and local and systemic infection.

(b) Change the insertion site dressing as prescribed.

(c) Clean the site with warm water and dry well; apply protective skin ointment or prescribed topical antibiotic to the site or according to protocol.

(d) Ensure that the bumper on a gastrostomy or jejunostomy tube is not too tightly pressed against the abdominal wall.

6. *Hyperglycemia.*

a. Caused by a formula with high glucose content.

b. Nursing care.

(1) Assess for clinical indicators of hyperglycemia, such as weakness, shakiness, anxiety, confusion, sweating, and tachycardia.

(2) Initiate feedings at a slow rate.

(3) Monitor blood glucose level every 4 hours.

(4) Administer hyperglycemia medications as prescribed.

(5) Consult with the primary health-care provider regarding the use of a low-carbohydrate formula.

7. *Tube obstruction.*

a. Occurs when tubing is inadequately flushed, crushed medication is not adequately crushed, a feeding is placed on hold to administer nursing care, and when a feeding tube "runs dry"; occurs more frequently with flexible, small-bore tubes.

b. Nursing care.

(1) Assess for a slowed or absent flow rate of formula.

(2) Prevent dependent loops in tubing and ensure that the tubing is not being compressed under the client.

(3) Shake cans of formula well before administering.

🛑 (4) Flush the tubing with 30 mL of water after completion of an intermittent feeding and after medication administration; flush the tubing of continuous or cyclic feedings with 30 mL of water every 4 hours or as prescribed.

(5) Use the liquid form of prescribed medications when possible.

(6) Crush medications if permitted and mix them with water; administer each medication separately, and flush the tube with 5 mL of water after each medication.

(7) Reposition the client and instruct the client to cough, which may promote a kink in the enteric tube to straighten.

(8) Withhold the feeding and notify the primary health-care provider if obstruction or paralytic ileus is a concern.

DID YOU KNOW?

To unclog an enteral nutrition tube, the nurse can employ several interventions that usually are included in agency protocols. Some protocols require in-service education.

1. First, fill a 60-mL syringe with lukewarm water and attach it to the enteral tube; gently push and pull the plunger of the syringe back and forth several times; clamp the enteral tube for several minutes to allow the warm water to "soak" the internal lumen; gently repeat this action several times until tube patency is reestablished. If this method is unsuccessful, employ one of the following methods.

2. Clog Zapper, by CORKAP: A multienzyme cocktail designed to reduce formula clogs; generally does not work on clogs caused by medications.

3. PEG Cleaning Brush, by BARD: A cleaning brush that is inserted into an enteral feeding tube using a twisting motion to penetrate and scrape a clog.

4. DeClogger, by BIONIX: A soft, flexible threaded device that is inserted into an enteral tube to clear the clog.

5. Tube Clear System, by Tube Clear Inc.: A cleaning stem is inserted into an enteral tube and is attached to power that generates a jackhammer-like motion inside the tube.

Evidence-based practice results are varied concerning the use of cranberry juice, carbonated beverages, and meat tenderizer to reestablish patency of an enteral feeding tube. Some findings do not advocate the use of these products because of their acidity or excessive sodium content. Most research demonstrates that gentle irrigation with warm water is most effective.

8. *Gastrointestinal disturbance.*

a. Occurs with situations such as decreased peristalsis, paralytic ileus, malabsorption problems, hypertonic or cold formulas. Cold formulas cause vasoconstriction, which decreases the flow of digestive solutions.

b. Nursing care.

(1) Assess for clinical indicators, such as excessive residual, distention, vomiting, diarrhea, reports of gas pains, decreased or increased bowel sounds, nausea, and abdominal cramping.

(2) Initiate and increase the flow rate slowly as tolerance is determined.

(3) Administer feedings at room temperature unless otherwise instructed by the manufacturer's directions.

(4) Assess for residual every hour for the first 4 hours and then every 4 hours, before administering medication, and when adding more formula.

(5) Administer prescribed medications, such as diphenoxylate/atropine (Lomotil) for diarrhea and Lactinex, a probiotic mixed culture of *Lactobacillus acidophilus* and *L. bulgaricus,* to restore

2. *Catheter occlusion:* Blockage of the lumen of the catheter; may be caused by a blood clot at the tip of the catheter.
   a. Indicated by a sluggish or an absent catheter flow rate.
   b. Stop the infusion.
   c. Attempt to relieve the obstruction following the prescription of the primary health-care provider or according to agency protocol.
     (1) Flush the catheter with heparin or saline solution.
     (2) If flushing is ineffective, attempt to aspirate the clot.
     (3) If attempts to aspirate the clot are ineffective, follow agency protocol using a thrombolytic agent, such as urokinase.
3. *Infection:* Entrance of pathogenic microorganisms into the blood via the catheter or catheter insertion site.
   a. Indicated by elevated vital signs, chills, and positive blood culture.
   b. Administer prescribed antipyretics and local and/or systemic antibiotics.
4. *Hyperglycemia and hypoglycemia:* Increased blood glucose level *(hyperglycemia)* or decreased blood glucose level *(hypoglycemia)* due to an excessive or inadequate intake of glucose respectively.
   a. Hyperglycemia is indicated by polyuria, polydipsia, headache, and lethargy.
   b. Hypoglycemia is indicated by diaphoresis, shakiness, confusion, and loss of consciousness.
   c. Initiate and maintain a consistent flow rate as prescribed.
   d. Assess blood glucose level every 6 hours.
   e. Administer insulin according to the primary health-care provider's prescription if the client experiences hyperglycemia.
   f. Administer glucose gel if the client experiences hypoglycemia.
D. Lipid emulsions and related nursing care
1. Review the primary health-care provider's history and physical for information indicating a history or presence of anemia; abnormal liver, biliary, or pancreatic function; or respiratory or coagulation impairments. Collaborate with the primary health-care provider about these conditions because they are associated with fat emboli and the administration of parenteral lipids.
2. Use a special administration set specific for lipids; use a new administration set for each bottle.
3. Place the client in the supine position and have the client perform the Valsalva maneuver when connecting a catheter to the circulatory access to prevent an air embolus.
4. Connect to the port below the filter if lipids are administered concurrently with PN because lipids will not pass through a PN filter because of their large particles.
5. Ensure that the solution is free from froth and separation into layers.
6. Ensure that lipids are at room temperature.
7. Initially infuse 1 mL/min.
8. Take the vital signs every 10 minutes for 30 minutes and assess for signs and symptoms of intolerance, indicted by fever, chills, flushing, nausea, vomiting, dyspnea, headache, and back pain.
9. If no clinical indicators of intolerance occur, increase the flow rate to the prescribed rate and retake the vital signs every 4 hours.
10. Complete the administration of lipids within 12 hours.

XII. Medications Associated With Nutrition

When a person is diagnosed with a nutritional problem, the primary health-care provider can prescribe a variety of medications depending on the client's need. The most common medications influencing a client's nutritional status include antacids, antiemetics, antilipidemics, antisecretory agents, hypoglycemics, and insulin. Nurses should know the mechanisms of action, therapeutic and nontherapeutic effects, and nursing care related to these medications. This information is necessary not only to provide direct client care but also for client teaching because these medications are often self-administered over prolonged periods of time.
A. Antacids and related nursing care: Decrease gastric acidity, protect stomach mucosa, and reduce epigastric pain (Table 20.7).
B. Antiemetics and related nursing care: Decrease nausea and vomiting; prevent and decrease motion sickness (Table 20.8).
C. Antilipidemics and related nursing care: Decrease low-density liproproteins (LDL),, triglycerides, and total cholesterol levels; increase high-density lipoproteins (HDL) levels (Table 20.9).
D. Antisecretory agents and related nursing rare: Decrease gastric acidity and pain (Table 20.10).
E. Oral hypoglycemics and related nursing care: Control blood glucose levels in type 2 diabetes (Table 20.11).
F. Insulins, their time action profiles, and related nursing care: Control the blood glucose level in type 1 diabetes (Table 20.12).

Table 20.7 Antacids and Related Nursing Care

Mechanisms of Action	Examples	Nontherapeutic Effects
• Bind with excess acid	• aluminum hydroxide • magnesium/aluminum hydroxide (Maalox, Mylanta)	• Aluminum salts contribute to constipation and hypophosphatemia

Related Nursing Care

- Teach the client to take the medication cautiously with a low-sodium diet because many antacids contain sodium.
- Shake liquids well; give with at least 2 oz of water to promote transit to the stomach.
- Teach the client to avoid foods that increase epigastric distress, such as spicy foods.
- Encourage the intake of foods high in calcium and iron.
- Assess emesis and feces for obvious and occult blood.
- Monitor serum phosphate and calcium levels with long-term use.
- Encourage the client to seek a medical evaluation if gastrointestinal signs and symptoms do not subside within 2 weeks.

Table 20.8 Antiemetics and Related Nursing Care

Mechanisms of Action	Examples	Nontherapeutic Effects
Phenothiazines • Inhibit chemoreceptor zone in the central nervous system	• prochlorperazine (Compazine) • promethazine (Phenergan)	• Confusion • Constipation • Photosensitivity • Sedation • Extrapyramidal responses
5-HT$_3$ antagonists • Inhibit serotonin at receptor sites in vagal nerve terminals • Inhibit chemoreceptor zones in the central nervous system	• ondansetron (Zofran)	• Dizziness • Headache • Diarrhea • Constipation
Nonphenothiazines • Inhibit chemoreceptor zones in the central nervous system • Increase gastrointestinal motility and gastric emptying	• metoclopramide (Reglan)	• Restlessness • Sleepiness • Anxiety • Depression • Extrapyramidal responses

Anticholinergics
• Correct imbalances of acetylcholine and norepinephrine in the central nervous system that produces motion sickness
	• scopolamine (Transderm Scop)
	• trimethobenzamide (Tigan)
		• Sleepiness
		• scopolamine:
		  • Blurred vision
		  • Dry mouth
		  • Tachycardia
		  • Urinary hesitancy
		• trimethobenzamide:
		  • Hypotension
		  • Local irritation

Related Nursing Care

- Administer before chemotherapy or movement that causes motion sickness.
- Provide for client safety because of depression of the central nervous system.
- Teach the client to avoid concomitant use of alcohol and other central nervous system depressants.
- Monitor for the presence of nontherapeutic responses, especially extrapyramidal responses, such as grimacing, rigidity, involuntary movements, and shuffling walk.

Phenothiazines

- Teach the client to use sunscreen and wear protective clothing.
- Assess for clinical indicators of neuroleptic malignant syndrome, such as hyperthermia, unstable blood pressure, diaphoresis, dyspnea, stupor, muscle rigidity, and urinary incontinence.

Table 20.9 **Antilipidemics and Related Nursing Care**

Mechanisms of Action	Examples	Nontherapeutic Effects

HMG-CoA reductase inhibitors (statins)
• *Inhibit the HMG-CoA enzyme, which promotes cholesterol synthesis*
	• *atorvastatin (Lipitor)*
	• *rosuvastatin (Crestor)*
	• *simvastatin (Zocor)*
		• *Nausea and vomiting*
		• *Diarrhea or constipation*
		• *Abdominal cramps*
		• *Muscle soreness*
		• *Hepatoxicity*
		• *Decreased absorption of fat-soluble vitamins*
		• Statins:
		  • *Muscle soreness*
		  • *Rhabdomyolysis: cola-colored urine, extreme muscle pain, and weakness*
		• ezetimibe: *Teratogenic, angioedema*
		• fenofibrate: *Pulmonary embolism*

Bile acid sequestrants • *Bind cholesterol in the GI tract*	• *cholestyramine (Questran)*	
Cholesterol absorption inhibitors • *Impede absorption of cholesterol in the small intestine*	• *ezetimibe (Zetia)*	
Fibrates • *Impede peripheral lipolysis* • *Decrease production and synthesis of triglycerides*	• *fenofibrate (Tricor)* • *gemfibrozil (Lopid)*	
Water-soluble vitamins • *Decrease hepatic lipoprotein synthesis* • *Impede release of free fatty acids from adipose tissue*	• *niacin*	

Related Nursing Care

- *Encourage the client to consume a diet low in cholesterol and fat and eat two to three servings of fish high in omega-3 fatty acids weekly.*
- *Teach the client to exchange vegetables oils with polyunsaturated fatty acids with those with monounsaturated fatty acids.*
- *Monitor liver function tests, lipid profile, hemoglobin (Hb) level, and red blood cell (RBC) count.*
- *Bile acid sequestrants: Teach the client to take the medication before meals with 8 oz of water.*
- **Statins:** *Teach the client to notify the primary health-care provider of the occurrence of cola-colored urine, extreme muscle pain, and weakness because these responses indicate rapid destruction of skeletal muscle (rhabdomyolysis).*
- **ezetimibe:** *Teach the client to avoid use during pregnancy and lactation.*
- **fenofibrate:** *Teach the client to notify the primary health-care provider of the occurrence of unilateral chest pain, difficulty breathing, or frothy sputum because these responses may indicate a pulmonary embolus.*

Table 20.10 **Antisecretory Agents and Related Nursing Care**

Mechanisms of Action	Examples	Nontherapeutic Effects
H₂ antagonists • *Decrease histamine at H_2 receptors in parietal cells, causing a decrease in gastric secretions*	• *famotidine (Pepcid)* • *ranitidine (Zantac)*	• *Decreased RBCs, WBCs, and platelets* • *Cardiac dysrhythmias* • *CNS concerns, such as confusion, dizziness, headache, sleepiness* • *Nephrotoxicity* • *Hypersensitivity responses*
Proton pump inhibitors • *Decrease entrance of hydrogen ions into the lumen of the gastrointestinal tract*	• *esomeprazole (Nexium)* • *lansoprazole (Prevacid)* • *omeprazole (Prilosec)* • *pantoprazole (Protonix)*	

Related Nursing Care

- *Teach the client to notify the primary health-care provider if clinical indicators of bleeding occur with concurrent use of warfarin.*
- *Be aware that these drugs may be given with an antacid, except ranitidine (Zantac), which must be given 1 to 2 hours before or after an antacid.*
- *Assess for clinical indicators of altered heart rate and rhythm and frank or occult blood in emesis or feces.*
- *Monitor complete blood count for signs of blood dyscrasias.*
- **H₂ antagonists:** *Teach the client to avoid smoking because it may inhibit therapeutic action and/or may cause diarrhea.*
- **Proton pump inhibitors:** *Teach the client not to crush or chew the medication; administer 30 minutes to 1 hour before meals depending on the specific drug.*

Table 20.11 Oral Hypoglycemics

Mechanisms of Action	Examples	Nontherapeutic Effects
Biguanides • *Increase sensitivity to insulin* • *Increase binding of insulin to its receptor*	• *metformin (Glucophage)*	• *Hypoglycemia* • *Lactic acidosis: Dyspnea, sleepiness, malaise, weakness, chills, hyperventilation, bradycardia, hypotension, myalgia, diarrhea*
Meglitinides • *Increase release of insulin from the pancreas*	• *repaglinide (Prandin)*	• *Hypoglycemia*
Sulfonylureas • *Stimulate beta cells to release insulin*	• *glimepiride (Amaryl)* • *glipizide (Glucotrol)* • *glyburide*	• *Hypoglycemia*
Thiazolidinediones • *Decrease insulin resistance* • *Decrease glyconeogenesis*	• *pioglitazone (Actos)* • *rosiglitazone (Avandia)*	• *Upper respiratory tract infection* • *Edema associated with heart failure: Crackles, dyspnea, peripheral edema, weight gain, jugular vein distension* • *Hepatotoxicity (rare)*
Incretin mimetics • *Mimic effects of GLP-1, an intestinal hormone* • *Increases secretion of insulin* • *Decreases glucose absorption from the gut* • *Decreases action of glucagon*	• *dulaglutide (Trulicity)* • *liraglutide (Victoza)*	• *N&V, abdominal pain, anorexia, indigestion* • *Fatigue* • *Diarrhea*
Dipeptidyl peptidase-4 inhibitor • *Prevents GLP-1 and GIP activation* • *Increases secretion of insulin* • *Decreases release of glucagon*	• *sitagliptin (Januvia)*	• *N&V* • *Common cold-like S&S* • *Photosensitivity*
Glifozin • *Inhibits renal glucose reabsorption*	• *canagliflozin (Invokana)*	• *Dizziness* • *Increased urination; pain or burning on urination* • *Allergic reaction* • *Genital discharge* • *Hyperkalemia* • *Ketoacidosis*

Related Nursing Care

- *Do not administer these drugs to clients with type 1 diabetes; serious burns or trauma; renal, hepatic, or endocrine disease; and uncontrolled infection or to clients who are pregnant or lactating.*
- Teach the client that therapy controls, not cures, type 2 diabetes; therapy is long-term; and the medication regimen should be followed as prescribed.
- Assess for clinical indicators of hyperglycemia, hypoglycemia, and hyperosmolar nonketotic coma.
- Assess blood glucose levels before meals, at bedtime, and whenever necessary if concerned about glucose status.
- Assess for ketones in urine if blood glucose level is 300 mg/dL or higher.
- Encourage the client to avoid alcohol due to potential for Antabuse-like response.
- *Teach the client not to crush sustained-release tables and to take these medications 30 minutes before meals or according to the primary health-care provider's instructions.*
- *Thiazolidinediones: Assess the client who has concurrent heart disease for peripheral edema, crackles, dyspnea, weight gain, and jugular vein distension; assess for clinical indicators of liver impairment, such as nausea, vomiting, abdominal pain, anorexia, fatigue, jaundice, and dark urine.*

Table 20.12 Insulins, Their Time Action Profiles, and Related Nursing Care

Insulin Type	Examples	Onset	Peak	Duration
Rapid acting	lispro (Humalog)	15–30 min	30 min–1.5 hr	3–4 hr
	aspart (NovoLog)	10–20 min	1–3 hr	3–5 hr
	glulisine (Apidra)	15–30 min	30 min–1.5 hr	3–4 hr
Short acting	regular (Novolin R)	30–60 min	2–5 hr	5–8 hr
	regular (Humulin R)	30–60 min	1–5 hr	6–10 hr
Intermediate acting	NPH (N) Novolin N Humulin N	1.5–4 hr	4–12 hr	18–24 hr

Table 20.12 Insulins, Their Time Action Profiles, and Related Nursing Care—cont'd

Insulin Type	Examples	Onset	Peak	Duration
Long acting	glargine (Lantus)	1–1.5 hr	Steadily delivered, no peak action	20–24 hr
	detemir (Levemir)	50 min–2 hr	Unknown	24 hr
Premixed	Novolin 70/30	30 min	2–12 hr	24 hr
	Humulin 70/30	30 min	2–4 hr	14–24 hr
	Novolog Mix 70/30	10–20 min	1–4 hr	24 hr
	Humulin 50/50	30 min	2–5 hr	18–24 hr
	Humalog 75/25	15 min	30 min–2.5 hr	16–20 hr

Related Nursing Care

- *Give only regular insulin intravenously; rapid-insulin analogs, such as aspart and glulisine, may be given IV in selective situations with medical supervision. Use only a dedicated IV line.*
- *Roll the vial to mix insulin; do not shake the vial, which could create bubbles and result in an inaccurate dose.*
- *Administer insulin using a calibrated insulin syringe to promote accuracy.*
- *Administer insulin as prescribed; generally before meals and at hour of sleep.*
- *Monitor blood glucose levels to determine amount of insulin to administer when providing insulin coverage; note that the primary health-care provider establishes dosages based on glucose levels.*
- *Monitor for clinical indicators of hyperglycemia and hypoglycemia.*
- *Follow appropriate sequence when mixing a short-acting and a long-acting insulin in the same syringe. (See "Mixing Insulin," Fig. 9.15, in Chapter 9, Medication.)*

Source: Vitale, B. (2017). *NCLEX-RN Notes: Content review and exam prep,* 3rd ed. Philadelphia: F. A. Davis Company, with permission.

CASE STUDY: Putting It All Together

A public health nurse makes a home visit to an obese woman whose infant son was just discharged from the hospital after a premature birth 1 month ago. The husband is serving in the military and recently left for a 6-month tour of duty on a ship going to the Middle East. In addition to the infant, the mother has another son who is 3 years of age, a 6-year-old daughter, and an adolescent daughter. The mother pumped her breasts and gave the nurses her bottled breast milk when she visited her son every other day while in the hospital. During the visit to the home, the mother asked the nurse, When the nurse explored the family's diet with the mother, the mother stated, "My three-year-old only wants to eat hot dogs, french fries, and peanut butter. I tell him that if he eats his vegetables he can have ice cream for dessert. My teenager is constantly on a diet even though she is thin as a rail and says she diets because she doesn't want to get fat like me." The mother voiced a concern about the belief that her adolescent "may have one of those eating problems because she is so thin." Also living in the home is a 75-year-old grandmother who is trying to help the mother with child care and chores around the house while the mother's husband is deployed. The woman shared that although the grandmother has been helpful around the house, the grandmother has problems with "bad teeth," uses too much salt when she cooks, and constantly depends on her for her social life. The woman's most serious concern about the grandmother is that because of the grandmother's "bad teeth" she has not been eating well and as a result is 20 pounds below her ideal body weight.

Case Study Questions

A. Compose the most appropriate response by the nurse to the mother's question, "Can I give my son regular milk now that he is 1 month old?"

_____

_____

_____

B. What are three things the nurse should encourage the mother to do to best meet her toddler's nutritional needs?

1. _____

continued.

CASE STUDY: Putting It All Together   *cont'd*

Case Study Questions

2. _____

3. _____

C. What nine clinical indicators of eating disorders should the nurse teach the mother to observe for when monitoring her adolescent's behavior and physical status?

1. _____

2. _____

3. _____

4. _____

5. _____

6. _____

7. _____

8. _____

9. _____

D. List six nursing interventions that may help the grandmother to meet her nutritional and social needs.

1. _____

2. _____

3. _____

4. _____

5. _____

6. _____

E. What are three important things the nurse should teach the mother about nutrition and breastfeeding?

1. _____

2. _____

3. _____

F. What are at least 10 things the nurse should teach the mother to do to achieve a more healthy weight?

1. _____

2. _____

3. _____

4. _____

5. _____

6. _____

7. _____

8. _____

9. _____

10. _____

REVIEW QUESTIONS

Be sure to read the Introduction for valuable test-taking tips.

1. What should a nurse do to prevent burns during meal-time in clients with mental and physical impairments?
   1. Assist clients with warm drinks.
   2. Use plastic instead of metal utensils.
   3. Serve unsteady clients only cold drinks.
   4. Wait until the food is cool before serving.

2. A nurse is caring for a client who is receiving bolus enteral feedings several times daily. Which nursing intervention is important to help prevent the client from experiencing diarrhea?
   1. Flush the tube after every feeding.
   2. Check the residual before each feeding.
   3. Elevate the head of the bed during the feeding.
   4. Discard the refrigerated opened cans of feeding formula after 24 hours.

3. A nurse is providing dietary teaching about a nutrition facts label to a client who recently began taking a diuretic daily. What information in the list of nutrients on a nutrition facts label is **most** important for the nurse to include in the teaching plan?

Nutrition Facts

8 servings per container
Serving size 2/3 cup (55g)

Amount per serving
Calories 230

	% Daily Value*
A → **Total Fat** 8g	**10%**
Saturated Fat 1g	**5%**
Trans Fat 0g	
B → **Cholesterol** 0mg	**0%**
C → **Sodium** 160mg	**7%**
Total Carbohydrate 37g	**13%**
Dietary Fiber 4g	**14%**
Total Sugars 12g	
Includes 10g Added Sugars	**20%**
D → **Protein** 3g	
Vitamin D 2mcg	10%
Calcium 260mg	20%
Iron 8mg	45%
Potassium 235mg	6%

* The % Daily Value (DV) tells you how much a nutrient in a serving of food contributes to a daily diet. 2,000 calories a day is used for general nutrition advice.

   1. A
   2. B
   3. C
   4. D

4. A nurse is caring for a client who is receiving continuous nutritional support via a nasogastric (NG) tube that is regulated by an enteral feeding pump. The nurse identifies that the client is having difficulty breathing and is restless. What should the nurse do **first**?
   1. Use a nasal cannula to provide oxygen.
   2. Activate the hold button on the feeding.
   3. Raise the bed to the high-Fowler position.
   4. Immediately notify the primary health-care provider.

5. A nurse is caring for a client who is receiving total parenteral nutrition. Which nursing actions are essential when providing care for this client? **Select all that apply.**
   1. Use tubing with an in-line filter.
   2. Obtain the vital signs every 8 hours.
   3. Monitor blood glucose every 4 hours.
   4. Compare the client's daily weight to fluid intake and output.
   5. Hang a 5% to 10% dextrose solution if the infusion is interrupted.

6. A nurse is caring for a client who had a large portion of the stomach surgically removed due to stomach cancer and is now experiencing dumping syndrome. For which clinical indicators of dumping syndrome should the nurse assess the client after the client completes a meal? **Select all that apply.**
   1. Hyperperistalsis
   2. Bradycardia
   3. Perspiration
   4. Palpitations
   5. Dyspnea
   6. Hypoxia

7. Blood glucose monitoring before meals and at bedtime is prescribed for a client. Place the following steps in the order in which they should be implemented.
   1. Wipe away the first drop of blood.
   2. Cleanse the area with alcohol and let it dry thoroughly.
   3. Place the hanging drop of blood gently on the end of the test strip.
   4. Put the client's finger in a dependent position in a cup of warm water.
   5. Prick the site with the lancet while holding it perpendicular to the client's finger.
   6. Check the code number on the strip and ensure that it compares with the code on the monitor screen.

   Answer: _____

8. A nurse is caring for a client who was admitted to the hospital from home. Family members reported having difficulty getting the client to eat. Which laboratory test should the nurse monitor because it is the **best** indicator of the client's nutritional status?
   1. Albumin
   2. Transferrin
   3. Blood urea nitrogen
   4. Total lymphocyte count

9. A nurse is caring for a debilitated client who is on bedrest and has been eating 50% of meals. What should the nurse plan to do to stimulate this client's appetite? **Select all that apply.**
   1. Serve small, frequent meals.
   2. Provide oral care before meals.
   3. Schedule procedures for after meals.
   4. Provide adequate pain medication before meals.
   5. Transfer the client to a comfortable chair for meals.

10. A nurse is caring for a client with gastroesophageal reflux disease. What should the nurse do? **Select all that apply.**
    1. Instruct the client to chew food thoroughly.
    2. Teach the client to avoid carbonated beverages.
    3. Serve food that has different textures and aromas.
    4. Offer fluids with food and at a preferred temperature.
    5. Teach the client to elevate the head of the bed on six-inch blocks.
    6. Encourage the client to avoid eating several hours before bedtime.

11. An older frail client is admitted to the hospital because of malnutrition and an inability to maintain weight. The nurse reviews the results of biochemical laboratory tests. Which laboratory results indicate a problem with nutrition? **Select all that apply.**
    1. Hematocrit 42%
    2. Hemoglobin 14 g/dL
    3. Transferrin 190 mg/dL
    4. Serum albumin 2.9 g/dL
    5. Blood urea nitrogen 18 mg/dL

12. A client is diagnosed with gluten intolerance. Which foods should the nurse encourage the client to avoid? **Select all that apply.**
    1. White rice
    2. Oatmeal cereal
    3. Steamed eggplant
    4. Veal cutlet parmesan
    5. Fruit thickened with tapioca

13. A nurse is providing dietary teaching to a person with a low fixed income. What should the nurse encourage the person to do when making meals on a limited budget? **Select all that apply.**
    1. Substitute eggs and beans for meat.
    2. Purchase luncheon meats for sandwiches.
    3. Buy fresh milk instead of powdered milk.
    4. Read the nutrition facts labels on prepared foods.
    5. Use store brand frozen meals over advertised brands.

14. A nurse is teaching a client about foods that should be avoided and foods that are acceptable on a lactose-free diet. Which foods selected by the client reflects an understanding of the teaching? **Select all that apply.**
    1. Yogurt
    2. Sherbet
    3. Fruit salad
    4. Hamburger
    5. Rice pudding

15. An older adult who lives alone is experiencing slow but steady weight loss over the past year. What should the nurse encourage the adult to do to address this concern? **Select all that apply.**
    1. Select nutrient-dense foods.
    2. Eat foods high in protein first.
    3. Purchase prepared frozen meals.
    4. Eat an extra meal before bedtime.
    5. Use bouillon powder for added flavor.

16. A nurse is planning a teaching program about atorvastatin (Lipitor) that was prescribed for a client who has high cholesterol. Which information is important for the nurse to emphasize? **Select all that apply.**
    1. Replace oils containing monosaturated fatty acids with oils containing polyunsaturated fatty acids.
    2. Notify the primary health-care provider if muscle pain, weakness, or fever occur.
    3. Crush and mix this medication with applesauce if it is hard to swallow the pill.
    4. Avoid drinking large amounts of grapefruit juice.
    5. Take this medication only with food.

17. A nurse is teaching a client who is a vegetarian about what food combinations make a complete protein. What food combinations should the nurse include in the teaching? **Select all that apply.**
    1. Lentils and tofu
    2. Cereal with milk
    3. Macaroni with cheese
    4. Back-eyed peas and rice
    5. Black and red bean soup

18. A nurse teaches a client how to follow a prescribed 2-g sodium diet. What client statement indicates that the client understands the teaching?
    1. "I can use as much salt substitutes as I want to season my food."
    2. "I must limit my intake of salt to two teaspoons of table salt daily."
    3. "I am allowed to drink diet cola because it has less salt than soda with sugar."
    4. "I should read nutrition facts labels for the amount of sodium that is in prepackaged foods."

19. A nurse is educating a client who is obese and on a calorie-restricted diet how to analyze a nutrition facts label. Which section of the nutrition facts label on a bag of snack food is **most** important for the obese client to consider?

    1. A
    2. B
    3. C
    4. D

20. A nurse is providing a class about foods to include and avoid when following a calorie-restricted 2-g sodium diet. A client with which cultural heritage should the nurse be **most** concerned about adjusting to a 2-g sodium diet?
    1. Asian
    2. Indian
    3. Puerto Rican
    4. Middle Eastern

21. A part-time evening nurse arrives on duty for a 6 p.m. to 12 midnight shift and is assigned to care for a client receiving peripheral parenteral nutrition (PPN) via a peripheral intravenous catheter inserted at 5 p.m. The nurse reviews the client's clinical record and completes a blood glucose test before the client's dinner at 6:10 p.m. In what order should the nurse implement the following interventions?
    1. Cover the glucose level with insulin according to the insulin prescription.
    2. Discuss the formula prescription with the primary health-care provider.
    3. Hang a bag of 20% dextrose and water and set it at 83 mL/hour.
    4. Contact the IV nurse to consider changing the IV site.
    5. Discontinue the PPN solution.
    Answer: _____

Client's Clinical Record

Nurse's Progress Note 1500

PPN infusion running as prescribed at 83 mL/hour. Slight erythema noted at PPN site. Client reports some "stinging" at the infusion site. Vital signs stable.

Primary Health-Care Provider's Prescriptions

Peripheral parenteral nutrition: 2,000 mL standard formula with 50% dextrose and 8.5% amino acids at 83 mL/hour. Weigh weekly.
VS every 8 hours. If temperature is greater than 100°F, notify primary health-care provider.
Soft diet as tolerated.
BGM a.c. and h.s.; cover as per insulin prescription.
If PPN is interrupted, start 20% dextrose and water at 83 mL/hour and notify the primary health-care provider.
Laboratory tests: Basic metabolic panel, magnesium, and phosphate daily for 3 days then MWF; triglyceride level in a.m.
Mondays CBC, INR, triglyceride level, and liver panel.

BGM at 6:10 p.m.

Glucose: 308

22. A nurse is preparing to administer a fat emulsion intravenously to an adult. What should the nurse do when administrating this solution? **Select all that apply.**
    1. Run the lipid solution at a rate of 1 mL/minute for the first 30 minutes.
    2. Administer the lipid solution within 15 minutes after removal from a refrigerator.
    3. Rotate the lipid solution bottle gently if the solution separates into layers or is cloudy.
    4. Stop the lipid solution immediately if the client demonstrates signs of respiratory distress.
    5. Connect the lipid solution infusion tubing to the port above the filter in the primary infusion line.

23. A nurse is caring for a client who is receiving a high-calcium diet. Which foods should the nurse teach the client to include in the diet? **Select all that apply.**
    1. Tuna fish
    2. Prune juice
    3. Whole milk
    4. Pinto beans
    5. Broccoli spears

24. Metformin 500 mg PO bid is prescribed for a client newly diagnosed with type 2 diabetes. What should the nurse teach the client to do when taking this medication? **Select all that apply.**
    1. Take medication between meals on an empty stomach.
    2. Increase the intake to three times a day when experiencing stress.
    3. Drink a glass of orange juice if experiencing signs of hyperglycemia.
    4. Be alert for nontherapeutic responses such as sleepiness, myalgia, and hyperventilation.
    5. Explain that it is acceptable to double a dose if a dose is missed, as long as this occurs infrequently.

25. A nurse is caring for a client who has diabetes and high cholesterol. Which foods should the nurse teach the client to avoid? **Select all that apply.**
    1. Eggs
    2. Celery
    3. Asparagus
    4. Calves liver
    5. Baked custard

26. A nurse is caring for a client who is weak and lethargic. Which actions are essential for the nurse to implement that address the most significant risk when feeding this client? **Select all that apply.**
    1. Record the intake of food as poor, good, or excellent on the daily activities form.
    2. Ask about preferences regarding the seasoning of food.
    3. Check the mouth for pocketed food after each bite.
    4. Encourage self-feeding.
    5. Thicken liquids.

27. A nurse is caring for a client who is recovering from abdominal surgery. The client reports experiencing "gas pains" and asks the nurse what can be done to prevent them in the future. Which should the nurse encourage the client to avoid until intestinal function fully returns? **Select all that apply.**
    1. Summer squash
    2. Chewing gum
    3. Onions
    4. Lentils
    5. Eggs

28. A Diabetic Nurse Educator teaches a client to limit the dietary intake of complex carbohydrates. The intake of which nutrient should the nurse teach the client to limit? **Select all that apply.**
    1. Milk
    2. Nuts
    3. Eggs
    4. Pasta
    5. Noodles

29. A nurse is teaching a client about what constitutes a healthy diet. Which client statement indicates that the teaching was effective?
    1. "I must eat a protein food daily to meet my vitamin C requirement."
    2. "I need to minimize my intake of foods containing trans fat."
    3. "I should ingest foods rich in nonessential amino acids."
    4. "I want one fifth of the foods on MyPlate to be grains."

30. A nurse is teaching a client how to calculate the kilocalories contained in an ounce of corn chips. The nutrition facts label indicates that a 1-ounce serving contains 10 g of fat, 16 g of carbohydrates, and 2 g of protein. The client accurately calculated the total number of kilocalories contained in 1 ounce of corn chips. How many kilocalories did the client calculate was contained in this snack? **Record your answer using a whole number.**
    Answer: _____ kilocalories

31. A nurse working in a primary care clinic is caring for a client who was diagnosed with a low vitamin D level. Vitamin D 5,000 units by mouth daily is prescribed. The nurse is teaching the client about foods high in vitamin D. The selection of which food by the client indicates to the nurse that the client can identify at least one food that is high in vitamin D?
    1. Nuts
    2. Eggs
    3. Liver
    4. Oranges

32. The proton pump inhibitor omeprazole is prescribed for a client. The prescription states to take 20 mg by mouth once a day. Which instructions should the nurse give the client regarding this medication? **Select all that apply.**
    1. "Take the capsule several hours before an antacid."
    2. "Report severe diarrhea, tarry stool, or headache."
    3. "Avoid taking nonsteroidal anti-inflammatories."
    4. "Sprinkle the capsule contents in applesauce."
    5. "Take the capsule with food."
    6. "Swallow the capsule whole."

33. A nurse is teaching a client how to calculate the kilocalories contained in one granola bar. The nutrition facts label indicates that one bar contains 1.5 g of fat, 19 g of carbohydrates, and 1 g of protein. How many kilocalories calculated by the client indicates the correct amount of kilocalories contained in this snack? **Record your answer using one decimal place.**
    Answer: _____ kilocalories

34. A nurse is teaching a client about nutrients that will increase the percentage of whole grains and fiber in the diet. Which nutrients selected by the client indicate that the teaching was effective? **Select all that apply.**
    1. Grits
    2. Noodles
    3. Broccoli
    4. Wild rice
    5. Corn bread
    6. Baked beans

35. Which information is essential for the nurse to include in a program supporting healthy eating habits? **Select all that apply.**
    1. Drink 8 glasses of fluid daily.
    2. Increase the intake of foods high in solid fats.
    3. Make 25% of your plate fruits and vegetables daily.
    4. Cream cheese and butter are included in the dairy circle on MyPlate.
    5. Two servings of seafood rich in omega-fatty acids should be included weekly.

REVIEW ANSWERS AND RATIONALES

1. ANSWER: 1.
Rationales:
1. Clients with mental and physical deficits need assistance with warm drinks to prevent oral trauma or burns from spills.
2. The use of plastic utensils does not prevent spilling hot liquids.
3. Clients have a right to have a variety of foods presented at different temperatures; serving only cold drinks violates a client's rights.
4. Warm foods should be served warm, and cold foods should be served cold.

TEST-TAKING TIP: Identify the option with the obscure clang association. The word *burns* is a key word in the stem that should direct the test-taker to the word *warm* in option 1. Identify options that deny the client's rights and that are equally plausible. Options 3 and 4 deny the client's right to have food and drinks served at warm temperatures and are equally plausible. Identify the option with a specific determiner. Option 3 contains the word *only,* which is a specific determiner. Identify the client-centered option. Option 1 is client centered.
Content Area: Nutrition
Integrated Processes: Nursing Process: Implementation
Client Need: Physiological Integrity; Basic Care and Comfort
Cognitive Level: Application
Concept: Safety

2. ANSWER: 4.
Rationales:
1. Flushing the tube after every feeding moves the formula into the stomach and helps maintain tube patency; it does not reduce the risk of diarrhea.
2. Checking the residual volume informs the nurse about the absorption of the last feeding. This step prevents the addition of more feeding than the client can digest; it does not prevent diarrhea. Generally, feedings are withheld when a certain residual volume (e.g., half the volume of the last feeding is identified.
3. Elevating the head of the bed 30° during a feeding helps to keep the formula in the stomach via the principle of gravity and helps to prevent aspiration; it does not prevent diarrhea.
4. Contaminated formula can cause diarrhea. Cans of opened formula support bacterial growth and must be discarded after 24 hours, even when refrigerated.

TEST-TAKING TIP: Identify the unique option. Option 4 is unique. It does not end in the word *feeding,* and it is the only option with a number.
Content Area: Nutrition
Integrated Processes: Nursing Process: Implementation
Client Need: Physiological Integrity; Basic Care and Comfort
Cognitive Level: Application
Concept: Safety

3. ANSWER: 3.
Rationales:
1. The intake of total fat is not as significant to monitor as is another nutrient when a client is taking a diuretic.

2. The intake of cholesterol is not as significant to monitor as is another nutrient when a client is taking a diuretic.
3. The client is taking a diuretic to limit or reduce excess fluid volume. This client should avoid excess dietary sodium because sodium helps to retain fluid, which is counterproductive.
4. The intake of protein is not as significant to monitor as is another nutrient when a client is taking a diuretic.

TEST-TAKING TIP: Identify the word in the stem that sets a priority. The word *most* in the stem sets a priority.
Content Area: Nutrition
Integrated Processes: Teaching/Learning; Nursing Process: Planning
Client Need: Physiological Integrity; Pharmacological and Parenteral Therapies
Cognitive Level: Analysis
Concept: Patient-Centered Care; Fluid and Electrolyte Balance

4. ANSWER: 2.
Rationales:
1. Oxygen should be initiated after other, more important interventions are implemented.
2. The client's respiratory distress may be due to NG tube migration into the respiratory tract. The feeding should be stopped until this is ruled out.
3. Raising the head of the bed to the high-Fowler position should be done after another more important nursing intervention.
4. The primary health-care provider should be notified of the client's change in status after emergency nursing actions are initiated.

TEST-TAKING TIP: Identify the word in the stem that sets a priority. The word *first* in the stem sets a priority. Identify the clang association. The word *feeding* in the stem and option 2 is a clang association.
Content Area: Nutrition
Integrated Processes: Nursing Process: Implementation
Client Need: Physiological Integrity; Basic Care and Comfort
Cognitive Level: Application
Concept: Oxygenation

5. ANSWER: 1, 5.
Rationales:
1. Using tubing with an in-line filter is necessary because of the high glucose concentration of parenteral nutrition solutions.
2. Vital signs should be monitored every 4 hours for signs of infection or sepsis.
3. Blood glucose should be monitored every 6 hours.
4. Assessment of daily weights in relation to intake and output is an intervention that assesses fluid balance. When a client is receiving total parenteral nutrition body weight should be assessed weekly.
5. A 5% to 10% dextrose solution should be administered when parenteral nutrition is interrupted to prevent hypoglycemia.

TEST-TAKING TIP: Identify the word in the stem that sets a priority. The word *essential* in the stem sets a priority. The question is asking, "What *must* be done when administering parenteral nutrition?"

Content Area: Nutrition
Integrated Processes: Nursing Process: Implementation
Client Need: Physiological Integrity; Pharmacological and Parenteral Therapies
Cognitive Level: Analysis
Concept: Nutrition

6. **ANSWER: 1, 3, 4.**
Rationales:
1. Hyperperistalsis occurs when food rapidly enters the intestine and water moves from the bowel wall into the intestinal lumen, causing osmotic diarrhea.
2. Tachycardia, not bradycardia, occurs in response to dumping syndrome. Tachycardia is a vasomotor reaction to rapid distention of the jejunal loop anastomosed to the stomach.
3. Perspiration is a sign of dumping syndrome. Perspiration is a vasomotor reaction to rapid distention of the jejunal loop anastomosed to the stomach.
4. Palpitations are a sign of dumping syndrome. Palpitations are a vasomotor reaction to rapid distention of the jejunal loop anastomosed to the stomach.
5. Dyspnea is not associated with dumping syndrome.
6. Hypoxia is not associated with dumping syndrome.
Content Area: Nutrition
Integrated Processes: Nursing Process: Evaluation
Client Need: Physiological Integrity; Basic Care and Comfort
Cognitive Level: Application
Concept: Nutrition

7. **ANSWER: 6, 4, 2, 5, 1, 3.**
Rationales:
6. Checking the code number on the strip and the monitor ensures that the blood glucose monitoring machine is calibrated accurately.
4. Holding the finger dependent and in warm water increases circulation and dilation of blood vessels at the intended puncture site.
2. Alcohol cleanses and limits the number of microorganisms at the puncture site limiting the risk of infection. Drying prevents the alcohol from inactivating the substance on the test strip that measures the level of glucose.
5. Holding the lance perpendicular to the client's finger facilitates skin penetration.
1. Wiping away the first drop of blood reduces the risk of using blood that may be contaminated with a cleaning product, which can alter test results.
3. Gently placing a droplet of blood on the end of the test strip avoids smearing blood on the test strip, which may contribute to an inaccurate test result.
Content Area: Nutrition
Integrated Processes: Nursing Process: Planning
Client Need: Physiological Integrity; Reduction of Risk Potential
Cognitive Level: Analysis
Concept: Metabolism

8. **ANSWER: 2.**
Rationales:
1. Although a decreased albumin level is an effective indicator of protein depletion, it is not the first laboratory value to change with protein depletion because its half-life is 21 days.

2. A transferrin level is an effective indicator of acute protein depletion because its half-life is only 8 days.
3. Blood urea nitrogen is not the best test to assess a client's nutrition level. Although a blood urea nitrogen level reflects an inadequate intake of dietary protein or malabsorption, it is more often monitored to assess the balance of urea production and excretion.
4. A total lymphocyte count is not the best test to assess nutrition level. Although a decreased level may indicate a decreased nutritional intake or malnutrition, it is more often monitored to assess a client's immune system.
TEST-TAKING TIP: Identify the word in the stem that sets a priority. The word *best* in the stem sets a priority.
Content Area: Nutrition
Integrated Processes: Nursing Process: Assessment
Client Need: Physiological Integrity; Reduction of Risk Potential
Cognitive Level: Analysis
Concept: Nutrition

9. **ANSWER: 1, 2, 4.**
Rationales:
1. Small, frequent meals are less likely to overwhelm (e.g., physically and visually) a client than large meals.
2. Oral care cleanses the mouth of debris and odors that can interfere with one's desire to eat.
3. Procedures should not be scheduled just after meals because this may cause nausea and vomiting. Procedures just before a meal may inhibit appetite. Procedures should be scheduled as far from meals as possible.
4. Adequate pain control will support comfort, which may enhance appetite.
5. The client has a prescription for bedrest and should not be transferred to a chair for meals.
Content Area: Nutrition
Integrated Processes: Nursing Process: Planning
Client Need: Physiological Integrity; Basic Care and Comfort
Cognitive Level: Application
Concept: Nutrition

10. **ANSWER: 2, 5, 6.**
Rationales:
1. Although chewing food thoroughly helps with the digestion of food, it does not help prevent gastroesophageal reflux.
2. Carbonated beverages overdistend the stomach, which precipitates gastric reflux.
3. Serving food with different textures and aromas addresses the needs of a client who has a decrease in the senses of smell and taste; it does not help prevent gastroesophageal reflux.
4. Fluids with meals will overdistend the stomach, which will increase the risk of gastroesophageal reflux.
5. Elevating the head of the bed on 6-inch blocks uses gravity to help keep fluid and food in the stomach when the client is in the supine position in bed.
6. Gastroesophageal reflux is less likely to occur if the stomach is empty when a person is in the supine position, such as when sleeping.

Content Area: Nutrition
Integrated Processes: Teaching/Learning; Nursing Process: Implementation
Client Need: Physiological Integrity; Basic Care and Comfort
Cognitive Level: Application
Concept: Patient-Centered Care; Nutrition

11. **ANSWER: 3, 4.**
Rationales:
1. A hematocrit level of 42% is within the expected range of 40% to 50%; a decrease in the hematocrit level indicates anemia.
2. A hemoglobin level of 14 g/dL is within the expected range of 12 to 16 g/dL for women and 14 to 18 g/dL for men; a decrease in the hemoglobin level indicates anemia.
3. A transferrin level of 190 mg/dL is below the expected range of 215 to 380 mg/dL; a decrease in the transferrin level indicates anemia and protein deficiency.
4. A serum albumin level of 2.9 g/dL is below the expected range of 3.3 to 5 g/dL; a decrease in the albumin level indicates malnutrition or malabsorption.
5. A blood urea nitrogen level of 18 mg/dL is within the expected range of 8 to 21 mg/dL; an increase in blood urea nitrogen level indicates starvation, diarrhea, or a high-protein intake.
Content Area: Nutrition
Integrated Processes: Nursing Process: Analysis
Client Need: Physiological Integrity; Reduction of Risk Potential
Cognitive Level: Analysis
Concept: Nutrition

12. **ANSWER: 2, 4.**
Rationales:
1. White rice is gluten free.
2. Oats is a nutrient that contains gluten and should be avoided when a person has intolerance to gluten. Malabsorption occurs in response to the sensitivity to the presence of the gliadin fraction of gluten.
3. Steamed eggplant is gluten free.
4. A veal cutlet is breaded and then fried when preparing veal cutlet parmesan; bread crumbs are made from wheat flour, which contains gluten. Malabsorption occurs in response to the sensitivity to the presence of the gliadin fraction of gluten.
5. Fruit thickened with tapioca is gluten free.
TEST-TAKING TIP: Identify the word in the stem that indicates negative polarity. The word *avoid* in the stem indicates negative polarity. This question is asking, "What should the nurse teach the client *not to eat?*"
Content Area: Nutrition
Integrated Processes: Teaching/Learning; Nursing Process: Implementation
Client Need: Physiological Integrity; Basic Care and Comfort
Cognitive Level: Analysis
Concept: Patient-Centered Care; Nutrition

13. **ANSWER: 1, 4.**
Rationales:
1. Eggs and beans are less expensive than meat; teach the client that rice with beans is a complete protein.
2. Luncheon meats should be avoided because they are expensive and less healthy because of their high sodium levels and the presence of nitrites in cured and smoked meat.
3. Powdered milk is less expensive than fresh milk.
4. By reading the nutrition facts label on prepared foods, the client can ensure the most nutrition for the cost.
5. Frozen meals should be avoided altogether because they are more expensive than food prepared at home and, generally, they are high in sodium and fat.
Content Area: Nutrition
Integrated Processes: Teaching/Learning; Nursing Process: Implementation
Client Need: Health Promotion and Maintenance
Cognitive Level: Application
Concept: Patient-Centered Care; Nutrition

14. **ANSWER: 3, 4.**
Rationales:
1. Yogurt is a milk product that contains lactose. The client has a deficiency of lactase, the enzyme necessary to digest the sugar in milk and milk products and therefore must avoid the intake of milk and milk products.
2. Sherbet is made with milk and milk contains lactose. The client has a deficiency of lactase, the enzyme necessary to digest the sugar in milk and milk products and therefore must avoid the intake of milk and milk products.
3. Fruit salad is a healthy choice from the menu because fruit does not contain lactose.
4. Hamburger is made with chopped beef. It does not contain milk and can be ingested by a person who is lactose intolerant. The person has a deficiency of lactase, the enzyme necessary to digest the sugar in milk and milk products.
5. Rice pudding is made with milk and milk contains lactose. The client has a deficiency of lactase, the enzyme necessary to digest the sugar in milk and milk products and therefore must avoid the intake of milk and milk products.
Content Area: Nutrition
Integrated Processes: Teaching/Learning; Nursing Process: Evaluation
Client Need: Physiological Integrity; Basic Care and Comfort
Cognitive Level: Analysis
Concept: Patient-Centered Care; Nutrition

15. **ANSWER: 1, 2.**
Rationales:
1. Nutrient-dense foods have a higher nutrient to calorie ratio. A nutrient-dense food provides the most nutrients for the fewest number of calories.
2. Protein is essential for building and repairing body tissue, regulating body functions, and providing energy when fats and carbohydrates are insufficient. Because of a decreased sense of taste, older adults often prefer concentrated sweets. Once sweets are ingested, older adults no longer feel hungry enough to eat essential nutrients.

3. Prepared frozen meals should be avoided because they are high in sodium and fat.

4. Four smaller meals a day may increase caloric intake because one is less overwhelmed and more likely to finish the meal. However, the fourth meal should be no closer than 2 to 3 hours before bedtime; this will reduce the risk of gastroesophageal reflux, which is common with older adults.

5. Bouillon powder is high in sodium and should be avoided. People should be encouraged to use lemon juice, vinegar, herbs, or spices free from sodium to flavor food.

Content Area: Nutrition
Integrated Processes: Teaching/Learning; Nursing Process: Implementation
Client Need: Health Promotion and Maintenance
Cognitive Level: Application
Concept: Patient-Centered Care; Nutrition

16. **ANSWER: 2, 3, 4.**
Rationales:
1. The opposite is encouraged. Vegetable oils with monosaturated fatty acids should replace vegetable oils with polyunsaturated fatty acids.
2. These nontherapeutic side effects, especially if accompanied by fever or malaise, indicate myopathy requiring immediate discontinuation of the medication.
3. Atorvastatin (Lipitor) is not enteric coated or a time-release capsule; it can be crushed and mixed with applesauce if necessary.
4. Large amounts of grapefruit juice should be avoided when taking atorvastatin (Lipitor) because this is associated with an increased risk of drug toxicity.
5. Atorvastatin (Lipitor) can be taken any time of day and can be taken with or without food.

TEST-TAKING TIP: Identify the option with a specific determiner. Option 5 contains the word *only* which is a specific determiner.

Content Area: Nutrition
Integrated Processes: Teaching/Learning; Nursing Process: Planning
Client Need: Physiological Integrity; Pharmacological and Parenteral Therapies
Cognitive Level: Application
Concept: Medication; Nutrition

17. **ANSWER: 2, 3, 4.**
Rationales:
1. Lentils and tofu are both legumes; legumes must be paired with a grain, nuts, or seeds to make a complete protein.
2. When cereal, which is made from a grain, and milk are served together, they make a complete protein.
3. When macaroni, which is made from a grain, and cheese, which is a milk product, are served together, they make a complete protein.
4. When black-eyed peas, a legume, and rice, a grain, are served together, make a complete protein.
5. Black and red beans are both legumes; legumes must be paired with a grain, nuts, or seeds to make a complete protein.

Content Area: Nutrition
Integrated Processes: Teaching/Learning; Nursing Process: Implementation
Client Need: Health Promotion and Maintenance

Cognitive Level: Analysis
Concept: Health Promotion; Nutrition

18. **ANSWER: 4.**
Rationales:
1. Salt substitutes are not free from salt; they should be used sparingly because they generally contain half as much salt as regular salt. In addition, large amounts of salt substitutes generally taste bitter rather than salty.
2. Two teaspoons of salt contain 4,000 mg (4 g) of sodium; this exceeds the 2-g sodium diet prescribed by the client's primary health-care provider.
3. Soda sweetened with aspartame generally has 50% more sodium than nonartificially sweetened soda.
4. Clients must learn how to read and interpret nutrition facts labels on prepared foods to ensure that they do not exceed 2,000 mg (2 g) of sodium daily when on a 2-g sodium diet.

TEST-TAKING TIP: Identify the option with a clang association. The word *sodium* in the stem and in option 4 is a clang association.

Content Area: Nutrition
Integrated Processes: Teaching/Learning; Nursing Process: Evaluation
Client Need: Physiological Integrity; Basic Care and Comfort
Cognitive Level: Application
Concept: Patient-Centered Care; Nutrition

19. **ANSWER: 1.**
Rationales:
1. Identifying the number of servings per container is critical to determining how many calories are contained in the entire package. A product may contain 4 servings and each serving is 90 calories. When clients ingest the entire product, thinking that they are eating only 90 calories, they are actually ingesting 360 calories.
2. Knowing the amount of calories that are in a serving size is the second, not first, most important piece of information when reviewing a nutrition facts label when receiving a calorie-restricted diet.
3. Although it is important to identify the amount of total fat in a product when receiving a calorie-restricted diet, another option is more important.
4. Sodium on a label is important because clients who are obese often experience hypertension and are receiving a 2-g sodium diet as well as a calorie-restricted diet. However, it is not the most important section on a label that an obese client should consider.

TEST-TAKING TIP: Identify the word in the stem that sets a priority. The word *most* in the stem sets a priority. Identify the unique option. Option 1 is unique because it is the only option that does not indicate an ingredient.

Content Area: Nutrition
Integrated Processes: Teaching/Learning; Nursing Process: Implementation
Client Need: Physiological Integrity; Basic Care and Comfort
Cognitive Level: Analysis
Concept: Patient-Centered Care; Nutrition

20. ANSWER: 1.

Rationales:

1. Soy sauce, which is very salty, is widely used to season food preferred by people with an Asian heritage. This may present a problem adjusting to a sodium-restricted diet.

2. Curry, which is not salty, is very popular in Indian recipes and should not pose a problem with a sodium-restricted diet.

3. People with Puerto Rican heritage often prefer such foods as rice and vegetables, which generally are not seasoned with excessive amounts of salt.

4. People with Middle Eastern heritage usually do not season their food with excessive amounts of salt. Grains, wheat, rice, and chickpeas in the form of hummus are popular.

TEST-TAKING TIP: Identify the word in the stem that sets a priority. The word *most* in the stem sets a priority.

Content Area: Nutrition

Integrated Processes: Teaching/Learning; Nursing Process: Assessment

Client Need: Health Promotion and Maintenance

Cognitive Level: Analysis

Concept: Culture

21. ANSWER: 5, 3, 1, 2, 4.

Rationales:

5. A PPN formula should not exceed 20% dextrose. Dextrose at 50% is too high a percentage for dilution by peripheral blood flow.

3. A 20% dextrose solution prevents rebound hypoglycemia and follows the primary health-care provider's prescription for the solution to be hung if the PPN is interrupted.

1. Cover the elevated glucose level with insulin which will cause the blood glucose level to decrease. The objective is to maintain the client's blood glucose level below 110 mg/dL.

2. The PPN prescription should be discussed with the primary health-care provider because the dextrose should be no more than 20% when administered in a PPN solution. Dextrose of 10% to 70% is permitted when total parenteral nutrition is provided via a central line.

4. Contacting the IV nurse who is an expert regarding IV intervention ensures evaluation of the site. The site may need to be changed given the presence of erythema.

Content Area: Nutrition

Integrated Processes: Communication and Documentation; Nursing Process: Planning

Client Need: Physiological Integrity; Pharmacological and Parenteral Therapies

Cognitive Level: Analysis

Concept: Patient-Centered Care; Nutrition

22. ANSWER: 1, 4.

Rationales:

1. Fat emulsions should be administered slowly over the first 30 minutes to provide time for adjustment to the higher glucose level and allow for observation of an allergic or adverse reaction (e.g., chills, fever, flushing, dyspnea, nausea, and vomiting). If a reaction occurs, the nurse should terminate the infusion and notify the primary health-care provider immediately.

2. Fat emulsions should be administered at room temperature to prevent pain, venous spasms, and hypothermia. It takes approximately 1 hour for the solution to warm to room temperature after removal from a refrigerator.

3. A lipid solution that is separated into layers or is cloudy should be discarded. Separation of the emulsion into layers, presence of fat globules, froth, or cloudy solution indicates contamination of the solution and should not be administered.

4. Respiratory distress may indicate a pulmonary embolus or interstitial pneumonitis due to an unseen precipitate of electrolytes in the product or an intravascular fat accumulation in the lungs.

5. The tubing of the lipid solution infusion set should be inserted into the total parenteral nutrition tubing below the filter because lipid solutions have an increased viscosity that will become trapped in the filter, obstructing the flow of the solution.

Content Area: Nutrition

Integrated Processes: Nursing Process: Implementation

Client Need: Physiological Integrity; Pharmacological and Parenteral Therapies

Cognitive Level: Application

Concept: Nutrition

23. ANSWER: 3, 5.

Rationales:

1. Three ounces of tuna fish contains 17 mg of calcium; it is not a generous source of calcium.

2. One cup of prune juice contains 700 mg of potassium and only 30 mg of calcium; it is not an adequate source of calcium.

3. One cup of whole milk contains 290 mg of calcium and should be encouraged when a client is receiving a high-calcium diet.

4. One cup of pinto beans contains approximately 882 mg of potassium and only 86 mg of calcium; they are an excellent source of potassium, not calcium.

5. A broccoli spear contains approximately 205 mg of calcium and should be encouraged when a client is receiving a high-calcium diet.

Content Area: Nutrition

Integrated Processes: Teaching/Learning; Nursing Process: Implementation

Client Need: Physiological Integrity; Basic Care and Comfort

Cognitive Level: Application

Concept: Patient-Centered Care; Nutrition

24. ANSWER: 1, 4.

Rationales:

1. Metformin (Glucophage) should be ingested with a meal to avoid gastrointestinal upset and to facilitate absorption.

2. A client should never increase the dose or frequency of any medication without being instructed to do so by the primary health-care provider. If the client is experiencing physical or emotional stress, the client's pattern of serum

glucose levels must be analyzed by the primary health-care provider. Increasing metformin (Glucophage) alone may not control the client's glucose level. The client may need to receive subcutaneously administered insulin temporarily until the stress and glucose levels subside.

3. Orange juice contains sugar and is ingested when a person has hypoglycemia, not hyperglycemia. Ingesting orange juice when experiencing hyperglycemia will cause the glucose level to increase even higher.

4. These responses indicate lactic acidosis, a serious nontherapeutic response to metformin (Glucophage), requiring its discontinuation. The risk of lactic acidosis increases with severe infection, dehydration, or severe or continuing diarrhea. Additional clinical indicators of lactic acidosis include chills, diarrhea, bradycardia, low blood pressure, dyspnea, and weakness. The client should notify the primary health-care provider immediately if any of these signs or symptoms occurs.

5. It is never acceptable to double a dose of metformin (Glucophage). If a dose is missed, it can be taken as long as it is not almost time for the next dose. A double dose can precipitate hypoglycemia.

Content Area: Nutrition
Integrated Processes: Teaching/Learning; Nursing Process: Implementation
Client Need: Physiological Integrity; Pharmacological and Parenteral Therapies
Cognitive Level: Application
Concept: Medication; Safety

25. **ANSWER: 1, 4, 5.**
    Rationales:
    1. One large egg contains approximately 275 mg of cholesterol and should be avoided by clients with diabetes when receiving a low-cholesterol diet. Egg consumption can increase the risk for cardiovascular disease in clients with diabetes. Research has not found a similar risk for clients without diabetes. Egg whites can be consumed because it is the yolk of the egg that contains cholesterol.
    2. One stalk of celery contains approximately 5 mg of cholesterol; celery is permitted on a low-cholesterol diet.
    3. Four spears of asparagus contain approximately 3 mg of cholesterol; asparagus is permitted on a low-cholesterol diet.
    4. Three ounces of calves liver contains 410 mg of cholesterol and should be avoided when receiving a low-cholesterol diet.
    5. One cup of baked custard contains approximately 280 mg of cholesterol and should be avoided when receiving a low-cholesterol diet.
    TEST-TAKING TIP: Identify the word in the stem that indicates negative polarity. The word *avoid* in the stem indicates negative polarity.
    Content Area: Nutrition
    Integrated Processes: Teaching/Learning; Nursing Process: Implementation
    Client Need: Physiological Integrity; Basic Care and Comfort
    Cognitive Level: Application
    Concept: Patient-Centered Care; Nutrition

26. **ANSWER: 3, 5.**
    Rationales:
    1. Food intake should be documented in the percentage of food ingested. The words poor, good, and excellent are relative and subjective.
    2. Although asking about seasoning preferences is something nurses should do, it is not as important as another intervention when caring for a client who is weak and lethargic.
    3. A person who is weak and lethargic may have difficulty chewing and swallowing, which increases the risk of pocketing food. Food pocketed between the gum and cheek increases the risk of aspiration, therefore, checking the mouth for pocketed food after each bite is one nursing action that reduces this risk.
    4. Generally, the nurse should encourage a client to participate in feeding himself or herself; however, in this situation, the client is weak and lethargic. Feeding the client helps the client to conserve energy for chewing, swallowing, and breathing.
    5. Thickened liquids are easier to manage and less likely to be aspirated than liquids without a thickening agent. This is a nursing action that can reduce the risk of aspiration when feeding a client.
    TEST-TAKING TIP: Identify the word in the stem that sets a priority. The word *essential* in the stem sets a priority. To answer this question the test-taker first has to identify the *most* important risk facing the client when eating. The most significant risk is aspiration when eating. Once this is identified, the test-taker then has to identify the *essential* nursing interventions that help to reduce this risk.
    Content Area: Nutrition
    Integrated Processes: Nursing Process: Implementation
    Client Need: Physiological Integrity; Safe and Effective Care Environment
    Cognitive Level: Application
    Concept: Safety

27. **ANSWER: 2, 3, 4.**
    Rationales:
    1. Summer squash is a low-carbohydrate food and, therefore, is less likely to produce as much intestinal gas as other vegetables that are high in sugar, starch, or fiber.
    2. A person chewing gum will swallow more frequently than when not chewing gum. Swallowed air will increase air in the gastrointestinal tract causing abdominal discomfort.
    3. Onions contain fructose, which is a monosaccharide. When not totally digested by the intestinal enzymes sucrase, lactase, and maltase, monosaccharides are acted upon by harmless intestinal bacteria, with gas being a by-product of this bacterial fermentation.
    4. Lentils, dried beans, and peas contain carbohydrates that are difficult to digest but are digested by harmless bacteria in the intestine. The harmless bacteria produce hydrogen, carbon dioxide and, in some people, methane, all of which exit the body as flatulence.
    5. Eggs are a nongassy protein.
    TEST-TAKING TIP: Identify the word in the stem that indicates negative polarity. The word *avoid* in the stem indicates negative polarity.

Content Area: Nutrition
Integrated Processes: Teaching/Learning; Nursing Process: Implementation
Client Need: Physiological Integrity; Basic Care and Comfort
Cognitive Level: Application
Concept: Patient-Centered Care; Nutrition

28. **ANSWER: 4, 5.**
Rationales:
1. Milk is a simple sugar, not a complex carbohydrate. A simple sugar contains a single sugar (saccharide) unit called a *monosaccharide.*
2. Nuts are incomplete proteins, not a complex carbohydrate. Incomplete proteins are nutrients that do not include all the essential amino acids required for protein synthesis. A complete protein can be made by combining two incomplete proteins, such as red beans and brown rice or peanut butter with whole-grain bread.
3. Eggs are a complete protein, not a complex carbohydrate. A complete protein is a nutrient that includes all of the essential amino acids required for protein synthesis; additional nutrients that are complete proteins include cheese and milk.
4. **Pasta is a complex carbohydrate. Complex carbohydrates consist of long chains of saccharides called polysaccharides. Additional nutrients that are complex carbohydrates include breads, cereals, grains, legumes, and vegetables.**
5. **Noodles are a complex carbohydrate. Complex carbohydrates consist of long chains of saccharides called polysaccharides. Additional nutrients that are complex carbohydrates include breads, cereals, grains, legumes, and vegetables.**
TEST-TAKING TIP: Identify the word in the stem that indicates negative polarity. The word *limit* in the stem indicates negative polarity.
Content Area: Nutrition
Integrated Processes: Teaching/Learning; Nursing Process: Implementation
Client Need: Physiological Integrity; Basic Care and Comfort
Cognitive Level: Application
Concept: Patient-Centered Care; Nutrition

29. **ANSWER: 2.**
Rationales:
1. Citrus fruits, such as oranges, grapefruits, and lemons, and green peppers, broccoli, apricot nectar, strawberries, and tomatoes provide vitamin C, not protein.
2. **Trans fat is a saturated fat that increases the LDH (low-density lipoprotein) level and should be avoided in a healthy diet.**
3. Nonessential amino acids can be synthesized by the body and do not need to be obtained from food or supplements.
4. MyPlate guidelines recommend that 30%, not 20%, of the food a person ingests daily should contain grains. Half of those grains should be whole grains.
TEST-TAKING TIP: Identify the unique option. Option 2 is unique. It is the only option that discusses a nutrient that should be minimized.

Content Area: Nutrition
Integrated Processes: Teaching/Learning; Nursing Process: Evaluation
Client Need: Health Promotion and Maintenance
Cognitive Level: Analysis
Concept: Health Promotion; Nutrition

30. **ANSWER: 162.**
Rationale:
Each gram of fat contains 9 kilocalories, each gram of carbohydrate contains 4 kilocalories, and each gram of protein contains 4 kilocalories. Nine kilocalories multiplied by 10 g of fat equals 90 kilocalories, 4 kilocalories multiplied by 16 g of carbohydrates equals 64 kilocalories, and 4 kilocalories multiplied by 2 g of protein equals 8 kilocalories, for a grand total of 162 kilocalories.
Content Area: Nutrition
Integrated Processes: Teaching/Learning; Nursing Process: Evaluation
Client Need: Physiological Integrity; Basic Care and Comfort
Cognitive Level: Application
Concept: Patient-Centered Care; Nutrition

31. **ANSWER: 2.**
Rationales:
1. Nuts are an excellent source of vitamin E, not D. Also, nuts are rich in vitamin B_6, thiamine, and niacin.
2. **Eggs are an excellent source of vitamin D and are also rich in vitamin A, vitamin B_{12}, pantothenic acid, biotin, riboflavin, and folic acid.**
3. Liver is an excellent source of vitamin K, not vitamin D. Also, liver is rich in vitamin A, folic acid, niacin, biotin, pantothenic acid, riboflavin, and thiamine.
4. Oranges are an excellent source of vitamin C, not D. Also, oranges are rich in folic acid.
Content Area: Nutrition
Integrated Processes: Teaching/Learning; Nursing Process: Evaluation
Client Need: Physiological Integrity; Basic Care and Comfort
Cognitive Level: Analysis
Concept: Patient-Centered Care; Nutrition

32. **ANSWER: 2, 3, 6.**
Rationales:
1. Omeprazole (Prilosec) can be taken concurrently with an antacid; no drug-to-drug interaction occurs that interferes with absorption of the medication.
2. **Diarrhea, tarry stools, or headache are nontherapeutic effects of omeprazole (Prilosec) and should be reported to the primary health-care provider.**
3. **Nonsteroidal anti-inflammatories may cause gastric irritation and should be avoided.**
4. A capsule of omeprazole (Prilosec) should not be opened, crushed, or chewed. The pellets in the capsule are designed for delayed absorption.
5. Omeprazole (Prilosec) should be given before food is eaten, preferably breakfast.
6. **A capsule of omeprazole (Prilosec) should be swallowed whole and should not be opened, crushed,**

or chewed. The pellets in the capsule are designed for delayed absorption.

TEST-TAKING TIP: Identify the options that are opposites. Options 4 and 6 are opposites. Examine these options carefully because oftentimes one of the options that is an opposite is the correct answer.

Content Area: Nutrition
Integrated Processes: Teaching/Learning; Nursing Process: Implementation
Client Need: Physiological Integrity; Pharmacological and Parenteral Therapies
Cognitive Level: Application
Concept: Medication; Nutrition

33. **ANSWER: 93.5.**

    Rationale:

    Each gram of fat contains 9 kilocalories, each gram of carbohydrate contains 4 kilocalories, and each gram of protein contains 4 kilocalories. Nine kilocalories multiplied by 1.5 g of fat equals 13.5 kilocalories, 4 kilocalories multiplied by 19 g of carbohydrates equals 76 kilocalories, and 4 kilocalories multiplied by 1 g of protein equals 4 kilocalories for a grand total of 93.5 kilocalories.

    Content Area: Nutrition
    Integrated Processes: Teaching/Learning; Nursing Process: Evaluation
    Client Need: Physiological Integrity; Basic Care and Comfort
    Cognitive Level: Application
    Concept: Patient-Centered Care; Nutrition

34. **ANSWER: 3, 4, 6.**

    Rationales:

    1. Grits are a food product made with refined grains. The milling process eliminates the bran and germ to make a finer texture; it also removes fiber, iron, and many B vitamins.
    2. Noodles are made with refined grains. The milling process eliminates the bran and germ to make a finer texture; it also removes fiber, iron, and many B vitamins.

    3. Broccoli is high in fiber and is an excellent nutrient for the client to choose.
    4. Wild rice is a whole-grain food product because it is made from the entire grain kernel.
    5. Cornbread is made with refined grains. The milling process eliminates the bran and germ to make a finer texture; it also removes fiber, iron, and many B vitamins.
    6. Baked beans are high in dietary fiber and an excellent choice by this client.

    Content Area: Nutrition
    Integrated Processes: Teaching/Learning; Nursing Process: Evaluation
    Client Need: Health Promotion and Maintenance
    Cognitive Level: Analysis
    Concept: Patient-Centered Care; Nutrition

35. **ANSWER: 1, 5.**

    Rationales:

    1. It is recommended that 8 glasses of fluid should be ingested daily. Water is essential because it is a component of circulating blood, is a basic solvent for the body's chemical processes, and helps maintain body temperature.
    2. Foods high in solid fats should be reduced, not increased, in a daily diet because they may contribute to atherosclerosis.
    3. Fruits and vegetables should be 50% of your plate daily, with slightly more vegetables than fruit. Fruits and vegetables provide essential nutrients for cellular growth and fiber for intestinal motility.
    4. Cream cheese and butter are not included in the dairy circle because they contain too little calcium.
    5. Two servings of seafood rich in omega-fatty acids should be included in the diet weekly. Omega-fatty acids help limit triglycerides, inflammation, hypertension, and cardiovascular and autoimmune diseases.

    Content Area: Nutrition
    Integrated Processes: Teaching/Learning; Nursing Process: Planning
    Client Need: Health Promotion and Maintenance
    Cognitive Level: Application
    Concept: Health Promotion; Nutrition

Chapter 21

Fluid, Electrolyte, and Acid-Base Balance

NURSING CONCEPTS

Acid/Base Balance
Collaboration
Communication
Fluid and Electrolyte Balance

Medication
Patient-Centered Care
Safety

KEY TERMS

Active transport—Active process whereby metabolic energy moves substances across a membrane from a less concentrated to a more concentrated solution

Anasarca—Massive generalized edema

Anions—Ions that have a negative charge

Buffer—Substance that combines with a strong acid or base to change it to a weaker acid or base

Cations—Ions that have a positive charge

Deficient fluid volume—Inadequate amount of body fluid.

Dehydration—Loss of fluid without a significant loss of electrolytes, resulting in a hyperosmolar imbalance

Diffusion—Passive process whereby molecules move across a membrane from a more concentrated solution to a less concentrated solution

Drop factor—Number of drops per milliliter that the tubing of an intravenous set delivers

Edema—Excessive amount of fluid in subcutaneous tissue

Electrolytes—Chemical substances that dissociate into electrically charged particles (ions) when dissolved in water

Excess fluid volume—Excessive amount of body fluid

Extracellular fluid (ECF)—Fluid outside of cells, which accounts for about 30% of body fluid and is further divided into *interstitial fluid* (fluid in the spaces between body cells), *intravascular fluid* (fluid within blood vessels [plasma]), and *transcellular fluid* (specific fluids, such as lymph, cerebrospinal, and peritoneal)

Filtration—Passive process whereby fluid and smaller molecules move from an area of higher pressure to an area of lower pressure

Hydrostatic pressure—Pressure exerted by a fluid within a closed system against the walls of the system

Hypertonic (concentrated)—Small amount of solvent contains a large amount of solute

Hypervolemia—Excessive amount of fluid and sodium in isotonic proportions

Hypotonic—Large amount of solvent contains a small amount of solute (dilute)

Hypovolemia—Loss of both fluids and electrolytes in equal or isotonic proportions

Insensible fluid loss—Fluid loss that is not perceived or easily measurable

Isotonic—Osmotic pressures of two liquids are equal

Intracellular fluid (ICF)—Fluid within cells, which accounts for about 70% of body fluid

Oncotic pressure (osmotic pressure)—Power of a solution to draw water across a semipermeable membrane

Osmosis—Passive process whereby water moves across a membrane from a less concentrated to a more concentrated solution.

Sensible fluid loss—Fluid loss that is perceived and measurable

Solute—Dissolved substance

Solvent—Substance in which a solute is dissolved

I. Concepts Related to Fluids and Electrolytes

More than 50% of the human body is composed of fluid, which is divided between the intracellular compartment and the extracellular compartment; the extracellular compartment is further divided into the intravascular, interstitial, and transcellular compartments. Fluid and electrolytes constantly move among these compartments via osmosis, diffusion, filtration, and active transport. Regulation of the body's fluid balance is more complex than just the amount of fluid taken into the body and the amount of fluid excreted from the body. It involves a variety of internal feedback mechanisms, including the thirst mechanism, antidiuretic hormone, renin-angiotensin-aldosterone system, and atrial natriuretic peptide. These basic concepts provide the foundation for understanding the balance of fluid within the human body.

A. Body fluids
   1. Constituents.
      a. Primarily water.
      b. Contains dissolved substances, such as gases (e.g., oxygen, carbon dioxide), electrolytes, glucose, and urea.
   2. Functions.
      a. Maintains blood volume.
      b. Controls body temperature.
      c. Transports substances to and from cells, such as nutrients, gases, and waste products.
      d. Serves as a medium for metabolic reactions within cells.
      e. Assists with digestion of nutrients.
      f. Lubricates joints.
   3. Distribution (Fig. 21.1).
      a. Intracellular and extracellular compartments are separated by selectively permeable membranes of cells and capillaries.

Fig 21.1 Distribution of body fluids. (From Wilkinson and Treas [2016]. *Fundamentals of nursing*, Vol. 1, 3rd ed. Philadelphia: F. A. Davis Company, with permission.)

      b. Total body fluid.
         (1) Full-term newborn: 70% to 80%.
         (2) 1-year-old: 64%.
         (3) Adult male: 55% to 60%.
         (4) Adult female: 45% to 55%.
         (5) Older adult: 45% to 50%.
      c. **Intracellular fluid (ICF)** is fluid within cells; about 70%.
      d. **Extracellular fluid (ECF)** is fluid outside of cells; about 30%.
         (1) *Interstitial:* Fluid in the spaces between body cells; about 22%.
         (2) *Intravascular:* Fluid within blood vessels (plasma); about 6%.
         (3) *Transcellular:* Specific fluids, such as lymph, cerebrospinal, peritoneal, synovial, pleural, intraocular, biliary, and pancreatic; about 2%.
      e. Third spacing: Accumulation and sequestration of fluid in extracellular spaces as a result of injury or disease, such as edema, ascites, and pleural effusion.
      f. Injury or inflammation: Increased capillary permeability permits fluid, electrolytes, and proteins to move into ECF compartment due to trauma, burns, and sepsis.
   4. Movement of fluid and electrolytes.
      a. Fluid intake.
         (1) Includes oral and intravenous (IV) intake.
         (2) Recommended oral intake.
            (a) 2,200 mL/day for women and 3,000 mL/day for men.
            (b) 80% from drinking fluids and 20% from food.
      b. Fluid output.
         (1) **Sensible fluid loss** is fluid loss that is perceived and measurable.
            (a) Urine: About 1,500 mL/day; varies based on intake and losses via other routes; at least 30 to 50 mL/hr.
            (b) Feces: 100 to 200 mL/day; soft stools contain more water than hard stools.
         (2) **Insensible fluid loss** is fluid loss that is not perceived or easily measurable.
            (a) Skin: 300 to 600 mL/day; extent of perspiration depends on body and environmental temperature, extent of muscle contraction, and metabolic activity.
            (b) Lungs: About 300 mL/day; increased respiratory rate increases amount lost.
      c. Osmosis (Fig. 21.2).
         (1) **Osmosis** is a passive process whereby water moves across a membrane from a less concentrated solution to a more concentrated solution.

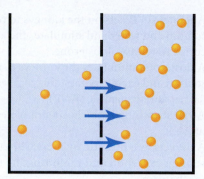

Fig 21.2 Osmosis. (From Wilkinson and Treas [2016]. *Fundamentals of nursing,* Vol. 1, 3rd ed. Philadelphia: F. A. Davis Company, with permission.)

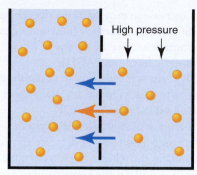

Fig 21.4 Filtration. (From Wilkinson and Treas [2016]. *Fundamentals of nursing,* Vol. 1, 3rd ed. Philadelphia: F. A. Davis Company, with permission.)

(2) **Oncotic pressure (osmotic pressure)** is the power of a solution to draw water across a semipermeable membrane.
  (a) For example: Plasma proteins and hypertonic IV solutions increase oncotic pressure because fluid moves from the interstitial compartment into the intravascular compartment.
  (b) For example: Low levels of protein in the blood, usually due to starvation or liver disease, decrease oncotic pressure because fluid moves from the intravascular compartment into the interstitial compartment.
d. Diffusion (Fig. 21.3).
  (1) **Diffusion** is a passive process whereby molecules move across a membrane from a more concentrated solution to a less concentrated solution.
  (2) For example: Oxygen moves from the alveoli into the pulmonary capillaries and carbon dioxide moves from the pulmonary capillaries into the alveoli.
e. Filtration (Fig. 21.4).
  (1) **Filtration** is a passive process whereby fluid and smaller molecules move from an

area of higher pressure to an area of lower pressure.
  (2) **Hydrostatic pressure** is the pressure exerted by a fluid within a closed system against the walls, such as the force exerted by blood against the vascular walls.
  (3) For example: Increased hydrostatic pressure associated with heart failure or kidney disease promotes movement of fluid out of the intravascular compartment into the interstitial compartment.
f. Active transport (Fig. 21.5).
  (1) **Active transport** is an active process whereby metabolic energy moves substances across a membrane from a less concentrated solution to a more concentrated solution.
  (2) For example: The sodium-potassium pump moves sodium out of cells and potassium into cells.
B. Maintenance of fluid balance
  1. Thirst mechanism.
    a. The thirst center in the hypothalamus is stimulated when an increase in the concentration of particles within the intravascular compartment (serum osmolarity) occurs.

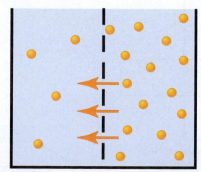

Fig 21.3 Diffusion. (From Wilkinson and Treas [2016]. *Fundamentals of nursing,* Vol. 1, 3rd ed. Philadelphia: F. A. Davis Company, with permission.)

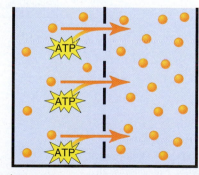

Fig 21.5 Active transport. (From Wilkinson and Treas [2016]. *Fundamentals of nursing,* Vol. 1, 3rd ed. Philadelphia: F. A. Davis Company, with permission.)

b. An increase in osmolality is caused by a decrease in fluid intake, excessive fluid loss, or excessive sodium intake via the diet or IV fluids.

2. Antidiuretic hormone (ADH).
   a. ADH causes the kidneys to retain fluid.
   b. Pressure sensors in the vascular system stimulate or inhibit the release of ADH.
3. Renin-angiotensin-aldosterone system (Fig. 21.6).
   a. Decreased blood flow or decreased blood pressure stimulates the release of renin from the kidneys.
   b. Renin stimulates the conversion of angiotensin I to angiotensin II.

c. Angiotensin II acts on the kidneys to retain sodium and water and stimulates the adrenal cortex to release aldosterone.
d. Aldosterone stimulates the kidneys to reabsorb sodium and excrete potassium.

4. Atrial natriuretic peptide (ANP).
   a. Atrial stretching in the heart stimulates release of ANP.
   b. ANP acts as a diuretic by increasing sodium excretion and inhibiting the thirst mechanism.

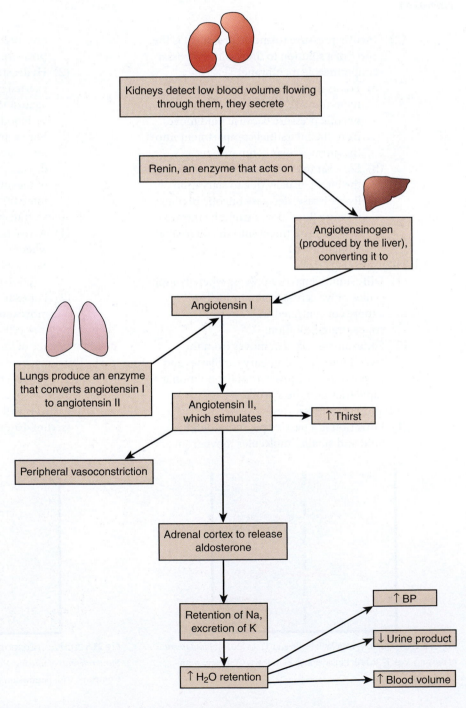

Fig 21.6 Renin-angiotensin-aldosterone system. (From Burton and Ludwig [2015]. *Fundamentals of nursing care: Concepts, connections & skill,* 2nd ed. Philadelphia: F. A. Davis Company, with permission.)

II. Alterations in Fluid Balance

Fluid imbalances include an inadequate amount of body fluid (*deficient fluid volume*) or an excessive amount of body fluid (*excess fluid volume*). These imbalances arise from a variety of conditions, and each has associated clinical manifestations. Nursing care for clients with alterations in fluid balance include many nursing interventions that pertain to both imbalances. However, some are specific to either deficit fluid volume or excess fluid volume. Nurses must have a thorough knowledge of all this information to provide comprehensive nursing care for clients with alterations in fluid balance.

A. Deficient fluid volume
1. **Deficient fluid volume** is an inadequate amount of body fluid.
2. **Hypovolemia** is the loss of both fluid and electrolytes in equal or isotonic proportions.
3. **Dehydration** is the loss of fluid without a significant loss of electrolytes, resulting in a hyperosmolar imbalance.
4. Causes.
   a. Decreased fluid intake.
   b. Loss of plasma or blood.
   c. GI losses by vomiting, diarrhea, or gastric decompression.
   d. Sweating.
   e. Adrenal insufficiency.
   f. Excessive urination (*polyuria*), possibly due to diuretics or diabetes.
5. Clinical manifestations.
   a. Weight loss.
   b. Flushed, dry skin and mucous membranes.
   c. Decreased tissue turgor; pinched skin on chest just below clavicle, on forehead, or over sternum takes several seconds to return to original position (*tenting*) (Fig. 21.7).

Fig 21.7 Tenting. (From Dillon [2016]. *Nursing health assessment: The foundation of clinical practice*, 3rd ed. F. A. Davis Company, with permission.)

   d. Thirst.
   e. Low-grade fever.
   f. Sunken eyeballs.
   g. Hypotension, orthostatic hypotension.
   h. Weak, thready, rapid pulse.
   i. Flat neck veins.
   j. Decreased capillary refill.
   k. Atonic muscles.
   l. Lethargy.
   m. Mental confusion.
   n. Decreased urine output (oliguria, anuria).
   o. Hemoconcentration results in increased hematocrit (>50%), blood urea nitrogen (>21 mg/dL), and urine specific gravity (>1.029).

B. Excess fluid volume
1. **Excess fluid volume** is an excessive amount of body fluid.
2. **Hypervolemia** is an excessive amount of fluid and sodium in isotonic proportions.
3. Causes.
   a. Excessive sodium intake via diet.
   b. Excessive IV fluids containing sodium.
   c. Congestive heart failure.
   d. Kidney disease.
   e. Cirrhosis of the liver.
   f. Increased aldosterone.
   g. Increased ADH.
4. Clinical manifestations.
   a. Weight gain.
   b. Pale, cool skin.
   c. **Edema** is excess fluid in subcutaneous tissue; can be dependent, generalized (**anasarca**), periorbital, pulmonary; increased tissue turgor; use scale for objective measurement of edema (Fig. 21.8A and Fig. 21.8B).
   d. Third heart sound (S_3 gallop) on auscultation of the heart.
   e. Increased, shallow respirations; dyspnea.
   f. Crackles on auscultation of the lungs.
   g. Hypertension.
   h. Full, bounding, rapid pulse.
   i. Distended neck veins.
   j. Muscle weakness, fatigue.
   k. Mental confusion.
   l. Diluted urine, possibly with increased volume.
   m. Hemodilution results in decreased hematocrit (<40%) and blood urea nitrogen (<8 mg/dL).

C. Commonalities of nursing care for clients with alterations in fluid balance
1. Obtain a health history to identify possible causes.
2. Obtain vital signs, including temperature, pulse, respirations, and blood pressure.
3. Assess breath sounds and characteristics of breathing; be aware that crackles and dyspnea indicate possible fluid overload.

Surface of skin

2 mm = 1+
4 mm = 2+
6 mm = 3+
8 mm
10 mm } = 4+

A

B

Fig 21.8 (A) Edema scale. (B) Pitting edema. ([A] From Nugent and Vitale [2016]. *Test success,* 7th ed. Philadelphia: F. A. Davis Company, with permission. [B] From Williams and Hopper [2015]. *Understanding medical surgical nursing,* 5th ed. Philadelphia: F. A. Davis Company, with permission.)

4. Assess mucous membranes, presence of thirst, and skin turgor; determine the extent of edema or presence of tenting.
5. Obtain a daily weight.
   a. Use the same scale every time; use a standing, chair, or bed scale, depending on the client's ability to stand, sit, or need to remain in bed.
   b. Weigh the client at same time every day, such as before breakfast after the first voiding.
   c. Weigh the client each day wearing similar clothes or use similar linens when using a bed scale.
   d. Notify the primary health-care provider of a change in weight of equal to or more than 2 lb (2.2 lb equal 2,000 mL of fluid) in a day or equal to or more than 5 lb in 1 to 2 weeks.

6. Monitor intake and output (I&O).
   a. Institute I&O for clients who are unstable, critically ill, or febrile; are receiving diuretics, continuous or intermittent IV infusions, or tube feedings; have had a procedure; or have fluid restrictions because of conditions such as deficient fluid volume, excessive fluid volume, or heart or kidney failure.
   b. Measure all fluid that goes into the body, such as oral, IV, tube feedings, and instillations into the GI tract or urinary bladder.
   c. Measure all fluid that exits from the body, such as urine, liquid feces, vomitus, wound drainage, and fluid from gastric decompression; and identify characteristics of output (e.g., color, clarity, and odor).

DID YOU KNOW?

A nurse can delegate the task of measuring amounts of I&O not requiring a sterile intervention to assistive nursing personnel. However, it is the responsibility of the delegating nurse to ensure that the intervention is within the person's job description and that the person has the knowledge and skill necessary to complete the skill accurately and safely. Tallying the results, determining the significance of the information, and notifying a primary health-care provider of results outside expectations also is the delegating nurse's responsibility.

   d. Use standard precautions when collecting certain body fluids, such as urine from a urinary retention catheter collection bag or liquid feces; use surgical asepsis when collecting certain body fluids, such as keeping the port of a wound drainage device sterile when collecting wound drainage.
   e. Measure volume in milliliters with an accurate measuring device and weigh diapers or incontinence pads; do not estimate volume.
   f. Record solid food that becomes a liquid at room temperature, such as ice cream and gelatin, in its entire volume.
   g. Record ice chips at half their volume; for example, 4 oz of ice chips equals 2 oz of fluid.
   h. Document immediately after administration or collection of fluid at the appropriate time on the I&O record (Fig. 21.9).
   i. Tally volumes of I&O as indicated, such as hourly, at the end of each shift, and at the end of a 24-hour period.
   j. Teach the client and family about monitoring fluid intake and output; encourage self-monitoring of I&O if the client is capable.
7. Assess level of consciousness, energy level, and changes in behavior.

DAILY INTAKE AND OUTPUT RECORD

DATE JUNE 5

	INTAKE							OUTPUT			
	L.V. FLUIDS						ORAL	URINE	EMESIS	N.G. TUBE	HEMOVAC
Time	Bottle	Amount	Solution	Medication and Dosage	*ABS	∓LIB					
8	1	1000	NS	20 mEq KCl				650			
8:30							360				
10:00							120				
11:30							240	150			
12:00									160		
1:40									90		60
2:15						↓		250			
3:00					525	475					45
7-8 TOTAL		8-HR TOTAL			525	475	720	1050	250		105
3-11 TOTAL		8-HR TOTAL									
11-7 TOTAL		8-HR TOTAL									
24 HOUR TOTAL											

INTAKE GRAND TOTAL ☐   OUTPUT GRAND TOTAL ☐

*ABS. = amount absorbed   ∓LIB = Left in bag

Fig 21.9 Daily I&O record. (From Nugent and Vitale [2016]. *Test success,* 7th ed. Philadelphia: F. A. Davis Company, with permission.)

8. Monitor laboratory results, such as hematocrit, blood urea nitrogen, serum electrolytes, creatinine clearance, and urine specific gravity.
9. Provide for safety, such as by assisting the client with getting out of bed.
10. Change position and massage dependent areas (except calves) every 2 hours to prevent pressure ulcers.
11. Facilitate oral fluid intake or restriction: Allot one-half during the day, two-thirds of the remaining fluid in the evening, and the rest during the night.

D. Specific nursing care for clients with deficient fluid volume
1. Administer IV fluids as prescribed.
🛑 2. Use an intravenous controller device when administering IV fluids.
3. Provide frequent mouth care.
4. Use assistive devices, such as sheep skin, gel cushion, and elbow and heel pads, to protect the skin over bony prominences.
5. Facilitate prescribed oral fluid intake (oral rehydration therapy).
   a. Set short-term goals, such as 4 oz/hr.
   b. Offer preferred fluids.
   c. Serve fluids at appropriate temperatures, such as cold beverages and hot tea and coffee.
   d. Encourage intake of foods that become liquid at room temperature, such as ice cream and custard.

E. Specific nursing care for clients with excess fluid volume
1. Assess the extent of third spacing by measuring with a centimeter tape over the umbilicus for abdominal girth with ascites and circumference of extremity with peripheral edema or compartment syndrome (mark the site on the extremity for continuity of assessments).
2. Maintain the client in a mid- or high-Fowler position to promote respirations.
3. Restrict dietary sodium as prescribed.
4. Administer prescribed diuretics.
5. Facilitate prescribed fluid restriction.
   a. Offer fluids between rather than with meals.
   b. Offer ice chips to relieve thirst; liquid volume is half frozen volume.
   c. Use a small container to promote perception of a larger volume when providing fluids.
   d. Suggest chewing sugarless gum to help keep the oral cavity moist.

III. Electrolytes

Electrolytes are chemical substances that dissociate into electrically charged particles (**ions**) when dissolved in water. **Cations** (e.g., sodium, potassium, calcium, and magnesium) have a positive charge. **Anions** (e.g., chloride, bicarbonate, and phosphate) have a negative charge. Electrolyte balance depends on normal kidney, hypothalamic, adrenocortical, and nervous system functioning. Imbalances can be identified by serum electrolyte levels and clinical manifestations.

A. Common electrolytes
 1. *Sodium* (Na^+): Normal serum level = 135 to 145 mEq/L.
    a. Major cation in ECF.
    b. Promotes fluid and acid-base balance, nerve impulse conduction, and cellular chemical reactions.
 2. *Potassium* (K^+): Normal serum level = 3.5 to 5.0 mEq/L.
    a. Major cation in ICF.
    b. Promotes nerve impulse conduction in cardiac, skeletal, and smooth muscles.
    c. Serves as a cofactor with enzymes in cellular metabolism.
 3. *Calcium* (Ca^{++}): Normal serum level = 8.5 to 10.5 mEq/L.
    a. Promotes bone health and cardiac and neuromuscular function.
    b. Serves as a factor in blood clotting.
    c. Has its level controlled by parathyroid gland secretion of parathyroid hormone.
    d. Has a reciprocal relationship with phosphorous; a decrease or increase in one results in the opposite reaction in the other.
 4. *Magnesium* (Mg^{++}): Normal serum level = 1.32 to 2.14 mEq/L.
    a. Essential for enzyme and neurochemical activities.
    b. Promotes cardiac and skeletal muscle excitability.
 5. *Chloride* (Cl^-): Normal serum level = 97 to 107 mEq/L.
    a. Major anion in ECF.
    b. Functions with sodium to regulate serum osmolality and blood volume.
    c. Component of hydrochloric acid (HCl) which is involved with regulating acid-base balance.
 6. *Bicarbonate* (HCO_3^-): Normal serum level = 22 to 26 mEq/L.
    a. Most important buffer in ECF.
    b. Helps regulate acid-base balance by neutralizing excess hydrogen ions as part of the carbonic-bicarbonate buffering mechanism.
 7. *Phosphate* (PO_4^-): Normal serum level = 2.5 to 4.5 mEq/dL.
    a. Most important buffer in ECF.
    b. Helps regulate acid-base balance by neutralizing excess hydrogen ions as part of the phosphate buffer system.
    c. Essential for functioning of red blood cells, nerves, and muscles.
    d. Involved in metabolism of proteins, carbohydrates, and fats.

B. Electrolyte imbalances and specific nursing care
 For common electrolyte imbalances and their serum values, causes, clinical manifestations, and specific nursing care see Table 21.1.
C. Commonalities of nursing care for clients with electrolyte imbalances
 1. Perform a history and physical to collect data that may help identify the cause of the imbalance.
 2. Monitor laboratory reports for serum electrolyte levels.
 3. Assess for clinical manifestations of each electrolyte imbalance.
 4. Monitor vital signs.
 5. Monitor cardiopulmonary status, particularly for impaired airway, respiratory depression, and dysrhythmias.

 6. Administer prescribed oral or IV fluids and electrolytes, using a volume controller for IV administration.
 7. Encourage intake or restriction of foods high in the electrolyte of concern, as appropriate.
 8. Maintain safety related to decreased level of consciousness, confusion, muscle weakness, and potential for seizures.

IV. Acid-Base Balance

pH reflects the strength of hydrogen ions in a solution. When a state of acid-base balance exists in the extracellular compartment, pH is 7.35 to 7.45. A pH less than 7.35 is acidic. A pH greater than 7.45 is alkaline. When in balance, body fluid has 27 mEq of bicarbonate (HCO_3^-) per liter and 1.35 mEq of carbonic acid (H_2CO_3) per liter; the bicarbonate-carbonic acid ratio is 20:1 (Fig. 21.10). This balance is fragile and is maintained through a variety of mechanisms. When this balance is disrupted, acid-base imbalances occur. Carbonic acid imbalances lead to respiratory acidosis or respiratory alkalosis, and bicarbonate and hydrogen imbalances lead to metabolic acidosis or metabolic alkalosis.

A. Components of acid-base balance
 1. Acid.
    a. Substance that has more hydrogen ions than bicarbonate ions.
    b. Yields hydrogen ions in solution.

Table 21.1 Electrolyte Imbalances and Specific Nursing Care

Imbalance	Causes	Clinical Manifestations	Specific Nursing Care
Sodium			
Hypernatremia *Serum level* >145 mEq/L.	• Increased intake of dietary sodium, such as foods high in salt or sodium bicarbonate. • Excessive IV saline solutions. • Deficient fluid volume. • Increased fluid retention, such as from cardiac, renal, and liver diseases. • Conditions in which fluid loss exceeds sodium loss, such as diaphoresis, diabetes mellitus, and diabetes insipidus.	• Thirst. • Dry, sticky mucous membranes. • Increased temperature, pulse, and blood pressure. • Agitation. • Confusion. • Nausea and vomiting. • Muscle weakness and cramps. • Lethargy.	• Maintain dietary sodium restrictions. • Give prescribed intravenous fluids, such as 5% dextrose in water or a hypotonic solution. • Teach the client to avoid foods high in sodium, such as cheese, condiments, canned foods, luncheon meat, salty snacks, and nonsalt substitutes.
Hyponatremia *Serum level* <135 mEq/L.	• Low-salt diet. • Excessive sweating. • Gastrointestinal (GI) losses via vomiting, diarrhea, or gastric decompression. • Excessive intake of sodium-free fluids (dilutional hyponatremia). • Burns. • Syndrome of inappropriate antidiuretic hormone (SIADH). • Adrenal insufficiency.	• Headache. • Confusion. • Personality changes. • Nausea and vomiting. • Muscle weakness and cramps. • Lethargy. • Seizures.	• Promote intake of dietary sodium. • *Maintain seizure precautions.* • Give prescribed IV fluids (e.g., normal saline). • Give prescribed osmotic diuretics if the client is hypervolemic.
Potassium			
Hyperkalemia *Serum level* >5 mEq/L.	• Deficient fluid volume. • Massive cellular damage, such as burns. • Medications, such as potassium-sparing diuretics. • Excessive intake of potassium supplements. • Acidosis, especially ketoacidosis. • Kidney disease. • Adrenal insufficiency.	• Muscle weakness. • Fatigue. • Flaccid paralysis. • Slow, weak, irregular pulse. • Dysrhythmias. • Peaked T waves, flattened P waves, prolonged PR internal and wide QRS complexes on electrocardiogram (ECG). • Nausea. • Abdominal cramps. • Diarrhea. • Increased bowel sounds.	• Maintain prescribed potassium-restricted diet. • Administer prescribed exchange resin to promote potassium excretion, such as sodium polystyrene sulfonate (Kayexalate) or hypertonic glucose IV solution with insulin to move potassium into cells. • *Monitor the heart rate for a dysrhythmia.*
Hypokalemia *Serum level* <3.5 mEq/L.	• GI losses via vomiting, diarrhea, or gastric decompression. • Decreased dietary intake of potassium. • Medications, such as laxatives and potassium-wasting diuretics. • Profuse diaphoresis. • Polyuria, diuretic phase of kidney failure.	• Muscle weakness. • Fatigue. • Decreased deep tendon reflexes. • Weak, irregular pulse. • Ventricular dysrhythmias. • Flattened T waves and elevated U waves on ECG. • Nausea and vomiting. • Abdominal distension. • Decreased bowel sounds.	• *Ensure adequate urinary output before giving IV potassium supplements.* • Assess for signs and symptoms of phlebitis at the infusion site. • Teach the client about foods high in potassium, such as bananas, cantaloupe, oranges, strawberries, potatoes, carrots, raisins, spinach, fish, pork, veal, and beef. • *Monitor the heart rate for a dysrhythmia.* • *Assess a client receiving digoxin because hypokalemia increases the risk of digitalis toxicity.*

Continued

Table 21.1 **Electrolyte Imbalances and Specific Nursing Care—cont'd**

Imbalance	Causes	Clinical Manifestations	Specific Nursing Care
Calcium			
Hypercalcemia *Serum level* *>10.5 mEq/L.*	• *Prolonged immobility.* • *Medications, such as thiazide diuretics or lithium.* • *Excessive intake of antacids, calcium, or vitamin D supplements.* • *Hyperparathyroidism.* • *Excessive intake of foods high in calcium.* • *Cancer of the bone or bone metastasis.* • *Osteoporosis.*	• *Deep bone pain.* • *Flank pain due to renal calculi.* • *Anorexia.* • *Nausea and vomiting.* • *Constipation.* • *Weak, relaxed muscles.* • *Lethargy.* • *Hypoactive reflexes.* • *Increased urine calcium (Sulkowitch test).* • *Confusion.* • *Decreased level of consciousness.* • *Dysrhythmias.* • *Shortened QT segment on ECG.*	• *Encourage fluid intake to prevent renal calculi.* • *Encourage dietary fiber to prevent constipation.* • *Teach the client to avoid foods high in calcium.* • *Prepare for hemodialysis, if prescribed.* • *Handle the client gently to prevent a pathological fracture.*
Hypocalcemia *Serum level* *<8.5 mEq/L.*	• *GI disturbances, such as diarrhea or malabsorption.* • *Inadequate vitamin D intake.* • *Medications, such as steroids, isoniazid (INH), furosemide, and cisplatin.* • *Hypoparathyroidism.* • *Kidney disease due to increased phosphorous.*	• *Paresthesia.* • *Hyperactive reflexes.* • *Muscle cramps.* • *Tetany.* • *Seizures.* • *Laryngeal spasms.* • *Stridor.* • *Hypotension.* • *Palpitations.* • *Dysrhythmias.* • *Prolonged QT segment on ECG.* • *Facial nerve twitching (Chvostek sign).* • *Carpopedal spasm (Trousseau sign).* 	• *Administer prescribed calcium supplements.* • *Maintain a patent airway.* • *Maintain seizure precautions.* • *Teach the client about foods high in calcium, such as dairy products; green, leafy vegetables; salmon; and sardines.* • *Encourage weight-bearing exercise.* • *Handle the client gently to prevent a pathological fracture.*
Magnesium			
Hypermagnesemia *Serum level* *>2.14 mEq/L.*	• *Medications, such as magnesium-containing antacids.* • *Excessive intake of magnesium supplements.* • *Kidney disease.* • *Adrenal insufficiency.*	• *Drowsiness.* • *Lethargy.* • *Hypoactive reflexes.* • *Muscle weakness.* • *Bradycardia.* • *Hypotension.* • *Flushed, warm skin.* • *Increased thirst.* • *Respiratory depression.* • *Bradypnea.*	• *Monitor respiratory status and reflexes.* • *Notify the primary health-care provider of absent patellar reflexes.* • *Teach the client to avoid foods high in magnesium.*

Table 21.1	Electrolyte Imbalances and Specific Nursing Care—cont'd		
Imbalance	**Causes**	**Clinical Manifestations**	**Specific Nursing Care**
Hypomagnesemia *Serum level* <1.32 mEq/L.	• GI disturbances such as diarrhea, malabsorption, and prolonged gastric decompression. • Medications, such as diuretics and aminoglycoside antibiotics. • Pancreatitis. • Liver cirrhosis. • Hyperparathyroidism.	• Disorientation. • Variability of mood. • Neuromuscular irritability. • Muscle weakness. • Seizures. • Dysrhythmias. • Nystagmus. • Diplopia.	• Teach the client about foods high in magnesium, such as whole grains; green, leafy vegetables; meat; and seafood. • Maintain seizure precautions. • Assess a client receiving digoxin because of the risk of digitalis toxicity.

(Figures from Wilkinson and Treas (2016). *Fundamentals of nursing*, Vol. 2, 3rd ed. Philadelphia: F. A. Davis Company, with permission.)

Fig 21.10 Acid-base balance. (From Phillips [2014]. *Manual of I.V. therapeutics: Evidenced-based practice for infusion therapy*, 6th ed. Philadelphia: F. A. Davis Company, with permission.)

2. Base.
   a. Substance that has more bicarbonate ions than hydrogen ions.
   b. Accepts hydrogen ions in solution.
3. Salt.
   a. Compound that results when an acid and a base are mixed.
   b. The acid releases H+ ions while the base releases OH− ions in a process called *hydrolysis*.
B. Mechanisms that maintain acid–base balance
   1. *Buffer mechanisms:* First line of defense; respond in seconds.
      a. Buffer.
         (1) A **buffer** is a substance that combines with a strong acid or base to change it to a weaker acid or base.
         (2) Substance that accepts or releases hydrogen ions to correct an acid-base imbalance.

   b. Bicarbonate buffer system.
      (1) Most important buffer in ECFs.
      (2) Neutralizes excess hydrogen ions.
   c. Phosphate buffer system.
      (1) Most important buffer in ICFs.
      (2) Neutralizes excess hydrogen ions.
   d. Plasma protein system.
      (1) Proteins can attract or release hydrogen ions.
      (2) Functions in both ICF and ECF.
   e. Hemoglobin system.
      (1) Chloride shifts into or out of cells, depending on the oxygen level; oxygen is carried in the hemoglobin molecule.
      (2) As chloride shifts into or out of cells, bicarbonate ions move in the opposite direction.
2. *Respiratory mechanisms:* Second line of defense; respond in minutes.
   a. When carbonic acid reaches the lungs, it breaks down into water (H_2O) and carbon dioxide (CO_2).
   b. Respiratory rate changes depending on the level of CO_2 in ECF under control of the medulla oblongata.
      (1) Rate increases with increased CO_2.
      (2) Rate decreases with decreased CO_2.
3. *Renal mechanisms:* Third line of defense; respond in hours to days.
   a. Kidneys control the buffer sodium bicarbonate ($NaHCO_3$) by excreting or conserving hydrogen ions.
   b. Kidneys also combine ammonia (NaH_3) with hydrochloric acid (HCl) to form ammonium (NH_4Cl), which is then excreted.
C. Acid-base imbalances and specific nursing care
   For acid-base imbalances and their serum values, causes, compensatory mechanisms, clinical manifestations, and specific nursing care see Table 21.2.
D. Commonalities of nursing care related to acid-base imbalances
   1. Perform a history and physical examination to collect data that may help identify the cause.

Table 21.2 Acid-Base Imbalances and Specific Nursing Care

Metabolic Acidosis

Blood Tests and Causes of Metabolic Acidosis	Compensatory Mechanisms and Clinical Manifestations	Specific Nursing Care
• pH <7.35. • HCO_3 <22 mEq/L. **Causes** • Base bicarbonate deficit due to severe diarrhea. • Increased acids resulting from lactic acidosis, ketoacidosis, aspirin poisoning, starvation, kidney disease, and terminal cancer.	• Hyperventilation occurs to blow off carbon dioxide. • Kidneys excrete hydrogen ions and retain bicarbonate. **Clinical manifestations** • Deep, rapid breathing (Kussmaul respirations). • Headache. • Confusion. • Coma. • Fruity odor to breath. • Nausea, vomiting, or diarrhea. • Weakness or drowsiness. • Hypotension. • Dysrhythmias. • Warm, flushed skin due to vasodilation.	• Administer sodium bicarbonate as prescribed. • Implement prescriptions directed at correcting the cause, such as administering insulin to correct ketoacidosis. • *Monitor for hypokalemia because, as the condition resolves, potassium moves back into cells.*

Respiratory Acidosis

Blood Tests and Causes of Respiratory Acidosis	Compensatory Mechanisms and Clinical Manifestations	Specific Nursing Care

• pH <7.35.
• $PaCO_2$ >42 mm Hg.
Causes
• Impaired gas exchange at the alveolar-capillary membrane due to conditions such as pneumonia, pulmonary edema, and emphysema.
• Respiratory obstructions such as:
  Mechanical: *For example, tumors and foreign objects.*
  Functional: *For example, cystic fibrosis and asthma.*
• Medications that depress respirations, such as opioids and anesthesia.
• Neuromuscular impairment, such as trauma to the medulla oblongata, spinal cord injury, and myasthenia gravis.
	• Respirations increase in rate and depth.
	• Kidneys excrete hydrogen ions.
	• Kidneys retain sodium to increase sodium bicarbonate.
	Clinical manifestations
	• Increased rate and depth of respirations.
	• Use of accessory muscles of respiration.
	• Dyspnea, shortness of breath.
	• Tachycardia.
	• Hypotension.
	• Warm, flushed skin due to vasodilation.
	• Restlessness.
	• Irritability.
	• Headache.
	• Disorientation.
	• Coma.
		• *Assess for signs of respiratory distress.*
		• *Maintain a patent airway, such as by administering prescribed bronchodilators and suctioning the airway.*
		• Maintain semi- to high-Fowler position.
		• Encourage the client to turn, cough, and deep breathe.
		• Encourage oral fluid intake as prescribed, usually 2 to 3 L/day to thin respiratory secretions.
		• Perform chest physiotherapy as prescribed, such as postural drainage and percussion.
		• Prepare for endotracheal intubation if prescribed.

Metabolic Alkalosis

Blood Tests and Causes of Metabolic Alkalosis	Compensatory Mechanisms and Clinical Manifestations	Specific Nursing Care
• pH >7.45. • HCO_3 >26 mEq/L. **Causes** • Loss of acid gastric secretions due to vomiting, gastric decompression, and lavage. • Medications, such as thiazide and loop diuretics and antacids with sodium bicarbonate.	• The rate and depth of respirations decrease. • Kidneys excrete excess sodium bicarbonate and retain hydrogen ions. **Clinical manifestations** • Paresthesia, tremors, and muscle hypertonicity. • Bradypnea. • Tachycardia. • Hypotension. • Dysrhythmias. • Dizziness. • Confusion. • Coma. • Decreased GI motility. • Hypotonic bowel sounds. • Decreased serum potassium.	• Administer prescribed IV fluids, such as sodium chloride. • *Monitor serum potassium levels.* • Implement prescriptions that address the underlying cause, such as discontinuing medications or correcting hypokalemia.

Table 21.2 Acid-Base Imbalances and Specific Nursing Care—cont'd

Respiratory Alkalosis

Blood Tests and Causes of Respiratory Alkalosis	Compensatory Mechanisms and Clinical Manifestations	Specific Nursing Care
• pH >7.45. • $PaCO_2$ <38 mm Hg. **Causes** • Hyperventilation due to anxiety or aggressive mechanical ventilation. • Fever. • Pain. • Hypoxia.	• Kidneys excrete excess bicarbonate. • Kidneys retain hydrogen ions. **Clinical manifestations** • Tachypnea. • Light-headedness, dizziness, confusion, and decreased level of consciousness. • Paresthesia. • Hyperreflexia. • Tetany. • Seizures. • Nausea and vomiting. • Epigastric pain. • Dysrhythmias related to hypokalemia.	• Stay with the client during an anxiety attack if present. • Encourage the use of appropriate breathing techniques, such as breathing more slowly. • Change the settings on the mechanical ventilator as prescribed, such as decreased rate or depth settings.

2. Obtain vital signs.

🛑 3. Assess for and maintain a patent airway.

🛑 4. Monitor cardiopulmonary status for respiratory impairment or dysrhythmias.

5. Monitor laboratory results for arterial blood gas and serum electrolyte levels.
6. Administer prescribed oral and IV fluids and electrolyte supplements.
7. Maintain client safety; institute seizure precautions when necessary.
8. Monitor I&O.

V. Administration of Intravenous (IV) Solutions

The administration of IV fluids may be necessary when oral rehydration therapy is not enough to correct a deficient fluid volume. A variety of IV solutions might be prescribed depending on the cause of the fluid imbalance. Nurses must be familiar not only with these solutions but also with the tubing used to administer IV fluids, the sites appropriate for insertion of IV access devices, and the various devices that control the flow of solution. Nurses must continuously assess and reassess clients for the desired outcomes of therapy as well as implement nursing care to prevent or treat the complications associated with the administration of IV fluids.

A. Intravenous solutions
  1. Liquids that contain a dissolved substance.
    a. **Solute:** Dissolved substance.
    b. **Solvent:** Substance in which a solute is dissolved.
  2. Concentration of solutions.
    a. *Isotonic.*
      (1) A solution is **isotonic** when osmotic pressures of two liquids are equal.

      (2) Solutions that have the same concentration of solutes as blood plasma, such as 0.9% sodium chloride, 5% dextrose in water (D_5W), and lactated Ringer's solution.
      (3) When infused, these solutions remain inside the intravascular compartment.
    b. *Hypotonic (dilute).*
      (1) A solution is **hypotonic** when a large amount of solvent contains a small amount of solute.
      (2) Solutions that have a lesser concentration of solutes than blood plasma, such as 0.45% sodium chloride and 0.33% sodium chloride.
      (3) When infused, these solutions pull body water from the intravascular compartment into the interstitial fluid compartment.
    c. *Hypertonic (concentrated).*
      (1) A solution is **hypertonic** when a small amount of solvent contains a large amount of solute.
      (2) Solutions that have a greater concentration of solutes than blood plasma, such as 5% dextrose in sodium chloride (D_5NS), 5% dextrose in 0.45% sodium chloride ($D_5\frac{1}{2}NS$), and 5% dextrose in lactated Ringer's solution (D_5LR).
      (3) When infused, these solutions move fluid from the interstitial compartment to the intravascular compartment.

B. Venipuncture sites for administration of intravenous infusions
  1. Selected based on the client's needs and the primary health-care provider's prescription.
  2. Depends on a multiplicity of factors.
    a. Age.
      (1) Adults: Use veins in hands and arms (Fig. 21.11A, B).
      (2) Infants: Use veins in scalp and dorsal foot.

Cephalic vein

Basilic vein

Dorsal venous arch

Metacarpal veins

Digital veins

A **Superficial veins of the hand**

Cephalic vein

Basilic vein

Median cubital vein

Accessory cephalic vein

Medial antebrachial vein

B **Superficial veins of the forearm**

Fig 21.11 Common venipuncture sites. (From Wilkinson and Treas [2016]. *Fundamentals of nursing*, Vol. 1, 3rd ed. Philadelphia: F. A. Davis Company, with permission.)

b. Type of solution: Large veins are used for parenteral nutrition and hypertonic, viscous, or irritating solutions because the infused solution is diluted faster than in small veins.

c. Rate of volume to be infused: Large veins can accommodate a larger volume of fluid and a faster rate of fluid administration than small veins can.

d. Duration of infusion therapy.

(1) Intermittent or short-term continuous infusions: Use metacarpal, basilic, and cephalic veins (Fig. 21.11).

(2) Long-term therapy using a central venous catheter: Most often use subclavian veins (Fig. 21.12A); the jugular or femoral veins also can be used. Central venous catheters can be tunneled through subcutaneous tissue to the chest wall (Fig. 21.12B).

(3) Long-term therapy using a peripherally inserted central venous catheter (PICC): Use basilic or cephalic vein (Fig. 21.13).

(4) Long-term therapy using an implanted venous access port: Use subclavian or jugular vein (Fig. 21.14).

C. Devices used for administration of intravenous infusions

1. *Gravity flow infusion sets.*

a. Used when a machine to control the flow of solution is unavailable or when a client is stable.

A

Cephalic vein

Entrance site

Basilic vein

Dacron cuff

Superior vena cava

Right atrium

Subcutaneous tunnel

Exit site

B

Fig 21.12 Central venous catheters. (A) Nontunneled central venous catheters are inserted into the jugular, subclavian, and, occasionally, femoral veins. (B) Tunneled central venous catheter is inserted through subcutaneous tissue in the chest wall into the jugular or subclavian vein. (From Wilkinson and Treas [2016]. *Fundamentals of nursing*, Vol. 1, 3rd ed. Philadelphia: F. A. Davis Company, with permission.)

Fig 21.13 Peripherally inserted central venous catheter (PICC). A PICC line is a long, soft, flexible catheter inserted through a vein in the arm and threaded into a central vessel. (From Wilkinson and Treas [2016]. *Fundamentals of nursing*, Vol. 1, 3rd ed. Philadelphia: F. A. Davis Company, with permission.)

Fig 21.14 Implanted venous access port: A central venous access device that enters the subclavian or jugular vein and is tunneled to a completely implanted subcutaneous reservoir (port) in the upper chest. (From Wilkinson and Treas [2016]. *Fundamentals of nursing*, Vol. 1, 3rd ed. Philadelphia: F. A. Davis Company, with permission.)

   b. Has tubing that connects an IV solution bag at one end to a client's venous access device at the other.

     (1) Primary administration set: Has a back-check valve and two or more injection ports (Fig. 21.15A).

       (a) The port most distal from the client is used for insertion of a secondary line

to administer an intermittent infusion (intravenous piggyback [IVPB]).

       (b) The port closest to the client is used for the administration of IV push medication.

     (2) Secondary administration set: Shorter tubing than a primary administration set and has no ports or check valve; connects a small volume intermittent infusion to the primary tubing (Fig. 21.15B).

   c. Flow regulated at drops per minute; a roller clamp or inline dial-a-flow device in a primary administration set is used to compress tubing to attain the prescribed rate.

   d. **Drop factor** is the number of drops per milliliter that the intravenous tubing delivers; usually 10, 15, or 60 drops per milliliter.

   e. Calculate flow rate using the following formula:

$$\text{drops per minute} = \frac{\text{total milliliters to be infused} \times \text{drop factor}}{\text{total time in minutes (hours} \times 60 \text{ minutes)}}$$

2. *Electronic infusion device.*

   a. Use when a client is physiologically fragile or a solution must be strictly controlled.

   b. Delivers a solution at a preset rate by exerting positive pressure.

   c. Has alarms that can detect factors such as an empty solution container, tube obstruction, air in the tubing, infiltration, or low battery.

   d. Set at milliliters per hour, using the following formula:

$$\text{mL/hr} = \frac{\text{total milliliters to be infused}}{\text{total time to be infused in hours}}$$

3. *Volume control device* (e.g., Volutrol, Buretrol, Soluset) (Fig. 21.16).

   a. Used for infants and children.

   b. Works on the principle of gravity.

   c. Drop factor usually is 60 gtt/mL (microdrip).

   d. Volume equal to the prescribed hourly rate is drained into the volume control chamber and then the upper roller clamp is closed; ensures excess fluid does not enter the volume control chamber and infuse.

   e. The air vent in the volume control chamber is opened during the infusion; ensures that solution flows toward client.

   f. Permits medication to be added by syringe to the chamber of the volume control device.

D. Nursing care related to administration of intravenous infusions

1. Verify the primary health-care provider's prescription.

2. Perform hand hygiene and then collect appropriate equipment.

A

Backcheck valve

Injection ports

Clamp

To IV solution bag

Spike

Roller clamp

Male luer-lok/hub

To venous access device

B

Fig 21.15 Intravenous administration sets. Intravenous administration sets: (A) Primary administration set; (B) Secondary administration set. (From Nugent & Vitale [2014]. *Fundamentals of nursing: Content review PLUS practice questions.* Philadelphia: F.A. Davis Company, with permission.)

Primary solution

Medication added by syringe

Volume control set

Fig 21.16 Volume control device. (From Phillips [2005]. *IV therapy notes: Nurse's pharmacology pocket guide,* Philadelphia: F. A. Davis Company, with permission.)

3. Identify the client and yourself, and explain the procedure.
4. Obtain the client's vital signs and assess status for selection of the insertion site and the presence of risk factors that may precipitate a complication,

such as age, physical instability, restlessness, and altered mental status.

5. Hang the prescribed solution. Apply a time tape to the IV solution container; attach a label with the date and time and your initials.
6. Prime the tubing to remove air and fill the drip chamber to half full.
7. Attach the IV administration tubing to the equipment accessing the client's vein (e.g., venous catheter or peripheral IV lock) while wearing clean gloves following agency protocol.
8. Secure the tubing with a transparent dressing and regulate the flow rate (Fig. 21.17A).
9. Label the equipment and dressing with the date and time and your initials, and on the dressing, add the venous access type and size (Fig. 21.17B).

10. Set parameters for alarms when using an electronic infusion device and ensure that alarms are activated (do not shut off alarms); respond to alarms immediately.
11. Promote patency and integrity of the line by coiling the tubing on the bed; avoiding dependent loops; keeping the tubing over rails, not through them; and ensuring the client is not lying on the tubing or excessively moving the involved extremity.

12. Monitor every hour or less; monitor more frequently if the solution contains a medication, such as potassium.
13. Change the IV solution bag, tubing, and dressing over the site according to agency protocols; for example, the solution is changed every 24 hours

and the tubing and dressing are changed every 72 hours.

14. Assess the client's response to the infusion, such as vital signs.
15. Assess for signs of complications as a result of the administration of an IV solution.
16. Document the specific fluid and amount absorbed on the I&O record.
17. Document the client's response in the clinical record.

E. Complications of intravenous infusions and related nursing care
1. Complications of IV therapy can be local or systemic and can cause minor discomfort or be life threatening.
2. Common complications associated with intravenous infusions, their causes, clinical manifestations, and related nursing care (see Table 21.3).

VI. Medications That Affect Excess Fluid Volume

The human body has compensatory mechanisms that help maintain fluid balance. However, when these mechanisms are inefficient or overwhelmed, the nurse can implement interventions prescribed by a primary healthcare provider. When clients have a deficient fluid volume, oral rehydration fluids or intravenous fluids usually are

Fig 21.17 (A) Applying a transparent occlusive dressing to an IV site. (B) Documenting important information on an IV site label. ([A] From Wilkinson and Treas [2016]. *Fundamentals of nursing*, Vol. 1, 3rd ed. Philadelphia: F. A. Davis Company, with permission. [B] From Burton and Ludwig [2015]. *Fundamentals of nursing care: Concepts, connections & skills*, 2nd ed. Philadelphia: F. A. Davis Company, with permission.)

Table 21.3 Complications of Intravenous Infusions and Related Nursing Care

Complication	Clinical Manifestations	Related Nursing Care
Fluid Overload		
• Excessive fluid within the intravascular compartment. **Causes** • Fluid is infused too rapidly. • Excess amount of fluid is infused. • IV volume overwhelms client's status.	• Sudden weight gain. • Edema. • Distended neck veins. • Hypertension. • Tachycardia. • Shortness of breath.	**Prevention** • Use an infusion device to regulate the flow rate. • Monitor the client and infusion frequently (e.g., every 30 to 60 minutes). **Intervention** • *Decrease the flow rate of the infusion to keep the vein open while awaiting medical direction.* • Place the client in the high-Fowler position. • Obtain and monitor the vital signs. • Administer oxygen. • Document the client's status and notify the primary healthcare provider.
Infiltration		
• IV fluid leaks into the interstitial compartment. **Causes** • IV catheter tip is displaced outside of the vein.	• Decreased flow rate. • Cessation of flow. • Coolness, pallor, swelling, and tenderness at site.	**Prevention** • Secure the catheter to limit movement in the vein. • Instruct the client to minimize movement and flexion of the involved extremity. **Intervention** • *Remove the catheter and restart one at another site.* • Elevate the affected arm on a pillow. • Document the event.

Continued

Table 21.3 Complications of Intravenous Infusions and Related Nursing Care—cont'd

Complication	Clinical Manifestations	Related Nursing Care
Phlebitis		
• Inflammation of a vein. **Causes** • Mechanical irritation. • Caustic solution, such as potassium chloride, antibiotics, and vitamin C. • Infection.	• Redness, warmth, swelling, and pain at site. • Decreased flow rate. • Palpable erythematous cord along vein.	**Prevention** • Use the smallest catheter practical. • Use a polyurethane catheter instead of a Teflon catheter. • Secure the catheter to limit movement in the vein. • Rotate the site every 72 hours. **Intervention** • *Remove the catheter and restart one at another site.* • Elevate the affected arm on a pillow. • Follow agency protocol (e.g., apply cold compress initially, apply warm compress every 4 to 6 hours for 20 minutes). • Document client's status and notify the primary health-care provider if erythema or streaking is present.
Infection		
• Invasion and multiplication of a pathogenic organism within the IV site. **Causes** *Local* • The cannula or IV site is contaminated. *Systemic* • Pathogens or their toxic products enter the intravascular compartment.	**Local** • Redness, swelling, and warmth at site. *Systemic* • Fluctuating fever. • Tachycardia. • Hypotension. • Chills. • Altered mental status. • Increased white blood cell count.	**Prevention** • Use sterile technique to insert and maintain integrity of the catheter and site. • Use sterile technique when changing IV solution bags and tubing. • Change the solution bag every 24 hours. • Change the tubing per agency protocol (e.g., every 48 to 72 hours); rotate site every 72 hours. • Examine the solution for clarity and presence of particulate matter; if present, discard. **Intervention** • *Remove the catheter, apply a sterile dressing, and restart one at another site.* • Notify the primary health-care provider of the client's status. • Obtain a blood specimen for culture and sensitivity testing if prescribed. • Administer antibiotics as prescribed.
Extravasation		
• Vesicant leaks into the interstitial compartment causing tissue damage. *Note:* A vesicant is an irritating solution that causes tissue to blister, slough, and become necrotic. **Causes** • IV catheter tip is displaced outside of the vein.	• Decreased flow rate. • Cessation of flow. • Pallor, coolness, swelling, and pain at the site. • Blanching and coolness of the surrounding skin. • Blistering of the skin. • Necrosis of the dermis.	**Prevention** • Use an infusion device to regulate flow. • Secure the catheter to limit movement in the vein. • Instruct the client to minimize movement and flexion of the involved extremity. *Intervention* • *Stop the infusion immediately.* • Elevate involved extremity on a pillow and apply a cool or warm compress as prescribed or per protocol. • Document the client's status and notify the primary health-care provider immediately. • Administer prescribed antidotes to alter the pH, alter DNA binding, and/or dilute or neutralize the drug.

prescribed because there are no medications that can promote fluid intake. However, when clients have an excess fluid volume medications can be prescribed that directly increase the excretion of urine (diuretics) or indirectly increase the excretion of urine by increasing cardiac output and interrupting the angiotensin I-angiotensin II cascade (cardiac medications).

A. Diuretics
  1. Increase excretion of urine.
  2. Examples: Table 21.4.

B. Cardiac medications
  1. Improved cardiac functioning increases renal blood flow, which increases fluid and electrolyte excretion and inhibits release of renin (precursor to the angiotensin I-angiotensin II cascade).
  2. Examples: Table 21.5.

C. Commonalities of nursing care for clients receiving medications that affect excess fluid volume
  1. Monitor I&O and daily weight.

Table 21.4 Diuretics That Affect Fluid Balance

Mechanism of Action	Examples	Nontherapeutic Effects
Thiazide and thiazide-like diuretics • *Promote excretion of sodium, potassium, and chloride in distal renal tubules.*	• *hydrochlorothiazide.* • *chlorothiazide (Diuril).* • *chlorthalidone (Hygroton).* • *metolazone (Zaroxolyn).*	• *Dehydration.* • *Hypokalemia.* • *Hyponatremia.* • *Hypomagnesemia.* • *Possible hyperglycemia in clients with diabetes.* • *Furosemide: Hearing problems if administered rapidly; aspirin toxicity if taken concurrently.*
Loop diuretics • *Inhibit reabsorption of sodium and chloride in the ascending loop of Henle and distal renal tubules.* • *Promote renal excretion of water, sodium, chloride, potassium, calcium, and magnesium.*	• *bumetanide (Bumex).* • *ethacrynic acid (Edecrin).* • *furosemide (Lasix).* • *torsemide (Demadex).*	
Potassium-sparing diuretics • *Inhibit sodium reabsorption in the distal tubules and collecting ducts.* • *Promote renal excretion of water and sodium, leading to potassium retention.*	• *amiloride (Midamor).* • *eplerenone (Inspra).* • *triamterene (Dyrenium).* • *spironolactone (Aldactone).*	• *Hyperkalemia.* • *Hypocalcemia.* • *Hypomagnesemia.*

Table 21.5 Cardiac Medications That Affect Fluid Balance

Mechanism of Action	Examples	Nontherapeutic Effects
Angiotensin-converting enzyme inhibiters (ACEIs) • *Block conversion of angiotensin I to angiotensin II.* • *Used for clients with hypertension.*	• *captopril (Capoten).* • *enalapril (Vasotec).* • *lisinopril (Prinivil).* • *quinapril (Accupril).*	• *Orthostatic hypotension.* • *Dizziness.* • *Headache.* • *Diarrhea.* • *Hyperkalemia.* • *Alterations in heart rate.* • *Teratogenic.* • *Erectile or ejaculation dysfunction.* • *ACEIs: Possible dry cough and angioedema.* • *Captopril: Possible agranulocytosis or neutropenia.*
Angiotensin II receptor blockers (ARBs) • *Block vasoconstriction and aldosterone-secreting effects of angiotensin II.* • *Used for clients with hypertension.*	• *candesartan (Atacand).* • *eprosartan (Teveten).* • *losartan (Cozaar).* • *valsartan (Divan).*	
Cardiac glycoside • *Inhibits ATPase, which increases intracellular calcium that ultimately slows and strengthens cardiac contractions.*	• *digoxin (Lanoxin).*	• *GI irritation.* • *Bradycardia.* • *Fatigue.* • *Weakness.* • *Toxicity: Anorexia, nausea, vomiting, diarrhea, yellow vision around lights, diplopia, abdominal distress, headache, dysrhythmias, disorientation.* *Note: Hypercalcemia and hypokalemia increase risk of toxicity.*

2. Monitor vital signs routinely, particularly for irregular heart rate; volume of pulse, such as bounding or thready; blood pressure, such as hypotension-hypovolemia or hypertension-hypervolemia.
3. Obtain vital signs before and after medication administration.
   a. Digoxin: Apical rate.
   b. Angiotensin-converting enzyme inhibiters (ACEIs) and angiotensin II receptor blockers (ARBs): Blood pressure and heart rate and rhythm; notify the primary health-care provider or follow agency protocol if results are outside predetermined parameters; for example, withhold drug if apical rate is <50 or >110 beats/minute; withhold drug if systolic BP is <100 mm Hg.
4. Assess skin turgor and location and extent of edema.
5. Assess for clinical manifestations of electrolyte imbalances, particularly hypokalemia and hyperkalemia.
6. Monitor serum electrolyte and blood glucose levels.

7. Encourage dietary intake of foods high in potassium, calcium, and magnesium, except if the client is taking a potassium-sparing diuretic.

8. Administer diuretics in the morning so their effects occur during waking hours; if needed, administer the second dose in early afternoon.

9. Maintain client safety, such as by teaching the client to rise slowly and teaching the client signs and symptoms of nontherapeutic drug effects.

🛑 10. **Digoxin (Lanoxin): Monitor blood levels of the drug, which should remain between 0.9 and 2.0 ng/mL; have digoxin-immune Fab, the antidote for digoxin toxicity, readily available.**

11. Monitor for therapeutic and nontherapeutic effects of medications.

12. Document medication administration and the client's response.

CASE STUDY: Putting It All Together

A 76-year-old man who lives alone since his wife died 6 months ago is admitted to the hospital from the emergency department with a 3-day history of nausea, vomiting, and diarrhea that the client attributes to a stomach virus. He states, "I feel weak and dizzy when I stand up, and I can't seem to keep anything down." He is currently receiving hydrochlorothiazide (HCTZ) daily for hypertension. When his symptoms did not subside after 3 days and he progressively "felt worse," he went to his primary health-care provider, who sent him to the emergency department for admission to the hospital.

Client's Clinical Record

Nursing Assessment
Sticky, dry oral mucosa.
Cracked lips.
Flushed face.
Tenting over the sternum.
50 mL of dark amber urine.
Weight loss of 5 lb from regular weight of 1 week ago.

Unsteadiness when transferring from chair to bed.
Orthostatic hypotension identified.

Vital Signs
Temperature: 99°F orally.
Blood pressure: 98/64 mm Hg.
Heart rate: 126 beats/minute, thready, regular rhythm.
Respiratory rate: 26 breaths/minute, regular rhythm.

Primary Health-Care Provider's Prescriptions
NPO.
Out of bed to chair for 1 hour twice daily.
Culture and sensitivity of stool and urine.
CBC, basic metabolic panel (BMP), and urinalysis.
IVF 1,000 mL 0.45% NaCl with 20 mEq KCl at 125 mL/hr.
I&O, daily weight.
Vital signs every 4 hours.
Discontinue hydrochlorothiazide (HCTZ).
Acetaminophen (Tylenol) 325 mg every 4 hours for temperature more than 101°F prn.
Ondasetron (Zofran) 8 mg sublingual every 8 hours prn for nausea.

Case Study Questions

A. Identify a cluster of subjective information that supports a concern about the client's fluid balance.

1. _____
2. _____
3. _____
4. _____

B. Identify a cluster of objective information that supports a concern about the client's fluid balance.

1. _____
2. _____
3. _____
4. _____
5. _____
6. _____

CASE STUDY: Putting It All Together

cont'd

Case Study Questions

C. What human response is the client exhibiting based on the nurse's initial collection of data?

_____

D. The following list includes the significant data collected by the nurse. How is each abnormal clinical indicator related to dehydration?

1. Temperature of 99°F

_____

2. Weak, thready pulse of 126 beats/minute with a regular rhythm

_____

3. Blood pressure of 98/64 mm Hg; orthostatic hypotension when moving from sitting to standing position

_____

4. Respirations of 26 breaths/minute with a regular rhythm

_____

5. Cracked lips, sticky and dry oral mucosa, and tenting

_____

6. Fatigue and weakness

_____

7. Oliguria and concentrated urine

_____

8. 5-lb weight loss in less than 1 week

_____

E. The following laboratory results support the nurse's conclusion that the client is dehydrated. What is the relationship of each of the abnormal findings to dehydration?

1. Elevated serum Na^+

_____

2. Elevated blood urea nitrogen

_____

3. Elevated urine specific gravity

_____

4. Elevated serum creatinine

_____

5. Elevated hemoglobin

_____

continued.

CASE STUDY: Putting It All Together   cont'd

Case Study Questions

6. Elevated hematocrit

_____

7. Decreased serum K+

_____

F. What independent and dependent nursing interventions should the nurse implement for this client in relation to the following areas?

1. Vital signs

_____

2. Diagnostic tests

_____

3. Nutrition

_____

4. Activity

_____

5. Hydration

_____

6. Hygiene

_____

7. Prescribed medications

_____

8. Health teaching

_____

G. Discuss the client's status associated with the following areas when evaluating the effectiveness of nursing care.

1. Vital signs

_____

2. Laboratory results

_____

3. Intake and output

_____

4. Complications of fluid overload

_____

REVIEW QUESTIONS

Be sure to read the Introduction for valuable test-taking tips.

1. How much fluid should a nurse teach a female client to consume during 24 hours to maintain normal fluid balance?
   1. 500 mL
   2. 1,000 mL
   3. 1,500 mL
   4. 2,200 mL

2. A client who is scheduled for chemotherapy is receiving 1 L of fluid over a 2-hour period before receiving nephrotoxic chemotherapy. The nurse assesses the client frequently for hypervolemia during this 2-hour period. For what signs of hypervolemia should the nurse assess the client? **Select all that apply.**
   1. Poor skin turgor
   2. Dyspnea on exertion
   3. Crackles in the lungs
   4. Jugular vein distention
   5. Decreased blood pressure

3. A nurse is caring for a client who is receiving a low-potassium diet. Which food should the nurse teach the client to avoid? **Select all that apply.**
   1. Chicken liver
   2. Tomato soup
   3. Lima beans
   4. Spinach
   5. Carrots

4. A client receiving furosemide (Lasix) daily is admitted with a diagnosis of dehydration and hypokalemia. The client's IV fluid is 1,000 mL 0.9% normal saline with 20 mEq of potassium chloride infusing at 125 mL/hr. What is **most** important for the nurse to assess?
   1. Food intake
   2. Intravenous site
   3. Respiratory rate
   4. Serum potassium

5. A nurse is completing a client's intake and output form for May 6. What is the total fluid intake for May 6?

Intake and Output

INTAKE	11-7	7-3	3-11	24 HR	11-
Oral/Tube	150	450	400		
Blood/Plasma					
I.V.	650	650	650		
Other					
Other					
TOTAL					
OUTPUT	11-7	7-3	3-11	24 HR	11-7
Liquid Stool					
Urine					
G.I. Suction					
Emesis					
Bowel Movement					
Other					
TOTAL					
INITIALS					

Answer: _____ mL

6. A nurse is monitoring the most recent laboratory results for a group of clients. Which result should cause the **most** concern?
   1. Serum potassium of 5.8 mEq/L for a client after cardiac surgery
   2. Hemoglobin level of 10 mg/dL for a client with a history of anemia
   3. Blood glucose of 124 mg/dL for a client with a history of type 1 diabetes
   4. White blood cell count of 10,000/mm³ for a client who had a colon resection 3 days ago

7. A nurse in the emergency department is caring for a variety of clients. Which clients should the nurse identify are at risk for a deficient fluid volume? **Select all that apply.**
   1. Man with chronic kidney disease
   2. Older adult with perfuse diaphoresis
   3. Adolescent experiencing ketoacidosis
   4. Infant experiencing diarrhea for 12 hours
   5. Woman who is in the 8th month of gestation

8. A nurse is caring for a client who is experiencing excess fluid volume evidenced by significant dependent edema. A 1,000-mL fluid restriction is prescribed. Which nursing intervention is **most** important?
   1. Offer ice chips frequently.
   2. Provide frequent mouth care.
   3. Assess extent of edema daily.
   4. Keep the legs lower than the heart.

9. A nurse is assessing a client for excess fluid volume. What questions should the nurse ask the client to obtain information specific to this problem? Select all that apply.
   1. "Do your rings feel tighter lately?"
   2. "How often do you need to urinate?"
   3. "How much water do you drink a day?"
   4. "Have you noticed an increase in thirst?"
   5. "Did you gain weight in the last few days?"

10. A nurse is caring for a client with a serum calcium level of 7.5 mEq/L. What nursing intervention is important when caring for this client? **Select all that apply.**
    1. Give the client the prescribed calcium supplement.
    2. Teach the client to avoid foods high in calcium.
    3. Prepare the client for hemodialysis.
    4. Protect the client from injury.
    5. Assess the client for tetany.

11. A client is receiving an intravenous infusion of 0.9% sodium chloride (NaCl) at 75 mL/hr. At 10 a.m. the client received an antibiotic diluted in 100 mL of NaCl; this solution was infused over 1 hour. At 2 p.m. the client received an antiemetic diluted in 50 mL of sterile water; this solution was infused over 30 minutes. Both medications were hung as IVPB infusions through a secondary line that interrupted the primary infusion of NaCl. How much intravenous solution did the client receive between 8 a.m. and 8 p.m.? **Record your answer using a whole number.**
    Answer: _____ mL

12. A nurse is caring for a client admitted to the hospital with a diagnosis of heart failure and is retaining fluid. For what clinical indicators should the nurse assess the client that supports the presence of this condition? **Select all that apply.**
    1. Dry skin
    2. Weight gain
    3. Hypertension
    4. Hemodilution
    5. Bounding pulse

13. An intravenous solution of 0.9% sodium chloride with 10 mEq of potassium chloride to be infused at 40 mL/hr is prescribed. The nurse has intravenous tubing with a drop factor of 60 gtt/mL. How many drops per minute should the nurse administer to deliver the prescribed amount of solution? **Record your answer using a whole number.**
    Answer: _____ drops/minute

14. A nurse is caring for a client who reports having severe diarrhea and vomiting for the last few days. Other than these problems the client does not have a concurrent medical diagnosis. The client's laboratory results indicate that the client has a serum sodium level of 147 mEq/L. For which clinical indicator unique to this serum sodium level should the nurse assess the client?
    1. Confusion
    2. Headache
    3. Agitation
    4. Thirst

15. A nurse is monitoring several clients for clinical manifestations of either hyperkalemia or hypokalemia. Which clinical manifestations can occur with both imbalances? **Select all that apply.**
    1. Irregular pulse
    2. Muscle weakness
    3. Facial nerve twitching
    4. Increased bowel sounds
    5. Flattened T wave on an electrocardiogram tracing

16. A nurse is obtaining a health history from a client who has a serum potassium level of 3.2 mEq. What client statements indicate a potential precipitating cause of this clinical manifestation? **Select all that apply.**
    1. "I've had diarrhea for several days."
    2. "We eat a lot of green leafy vegetables in our house."
    3. "I take electrolyte supplements because I'm on a diuretic."
    4. "I have been vomiting everything I drank or ate yesterday and today."
    5. "My blood glucose has been very high lately because I have diabetes."

17. A nurse is assessing a client with a diagnosis of hypocalcemia. Which client clinical manifestations support this diagnosis? **Select all that apply.**
    1. Hypoactive reflexes
    2. Carpopedal spasm
    3. Relaxed muscles
    4. Deep bone pain
    5. Muscle cramps
    6. Paresthesia

18. A nurse is caring for a client who is experiencing impaired venous return secondary to immobility. Furosemide 40 mg PO daily is prescribed. Place the following statements in order of application of the nursing process.
    1. Excess fluid volume is related to impaired venous return secondary to immobility.
    2. The client's potassium level remains within the expected range.
    3. The client has 2+ edema of the lower extremities.
    4. Administer furosemide 40 mg PO daily.
    5. The client will lose 1.5 lb daily.
    Answer:_____

19. A nurse is caring for a client who has a cardiac monitor. The client's serum potassium level is 5.9 mEq/L. The nurse should check the cardiac monitor for the presence of which altered cardiac tracing related to this client's potassium level?
    1. Peaked P wave
    2. Peaked T wave
    3. Narrow QRS complex
    4. Shortened PR interval

20. A nurse working on the 8 a.m. to 4 p.m. shift is monitoring the intake and output of a client. In the morning, the client voids 640 mL, drinks 4 oz of orange juice and 6 oz of coffee, and consumes 6 oz of milk in cereal. For lunch, the client has 3 oz of cream of chicken soup, a chicken breast with a portion of rice, and a 12-oz can of ginger ale. After lunch, the client reports feeling nauseated and ultimately vomits 280 mL of greenish-yellow fluid containing food particles from lunch. The primary health-care provider prescribes NPO with ice chips to help relieve thirst. The nurse gives the client an 8-oz cup of ice chips that the client consumes by the end of the shift. The client voids 320 mL at 3 p.m. The client vomits another 130 mL of fluid just before the end of the shift. What is the client's oral intake for the 8 a.m. to 4 p.m. shift?
    Answer: _____ mL

21. A nurse is caring for two clients, one with a diagnosis of excess fluid volume and one with deficient fluid volume. Which nursing interventions are unique to excess fluid volume that are unrelated to deficient fluid volume? **Select all that apply.**
    1. Obtain a daily weight.
    2. Record intake and output.
    3. Auscultate for breath sounds.
    4. Place the client in the mid-Fowler position.
    5. Monitor laboratory values for renal function and electrolytes.

22. A nurse is caring for a client receiving digoxin to improve cardiac function. For the past few days, the client has been experiencing diarrhea and vomiting because of a gastrointestinal infection. For which clinical manifestations should the nurse assess the client? **Select all that apply.**
    1. Orthostatic hypotension
    2. Irregular heart rhythm
    3. Visual disturbances
    4. Increased pulse
    5. Muscle cramps

23. An older adult is admitted to the hospital via the emergency department for unexplained episodes of fainting. When the client arrives on the unit, the nurse reviews the primary health-care provider's prescriptions, obtains the client's vital signs, and performs a physical assessment. Which is most important for the nurse to do based on this information?
    1. Offer a variety of fluids to keep at the client's bedside.
    2. Hold the lunch tray until the client talks with the dietitian.
    3. Teach the client how to collect a midstream urine specimen.
    4. Have the client sit on the side of the bed for a minute before standing.

Client's Clinical Record

Vital Signs

Temperature: 99.9°F, temporal.
Pulse: 104 beats/minute.
Respirations: 16 breaths/minute, regular rhythm.
Blood pressure: 96/64 mm Hg.

Primary Health-Care Provider's Prescriptions

Regular diet.
Encourage PO fluids.
OOB to a chair with assist.
Vital signs every 8 hours.
I&O.
Daily weight.
Midstream urine specimen for C&S.
IVF 1,000 mL 0.9% normal saline bolus X 1.

Physical Assessment

Voiding dark amber urine.
Tenting of skin over sternum.
Weight 116 lb. Client states a loss of 3 lb in the last 2 days.

24. A client is receiving a potassium-sparing diuretic. For which nontherapeutic effect should the nurse assess the client?
    1. Muscle weakness
    2. Hypoactive reflexes
    3. Respiratory depression
    4. Dry sticky mucous membranes

25. A client is admitted to the hospital after several days of diarrhea, nausea, and vomiting. Which clinical indicators should the nurse expect to identify when completing an admission nursing assessment? **Select all that apply.**
    1. Adventitious breath sounds
    2. Nonelastic skin turgor
    3. Weak, thready pulse
    4. Frothy sputum
    5. Weight gain

26. A nurse is caring for an older adult and suspects that the client may be experiencing hypovolemia. For which clinical indicators should the nurse assess the client that supports this conclusion? **Select all that apply.**
    1. Decreased capillary refill
    2. Distended neck veins
    3. Amber colored urine
    4. Bradycardia
    5. Weak pulse

27. Which independent nursing actions are appropriate for a client with deficient fluid volume? **Select all that apply.**
    1. Lubricating the lips
    2. Assessing skin turgor
    3. Discontinuing diuretics
    4. Increasing oral fluid intake
    5. Providing intravenous fluids

28. A nurse is caring for a client who has a prescription for a fluid restriction of 1,400 milliliters in 24 hours. The client is receiving medication in 50 milliliters of solution IVPB four times a day. How much fluid should the nurse allocate for oral intake during the day?
    1. 400 milliliters
    2. 800 milliliters
    3. 1,000 milliliters
    4. 1,300 milliliters

29. A nurse is implementing a medication prescription that is to be delivered using a hard plastic intravenous volume-controlled infusion set. Which nursing action is **most** important when providing a medication using this IV set?
    1. Keep the upper fluid flow roller/slide clamp above the volume-control chamber in the open position throughout the infusion.
    2. Drain solution from the primary container into the volume-control chamber equal in volume to the prescribed hourly rate.
    3. Make certain that the volume-control chamber does not empty completely during the infusion.
    4. Ensure that the air vent in the volume-control chamber is closed during the infusion.

30. A nurse is caring for a client who is receiving a 2-g sodium diet. Which food should the nurse teach the client to avoid? **Select all that apply.**
    1. Processed cheese
    2. Italian sausage
    3. Canned soup
    4. Tomatoes
    5. Bananas
    6. Eggs

31. A nurse is caring for a client who is hyperventilating. What should the nurse do to reduce the risk of respiratory alkalosis?
    1. Teach the client breathing techniques.
    2. Have the client breathe into a paper bag.
    3. Encourage the client to try to remain calm.
    4. Position the client in a high-Fowler position.

32. A nurse is caring for a client who reports having an "upset stomach" with vomiting and a low-grade fever for several days. The nurse collects the following vital signs: Blood pressure 100/72 mm Hg, pulse 92 beats/minute and thready, respirations 24 breaths/minute, and temperature 100.6°F. Which additional clinical indicators are consistent with this cluster of data? **Select all that apply.**
    1. Flat neck veins
    2. Increased thirst
    3. Peripheral edema
    4. Dry mucous membranes
    5. Red tongue with furrows
    6. Decreased blood urea nitrogen

33. A 58-year-old woman comes to the emergency department reporting multiple vague discomforts. The nurse obtains the client's history and performs an intake interview. The primary health-care provider performs a physical assessment and prescribes x-rays, an electrocardiogram, a complete blood count, a urinalysis, a metabolic panel, and a high-fiber diet. What is the **most** important nursing intervention while caring for this client?
    1. Encouraging the client to increase the fiber in her diet
    2. Handling the client carefully when completing the prescribed tests
    3. Obtaining the blood specimens before sending the client for x-rays
    4. Scheduling the electrocardiogram after determining if the client has a pacemaker

Client's Clinical Record

Medical/Surgical History

Client is a 58-year-old woman who was diagnosed with cancer of the breast 8 years ago. Initially had a mastectomy, radiation, and chemotherapy. Had a hysterectomy 10 years ago for multiple fibroids.

Client Interview

Client reports experiencing a decreased appetite and chronic constipation. States she has been feeling very tired, weak, and achy all over for several weeks. A family member states that the client has become a little confused lately.

Physical Assessment

Temperature: 99.4°F, oral.
Pulse: 88 beats/minute, irregular rhythm.
Respirations: 22 breaths/minute.
Deep tendon reflexes: Hypoactive.
Movement of extremities through range of motion increases achy feeling.

---

34. A nurse in the emergency room is caring for a client with a diagnosis of respiratory acidosis due to an asthma attack. Which medication should the nurse anticipate that the primary health-care provider probably will prescribe?
1. Diuretic
2. Bronchodilator
3. Sodium chloride
4. Sodium bicarbonate

35. A nurse is taking a client's blood pressure. After the blood pressure cuff was inflated above the client's systolic pressure, the client's hand and wrist appeared as in the illustration. For which additional clinical indicator should the nurse assess the client? **Select all that apply.**

1. Irregular heart rate
2. Nonelastic skin turgor
3. Facial nerve twitching
4. Sticky mucous membranes
5. Decreased deep tendon reflexes

36. A client is receiving hydrochlorothiazide. When evaluating the client's response to hydrochlorothiazide, which common nontherapeutic response is important for the nurse to monitor?
1. Dysrhythmias
2. Impaired airway
3. Elevated glucose
4. Elevated blood pressure

37. A nurse is inserting a catheter to provide short-term intravenous therapy. Which site should the nurse use that is appropriate for short-term therapy but is not appropriate for long-term therapy?
1. Basilic vein
2. Cephalic vein
3. Subclavian vein
4. Metacarpal vein

38. A nurse is preparing a class for a group of clients about what foods to eat when receiving a non-potassium sparing diuretic. Which foods should the nurse discuss in the class? **Select all that apply.**
1. Apples
2. Potatoes
3. Skim milk
4. Nonfat yogurt
5. Cranberry juice
6. Salad dressings

39. A nurse is caring for a client who is receiving an intravenous piggyback medication intermittently via a primary intravenous infusion line. Which nursing intervention is **most** important to prevent infection associated with this therapy?
1. Wipe the port on the primary intravenous set with an alcohol sponge before connecting the intravenous piggyback.
2. Prime the tubing of an intravenous piggyback until a drop of solution appears at the distal end of the tubing.
3. Set the alarm on the electronic infusion device to alert the nurse if the tubing becomes obstructed.
4. Wear sterile gloves when preparing and administering parenteral solutions.

40. A nurse monitors the laboratory reports of a client with a fluid and electrolyte imbalance. Which laboratory value should the nurse report to the primary health-care provider?
1. 2.5 mEq/L magnesium
2. 4.5 mEq/L potassium
3. 158 mEq/L sodium
4. 5 mEq/L calcium

41. A client has a prescription for IVF: 0.9% sodium chloride to infuse at 80 mL/hr. The nurse has an infusion set that has a drop factor of 10 drops/mL. At how many drops per minute should the nurse set the infusion rate? **Record your answer using a whole number.**

    Answer: _____ drops per minute

42. A nurse is monitoring a client's IV located on the forearm just below the antecubital fossa. Which clinical manifestations alert the nurse that an infiltration may have occurred? **Select all that apply.**
    1. A blood return does not occur when the insertion site is below the level of the intravenous solution bag.
    2. A red line under the skin extends several inches above the insertion site.
    3. The insertion site is surrounded with tissue swelling.
    4. The skin feels cool around the insertion site.
    5. A decrease in the flow rate.

43. A nurse is assessing skin turgor in an older adult. Which site should the nurse use to assess for tenting?
    1. Hand
    2. Ankle
    3. Forearm
    4. Sternum

44. A client has a prescription for IVF: 1,000 mL of 5% dextrose in water every 12 hours. At what rate should the nurse set the volume infusion device? **Record your answer using a whole number.**

    Answer: _____ mL/hr

45. A nurse is monitoring a client's intravenous insertion site that is in the right forearm just below the antecubital fossa. The nurse identifies that an infiltration has occurred and removes the intravenous catheter. What should the nurse do **next**?
    1. Keep the right arm dependent.
    2. Restart the infusion in the client's left forearm.
    3. Apply the standing prescribed warm soak to the right forearm.
    4. Reinsert the infusion distal to the previous site in the client's right arm.

REVIEW ANSWERS AND RATIONALES

1. ANSWER: 4.
Rationales:
1. 500 mL is an inadequate amount of intake to maintain normal fluid balance.
2. 1,000 mL is an inadequate amount of intake to maintain normal fluid balance.
3. 1,500 mL is an inadequate amount of intake to maintain normal fluid balance.
4. 2,200 mL is an average daily intake necessary for a female to maintain fluid balance. Fluid, along with electrolytes, acids, and bases, keeps the body in chemical balance through the processes of osmosis, filtration, diffusion, and active transport.
Content Area: Fluid, Electrolyte, and Acid-Base Balance
Integrated Processes: Teaching/Learning; Nursing Process: Implementation
Client Need: Physiological Integrity; Basic Care and Comfort
Cognitive Level: Knowledge
Concept: Patient-Centered Care; Fluid and Electrolyte Balance

2. ANSWER: 2, 3, 4.
Rationales:
1. Skin turgor does not provide critical information regarding a client's hypervolemic status; it is a better indicator of dehydration. With normal fluid balance the skin will return to its prepinch position immediately when released. With dehydration, the skin will remain elevated for a few seconds once the pinch is released, reflecting less fluid in cells and the interstitial space.
2. Dyspnea on exertion occurs in response to excess fluid in the lungs. Excess fluid accumulates in the parenchyma of the lungs and alveoli.
3. The client's respiratory status is the best indicator of the client's tolerance for a large amount of fluid given intravenously. Crackles in the lungs usually are a sign of hypervolemia because fluid leaves the low-pressure pulmonary system and moves into the lungs.
4. Jugular vein distention occurs with an increase in fluid in the intravascular compartment (hypervolemia).
5. The blood pressure increases, not decreases, with excess fluid volume because of hypervolemia.
Content Area: Fluid, Electrolyte, and Acid-Base Balance
Integrated Processes: Nursing Process: Evaluation
Client Need: Physiological Integrity; Pharmacological and Parenteral Therapies
Cognitive Level: Application
Concept: Fluid and Electrolyte Balance

3. ANSWER: 2, 3, 4.
Rationales:
1. Three chicken livers contain only approximately 90 mg of potassium.
2. One cup of canned tomato soup contains approximately 450 mg of potassium and should be avoided when receiving a low-potassium diet.
3. A half cup of lima beans contains 550 mg of potassium and should be avoided when receiving a low-potassium diet.

4. A half cup of cooked spinach contains approximately 420 mg of potassium and should be avoided when receiving a low-potassium diet.
5. A half cup of cooked frozen carrots contains only approximately 115 mg of potassium.
TEST-TAKING TIP: Identify the word in the stem that indicates negative polarity. The word *avoid* in the stem indicates negative polarity. The question is asking, "Which foods should a client *not eat* when receiving a low-potassium diet?"
Content Area: Fluid, Electrolyte, and Acid-Base Balance
Integrated Processes: Teaching/Learning; Nursing Process: Implementation
Client Need: Physiological Integrity; Basic Care and Comfort
Cognitive Level: Application
Concept: Patient-Centered Care; Fluid and Electrolyte Balance

4. ANSWER: 4.
Rationales:
1. Although monitoring how much high-potassium food the client is ingesting is important, it is not as important as another option.
2. Although monitoring the IV site for infiltration or irritation is important, it is not as critical as another option.
3. Although monitoring the respirations will reflect tolerance of IV fluid intake, it is not as significant as another option. Fluid intake of 125 mL/hr intravenously is appropriate for a client who is dehydrated and is unlikely to cause hypervolemia early in treatment.
4. Measuring the serum potassium level is essential when administering IV potassium because hyperkalemia can occur rapidly. Hyperkalemia can cause cardiac dysrhythmias.
TEST-TAKING TIP: Identify the word in the stem that sets a priority. The word *most* in the stem sets a priority. Identify the clang association. The word *potassium* in the stem and in option 4 is a clang association. Examine option 4 carefully.
Content Area: Fluid, Electrolyte, and Acid-Base Balance
Integrated Processes: Nursing Process: Evaluation
Client Need: Physiological Integrity; Pharmacological and Parenteral Therapies
Cognitive Level: Application
Concept: Medication; Fluid and Electrolyte Balance

5. ANSWER: 2,950.
Rationale:
The nurse should total the oral/tube intake for 11 p.m. to 7 a.m., 7 a.m. to 3 p.m., and 3 p.m. to 11 p.m. for a total of 1,000 mL and then total the IV intake for 11 p.m. to 7 a.m., 7 a.m. to 3 p.m., and 3 p.m. to 11 p.m. for a total of 1,950 mL. The total oral/tube intake (1,000) should be added to the total IV intake (1,950) for a grand total of 2,950 mL.
Content Area: Fluid, Electrolyte, and Acid-Base Balance
Integrated Processes: Nursing Process: Evaluation
Client Need: Physiological Integrity; Basic Care and Comfort
Cognitive Level: Analysis
Concept: Fluid and Electrolyte Balance

6. **ANSWER: 1.**

Rationales:

1. **A serum potassium level of 5.8 mEq/L is higher than the expected range of 3.5 to 5.0 mEq/L and should be reported to the primary health-care provider immediately. A high serum potassium level can cause dysrhythmias and cardiac arrest.**
2. A hemoglobin level (Hb) of 10 g/dL for a client with anemia is not unexpected. The expected range for a male is 14 to 18 g/dL and for a female 12 to 16 g/dL.
3. A blood glucose level of 124 mEq/dL is close to the expected range of 70 to 100 mg/dL. It is not unusual for a client with diabetes to have a slightly elevated blood glucose level.
4. A white blood cell count of 10,000/mm³ is within the expected range of 4,500 to 10,000/mm³.

TEST-TAKING TIP: Identify the word in the stem that sets a priority. The word *most* in the stem sets a priority.
Content Are: Fluid, Electrolyte, and Acid-Base Balance
Integrated Processes: Nursing Process: Analysis
Client Need: Physiological Integrity; Reduction of Risk Potential
Cognitive Level: Analysis
Concept: Fluid and Electrolyte Balance

7. **ANSWER: 2, 3, 4.**

Rationales:

1. People with chronic kidney problems usually experience excess fluid volume, not deficient fluid volume, because the kidneys are unable to maintain the balance of fluids, minerals, and organic substances in the body.
2. **Fluid is lost with profuse diaphoresis. Physiological responses to alterations in fluid balance, such as the thirst mechanism, in older adults are diminished resulting in older adults not drinking when dehydrated. Fluid loss and a lack of drinking increase the risk of deficient fluid volume in older adults.**
3. **The passage of a large volume of urine in a short period of time (polyuria) and insensible fluid loss related to the deep, rapid respirations associated with ketoacidosis will precipitate a deficient fluid volume.**
4. **A large volume of fluid can be lost with frequent watery stools (diarrhea); infants are particularly vulnerable to fluid balance problems because 65% to 80% of their body weight is related to fluid.**
5. Deficient fluid volume usually is not associated with pregnancy. Toward the latter part of pregnancy, women may experience dependent edema at the end of the day because pressure of the gravid uterus impedes venous return.
Content Area: Fluid, Electrolyte, and Acid-Base Balance
Integrated Processes: Nursing Process: Analysis
Client Need: Physiological Integrity; Physiological Adaptation
Cognitive Level: Analysis
Concept: Fluid and Electrolyte Balance

8. **ANSWER: 3.**

Rationales:

1. Offering ice chips frequently is a dependent function of the nurse. If the client is receiving a restricted fluid intake, the prescription should include if and how often ice chips can be given to the client to keep the mucous membranes of the mouth moist.
2. Although providing frequent mouth care is important when a client has a fluid restriction, it is not the priority.
3. **The nurse should assess the extent of edema daily by using an objective measure, such as a 1+, 2+, 3+ and 4+ scale or, if the edema is extending up the legs, measuring the circumference of the calves at the same place daily. In addition, a daily weight is an objective measure of fluid retained in the body. A 2.2-lb weight gain is equal to 1 L of fluid.**
4. Keeping the legs lower than the heart inhibits venous return, which will promote venous stasis and exacerbate the dependent edema in the legs.

TEST-TAKING TIP: Identify the word in the stem that sets a priority. The word *most* in the stem sets a priority. Identify the equally plausible options. Options 1 and 2 are associated with keeping the mucous membranes of the mouth moist. One of these is no better than the other. Eliminate options 1 and 2 from further consideration. Identify the clang association. The word *edema* in the stem and in option 3 is a clang association. Examine option 3 carefully.
Content Area: Fluid, Electrolyte, and Acid-Base Balance
Integrated Processes: Nursing Process: Implementation
Client Need: Physiological Integrity; Physiological Adaptation
Cognitive Level: Application
Concept: Fluid and Electrolyte Balance

9. **ANSWER: 1, 5.**

Rationales:

1. **Excess fluid volume results in an increase in interstitial fluid; swelling in the hands and feet can result in rings and shoes feeling tighter.**
2. The volume of urine excreted per day is more important than the number of times a person urinates. An increase in the number of times a person urinates (frequency) is related to a urinary tract infection or retention with overflow.
3. Asking "How much water do you drink a day?" is information that by itself is useless. Fluid balance is assessed by comparing the amount of fluid taken into the body and the amount of fluid exiting the body.
4. Thirst is associated with deficient, not excess, fluid volume.
5. **One liter of fluid is equal to 2.2 lb. Retained fluid will cause weight gain.**
Content Area: Fluid, Electrolyte, and Acid-Base Balance
Integrated Processes: Communication and Documentation; Nursing Process: Assessment
Client Need: Physiological Integrity; Physiological Adaptation
Cognitive Level: Analysis
Concept: Fluid and Electrolyte Balance

10. **ANSWER: 1, 4, 5.**

Rationales:

1. **The client is experiencing hypocalcemia because the client's serum calcium level is less than the expected range of 8.5 to 10.5 mEq/L. Calcium supplements are necessary to prevent cardiac dysrhythmias, a major concern with hypocalcemia.**
2. The client should be ingesting, not avoiding, foods high in calcium.

3. A client with hypercalcemia, not hypocalcemia, may receive hemodialysis.

4. The client must be protected from injury because of paresthesia, hyperactive reflexes, muscle spasms/cramps (tetany), and the potential for seizures associated with hypocalcemia.

5. Tetany, intermittent tonic muscular spasms of the arms or legs, is associated with a low serum calcium level. Sodium moves into excitable cells in the presence of low calcium levels; this decreases the threshold of action potentials with subsequent depolarization of cells resulting in nerve excitability and muscle contraction (tetany).

TEST-TAKING TIP: Identify the clang associations. The word *calcium* in the stem and in options 1 and 2 are clang associations. Examine these options carefully. Option 1 is a correct answer and option 2 is a distractor. An option with a clang association is more often than not, but *not always*, the correct answer. Identify the options that are opposites. Options 1 and 2 are opposites. Option 1 addresses increasing calcium intake, and option 2 addresses avoiding foods high in calcium. Examine options 1 and 2 carefully because, more often than not, an option that is an opposite is the correct answer.

Content Area: Fluid, Electrolyte, and Acid-Base Balance
Integrated Processes: Nursing Process: Implementation
Client Need: Physiological Integrity; Reduction of Risk Potential
Cognitive Level: Application
Concept: Fluid and Electrolyte Balance

11. **ANSWER: 638.**
    Rationale:
    For 6 hours, the client received the prescribed infusion of NaCl, which totaled 450 mL. The antibiotic infusion interrupted the primary infusion of NaCl; therefore, 100 mL of NaCl containing the antibiotic infused over 1 hour. The antiemetic interrupted the primary infusion of NaCl for half an hour; therefore, 50 mL of sterile water containing the antiemetic infused for half an hour, and the original infusion of NaCl infused for half an hour. The total amount of intravenous solution that infused was 450 + 100 + 50 + 38 (half of 75 is 37.5, but it must be rounded up to 38) = 638 mL.
    Content Area: Fluid, Electrolyte, and Acid-Base Balance
    Integrated Processes: Nursing Process: Evaluation
    Client Need: Physiological Integrity; Pharmacological and Parenteral Therapies
    Cognitive Level: Application
    Concept: Medication; Fluid and Electrolyte Balance

12. **ANSWER: 2, 4, 5.**
    Rationales:
    1. Deficient, not excess, fluid volume is associated with dry skin. Dry skin with deficient fluid volume is because of inadequate fluid in tissue.
    2. Heart failure is associated with excess fluid volume (hypervolemia). Each liter of fluid retained adds 2.2 pounds of weight to the body.
    3. Hypotension is associated with deficient fluid volume, not excess fluid volume. Heart failure is associated with excess fluid volume (hypervolemia).

4. Heart failure is associated with excess fluid volume (hypervolemia). An increase in the fluid content of the blood results in a decrease in the concentration of formed elements in the blood. This can be monitored via laboratory blood tests.

5. A bounding pulse is associated with excess fluid volume within the intravascular compartment.
Content Area: Fluid, Electrolyte, and Acid-Base Balance
Integrated Processes: Nursing Process: Assessment
Client Need: Physiological Integrity; Physiological Adaptation
Cognitive Level: Application
Concept: Fluid and Electrolyte Balance

13. **ANSWER: 40.**
    Rationale:
    The drops per minute are determined by multiplying the total number of milliliters prescribed by the drop factor divided by 60 minutes.

$$\text{Drops per minute} = \frac{40\ (\text{mL}) \times 60\ (\text{gtt})}{60\ \text{minutes}} = \frac{2,400}{60} = 40\ \text{drops/minute}$$

Content Area: Fluid, Electrolyte, and Acid-Base Balance
Integrated Processes: Nursing Process: Planning
Client Need: Physiological Integrity; Pharmacological and Parenteral Therapies
Cognitive Level: Application
Concept: Medication; Fluid and Electrolyte Balance

14. **ANSWER: 4.**
    Rationales:
    1. Increased and decreased serum sodium levels can cause confusion because of interference with nerve impulse conduction and cellular chemical reactions.
    2. The client's serum sodium level is higher than the expected range of 135 to 145 mEq/L. Decreased, not increased, serum sodium levels cause a headache due to cerebral edema.
    3. Decreased and increased serum sodium levels can cause agitation because of interference with nerve impulse conduction and cellular chemical reactions.
    4. The sensation of thirst is triggered when plasma osmolarity increases due to inadequate fluid intake in the presence of excessive fluid loss and no other concurrent medical diagnosis.

TEST-TAKING TIP: Identify the equally plausible options. Options 1 and 3 are equally plausible. One is no better than the other. Eliminate both from further consideration. Identify the unique option. Option 4 is unique because it is the only clinical indicator that does not occur with both an increase and decrease in the serum sodium level; it occurs only with increased serum sodium.

Content Area: Fluid, Electrolyte, and Acid-Base Balance
Integrated Processes: Communication and Documentation; Nursing Process: Assessment
Client Need: Physiological Integrity; Physiological Adaptation
Cognitive Level: Analysis
Concept: Fluid and Electrolyte Balance

15. ANSWER: 1, 2.

Rationales:

1. Potassium is a component of the sodium-potassium pump that is involved with muscle contraction. The heart is a muscle; therefore, an increase or decrease in serum potassium will result in dysrhythmias and abnormalities evident on an electrocardiogram.

2. Potassium is a component of the sodium-potassium pump that is involved with muscle contraction. An increase or decrease in serum potassium will result in muscle weakness and fatigue.

3. Facial nerve twitching (Chvostek sign) is associated with hypocalcemia, not hyperkalemia.

4. Increased bowel sounds, diarrhea, and abdominal cramps are associated with hyperkalemia. Abdominal distention, decreased bowel sounds, and constipation are associated with loss of muscle tone related to hypokalemia.

5. On an electrocardiogram tracing, the T wave will be flattened with hypokalemia (due to delayed repolarization) and peaked with hyperkalemia (due to rapid repolarization).

Content Area: Fluid, Electrolyte, and Acid-Base Balance
Integrated Processes: Nursing Process: Assessment
Client Need: Physiological Integrity; Physiological Adaptation
Cognitive Level: Analysis
Concept: Fluid and Electrolyte Balance

16. ANSWER: 1, 4.

Rationales:

1. The expected serum potassium level is 3.5 to 5.0 mEq; a level of 3.2 mEq indicates hypokalemia. Potassium is an ion found in gastrointestinal fluids, such as gastric and intestinal contents. Prolonged diarrhea can result in hypokalemia.

2. This should not result in hypokalemia. Green leafy vegetables, such as spinach, contain potassium.

3. Excessive intake of potassium chloride can result in hyperkalemia, not hypokalemia.

4. The expected serum potassium level is 3.5 to 5.0 mEq; a level of 3.2 mEq indicates hypokalemia. Potassium is an ion found in gastrointestinal fluids, such as gastric and intestinal contents. Vomiting and gastric decompression can result in hypokalemia.

5. Diabetic ketoacidosis precipitates hyperkalemia; potassium, an intracellular ion, is released when cells break down to meet energy needs.

Content Area: Fluid, Electrolyte, and Acid-Base Balance
Integrated Processes: Communication and Documentation; Nursing Process: Analysis
Client Need: Physiological Integrity; Physiological Adaptation
Cognitive Level: Analysis
Concept: Fluid and Electrolyte Balance

17. ANSWER: 2, 5, 6.

Rationales:

1. Hypoactive reflexes are associated with hypercalcemia, not hypocalcemia, because of loss of cell membrane excitability.

2. Carpopedal spasm (Trousseau's sign) is a classic indicator of hypocalcemia. When a sphygmomanometer is inflated above the systolic pressure and flexion of the wrist and hand occurs, it indicates hypocalcemia. This occurs in response to increased neuromuscular excitability associated with hypocalcemia.

3. Weak, relaxed muscles and hypoactive reflexes are associated with hypercalcemia, not hypocalcemia because of decreased neuromuscular excitability.

4. Deep bone pain is associated with hypercalcemia, not hypocalcemia, as calcium moves out of bones and into the intravascular compartment.

5. Calcium is involved with neuromuscular functioning; therefore, a decrease in serum calcium results in muscle cramps.

6. Calcium is involved with neuromuscular functioning; therefore, a decrease in serum calcium results in paresthesia (unpleasant numbness, prickly, stinging, or burning feeling).

TEST-TAKING TIP: Identify options that are opposites. Options 3 and 5 are opposites. Consider these options carefully.

Content Area: Fluid, Electrolyte, and Acid-Base Balance
Integrated Processes: Nursing Process: Analysis
Client Need: Physiological Integrity; Physiological Adaptation
Cognitive Level: Application
Concept: Fluid and Electrolyte Balance

18. ANSWER: 3, 1, 5, 4, 2.

Rationales:

3. Two plus edema of the lower extremities is a nursing assessment and is the first step of the nursing process.

1. Excess fluid volume that is related to impaired venous return secondary to immobility is the identification of the client's problem and is the second step of the nursing process.

5. Stating that the client will lose 1.5 pounds daily is an expected outcome and is the first part of the third step of the nursing process, planning. The second half of the planning step involves identifying planned nursing interventions.

4. Administering furosemide (Lasix) 40 mg PO daily is an intervention implemented by the nurse in relation to the data in this scenario. Implementation of a planned nursing intervention is the fourth step of the nursing process.

2. When evaluating outcomes associated with administration of furosemide (Lasix), it is not only weight loss and a decrease in blood pressure that is expected, but also that the potassium level will return and remain within the expected range. Clients receiving furosemide (Lasix) are at risk for hypokalemia. Therefore, monitoring serum potassium levels is important when a client is receiving furosemide (Lasix).

Content Area: Fluid, Electrolyte, and Acid-Base Balance
Integrated Processes: Nursing Process: Analysis
Client Need: Safe and Effective Care Environment; Management of Care
Cognitive Level: Analysis
Concept: Medication; Fluid and Electrolyte Balance

19. **ANSWER: 2.**
Rationales:
1. P waves are flattened, not peaked, with hyperkalemia.
2. Peaked T waves are associated with an elevated serum potassium level higher than 5 mEq/L. Peaked T waves occur because of a longer cell membrane action potential in myocardial tissue.
3. QRS complexes are widened, not narrowed, with hyperkalemia due to fusion of the T and U waves.
4. The PR interval will be prolonged because excess potassium reduces myocardial excitability including conductive tissues.
Content Area: Fluid, Electrolyte, and Acid-Base Balance
Integrated Processes: Nursing Process: Assessment
Client Need: Physiological Integrity; Physiological Adaptation
Cognitive Level: Analysis
Concept: Fluid and Electrolyte Balance

20. **ANSWER: 1,050.**
Rationale:
The client's intake is 120 mL (4 oz of orange juice); 180 mL (6 oz of coffee); 180 mL (6 oz of milk); 90 mL (3 oz of soup); 360 mL (12 oz of ginger ale); 120 mL (8 oz of ice chips; liquid volume of ice chips is equal to half the volume of the frozen volume of ice chips). The total oral intake is 1,050 mL.
Content Area: Fluid, Electrolyte, and Acid-Base Balance
Integrated Processes: Nursing Process: Assessment
Client Need: Physiological Integrity; Basic Care and Comfort
Cognitive Level: Application
Concept: Fluid and Electrolyte Balance

21. **ANSWER: 3, 4.**
Rationales:
1. A daily weight provides valuable information whether the client has excess fluid volume or deficient fluid volume. Weight loss or gain is an objective measure of fluid loss or fluid gain. One liter of fluid is equal to 2.2 lb.
2. Monitoring intake and output should be done for clients with excess fluid volume or deficient fluid volume. The intake and output should be relatively balanced. If the intake is greater than the output, then the client may develop excess fluid volume. If the output is greater than the intake, then the client may develop deficient fluid volume.
3. The lungs are a low-pressure system. The blood pressure increases with excess fluid volume because of hypervolemia; with hypervolemia, fluid moves into the lungs causing crackles and dyspnea.
4. A client with excess fluid volume should be positioned with the head of the bed elevated. This minimizes the movement of fluid from the vascular system to the lungs, which is a low-pressure system. A mid-Fowler position is not necessary for clients with a diagnosis of deficient fluid volume because this would place excess pressure on the sacral area, which should be avoided. The integrity of the skin is compromised in a person with dehydration, which increases the risk of pressure ulcers.
5. Laboratory values for renal function and electrolytes will reflect the physiological status of clients whether they are experiencing a deficient or excess fluid volume.

Content Area: Fluid, Electrolyte, and Acid-Base Balance
Integrated Processes: Nursing Process: Implementation
Client Need: Physiological Integrity; Physiological Adaptation
Cognitive Level: Analysis
Concept: Fluid and Electrolyte Balance

22. **ANSWER: 2, 3.**
Rationales:
1. Orthostatic hypotension is a side effect of diuretics, angiotensin-converting enzyme inhibitors, and angiotensin II receptor blockers, not digoxin (Lanoxin).
2. An irregular heart rhythm indicating a cardiac dysrhythmia occurs with digoxin (Lanoxin) toxicity because of the effects of digoxin on cardiac function. Digoxin increases the force of cardiac contraction, slows the heart rate, and decreases conduction through the SA and AV nodes. Excessive amounts of digoxin can cause serious alterations in cardiac function.
3. Yellow vision around lights and diplopia are classic signs of digoxin (Lanoxin) toxicity. Hypokalemia caused by vomiting and diarrhea increases the risk of digoxin (Lanoxin) toxicity.
4. Bradycardia, not tachycardia, is a nontherapeutic response to digoxin. An increased pulse rate is associated with hypernatremia, not digoxin (Lanoxin) toxicity.
5. Muscle cramps are associated with hypocalcemia, not digoxin (Lanoxin) toxicity.
Content Area: Fluid, Electrolyte, and Acid-Base Balance
Integrated Processes: Nursing Process: Evaluation
Client Need: Physiological Integrity; Pharmacological and Parenteral Therapies
Cognitive Level: Application
Concept: Medication; Fluid and Electrolyte Balance

23. **ANSWER: 4.**
Rationales:
1. Although providing a variety of fluids to keep at the bedside should be done, it is not the priority. Because the client is receiving a 1,000-mL bolus of IV fluid, the oral intake at this time is not as critical as the action in another option.
2. There is no indication to hold the client's lunch.
3. Although a midstream urine sample should be collected because it is prescribed by the primary health-care provider, the nurse should collect the specimen and not expect an older adult with a history of fainting to collect the specimen independently.
4. Safety is a priority. The client who is dehydrated generally is hypovolemic, which can precipitate orthostatic hypotension. Having the client sit for a minute after raising the head of the bed and then having the client sit on the side of the bed with the legs resting on the floor (dangle) for a minute before standing allows time for the blood pressure to equalize, which minimizes the risk of orthostatic hypotension and a fall.
TEST-TAKING TIP: Identify the word in the stem that sets a priority. The word *most* in the stem sets a priority.
Content Area: Fluid, Electrolyte, and Acid-Base Balance
Integrated Processes: Communication and Documentation; Nursing Process: Implementation
Client Need: Physiological Integrity; Physiological Adaptation
Cognitive Level: Analysis
Concept: Patient-Centered Care; Safety

24. ANSWER: 1.
Rationales:
1. Muscle weakness is a classic nontherapeutic response to a potassium-sparing diuretic that indicates hyperkalemia. The amount of potassium accumulating in the blood eventually causes hyperkalemia.
2. Hypoactive reflexes indicate hypercalcemia. Hypocalcemia, not hypercalcemia, is a nontherapeutic response to a potassium-sparing diuretic.
3. Respiratory depression indicates hypermagnesemia. Hypomagnesemia, not hypermagnesemia, is a nontherapeutic response to a potassium-sparing diuretic.
4. Dry, sticky mucous membranes indicate hypernatremia, which is not a nontherapeutic response to a potassium-sparing diuretic.
TEST-TAKING TIP: Identify the word in the stem that indicates negative polarity. The word *nontherapeutic* in the stem indicates negative polarity. The question is asking, "What effect is not a therapeutic response to the drug?"
Content Area: Fluid, Electrolyte, and Acid-Base Balance
Integrated Processes: Nursing Process: Evaluation
Client Need: Physiological Integrity; Pharmacological and Parenteral Therapies
Cognitive Level: Application
Concept: Fluid and Electrolyte Balance

25. ANSWER: 2, 3.
Rationales:
1. Diarrhea and vomiting can cause deficient, not excess, fluid volume. Adventitious breath sounds, such as moist crackles, are associated with excess fluid volume as fluid moves into the lungs because of the low pressure of the pulmonary system.
2. Diarrhea and vomiting can cause deficient fluid volume. Nonelastic skin turgor occurs with deficient fluid volume because fluid has moved from the intracellular and interstitial compartments into the intravascular compartment; the pinch of skin does not return to its original position in less than 3 seconds (tenting).
3. Diarrhea and vomiting can cause deficient fluid volume. A weak, thready pulse results from a decrease in the volume of fluid in the intravascular compartment (hypovolemia).
4. Diarrhea and vomiting can cause deficient, not excess, fluid volume. Frothy sputum is associated with excess fluid volume. The elevated blood pressure associated with hypervolemia can cause movement of fluid into the lung (pleural effusion), resulting in frothy sputum.
5. Diarrhea and vomiting can cause deficient, not excess, fluid volume. Weight loss, not weight gain, is associated with deficient fluid volume. Every liter of fluid is equal to 2.2 lb.
Content Area: Fluid, Electrolyte, and Acid-Base Balance
Integrated Processes: Nursing Process: Assessment
Client Need: Physiological Integrity; Basic Care and Comfort
Cognitive Level: Application
Concept: Fluid and Electrolyte Balance

26. ANSWER: 1, 3, 5.
Rationales:
1. Decreased capillary refill is associated with deficient fluid volume due to a decrease in the circulating blood volume (hypovolemia).
2. Distended neck veins are associated with hypervolemia, not hypovolemia. Flat neck veins are associated with hypovolemia due to the decrease in intravascular fluid volume.
3. With hypovolemia, urine is concentrated, which causes the amber color.
4. Tachycardia (more than 100 beats/minute), not bradycardia (less than 60 beats/minute), is associated with hypovolemia. The heart rate increases to transport more oxygen to meet the oxygen needs of body cells.
5. A weak pulse is associated with hypovolemia because of the decrease in intravascular fluid volume; it is referred to as a weak, thready pulse.
Content Area: Fluid, Electrolyte, and Acid-Base Balance
Integrated Processes: Nursing Process: Assessment
Client Need: Physiological Integrity; Basic Care and Comfort
Cognitive Level: Analysis
Concept: Fluid and Electrolyte Balance

27. ANSWER: 1, 2.
Rationales:
1. Lubricating the lips of a client is an independent nursing action because a nurse has a license to treat human responses. It does not require a prescription from a primary health-care provider. Clients with a deficient fluid volume have dry mucous membranes.
2. Assessing skin turgor is an independent nursing action. It does not require a prescription from a primary health-care provider. Clients with deficient fluid volume will exhibit tenting when the skin is pinched; this results from decreased fluid in the intracellular and interstitial fluid compartments.
3. Discontinuing a drug is a dependent function of the nurse. It requires a prescription from a primary health-care provider.
4. Increasing oral fluid intake is a dependent function of the nurse. The nurse must have a diet prescription with no fluid restrictions before encouraging an increase in oral fluid intake.
5. Providing intravenous fluids is a dependent function of the nurse. Providing intravenous fluids requires a prescription from a primary health-care provider.
Content Area: Fluid, Electrolyte, and Acid-Base Balance
Integrated Processes: Nursing Process: Implementation
Client Need: Physiological Integrity; Physiological Adaptation
Cognitive Level: Analysis
Concept: Fluid and Electrolyte Balance

28. ANSWER: 2.
Rationales:
1. Although at first it may seem appropriate to divide fluid intake equally over the entire course of the day, it is inappropriate. Less fluid is needed at night when the client generally is sleeping.

2. Fluids administered intravenously must be accounted for in a restricted fluid diet. Therefore, 200 milliliters should be subtracted from the 1,400 milliliters allocated for fluid intake before dividing the remaining fluid across 24 hours. Eight hundred milliliters allocated for the daylight hours, with 300 milliliters for evenings and 100 milliliters for nights, is an appropriate division of 1,200 milliliters of fluid over 24 hours. More fluid should be allocated in the daylight hours because the client is awake.

3. One thousand milliliters is too large an amount of fluid to be allocated to the daylight hours. One thousand milliliters of fluid during the day leaves only 200 milliliters to be divided between the evening and night hours, which is too small a volume for these time frames.

4. Oral fluid in the daylight hours of 1,300 milliliters, in addition to the 200 milliliters for the four intravenous piggybacks, total 1,500 milliliters in 24 hours; this exceeds the 1,400 milliliters of fluid restriction.

Content Area: Fluid, Electrolyte, and Acid-Base Balance
Integrated Processes: Nursing Process: Planning
Client Need: Physiological Integrity; Pharmacological and Parenteral Therapies
Cognitive Level: Analysis
Concept: Fluid and Electrolyte Balance

29. **ANSWER: 2.**
    Rationales:
    1. Keeping the fluid flow roller/slide clamp above the volume-control chamber in the open position during the infusion is contraindicated. This action will cause the volume-control chamber to continually fill with solution from the primary infusion container. This may place the client at risk for receiving a larger volume of fluid than the volume of fluid prescribed. Instead, once the volume-control chamber is filled with the prescribed hourly volume the upper roller/slide clamp is closed. This prevents additional solution from entering the volume-control chamber.
    2. This action is the most important of the options presented because it ensures that fluid beyond the hourly volume is not available to infuse by accident. Only 1 hour's worth of solution is available for infusion via the volume-control chamber.
    3. Although it is important not to let the volume-control chamber run out because doing so may result in an occlusion, it is not the most important action associated with administering an infusion using a volume-control administration set.
    4. The air vent associated with a hard plastic volume-control infusion set should be open, not closed. The volume-controlled chamber can develop negative pressure, which will prevent solution from infusing.
    Content Area: Fluid, Electrolyte, and Acid-Base Balance
    Integrated Processes: Nursing Process: Implementation
    Client Need: Physiological Integrity; Pharmacological and Parenteral Therapies
    Cognitive Level: Analysis
    Concept: Fluid and Electrolyte Balance

30. **ANSWER: 1, 2, 3.**
    Rationales:
    1. One slice (1 oz) of processed cheese has 380 to 400 mg of sodium and should be avoided when receiving a 2-g sodium diet.
    2. A large amount of salt is used in the recipe for Italian sausages; one average size Italian sausage contains approximately 820 mg of sodium and should be avoided when on a 2-g sodium diet.
    3. One cup of canned soup on average contains 900 to 1,000 mg of sodium and should be avoided when receiving a 2-g sodium diet.
    4. One tomato contains approximately 10 mg of sodium.
    5. One banana has 1 mg of sodium.
    6. One large egg contains 69 mg of sodium.
    TEST-TAKING TIP: Identify the word in the stem that indicates negative polarity. The word *avoid* in the stem indicates negative polarity. The question is asking, "What food should the client *not eat* when receiving a 2-g sodium diet?"
    Content Area: Fluid, Electrolyte, and Acid-Base Balance
    Integrated Processes: Teaching/Learning; Nursing Process: Implementation
    Client Need: Physiological Integrity; Basic Care and Comfort
    Cognitive Level: Application
    Concept: Patient-Centered Care; Fluid and Electrolyte Balance

31. **ANSWER: 1.**
    Rationales:
    1. Breathing techniques help to rebalance the oxygen and carbon dioxide levels in the blood. Breathing techniques involve slowing the rate of respirations. For example, inhale slowly using abdominal breathing for 5 seconds, hold the breath for 2 seconds and then exhale slowly over 5 seconds, repeat for two cycles and then breathe regularly for five cycles and then repeat. This engages the client in focusing on the breathing and relaxing.
    2. Breathing into a paper bag is controversial and should be avoided. While it may not hurt a person who is hyperventilating due to a panic attack, it has not proven to be that beneficial. However, if the hyperventilation is due to an underlying medical problem, such as asthma or cardiac ischemia, breathing into a paper bag can make the condition worse and may even be fatal.
    3. Telling the client to remain calm in the midst of an episode of hyperventilation is inappropriate. This is not client centered.
    4. Although the high-Fowler position may be comfortable for a client experiencing hyperventilation, it will not prevent respiratory alkalosis. The high-Fowler position generally is used to facilitate thoracic excursion when a client is experiencing respiratory acidosis.
    TEST-TAKING TIP: Identify options with obscure clang associations. The word *hyperventilating* in the stem and the word *breathing* in option 1 and *breathe* in option 2 are obscure clang associations. Examine options 1 and 2 carefully. In this question, option 1 is the correct answer and option 2 is a distractor. Identify the option that denies the client's feelings and concerns. Option 3 denies the client's feelings and concerns.

Content Area: Fluid, Electrolyte, and Acid-Base Balance
Integrated Processes: Teaching/Learning; Nursing Process: Implementation
Client Need: Physiological Integrity; Physiological Adaptation
Cognitive Level: Application
Concept: Acid-Base Balance

32. ANSWER: 1, 2, 4, 5.
Rationales:
1. Flat neck veins indicate deficient fluid volume due to hypovolemia, which is the client's problem.
2. The thirst center in the hypothalamus is stimulated when an increase in the concentration of particles within the intravascular compartment occurs with deficient fluid volume.
3. Peripheral edema is related to excess fluid volume, which is not the client's problem.
4. The cluster of data in the stem indicates that the client is experiencing deficient fluid volume. Dry mucous membranes are a clinical manifestation of deficient fluid volume due to a decrease of fluid in the intracellular and interstitial compartments.
5. The cluster of data in the stem indicates that the client is experiencing a deficient fluid volume. A red tongue with furrows supports the conclusion that the client is dehydrated; fluid from the intracellular and interstitial compartments moves to the intravascular compartment in an attempt to maintain the circulating blood volume.
6. The blood urea nitrogen will be increased, not decreased, with deficient fluid volume. The urea nitrogen becomes more concentrated as the intravascular fluid volume decreases.
Content Area: Fluid, Electrolyte, and Acid-Base Balance
Integrated Processes: Nursing Process: Assessment
Client Need: Physiological Integrity; Basic Care and Comfort
Cognitive Level: Analysis
Concept: Fluid and Electrolyte Balance

33. ANSWER: 2.
Rationales:
1. Although encouraging an increase in fiber in the diet may be done eventually, it is not the priority at this time.
2. The client's clinical manifestations (e.g., anorexia, constipation, fatigue, weakness, confusion, and depressed deep tendon reflexes) are consistent with the signs and symptoms of hypercalcemia. Metastasis to the bone precipitates hypercalcemia. The demineralization of bone, resulting in osteoporosis, causes achy bone pain. This client is at high risk for pathologic fractures. Extreme caution should be used when moving the client, and the extremities should be supported above and below joints.
3. Obtaining blood specimens before sending the client for x-rays is unnecessary.
4. Although scheduling the electrocardiogram after determining if the client has a pacemaker may be done as part of the client's assessment, it is not the priority at this time.
TEST-TAKING TIP: Identify the word in the stem that sets a priority. The word *most* in the stem sets a priority. Identify the unique option. Option 2 is unique because it is the only option that does not contain a clang association.

The word *fiber* in the stem and in option 1, the word *x-rays* in the stem and in option 3, and the word *electrocardiogram* in the stem and in option 4 are clang associations.
Content Area: Fluid, Electrolyte, and Acid-Base Balance
Integrated Processes: Communication and Documentation; Nursing Process: Implementation
Client Need: Safe and Effective Care Environment; Safety and Infection Control
Cognitive Level: Analysis
Concept: Patient-Centered Care; Fluid and Electrolyte Balance

34. ANSWER: 2.
Rationales:
1. Diuretics cause diuresis of excess fluid in the body. Excess fluid in the body is not the cause of respiratory acidosis in a client with asthma.
2. Asthma causes airway obstruction due to inflammation of the respiratory passages. A bronchodilator offers some relief of the clinical manifestations of acute asthma by quickly dilating and opening respiratory passages. Improved breathing will bring more oxygen into the alveoli and subsequently the circulation resolving the respiratory acidosis.
3. Administration of sodium chloride is associated with the treatment of metabolic alkalosis, not respiratory acidosis.
4. Administration of sodium bicarbonate is associated with the treatment of metabolic acidosis, not respiratory acidosis.
Content Area: Fluid, Electrolyte, and Acid-Base Balance
Integrated Processes: Nursing Process: Planning
Client Need: Physiological Integrity; Pharmacological and Parenteral Therapies
Cognitive Level: Analysis
Concept: Medication; Acid-Base Balance

35. ANSWER: 1, 3.
Rationales:
1. Flexion of the wrist and hand when a blood pressure cuff is inflated above the client's systolic level (Trousseau's sign) indicates hypocalcemia. Cardiac irregularity is a serious consequence of a decrease in serum calcium (hypocalcemia).
2. Nonelastic skin turgor is not associated with the problem related to the client's manifestation in the illustration.
3. Facial nerve twitching is associated with hypocalcemia, which is the client's problem. A low serum calcium level causes sodium to move into excitable cells, which decreases the threshold of action potentials; this causes subsequent depolarization of cells resulting in nerve excitability and facial nerve twitching (Chvostek sign).
4. Sticky mucous membranes are associated with an increase in serum sodium (hypernatremia). The clinical manifestation reflected in the illustration is not related to hypernatremia.
5. Deep tendon reflexes increase, not decrease, with the client's physical problem. A decrease in deep tendon reflexes occurs with a decrease in serum potassium (hypokalemia) and with an increase in serum calcium (hypercalcemia).

Content Area: Fluid, Electrolyte, and Acid-Base Balance
Integrated Processes: Nursing Process: Assessment
Client Need: Physiological Integrity; Physiological Adaptation
Cognitive Level: Analysis
Concept: Fluid and Electrolyte Balance

36. **ANSWER: 1.**
    Rationales:
    1. **A dysrhythmia is a serious nontherapeutic effect associated with hydrochlorothiazide (HydroDIURIL) therapy. It indicates a low-potassium level (hypokalemia).**
    2. An impaired airway is unrelated to hydrochlorothiazide (HydroDIURIL) therapy.
    3. An elevated glucose level is unrelated to hydrochlorothiazide (HydroDIURIL) therapy.
    4. A decreased, not increased, blood pressure is related to hypovolemia, which is a nontherapeutic response to diuretic therapy.
    TEST-TAKING TIP: Identify the word in the stem that indicates negative polarity. The word *nontherapeutic* in the stem indicates negative polarity.
    Content Area: Fluid, Electrolyte, and Acid-Base Balance
    Integrated Processes: Nursing Process: Implementation
    Client Need: Physiological Integrity; Pharmacological and Parenteral Therapies
    Cognitive Level: Application
    Concept: Medication; Fluid and Electrolyte Balance

37. **ANSWER: 4.**
    Rationales:
    1. A basilica vein is a larger vein used for long-term therapy. Larger veins accommodate hypertonic, viscous, or irritating solutions because the infused solution is diluted by a greater volume of blood than in smaller veins. Also, larger veins can accommodate a larger volume of fluid and at a faster rate than fluid administered via a small vein.
    2. A cephalic vein is a large vein used for long-term therapy. Larger veins accommodate hypertonic, viscous, or irritating solutions because the infused solution is diluted by a greater volume of blood than in smaller veins. Also, larger veins can accommodate a larger volume of fluid and at a faster rate than fluid administered via a small vein.
    3. A subclavian vein is a large vein used for long-term therapy. Larger veins accommodate hypertonic, viscous, or irritating solutions because the infused solution is diluted by a greater volume of blood than in smaller veins. Also, larger veins can accommodate a larger volume of fluid and at a faster rate than fluid administered via a small vein.
    4. **A metacarpal vein is a small vein that can be used for short-term intravenous therapy.**
    Content Area: Fluid, Electrolyte, and Acid-Base Balance
    Integrated Processes: Nursing Process: Planning
    Client Need: Physiological Integrity; Pharmacological and Parenteral Therapies
    Cognitive Level: Analysis
    Concept: Medication; Fluid and Electrolyte Balance

38. **ANSWER: 2, 3, 4.**
    Rationales:
    1. One apple contains only 65 mg of potassium and is not an adequate source of potassium in the diet.
    2. **One baked potato with the skin contains approximately 845 mg of potassium, which, if ingested, can replace potassium lost because of the diuretic.**
    3. **One cup of skim milk contains approximately 400 mg of potassium, which, if ingested, can replace potassium lost because of the diuretic.**
    4. **Eight ounces of nonfat yogurt contains approximately 580 mg of potassium, which, if ingested, can replace potassium lost because of the diuretic.**
    5. One cup of cranberry juice contains approximately 60 mg of potassium and is not a generous source of potassium in the diet.
    6. One tablespoon of salad dressing contains 2 to 20 mg of potassium and is not a generous source of potassium in the diet.
    Content Area: Fluid, Electrolyte, and Acid-Base Balance
    Integrated Processes: Teaching/Learning; Nursing Process: Planning
    Client Need: Physiological Integrity; Pharmacological and Parenteral Therapies
    Cognitive Level: Application
    Concept: Medication; Fluid and Electrolyte Balance

39. **ANSWER: 1.**
    Rationales:
    1. **Wiping the intravenous port with an alcohol sponge before connecting the intravenous piggyback is essential to prevent the introduction of pathogens into an intravenous line.**
    2. Priming the tubing of the intravenous piggyback set prevents air from entering the primary intravenous line; it does not prevent infection.
    3. Although setting the alarm on the electronic infusion device may be done, it alerts the nurse of an obstruction, not the presence of infection.
    4. Sterile gloves are not necessary to maintain sterility of equipment when preparing and attaching an IVPB to a primary intravenous infusion line. If there is a risk of coming into contact with a client's blood or body fluids, the nurse should wear clean gloves.
    TEST-TAKING TIP: Identify the word in the stem that sets a priority. The word *most* in the stem sets a priority. Identify the clang associations. The words *intravenous piggyback* in the stem and in options 1 and option 2 are clang associations. Examine options 1 and 2 carefully.
    Content Area: Fluid, Electrolyte, and Acid-Base Balance
    Integrated Processes: Nursing Process: Implementation
    Client Need: Physiological Integrity; Reduction of Risk Potential
    Cognitive Level: Application
    Concept: Safety

40. **ANSWER: 3.**
    Rationales:
    1. A level of 2.2 mEq/L is within the expected range of 1.5 mEq/L to 2.5 mEq/L for a serum magnesium level.

2. A level of 4.5 mEq/L is within the expected range of 3.5 mEq/L to 5.3 mEq/L for a serum potassium level.

3. A level of 158 mEq/L is above the expected range of 136 mEq/L to 148 mEq/L, indicating hypernatremia.

4. A level of 5 mEq/L is within the expected range of 4.5 mEq/L to 5.5 mEq/L for a serum calcium level.

Content Area: Fluid, Electrolyte, and Acid-Base Balance
Integrated Processes: Communication and Documentation; Nursing Process: Implementation
Client Need: Physiological Integrity; Reduction of Risk Potential
Cognitive Level: Analysis
Concept: Fluid and Electrolyte Balance

41. ANSWER: 13.

Rationale:

Arrive at the answer to this question using the following formula.

$$\frac{\text{Total mL to be infused} \times \text{drop factor}}{\text{Total time in minutes}}$$

$$\frac{80 \ (\text{mL}) \times 10 \ (\text{drop factor})}{60 \ (\text{minutes})} = \frac{800}{60} = 13.33$$

Round down to 13 drops per minute because 0.3 is less than 0.5.

Content Area: Fluid, Electrolyte, and Acid-Base Balance
Integrated Processes: Nursing Process: Planning
Client Need: Physiological Integrity; Pharmacological and Parenteral Therapies
Cognitive Level: Application
Concept: Fluid and Electrolyte Balance

42. ANSWER: 1, 3, 4, 5.

Rationales:

1. Failure of blood to return in an intravenous catheter when the intravenous solution bag is lowered below the insertion site indicates that the catheter is outside the vein. A blood return when the intravenous solution bag is lowered below the insertion site is an expected response when an intravenous catheter is in a vein.

2. A red line under the skin extending several inches above the insertion site of an intravenous needle is a sign of inflammation of a vein (phlebitis), not infiltration.

3. Swelling of tissue around the insertion site occurs with an infiltration because the intravenous solution is entering the interstitial compartment.

4. The site will be cool to the touch with an infiltration because the solution infusing into the subcutaneous tissue is at room temperature, which is lower than body temperature. Warmth may indicate the presence of inflammation or infection.

5. The flow rate will slow down because the cannula is displaced outside of the vein.

TEST-TAKING TIP: Identify the clang association. The letters *IV* in the stem is a clang association with the word *intravenous* in option 1. Examine option 1 carefully. Identify the unique option. Option 5 is the only option without the word *insertion*. Examine option 5 carefully.

Content Area: Fluid, Electrolyte, and Acid-Base Balance
Integrated Processes: Nursing Process: Evaluation

Client Need: Physiological Integrity; Pharmacological and Parenteral Therapies
Cognitive Level: Application
Concept: Tissue Integrity

43. ANSWER: 4.

Rationales:

1. The hands in older adults have a decrease in subcutaneous tissue resulting in numerous wrinkles that interfere with assessment of skin turgor.

2. Many older adults have less efficient venous return or cardiac disease that results in dependent edema of the ankles. Edema interferes with assessment of skin turgor.

3. The forearms in older adults have a decrease in subcutaneous tissue resulting in numerous wrinkles that interfere with assessment of skin turgor.

4. Pinching the skin over the sternum, anterior chest below the clavicle, or forehead are the preferred sites for assessing tenting. These sites are less likely to have wrinkles or edema that interfere with assessment of skin turgor.

Content Area: Tissue Integrity and Hygiene
Integrated Processes: Nursing Process: Assessment
Client Need: Physiological Integrity; Basic Care and Comfort
Cognitive Level: Application
Concept: Fluid and Electrolyte Balance

44. ANSWER: 83.

Rationale:

A volume control device is programmed at milliliters per hour. Therefore, to answer the question, divide 12 hours into 1,000 milliliters to determine the hourly rate. 1000 ÷ 12 = 83.33 milliliters per hour. Round the answer down to 83 because 0.3 is less than 0.5.

Content Area: Fluid, Electrolyte, and Acid-Base Balance
Integrated Processes: Nursing Process: Planning
Client Need: Physiological Integrity; Pharmacological and Parenteral Therapies
Cognitive Level: Application
Concept: Fluid and Electrolyte Balance

45. ANSWER: 2.

Rationales:

1. The arm should be elevated on a pillow above the level of the heart. This will promote venous return and facilitate resorption of the intravenous solution in the interstitial compartment.

2. Restarting the infusion in the client's left arm allows the right arm to recover from the trauma of the infiltration. Also, the infusion should be restarted as soon as possible to limit the interruption of the IV fluid prescription. Once the infusion is restarted, the flow rate should be set at the prescribed rate. It should not be increased to make up the amount of solution that was not administered. An increased flow rate could cause an excessive amount of fluid in the intravascular compartment (hypervolemia).

3. The preparation of a warm soak will take time, causing a delay in meeting the client's primary need. This is a dependent function of the nurse and requires a prescription

from a person with a prescriptive license or a standing protocol of the facility.

4. When an infusion is restarted in an extremity that had an infiltration, the site should be proximal to the site of the infiltration; this prevents trauma at the site of the infiltration. The use of the same arm is discouraged but may be used when an alternate site is unavailable.

TEST-TAKING TIP: Identify the word in the stem that sets a priority. The word *next* in the stem sets a priority. Identify the options that are opposites. Options 2 and 4 are opposites. In option 2, the infusion is restarted in the left arm and in option 4 the infusion is restarted in the right arm. Consider these options carefully. Often, when there are opposites, one of them is the correct answer. Identify the options that have a clang association. The stem contains the word *forearm* and options 2 and 3 both contain the word *forearm*. Identify the option that is unique. Option 2 is the only option that addresses the left arm. Options 1, 3, and 4 address the right arm.

Content Area: Fluid, Electrolyte, and Acid-Base Balance
Integrated Processes: Nursing Process: Implementation
Client Need: Physiological Integrity; Pharmacological and Parenteral Therapies
Cognitive Level: Application
Concept: Tissue Integrity

Chapter 22

Urinary Elimination

NURSING CONCEPTS

Cellular Regulation
Collaboration
Comfort
Communication
Elimination

Fluid and Electrolyte Balance
Growth and Development
Infection
Patient-Centered Care
Safety

KEY TERMS

Anuria—Absence of urine output or output less than 200 mL daily

Blood urea nitrogen (BUN)—Reflects the blood level of urea, which is a by-product of protein metabolism

Clean-catch urine specimen—Provides a urine specimen with minimal introduction of microorganisms from the perineal area

Continuous bladder irrigation—Constant instillation of a genitourinary (GU) irrigant (e.g., normal saline solution) into the bladder via a three-lumen urinary catheter to maintain tube patency when clots and debris are expected after urinary system surgery

Creatinine level—Amount of creatinine in blood, which is a by-product of muscle catabolism.

Credé maneuver—Application of manual pressure over the bladder to initiate voiding

Cystoscopy—Insertion of a fiberoptic instrument through the urethra to examine the bladder

Dysuria—Painful or difficulty voiding

Enuresis—Involuntary passage of urine when awake

Hematuria—Blood in the urine

Ileal conduit—Use of a segment of the ileum as a reservoir in which the ureters are implanted and the end is brought through the abdominal wall to form a stoma from which urine drains continuously

Incontinence (urinary)—Involuntary passage of urine

Intermittent bladder irrigation—Periodic instillation of a solution into the urinary bladder to administer medication, flush the bladder, or to maintain patency of a urinary retention catheter

Kock pouch—Pocket formed by connecting the ureters to a reservoir made from a portion of the ileum, which is connected to the skin and emptied via a surgically created nipple valve

Nephrostomy tube—Tube placed into the pelvis of a kidney to drain urine

Nocturia—Awakening at night to void

Nocturnal enuresis—Involuntary passage of urine when sleeping

Oliguria—Urine output less than 500 mL daily

Overflow incontinence—Involuntary frequent passage of a small amount of urine in conjunction with a distended bladder

Polyuria—Abnormally large volume of urine output daily

Pyuria—Pus in the urine

Residual urine—Amount of urine left in the bladder after voiding

Suprapubic tube—Catheter surgically inserted through a small incision above the symphysis pubis to drain urine from the bladder

Urinalysis—Physical, chemical, and microscopic examination of urine to aid in the medical diagnosis of disease

Urinary frequency—Voiding that occurs more often than usual

Urinary hesitancy—Delay in initiating voiding

Urinary retention—Accumulation of urine in the bladder

Urinary urgency—Strong desire to void

I. Structures and Functions of the Urinary System

The ability to produce and eliminate waste in the form of urine is essential for life. The mechanisms of glomerular filtration and the production of urine are complex and require an integration of factors, involving effective functioning of the kidneys, ureters, urinary bladder, and urethra. In addition, elimination of urine in the male is influenced when an enlarged prostate gland causes obstruction of the urethra. Knowledge of anatomy and physiology that influences urinary elimination is the basis for understanding how to best care for clients with urinary elimination problems (Fig. 22.1).

A. Kidneys
   1. Filter metabolic waste, excess ions, bacterial toxins, water-soluble drugs, drug metabolites, and water from the blood and excrete them as urine.
   2. Form urine by filtration, reabsorption, and secretion.
   3. Regulate blood volume, blood pressure (BP), fluid and electrolyte balance, and acid-base balance.
   4. Secrete rennin that causes the conversion of angiotensinogen to angiotensin I, which is subsequently converted to angiotensin II, which stimulates the nephrons to promote sodium and water retention.
   5. Secrete erythropoietin, which acts on the bone marrow to produce red blood cells.
   6. Converts part of calcidiol, a vitamin D metabolite, to calcitriol, the biologically active form of vitamin D, which travels in the blood to control the concentration of calcium and phosphate and promote growth and remodeling of bone.
   7. Produce a volume of filtrate in 1 minute (glomerular filtration rate [GFR]).

B. Ureters
   1. Transport urine produced by the kidneys to the bladder.
   2. Funnel shaped at the renal pelvis.
   3. Are 10 to 12 inches (25 to 30 cm) in length.
   4. Enter the bladder at the posterior corners of the bladder floor.

C. Bladder
   1. Receives urine from the ureters.
   2. Stores urine (600 to 1,000 mL) until it is eliminated.
   3. Urge to eliminate is stimulated by 200 to 250 mL of urine.

D. Urethra
   1. Transports urine from the bladder and semen from the prostate gland in males to outside the body.

MAKING THE CONNECTION

Glomerular Filtration Rate (GFR) and the Production of Urine

Each kidney contains over a million nephrons. Each nephron has six structures: glomerulus, Bowman's capsule, proximal convoluted tubule, loop of Henle, distal convoluted tubule, and collecting duct. Each structure has its own role in filtering the blood, removing metabolic waste, and controlling the excretion and retention of fluids and solutes based on the needs of the body. Approximately 1,200 mL of blood is routed through the kidneys every 60 seconds. The GFR is the amount of glomerular filtrate (a substance with a composition similar to plasma containing water, electrolytes, glucose, amino acids, and metabolic wastes) formed by the kidneys every minute. When the kidneys are diseased, the GFR decreases because the ability of the nephrons to produce urine is impaired and metabolic waste, toxins, excess ions, and water accumulate to toxic levels that, in turn, can cause damage to the cells of the body. A GFR below 60% indicates impaired kidney function and a decreased ability to produce urine. In addition, the appearance of clinical manifestations of impaired kidney function occur, such as an elevation in BP, presence of blood or protein in the urine, elevation of toxic substances in the blood (e.g., BUN and creatinine), and fluid retention, resulting in edema and weight gain.

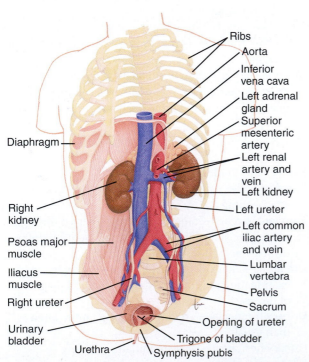

Fig 22.1 Structures of the urinary system. The organs of the urinary system include the kidneys, ureters, bladder, and urethra. (From Scanlon [2015]. *Essentials of anatomy and physiology*, 7th ed. Philadelphia: F. A. Davis Company, with permission.)

2. Is 1.5 to 2 inches long in a female and 8 inches in a male.
3. Opens at the urinary meatus.

E. Prostate gland (male)
1. Ring-like gland through which the urethra passes.
2. Contracts rhythmically and secretes prostatic fluid with male ejaculate, which has an alkaline pH that helps sperm to survive in the acid environment of the female reproductive tract and mobilizes sperm after ejaculation.

II. Urination

After urine is produced, it is stored in the bladder until voiding occurs. The ability to void requires an integrated operative functioning of the bladder, urethra, brain, spinal cord, and peripheral nerves supplying the bladder and urethra. In addition, a person must be able to recognize and respond to the urge to void. A nurse must understand the integrated operative function of urination and identify the expected characteristics of a client's urine and common problems associated with the urinary system to better meet a client's urinary elimination needs.

A. Process of urination
1. Urination (*voiding, micturition*) is the act of emptying the urinary bladder.
2. The detrusor muscle in the bladder contracts, urging stored urine through the relaxed internal urethral sphincter into the urethra, which results in a conscious urge to void.
3. The external urethral sphincter inhibits the release of urine until a person is ready to urinate; once ready, the brain signals the external sphincter to relax and further detrusor muscle contraction empties the bladder.

B. Urine characteristics
1. Color.
   a. Indicates the degree of concentration.
   b. Usually straw colored, pale to amber.
2. Clarity or turbidity.
   a. Usually transparent or translucent.
   b. Cloudiness indicates the presence of abnormal constituents.
3. Amount.
   a. Indicates the volume of production and excretion of urine.
   b. Usually 1,200 to 1,500 mL daily.

DID YOU KNOW?

The body produces approximately 60 mL of urine per hour. Because the bladder stimulates the urge to void every 200 to 250 mL, voiding typically occurs every 3 to 6 hours. In addition, the volume of urinary output should be close to that of fluid intake.

4. Odor.
   a. Is aromatic.
   b. Can indicate the presence of certain foods and constituents related to infection.
5. Specific gravity.
   a. Reflects the kidneys' ability to concentrate urine.
   b. Usually 1.001 to 1.029.
6. pH.
   a. Reflects the kidneys' ability to maintain a balanced hydrogen ion concentration in the blood.
   b. Usually between 4.6 and 8; average is 6.
7. Protein.
   a. Exists in molecules that generally are too large to leak into the glomerular filtrate, but leakage can occur in the presence of glomerular damage or impaired tubular reabsorption.
   b. A random urine specimen for protein more than 6 mg/dL when tested with a dipstick indicates renal disease.
   c. The amount of protein in a 24-hour specimen indicates the severity of kidney disease; an expected 24-hour result is 25 to 150 mg.

C. Abnormal characteristics of urine and their implications. (See Table 22.1.)

III. Factors Affecting Urinary Function

Age, psychosociocultural influences, nutrition, hydration, activity, position, mobility, medical problems, surgical and diagnostic procedures, ability to communicate, and medications can dramatically affect urinary function. Understanding these factors will aid nurses in assessing clients, maintaining a nonjudgmental attitude when working with diverse individuals, and planning individualized nursing care.

A. Developmental
1. Infants.
   a. Generally produce 8 to 10 wet diapers daily.
   b. Develop voluntary control at 18 to 24 months of age.
2. Children: May experience involuntary passage of urine when awake (**enuresis**) or when sleeping (**nocturnal enuresis**).
3. Older adults.
   a. Experience a decline in urinary system function.
   b. Are less able to filter waste and maintain acid-base and fluid and electrolyte balance.
   c. Experience a loss of bladder tone, contributing to urgency, frequency, and incomplete emptying of the bladder.
   d. Older women: Experience additional weakening of pelvic floor muscles due to childbearing and genitourinary atrophy.

Table 22.1 Abnormal Characteristics of Urine and Their Implications

Characteristic	Implication
Color	
Dark amber.	Concentrated urine. Related to decreased fluid intake or excessive fluid loss.
Clear color.	Dilute urine. Related to excessive fluid intake.
Red, pink, or rusty brown.	Related to blood cells in the urine *(hematuria)*.
Dark orange.	Related to medication use. For example: Rifampin, an antibiotic for tuberculosis, can turn urine reddish orange; metronidazole (Flagyl), an antibiotic for a wide range of infections, can turn urine dark brown; indomethacin (Indocin) for arthritis can turn urine blue or green.
Clarity	
Cloudiness in fresh specimen.	Indicates presence of mucus, bacteria, white blood cells, pus, prostatic fluid, or products of vaginal discharge.
Amount	
Urine output less than 30 mL/hr in absence of obstruction.	Generally indicates a decrease in circulation to the kidneys.
Excessive urine output beyond fluid intake.	Associated with diuretic therapy, inadequate level of antidiuretic hormone, and liquids that increase the secretion of urine, such as alcohol, caffeine, tea, and coffee.
Odor	
Ammonia-like or fetid odor.	Indicates infection.
Sweet odor.	Indicates an elevated glucose content.
Syrup odor.	Indicates a congenital metabolic disorder.
Other characteristic odors.	Indicates intake of certain foods that can cause characteristic odors (e.g., garlic, asparagus, and onions).
Specific Gravity	
More than 1.029.	Indicates concentrated urine due to decreased fluid intake, dehydration after excess fluid loss, or kidney disease.
Less than 1.001.	Indicates dilute urine usually due to increased fluid intake.
pH	
Less than 4.5 (acidic).	Associated with acidosis, starvation, and diarrhea. Associated with a diet high in protein foods or cranberry juice.
More than 8 (alkaline).	Associated with alkalosis and UTI. Associated with a high intake of fruits and vegetables (e.g., vegetarian diet).
Other Findings	
Presence of protein: More than 8 mg/dL.	Associated with renal disease, diabetic disease of the kidney, toxemia of pregnancy, inflammation of the glomeruli *(glomerulonephritis)*, and degenerative changes in the kidneys, especially in the renal tubules *(nephrosis)*.
Presence of glucose.	Associated with undiagnosed or uncontrolled diabetes.
Presence of ketone bodies, the end-products of fatty acid breakdown.	Associated with diabetes, fasting/starvation, high-protein diet, vomiting, and being on nothing-by-mouth without nutritional support.
Hemoglobin: Red blood cells via microscopic exam more than 5/higher power field (hpf).	Associated with bleeding from the urinary tract, UTI, glomerulonephritis, inflammation of the kidney and renal pelvis *(pyelonephritis)*, trauma, kidney stones *(nephrolithiasis)*, or hemolytic reactions.

e. Older men: May experience an enlarged prostate, causing urine leakage, awakening at night to void *(nocturia)*, and urine retention.

B. Psychosociocultural

1. Lack of privacy or an unfamiliar environment may lead to an inability to void in public (bashful bladder).

2. Loss of dignity related to toileting activities in a health-care environment, especially if the client is catheterized, can cause emotional distress.

3. Cultural influences may cause a person to insist on a caregiver of the same gender to provide toileting assistance.

4. Muslims use the left hand for toileting activities and the right hand for eating and praying.

C. Nutrition and hydration
1. As fluid intake increases, a corresponding increase in urine output occurs; as fluid intake decreases, a corresponding decrease in urine output occurs.
2. Some substances increase urine production (e.g., coffee, tea, cola, alcohol, and chocolate) by inhibiting the release of antidiuretic hormone.
3. Sodium intake produces water retention, causing decreased urine production.

D. Activity and position
1. Exercise maintains detrusor and pelvic floor muscle tone, which helps the bladder to empty completely.
2. Heavy exercise can precipitate dehydration via sweating, causing the kidneys to retain water, reducing urine output.
3. Gravity assists in the flow of urine and the ability to empty the bladder completely; typically, the sitting position is best for women and the standing position is best for men.
4. The bladder may not empty completely when on a bed pan or when using a urinal while lying flat; the side-lying position may facilitate urination for men who are on bedrest.

E. Medications and anesthetic agents
1. Many classifications of drugs can damage kidney cells (nephrotoxic) or cause urinary retention, such as antispasmodics, antihistamines, tricyclic antidepressants, anticholinergics, antihypertensives, antiparkinsonism drugs, and chemotherapeutic agents for cancer.
2. Diuretics cause an increase in urine production; if urine output is excessive in relation to fluid intake, dehydration occurs; urine output decreases when a client is dehydrated.
3. Some drugs change the color of urine; for example, phenazopyridine causes the urine to appear reddish orange.
4. Anesthetic agents generally decrease BP and GFR, causing a decrease in urine production; spinal anesthesia reduces the perception of the need to void, leading to bladder distention.

F. Physiological problems
1. Problems can interfere with the production of urine; for example, cardiovascular and metabolic disorders that reduce blood flow through the kidneys (e.g., hypertension, heart failure, shock, and diabetes mellitus).
2. Problems can impair the nervous system that innervates the urinary system; for example, brain attack (stroke) or spinal cord injury.
3. Problems can interfere with the flow of urine; for example, calculi and enlargement of the prostate gland.

4. Problems can cause inflammation of the structures of the urinary system; for example, urinary tract infection (UTI).
5. Impaired cognition (e.g., delirium, dementia) or a mental health problem may alter a person's perception of the need to void.

G. Surgical and diagnostic procedures
1. Rectal, vaginal, and pubic surgery and childbirth can result in trauma to and edema of local tissues, causing pressure on the structures of the urinary system and loss of pelvic floor muscle control.
2. Some surgical procedures (e.g., hysterectomy, transurethral resection of the prostate) require insertion of a temporary indwelling urinary catheter postoperatively.
3. Insertion of a fiberoptic instrument (cystoscope) through the urethra to examine the bladder (**cystoscopy**) can cause urethral swelling, obstructing urinary excretion.

H. Communication or mobility problems
1. An inability to communicate the need to void can result in what appears to others to be an episode of incontinence when in fact the client cannot indicate personal needs to others.
2. An inability to engage in toileting activities, such as undressing, can result in episodes of urination before reaching a toilet.
3. An inability to be mobile, such as with clients who are bed- or chair-bound, may prevent a client from obtaining assistance in time to make it to the bathroom.

IV. Assessment of the Urinary System

The first step of the nursing process is assessment. When collecting information relative to a client's urinary function, the nurse obtains a client history, performs a physical assessment, and assesses the volume and characteristics of urine. Data collected from these assessments help determine whether the client's urinary system is functioning adequately or further action is required by a nurse or the primary health-care provider.

A. Obtain a health history
1. Identify any change in urination habits or urine characteristics.
2. Ask questions about the presence of clinical manifestations that indicate infection.
   a. **Urinary urgency** is a strong desire to void.
   b. **Urinary frequency** is voiding that occurs more often than usual.
   c. **Dysuria** is painful or difficulty voiding.
   d. **Hematuria** is blood in the urine.
3. Ask questions about the clinical manifestations of urine flow.
   a. **Urinary hesitancy** is a delay in initiating voiding.

b. **Nocturia** is the awakening at night to void.

c. **Overflow incontinence** is the involuntary frequent passage of a small amount of urine in conjunction with a distended bladder.

d. **Urinary incontinence** is the involuntary passage of urine.

4. Ask about daily urine volume.

a. **Oliguria** is when urine output is less than 500 mL daily (oliguria).

b. **Polyuria** is an abnormally large volume of urine output daily.

c. **Anuria** is the absence of urine output or urine output of less than 100 mL daily.

5. Assess for flank pain that indicates a problem with the kidneys.

6. Identify a history of urinary system problems (e.g., infection, kidney or bladder problems, urinary tract surgery or urinary system diagnostic procedures or tests).

7. Assess lifestyle factors that can affect the urinary system (e.g., daily caffeine and fluid intake, smoking history, management of activities of daily living, emotional stress, and access to a bathroom).

8. Identify any medications the client is currently taking that may impact the urinary system.

9. Ask how long the client has been experiencing any identified problems; how the client manages the problem; and what has been done medically.

B. Perform a physical assessment

1. Assess the characteristics of urine. (See "Urine Characteristics" in this chapter.)

2. Measure intake and output (I&O).

3. Assess for weight gain and edema.

4. Palpate the suprapubic area for bladder distention if the client is unable to void.

a. **Urinary retention** is the accumulation of urine in the bladder; more than 500 mL of urine produces a bulge in the central lower abdomen just above the symphysis pubis when the client is in the supine position.

b. May be difficult to identify in an obese client.

5. Use a bladder ultrasonic scanner to assess for the amount of urine retained in the bladder after voiding (**residual urine**); this assessment is more objective than palpation and percussion.

6. Auscultate the abdominal aorta and renal arteries for an adventitious sound of arterial blood flow; presence indicates a vascular problem.

7. Assess perineal skin integrity.

a. Assess for presence of a perineal rash with macerated skin (ammonia contact dermatitis), which may extend to the thighs and usually is caused by urinary incontinence.

b. Assess for the presence of a perineal red rash with satellite lesions, which may extend to the thighs and is related to a fungal infection (*Candida* rash).

8. Assess the vaginal vault for clinical manifestations of atrophic vaginitis (e.g., dry, thin mucosa; tenderness; pallor; easy bleeding).

9. Assess the client's mental status, mobility, dexterity, and visual acuity to determine ability to self-toilet.

10. Assess for the presence of a urinary diversion.

V. Urinary System Diagnostic Tests and Related Nursing Care

A history and physical may need to be supplemented with data collected via diagnostic tests prescribed by the primary health-care provider. Some tests are essential to arrive at a medical diagnosis (e.g., urine culture and sensitivity, cystoscopy), whereas others are employed to identify specific information about a client's urinary function (e.g., blood chemistry tests, urodynamic studies). Nurses must understand these tests because some of them are performed by the nurse, some require specific nursing interventions before and after the test, and all of them require client teaching.

A. Urine specimens

1. Commonalities of nursing care when collecting a urine specimen.

a. Wash your hands and collect the necessary equipment.

b. Explain the procedure to the client.

c. Wear clean gloves to prevent exposure to the client's body fluids.

2. *Urinalysis.*

a. A **urinalysis** is the physical, chemical, and microscopic examination of urine to aid in the medical diagnosis.

b. Macroscopic and microscopic analysis of urine for normal and abnormal constituents (physical and chemical); includes color, turbidity, pH, specific gravity, protein, glucose, ketones, red blood cells, white blood cells, bacteria/yeast, and casts (precipitation of protein substances).

c. Specific nursing care.

(1) Instruct the client to void into a clean bed pan, urinal, or specimen hat positioned under the toilet seat if transferring 30 mL of urine to a traditional clean urine specimen cup.

(2) Teach to avoid contaminating the specimen with feces, toilet tissue, or menstrual blood; if the client is menstruating, note it on the laboratory slip.

(3) For infants, wash the genital area, allow the area to dry, and then place a collection device over the infant's genital area.

(4) Move urine to a transfer container if a bed-pan, urinal, or hat is used to collect urine.
  (a) Use a urine transfer "straw" with adaptor to transfer the specimen to an evacuated urine collection tube.
  (b) Pour 30 mL into a traditional specimen container carefully.
(5) If a urine collection container with an integrated port in the lid was used to collect the urine, insert a collection tube into the special access port. The closed system automatically transfers the urine to the collection tube via a vacuum.
(6) Label the container (specimen cup or collection tube) with the client's name, date, and time of collection according to agency policy and place it in a biohazardous bag to reduce the transmission of infection.
(7) Assist the client with perineal and hand hygiene.
(8) Clean or dispose of supplies.
(9) Remove gloves and then wash hands.
(10) Document the procedure in the client's clinical record.
(11) Send the specimen to the laboratory with the appropriate laboratory slip within 15 minutes; place the specimen in a specimen refrigerator if a delay occurs.

3. *Clean-catch (midstream) specimen.*
  a. A **clean-catch urine specimen** provides a specimen with minimal introduction of microorganisms from the perineal area.
  b. Specific nursing care.
    (1) Maintain sterility of the urine specimen cup by turning the inside of the lid of the cup toward the ceiling when placing it on a clean surface, avoiding touching the perineum with the cup, and closing the lid without touching the inside of the cup or lid.
    (2) Collect urine or teach the client how to collect the urine.
      (a) For males: Retract the foreskin to expose the urinary meatus if the client is uncircumcised; clean the urinary meatus in a circular motion with three different swabs; have the client begin voiding; after some urine is voided, position the sterile container under the stream and collect the specimen; allow the client to finish voiding; return the foreskin to the expected position if necessary; and close the container without contaminating the inside of the cup or lid.
      (b) For females: Separate the labia minora and cleanse the area from the pubis to the rectum with three different swabs; have the client begin to void while keeping the labia separated; allow urine to flow and then hold the sterile specimen cup under the stream and collect the specimen; remove the container; release the hand from the labia; allow the client to finish voiding; and close the container without contaminating the inside of the cup or lid.

4. *Twenty-four-hour urine specimen.*
  a. Measures kidneys' excretion of substances, such as protein, uric acid, creatinine, selected hormones, urobilinogen, and other substances, that the body does not excrete at an even rate throughout the day.
  b. Specific nursing care.
    (1) Explain the need to collect all urine for the next 24 hours.
    (2) Post reminders for the client and staff on the bathroom door if permitted by policy.
    (3) Check with the laboratory whether the specimen container has a preservative or needs to be kept in a basin of ice.
    (4) Begin by having the client void, discard this urine, and record the time.
    (5) Collect all voided urine during the next 24 hours.
    (6) Have the client void at the end of the 24 hours and add this urine to the container.

🛑 (7) If the client fails to collect a voiding, have the client empty the bladder and begin the 24 hours again.

5. *Culture and sensitivity.*
  a. Identifies the causative microorganism and the most effective antibiotic to eradicate the microorganism; takes 24 to 72 hours for organisms to multiply and be identified.
  b. Specific nursing care.
    (1) Collect a clean-catch urine specimen or a specimen from a urinary catheter.
    (2) Maintain surgical asepsis to prevent contamination of the specimen.

🛑 (3) Obtain the urine specimen before the client takes a prescribed antibiotic.

6. *Dipstick testing of urine.*
  a. Provides a quick, bedside assessment of specific constituents of urine (e.g., pH, specific gravity, protein, glucose, ketones, and occult blood).
  b. Specific nursing care.
    (1) Ensure that the correct strip is used and that it has not expired.

(2) Dip the test strip into the urine, tap the strip to dislodge excess urine, and place the strip horizontally across the top of the urine cup to prevent urine from flowing down the strip or collecting at one site on the strip, causing inaccurate results.

(3) Begin timing according to the manufacturer's directions and at the correct time; compare the results to the color chart on the dipstick bottle.

(4) Document the results in the client's clinical record and report any abnormalities to the primary health-care provider.

7. *Collecting a urine specimen from a urinary catheter.*

a. Specific nursing care when collecting a specimen via a single-lumen catheter.

(1) Insert a single-lumen urinary catheter into the bladder following all the principles associated with surgical asepsis. (See "Inserting a Urinary Catheter" in this chapter.)

(2) Collect the specimen and then immediately remove the catheter.

b. Specific nursing care when collecting a specimen from an indwelling urinary catheter (Fig. 22.2).

(1) Ensure that the drainage tube is free from urine and then clamp it below the level of the specimen port on the drainage tubing for 15 to 30 minutes, allowing fresh urine to collect.

(2) Wash your hands and don clean gloves.

Fig 22.2 Obtaining a specimen from an indwelling urinary catheter. (From Burton and Ludwig [2015]. *Fundamentals of nursing care: Concepts, connections & skills,* 2nd ed. Philadelphia: F. A. Davis Company, with permission.)

(3) Clean the specimen port with an alcohol swab.

(4) Insert the needle of a sterile syringe into the port and aspirate the required amount of urine.

(5) Transfer the specimen to a sterile specimen cup.

(6) Discard the needle and syringe into a sharps disposal container.

(7) Close the lid tightly on the specimen cup without contaminating the inside of the cup or lid. Transfer the urine to a collection tube if it is the protocol of the agency.

🛑 (8) Maintain the closed drainage system; never separate the catheter from the drainage tubing to collect a specimen because it creates a portal of entry for microorganisms, and never collect a specimen from the collection bag because the urine is not fresh.

🛑 (9) Remove the clamp from the drainage tubing.

B. Blood chemistry tests

1. *Blood urea nitrogen (BUN).*

a. **Blood urea nitrogen** reflects the level of urea nitrogen, a by-product of protein metabolism, in blood.

b. Expected level is 10 to 20 mg/dL.

c. Increased levels.

(1) Occur in kidney disease because urea excretion is decreased.

(2) Can also occur due to digested blood from gastrointestinal (GI) bleeding, dehydration, high-protein diet, steroids, strenuous activity, and nephrotoxic drugs.

d. Decreased levels.

(1) Generally indicate overhydration.

(2) Can also be caused by severe liver damage, a low-protein diet, malnutrition, phenothiazine medications, and IV glucose without protein intake.

e. Specific nursing care.

(1) Keep the client on nothing-by-mouth (NPO) status for 8 hours.

(2) Avoid hemolysis of the specimen (e.g., avoid shaking the specimen tube and send the specimen to the lab immediately).

(3) Identify drugs the client is taking that may increase BUN (e.g., antibiotics, diuretics, antihypertensives, nephrotoxic drugs, sulfonamides, morphine, and salicylates).

2. *Creatinine level.*

a. **Creatinine level** reflects the level of creatinine, a by-product of muscle catabolism, in blood.

b. Expected level is 0.5 to 1.5 mg/dL.

c. More than 2.5 mg/dL is indicative of kidney impairment.

d. Is more reliable than BUN in determining kidney function because the level is not affected by diet or fluid intake.

e. Specific nursing care.

   (1) Instruct the client to avoid eating red meat the night before the test.

   (2) Identify drugs that the client is taking that may increase levels (e.g., cefazolin [Ancef], methyldopa [Aldomet], cephalothin [Keflin], gentamicin, ascorbic acid, barbiturates, and lithium).

C. Intravenous pyelogram (IVP)

1. Radiopaque dye injected intravenously concentrates in urine.

2. Facilitates x-ray visualization of kidneys, ureters, and bladder.

3. Is risky when a client has kidney failure because it requires use of a dye that can stress the kidneys.

4. Specific nursing care.

  a. Obtain an informed consent.

  b. Explain that the client may experience a warm, flushed sensation or a salty taste when the dye is injected.

  c. Explain that it takes about 1 hour to complete; x-ray films are taken at various intervals as the dye moves through the urinary system.

  d. Ensure that an enema or a laxative is taken before the procedure, as prescribed, to ensure that stool and gas do not interfere with the test.

  e. Explain food and fluid restrictions if prescribed.

  f. Encourage the client to void before the examination.

  g. Encourage increased fluid intake after the procedure to facilitate excretion of the contrast/radioactive substance.

  h. Monitor I&O after the procedure to assess kidney function.

  i. Assess for reactions to the contrast media (e.g., rash, nausea, and hives) during and after the test.

DID YOU KNOW?

People who are allergic to shellfish generally are allergic to the protein it contains rather than iodine. People who are allergic to shellfish are at a no greater risk of an allergic reaction to the contrast dye than someone who is not allergic to shellfish.

D. Ultrasound tests

1. Noninvasive tests using high-frequency sound waves to create an image of the urinary system. Conducted by a certified ultrasound technician.

2. Can identify the amount of urine in the bladder, masses, cysts, edema, and stones.

3. Safe for clients with kidney failure because they do not require dye.

4. Commonalities of nursing care for clients having ultrasound tests.

  a. Explain the test, including the fact that it will be painless.

  b. Provide privacy.

  c. Explain that a conductive gel is applied to the skin and that a transducer is moved smoothly back and forth over the gelled site while a machine visualizes structures of the urinary system.

  d. Provide hygiene after the test to remove the conductive gel.

5. Bladder ultrasound scan (Fig. 22.3).

  a. Noninvasive test using sound waves to detect the amount of urine in the bladder.

  b. Provides data for determining the need for catheterization.

  c. Can be done at the bedside by trained caregivers, including nurses educated in this procedure.

  d. Specific nursing care.

    (1) Place the client in the supine position.

    (2) Expose only the lower abdomen and suprapubic area.

    (3) Turn the scan device on to female or male; use male if the client had a hysterectomy.

    (4) Use an ultrasound gel pad or 5 mL of conducting gel to improve ultrasound conduction.

    (5) Place the scan head approximately 1.5 inches (4 cm) above the pubic bone midline below the umbilicus (symphysis pubis), aiming the scan head toward the client's coccyx.

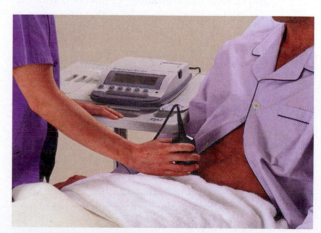

Fig 22.3 Bladder ultrasound scanner. (From Williams and Hopper [2015]. *Understanding medical surgical nursing*, 5th ed. Philadelphia: F. A. Davis Company, with permission.)

(6) Press the scan head button, wait until it beeps, and release the button.

(7) Look for bladder volume to be displayed.

(8) Repeat the measurement because several measurements ensure accuracy.

(9) Clean the client's abdomen and suprapubic area after the procedure to remove conducting gel.

(10) Clean the scan head with isopropyl alcohol.

(11) Wash your hands.

(12) Document the results and client responses in the client's clinical record.

E. Cystoscopy

1. Insertion of a fiberoptic tube through the urethra to directly visualize the inside of the bladder (*cystoscopy*) to identify stones, lesions, tumors, irritation, or structural problems.

2. Allows specialized instruments to be passed through the tube to take a biopsy or remove small stones or to provide local treatment.

3. Nursing care.

a. Obtain a signed consent form.

b. Explain that urine may be pink initially after the procedure because of slight bleeding due to irritation of the mucous membranes of the urinary tract.

c. Encourage increased fluid intake before and after the procedure.

d. Administer antibiotics before and after procedure if prescribed; increasing evidence indicates antibiotics are not necessary for most clients.

e. Maintain bed rest initially after the procedure because orthostatic hypotension may occur.

f. Assess I&O after the procedure because urinary retention may occur.

g. Assess for hematuria, dysuria, bladder spasms, and clinical manifestations of infection after the test. Report these responses to the primary health-care provider.

F. Urodynamic studies

1. Measure stored urine, its flow and elimination in the lower urinary tract, bladder and urethra pressure, and muscle activity.

2. Include the use of uroflowmetry, cystometrograms, and urethra pressure profile measuring devices.

3. Nursing care.

a. Encourage the client to drink fluid so that the bladder is full before the test.

b. Explain to the client that a catheter will be inserted through the urethra into the bladder as part of the test.

c. Encourage the client to drink 8 to 10 glasses of fluid after the test to flush the urinary structures; administer STAT antibiotic if prescribed.

d. Teach the client clinical manifestations of UTI and instruct the client to notify the primary health-care provider if any occur.

VI. Nursing Care to Assist Clients With Urinary Elimination

Nursing interventions related to the urinary system involve activities concerning the assessment of a client's urinary status, collection of specimens for diagnostic tests, promotion of efficient urinary functioning, and the prevention and treatment of urinary problems. Many of these interventions are independent functions of the nurse; however, some require a primary health-care provider's prescription. Nurses must have a thorough understanding of when and how to implement these interventions.

A. Independent nursing interventions

1. Assess the client's urinary functioning and the amount and characteristics of urinary output. (See "Assessment of the Urinary System" in this chapter.)

2. Encourage the client to follow consistent daily routines.

3. Encourage the client to engage in regular exercise to help maintain pelvic floor and bladder muscle tone.

4. Encourage the client to drink 8 to 10 glasses of fluid daily.

a. Provide hourly goals for intake.

b. Keep fluids in easy reach.

c. Provide fluids that the client prefers.

5. Assist the client with toileting as soon as the need to void is indicated by the client.

6. Provide privacy during toileting.

7. Encourage the client to void (e.g., when the urge to void is felt; on awakening, after meals, and at bedtime; every 2 hours when awake).

8. Encourage the client to completely empty the bladder when voiding to prevent urinary stasis.

9. Assist with positioning.

a. Female: Sitting.

b. Male: Standing or side lying.

10. Provide a commode at the bedside for clients who are unable to ambulate to a bathroom.

11. Assist bed-bound clients to use a bedpan; remove the bedpan as soon as the client is done voiding; provide perineal care. (See Fig. 23.6 in Chapter 23, Bowel Elimination.)

12. Promote urination.

a. Put the client's hands in warm water.

b. Turn on a sink faucet so that the client can hear the sound of running water.

c. Pour warm water over the client's perineum.

d. Place a warm moist wash cloth over the client's perineum.

e. Apply manual pressure over the client's bladder (**Credé maneuver**).

13. Teach the client techniques to prevent UTIs. (See "Urinary Tract Infection" in this chapter.)

14. Provide nursing care for clients who are incontinent of urine. (See "Urinary Incontinence" in this chapter.)

15. Teach the client about prescribed diagnostic tests and the interventions to self-perform in relation to various tests.

B. Dependent nursing interventions

1. Implement care that prepares a client for a test that requires a prescription (e.g., NPO, medications, enema).

2. Obtain urine specimens for prescribed diagnostic tests. (See "Urinary System Diagnostic Tests and Related Nursing Care" in this chapter.)

3. Insert and maintain urinary catheters as prescribed. (See "Urinary Catheters" in this chapter.)

4. Provide nursing care for clients with a urinary diversion. (See "Nursing Care for Clients With a Urinary Diversion" in this chapter.)

5. Administer prescribed kidney-specific anti-infectives, urinary antispasmodics, and estrogen; teach the client information about the medications and self-administration of the medication

regimen. (See "Medications That Affect the Urinary System" in this chapter.)

VII. Nursing Care for Clients With Urinary Elimination Problems

Urinary incontinence, UTI, nocturnal enuresis, and urinary retention are common problems related to the urinary system. It is essential that nurses understand the clinical manifestations, precipitating factors, and nursing care associated with each problem. Nursing interventions include activities concerned with promotion of efficient urinary functioning and the prevention and treatment of urinary problems. Many of these interventions are independent functions of the nurse; however, some require a primary health-care provider's prescription or a standing protocol.

A. Urinary incontinence

1. Overview.

a. **Urinary incontinence** is the inability to control the passage of urine.

b. May be acute and reversible (e.g., when due to infection or medication side effect) or chronic and nonreversible (e.g., when due to neurological problems, such as spinal cord injury).

2. Clinical manifestations. (See Table 22.2 for types, clinical manifestations, and precipitating factors of urinary incontinence.)

Table 22.2 Types of Urinary Incontinence

Type of Incontinence	Clinical Manifestations	Precipitating Factors
Total Continuous and unpredictable passage of urine.	• Lack of awareness of bladder filling. • Nocturia. • Absence of bladder contraction or distention.	• Neurological dysfunction causing micturition at unpredictable times. • Diseases or trauma affecting the spinal cord nerves.
Urge Passage of urine after a strong need to void.	• Urgency and frequency more often than every 2 hours. • Voiding <100 mL at each voiding. • Bladder spasms. • Nocturia.	• Overactive bladder tone. • Decreased bladder capacity. • Bladder spasms. • Bladder infection. • Intake of irritating fluids or foods, such as caffeine or alcohol. • History of conditions such as pelvic inflammatory disease, genitourinary atrophy; abdominal surgery; presence of an indwelling urinary catheter.
Stress Passage of urine when intra-abdominal pressure increases.	• Urgency or frequency more often than every 2 hours. • Precipitated by a behavior that increases intra-abdominal pressure. • Passage of <50 mL of urine (dribbling) with each episode of incontinence.	• Activities that increase intra-abdominal pressure, such as exercise, laughing, coughing, sneezing, bending, and lifting. • Degenerative changes in pelvic muscles and structural supports due to pregnancy, childbirth, aging, or chronic constipation. • Incompetent bladder outlet. • Overdistention between voidings. • Obesity.

Continued

Table 22.2 Types of Urinary Incontinence—cont'd

Type of Incontinence	Clinical Manifestations	Precipitating Factors
Overflow Passage of urine related to a distended bladder.	• Frequent loss of small amounts of urine.	• Urinary retention. • Fecal impaction. • Neurological disorders. • Prostate enlargement.
Reflex Passage of urine occurring at approximate predictable times when a certain bladder volume is achieved.	• Absence of urge or sense of bladder fullness. • Inability to inhibit or initiate urine flow voluntarily. • Absence of voiding sensation.	• Spinal cord lesion interfering with messages above the level of the sacral reflex arc. • Inflammation of the bladder. • Radical pelvic surgery.
Transient Short-term incontinence precipitated by a situation that, once addressed, will resolve the incontinence spontaneously.	• With diuretics: Urgency, frequency, and large urine volume. • With UTI: Burning on urination, dysuria, bladder spasms, pyuria, hematuria, foul odor to urine, chills, fever, back pain, nausea, and vomiting.	• Medications, such as diuretics. • UTI.
Functional Inability of a usually continent person to reach the bathroom or remove clothing in time to prevent incontinence.	• Incontinent of urine before being able to void in a bathroom.	• Impaired lower extremities that interfere with the ability to get to a bathroom or transfer to a toilet. • Impaired mobility of the hands to manage clothing, such as buttons and zippers. • Fatigue or activity intolerance that interferes with the ability to tolerate toileting activities. • Dependence on another to help with transfer to the bathroom or removal of clothing; often a problem in an institutional setting. • Lack of access to a bathroom, such as a shared bathroom or long distance to the bathroom.

3. Commonalities of nursing care for clients with urinary incontinence.
   a. Independent nursing care.
      (1) Provide perineal care immediately after voiding or on a regular schedule.
      (2) Encourage the use of/or apply an appropriate incontinence device (e.g., pads, Depends, external condom catheter); avoid the use of the word "diaper."
      (3) Apply an external condom catheter for a male client.
         (a) Provide perineal care; rinse and dry thoroughly.
         (b) Avoid lubricants or the catheter will slide off.
         (c) Measure the circumference of the penis to ensure correct catheter size.
         (d) Hold the penis and place the condom over and beyond the glans penis (Fig. 22.4A); unroll the condom the full length of the penis, leaving 1 to 2 inches between the glans penis and drainage tubing of the catheter (Fig. 22.4B).
         (e) Do not retract the foreskin if the client is uncircumcised.
         (f) Secure the condom: For a condom with internal adhesive, grasp the penis and gently compress so the entire condom comes into contact with the penile shaft; for a condom with an external adhesive strip, wrap the strip in a spiral along the shaft but do not overlap the ends or use surgical tape because these actions can act as a tourniquet.
         (g) Ensure that the condom is not twisted to prevent trauma (e.g., obstruction of urine flow, irritation at meatus, skin breakdown).
         (h) Secure the catheter to the thigh to prevent tissue trauma.
      (4) Encourage necessary lifestyle changes, such as cessation of smoking, weight management, and dietary changes.
      (5) Assess for clinical manifestations of a vaginal infection or UTI, such as hematuria, dysuria, and vaginal irritation.

Fig 22.4 Condom catheter. (A) Placing a condom catheter over and beyond the glans penis. (B) Leaving 1 to 2 inches between the glans penis and drainage tubing. (From Wilkinson and Treas [2016]. *Fundamentals of nursing,* Vol. 2, 3rd ed. Philadelphia: F. A. Davis Company, with permission.)

    b. Dependent nursing care.
      (1) Apply a perineal skin barrier as per agency protocol.
      (2) Administer medications as prescribed.
      (3) Teach the client how to use a prescribed anti-incontinence device (e.g., intravaginal support [pessary], penis clamp, internal urethral meatus plug).
  4. Specific nursing care for clients with stress and/or urge incontinence.
    a. Teach the client to avoid constipation: Increase fluid intake, eat high-fiber foods, and increase activity.
    b. Teach the client to limit activities that increase intra-abdominal pressure (e.g., high-impact exercises, lifting, bending).
    c. Encourage the client to perform Kegel exercises to strengthen the pelvic floor.
      (1) Tighten the pelvic muscles as if to stop urination or passing of gas.
      (2) Hold for 5 to 10 seconds and then rest 5 to 10 seconds.
      (3) Repeat two to four times a day with 15 repetitions per session.

      (4) Explain to the client that it may take 6 to 12 months for positive results.
    d. Teach vaginal weight training to females if prescribed.
      (1) Insert a small cone-shaped weight into the vagina and contract the pelvic floor muscles to keep it in place.
      (2) Keep the cone-shaped weight in the vagina for 15 minutes twice a day.
    e. Employ a bladder retraining program, particularly for clients with urge incontinence (e.g., using a voiding diary; scheduling regular times for voiding; using distraction and relaxation techniques to relax the detrusor muscle, thereby increasing bladder capacity).
    f. Administer prescribed medications to relax the detrusor muscle and increase bladder capacity (e.g., anticholinergics, smooth-muscle relaxants, calcium channel blockers, antidepressants) and estrogen for women who have genital atrophy.
  5. Specific nursing care for clients with overflow incontinence.
    a. Identify distension of the urinary bladder: Bladder scan indicates urinary volume; palpation reveals smooth, round, tense mass in suprapubic area.
    b. Insert a single-lumen or indwelling urinary catheter if prescribed.
  6. Specific nursing care for clients with reflex incontinence.
    a. Precipitate urination: Stroke inner thigh, pull on pubic hair.
    b. Insert a single-lumen urinary catheter if prescribed.
    c. Administer prescribed medications to relax the urinary sphincter such as diazepam (Valium).
  7. Specific nursing care for clients with functional incontinence.
    a. Teach the client to schedule routine toileting, especially 15 minutes before the identified pattern of incontinence.
    b. Teach the client methods to facilitate toileting: Velcro clothing closures, bedside commode or urinal, gait and strength training, raised toilet seat, and bathroom grab bars.
B. Urinary tract infection
  1. Overview.
    a. Urinary tract infection occurs when there is an invasion of the bladder by bacteria, viruses, or fungi; *Escherichia coli,* which normally resides in the colon, most commonly invades the urinary tract.
    b. May occur in the urethra *(urethritis),* bladder *(cystitis),* ureters, kidneys *(pyelonephritis).*

2. Clinical manifestations.
   a. Burning on urination (**dysuria**).
   b. Bladder spasms or back pain.
   c. Frequency.
   d. Hematuria.
   e. Chills; fever.
   f. Pus in the urine *(pyuria)*.
   g. Foul odor to urine.
   h. Positive urine culture.
3. Precipitating factors.
   a. Sexual activity; use of spermicidal contraceptive gel.
   b. Dryness of the mucosa and decrease in normal flora due to aging.
   c. Presence of an indwelling urinary catheter.
   d. Illnesses that affect the kidneys (e.g., diabetes mellitus, renal calculi).
   e. Conditions that cause urinary stasis (e.g., prostate gland enlargement, hypotonic bladder).
4. Independent nursing care.
   a. Teach the client clinical manifestations of UTI.
   b. Provide perineal care immediately after voiding or on a regular schedule.
   c. Encourage the use of or apply an incontinence device (e.g., pads, Depends, external condom catheter).
   d. Teach the client preventative measures.
      (1) Void every 2 to 4 hours, not just in response to the urge.
      (2) Avoid food and beverages that can irritate the bladder (e.g., citrus fruits, caffeinated beverages, alcohol, and some spices).
      (3) For women: Wear cotton underwear; void before and after intercourse; avoid bubble and baking soda baths, perineal deodorant sprays, and douches.
      (4) Drink at least 24 oz of cranberry juice daily.
5. Dependent nursing care.
   🛑 a. Collect a urine specimen before initiating antibiotic therapy.

   b. Apply a topical barrier to maintain skin integrity per agency protocol.
   c. Administer prescribed medications.
      (1) Antibiotics, such as cephalexin (Keflex), nitrofurantoin (Macrobid), and sulfonamides (e.g., Bactrim, Septra), to eradicate the causative organism.
      (2) Urinary analgesics, such as phenazopyridine, to limit discomfort.
      (3) Anticholinergic drugs, such as oxybutynin (Ditropan, Oxytrol), to inhibit involuntary bladder contractions.

MAKING THE CONNECTION

Cranberry Juice and Decreased Incidence of Urinary Tract Infections

Research data indicate that the ingestion of cranberry juice or cranberry extract tablets is related to a significant decrease in the incidence of symptomatic UTIs. Constituents in cranberries prevent bacteria from adhering to a person's cell surface membranes, thereby impairing colonization and subsequent infection, rather than by the historical premise that acidification of urine provides an antibacterial effect. Cranberry intake has been found to be a safe, herbal choice for *preventing* a UTI. However, it should be used cautiously in long-term use for clients who have a propensity to form urinary oxalate stones. Interestingly, conclusions of randomized trials reported no evidence demonstrating that cranberry is effective in *treating* a UTI. Therefore, ingestion of cranberry juice (24 oz daily) or extract tablets (300 to 400 mg twice a day) is recommended in the prophylaxis of a UTI but is not recommended for its treatment.

C. Nocturnal enuresis
   1. Overview.
      a. **Nocturnal enuresis** is the involuntary passage of urine when asleep.
      b. Occurs after voluntary control should have been established.
   2. Clinical manifestations.
      a. Urinating when asleep.
      b. Person fails to awaken when the bladder empties.
   3. Precipitating factors.
      a. Health problems that interfere with the ability to concentrate urine.
      b. Health problems associated with excessive urine output (e.g., diabetes mellitus, diabetes insipidus).
      c. UTIs.
      d. Trauma or diseases of the spinal cord.
      e. Structural defects of the urinary tract.
      f. Misguided attempts at toilet training.
      g. Emotional stressors (e.g., birth of sibling, illness or death in the family, separation from family).

DID YOU KNOW?

Up to 25% of 5-year-old children experience nighttime bedwetting. It occurs three times more frequently in males than in females and is more common in first-born children. It decreases to 8% of male children and 4% of female children by the age of 12, and less than 3% of adolescents still experience nighttime bedwetting. To be diagnosed with nocturnal enuresis, a child 5 to 6 years of age must have two or more episodes per month, and a child older than 6 years of age must have one or more episodes per month. There is no single explanation for nocturnal enuresis; it is believed to be multifactorial, including a familial tendency. Medical causes are ruled out first before addressing psychological factors because they generally are believed to be the result, not the cause, of nocturnal enuresis. In fact, research demonstrates that children with nocturnal enuresis do not have an increased incidence of emotional problems, and for most children, it is not a rebellious act.

4. Independent nursing care.
   a. Include the client in formulating a plan of care; offer hope and encouragement that the plan will work.
   b. Train the bladder to hold larger amounts of urine when awake (e.g., gradually increase time between voidings).
   🛑 c. **Teach family members not to make the client feel guilty or ashamed.**
   d. Encourage the client to avoid fluid intake after the evening meal.
   e. Encourage the client to empty the bladder just before going to bed.
5. Dependent nursing care.
   a. Administer prescribed medications.
      (1) Tricyclic antidepressants, such as imipramine (Tofranil); administer at bedtime; ensure monthly blood tests to assess for granulocytosis; question the prescription for a child younger than age 6 years; must be gradually reduced over 6 days to prevent withdrawal.
      (2) Anticholinergics, such as oxybutynin (Ditropan); teach parents to assess for clinical manifestations of urinary retention.
   b. Teach the client to use a bed alarm, which awakens the client when voiding, only if prescribed by a primary health-care provider trained in the treatment of enuresis; its use is controversial

D. Urinary retention
1. Overview.
   a. **Urinary retention** is the accumulation of urine in the bladder due to an inability to empty the bladder completely.
   b. Excessive distention of the urinary bladder impairs contractility of the detrusor muscle, further impairing urination.
2. Clinical manifestations.
   a. Suprapubic distention.
   b. Reported feeling of bladder fullness and discomfort; inability to void despite presence of urge.

   c. Overflow incontinence exhibited as frequent urination of small amounts of urine.
3. Precipitating factors.
   a. Factors that cause inflammation and swelling of the genitourinary tract (e.g., infection, childbirth, and pelvic surgery).
   b. Neurological problems that affect the brain, spinal cord, or peripheral nerves (e.g., brain attack, tumors, and blunt trauma to neurological tissue).
   c. Infection (e.g., genital herpes).
   d. Obstructions (e.g., enlarged prostate, strictures, tumor, urinary calculi, and fecal impaction).
   e. Medications (e.g., antihistamines, tricyclic antidepressants, beta-adrenergic blockers, monoamine oxidase inhibitors, antispasmodics, antiparkinsonism medications, opioids, and anesthetic agents).
4. Independent nursing care.
   a. Monitor I&O.
   b. Palpate the suprapubic area for bladder distention.
   c. Encourage the client to use a position that facilitates voiding by the use of gravity.
   d. Provide privacy when toileting.
   e. Use techniques to encourage voiding (e.g., warm washcloth on perineum, placing hands in warm water, running a faucet).
5. Dependent nursing care.
   a. Assist the client with a warm-water bath that exposes just the perineal area to the water (*sitz bath*).
   b. Measure postvoiding residual (e.g., catheterization with a single-lumen tube, bladder ultrasound).
   c. Insert a single-lumen catheter or indwelling urinary catheter as prescribed.
   d. Provide preoperative and postoperative care for a client having surgery to remove an obstruction, such as prostate surgery.
   e. Teach intermittent self-catheterization to drain the bladder for clients with spinal cord injuries or neurological disorders.

VIII. Urinary Catheters

A urinary catheter may be inserted into the urinary bladder via the urethra to collect a specimen, empty the urinary bladder and then be removed, or remain in place to mitigate a problem. The insertion of a urinary catheter is a dependent function of the nurse and requires a prescription. There are various types of urinary catheters, each with its own distinct purpose. The nurse must know the principles associated with urinary catheter insertion, nursing care common to all types of urinary catheters, and nursing care specific to each type of catheter to ensure that the client's urinary elimination needs are met based on established standards of nursing practice.

A. Purpose
1. Obtain a sterile specimen.
2. Maintain an empty bladder during diagnostic tests and during or after surgical procedures.
3. Treat or prevent urinary retention.
4. Measure the volume of residual urine.

B. Types (Fig. 22.5)
1. Single-lumen (straight) catheter.
   a. Single-lumen tube inserted through urethra; used to obtain a sterile urine specimen, to measure residual urine after voiding, or for the immediate relief of urinary retention.
   b. Immediately removed when bladder is emptied of urine.
2. Indwelling catheter (retention catheter).
   a. Double-lumen tube inserted through urethra; used for continuous bladder drainage.
   b. One lumen to inflate the balloon to keep the tube in place and a second lumen to drain urine.
3. Triple-lumen catheter.
   a. Triple-lumen tube inserted through urethra or suprapubic area; used for continuous bladder irrigation.
   b. One lumen to inflate the balloon, second lumen to continuously instill a GU irrigant, and third lumen to drain urine and irrigant into a collection container.
4. Suprapubic catheter.
   a. Double-lumen tube inserted through suprapubic area; used for continuous bladder drainage when the urethral route is contraindicated.
   b. One lumen to inflate the balloon to keep the tube in place and a second lumen to drain urine.

C. Insertion of a urinary catheter
1. Explain what is going to be done and why, provide privacy, and wash your hands.
2. Position the client in the supine position, and drape the client, exposing only the perineal area.
   a. *Women:* Flex the knees, and allow the thighs to externally rotate; Sims' position with the upper leg flexed is also acceptable.
   b. *Men:* Slightly separate the legs with the knees and hips extended.
3. Don clean gloves, wash the perineal area, remove your gloves, and wash your hands.
4. Arrange the work area.
   a. Open a sterile catheter kit on a clean bedside table without contaminating the inside.
   b. Arrange a trash receptacle impervious to liquid in easy reach.
5. Don sterile gloves and maintain their sterility throughout the procedure.
6. Place the first sterile drape in position without contaminating the drape.
   a. *Women:* Under the perineal area.
   b. *Men:* Across the thighs.

Fig 22.5 Types of urinary catheters. (A) A single-lumen catheter is used to obtain a urine sample or immediately drain the bladder. (B) A double-lumen catheter is the most commonly used indwelling catheter. (C) A triple-lumen catheter is inserted when the client requires irrigation of the bladder. (From Wilkinson and Treas [2016]. *Fundamentals of nursing,* Vol. 1, 3rd ed. Philadelphia: F. A. Davis Company, with permission.)

7. Position the second sterile drape with the opening (fenestrated drape) arranged so that the urinary meatus is visible.
   a. *Women:* Over the perineum with the hole over the labia.
   b. *Men:* Over the thighs with the hole over the penis.
8. Organize the sterile supplies in the catheter kit.
   a. Pour the antiseptic solution over the cotton balls.
   b. Arrange the forceps near the cotton balls.
   c. Squeeze sterile lubricant into the kit tray.
   d. Connect the syringe to the catheter port.
   e. Roll the catheter tip in the lubricant (a length of 2 inches for women and 8 inches for men).
9. Position the catheter kit on the sterile field.
   a. *Women:* Between the client's legs.
   b. *Men:* On top of the thighs or between the client's legs.
10. Place the collection bag on the field or nearby if it is preattached to the catheter and tubing.
11. Cleanse the urinary meatus.
    a. *Women:* With one hand, spread and gently pull the labia majora and minora upward, exposing the urinary meatus, and hold this position throughout the procedure (see the black arrow in Fig. 22.6); with the other hand, hold an antiseptic-soaked cotton ball with the forceps and wipe from the pubis to the rectum along the far labia and then discard the cotton ball in the trash receptacle; repeat this along the near labia and then down the middle using a new cotton ball each time (see the red arrows in Fig. 22.6).

Fig 22.7 Cleansing the male urinary meatus. (From Wilkinson and Treas [2016]. *Fundamentals of nursing,* Vol. 2, 3rd ed. Philadelphia: F. A. Davis Company, with permission.)

   b. *Men:* Reach through the fenestrated drape and grasp the penis (retract the foreskin if the client is uncircumcised) and hold this position throughout the procedure; with the other hand, hold an antiseptic-soaked cotton ball with the forceps and wipe in a circular motion from the center of the urinary meatus outward and down the penis and then discard the cotton ball in the trash receptacle; repeat this two more times using a new cotton ball each time (Fig. 22.7).
12. Insert the catheter.
    a. *Women:* Insert the lubricated end of the catheter 2 to 3 inches into the urinary meatus until urine begins to flow into the tubing and then advance it 1 more inch (this ensures that the catheter has completely passed through the urethra); encourage the client to take deep breaths to facilitate relaxation; if the catheter touches unsterile linen or the labia or vagina, it is no longer sterile and a new sterile catheter must be used.
    b. *Men:* Insert the lubricated end of the catheter 7 to 9 inches into the urinary meatus until urine begins to flow and then advance 1 more inch to ensure that the catheter has completely passed through the urethra (Fig. 22.8); do not force catheter insertion if resistance is felt; lower the penis when the bladder is empty; replace the foreskin if the client is uncircumcised.

Clitoris

Labia majora

Urinary meatus

Labia minora

Vagina

Fig 22.6 Female catheterization. (From Nugent & Vitale [2014]. *Fundamentals of nursing: Content review PLUS practice questions.* Philadelphia: F. A. Davis Company, with permission.)

Fig 22.8 Inserting a urinary catheter into the penis. (From Wilkinson and Treas [2016]. *Fundamentals of nursing,* Vol. 2, 3rd ed. Philadelphia: F. A. Davis Company, with permission.)

A   Catheter placement, male

B   Catheter placement, female

Fig 22.9 Catheter placement. (A) Male. (B) Female. (From Wilkinson and Treas [2016]. *Fundamentals of nursing,* Vol. 2, 3rd ed. Philadelphia: F. A. Davis Company, with permission.)

13. Hold the catheter in place and, with the other hand, inflate the balloon using the attached saline-filled syringe (Fig. 22.9); if the client complains of discomfort, deflate the balloon, advance the catheter 1 inch, and reinflate the balloon because the catheter may be in the urethra.

14. Discard used supplies, remove your gloves, and wash your hands.

🛑 15. Hang the urine collection bag on the bed frame rather than on a side rail to prevent trauma to the urinary meatus and bladder when the side rail is moved.

   a. Always hang a urine collection bag below the level of the bladder to promote urine flow by gravity and prevent back flow of urine into the bladder.

   b. Keep the urine collection bag off the floor and coil the loops of the tubing on the bed to avoid dependent loops.

🛑 16. Secure the catheter to the client's thigh for females or abdomen for males (e.g., using catheter strap, tape) to prevent tension on the tubing and trauma to the bladder and urinary meatus (Fig. 22.10).

17. Don clean gloves, cleanse the perineal area, and remove your gloves.

18. Return the client to a comfortable position and wash your hands.

19. Document the amount and characteristics of urine and the client's response to the procedure.

D. Nursing care for clients with an indwelling urinary catheter

  1. Perform routine assessments.

    a. Monitor I&O.

    b. Monitor urine characteristics.

    c. Assess the perineal area for clinical manifestations of an infection of skin and mucous membranes.

    d. Assess for clinical manifestations of a UTI.

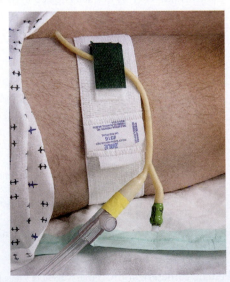

Fig 22.10 Securing a urinary catheter. (From Wilkinson and Treas [2016]. *Fundamentals of nursing,* Vol. 2, 3rd ed. Philadelphia: F. A. Davis Company, with permission.)

2. Provide care to prevent a UTI.
   a. Keep the collection bag below the level of the bladder by attaching it to the bed frame and coiling the tubing on the bed to prevent dependent loops.
   b. Maintain a closed system to prevent the introduction of pathogens by maintaining the integrity of all connections; if the tubing becomes disconnected, wipe both ends of the tubing with an antiseptic solution before reconnecting them.
   c. Secure the tubing to the client's anterior thigh for females and lower abdomen in males; this limits tension on tubing and helps to prevent lying on the tubing.
   d. Wash the perineal area and around and down the catheter with mild soap and water and rinse and dry thoroughly every 8 hours; avoid using powders and lotions after perineal care because these products provide a medium for the growth of microorganisms.
   e. Encourage ambulation and the upright position to facilitate bladder emptying if permitted.
   f. Encourage the intake of 3 L of fluid daily, if permitted, to help flush the urinary tract.
   g. Encourage the intake of foods that increase urine acidity (e.g., cranberry juice, eggs, meat, poultry, whole grains, plums, prunes, and tomatoes); acidic urine discourages the growth of microorganisms.
   h. Discourage the intake of foods that increase urine alkalinity (e.g., most fruits, vegetables, legumes, milk, and milk products); alkaline urine favors the growth of microorganisms.
   i. Maintain aseptic technique when emptying the collection bag (e.g., keep the drainage bag off the floor; ensure the spout does not touch the collection graduate or floor).
   j. Teach the client the importance of meticulous perineal care after a bowel movement.
   k. Administer a prescribed oral or intravenous antibiotic and a prescribed topical antibiotic or antifungal ointment to the perineal area.
3. Specific nursing care to prevent obstruction of the catheter.
   a. Ensure the catheter has no mechanical obstructions (e.g., kinks in the tubing, client lying on the tubing).
   b. Monitor the patency of the tubing every 2 hours, especially if sediment or hematuria is present.
   c. Ensure that if a clamp is used during a procedure that it is removed promptly after the procedure (e.g., obtaining a urine specimen,

instilling a medication into the bladder for a prescribed time frame).
   d. Instill or irrigate the catheter with sterile normal saline solution as prescribed, especially if the client's urine has blood clots or large amounts of sediment.
   e. Change the catheter if drainage is impaired.
E. Removal of a urinary catheter
   a. Prepare client for removal of the catheter if prescribed: Clamp the drainage tubing distal to the French catheter as specified (e.g., clamp for 2 hours and release for 15 minutes three times a day); this increases bladder tone in preparation for discontinuation of the urinary catheter.

   🛑 b. Use a needleless syringe to remove the fluid in the balloon before removal of the urinary catheter; never use scissors to cut a urinary catheter to drain the balloon because it can compress the lumen preventing removal of the fluid.

IX. Urinary Diversions

Because of a disease process or injury to the urethra, bladder, or ureter, a client may require the creation of a urinary diversion to permit evacuation of urine. An ileal conduit, Kock pouch, nephrostomy tube, suprapubic tube, and ureterostomy tube are types of urinary diversions created for the elimination of urine. To best meet clients' urinary elimination needs, the nurse must understand each type of diversion, including the way in which it is formed and the way in which it works; the general physical and psychological nursing care of a client with a urinary diversion; and the specific nursing care related to each type of urinary diversion.

A. Types
   1. *Ileal conduit* (Fig. 22.11).
      a. An **ileal conduit** is when a segment of the ileum is removed and used as a pouch reservoir.

Fig 22.11 Ileal conduit. (From Williams and Hopper [2015]. *Understanding medical surgical nursing*, 5th ed. Philadelphia: F. A. Davis Company, with permission.)

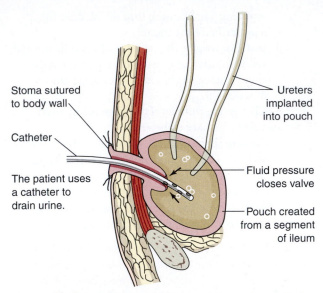

Fig 22.12 Kock pouch. (From Williams and Hopper [2015]. *Understanding medical surgical nursing,* 5th ed. Philadelphia: F. A. Davis Company, with permission.)

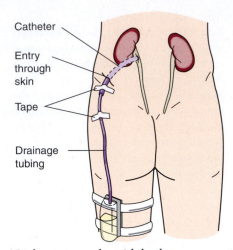

Fig 22.13 Nephrostomy tube with leg bag. (From Williams & Hopper [2015]. *Understanding medical surgical nursing,* 5th ed. Philadelphia: F. A. Davis Company, with permission.)

   b. One end is brought through the abdominal wall to form a stoma.
   c. Ureters are implanted into the pouch.
   d. Urine drains continuously.
2. *Kock pouch* (Fig. 22.12).
   a. A **Kock pouch** is formed when a portion of the ileum is used to form a pouch reservoir, which is connected to the skin.
   b. Ureters empty into the pouch.
   c. A nipple valve is created surgically and the pouch is emptied by inserting a clean catheter every few hours.
   d. A small dressing is worn over the nipple stoma between emptying.
3. *Nephrostomy tube* (Fig. 22.13).
   a. A **nephrostomy tube** is a tube placed into the pelvis of a kidney to drain urine into a collection container.
   b. Prevents accumulation of urine and stretching of the renal pelvis *(hydronephrosis)* due to an obstructed ureter.
4. *Suprapubic tube* (Fig. 22.14).
   a. A **suprapubic tube** is a catheter that is surgically inserted through a small incision above the symphysis pubis to drain urine into a collection container.
   b. It diverts urine when flow of urine through the urethra is impaired.
   c. It may be temporary or permanent.
B. Nursing care for clients with a urinary diversion
   1. Monitor I&O.
   2. Assess site for clinical manifestations of inflammation or infection.

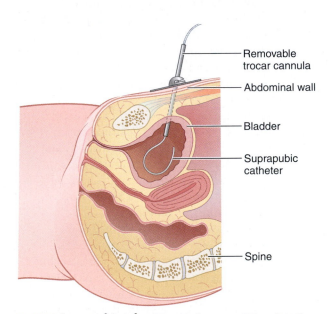

Fig 22.14 Suprapubic tube. (From Wilkinson and Treas [2016]. *Fundamentals of nursing,* Vol. 1, 3rd ed. Philadelphia: F. A. Davis Company, with permission.)

   3. Provide emotional support and teach self-care.
   4. Keep the skin around the site clean and dry; apply a moisture-proof skin barrier as prescribed to reduce risk of maceration of skin.
   5. Apply a prescribed topical antibiotic (e.g., bacitracin) or antifungal (e.g., nystatin) ointment on the skin around the tube entry site.
   6. Secure the tubing to the body (e.g., abdomen or flank area) depending on the entry site to reduce tension on the tube.
   7. Keep the tubing and collection bag(s) dependent to the site being drained.

8. Empty smaller urine collection devices (e.g., leg bag) frequently; leg bag is used under clothing during the day to facilitate ambulation; attach the tubing to a larger collection device when the client is in bed or at night.

9. Suprapubic tube: In preparation for removal of a temporary tube, clamp the catheter for 3- to 4-hour periods during the day as prescribed to assess whether the client is voiding a satisfactory volume through the urethra; residual is measured to determine what is satisfactory.

X. Bladder Irrigations

Instillation of a solution into the urinary bladder may be prescribed to flush the bladder, instill medication into the bladder, or maintain patency of a urinary catheter. Instillations may be intermittent or continuous. The nurse must know the principles of and implement actions related to nursing care associated with both intermittent and continuous bladder irrigations to best meet clients' urinary elimination needs.

A. Types
1. Intermittent bladder irrigation.
   a. An **intermittent bladder irrigation** is used to instill medication.
   b. Used to flush the bladder or to restore catheter patency.
2. Continuous bladder irrigation.
   a. A **continuous bladder irrigation** is the constant instillation of an irrigant into the bladder via a three-lumen urinary catheter to maintain catheter patency when hematuria, clots, or debris are anticipated, generally after surgery (e.g., resection of the prostate).
   b. **Requires** a triple-lumen catheter: One to inflate the balloon to hold the catheter in the bladder, the second to continuously instill the genitourinary (GU) irrigant, and the third to drain urine and irrigant to a collection device.

B. Nursing care for clients receiving a bladder irrigation
1. Commonalities of nursing care when implementing a bladder irrigation.
   a. Provide for privacy.
   b. Assess the client's comfort, including the presence of painful bladder spasms.
   c. Assess the urinary catheter often for tube patency.
   d. Calculate urine output by deducting the volume of irrigant from the total output.
   e. Document the nursing care provided and client responses in the clinical record.

2. Specific nursing care for clients with a prescription for intermittent bladder irrigation.
   a. Wash hands and then don clean gloves.
   b. Cleanse the catheter port with an alcohol swab.
   c. Compress the drainage tube with the fingers of one hand; this permits the irrigant to flow into the bladder rather than down the tube into the collection bag.
   d. Instill the irrigant into the port slowly to facilitate the flow of the irrigant into the bladder and limit trauma to the mucous membranes of the urinary tract (Fig. 22.15).
   e. Allow the solution to return via gravity.
3. Specific nursing care for clients with a prescription for continuous bladder irrigation (Fig. 22.16).
   a. Connect a 3-L bag of the prescribed solution to the input port of the three-way catheter.
   b. Adjust the flow rate as prescribed; a specific rate may be prescribed (e.g., 40 to 60 drops per minute) or the rate may be left to the discretion of the nurse to keep output pink and clot free.
   c. Assess output every 15 minutes to ensure patency of the tubing; if the tubing becomes occluded, bladder distention and fluid backup

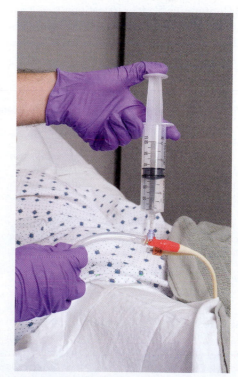

Fig 22.15 Intermittent bladder irrigation. (From Wilkinson and Treas [2016]. *Fundamentals of nursing*, Vol. 2, 3rd ed. Philadelphia: F. A. Davis Company, with permission.)

Fig 22.16 Continuous bladder irrigation. (From Burton and Ludwig [2015]. *Fundamentals of nursing care: Concepts, connections & skills,* 2nd ed. Philadelphia: F. A. Davis Company, with permission.)

can cause distention of the pelvis of the kidney and impede kidney function.

d. Ensure that the 3-L bag of irrigant is replaced when the previous bag is low on fluid so it does not run out because the flow must be uninterrupted to ensure catheter patency.

XI. Medications That Affect the Urinary System

When a person is diagnosed with a urinary system problem, the primary health-care provider can prescribe medication, such as kidney-specific anti-infectives to treat a UTI; urinary antispasmodics to reduce bladder spasms, increase bladder capacity and decrease incontinence; or estrogen to decrease vaginal and vulvar itching, inflammation, and dryness, which impact the urinary system. Nurses should know the mechanisms of action, therapeutic and nontherapeutic effects, and nursing care related to the common medications prescribed to treat urinary system problems.

A. Kidney-specific anti-infectives and related nursing care (Table 22.3).

B. Urinary antispasmodics and related nursing care (Table 22.4).

C. Estrogen and related nursing care (Table 22.5).

Table 22.3 Kidney-Specific Anti-infectives and Related Nursing Care

Mechanism of Action	Examples	Nontherapeutic Effects
• Have a bactericidal or bacteriostatic effect on kidney, ureter, bladder, and urethral infections. • Used for local UTI. • Administered PO or IV. **Sulfonamides** • Have a bacteriostatic effect. • Used to treat UTI. • Administered PO, IM, IV.	• nitrofurantoin (Macrobid) **Sulfonamides** • sulfamethoxazole (Bactrim) • trimethoprim/ sulfamethoxazole (Septra)	• Irritation of GI mucosa, such as anorexia, nausea, vomiting, abdominal pain, diarrhea, and pseudomembranous colitis. • Allergic responses, such as skin rash and exfoliative dermatitis. • Neurotoxicity, such as headache and peripheral neuropathy. • Nephrotoxicity. • Decreased white blood cell, red blood cell, and platelet counts. • Photosensitivity. • Staining of teeth. **Sulfonamides** • Same as above plus hepatic necrosis, toxic epidermal necrolysis, agranulocytosis, aplastic anemia, erythema multiforme, and Stevens-Johnson syndrome.

Nursing Care

• *Obtain a specimen for urine culture and sensitivity before initiating antibiotics.*
• Administer with food and encourage the client to rinse the mouth to minimize GI irritation.
• Monitor I&O and blood work for signs of therapeutic and nontherapeutic effects.
• Increase oral fluid intake to facilitate drug excretion and minimize risk of toxicity and crystalluria.
• Protect from sunlight.
• Nitrofurantoin: *Dilute oral solutions in milk or juice, use a straw, and have the client rinse the mouth to minimize staining of teeth; do not open capsules or crush tablets; explain that urine will be brown or rust in color.*

Table 22.4 **Urinary Antispasmotics and Related Nursing Care**

Mechanism of Action	Examples	Nontherapeutic Effects
• *Have antispasmodic action on smooth muscle of the urinary tract.* • *Increase bladder capacity.* • *Decrease frequency, urgency, and urge incontinence.*	• *oxybutynin (Ditropan)* • *tolterodine (Detrol)*	• *Anticholinergic effects, such as palpitations, tachycardia, headache, dizziness, dry mouth, urinary retention, allergic reaction, drowsiness, blurred vision, and constipation.* • *Sedation and weakness in older adults.*

Nursing Care

• *Monitor I&O and for clinical manifestations of therapeutic and nontherapeutic effects.*
• *Administer 30 to 60 minutes before meals and at hour of sleep.*
• *Teach the client to avoid driving or activities requiring alertness if drowsiness occurs.*
• *Encourage the client to chew gum or suck on hard candy or ice chips to relieve dry mouth.*
• *Oxybutynin: Teach the client to avoid hot environments because the ability to perspire may be impaired.*

Table 22.5 **Estrogen and Related Nursing Care**

Mechanism of Action	Examples	Nontherapeutic Effects
• *Decreases vaginal and vulvar itching, inflammation, and dryness.* • *Used to treat atrophic vaginitis.* • *Inserted with a vaginal applicator.*	• *estropipate vaginal cream (Ogden)* • *estradiol vaginal ring (Femring, Estring)*	• *Femring: Risk of endometrial carcinoma in clients with an intact uterus.*

Nursing Care

• *Teach the client the method for using the vaginal applicator; explain that the dose is marked on the applicator and the client should wash the applicator with soap and water and dry it after each use.*
• *Encourage the client to remain in the supine or recumbent position for 30 minutes after insertion.*
• *Teach the client to avoid the use of tampons and to use a sanitary pad to protect clothing.*

CASE STUDY: Putting It All Together

A 67-year-old man visits his primary health-care provider because of an inability to urinate and lower abdominal distension. The provider diagnoses urinary retention and sends the client immediately to the hospital for the insertion of a urinary retention catheter. At the hospital, a urinary retention catheter is inserted and the client is admitted to a surgical unit for diagnostic tests in preparation for surgery to remove obstructing prostate tissue. The nurse completes an admission interview, identifies the client's home medications, and reviews the primary health-care provider's prescriptions, which were faxed to the hospital from the provider's office. The nurse reads the client's clinical record.

Client's Clinical Record

Admission Interview

This 67-year-old male explained that he rents a room in a boarding house and shares a bathroom with three other men. He stated, "I am being treated for heart disease, allergies in the spring, and depression. I smoke two packs of cigarettes a day, love my four cups of coffee in the morning, and enjoy a six-pack of beer and bag of potato chips every night while watching TV. There is not much to do since my third heart attack 10 months ago." He explained that over the past year he had two UTIs and more frequent nighttime awakenings to urinate. He described urinary hesitancy, frequency, a slow urinary stream, and discomfort when urinating. When asked what brought him to his primary health-care provider today, he stated, "For 24 hours, I couldn't urinate. When my lower belly started to get bigger and I felt a lot of pressure down there (pointing to his suprapubic area), I went to the doctor. The doctor said that I had to go to the hospital because I had an enlarged prostate and that I needed surgery."

Primary Health-Care Provider's Prescriptions
2-gram sodium diet.
OOB to chair with assistance.
Vital signs every shift.
Urinary retention catheter to gravity.
I&O.
Pelvic and renal sonogram.

continued.

CASE STUDY: Putting It All Together

cont'd

Urinalysis, urine C&S.
CBC, metabolic profile.
tamsulosin (Flomax) 0.4 mg PO every a.m.
IV 0.9% sodium chloride 75 mL per hour for 2 L.

Medication Reconciliation Form
Hydrochlorothiazide 50 mg PO daily in a.m.; for
  hypertension; last taken this a.m.

Loratadine (Claritin) 10 mg PO daily; for seasonal
  allergies; last taken this a.m.
Sertraline (Zoloft) 50 mg PO a.m.; for depression; last
  taken this a.m.

Case Study Questions

A. Identify at least eight factors in this scenario that may have impacted the client's urinary elimination and explain your answer.

  1. _____
  2. _____
  3. _____
  4. _____
  5. _____
  6. _____
  7. _____
  8. _____

B. Identify at least five additional clinical indicators of urinary retention the nurse should explore with the client to ensure a complete history.

  1. _____
  2. _____
  3. _____
  4. _____
  5. _____

C. Identify medications that the client was taking at home that may have had an impact on the client's urinary system and explain your answer.

  1. _____
  2. _____
  3. _____

D. After surgery, the client is expected to have a triple-lumen urinary catheter for continuous bladder irrigation. Identify at least 10 nursing interventions that should be implemented for clients with any type of urinary tube, and three nursing interventions that are specific to caring for clients with a triple-lumen urinary catheter for continuous bladder irrigation.
Common principles associated with caring for clients with any type of urinary tube:

  1. _____
  2. _____
  3. _____
  4. _____
  5. _____

CASE STUDY: Putting It All Together

cont'd

_____ **Case Study Questions** _____

6. _____

7. _____

8. _____

9. _____

10. _____

Specific principles when caring for a client with a triple-lumen urinary catheter for continuous bladder irrigation:

1. _____

2. _____

3. _____

REVIEW QUESTIONS

Be sure to read the Introduction for valuable test-taking tips.

1. A hospitalized 70-year-old adult had a computed tomography (CT) scan with contrast at 11 a.m. The client has an IV running at 125 mL per hour and ingested 50% of lunch with an 8-oz cup of coffee and 4 oz of soup at 12 noon. The nurse is going on a break at 1 p.m. and provides the following information to the nurse accepting responsibility for the client. Which information about the client is of **most** concern to the nurse accepting responsibility for the client?
   1. Presence of slight nausea
   2. Urine output 100 mL at 12:45
   3. Blood pressure 148/84 mm Hg
   4. Medicated for a mild headache

2. A nurse is assisting a female client who is experiencing numerous daily episodes of urge incontinence to gain better control of urination. Which outcome reflects achievement of a goal associated with this client's urge incontinence?
   1. Urinates every two hours while remaining dry between voiding
   2. Wears an adult incontinence brief only when venturing outside the home
   3. Empties the bladder every time before leaving the house, limiting incontinence
   4. Uses deep, slow breathing until the sensation to void subsides, increasing intervals between voiding

3. A nurse identifies that a client may be experiencing urinary retention. Which clinical indicators support this inference? **Select all that apply.**
   1. Voiding small amounts of urine several times hourly
   2. Abdominal palpation indicating bladder distention
   3. Tenderness over the symphysis pubis on palpation
   4. Dysuria on voiding
   5. Blood-tinged urine

4. A nurse is caring for an older adult female who says, "Why am I always getting bladder infections?" How should the nurse respond?
   1. "Women have a shorter urethra than men do, and that makes women more susceptible than men to bladder infections."
   2. "Older adults may experience retained urine, which becomes more acidic and promotes the development of bladder infections."
   3. "It is hard for women to cleanse the urinary meatus, which increases the risk of bladder infections."
   4. "Infrequent sexual intercourse predisposes women to bladder infections."

5. A nurse is caring for a client who has a urinary retention catheter. A urine culture and sensitivity is prescribed. Which step ensures that the collected specimen is sterile?
   1. Swab the specimen port with an antiseptic swab.
   2. Don sterile gloves when obtaining the specimen.
   3. Use a urinalysis container to collect the specimen.
   4. Collect the specimen early in the morning before breakfast.

6. Nitrofurantoin (Macrodantin) 100 mg by mouth twice a day is prescribed for a client with a urinary tract infection. The pharmacy sends unit dose packages labeled 25 mg per capsule. The primary nurse on the 12-hour day shift checks the medication drawer to ensure that there are enough capsules for the next 24 hours. How many tablets should be available for disbursement to the client? **Record your answer using a whole number.**
   Answer: _____ capsules

7. While all of the following clinical manifestations are important to report to a primary health-care provider, which is **most** important?
   1. Anuria
   2. Dysuria
   3. Polyuria
   4. Nocturia

8. A client reports concern about not having urinated in several hours, having the sensation of the need to void, and having moderate abdominal distention. What should the nurse do **first**?
   1. Encourage the client to drink more fluid.
   2. Stroke the inner aspect of the client's thigh.
   3. Pour warm water over the client's perineal area.
   4. Have the client assume an upright position for voiding.

9. A client with a history of urinary tract infections asks the nurse for suggestions to limit their occurrence. Which should the nurse encourage the client to ingest to inhibit the growth of microorganisms that can cause a bladder infection? **Select all that apply.**
   1. Eggs
   2. Meats
   3. Apple juice
   4. Whole-grain breads
   5. Concentrated cranberry juice

10. Which nursing intervention is **most** effective when assisting a client to completely empty the bladder?
    1. Place the client's hands in warm water.
    2. Place a warm, wet washcloth over the genital area.
    3. Encourage the client to wait a minute and attempt to urinate again.
    4. Turn a faucet on in the client's room to produce sounds of flowing water.

11. A client reports signs and symptoms associated with urge incontinence. Which actions should the nurse teach the client to employ to gain better bladder control? **Select all that apply.**
    1. Practice Kegel exercises.
    2. Avoid lifting heavy objects.
    3. Avoid products with caffeine.
    4. Attend a bladder retraining program.
    5. Use the Credé maneuver when voiding.
    6. Urinate immediately when feeling the sensation to void.

12. A home-care nurse is caring for a cognitively intact woman who has arthritis that affects her hands, hips, and knees and slows her mobility. The client tells the nurse about having a few episodes of urinary incontinence that were upsetting. The nurse identifies that the client is experiencing functional incontinence. Which nursing interventions in the plan of care are specific to limiting episodes of incontinence in this client? **Select all that apply.**
    1. Encourage wearing clothing with Velcro closures instead of buttons and zippers.
    2. Suggest purchasing a lift chair if economics permit.
    3. Encourage avoiding products with caffeine.
    4. Teach to position a commode nearby.
    5. Teach the client Kegel exercises.
    6. Suggest voiding every 2 hours.

13. A nurse is caring for a female client who has a history of frequent urinary tract infections. What should the nurse teach the client to do? **Select all that apply.**
    1. Wear nylon underwear.
    2. Avoid artificial sweeteners.
    3. Void before having intercourse.
    4. Take a bubble bath rather than showering.
    5. Urinate when the urge to urinate is perceived.
    6. Encourage the intake of concentrated cranberry juice daily.

14. A client has a urinary retention catheter in place. The nurse must obtain a sterile urine specimen for culture and sensitivity. Where should the nurse place the clamp to allow urine to collect in the tubing so that the nurse can collect the specimen?
    1. A
    2. B
    3. C
    4. D

15. A nurse is caring for a group of clients. Which client should cause a concern about potential urinary retention?
    1. The client who is immobile in bed
    2. The client who just had a retention catheter removed
    3. The client who is disoriented to time, place, and person
    4. The client who just was placed on a fluid restricted diet

16. A nurse is caring for a postoperative client with a urinary retention catheter. The nurse reviews the surgeon's prescriptions, reviews the last nursing progress note, and performs a physical assessment of the client. Which action should the nurse perform **first**?
    1. Ambulate the client in the room.
    2. Encourage coughing and deep breathing.
    3. Empty the client's urine collection chamber hourly.
    4. Turn off the compression device during ankle pumping exercises.

Client's Clinical Record

Surgeon's Postoperative Prescriptions 0900

IVF 0.9% sodium chloride at 50 mL/hour.
Full liquid diet progress to 2-g Na diet as tolerated.
I&O.
Ambulate in room this p.m. and progress to 50 feet bid in a.m.
Apply sequential compression devices when in bed.
OOB in chair for meals starting noon tomorrow.
Maintain urinary retention catheter to bedside collection bag.
Heparin 5,000 units Sub-Q bid.
PCA: Hydromorphone (Dilaudid) 1 mg/hr with 0.2 mg/15 min
    lockout, not to exceed 7.2 mg in 4 hours.
Docusate sodium (Colace) 100 mg PO daily.

Progress Notes 0900

Client received from the PACU at 0900; vital signs stable.
Alert to time, place, and person. States that pain is a level 2
and tolerable. Abdominal dressing dry and intact. IVF 0.9%
NaCl in right antecubital space; site dry, and intact; running
at 50 mL/hr. PCA infusion site is dry and intact and infusion
pump is set at prescribed rate. 60 mL noted in hourly urine
collection chamber and emptied into the main collection
chamber. Urine is straw colored, no sediment noted.

Nurse's Physical Assessment 1000

Client resting in bed; vital signs stable; client states pain is
tolerable on a level 3 and it was unnecessary to push the PCA
pump during the last hour. Dressing dry and intact; 70 mL
urine noted in hourly urine chamber. 100 mL oral fluids tolerated. IVF 0.9% NaCl running at 50 mL/hour. States a desire
to engage in ankle pumping exercises.

17. A female client is scheduled for thoracic surgery and
is told by the surgeon that a urinary catheter will be
placed in the bladder in the operating room. After
the surgeon leaves, the client asks the nurse, "Why
am I going to have a tube in my bladder when I am
having surgery in my chest?" Which response by the
nurse is appropriate?
    1. "It is more convenient to control urine flow
       rather than having to clean a client after being
       incontinent."
    2. "We want clients to rest after your type of sur-
       gery. You will not be burdened with having to
       use a bedpan."
    3. "A urinary catheter enables us to easily secure a
       urine specimen for laboratory tests that generally
       are prescribed after surgery."
    4. "Hourly urine production is monitored with a
       urinary catheter. It is an effective way to assess
       kidney and circulatory function."

18. A nurse is caring for a 3-week-old infant. Which assessment regarding the number of diapers the infant
soils daily should cause concern?
    1. 7
    2. 8
    3. 9
    4. 10

19. A nurse is caring for a group of clients with a variety
of urinary retention catheters. Which of the following nursing interventions are common to all types of
urinary catheters? **Select all that apply.**
    1. Provide perineal care three times a day and when-
       ever necessary.
    2. Position the collection container below the level of
       the pelvis.
    3. Ensure that the balloon is filled with sterile saline.
    4. Hang the collection bag on the frame of the bed.
    5. Tape the collection tubing to the inner thigh.

20. Place these interventions in the order that they
should be performed when collecting a urine
specimen from an infant.
    1. Wash the hands and don clean gloves.
    2. Apply a collection device over the genitals.
    3. Wash the genital area and allow the area to dry.
    4. Remove the collection bag once the infant
       urinates.
    5. Send the entire bag in a specimen container to the
       laboratory.
    Answer: _____

21. Which of the following is essential to ensure reliable
bedside dipstick testing of urine? **Select all that
apply.**
    1. Use the correct reagent.
    2. Ensure adequate lighting.
    3. Ensure that the kit is not past the expiration date.
    4. Avoid delegating the procedure to another nursing
       team member.
    5. Read the test results immediately after removing
       the test strip from the urine.

22. A client's specific gravity is 1.032. For what additional clinical indicators should the nurse assess the
client? **Select all that apply.**
    1. Weight loss
    2. Hypertension
    3. Peripheral edema
    4. Decreased skin turgor
    5. Rapid, weak pulse rate

23. A nurse is caring for a client who is having urine
collected for a 24-hour urine test. During the
afternoon of the testing period, the client forgets
and accidentally voids into the toilet but tells
the nurse right away. What should the nurse
do next?
    1. Start the test again in the morning.
    2. Identify the time and begin a new test.
    3. Add the time since the previous voiding to the end
       of the test.
    4. Notify the delay of the test to the primary health-
       care provider.

24. A nurse is assessing a client with the diagnosis of urinary tract infection (UTI). Which clinical indicators identified by the nurse support this medical diagnosis? **Select all that apply.**
    1. Sweet, fruity odor to the urine
    2. Dark amber color of urine
    3. Blood-tinged urine
    4. Cloudy urine
    5. Foamy urine

25. A nurse is caring for a client with a diagnosis of UTI. Which clinical indicators identified during a nursing assessment support this medical diagnosis? **Select all that apply.**
    1. Dysuria
    2. Hematuria
    3. Urinary retention
    4. Urgent sensation to void
    5. Distended suprapubic area

26. A nurse is assessing a client and is concerned that the client may be experiencing urinary retention. Which clinical indicators support this conclusion? **Select all that apply.**
    1. Blood-tinged urine
    2. Amber-colored urine
    3. Reports of abdominal pressure
    4. Lower abdominal distention on palpation
    5. Voiding small amounts of urine at a time

27. A straight catheterization is prescribed for a client who has urinary retention. The draining volume reaches 750 mL without completely emptying the bladder. What alternative does the nurse have to help prevent bladder spasms?
    1. Remove the catheter and reinsert a retention catheter.
    2. Continue the complete emptying of the client's bladder.
    3. Release the remaining urine in the bladder slowly over 20 minutes.
    4. Take the catheter out and then recatheterize the client in 20 minutes.

28. A nurse is caring for a client who has an indwelling urinary catheter. Which nursing actions are important to include in this client's plan of care? **Select all that apply.**
    1. Obtain the vital signs routinely.
    2. Cleanse the perineal area several times a day.
    3. Monitor the tubing for kinks and obstructions.
    4. Assess the urine for color, cloudiness, and volume.
    5. Attach the drainage collection bag to the bed railing.
    6. Position the drainage bag above the level of the bladder.

29. A nurse receives a prescription to initiate continuous bladder irrigation. Which catheter should the nurse choose to perform the procedure correctly?
    1. Straight catheter
    2. Indwelling catheter
    3. Triple-lumen catheter
    4. Double-lumen catheter

30. A nurse is to perform a onetime bladder catheterization. The nurse verifies the prescription, washes the hands, and identifies the client. Place the following steps of the procedure in the order in which they should be performed.
    1. Don sterile gloves.
    2. Lubricate the catheter tip.
    3. Unwrap the catheter kit creating a sterile field.
    4. Advance the catheter 1 inch after urine begins to flow.
    5. Clean the urethral meatus with the solution provided in the kit.
    Answer: _____

31. A postoperative client has an indwelling catheter that has not drained urine in 2 hours. What should the nurse do **first?**
    1. Ask the primary health-care provider for a prescription to irrigate the catheter.
    2. Milk the tubing to dislodge any mucus or sediment in the catheter.
    3. Palpate the client's suprapubic area to assess for distention.
    4. Recognize the client's status is within expected limits.

32. A nurse is caring for a client receiving continuous bladder irrigation (CBI) after prostate surgery. Which nursing action is essential when caring for this client?
    1. Check the volume of the client's output every hour to ensure tube patency.
    2. Increase the irrigation solution flow rate until the return flow is pink and free from clots.
    3. Irrigate the double-lumen catheter according to the primary health-care provider's prescription.
    4. Turn the client from side to side to promote output, which helps to minimize clot formation in the urine.

33. A 24-hour urine test is prescribed. Which actions should be implemented by the nurse when conducting this test? **Select all that apply.**
    1. Have the client void one last time at the end of the 24 hours and add it to the volume being collected.
    2. Have the client void one last time at the end of the 24 hours and discard this urine.
    3. Collect the first voiding and then add subsequent voidings for the next 24 hours.
    4. Discard the first voiding and then collect the urine for the next 24 hours.
    5. Store the collected urine during the 24 hours in a collection container.

34. A nurse is caring for a client with a history of experiencing residual urine after voiding. The nurse uses a bladder ultrasound scanner (BUS) to detect the amount of urine that remains in the bladder after the client voids. Which actions should the nurse implement that are essential to this test? **Select all that apply.**
    1. Repeat the measurement several times.
    2. Provide perineal hygiene before the procedure is initiated.
    3. Position the client in the supine position for the duration of the procedure.
    4. Explain that no discomfort will be experienced as the transducer is moved on the surface of the skin.
    5. Place the scan head on the abdomen, midline four inches above the pubic bone, aiming the scan head toward the coccyx.

35. A nurse is caring for a client who is scheduled for a cystoscopy. Which information should the nurse include when telling the client about what to expect after the procedure?
    1. Urinary retention may occur after the procedure.
    2. Urine may be dark red initially after the procedure.
    3. Bedrest is necessary for several days after the procedure.
    4. A clear liquid diet generally is prescribed for a few days after the procedure.

36. A nurse is applying a condom urinary catheter. Place the following steps in the order in which they should be implemented.
    1. Hold the penis and place the catheter beyond the glans, leaving at least a 1-inch space at the tip of the penis.
    2. Unroll the condom along the full length of the shaft of the penis.
    3. Apply the adhesive strip supplied by the manufacturer.
    4. Secure the condom with gentle compression.
    5. Hang the collection bag from the bed frame.
    6. Provide perineal care and dry thoroughly.
    Answer: _____

37. A nurse is obtaining a health history from a client. The client states that she is embarrassed about episodes of incontinence when she sneezes or exercises and that she no longer attends an exercise program for this reason. She now walks several miles a day to lose the 50 lb she gained when pregnant with her fifth child. Based on this information, which nursing intervention will **best** help the client to address the underlying cause of her lack of urine control?
    1. Teach the client foods to avoid that irritate the bladder mucosa.
    2. Encourage the client to return to her exercise class.
    3. Have the client prepare a toileting schedule.
    4. Teach the client Kegel exercises.

38. The nurse is caring for an older adult who is receiving oxybutynin to reduce the occurrence of bladder spasms related to a UTI. For which side effects should the nurse assess the client? **Select all that apply.**
    1. Dizziness
    2. Diaphoresis
    3. Gastric irritation
    4. Urinary retention
    5. Orange-colored urine

39. A nurse is caring for a client with an indwelling urinary catheter. A urine specimen for culture and sensitivity is prescribed. What should the nurse do when collecting this specimen?
    1. Place the urine specimen in a sterile urine container.
    2. Obtain the urine specimen from the hourly urine chamber of the collection bag.
    3. Collect the urine specimen from the drainage port at the bottom of the collection bag.
    4. Take the urine specimen directly from the distal end of the catheter after separating it from the tubing.

40. A nurse receives a prescription to collect a clean-catch urine. What specific techniques should the nurse use that are different from those used to obtain urine for a urinalysis? **Select all that apply.**
    1. The urine specimen should be sent to the laboratory as soon as possible after it is obtained.
    2. The urine should be collected in the middle of a free-flowing stream of urine.
    3. The urinary meatus must be cleansed three times with an antiseptic swab.
    4. The urine specimen should be obtained first thing in the morning.
    5. The urine specimen should be collected in a sterile container.

REVIEW ANSWERS AND RATIONALES

1. ANSWER: 2.
Rationales:
1. Slight nausea is a mild, not critical, reaction to the contrast dye; however, continued monitoring of this symptom should occur.
2. A urine output of 100 mL is too little output with an intake of 610 mL over 2 hours (125 + 125 + 240 + 120 = 610) and may reflect reduced kidney efficiency in reaction to the contrast dye. This is a serious concern and should be reported to the primary health-care provider.
3. A blood pressure of 148/84 mm Hg is within the expected range of <150 systolic and <90 diastolic for a client who is ≥60 years of age.
4. A headache is a mild, not critical, reaction to the contrast dye; however, ongoing monitoring should occur to ensure that the client obtains relief.
TEST-TAKING TIP: Identify the word in the stem that sets a priority. The word *most* in the stem sets a priority. All the options reflect important information, but one is *most* essential and should be communicated to the primary health-care provider.
Content Area: Urinary Elimination
Integrated Processes: Communication and Documentation; Nursing Process: Evaluation
Client Need: Safe and Effective Care Environment; Management of Care
Cognitive Level: Application
Concept: Elimination

2. ANSWER: 4.
Rationales:
1. Although scheduled voiding may be done initially, it does not specifically address overcoming the urge to void.
2. Although wearing an incontinence brief may provide a client with a sense of security, it will not help reduce the urge to void.
3. People with urge incontinence often void every time they leave the house and stay close to a bathroom to minimize the risk of incontinence. While this action may prevent incontinence, it does not help to reduce the urge to void.
4. Deep, slow breathing helps to progressively relax a person and has proven successful in reducing the urge sensation. Additional interventions include strengthening perineal muscles (Kegel exercises), biofeedback, lifestyle modifications (e.g., avoidance of caffeine, weight reduction, and fluid modifications), and intake of prescribed antimuscarinic agents.
TEST-TAKING TIP: Identify the options with specific determiners. The words *every* in options 1 and 3 and *only* in option 2 are specific determiners. Rarely are options with specific determiners the correct answer. Examine option 4 carefully.
Content Area: Urinary Elimination
Integrated Processes: Teaching/Learning; Nursing Process: Evaluation
Client Need: Physiological Integrity; Basic Care and Comfort
Cognitive Level: Application
Concept: Elimination

3. ANSWER: 1, 2, 3.
Rationales:
1. Voiding small amounts of urine several times hourly is characteristic of urinary retention. Pressure within the bladder increases as urine collects until the external urethral sphincter is unable to hold back the urine and voiding of small amounts of urine occurs (retention with urinary overflow).
2. When the bladder fills to capacity, it rises up out of the pelvis and can be palpated over the symphysis pubis; this is characterized as bladder distention.
3. Retained urine causes stretching of the bladder wall, which precipitates a feeling of pressure, discomfort, and tenderness over the symphysis pubis, especially during palpation.
4. Dysuria or pain on urination most often is associated with bladder infection, not urinary retention.
5. Blood-tinged urine most often is associated with irritation of or trauma to the bladder and urethral mucosa (e.g., bladder infection, bladder cancer, physical trauma).
TEST-TAKING TIP: Identify the obscure clang associations. The word *urinary* in the stem and *urine* in options 1 and 5 are obscure clang associations. In this question option 1 is a correct answer and option 5 is a distractor.
Content Area: Urinary Elimination
Integrated Processes: Nursing Process: Assessment
Client Need: Physiological Integrity; Basic Care and Comfort
Cognitive Level: Application
Concept: Elimination

4. ANSWER: 1.
Rationales:
1. This statement is true. The shorter urethra in women makes them more susceptible to bladder infections than men who have a longer urethra. Also, the female urinary meatus is close to the anus, which increases the risk of transmission of microorganisms from the intestinal tract to the urinary meatus.
2. Retained urine associated with aging becomes more alkaline, not acidic, which is an ideal site for bacterial growth.
3. As long as a woman cleanses the perineal area when bathing daily, perineal cleanliness should not be an issue.
4. Frequent, not infrequent, sexual intercourse predisposes women to bladder infections.
Content Area: Urinary Elimination
Integrated Processes: Communication and Documentation; Nursing Process: Implementation
Client Need: Health Promotion and Maintenance
Cognitive Level: Application
Concept: Elimination

5. ANSWER: 1.
Rationales:
1. Swabbing the specimen port with an antiseptic swab is necessary to remove microorganisms from the port that may contaminate the specimen. In addition, it reduces the risk of introducing microorganisms into the closed urinary retention catheter and collection bag system.
2. Sterile gloves are not necessary to maintain sterility of the specimen. Clean gloves protect the nurse from the client's blood and body fluids.

3. The urine collection container must be a sterile urine collection container, not the clean container used for specimens for unsterile urinalysis specimens.

4. The time of day a specimen is collected from a urinary retention catheter will not alter the sterility of the specimen.

Content Area: Urinary Elimination
Integrated Processes: Nursing Process: Implementation
Client Need: Physiological Integrity; Reduction of Risk Potential
Cognitive Level: Application
Concept: Elimination

6. **ANSWER: 8.**
Rationale:
Use ratio and proportion to identify the number of capsules required for each dose. Then multiply the product of this calculation by 2 because the prescribed dose is to be administered twice a day.

$$\frac{\text{Desire } 100 \text{ mg}}{\text{Have } 25 \text{ mg}} = \frac{x \text{ capsules}}{1 \text{ capsule}}$$

$$25x = 100 \times 1$$
$$25x = 100$$
$$x = 100 \div 25$$
$$x = 4 \text{ capsules}$$

Multiply 4 capsules by 2 (the number of times the dose is to be administer in a 24-hour period) to arrive at 8 capsules required for the client in a 24-hour period.

Content Area: Urinary Elimination
Integrated Processes: Nursing Process: Planning
Client Need: Physiological Integrity; Pharmacological and Parenteral Therapies
Cognitive Level: Application
Concept: Medication; Elimination

7. **ANSWER: 1.**
Rationales:
1. **Anuria describes urine output of less than 100 mL in 24 hours. Anuria is associated with kidney disease or congestive heart failure; both can be life-threatening situations.**
2. Dysuria refers to painful or difficult urination. Although this is serious and may be associated with infection or partial obstruction of the urinary tract, generally it is not as critical as another clinical manifestation.
3. Polyuria refers to excessive urination. Although serious and may be caused by excessive hydration, diabetes mellitus, diabetes insipidus, or kidney disease, generally it is not as critical as another clinical manifestation.
4. Nocturia is defined as awakening at night to void. Although a concern because it may be associated with excessive fluid intake and a variety of urinary tract and cardiovascular problems, it generally is not as critical as another clinical manifestation.

TEST-TAKING TIP: Identify the word in the stem that sets a priority. The word *most* in the stem sets a priority.
Content Area: Urinary Elimination
Integrated Processes: Communication and Documentation; Nursing Process: Analysis

Client Need: Safe and Effective Care Environment; Management of Care
Cognitive Level: Analysis
Concept: Elimination

8. **ANSWER: 4.**
Rationales:
1. Although encouraging an increase in oral fluid intake may be implemented, it does not immediately address the client's need to void. Also, the client's bladder already is moderately distended.
2. Stroking the inner aspect of the client's thigh may stimulate sensory nerves and promote the micturition reflex. However, this action should not be the first intervention.
3. Although pouring warm water over the perineal area may stimulate voiding, it is not the first action the nurse should take.
4. **Assuming an upright position for voiding uses gravity to move urine downward toward the urinary meatus. Also, it is the most common position that people use to urinate. Assuming this position psychologically may facilitate voiding.**

TEST-TAKING TIP: Identify the word in the stem that sets a priority. The word *first* in the stem sets a priority. Identify the clang association. The word *void* in the stem and *voiding* in option 4 is a clang association.
Content Area: Urinary Elimination
Integrated Processes: Communication and Documentation; Nursing Process: Implementation
Client Need: Physiological Integrity; Basic Care and Comfort
Cognitive Level: Application
Concept: Elimination

9. **ANSWER: 1, 2, 4, 5.**
Rationales:
1. **Eggs increase urine acidity, which tends to inhibit the growth of microorganisms.**
2. **Meats increase urine acidity, which tends to inhibit the growth of microorganisms.**
3. Apple juice does not increase urine acidity. Pathogenic microorganisms exist and multiply more readily in alkaline environments.
4. **Whole-grain breads increase urine acidity, which tends to inhibit the growth of microorganisms.**
5. **Concentrated cranberry juice increases urine acidity, which tends to inhibit the growth of microorganisms. Other theories are that the antioxidants in cranberries change bacteria so they cannot stick to the urinary tract walls and that a component of cranberries creates a Teflon-like coating on the walls of the urinary tract that prevents *Escherichia coli* from sticking.**
Content Area: Urinary Elimination
Integrated Processes: Teaching/Learning; Nursing Process: Implementation
Client Need: Health Promotion and Maintenance
Cognitive Level: Application
Concept: Patient-Centered Care; Elimination

10. ANSWER: 3.

Rationales:

1. Although placing a client's hands in warm water may initiate micturition, it is not the most effective intervention to facilitate complete bladder emptying.

2. Although stroking the inner aspect of a client's thigh may initiate micturition, it is not the most effective intervention to facilitate complete bladder emptying. Although a warm, wet washcloth placed over the genital area may help initiate urination, it may not facilitate complete bladder emptying.

3. Encouraging a client to wait until urine stops flowing, wait a minute, and then attempt to void again (double void) may facilitate complete bladder emptying. A small amount of urine remains in the bladder after voiding (residual urine), which can support bacterial growth; therefore, complete bladder emptying contributes to a decreased risk of bladder infection.

4. Although sounds of flowing water may initiate micturition, it is not the most effective intervention to facilitate complete bladder emptying.

TEST-TAKING TIP: Identify the word in the stem that sets a priority. The word *most* in the stem sets a priority. Identify the unique option. Option 3 is unique because the actual action used to completely empty the bladder is performed by the client, not the nurse.

Content Area: Urinary Elimination
Integrated Processes: Nursing Process: Implementation
Client Need: Physiological Integrity; Basic Care and Comfort
Cognitive Level: Application
Concept: Elimination

11. ANSWER: 1, 3, 4.

Rationales:

1. Kegel exercises strengthen the muscles in the pelvic floor, which should help to minimize the urge-to-void.

2. Avoiding lifting heavy objects is an intervention to reduce incontinence associated with stress, not urge, incontinence.

3. Caffeine irritates the mucosa of the bladder and should be avoided to reduce bladder irritability and urge incontinence.

4. A bladder retraining program includes such activities as practicing holding larger amounts of urine between voidings, scheduling voiding times, and using distraction and relaxation techniques to reduce the urge sensation, thereby improving bladder control.

5. The Credé maneuver, application of pressure over the bladder, is used to promote emptying of the bladder, not to gain bladder control as a result of urge incontinence.

6. Urinating immediately when feeling the sensation to void will reinforce urge incontinence. Specific techniques must be used to ignore the urge to void.

TEST-TAKING TIP: Identify the clang association. The word *bladder* in the stem and in option 4 is a clang association.

Content Area: Urinary Elimination
Integrated Processes: Teaching/Learning; Nursing Process: Implementation
Client Need: Physiological Integrity; Basic Care and Comfort
Cognitive Level: Analysis
Concept: Patient-Centered Care; Elimination

12. ANSWER: 1, 2, 4, 6.

Rationales:

1. This client is experiencing functional incontinence. Functional incontinence involves the inability to get to the bathroom in time because of environmental factors or sensory, cognitive, or mobility issues. This client has impaired mobility and dexterity of the hands. Velcro closures, instead of buttons and zippers, may facilitate quicker disrobing to urinate.

2. A lift chair will facilitate moving from a sitting to standing position shortening the time it takes to move to a bathroom to void.

3. Avoiding products with caffeine is encouraged to reduce bladder irritability associated with urge, not functional, incontinence.

4. A commode positioned nearby will reduce the distance a person with a mobility problem has to move to get to a toilet.

5. Kegel exercises are recommended to strengthen weak pelvis muscles associated with stress and urge, not functional, incontinence.

6. Voiding at timed intervals avoids waiting until a bladder is full and, as a result, enables more time to move to the bathroom or commode.

Content Area: Urinary Elimination
Integrated Processes: Communication and Documentation; Nursing Process: Planning
Client Need: Physiological Integrity; Basic Care and Comfort
Cognitive Level: Analysis
Concept: Patient-Centered Care; Elimination

13. ANSWER: 2, 5, 6.

Rationales:

1. Cotton underwear should be worn because nylon prevents evaporation of moisture. Bacteria multiply in a warm, moist, dark environment.

2. Artificial sweeteners are a bladder irritant. When the bladder mucosa is irritated, it is more vulnerable to invasion of pathogens.

3. The client should urinate after, not before, intercourse to flush away bacteria that may have entered the urethra during sexual activity.

4. Bubble baths and baking soda baths should be avoided because the urethra is exposed to pathogens in the bath water. This may increase the risk of a UTI.

5. Voiding immediately when the urge is perceived helps to avoid stagnant urine in the bladder. Bacteria multiply in stagnant urine.

6. Concentrated cranberry juice acidifies the urine, which inhibits the growth of pathogens in the bladder. Other theories include that the antioxidants in cranberries change bacteria so they cannot stick to the urinary tract walls and that a component of cranberries creates a Teflon-like coating on the walls of the urinary tract that prevents *Escherichia coli* from sticking.

TEST-TAKING TIP: Identify the clang association. The word *urinary* in the stem and the word *urinate* in option 5 is a clang association. Examine this option carefully when considering which options are correct answers.

Content Area: Urinary Elimination
Integrated Processes: Teaching/Learning; Nursing Process:
Implementation
Client Need: Health Promotion and Maintenance
Cognitive Level: Application
Concept: Patient-Centered Care; Elimination

14. **ANSWER: 4.**
Rationales:
1. Compression along the catheter itself may permanently compromise the patency of the lumen that drains urine from the bladder and the lumen that permits inflation and deflation of the balloon.
2. Compression along the catheter itself may permanently compromise the patency of the lumen that drains urine from the bladder.
3. Compression along the catheter extension that leads to the inflation port may permanently compromise the patency of the lumen that permits inflation and deflation of the balloon.
4. **Compression of the collection tubing immediately distal to the collection port will interrupt the flow of urine from the urinary bladder to the urine collection bag. Urine will collect above the specimen port in the drainage tubing without compromising the integrity of the urinary catheter.**
TEST-TAKING TIP: Identify the unique option. Option 4 is unique. Options 1, 2, and 3 are related to the catheter. Option 4 is related to the collection bag tubing. Examine option 4 carefully.
Content Area: Urinary Elimination
Integrated Processes: Nursing Process: Implementation
Client Need: Physiological Integrity; Reduction of Risk
Potential
Cognitive Level: Analysis
Concept: Elimination

15. **ANSWER: 2.**
Rationales:
1. Immobility is more likely to contribute to urinary incontinence than urinary retention because of a decrease in bladder tone.
2. **The bladder loses tone while a urinary retention catheter is in place. Intake and output should be monitored after its removal because urinary retention is a potential problem. If urinary retention occurs, the primary health-care provider will either prescribe that the client be straight catheterized and output monitored for another 8 hours or the urinary retention catheter will be represcribed.**
3. Disorientation to time, place, and person is more likely to contribute to urinary incontinence than urinary retention because of a decreased ability to comprehend and react to the sensation of a full bladder.
4. Urinary retention is not a complication associated with a fluid-restricted diet.
TEST-TAKING TIP: Identify the option with the clang association. The word *retention* in the stem and in option 2 is a clang association. More often than not, an option with a clang association is the correct answer. Examine option 2 carefully.

Content Area: Urinary Elimination
Integrated Processes: Nursing Process: Assessment
Client Need: Physiological Integrity; Reduction of Risk
Potential
Cognitive Level: Analysis
Concept: Elimination

16. **ANSWER: 3.**
Rationales:
1. Ten in the morning is too early to ambulate the client. The surgeon's prescription indicates that the client should be ambulated around the room during the p.m. hours.
2. Although encouraging coughing and deep breathing is an independent function of the nurse and should be encouraged when caring for postoperative clients, it is not the first thing the nurse should do from among the options presented.
3. **It is 1 hour since the last assessment, and the hourly urine collection container should be emptied into the large chamber of the collection device. Monitoring hourly urine output helps to assess cardiac and renal status and accuracy is essential.**
4. The sequential compression devices should be turned off and removed only when the client is out of bed.
TEST-TAKING TIP: Identify the word in the stem that sets a priority. The word *first* in the stem sets a priority.
Content Area: Urinary Elimination
Integrated Processes: Communication and Documentation;
Nursing Process: Implementation
Client Need: Physiological Integrity; Physiological Adaptation
Cognitive Level: Analysis
Concept: Patient-Centered Care; Elimination

17. **ANSWER: 4.**
Rationales:
1. Urinary retention catheters are not used to make it more convenient for the nursing staff to care for a client. A urinary retention catheter increases the risk for a bladder infection; therefore, it is used only when absolutely necessary.
2. Occasionally a urinary retention catheter may be used to make it more convenient for the client. However, this is not the reason why a urinary retention catheter is being inserted for this client. The risk of infection outweighs the benefit to a client when a urinary retention catheter is used just for convenience. Exceptions include when a urinary retention catheter is used to protect a client from urinary incontinence when a person is actively dying or when a client has a large sacral pressure ulcer.
3. Urinary retention catheters are never used to make it more convenient for the nursing staff to contain or collect urine.
4. **After abdominal or thoracic surgery, assessing hourly urine production is an effective way to assess kidney and circulatory function. Also, hourly urine production may be monitored to assess a nonsurgical client who is in critical condition.**
TEST-TAKING TIP: Identify the options that are equally plausible. Options 1 and 2 are both concerned with care being more convenient. Option 1 is no better than option 2. Eliminate options 1 and 2 from further consideration. Identify the options with a clang association. The words *urinary*

and *catheter* in the stem and in options 3 and 4 are clang associations. Examine options 3 and 4 carefully.
Content Area: *Urinary Elimination*
Integrated Processes: *Communication and Documentation; Nursing Process: Implementation*
Client Need: *Physiological Integrity; Reduction of Risk Potential*
Cognitive Level: *Application*
Concept: *Elimination*

18. ANSWER: 1.
Rationales:
1. Seven diapers is too small a number of soiled diapers daily for an infant who is several weeks old.
2. Eight soiled diapers daily is expected for a 3-week-old infant. A well-hydrated infant who is several weeks old produces enough urine to soil 8 to 10 diapers daily.
3. Nine soiled diapers daily is expected for a 3-week-old infant. A well-hydrated infant who is several weeks old produces enough urine to soil 8 to 10 diapers daily.
4. Ten soiled diapers daily is expected for a 3-week-old infant. A well-hydrated infant who is several weeks old produces enough urine to soil 8 to 10 diapers daily.
TEST-TAKING TIP: Identify the words in the stem that establish negative polarity. The words *cause the most concern* asks the test-taker to identify an assessment that is unexpected.
Content Area: *Urinary Elimination*
Integrated Processes: *Nursing Process: Assessment*
Client Need: *Physiological Integrity; Reduction of Risk Potential*
Cognitive Level: *Application*
Concept: *Elimination*

19. ANSWER: 1, 2, 4.
Rationales:
1. Perineal care should be provided three times a day and whenever necessary, such as after passing of stool, for all clients with urinary retention catheters.
2. Positioning the collection container below the level of the pelvis is common for all types of urinary retention catheters. This promotes urine flow from the client to the collection bag and prevents the flow of urine back into the bladder, which can cause an infection.
3. All urinary retention catheter balloons should be filled with sterile water because saline will crystallize, resulting in partial deflation of the balloon when it is removed. A partially deflated balloon will cause trauma to the urethral mucosa during removal.
4. The collection bag should be hung on the bed frame, not the side rail, for all types of urinary retention catheters. A bed rail should not be used because when the rail is raised, it could raise the collection bag higher than the pelvis. When the rail is lowered, it could cause strain on the catheter or pull the catheter out, causing trauma to the urethra.
5. A catheter, not collection tubing, should be taped to the abdomen, not the thigh, of a male client. A catheter can be taped to the inner thigh of a female client.

Content Area: *Urinary Elimination*
Integrated Processes: *Nursing Process: Implementation*
Client Need: *Physiological Integrity; Reduction of Risk Potential*
Cognitive Level: *Analysis*
Concept: *Elimination*

20. ANSWER: 1, 3, 2, 4, 5.
Rationales:
1. First: Washing the hands limits the presence of microorganisms. The nurse should don clean gloves because they protect the nurse from blood and body fluids.
3. Second: Washing the genital area and allowing it to dry to remove soiled matter, prevent specimen contamination, and prepare the skin for adhesion of the collection bag.
2. Third: Apply the collection device to enable the collection of a urine specimen.
4. Fourth: Remove the bag immediately after the infant voids to ensure that a fresh sample of urine is tested.
5. Fifth: The entire bag should be sent to the laboratory because it is difficult to remove urine from an infant collection bag. In addition, it protects the specimen from contamination by environmental elements.
Content Area: *Urinary Elimination*
Integrated Processes: *Nursing Process: Planning*
Client Need: *Safe and Effective Care Environment; Management of Care*
Cognitive Level: *Analysis*
Concept: *Elimination*

21. ANSWER: 1, 2, 3.
Rationales:
1. The correct reagent must be used to ensure reliable results.
2. Adequate lighting facilitates accurate interpretation of the color chart with the dipstick.
3. The kit must not be past the expiration date to ensure reliable results.
4. The procedure may be delegated to unlicensed assistive personnel as long as the individual knows how to perform the skill. Have the person report the results, but save the specimen in case the urine has to be retested.
5. The strip should be read after removing the test strip from the urine at the exact time indicated on the bottle label; waiting times may vary depending on the manufacturer's instructions.
Content Area: *Urinary Elimination*
Integrated Processes: *Nursing Process: Implementation*
Client Need: *Physiological Integrity; Reduction of Risk Potential*
Cognitive Level: *Application*
Concept: *Elimination*

22. ANSWER: 1, 4, 5.
Rationales:
1. Weight loss is sign of deficient fluid volume as is a specific gravity of 1.032. The loss of 1 liter of fluid is reflected in a weight loss of 2.2 pounds.
2. Hypertension is a sign of excess, not deficient, fluid volume because of hypervolemia.

3. Peripheral edema is a sign of excess, not deficient, fluid volume as fluid is retained in the interstitial compartment.

4. Decreased skin turgor is a sign of deficient fluid volume, as is a specific gravity of 1.032. Fluid moves from the intracellular and interstitial compartments into the intravascular compartment, causing decreased skin turgor and dry skin and mucous membranes.

5. A rapid, weak pulse is a sign of deficient fluid volume, as is a specific gravity of 1.032. The heart rate increases as blood vessels constrict in response to less fluid in the circulation and in an attempt to meet the body's peripheral cellular needs. The volume of the pulse is weak (thready) because of hypovolemia.

Content Area: Urinary Elimination
Integrated Processes: Nursing Process: Assessment
Client Need: Physiological Integrity; Reduction of Risk Potential
Cognitive Level: Analysis
Concept: Fluid and Electrolyte Balance

23. ANSWER: 2.
Rationales:
1. It is not necessary to wait until the morning to begin the test again.
2. Starting the test again is the most appropriate action by the nurse. The test is based on urine collected during any 24-hour time period.
3. Adding the time since the previous voiding to the end of the test is inappropriate and will cause inaccurate test results.
4. Although the primary health-care provider should be notified of the delay in the test, it is not the priority at this time.
TEST-TAKING TIP: Identify the word in the stem that sets a priority. The word *next* in the stem sets a priority.
Content Area: Urinary Elimination
Integrated Processes: Nursing Process: Implementation
Client Need: Physiological Integrity; Reduction of Risk Potential
Cognitive Level: Application
Concept: Elimination

24. ANSWER: 3, 4.
Rationales:
1. A sweet, fruity odor to urine is associated with incomplete fat metabolism related to diabetes mellitus or starvation, not a UTI. The sweet, fruity odor is caused by excess glucose in the urine.
2. Dark, amber urine is caused by high levels of bilirubin in the urine associated with liver dysfunction, not a UTI. Urine may also be dark amber if the urine is very concentrated.
3. Hematuria (blood-tinged urine) is associated with a urinary tract infection as a result of irritation of the bladder and urethral mucosa.
4. Cloudy urine is caused by the presence of bacteria, white blood cells, and/or red blood cells associated with a UTI.
5. Foamy urine is caused by protein in the urine and is associated with renal disease, not a UTI.

Content Area: Urinary Elimination
Integrated Processes: Nursing Process: Assessment
Client Need: Physiological Integrity; Physiological Adaptation
Cognitive Level: Application
Concept: Elimination

25. ANSWER: 1, 2, 4.
Rationales:
1. Dysuria (pain or burning on urination) is caused by urine flowing over inflamed mucosal tissue and is associated with a UTI.
2. Hematuria (blood-tinged urine) is caused by irritation of the bladder and urethral mucosa and is associated with a UTI.
3. Urinary frequency, not retention, is associated with a UTI. Urinary retention is associated with the inability of the bladder to empty because of obstruction, inflammation and swelling, neurological problems, anxiety, or an adverse effect of a medication.
4. Urgency (an overwhelming sensation of the need to void) is caused by bladder irritability secondary to a UTI.
5. A distended suprapubic area is associated with urinary retention, not a UTI.
Content Area: Urinary Elimination
Integrated Processes: Nursing Process: Assessment
Client Need: Physiological Integrity; Physiological Adaptation
Cognitive Level: Application
Concept: Elimination

26. ANSWER: 3, 4, 5.
Rationales:
1. Blood-tinged urine is caused by irritation of the bladder and urethral mucosa associated with a urinary tract infection, not retention.
2. Amber-colored urine is associated with concentrated urine related to dehydration or high levels of bilirubin related to liver dysfunction.
3. Abdominal pressure occurs as the bladder fills beyond a comfortable level of stretch, which is associated with urinary retention.
4. When the bladder is distended, it rises up out of the pelvis and is identified when the lower abdomen is palpated.
5. With urinary retention, pressure builds in the bladder to where the external urethral sphincter is unable to maintain closure. It opens temporarily and a small amount of urine escapes until pressure subsides and the sphincter closes. This can happen several times every hour and is a classic sign of urinary retention. It is called urinary retention with overflow.
Content Area: Urinary Elimination
Integrated Processes: Nursing Process: Assessment
Client Need: Physiological Integrity; Basic Care and Comfort
Cognitive Level: Application
Concept: Elimination

27. ANSWER: 3.
Rationales:
1. Removing the catheter and inserting a retention catheter is contraindicated because it increases the risk of a bladder infection. In addition, the retention catheter will continue

to empty the bladder, which may precipitate bladder spasms. Inserting a urinary retention catheter is a dependent function of the nurse and requires a prescription.

2. Continuing to empty the client's bladder after 750 mL has been removed may precipitate bladder spasms.

3. Releasing the urine over 20 minutes decreases irritability as the bladder distention is relieved; this will help reduce bladder spasms.

4. Removing the catheter and recatheterizing the client is contraindicated because doing so increases the risk of a bladder infection.

TEST-TAKING TIP: Identify equally plausible options. Options 1 and 4 are equally plausible. They both involve inserting a urinary catheter. Identify the options that are opposites. Options 2 and 3 are opposites. Examine options 2 and 3 carefully. The tip identifying clang associations will not help in focusing on a potential correct answer because the words *urine, bladder,* and *catheter* in the stem are in one or more of the options.

Content Area: Urinary Elimination
Integrated Processes: Nursing Process: Implementation
Client Need: Physiological Integrity; Reduction of Risk Potential
Cognitive Level: Application
Concept: Elimination

28. **ANSWER: 1, 2, 3, 4.**
    Rationales:

1. **A foreign body in a body cavity, such as an indwelling urinary catheter, increases the risk for an infection. Vital signs will increase when the client has an infection.**

2. **Cleansing the perineal area reduces the risk of a urinary tract infection. It removes debris and microorganisms away from the urinary meatus.**

3. **When a urinary drainage tube is kinked or compressed, it interferes with drainage of urine and urine will back up into the bladder. Stasis of urine increases the risk of a bladder infection.**

4. **Assessing urine for color, cloudiness, and volume is necessary for identifying the presence of a urinary tract infection. Urine that is cloudy or pink may indicate the presence of an infection.**

5. Attaching the drainage bag to the bed railing is contraindicated because, if the railing is raised, urine may flow back into the bladder. Also, if the rail is raised or lowered with the bag attached, it may cause trauma to the urinary meatus.

6. Positioning the urinary drainage bag above the bladder is contraindicated; this will cause urine to flow back into the bladder.

TEST-TAKING TIP: Identify the obscure clang association. The word *urinary* in the stem and the word *urine* in option 4 is a clang association. Examine option 4 carefully.

Content Area: Urinary Elimination
Integrated Processes: Nursing Process: Planning
Client Need: Physiological Integrity; Reduction of Risk Potential
Cognitive Level: Application
Concept: Elimination

29. **ANSWER: 3.**
    Rationales:

1. A straight catheter has one lumen and is used for one-time bladder drainage.

2. An indwelling catheter is a double-lumen catheter used for ongoing bladder drainage. One lumen permits passage of sterile water for balloon inflation and the other for urinary drainage.

3. A triple-lumen catheter is used for continuous bladder irrigation. One lumen permits passage of sterile water for balloon inflation, another for instilling a GU irrigant into the bladder, and the third for bladder drainage (combination of urine and GU irrigant).

4. A double-lumen catheter is used as an indwelling catheter.

TEST-TAKING TIP: Identify the options that are equally plausible. Options 2 and 4 are equally plausible because they both have two lumens. These options can be deleted from further consideration.

Content Area: Urinary Elimination
Integrated Processes: Nursing Process: Planning
Client Need: Physiological Integrity; Basic Care and Comfort
Cognitive Level: Application
Concept: Elimination

30. **ANSWER: 3, 1, 5, 2, 4.**
    Rationales:

3. The outside of a sterile package is not sterile and can be touched with the hands.

1. After a sterile field is established, sterile gloves must be worn to maintain sterility of the field and the equipment touched during the procedure.

5. Cleaning the urethral meatus with the provided antiseptic removes debris and microorganisms; this limits the risk of a bladder infection.

2. A lubricated catheter tip limits trauma to the urinary meatus and mucous membranes of the urinary tract.

4. Advancing the catheter 1 inch after urine flows ensures that the catheter is past the internal and external urinary sphincters.

Content Area: Urinary Elimination
Integrated Processes: Nursing Process: Planning
Client Need: Physiological Integrity; Reduction of Risk Potential
Cognitive Level: Analysis
Concept: Elimination

31. **ANSWER: 2.**
    Rationales:

1. An attempt should be made to reestablish patency of the catheter lumen before obtaining a prescription to irrigate the catheter.

2. Two hours should produce a minimum of 60 mL of urine, even if the client had no fluid intake. Milking the tubing should be performed first to dislodge sediment or a mucus plug that may be interfering with the flow of urine.

3. Palpating the client's suprapubic area may not reveal distention after only 3 hours. As much as 500 or more milliliters of urine may need to accumulate before abdominal distention is palpable.

4. Some action is required because urine output over three hours should be at least 90 mL (i.e., 30 mL/hr).
TEST-TAKING TIP: Identify the word in the stem that sets a priority. The word *first* in the stem sets a priority. Identify the clang associations. The word *catheter* in the stem and in options 1 and 2 are clang associations. Examine options 1 and 2 carefully. More often than not, an option with a clang association is the correct answer.
Content Area: Urinary Elimination
Integrated Processes: Nursing Process: Implementation
Client Need: Physiological Integrity; Reduction of Risk Potential
Cognitive Level: Application
Concept: Elimination

32. ANSWER: 2.
Rationales:
1. One hour is too long a period of time to wait between assessments of tube patency with a CBI. The volume of output should be checked every 15 minutes. The faster the flow rate, the more frequently the nurse should assess the output. If the tube becomes obstructed soon after being checked and it is not reassessed for a long period of time, then a large volume of urine and solution can collect in and distend the bladder; this increases the potential of injury to the operative site as well as results in reflux to the kidneys.
2. Increasing the flow rate of the irrigating solution helps to dilute the effluent from the bladder, thereby minimizing the formation of clots in the urine. A pink effluent, without the presence of clots, is the clinical sign that indicates that the irrigating solution flow rate is sufficient to maintain patency.
3. A CBI requires a triple-lumen, not a double-lumen, urinary retention catheter. One lumen is attached to the urine collection bag, a second lumen is used to inflate the balloon that holds the catheter in the bladder, and a third lumen is attached to the tubing from the irrigation solution bag.
4. A client may be encouraged to turn from side to side to facilitate respirations, relieve pressure on bony prominences, and promote venous return from the lower extremities, not to minimize clot formation.
TEST-TAKING TIP: Identify the word in the stem that sets a priority. The word *essential* in the stem sets a priority. Identify the clang association. The word *irrigation* in the stem and in option 2 is a clang association. More often than not, an option with a clang association is the correct answer. Examine option 2 carefully.
Content Area: Urinary Elimination
Integrated Processes: Nursing Process: Implementation
Client Need: Physiological Integrity; Reduction of Risk Potential
Cognitive Level: Application
Concept: Elimination

33. ANSWER: 1, 4, 5.
Rationales:
1. Having the client void one last time at the end of the 24-hour period and adding it to the large collection container completes the test. It accurately includes the urine being produced within the specified 24-hour period.

2. The last urine collected at the end of the test is not discarded but is added to the volume being collected.
3. The first voiding is discarded, not collected, and then all additional urine voided within 24 hours is collected.
4. Discarding the first voiding is the correct way to initiate a 24-hour urine test. If the first voiding is included, the urine volume will incorporate more hours of urine produced than should be included in 24 hours. The test results will be altered by excessive amounts of constituents in the greater volume of urine collected. This test can test for levels of adrenocortical steroids, hormones, protein, and creatinine clearance.
5. All voided urine for 24 hours is collected and then stored in a large collection container.
TEST-TAKING TIP: Identify opposite options. Options 1 and 2 are opposites. One of these options is correct and the other is a distractor. Options 3 and 4 are opposites. One of these options is correct and the other is a distractor.
Content Area: Urinary Elimination
Integrated Processes: Nursing Process: Implementation
Client Need: Physiological Integrity; Reduction of Risk Potential
Cognitive Level: Application
Concept: Elimination

34. ANSWER: 1, 3, 4.
Rationales:
1. Repeating the measurement several times ensures accuracy of the measurement.
2. Perineal hygiene is not necessary before implementing the procedure. However, washing the conducting gel from the abdomen and suprapubic area is necessary after completing the procedure.
3. The client is placed in the supine position so that the lower abdomen and suprapubic areas are exposed.
4. Explaining that no discomfort will be experienced as the transducer is moved on the surface of the skin is accurate information. This is a painless noninvasive procedure that should cause no discomfort.
5. The transducer is applied midline 1.5 inches, not 4 inches, above the pubic bone, aiming the scan head toward the client's coccyx for an accurate reading.
Content Area: Urinary Elimination
Integrated Processes: Nursing Process: Implementation
Client Need: Physiological Integrity; Reduction or Risk Potential
Cognitive Level: Application
Concept: Elimination

35. ANSWER: 1.
Rationales:
1. Urinary retention may occur after the procedure due to urethral edema.
2. It is not uncommon to experience pink, not red, urine after the procedure. The instrumentation may irritate the mucosal lining of the urinary tract, resulting in minor bleeding.
3. It is not necessary to maintain bedrest for several days after the procedure. Bedrest may be encouraged on the day of the procedure because hypotension may occur immediately after the procedure.

4. The client can resume a regular diet immediately after the procedure. The client will be advised to increase fluid intake for several days. A large amount of dilute urine decreases dysuria, prevents urinary stasis, and limits the accumulation of bacteria in the bladder.
Content Area: Urinary Elimination
Integrated Processes: Communication and Documentation; Nursing Process: Planning
Client Need: Physiological Integrity; Reduction of Risk Potential
Cognitive Level: Application
Concept: Elimination

36. **ANSWER: 6, 1, 2, 4, 3, 5.**
Rationales:
6. The first step is providing perineal hygiene and drying the penis thoroughly. A penis that is clean and free from debris and moisture reduces the risk of infection, skin breakdown, and nonadherence of the condom.
1. The second step ensures that the catheter does not compress the glans and that there is a 1- to 1 and a 1/2-inch distance between the glans penis and the drainage tubing. These actions prevent pressure against the glans and tissue at the distal end of the penis.
2. The third step is applying the condom to the full length of the shaft of the penis. Holding the penis firmly, perpendicular to the abdomen, extends the penis and facilitates the unrolling of the condom down the shaft of the penis.
4. The fourth step is securing the condom to the shaft by grasping the penis and gently compressing it so that the entire condom comes into contact with the shaft of the penis.
3. The fifth step is taping the external adhesive strip over the condom in a spiral along the length of the shaft. Applying it in a spiral reduces the risk of obstructing circulation, which can occur when it is applied around the condom at the proximal end of the penis. Some condom catheters have a sticky inner surface so that when it is unrolled and gently compressed against the shaft of the penis it adheres to the shaft of the penis.
5. The last step in the procedure is hanging the urine collection bag on the bed frame below the level of the bladder.
Content Area: Urinary Elimination
Integrated Processes: Nursing Process: Planning
Client Need: Safe and Effective Care Environment; Management of Care
Cognitive Level: Analysis
Concept: Elimination

37. **ANSWER: 4.**
Rationales:
1. An irritated bladder is associated with urge, not stress, incontinence.
2. Returning to her exercise class will help her continue to lose weight because obesity is a contributing factor for stress incontinence; however, the information in another option is a more effective intervention that will improve the underlying cause of her problem.

3. Although a toileting schedule may help keep the bladder less full just before exercise or other planned strenuous activity, it will not help correct the underlying cause of stress incontinence.
4. **The client is experiencing stress incontinence, most likely due to weakened pelvic floor muscles as result of five pregnancies and obesity. Stress incontinence occurs when intra-abdominal pressure increases related to such activities as exercise, laughing, coughing, sneezing, bending, and lifting. Kegel exercises help to increase pelvic floor muscle tone and should help the client regain control of urine.**
TEST-TAKING TIP: Identify the word in the stem that sets a priority. The word *best* in the stem sets a priority. Identify the clang associations. The word *exercise* in the stem and in options 2 and 4 are clang associations. Examine options 2 and 4 carefully.
Content Area: Urinary Elimination
Integrated Processes: Teaching/Learning; Nursing Process: Implementation
Client Need: Physiological Integrity; Basic Care and Comfort
Cognitive Level: Analysis
Concept: Patient-Centered Care; Elimination

38. **ANSWER: 1, 4.**
Rationales:
1. **Dizziness is associated with oxybutynin (Ditropan) because of its effect on the central nervous system.**
2. Decreased sweating, not diaphoresis, is associated with oxybutynin (Ditropan).
3. Gastric irritation is not associated with oxybutynin (Ditropan); however, it can precipitate constipation.
4. **Urinary retention is associated with oxybutynin (Ditropan) because it has direct spasmolytic action on smooth muscle, including smooth muscle lining the genitourinary tract.**
5. Orange-colored urine is associated with the drug phenazopyridine, a urinary tract analgesic, not oxybutynin (Ditropan).
TEST-TAKING TIP: Identify words in the stem that indicate negative polarity. The words *side effect* in the stem indicate negative polarity. The question is asking, "*What is not a therapeutic effect of oxybutynin?*"
Content Area: Urinary Elimination
Integrated Processes: Nursing Process: Evaluation
Client Need: Physiological Integrity; Pharmacological and Parenteral Therapies
Cognitive Level: Application
Concept: Medication; Elimination

39. **ANSWER: 1.**
Rationales:
1. **The urine specimen should be collected and contained following the principles of sterile technique. A sterile container will not introduce environmental microorganisms into the specimen. This ensures that the results of the culture and sensitivity reflect the microorganisms present in the client's urinary tract.**
2. Urine collected from the hourly urine section of the urinary collection device may be as long as 1 hour old

and, therefore, not current. The hourly urine section of the collection bag moves collected urine into the main portion of the urine collection container when it is lifted. Generally, it does not have its own port.

3. Collecting urine from the drainage port at the bottom of the collection bag is contraindicated because the urine in this section of a urinary collection device may be many hours old.

4. Urinary retention catheters and collection bags generally are designed as closed drainage systems so they cannot be separated; this avoids unnecessary separation of tubing that may permit introduction of pathogenic microorganisms.

TEST-TAKING TIP: Identify the unique option. Option 1 is unique. Options 2, 3, and 4 all relate to the removal of urine from the drainage system. Option 1 is the only option that contains an intervention that is performed after the urine is actually collected.

Content Area: Urinary Elimination
Integrated Processes: Nursing Process: Implementation
Client Need: Physiological Integrity; Reduction of Risk Potential
Cognitive Level: Application
Concept: Elimination

40. ANSWER: 2, 3, 5.

Rationales:

1. All specimens should be sent to the laboratory as soon as they are obtained to limit the degradation of constituents.

2. A client should begin to urinate and after some urine has passed the collection container then is placed under the stream of urine. The initial stream of urine helps to flush the urinary meatus of debris or microorganisms that may contaminate the urine specimen; hence the name "clean catch."

3. In a male, the foreskin, if present, and in the female the labia majora and minora, are retracted to expose the urinary meatus. The meatus is then swabbed three times with an antiseptic solution to remove microorganisms on the skin and mucous membranes that may contaminate the urine specimen.

4. A clean-catch urine specimen and a specimen for a urinalysis can be obtained at any time.

5. A clean-catch urine specimen, although not a specimen obtained using sterile technique, is a specimen with the minimal introduction of microorganisms from the perineal area. A sterile container is used to further limit contamination of the specimen.

TEST-TAKING TIP: Identify the unique option. Option 3 contains the word *urinary* whereas all the other options contain the word *urine*. Examine option 3 carefully.

Content Area: Urinary Elimination
Integrated Processes: Nursing Process: Planning
Client Need: Physiological Integrity; Reduction of Risk Potential
Cognitive Level: Analysis
Concept: Elimination

Chapter 23

Bowel Elimination

NURSING CONCEPTS

Comfort
Elimination
Fluid and Electrolyte Balance
Growth and Development
Infection
Inflammation

Medication
Metabolism
Mobility
Patient-Centered Care
Perioperative
Safety

KEY TERMS

Anabolism—Synthesis of larger compounds from smaller compounds

Catabolism—The breakdown of complex compounds into simple compounds, releasing energy for other body processes

Colostomy—Formation of an opening (stoma) between the colon and the surface of the abdomen to permit feces to exit the body

Constipation—Intestinal hypomotility that precipitates two or fewer stools a week and hard, dry feces

Diarrhea—Intestinal hypermotility that precipitates passage of fluid and unformed stool three or more times a day

Fecal impaction—Hard, dry stool firmly wedged in the rectal vault that cannot be passed

Fecal incontinence—Involuntary passage of feces and flatus from the anus

Flatulence—Excessive gas in the stomach and intestines that leads to distention of these organs precipitating physical discomfort

Flatus—Gas in the stomach and intestines as a natural by-product of digestion

Gluconeogenesis—The conversion of protein or fat into glucose by the liver

Glycogenolysis—The breakdown of glycogen from the liver when the blood glucose decreases, releasing glucose

Glycogenesis—The conversion of excess glucose to glycogen, which is stored in the liver

Hemorrhoid—Engorged, painful, bleeding vein in the lining of the rectum or anus

Hydrolysis—Splitting of a compound into small segments in preparation for GI absorption and metabolism

Ileostomy—Formation of an opening (stoma) between the ileum and the surface of the abdomen to permit feces to exit the body

Mastication—Process of chewing

Obstipation—Intractable constipation

Perceived constipation—Self-diagnosed constipation

I. Structures and Functions Related to Bowel Elimination

The structures and functions of bowel elimination are associated with the ingestion of food and elimination of the waste products of digestion in the form of feces. Many factors can affect a person's bowel elimination, including developmental level, emotional and cultural factors, dietary and fluid intake, activity, medications, perioperative issues, and physiological problems. Nurses must understand the basic anatomy and physiology of the gastrointestinal system and the issues that impact a client's bowel elimination to better meet clients' nursing needs.

(4) When blood glucose decreases, gluconeo-genesis increases and glycogen from the liver breaks down releasing glucose (**glycogenolysis**).

C. Factors affecting bowel elimination
1. Developmental level.
   a. Toddlers: Develop intestinal control at about 2 to 3 years of age.
   b. Pregnant women: Enlarged uterus imposes on intestinal structures, resulting in decreased peristalsis.
   c. Older adults: Experience decreased peristalsis.
2. Emotional and cultural factors.
   a. Lack of privacy: Some cultures are open and others prefer privacy when attending to bodily functions.
   b. Inadequate amount of time to defecate.
   c. Embarrassment: Fecal elimination is often asso-ciated with sights and odors that may be offen-sive to others and make the client self-conscious.
3. Nutrition.
   a. Lack of fiber and excessive milk: Results in a decrease in peristalsis.
   b. Irregular eating patterns: Can interfere with regu-larity of bowel movements or decrease peristalsis.
   c. Caffeine and fiber promote peristalsis.
4. Fluid intake.
   a. Need 6 to 8 glasses of water daily.
   b. Decreased fluid intake causes constipation.
5. Activity.
   a. Activity increases muscle tone and stimulates peristalsis.
   b. Inactivity contributes to decreased muscle tone and constipation.
6. Medications.
   a. Antibiotics destroy normal intestinal flora.
   b. Antacids often slow peristalsis.
   c. Iron causes constipation.
   d. Analgesics, opioids, and antimotility drugs slow peristalsis.
   e. Laxatives and cathartics increase peristalsis.
7. Perioperative issues: Anesthesia and handling of the bowel during surgery may slow motility and cause cessation of peristalsis (*adynamic ileus, postoperative ileus, paralytic ileus*).
8. Physiological problems: Common problems include GI infections, food allergies, cancer, diverticulosis and diverticulitis, irritable bowel syndrome, and malabsorption syndromes.

II. Nursing Assessment of Bowel Elimination

The first step of the nursing process is assessment. When col-lecting information relative to a client's GI status, the nurse obtains a client history, performs a physical assessment and assesses the characteristics of stool. This section provides guidelines to facilitate a comprehensive assessment of a client's gastrointestinal status.

A. Obtain a health history regarding bowel habits and patterns
1. Previous bowel habits and patterns and any changes.
2. Dietary habits, use of supplements, change in appetite, and daily fluid intake.
3. Level of activity, mobility, and exercise.
4. Presence of pain or discomfort.
5. Past and present illnesses, injury, and surgery that might affect GI function.
6. Use of medications that can affect GI function, such as antibiotics, iron, laxatives, cathartics, antacids, and analgesics.
7. Ability to self-toilet.
8. Emotional status and current stressors.
9. Social history (e.g., number of people using one bathroom, cultural background).

B. Physical assessment related to bowel elimination
1. Follow a systematic pattern when assessing the abdomen; four abdominal quadrants (Fig. 23.2).
2. Assess color and integrity of the abdomen via inspection.
   a. Normal findings.
      (1) Uniform color.
      (2) Unblemished; silverfish white stretch marks (*striae*); possible surgical scars.
   b. Deviations.
      (1) Tense, glistening skin, possibly indicating edema, ascites, or flatulence.
      (2) Purple striae, possibly indicating rapid weight loss or gain or Cushing's syndrome; rashes; other lesions.

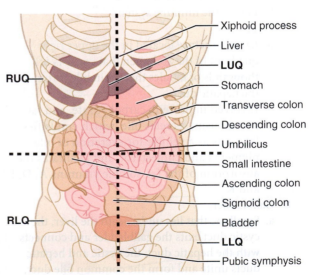

Fig 23.2 Four abdominal quadrants. (From Wilkinson and Treas [2016]. *Fundamentals of nursing*, Vol. 1, 3rd ed. Philadelphia: F. A. Davis Company, with permission.)

3. Assess contour of the abdomen via inspection.
   a. Normal findings: Flat; round (convex); scaphoid (concave).
   b. Deviations.
      (1) Abdominal distension.
      (2) Requires a further focused assessment.
         (a) Measure the abdominal girth with a centimeter tape measure around the body at the level of the umbilicus to obtain base line measurement.
         (b) Assess for ascites by placing the hands on each side of the abdomen while pushing against the abdomen with one hand and feeling for the presence of fluid exerting pressure against the other side of the abdomen (fluid wave test).
         (c) Assess for hypoactive bowel sounds via auscultation.
4. Assess symmetry of the abdomen via inspection.
   a. Instruct client to take a deep breath.
   b. Normal findings: Symmetrical appearance.
   c. Deviations.
      (1) Enlarged liver and spleen become more prominent.
      (2) Localized protrusions may indicate an umbilical or inguinal hernia or a tumor.
5. Assess for presence of vascular patterns on abdomen.
   a. Normal findings: No visible prominent veins.
   b. Deviations: Dilated veins visible, particularly around umbilicus *(caput medusa)*; associated with ascites, liver disease, and portal hypertension.
6. Auscultate the abdomen for bowel sounds.
   a. Disconnect nasogastric tube suction if present.
   b. Follow a logical sequence.
   c. Listen in each area for 1 minute.
   d. Normal findings.
      (1) High-pitched, irregular musical sounds or gurgles *(borborygmi).*
      (2) Occur every 5 to 15 seconds and last 1 to several seconds.
   e. Deviations.
      (1) Hyperactive: Loud, frequent sounds occurring about every 2 to 3 seconds; caused by increased peristalsis associated with diarrhea, gastroenteritis, and early bowel obstruction.
      (2) Hypoactive: Soft, infrequent sounds occurring about one per minute; caused by decreased intestinal peristalsis associated with anesthesia, abdominal surgery, or conditions such as bowel infections, obstruction, or impaired innervation.
      (3) Absent: No sounds heard after listening for 5 minutes.

7. Auscultate the abdomen for vascular sounds (see Fig. 14.10 in Chapter 14, Physical Assessment.)
8. Percuss the abdomen to determine position, size, and/or density of underlying structures.
   a. Percuss several areas in each quadrant of the abdomen using a systematic sequence (Fig. 23.3).
   b. Normal findings.
      (1) Tympany over the stomach and gas-filled intestine.
      (2) Dullness over the liver, spleen, and full bladder; no tenderness.
   c. Deviations.
      (1) High-pitched tympany heard with distention.
      (2) Large dull areas associated with organ enlargement, tumors, and presence of fluid.
9. Palpate the abdomen to determine the position and size of underlying structures.
   a. Do not palpate the abdomen when pulsations are present, in a client who had an organ transplant, or when a Wilm's tumor is suspected.
   b. Palpate several areas in each quadrant of the abdomen using a systematic sequence.
   c. Use light palpation; press down 1 to 2 cm with a slight circular motion.
   d. Normal findings: Abdomen is soft, not tender, and without palpable masses.
   e. Deviations: Tenderness, guarding, and rigidity may indicate peritonitis; presence of masses.
10. Assess the anus and perianal area via inspection for color, intactness, and presence of lesions and via touch for the anal reflex.
   a. Normal findings.
      (1) Color slightly darker than color of buttocks.
      (2) Intact skin that is coarser and moister than perianal skin; absence of lesions.
      (3) Puckering of anus when touched with gloved finger (anal reflex).

Fig 23.3 Percussion of abdomen. (From Dillon [2016]. *Nursing health assessment: The foundation of clinical practice,* 3rd ed. Philadelphia: F. A. Davis Company, with permission.).

b. Deviations.
   (1) Fissures, lesions, warts, hemorrhoids, bleeding, or rectal prolapse.
   (2) Lack of anal tone.

C. Characteristics of stool
   1. Characteristics of stool are influenced by factors such as dietary and fluid intake, exercise, medications, and disease processes.
   2. Characteristics of stool include color, consistency, quantity, shape, odor, and constituents (Table 23.1).

III. Diagnostic Tests and Related Nursing Care

Diagnostic tests may be prescribed by the primary healthcare provider to provide information regarding a client's gastrointestinal functioning. The tests presented mainly are prescribed to support a medical diagnosis. Nurses must understand these tests because some of them require the nurse to collect a specimen, others require nursing interventions before and after the test, and all of them require client teaching.

A. Stool examination
   1. Commonalities of nursing care for obtaining stool specimens.
      a. Perform hand hygiene, and wear clean gloves.
      b. Instruct the client to defecate in a clean, dry bedpan or container under the toilet seat.
      c. Use medical aseptic technique to collect 1 inch of formed stool or 15 to 30 mL of liquid stool.
      d. Ensure that the specimen is not contaminated with urine, water, or toilet paper.
      e. Use a preservative if required.
      f. Place the labeled container with the specimen into a biohazard, fluid-impervious bag; include appropriate label and laboratory forms.
      g. Note on the label if the client is menstruating.
      h. Send the specimen to the laboratory promptly because bacteriological changes may alter test results if testing is delayed.
   2. Gross and microscopic stool examination in the laboratory.
      a. Gross examination: Assesses stool for consistency, color, presence of blood, mucus, excess fat, and pus.
      b. Microscopic examination: Identifies constituents, such as WBCs, unabsorbed fat, and parasites.
   3. Culture and sensitivity.
      a. Culture assesses stool for presence of pathogens.
      b. Sensitivity identifies the most effective antibiotics.
      c. Obtain a specimen using sterile technique.
      d. Place the specimen in a sterile container.
   4. Occult blood (guaiac, Hemoccult).
      a. Assesses stool for microscopic amounts of blood in feces.
      b. Teach the client to avoid red meat, poultry, fish, vitamin C, aspirin, and nonsteroidal anti-inflammatory drugs before the test because these substances can cause false-positive results.

Table 23.1 Characteristics of Normal and Abnormal Stool

Expected Features	Abnormal Features and Precipitating Factors
Color • Adult: Brown. • Infant: Yellow.	• *Clay colored: Lack of bile due to biliary obstruction; barium used for diagnostic tests.* • *White: Undigested fat (steatorrhea); barium used for intestinal diagnostic tests.* • *Red: Lower GI bleeding; foods such as beets.* • *Black, tarry: Digested blood from upper GI tract; stool darkened by blood pigments (melena).* • *Pale brown: Malabsorption; diet high in milk or low in meat.* • *Green: Intestinal infection, such as C. difficile.*
Consistency • Formed, soft, moist, liquid.	• *Unformed, liquid: Increased intestinal motility (see "Diarrhea," in this chapter).* • *Hard, dry: Decreased intestinal motility (see "Constipation," in this chapter).*
Quantity • 100 to 400 g produced daily, evacuated every 1 to 3 days. • Amount depends on oral intake.	• *Excessive: Excessive intake of high-fiber foods, diarrhea.* • *Absent or small amount: Inadequate intake of food, especially foods high in fiber; GI obstruction; constipation.*
Shape • Tubular, about 1 inch in diameter.	• *Pencil shaped: Inflamed mucosa.* • *Ribbon shaped: Intestinal obstruction.*
Odor • Aromatic; depends on foods eaten and client's intestinal flora.	• *Pungent: Intestinal infection; blood in stool.*
Constituents • Undigested roughage, epithelial cells, protein, bile pigments, inorganic matter, dead bacteria.	• *Mucus: Intestinal inflammation.* • *Pus: Bacterial infection.* • *Blood (GI bleeding): Black—upper GI bleeding; red—lower GI bleeding.* • *Fat in large amounts: Malabsorption syndrome, enteritis, pancreatic disease.*

c. Ensure that the specimen is not contaminated with menstrual blood.

d. Use a commercial kit.

    (1) Apply a thin smear of stool on the designated window of the test packet.

    (2) Apply a reagent on the area following the specific times indicated by the manufacturer.

    (3) Note that a blue color in response to the reagent indicates the presence of occult blood.

    (4) Repeat the test for three consecutive defecations of stool.

5. Ova and parasites.

a. Assessment via a stool specimen.

    (1) Assesses stool for the presence of parasites and their eggs.

    (2) Collect several specimens from various sections of the stool.

    (3) Transport the specimen to the laboratory while still warm to maintain viability of the parasites and eggs.

b. Tape test for obtaining specimen for presence of pinworm eggs.

    (1) Assesses for pinworm eggs from around the anus.

    (2) Wear clean gloves to protect self from the client's body fluids and parasites.

    (3) Collect the specimen in the morning as soon as the client awakens.

    (4) Spread the buttocks, press clear cellophane tape against the skin surrounding the anal opening, remove tape immediately, and place it on a slide.

DID YOU KNOW?

Pinworms migrate at night from the rectum to the perianal area to deposit eggs and then return to the rectum before the morning. This is the reason why test tape specimens should be obtained in the morning before the client has a bowel movement or performs perineal hygiene.

B. Lower GI series (barium enema)

1. Fluoroscopic radiologic examination of the colon after a contrast medium is instilled rectally.

2. Secure consent for the procedure.

3. Teach about and maintain prescribed dietary restrictions, such as providing a clear liquid diet for 24 hours before the test and maintaining nothing-by-mouth (NPO) status for 8 hours before the test.

4. Teach about and/or implement bowel prep, such as a laxative, enema, or suppository, the evening before and/or the morning of the test.

5. Explain what will be done in the x-ray department: Positioned on left side and barium will be inserted into the rectum; position will be changed from left side, to back, and then prone; fluoroscopy follows progress of the barium and x-rays are taken.

6. Encourage increased fluid intake for 24 hours after the procedure to facilitate defecation of barium.

7. Administer laxatives or cathartics as prescribed to facilitate expulsion of the barium.

8. Monitor stool, which will be chalky white for 24 to 48 hours or until the barium is completely evacuated.

C. Endoscopy

1. Commonalities of nursing care associated with an endoscopy.

a. Teach the client about the procedure, and secure consent for the procedure.

b. Teach about bowel prep, such as medications, cathartics, and enemas the day before and morning of the procedure to cleanse the bowel.

c. Teach about a clear liquid diet for 48 hours before and NPO after midnight the night before the procedure.

d. Administer prescribed medications, such as a sedative or anxiolytic, before the procedure.

2. Sigmoidoscopy.

a. Insertion of a tubular speculum for examination of the sigmoid colon and rectum.

b. Position the client in the knee chest position or on the left side.

c. Encourage the client to take deep breaths to reduce discomfort and relax muscles.

d. Sit the client up slowly to avoid hypotension after the procedure.

3. Colonoscopy.

a. Insertion of a flexible endoscope through the anus to visualize the entire colon.

b. Instruct client to arrange transportation home after the procedure and to avoid driving for 24 hours because conscious sedation is used.

c. Explain that the scope will be inserted through the anus into the colon and that polyps may be excised, feces suctioned, and a biopsy taken.

d. Explain that increased flatus and abdominal cramping may occur after the test because air is inflated into the bowel during the test to promote visualization.

e. Monitor vital signs after the procedure because conscious sedation is used during the procedure.

f. Instruct client to notify the primary health-care provider if abdominal pain, fever, chills, muco-purulent discharge, or rectal bleeding occur after the test because these signs may indicate bowel perforation, hemorrhage, or infection.

g. Instruct client to avoid heavy lifting for a week and high-fiber foods for 48 hours if a polyp was excised or biopsy was taken during the procedure.

IV. Common Human Responses Associated With Bowel Elimination and Related Nursing Care

Diarrhea, constipation, fecal incontinence, hemorrhoids, and flatulence are common human responses related to bowel elimination. It is essential that the nurse understand the clinical manifestations, precipitating factors, and nursing care associated with each human response to better meet clients' needs associated with each of these responses.

A. Diarrhea

1. Description.
   a. **Diarrhea** is when intestinal hypermotility precipitates passage of fluid and unformed stool.
   b. Frequency of stool occurs three or more times a day.
2. Clinical manifestations.
   a. Frequent loose stools.
   b. Abdominal cramps, pain, or urgency.
   c. Abdominal distention.
   d. Hyperactive bowel sounds or flatus.
   e. Anorexia, nausea, and vomiting.
   f. Blood in the stool (frank, occult).
   g. Deficient fluid volume: Weight loss; thready pulse; hypotension; decreased tissue turgor; furrows of the tongue; flushed, dry skin and mucous membranes; sunken eyeballs; decreased urine output; atonic muscles; and mental confusion.
   h. Electrolyte imbalances, such as hyponatremia and hypokalemia.
   i. Stool possibly positive for causative pathogen or helminthic.
   j. With *Clostridium difficile,* characteristic odor and green-colored stool.
3. Precipitating factors.
   a. Viral, bacterial, or parasitic gastroenteritis.
   b. Spicy or greasy food.
   c. Raw seafood.
   d. Contaminated food and water.
   e. Excessive dietary fiber.
   f. Anxiety or other emotional disturbance.
   g. Drug side effects: Antibiotics suppress normal GI flora; antineoplastics and laxatives irritate the mucous membranes of the intestines, increasing peristalsis.
   h. Enteral nutrition (nasogastric or gastrostomy); hypertonic formula or too-rapid administration precipitates peristalsis. (For additional information about enteral nutrition, see "Enteral Nutrition" in Chapter 20, Nutrition.)
   i. Health problems, such as lactose intolerance, irritable bowel syndrome, malabsorption syndrome, and celiac disease.
   j. Ingestion of heavy metals, such as lead or mercury.
   k. Inflammatory bowel diseases, such as ulcerative colitis or Crohn's disease.
4. Nursing care for clients who have diarrhea.
   a. Assess the client.
      (1) Stool frequency, amount, and characteristics, such as consistency, color, and odor.
      (2) Signs and symptoms of deficient fluid volume and electrolyte imbalances.
      (3) Recent foreign travel and dietary intake.
   b. Obtain a stool specimen (e.g., culture and sensitivity, ova and parasite).
   c. Maintain standard precautions, such as frequent hand hygiene and gloves for perineal care, when assisting with fecal elimination. Institute contact precautions if diarrhea is caused by infection or infestation; wear a gown and gloves.
   d. Assist with elimination, such as providing privacy and transferring the client to the toilet, commode, or bedpan; use air fresheners discretely.
   e. Provide perineal care, such as assessing skin for breakdown and using a protective skin barrier.
   f. Maintain the prescribed diet, such as NPO, clear liquid, full liquid, bland, low fiber, or dairy- or gluten-free.
   g. Increase oral fluid intake gradually because a large amount can precipitate peristalsis.
   h. Administer prescribed medications, such as antibiotics, antidiarrheals, antihelminthics, enteric bacterial replacements, and electrolytes.
   i. Administer prescribed IV fluids.
   j. Provide health teaching.
      (1) Discourage intake of spicy and fatty foods; caffeine; and high-fiber foods, such as whole grains, raw fruits and vegetables, figs, and prunes.
      (2) Discourage intake of hot and cold fluids because they stimulate peristalsis.
      (3) Encourage foods high in sodium, such as tomatoes and bouillon, and potassium, such as bananas, oranges, apricots, and potatoes.
      (4) Teach correct handling and refrigeration of food.
         (a) Clean surfaces with hot water and soap after preparing raw chicken.

(b) Provide adequate refrigeration of perishable foods, such as milk and dairy products and foods containing mayonnaise; discard expired eggs

k. Document assessments, interventions, and client responses.

B. Constipation

1. Description.

a. **Constipation** is intestinal hypomotility that precipitates two or fewer stools a week and hard, dry feces.

b. **Obstipation** is intractable constipation.

c. **Perceived constipation:** Self-diagnosed constipation.

d. **Fecal impaction** is hard, dry stool firmly wedged in the rectal vault that cannot be passed.

2. Clinical manifestations.

a. Hypoactive bowel sounds.

b. Distended abdomen.

c. Rectal pressure or back pain.

d. Straining at stool.

e. Anorexia.

f. Blood-streaked stool.

g. Possible fluid and electrolyte imbalances.

h. For fecal impaction: Oozing diarrhea around an impaction; fecal mass confirmed by digital examination.

3. Precipitating factors.

a. Elimination habits.

(1) Laxative or enema misuse.

(2) Urge ignored because of inaccessible bathroom or anticipation of pain because of hemorrhoids, rectal or anal fissures, or other rectal or anal problems.

b. Inadequate fluid intake (less than 2 L/day).

c. Inadequate intake of fiber (e.g., whole grains, fruits, vegetables) in diet.

d. Side effects of opioids, iron, or anesthesia.

e. Developmental level.

(1) Child: Stool withholding behavior.

(2) Pregnant woman: Uterine compression of intestine, decreasing peristalsis.

(3) Older adult: Decreased peristalsis.

f. Inadequate physical activity.

g. Presence of mechanical obstruction or anal lesion.

h. Weak abdominal muscles; pelvic floor dysfunction or damage.

i. Anxiety or other emotional disturbance.

j. Cultural and family health beliefs, such as daily use of a laxative or cathartic.

4. Nursing care for clients who have constipation.

a. Assess stool for frequency, amount, color (e.g., greenish black due to iron intake), and shape (e.g., ribbon shape due to obstruction, pencil shape due to mucosal inflammation).

b. Assess for perceived constipation by asking if laxatives or cathartics are used daily.

c. Maintain standard precautions, such as performing frequent hand hygiene and wearing gloves when providing perineal care and assisting with fecal elimination.

d. Assist with elimination, such as providing privacy and encouraging the client to sit in an upright position, lean forward at the hips, apply manual pressure over the abdomen, and bear down while exhaling to prevent straining.

🛑 e. Encourage toileting after meals or offer a warm drink before a client's attempt to defecate to take advantage of the gastrocolic reflex. The gastrocolic reflex is the initiation of peristaltic waves when food enters the stomach, particularly when the stomach is empty.

f. Administer prescribed medications, such as laxatives and cathartics.

g. Administer prescribed enemas, such as oil retention, small-volume hypertonic solution, tap water, or soapsuds.

h. Provide health teaching.

(1) Encourage intake of high-fiber foods, such as whole grains, fruits, and vegetables.

(2) Discourage intake of binding foods, such as bananas and rice.

(3) Encourage increased fluid intake, activity, and exercise.

(4) Encourage consistent bowel habits, and teach the client to respond to the urge to defecate.

(5) Teach that a daily bowel movement is not always realistic and laxatives and cathartics are not advised because it causes dependence.

i. Provide perioperative nursing care if surgery is necessary to remove a fecal impaction.

j. Document assessments, interventions, and client responses.

DID YOU KNOW?

Perceived constipation is identified when a person uses enemas, laxatives, and/or suppositories to achieve a daily bowel movement. Some people believe that they are constipated if they do not have a bowel movement every day. However, a "normal" bowel pattern is highly individualized. Bowel movements may be as often as one to three movements every day to only three times a week. Nursing interventions for a client with perceived constipation are the same as for those with constipation. In addition, education is essential to help the client identify and achieve the goal of a pattern of elimination without the assistance of laxatives, enemas, or suppositories that is "normal" for them. This requires learning in the affective domain because the client must change a belief regarding what represents regularity of bowel function.

C. Fecal incontinence
1. Description.
   a. **Fecal incontinence** is the involuntary passage of feces and flatus from the anus.
   b. Extent of incontinence ranges from occasional episodes of seepage of stool to total loss of control of the passage of stool.
2. Clinical manifestations.
   a. Inability to control exit of feces from the body.
   b. Embarrassment due to soiling.
3. Precipitating factors.
   a. Inability to recognize the urge to defecate or the presence of rectal fullness due to altered thought processes.
   b. Impaired anal sphincter control or its nerve supply (e.g., brain attack and spinal cord damage).
   c. Decreased muscle tone.
   d. Diarrhea.
4. Nursing care for clients who have fecal incontinence.

🛑 a. Maintain a nonjudgmental environment; understand that incontinence may be viewed by the client as regression.

   b. Provide privacy and positive reinforcement.
   c. Provide prompt hygiene care.
   d. Use an incontinence device, such as Depends; avoid using the word "diaper," which is demeaning.
   e. Encourage attempts to defecate (e.g., in the morning, evening, and after meals to take advantage of the gastrocolic reflex).
   f. Implement and teach the client about a bowel retraining program.
      (1) Follow the client's usual pattern.
      (2) Follow the schedule exactly.
      (3) Increase fiber in the diet gradually.
      (4) Encourage the intake of eight or more glasses of water daily.
      (5) Administer a prescribed suppository or cleansing enema to empty the bowel to help promote eventual regularity.

D. Hemorrhoids
1. Description.
   a. **Hemorrhoids** are engorged, painful, bleeding veins in the lining of the rectum and anus.
   b. Can be internal or external.

2. Clinical manifestations.
   a. Rectal pressure, burning, and pain.
   b. Frank red blood from the anus.
3. Precipitating factors.
   a. Constipation or straining on defecation.
   b. Situations that increase venous pressure, such as pregnancy, weightlifting, standing for long periods of time, heart failure, and chronic liver disease.
4. Nursing care for clients who have hemorrhoids.
   a. Assess the anal area for the extent of swelling.
   b. Assess levels of rectal pain.
   c. Provide meticulous perianal hygiene, especially after defecation.
   d. Administer prescribed medications, such as stool softeners, local anesthetics, and anal lubricants.
   e. Administer prescribed thermal therapy to the perianal area, such as cold (e.g., cold packs) or heat (e.g., warm compresses and sitz baths).
   f. Provide health teaching.
      (1) Encourage the intake of high-fiber foods after acute episodes have subsided.
      (2) Encourage the intake of at least 2 L of fluid daily.
      (3) Teach the client to avoid standing or sitting for long periods.
   g. Provide care related to band ligation, hemorrhoidectomy, sclerotherapy, cryosurgery, infrared photocoagulation, or laser surgery.

E. Flatulence
1. Description.
   a. **Flatus** is gas in the stomach and intestines as a natural by-product of digestion that is expelled through the anus.
   b. **Flatulence** is excessive gas in the stomach and intestines that leads to distention of these organs precipitating physical discomfort.
2. Clinical manifestations of flatulence.
   a. Hyperactive bowel sounds.
   b. Cramping and/or abdominal pain.
   c. Abdominal distention.
3. Precipitating factors.
   a. Absent or decreased GI motility due to such factors as inadequate fiber in the diet, immobility, anesthesia, and opioids.
   b. Gas-forming foods and fluids, such as beans, peas, cabbage, onions, cauliflower, highly spicy foods, milk and milk products, and carbonated beverages.
   c. Swallowing of air that accompanies the intake of food and fluid.
4. Nursing care for clients who have flatulence.
   a. Inspect the abdomen for abdominal distention.
   b. Auscultate bowel sounds for hypoactivity or hyperactivity; be aware that the absence of

bowel sounds may indicate cessation of peristalsis (such as from adynamic ileus, postoperative ileus, or paralytic ileus).

c. Encourage activity.
   (1) Encourage in-bed activity when on bedrest, such as turning from side to side.
   (2) Increase ambulation; progressive ambulation after surgery.
d. Administer prescribed medications, such as antiflatulents or bulk cathartics.
e. Insert a lubricated rectal tube as prescribed (4 to 5 inches for 15 to 20 minutes every 3 to 4 hours) to promote the expulsion of gas.
f. Administer a return-flow enema (Harris flush, Harris drip).
g. Teach to avoid gas-forming foods and fluids.

Fig 23.4 Small-volume enema. (From Burton and Ludwig [2015]. *Fundamentals of nursing care: Concepts, connections & skills,* 2nd ed. Philadelphia: F. A. Davis Company, with permission.)

V. Enemas

An *enema* is the instillation of solution into the intestine via the anus and rectum. The administration of an enema is a dependent function of the nurse that requires a prescription from a primary health-care provider. There are various types of enemas, each with its own distinct purpose because of the way in which it precipitates a response in the body. Commonalities of nursing care for clients receiving an enema are presented here as well as nursing care specific to each type of enema.

A. Commonalities of nursing care for clients receiving an enema
   1. Maintain standard precautions, such as performing hand hygiene and wearing gloves.
   2. Explain the procedure to the client.
   3. Prepare the equipment.
      a. Fill the enema container with solution that is 105°F or obtain a prefilled hypertonic enema product.
      b. Flush the tubing or nozzle to remove air.
      c. Lubricate the tip of the tube or nozzle with water-soluble jelly.
   4. Provide privacy, such as by closing the door, pulling the curtain, draping the client, and ensuring that the bathroom is accessible and reserved.
   5. Place the client in left-lateral or left Sims' position to allow the solution to flow by gravity along the natural curve of the sigmoid.
      a. For small-volume enemas (e.g., hypertonic, oil retention): Insert the probe attached to the container its full length into the anus slowly (Fig. 23.4).
      b. Large-volume enemas (e.g., tap water, soapsuds): Insert the rectal tube into the anus slowly, 3 to 4 inches for an adult (Fig. 23.5).

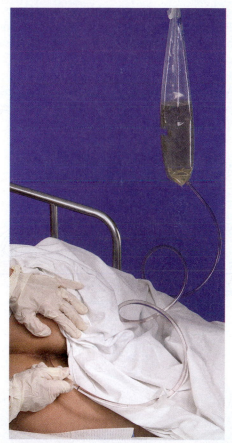

Fig 23.5 Tap-water enema. (From Wilkinson and Treas [2016]. *Fundamentals of nursing,* Vol. 2, 3rd ed. Philadelphia: F. A. Davis Company, with permission.)

   6. Interrupt the flow of solution if abdominal pain or cramping occurs; resume the flow when the client states the feeling has subsided.
   7. Encourage the client to retain the fluid as long as possible to promote maximum evacuation.

8. Assist the client to a commode or toilet or assist the client onto a bedpan (regular or fracture bedpan) when a client is on bedrest or is unable to exit the bed.
   a. Begin with the client in the supine position.
   b. Turn the client on the side or have the client flex the hips and knees and lift the pelvis up off the bed.
   c. Position the closed end of a regular bedpan or the closed, flat end of a fracture bedpan against the buttocks (Fig. 23.6).
   d. Assist the client to return to the supine position while the nurse holds the bedpan in place.
   e. Raise the side rails.
   f. Raise the head of the bed to a comfortable height for the client.
   g. Position a call bell within easy reach.
9. Remain close to the client during evacuation because it may cause dizziness, which is a safety concern.
10. Provide perineal hygiene care after the procedure.
11. Monitor for therapeutic effect (fecal returns) and untoward results (abdominal distension, rectal bleeding); notify the primary health-care provider if untoward effects occur.
12. Document client responses.
B. Types of enemas and related nursing care (Table 23.2)

VI. Bowel Diversions

Because of a disease process or injury to the bowel, a client may require partial or total, temporary or permanent, surgical removal of the bowel and the creation of a bowel diversion to permit evacuation of intestinal wastes. There are many commonalities of nursing care for clients with bowel diversions, but specific nursing care relates to the differences in the consistency of the fecal discharge (effluent), the type of appliance required, and factors that determine the need for intestinal irrigation.

A. Types of bowel diversions (Fig. 23.7)
   1. Colostomy.
      a. A **colostomy** is the formation of an opening (stoma) between the colon and the surface of the abdomen to permit feces to exit the body from the large intestine.
      b. Stoma in ascending colon: Liquid stool collected in an appliance.
      c. Stoma in transverse colon: Semisolid stool collected in an appliance.
      d. Stoma in descending or sigmoid colon: Solid stool collected in an appliance; may be controlled by daily intestinal irrigations with effluent eliminated in the toilet.
   2. Ileostomy.
      a. An **ileostomy** is the formation of an opening (stoma) between the ileum and the surface of the abdomen to permit feces to exit the body from the small intestine.
      b. Typical ileostomy: Liquid stool collected in an appliance.
      c. Continent Kock pouch: Tube inserted into an external stoma empties an internal reservoir of liquid stool; external pouch unnecessary.
      d. Ileal-anal anastomosis: Procedure that preserves evacuation through the anus, but evacuation is spontaneous rather than voluntary; liquid stool.
B. Nursing care for clients with a bowel diversion
   1. Assess the stoma, which should be deep pink or brick red, shiny, and moist (Fig. 23.8); a pale, purple, or black stoma indicates ischemia and the primary health-care provider should be notified immediately.
   2. Assess for bowel sounds and the presence of distention; motility generally returns 3 to 6 days after surgery.

Fig 23.6 Placing a client on a bedpan: (A) Regular bedpan. (B) Fracture bedpan.

Table 23.2 Types of Enemas and Related Nursing Care

Type	Description	Related Nursing Care
Tap water	• Involves induction of water into the colon. • Causes distention, which initiates the defecation reflex, stimulating peristalsis.	• Use 500 to 1,000 mL of tap water. • Raise the bag 12 inches above the anus or 18 inches above the anus for a "high" enema. • *Assess for signs and symptoms of water toxicity or circulatory overload, such as hypertension, bounding pulse, tachycardia, and tachypnea; may progress to restlessness, anxiety, moist breath sounds, crackles, and dyspnea.*
Soapsuds	• Involves induction of soapy water into the colon. • Irritates the bowel, which initiates the defecation reflex, stimulating peristalsis.	• Use 500 to 1,000 mL of solution. • Raise the bag 12 inches above the anus or 18 inches above the anus for a "high" enema. • *Give a maximum of three times when prescription includes "enemas until clear."* • *Use only the liquid castile soap included in the enema kit because other soaps and detergents can cause bowel irritation and damage.*
Hypertonic (Fleet)	• Involves induction of a small volume of commercially prepared hypertonic solution into the colon. • Pulls fluid out of interstitial spaces via osmosis filling the colon with fluid. • Causes distention, initiating the defecation reflex stimulating peristalsis.	• Insert prelubricated rectal tube of the 4 to 6 ounce container 3 to 4 inches into rectum. • Squeeze and roll the container slowly from distal to proximal end until empty. • Remove rectal tube and container while still compressed. • Encourage retention for as long as possible for best results. • *Assess for signs and symptoms of dehydration and electrolyte imbalances.*
Oil-retention enema	• Involves induction of mineral oil into the colon, which lubricates the rectum and sigmoid colon and softens stool. • A tap-water or soapsuds enema often follows an oil-retention enema according to manufacturer's directions.	• Insert a prelubricated rectal tube of the 30 to 60 mL container 3 to 4 inches into the rectum. • Squeeze and roll the container slowly from the distal to proximal end until empty. • Remove rectal tube and container while still compressed. • *Encourage retention for as long as possible for best results.*
Return-flow enema (Harris flush, Harris drip)	• Involves slow induction and exit of solution to facilitate expulsion of flatus. • Commonly used after surgery to relieve flatulence. • Reduces abdominal distention.	• Instill 100 to 200 mL of solution slowly into the colon. • Lower the solution container slightly below the anus to withdraw fluid and gas into the collection container via the same tubing. • Repeat the raising and lowering process five or six times. • Evaluate the results, such as bubbles returning into the collection container and reduction of abdominal distention and cramping.
Medicated enemas	• Involves instillation of a solution containing a drug to achieve a specific result. *Sodium polystyrene sulfonate (Kayexalate)* • Exchanges sodium ions for potassium ions, promoting the excretion of potassium. *Antibiotic solution (e.g., neomycin)* • Reduces bacteria in the colon before bowel surgery to decrease the risk of infection.	• Administer according to the primary health-care provider's prescription and manufacturer's directions. • Evaluate the results and side effects of the medication.

A. Sigmoid colostomy

B. Descending colostomy

C. Transverse colostomy, double-barreled

D. Ascending colostomy

E. Ileostomy

Fig 23.7 Location of various bowel diversion ostomies. Shaded areas indicate sections of the bowel that are removed or being "rested." The closer the colostomy is to the ascending colon ("higher"), the more liquid and continuous the drainage will be. (From Wilkinson and Treas [2016]. *Fundamentals of nursing,* Vol. 1, 3rd ed. Philadelphia: F. A. Davis Company, with permission.)

Fig 23.8 Healthy ileostomy stoma. (From Wilkinson and Treas [2016]. *Fundamentals of nursing,* Vol. 1, 3rd ed. Philadelphia: F. A. Davis Company, with permission.)

Fig 23.9 Ostomy supplies. (From Wilkinson and Treas [2016]. *Fundamentals of nursing,* Vol. 2, 3rd ed. Philadelphia: F. A. Davis Company, with permission.)

3. Assess the amount, consistency, and characteristics of stool.
4. Change the appliance every 3 to 5 days or as needed; note that many ostomy supplies are available on the market (Fig. 23.9).
   a. Clean the area with soap and water.
   b. Use a protective barrier on the skin under the appliance.
   c. Apply an antifungal agent on the skin under the appliance if prescribed.
   d. Measure and then apply the appliance with a 1/8-inch clearance to avoid stoma damage or skin exposure to stool (Fig. 23.10A and Fig. 23.10B).
5. Empty the bag when it is half full to avoid excessive tension on the appliance interfering with the integrity of the adhesive resulting in leakage of stool.
6. Refer the client to the United Ostomy Association or an enterostomal therapist.
7. Irrigate a distal colostomy (Fig. 23.11).
   a. Irrigate at the same time every day; note that the procedure may take as long as 60 minutes.
   b. Ensure privacy and adequate access to the bathroom.
   c. Prepare the irrigating bag with 300 to 1,000 mL of irrigating solution, as prescribed.
   d. Ensure the irrigating solution is at or slightly above body temperature.

Measuring stoma size

Applying a stoma appliance

Fig 23.10 (A) Measuring stoma size. (B) Applying a stoma appliance. ([A] From Wilkinson and Treas [2016]. *Fundamentals of nursing,* Vol. 2, 3rd ed. Philadelphia: F. A. Davis Company, with permission; [B] From Burton and Ludwig [2015]. *Fundamentals of nursing care: Concepts, connections & skills,* 2nd ed. Philadelphia: F. A. Davis Company, with permission.)

Irrigation solution

Irrigation cone inserted into stoma

Fig 23.11 Colostomy irrigation. (From Wilkinson and Treas [2016]. *Fundamentals of nursing,* Vol. 2, 3rd ed. Philadelphia: F. A. Davis Company, with permission.)

e. Flush the solution through the tubing to expel air (priming).

f. Lubricate the cone at the end of the tubing.

g. Position the client on a toilet or in a side-lying position in bed.

h. Place the irrigating sleeve over the stoma.

i. Insert the lubricated cone through the opening of the sleeve and gently into the stoma in the direction of the lumen; hold the cone in place during the inflow of solution.

🛑 j. Stop the procedure and notify the primary health-care provider if resistance occurs when inserting the cone.

❗ k. Shut off the flow of solution if the client experiences cramping; restart the flow once cramping subsides.

l. Remove the cone and tubing when the inflow of solution is complete; allow at least 30 minutes for evacuation through the sleeve into the toilet or bedpan.

m. Provide hygiene.

n. Apply an appliance.

o. Document the results and the client's response.

VII. Medications That Affect Bowel Elimination

When a person is diagnosed with a GI problem, the primary health-care provider can prescribe appropriate medications, depending on the client's need. The most common medications affecting fecal elimination include antidiarrheals, cathartics and laxatives, and antiflatulents. Additional medications, such as antacids, antiemetics, and antisecretory agents, usually are prescribed for problems interfering with nutrition, but they indirectly influence the GI tract. Nurses should know the mechanisms of action, therapeutic and nontherapeutic effects, and nursing care related to the common medications that are specifically designed to address a client's GI needs.

A. Antidiarrheals and related nursing care: decrease diarrhea and increase the production of formed stool (Table 23.3).

B. Laxatives and cathartics and related nursing care: prevent or treat constipation; evacuate the bowel for diagnostic tests or surgery (Table 23.4).

C. Antiflatulent and related nursing care: decrease the amount of intestinal gas (flatus) (Table 23.5).

D. Antacids (Table 20.7), antiemetics (Table 20.8), and antisecretory agents (Table 20.10): See Chapter 20, Nutrition, for information and nursing care related to these agents.

Table 23.3 Antidiarrheals and Related Nursing Care

Mechanism of Action	Examples	Nontherapeutic Effects
Motility suppressants • Inhibit mucosal receptors responsible for peristalsis.	• diphenoxylate HCl with atropine sulfate (Lomotil) • loperamide (Imodium)	• Tachycardia. • Respiratory depression. • Ileus. • Urinary retention. • Dry mouth. • Sedation, lethargy, and drowsiness. • Dizziness and weakness.
Enteric bacterial replacement • Reestablishes the intestinal flora.	• lactobacillus acidophilus (Bacid)	• Abdominal cramps. • Increased flatulence.

Nursing Care

• Assess for frequency of bowel movements and the color and characteristics of stool.
• Auscultate bowel sounds for a decrease in intestinal hypermotility, indicating a therapeutic effect.
• Monitor for signs and symptoms of fluid and electrolyte imbalances, such as deficient fluid volume, hypokalemia, and hyponatremia.
• Encourage increased fluid intake.
• Assess for therapeutic and nontherapeutic effects.
• Diphenoxylate HCl with atropine sulfate: Encourage the client to suck on hard candy to stimulate salivation associated with dry mucous membranes.

Table 23.4 Laxatives and Cathartics and Related Nursing Care

Mechanism of Action	Examples	Nontherapeutic Effects
Bulk forming • Increases bulk to stimulate peristalsis.	• methylcellulose (Citrucel) • psyllium (Metamucil)	• Diarrhea. • Fluid passed with feces.
Stool softeners • Promote entry of water and fat into feces to soften and decrease drying of stool. • May take several days to act.	• docusate sodium (Colace)	• Diarrhea • Mild cramps
Stimulants and irritants • Irritate bowel, causing propulsion of contents out of the body. • Are rapid acting.	• bisacodyl (Dulcolax) • cascara/senna (Senokot, Ex-Lax)	• Diarrhea. • Fluid passed with feces.
Lubricants • Soften feces.	• mineral oil	• Diarrhea. • Decreased absorption of fat-soluble vitamins.
Saline osmotics • Draws water into intestinal lumen, distending the bowel and stimulating peristalsis.	• magnesium salts (Milk of Magnesia)	• Diarrhea. • Dehydration. • Hypernatremia. • Decreased absorption of fat-soluble vitamins.

Nursing Care

• Assess frequency of bowel movements and color and characteristics of stool.
• Identify situations when these medications are contraindicated (e.g., in the presence of nausea and vomiting, abdominal pain, or additional signs and symptoms of acute abdomen because these may indicate bowel obstruction).
• Avoid administering saline osmotics to older adults or children because of the risk of fluid and electrolyte imbalances.
• Administer at bedtime.
• Encourage increased fluid intake, activity, and dietary fiber.
• Auscultate bowel sounds for an increase in intestinal motility.
• Assess for therapeutic and nontherapeutic effects.

Table 23.5 Antiflatulent and Related Nursing Care

Mechanism of Action	Example	Nontherapeutic Effects
• Causes coalescence of gas bubbles.	• simethicone (Gas-X)	• None known.

Nursing Care

- Assess bowel sounds and extent of abdominal distention before and after administration.
- Administer after meals and at bedtime.
- Shake liquid preparations well.
- Teach the client to avoid gas-forming liquids and foods, such as carbonated beverages, beans, and cabbage.
- Assess for therapeutic effects.

CASE STUDY: Putting It All Together

A nurse is admitting a middle-aged adult man to the hospital with a diagnosis of dehydration due to increasing GI distress and diarrhea. The client was recently discharged from the hospital after being treated with antibiotics for a mild superficial skin infection involving the suture line following a total knee replacement. The client tells the nurse, "Within a few days after discharge from the hospital, I got diarrhea and I thought it was due to something I ate. I took Lomotil for a few days, but it didn't help, so I went to my doctor. Now I am being put in the hospital for IV fluids and tests to find out what's causing the diarrhea." The nurse reviews the client's clinical record for the admission history and physical assessment and the primary health-care provider's prescriptions and then obtains the client's vital signs.

Client's Clinical Record

Admission History and Physical Assessment

Client stated, "I have been having loose bowel movements for about a week and then they became watery and increased to four to five times a day. When I got severe abdominal cramps, I finally went to my doctor."

Reports 3-lb weight loss in the past few days.
Reports thirst and fatigue.
Abdominal distention present.

Stool greenish in color and malodorous.
Perianal irritation and excoriation.
Flat neck veins.

Primary Health-Care Provider's Prescriptions

Contact precautions.
CBC.
Basic metabolic panel and magnesium and phosphorous levels.
Test stools for culture and sensitivity, ova and parasites, and *Clostridium difficile*.
Guaiac stool for occult blood × 3.
Vital signs and BP every 4 hours.
I&O.
Daily weight.
NPO.
OOB in room as tolerated.
IVF: D_5 0.45% sodium chloride 125 mL/hr.
Metronidazole (Flagyl) 500 mg, IVPB over 60 minutes, every 8 hours.

Vital Signs

Pulse: 98 beats/minute, regular rhythm, thready.
Temperature: 101.2°F, orally
Respirations: 20 breaths/minute.
Blood pressure: 108/68 mm Hg.

Case Study Questions

A. Identify at least five additional indicators of GI distress the nurse should monitor that are not included in the scenario.

1. _____
2. _____
3. _____
4. _____
5. _____

continued.

CASE STUDY: Putting It All Together

cont'd

Case Study Questions

B. Identify at least six clinical indicators of dehydration, a complication of diarrhea, the nurse should assess that are not included in the scenario.

1. _____

2. _____

3. _____

4. _____

5. _____

6. _____

C. After interviewing the client and completing a physical assessment, identify the most likely precipitating factor causing the client's diarrhea and explain your answer.

_____

D. Which prescription by the primary health-care provider should the nurse implement first? Explain your answer.

_____

E. Identify at least 10 nursing interventions that are associated with caring for this client with diarrhea caused by the presence of *C. difficile.*

1. _____

2. _____

3. _____

4. _____

5. _____

6. _____

7. _____

8. _____

9. _____

10. _____

REVIEW QUESTIONS

Be sure to read the Introduction for valuable test-taking tips.

1. A nurse is caring for a client who has a prescription for a fleet enema to be self-administered at home the morning of ambulatory surgery. What is important for the nurse to teach the client about this enema? **Select all that apply.**
   1. "Insert the nozzle its full length into the rectum to ensure it is beyond the internal rectal sphincter."
   2. "Retain the enema solution as long as possible to promote evacuation."
   3. "Lay on the right side as the solution is administered for best results."
   4. "Warm it in the microwave for 1 minute to promote comfort."
   5. "Squeeze the container until the solution container is empty."

2. A client comes to the clinic reporting abdominal bloating. It is identified that the client has slowed intestinal peristalsis. Which should the nurse encourage the client to do to increase intestinal peristalsis and minimize abdominal bloating? **Select all that apply.**
   1. Eat a high-fiber diet.
   2. Increase fluid intake.
   3. Use laxatives sparingly.
   4. Drink prune juice every morning.
   5. Raise the head of the bed 30° when sleeping.

3. A client is scheduled for an esophagogastroduodenoscopy. Which information should the nurse include when teaching the client about this procedure? **Select all that apply.**
   1. Mild bloating and flatulence is common after the procedure.
   2. A scope will be inserted via the nose and into the stomach and duodenum.
   3. Once you go home you can use saline gargles to relieve any throat discomfort.
   4. Call the primary health-care provider if vomiting blood occurs after the procedure.
   5. Drinking a small amount of water after awakening from the anesthesia is acceptable.

4. A client is admitted to the hospital for surgery for a gastric ulcer. What color should the nurse expect when assessing the client's stool?
   1. Pink to red
   2. Black, tarry
   3. Clay colored
   4. White, frothy

5. A nurse is to administer a premixed hypertonic disposable enema. The nurse verifies the prescription and performs all nursing interventions necessary before actually administering the enema. Place the remaining steps of the procedure in the order in which they should be implemented.
   1. Don clean gloves.
   2. Drape the client with the top sheet so that only the buttocks are exposed.
   3. Position the client in the left side-lying position with the right leg flexed.
   4. Remove the enema tip from the client's rectum while holding the container in the rolled-up position.
   5. Squeeze the enema container, maintaining slow, steady pressure from the bottom while rolling it up until all fluid is delivered.
   6. Insert the prelubricated enema tip beyond the internal sphincter slowly while directing the enema tip toward the umbilicus.
   Answer: _____

6. A client reports a long-term problem with constipation. Which should the nurse instruct the client to do to help minimize this problem? **Select all that apply.**
   1. "Include more bananas in your diet."
   2. "Drink a minimum of one quart of fluid a day."
   3. "Hold your breath when bearing down to have a bowel movement."
   4. "Increase the amount of fruits and vegetables that you eat on a daily basis."
   5. "Attempt to have a bowel movement after drinking a warm liquid in the morning."

7. A nurse is caring for a client who was admitted to the hospital with upper gastrointestinal bleeding. For which clinical indicator associated with upper gastrointestinal bleeding should the nurse assess the client?
   1. Pale, clay-colored stool
   2. Yellow, greenish stool
   3. Hard, dry brown stool
   4. Black, tarry stool

8. A client reports frequent episodes of constipation. Which should the nurse teach the client to do to help relieve this problem? **Select all that apply.**
   1. Use a prepackaged 4 oz enema once a week.
   2. Drink at least 3 quarts of fluid every day.
   3. Exercise at least 30 minutes every day.
   4. Eat 3 cups of vegetables a day.
   5. Take a laxative 3 times a week.

9. A nurse is caring for an outpatient client who is prescribed diphenoxylate HCl with atropine sulfate for diarrhea. Which information should the nurse include when teaching the client about nontherapeutic effects of this medication? **Select all that apply.**
   1. Monitor your pulse for a fast heart rate.
   2. You may experience some nausea and vomiting.
   3. Suck on hard candy when experiencing a dry mouth.
   4. Report abdominal cramps to the primary health-care provider immediately.
   5. Avoid engaging in hazardous activity until the response to the medication is known.

10. A nurse identifies that a client may have perceived constipation. What specific questions related to perceived constipation should the nurse ask the client? **Select all that apply.**
    1. "How often do you take a laxative?"
    2. "What is the consistency of your stools?"
    3. "Do you have a sensation of rectal fullness?"
    4. "When was the last time you had a bowel movement?"
    5. "Do you feel the need to have a bowel movement every day?"

11. Which independent nursing actions are associated with caring for a client with diarrhea? **Select all that apply.**
    1. Suggesting eating the banana from the breakfast tray
    2. Providing perineal care after each defecation
    3. Monitoring the client's hematocrit level
    4. Administering intravenous fluids
    5. Administering an antidiarrheal

12. A nurse is caring for a client who just had surgery 6 hours ago to remove a portion of the intestine and the surgical creation of a stoma. Which actions should be implemented by the nurse when caring for this client? **Select all that apply.**
    1. Auscultate for bowel sounds.
    2. Assess the color of the stoma.
    3. Explain that bowel function will return in two days.
    4. Empty the fecal collection bag when it is completely full.
    5. Clean the peristomal area with gentle soap and warm water.

13. A nurse is caring for a client who is menstruating and has a prescription for a stool specimen. What should the nurse do when collecting this specimen? **Select all that apply.**
    1. Wear sterile gloves to maintain sterility of the stool sample.
    2. Note on the specimen label that the client was menstruating.
    3. Collect one inch of formed feces to ensure an adequate sample.
    4. Send it to the laboratory promptly to avoid a degraded specimen.
    5. Flush the toilet first so that the water is clean and free from debris.

14. A nurse is caring for an older adult who was admitted to the hospital from the emergency department for rehydration therapy. The nurse reviews the client's clinical record and interviews the client. Which nursing intervention is the **most** important for this client regarding self-health management after discharge?
    1. Discuss the client's reason for taking a cathartic daily.
    2. Schedule monthly checkups with the primary health-care provider.
    3. Have a social worker assist the client with transportation to the local senior center for socialization.
    4. Teach the need to change position slowly to allow time for the body to adjust to the change in position.

Client's Clinical Record

Client Interview

An older adult female stated that she fainted in the yard while gardening and a neighbor called 911 for an ambulance, which took her to the emergency department. She said that she has been following all of her doctor's orders, but she has been taking milk of magnesia daily because she likes having a bowel movement every day. She shared that her stools have been very loose lately, but she would rather have them loose than to be constipated and bloated. She stated that she is very lonely because she has no family living nearby and does not drive anymore, so she watches a lot of television and works in her garden. She said that she just got up too quickly after weeding and that was why she fainted.

Laboratory Results

Hb: 16.8 g/dL.
Hct: 47%.
Creatinine: 1.3 mg/dL.
BUN: 46 mg/dL.
Potassium: 3.4 mEq/L.
Sodium: 147 mEq/L.

Medication Reconciliation Form (medications taken at home)

Centrum Silver vitamin daily.
Calcium 600 mg twice a day.
Magnesium hydroxide (MOM) 2 tablespoons at bedtime daily.
Ibuprofen (Advil) 400 mg every 6 hours when needed for joint pain, not to exceed 1,600 mg daily.

15. A nurse is caring for a client who is constipated. Which food is **most** appropriate for the nurse to teach the client to eat?
    1. Celery
    2. Grapefruit
    3. Bran cereal
    4. Sunflower seeds

16. A nurse is caring for a client who is scheduled for a lower GI series. Which information about this test should the nurse include in a discussion with the client? **Select all that apply.**
    1. "You will have to take a laxative the night before the test."
    2. "You will have chalky white-colored stool for 1 to 2 days after the test."
    3. "You will have to increase your fluid intake to 3 quarts after the test."
    4. "You will remain in the supine position for the duration of the test."
    5. "You will drink 8 ounces of barium just before the test."

17. The attached graphics illustrate bowel diversions with the stoma site and intestinal structures removed. Which intestinal diversion should the nurse anticipate will have the most formed stool?

A   B

C   D

    1. A
    2. B
    3. C
    4. D

18. A nurse is teaching a client about the best foods to eat to avoid constipation. Which vegetable selected by the client from the hospital menu indicates that the teaching was effective?
    1. Carrots
    2. Spinach
    3. Cabbage
    4. Zucchini

19. A nurse is teaching a client with diarrhea about foods that should be avoided. Which foods eliminated from the diet by the client indicates that the teaching was effective? **Select all that apply.**
    1. Graham crackers
    2. Chicken breast
    3. Kidney beans
    4. Scallops
    5. Yogurt

20. A nurse is teaching a client about high-fiber foods to eat when constipated. Which food should the nurse expect the client will select that indicates that the teaching was effective?
    1. Peas
    2. Apples
    3. Cherries
    4. Asparagus

21. A nurse is caring for a client with a transverse colostomy who has a two-piece ostomy appliance. Which actions are important for the nurse to do when caring for this client? **Select all that apply.**
    1. Tuck some gauze into the stoma after cleaning it until the new faceplate and bag is applied.
    2. Cut an opening in the faceplate so that it is at least ⅛ inch away from around the stoma.
    3. Empty the bag from the bottom, avoiding disconnecting the bag from the faceplate.
    4. Change the faceplate of the appliance every 3 to 5 days or when necessary.
    5. Teach the client how to implement a daily irrigation of the bowel.

22. A nurse working in a nursing home identifies that a client may have a fecal impaction. Which clinical manifestation is **most** specific to this problem?
    1. Passage of a small amount of brown liquid from the rectum
    2. Lack of a bowel movement for several days
    3. Distension of the abdomen
    4. Feeling of rectal fullness

23. A nurse is teaching a client with diarrhea about what foods to select from a menu. Which foods selected by the client indicate that the teaching was effective? **Select all that apply.**
   1. Shrimp
   2. Chickpeas
   3. Rye bread
   4. Milk shake
   5. Cottage cheese

24. A tap-water enema is prescribed for a client. The client says, "How does this type of enema work?" Which rationale should the nurse include in words the client will understand when answering the client's question?
   1. Water causes excessive interstitial fluid loss.
   2. Instilled water stimulates a bowel movement.
   3. Surface tension of water is reduced by soapsuds.
   4. Hypertonic nature of the water irritates the intestinal mucosa.

25. The nurse is caring for a client who is constipated. Bisacodyl (Dulcolax) 15 mg PO h.s. is prescribed. Bisacodyl is supplied in 5-mg tablets. How many tablets should the nurse administer? **Record your answer using a whole number.**
   Answer: _____ tablets

26. A parent brings a child to the clinic because the child has been reporting rectal itching. A specimen must be obtained so that the standard test for pinworms can be performed. What should the nurse instruct the parent to do? **Select all that apply.**
   1. Wash the anal area and then attempt to collect the sample.
   2. Collect the specimen as soon as the child awakens in the morning.
   3. Press cellophane tape to the area around the anus and place it on a slide.
   4. Insert a cotton-tipped swab into the anus and smear the sample on a slide.
   5. Pick up any worms found around the anus at night and put them in a sterile container.

27. A nurse is caring for a client adjusting to a colostomy in the descending colon. The client is concerned about eating foods that may cause an intestinal blockage. What foods should the nurse teach the client to avoid? **Select all that apply.**
   1. Cranberry juice
   2. Green beans
   3. Fresh pears
   4. Popcorn
   5. Rice

28. A nurse is teaching a client what to expect regarding a colonoscopy. Which information is **most** important to include in this discussion with the client?
   1. "You can expect flatus after the test because air is inflated into the bowel during the test."
   2. "Report abdominal pain, fever, chills, or bleeding to the primary health-care provider."
   3. "Avoid high-fiber food for a week if a polyp or biopsy is taken during the procedure."
   4. "Do not lift anything for a week if a polyp or biopsy is taken during the procedure."

29. A nurse is caring for a client who has an episode of diarrhea with frothy, odorous stool, containing an excessive amount of fat. Which word should the nurse use when documenting this type of stool?
   1. Chyme
   2. Melena
   3. Meconium
   4. Steatorrhea

30. Which dependent nursing interventions are associated with caring for a client who is constipated? **Select all that apply.**
   1. Assisting the client with ambulation 3 times a day
   2. Administering docusate sodium 100 mg twice a day
   3. Encouraging the intake of prunes from the meal tray
   4. Encouraging the client to turn from side to side in bed
   5. Responding immediately to the client's urge to defecate

31. A client self-administers a bowel prep consisting of NuLYTELY and bisacodyl the night before a colonoscopy and additional NuLYTELY in the morning. For what **most** serious adverse effect should the nurse assess the client?
   1. Deficient fluid volume
   2. Electrolyte imbalances
   3. Intestinal cramping
   4. Severe diarrhea

32. A nurse is teaching a client how to test stool for the presence of occult blood. Which information is important to teach the client about this test to achieve accurate results? **Select all that apply.**
   1. Repeat the test three consecutive defecations in a row.
   2. Collect the specimen in the morning on three successive days.
   3. Apply a thick layer of feces on the designated window of the packet.
   4. Defecate into a dry clean container inserted under the seat of the toilet.
   5. Avoid taking nonsteroidal anti-inflammatory medications before the test.

33. A client reports not having a bowel movement for several days. Place the nurse's actions in order of priority.
    1. Obtain a prescription for an enema.
    2. Request a prescription for a laxative.
    3. Encourage the client to drink more fluids.
    4. Ask the client when the last bowel movement occurred.
    5. Explore with the client how much fiber is being consumed in the diet.
    Answer: _____

34. A client has multiple fixation devices for fractures of the extremities because of trauma experienced in a motor vehicle collision. Bedrest and a regular diet are prescribed, and morphine sulfate 10 mg every 4 hours prn for moderate pain is prescribed. Which action by the nurse can help limit a common side effect of this medication?
    1. Prolong the times between the administrations of pain medication.
    2. Explain why ingesting yogurt daily is helpful.
    3. Teach the client to increase dietary fiber.
    4. Place the client on oxygen therapy.

35. A nurse is caring for a client with a nasogastric tube to intermittent wall suction. What should the nurse do to ensure that it is functioning effectively?
    1. Verify that the tubing is intact and patent.
    2. Position the client below the level of the collection bottle.
    3. Elevate the head of the client's bed to a semi-Fowler position.
    4. Ensure that the collection bottle is attached to a humidification adaptor.

REVIEW ANSWERS AND RATIONALES

1. ANSWER: 1, 2, 5.
Rationales:
1. The nozzle on a Fleet enema should be inserted its full length into the rectum to clear the internal rectal sphincter.
2. A Fleet enema is a hypertonic solution that draws fluid out of interstitial spaces via osmosis, filling the colon with fluid. This causes distention, which stimulates peristalsis, initiating the defecation reflex. The longer it is retained, the more time the hypertonic solution has to draw fluid out of the interstitial spaces and to fill the colon with fluid.
3. The left, not right, lateral or Sims' position allows solution to flow by gravity along the natural curve of the sigmoid.
4. An enema solution should never be warmed in a microwave. The water may become too hot and cause damage to the intestinal mucosa.
5. Squeezing the enema container until all the solution is instilled is important because the appropriate amount of hypertonic solution will achieve the best result.

TEST-TAKING TIP: Identify the clang association. The word *enema* in the stem and in option 2 is a clang association. Examine option 2 carefully.
Content Area: Bowel Elimination
Integrated Processes: Teaching/Learning; Nursing Process: Implementation
Client Need: Physiological Integrity; Reduction of Risk Potential
Cognitive Level: Application
Concept: Elimination

2. ANSWER: 1, 2, 4.
Rationales:
1. High-fiber foods increase bulk in fecal material, thereby facilitating intestinal peristalsis; bulkier feces increase pressure against the intestinal wall, which moves feces more rapidly through the colon. Instruct the client to increase fluid intake when ingesting high-fiber foods to prevent a bowel obstruction.
2. Two thousand to 3,000 mL of fluid daily provides enough fluid to be reabsorbed in the large intestine as well as promote a looser stool. Fluid in the colon mixes with the feces, increasing bulk; the increase in bulk stimulates intestinal peristalsis.
3. The use of laxatives, even sparingly, should be avoided because they weaken the bowel's usual response to pressure against the walls of the bowel.
4. Prune juice is high in fiber and is recommended to increase intestinal peristalsis.
5. Elevating the head of the bed 30° when sleeping helps reduce the risk of gastric reflux; it does not increase intestinal peristalsis.
Content Area: Bowel Elimination
Integrated Processes: Teaching/Learning; Nursing Process: Implementation
Client Need: Physiological Integrity; Basic Care and Comfort
Cognitive Level: Application
Concept: Patient-Centered Care; Elimination

3. ANSWER: 1, 3, 4.
Rationales:
1. Mild bloating and flatulence are common after the procedure. During the procedure carbon dioxide is introduced into the intestine to distend the lumen so that the instrument can be advanced safely and to maximize visualization of the intestinal mucosa.
2. Insertion of a scope via the nose and into the stomach and duodenum is incorrect information. The scope is introduced via the mouth, not the nose.
3. The client can use saline gargles to relive any throat discomfort upon returning home after the procedure. Saline is an isotonic solution that is soothing to the mucous membranes of the pharynx.
4. If the client is vomiting blood; has epigastric, substernal or shoulder pain; has black, tarry stools; or a fever, the gastrointestinal tract may have been perforated during the procedure. Immediate medical attention is necessary to treat this complication.
5. The client should not eat or drink until after the gag reflex and the ability to swallow return.

TEST-TAKING TIP: Identify the clang associations. The word *procedure* in the stem and in options 1 and 4 are clang associations.
Content Area: Bowel Elimination
Integrated Processes: Teaching/Learning; Nursing Process: Implementation
Client Need: Physiological Integrity; Reduction of Risk Potential
Cognitive Level: Application
Concept: Patient-Centered Care; Elimination

4. ANSWER: 2.
Rationales:
1. Pink- to red-colored stool indicates the presence of lower gastrointestinal bleeding such as hemorrhoids, anal fissures, and mucosal erosion.
2. Black, tarry stool (melena) indicates upper gastrointestinal bleeding. The black color is caused by hemoglobin in the blood being changed by digestive enzymes and intestinal bacteria.
3. Clay-colored stool is caused by lack of bile due to biliary obstruction.
4. White, frothy stool (steatorrhea) contains undigested fat related to diseases of the biliary tract or pancreas. Fat absorption is dependent on bile and pancreatic lipases.
Content Area: Bowel Elimination
Integrated Processes: Nursing Process: Assessment
Client Need: Physiological Integrity; Physiological Adaptation
Cognitive Level: Application
Concept: Elimination

5. ANSWER: 3, 2, 1, 6, 5, 4.
Rationales:
3. Positioning the client in the left side-lying position facilitates the flow of solution by gravity into the sigmoid and descending colons. Flexing the right leg allows exposure of the anus.
2. Draping the client supports privacy and dignity.

1. Donning clean gloves protects the nurse from the client's body fluids.

6. Slow insertion of the enema tip helps prevent sphincter spasm and inserting it beyond the internal sphincter helps minimize outflow of enema solution while it is being instilled. Directing the enema tip toward the umbilicus follows the normal contour of the rectum.

5. Squeezing the container from the bottom and rolling it up toward the tip while maintaining steady pressure prevents fluid from being suctioned back into the container.

4. Removing the container while firmly holding the container in the rolled-up position prevents fluid from being suctioned back into the container.

Content Area: Bowel Elimination
Integrated Processes: Nursing Process: Planning
Client Need: Physiological Integrity; Basic Care and Comfort
Cognitive Level: Analysis
Concept: Elimination

6. **ANSWER: 4, 5.**
Rationales:

1. Bananas should be avoided because they promote constipation.

2. A minimum of 2 to 3 quarts of fluid should be ingested to promote a soft stool.

3. Bearing down while holding the breath (Valsalva maneuver) should be avoided because it places a strain on the heart and can precipitate a cardiac dysrhythmia.

4. Fruits and vegetables contain fiber that adds bulk to stool, facilitating defecation.

5. Warm fluid or food entering an empty stomach precipitates the gastrocolic reflex, which precipitates intestinal peristalsis. Intestinal peristalsis moves fecal material toward the rectum where it can be evacuated.

Content Area: Bowel Elimination
Integrated Processes: Teaching/Learning; Nursing Process: Implementation
Client Need: Physiological Integrity; Basic Care and Comfort
Cognitive Level: Application
Concept: Patient-Centered Care; Elimination

7. **ANSWER: 4.**
Rationales:

1. Pale, clay-colored stool indicates a lack of bile, generally due to biliary obstruction. Also, it is associated with barium used for intestinal diagnostic tests.

2. Yellow, greenish stool is associated with intestinal infection, such as *C. difficile*.

3. Hard, dry, brown stool indicates decreased intestinal motility (constipation).

4. Black, tarry stool indicates digested blood emanating from the upper gastrointestinal tract. Stool darkened by blood pigments is call melena.

Content Area: Bowel Elimination
Integrated Processes: Nursing Process: Assessment
Client Need: Physiological Integrity; Physiological Adaptation
Cognitive Level: Application
Concept: Elimination

8. **ANSWER: 2, 3, 4.**
Rationales:

1. The consistent use of enemas is contraindicated. Frequent use of enemas will precipitate a reliance on this method to evacuate the bowel.

2. Three liters of fluid will provide enough fluid to meet metabolic needs and enough fluid to promote a softer stool.

3. Exercise promotes intestinal peristalsis, which helps propel fecal material toward the rectum.

4. Vegetables contain fiber, which creates a larger fecal mass as well as promotes intestinal peristalsis.

5. The consistent use of laxatives is contraindicated. Excessive laxative use will precipitate a reliance on this method to evacuate the bowel.

Content Area: Bowel Elimination
Integrated Processes: Teaching/Learning; Nursing Process: Implementation
Client Need: Physiological Integrity; Basic Care and Comfort
Cognitive Level: Application
Concept: Patient-Centered Care; Elimination

9. **ANSWER: 1, 3, 5.**
Rationales:

1. Tachycardia is a nontherapeutic response to diphenoxylate HCL with atropine sulfate (Lomotil). The drug should be discontinued, and the fast pulse rate should be reported to the primary health-care provider.

2. Nausea and vomiting are not nontherapeutic effects of diphenoxylate HCL with atropine.

3. Sucking on hard candy will stimulate salivation to moisten a dry mouth, which is a manageable side effect associated with diphenoxylate HCL with atropine sulfate (Lomotil).

4. Abdominal cramps are not a side effect of diphenoxylate HCL with atropine sulfate (Lomotil). Abdominal cramps are a side effect of enteric bacterial replacement therapy (*lactobacillus acidophilus* [Bacid]).

5. Diphenoxylate is a synthetic narcotic that can cause sedation, drowsiness, dizziness, lethargy, and weakness. Hazardous activities should be avoided until the client's response to the medication is evaluated.

TEST-TAKING TIP: Identify the word in the stem that indicates negative polarity. The word *nontherapeutic* indicates negative polarity.

Content Area: Bowel Elimination
Integrated Processes: Teaching/Learning; Nursing Process: Planning
Client Need: Physiological Integrity; Pharmacological and Parenteral Therapies
Cognitive Level: Application
Concept: Medication; Elimination

10. **ANSWER: 1, 5.**
Rationales:

1. "How often do you take a laxative?" is a question that should be asked of clients suspected of having perceived constipation because these individuals frequently self-prescribe the daily use of laxatives, suppositories, or enemas to ensure a bowel movement every day.

2. "What is the consistency of your stools?" is a question that should be asked of all clients with constipation; it is not specific to perceived constipation.

3. "Do you have a sensation of rectal fullness?" is a question that should be asked of all clients with constipation; it is not specific to perceived constipation.

4. "When was the last time you had a bowel movement?" is a question that should be asked of all clients with constipation; it is not specific to perceived constipation.

5. When a person believes that they should have a bowel movement every day the person will often take measures to facilitate daily bowel movements. This is a classic symptom of perceived constipation.

Content Area: Bowel Elimination
Integrated Processes: Communication/Documentation; Nursing Process: Assessment
Client Need: Physiological Integrity; Basic Care and Comfort
Cognitive Level: Analysis
Concept: Elimination

11. **ANSWER: 1, 2, 3.**
    Rationales:
    1. Although providing a diet is based on a prescription by a primary health-care provider and therefore a dependent function of the nurse, suggesting a food within the diet that is best for a client with diarrhea is associated with client teaching. Client teaching is an independent function of the nurse.
    2. Providing for hygiene needs of a client is an independent function of the nurse and does not require a prescription from a primary health-care provider.
    3. Monitoring the results of laboratory tests is an independent function of the nurse that does not require a prescription from the primary health-care provider. When a person has diarrhea, the hematocrit level generally is elevated due to hypovolemia. A nurse should notify the primary health-care provider if a level is outside the expected range.
    4. Administering intravenous fluids requires a prescription from a primary health-care provider and, therefore, is a dependent function of the nurse.
    5. Administering an antidiarrheal requires a prescription from a primary health-care provider and, therefore, is a dependent function of the nurse.

Content Area: Bowel Elimination
Integrated Processes: Nursing Process: Implementation
Client Need: Physiological Integrity; Basic Care and Comfort
Cognitive Level: Application
Concept: Elimination

12. **ANSWER: 2, 5.**
    Rationales:
    1. Intestinal motility generally returns 3 to 5 days after intestinal surgery. It is not necessary to assess for bowel sounds 6 hours after surgical creation of a bowel diversion.
    2. A stoma should be deep pink/brick red, shiny, and moist. This indicates that the stoma is receiving adequate circulation. If the stoma is pale, purple, or

black it indicates ischemia; this should be reported to the primary health-care provider immediately.
3. Bowel motility returns 3 to 5 days, not 2 days, after bowel diversion surgery.
4. It is too early to expect any fecal elimination. Once bowel function returns, the bag should be emptied when it is half full to avoid the weight of the bag from pulling the appliance away from the surface of the skin. If the bag is full it can cause unnecessary stress and strain on surrounding tissue as well as cause leakage under the seal of the appliance.
5. The peristomal area should be cleaned with gentle soap and warm water. Any solution stronger will interfere with tissue integrity and healing.

TEST-TAKING TIP: Identify the clang association. The word *stoma* in the stem and in option 2 is a clang association.

Content Area: Bowel Elimination
Integrated Processes: Nursing Process: Implementation
Client Need: Physiological Integrity; Basic Care and Comfort
Cognitive Level: Application
Concept: Elimination

13. **ANSWER: 2, 3, 4.**
    Rationales:
    1. Clean, not sterile, gloves should be worn when collecting a stool specimen to protect the caregiver from the client's blood or body fluids.
    2. The specimen label should indicate when a client is menstruating because if blood contaminates the stool specimen it will alter some of the test results.
    3. One inch of formed stool or 15 to 30 mL of liquid stool is necessary to complete commonly prescribed tests on stool.
    4. A stool specimen should be transported to the laboratory promptly because bacteriological changes may alter test results if testing is delayed.
    5. The client should be encouraged to defecate into a clean, dry bedpan and should be taught not to contaminate the stool specimen with urine, water, or toilet paper, which may alter test results.

TEST-TAKING TIP: Identify the clang associations. The word s*pecimen* in the stem and in options 2 and 4 are clang associations. The word *menstruating* in the stem and in option 2 is a clang association.

Content Area: Bowel Elimination
Integrated Processes: Nursing Process: Implementation
Client Need: Physiological Integrity; Reduction of Risk Potential
Cognitive Level: Application
Concept: Elimination

14. **ANSWER: 1.**
    Rationales:
    1. The client is experiencing perceived constipation and believes she needs to take milk of magnesia to ensure a daily bowel movement. This practice most likely caused the client to become dehydrated. Hypovolemia most likely precipitated the "fainting" episode. All of the laboratory results indicate dehydration. The Hb of 16.8 g/dL is higher than the expected range of 12 to 16 g/dL for an

older adult female. This is because the total blood volume is decreased with dehydration, but the red blood cell count remains the same. The Hct of 47% is higher than the expected range of 34 to 46% for an older adult female. This is because the total blood volume is decreased with dehydration, but the red blood cell count remains the same. A creatinine of 1.3 mg/dL is higher than the expected range of 0.5 to 1.2 mg/dL, indicating dehydration secondary to hemoconcentration. A BUN of 46 mg/dL is higher than the expected range of 8 to 21 mg/dL, indicating dehydration secondary to hemo-concentration. The potassium level of 3.4 mEq/L is lower than the expected range of 3.5 to 5.0 mEq/L for an older adult. This occurs when a client abuses laxatives, causing potassium wasting. The sodium level of 147 mEq/L is higher than the expected range of 135 to 145 mEq/L for an older adult. This occurs with diarrhea because water is lost in excess of the loss of sodium.

2. Scheduling monthly checkups with the primary health-care provider will not prevent this event from occurring again in the future. The underlying cause of the client's fainting must be identified.

3. Although the client's psychosocial integrity is important, it is not the priority. The underlying cause of the client's fainting must be identified.

4. Although teaching the need to change position slowly is important for safety reasons, it is not the priority. The underlying cause of the client's fainting must be identified.

TEST-TAKING TIP: Identify the word in the stem that sets a priority. The word *most* in the stem sets a priority. Identify the unique option. Option 1 is unique because it is the only option that attempts to collect more information from the client.

Content Area: *Bowel Elimination*
Integrated Processes: *Communication/Documentation; Nursing Process: Assessment*
Client Need: *Health Promotion and Maintenance*
Cognitive Level: *Analysis*
Concept: *Patient-Centered Care; Elimination*

15. ANSWER: 3.
Rationales:
1. One stalk of celery has 1.1 g of fiber, which is significantly less than the amount of fiber in the correct answer.
2. One-half of a medium-size grapefruit has 3.1 g of fiber, which is significantly less than the amount of fiber in the correct answer.
3. One cup of bran cereal has 19.9 g of fiber. This food has the highest amount of fiber from among the foods in the options presented.
4. One-quarter cup of sunflower seeds has 3 g of fiber, which is significantly less than the amount of fiber in the correct answer.

TEST-TAKING TIP: Identify the word in the stem that sets a priority. The word *most* in the stem sets a priority.

Content Area: *Bowel Elimination*
Integrated Processes: *Teaching/Learning; Nursing Process: Implementation*

Client Need: *Physiological Integrity; Basic Care and Comfort*
Cognitive Level: *Application*
Concept: *Patient-Centered Care; Elimination*

16. ANSWER: 1, 2, 3.
Rationales:
1. A bowel prep for a lower GI series (barium enema) generally includes a laxative the night before the test to help clear the bowel of feces. Also, a small hypertonic enema may be prescribed the morning of the test.
2. Stool will be chalky white for 24 to 48 hours after the test. After the barium is completely evacuated, stool returns to its characteristic brown color.
3. An increase in fluids after the test facilitates defecation of the barium.
4. The client starts on the left side, then moves to the back, and then prone during the test; the fluoroscope follows the progress of the barium and x-rays are taken.
5. The client does not drink barium. Barium is instilled rectally via a rectal tube.

Content Area: *Bowel Elimination*
Integrated Processes: *Communication/Documentation; Nursing Process: Implementation*
Client Need: *Physiological Integrity; Reduction of Risk Potential*
Cognitive Level: *Application*
Concept: *Elimination*

17. ANSWER: 1.
Rationales:
1. This stoma is in the sigmoid colon. The fecal matter (effluent) has passed through most of the large intestine. Fluid within the effluent is reabsorbed in the large intestine, leaving a formed to solid fecal matter.
2. This stoma is in the descending colon. Some fluid in the fecal matter has been reabsorbed in the large intestine. The consistency of fecal matter will be soft to formed.
3. This stoma is in the ascending colon. The fecal matter has not passed through enough of the large intestine for fluid to be reabsorbed. The fecal matter will have a liquid consistency.
4. This stoma is in the ileum of the small intestine (ileostomy). The fecal matter has not yet reached the large intestine where fluid within the fecal matter is reabsorbed; therefore, the fecal matter will have a liquid consistency.

Content Area: *Bowel Elimination*
Integrated Processes: *Nursing Process: Evaluation*
Client Need: *Physiological Integrity; Physiological Adaptation*
Cognitive Level: *Analysis*
Concept: *Elimination*

18. ANSWER: 2.
Rationales:
1. One-half cup cooked carrots has 3.4 g of fiber; this is about half the fiber of the vegetable that is the correct answer.
2. One-half cup cooked spinach has 7 g of fiber; this is twice as much fiber as the vegetables in the options that are distractors.

3. Two-thirds cup cooked cabbage has 3 g of fiber; this is less than half the fiber of the vegetable that is the correct answer.

4. One-half cup cooked zucchini has 3 g of fiber; this is less than half the fiber of the vegetable that is the correct answer.

TEST-TAKING TIP: Identify the word in the stem that indicates negative polarity. The word *avoid* in the stem indicates negative polarity.

Content Area: Bowel Elimination
Integrated Processes: Teaching/Learning; Nursing Process: Evaluation
Client Need: Physiological Integrity; Basic Care and Comfort
Cognitive Level: Application
Concept: Patient-Centered Care; Elimination

19. **ANSWER: 1, 3.**
   Rationales:
   1. Three graham crackers contain 3.1 g of fiber and should be avoided when experiencing diarrhea; fiber provides bulk that probably will prolong the diarrhea.
   2. Chicken breasts contain a small amount of fiber.
   3. One-half cup of cooked kidney beans contains 9.7 g of fiber and should be avoided when experiencing diarrhea; fiber provides bulk that is likely to prolong the diarrhea.
   4. Scallops contain no fiber.
   5. Yogurt contains no fiber.

   TEST-TAKING TIP: Identify the words in the stem that indicate negative polarity. The words *avoid* and *eliminated* in the stem indicate negative polarity.

   Content Area: Bowel Elimination
   Integrated Processes: Teaching/Learning; Nursing Process: Evaluation
   Client Need: Physiological Integrity; Basic Care and Comfort
   Cognitive Level: Application
   Concept: Patient-Centered Care; Elimination

20. **ANSWER: 1.**
   Rationales:
   1. One-half cup of cooked peas has 6.7 g of fiber; this food contains the greatest amount of fiber of the foods presented in the options.
   2. One small apple has 3 g of fiber; this food contains less fiber than the food that is the correct answer.
   3. Ten cherries have 1.2 g of fiber; this food contains less fiber than the food that is the correct answer.
   4. One-half cup of cooked asparagus has 1.7 g of fiber; this food contains less fiber than the food that is the correct answer.

   Content Area: Bowel Elimination
   Integrated Processes: Teaching/Learning; Nursing Process: Evaluation
   Client Need: Physiological Integrity; Basic Care and Comfort
   Cognitive Level: Application
   Concept: Patient-Centered Care; Elimination

21. **ANSWER: 2, 3, 4.**
   Rationales:
   1. The nurse can lay a 4 × 4 gauze over, not tucked into, the stoma to help absorb any leaking effluent; this will help keep the skin clean and dry. Tucking gauze into the stoma may damage the mucous membranes and should be avoided.
   2. The flange opening should be no more than ⅛-inch to ¼-inch clearance around the stoma. This distance does not infringe on the stoma and yet protects as much skin as possible around the stoma from digestive enzymes contained in stool.
   3. The bag can be emptied from the bottom.
   4. A faceplate changed every 3 to 5 days ensures adherence of the faceplate to the skin. The adhesive backing may loosen from the skin beyond 3 to 5 days, allowing leakage underneath the faceplate, resulting in skin excoriation.
   5. A transverse colostomy will not achieve regularity because stool is too soft in the transverse colon. Colostomy irrigations generally are used for stomas located in the sigmoid colon where stool is more formed and control with a daily irrigation may be possible.

   TEST-TAKING TIP: Identify the clang association. The word *appliance* in the stem and in option 4 is a clang association. More often than not, the option with the clang association is a correct answer. Examine option 4 carefully.

   Content Area: Bowel Elimination
   Integrated Processes: Nursing Process: Implementation
   Client Need: Physiological Integrity; Physiological Adaptation
   Cognitive Level: Application
   Concept: Elimination

22. **ANSWER: 1.**
   Rationales:
   1. Intestinal peristalsis increases behind a fecal impaction in an attempt to move the fecal mass toward the rectum. As pressure builds behind the impaction, fluid moves around the mass toward the rectum, resulting in the passage of brown liquid.
   2. Although there is a lack of a bowel movement with a fecal impaction, this occurs also with constipation without a fecal impaction.
   3. Although abdominal distension occurs with a fecal impaction, this occurs also with constipation without a fecal impaction.
   4. The client may not have a feeling of rectal fullness with a fecal impaction; this depends on where the impaction is located.

   TEST-TAKING TIP: Identify the word in the stem that sets a priority. The word *most* in the stem sets a priority.

   Content Area: Bowel Elimination
   Integrated Processes: Nursing Process: Assessment
   Client Need: Physiological Integrity; Basic Care and Comfort
   Cognitive Level: Application
   Concept: Elimination

23. ANSWER: 1, 4, 5.

Rationales:

1. Shrimp contains no fiber.

2. One-half cup of cooked chickpeas contains 6 g of fiber and should be avoided when experiencing diarrhea. Chickpeas will provide bulk that may prolong the diarrhea.

3. Two slices of rye bread contain approximately 5.8 g of fiber and should be avoided when experiencing diarrhea. Rye bread will provide bulk that may prolong the diarrhea.

4. A milk shake contains no fiber.

5. Cottage cheese contains no fiber.

Content Area: Bowel Elimination
Integrated Processes: Teaching/Learning; Nursing Process: Evaluation
Client Need: Physiological Integrity; Basic Care and Comfort
Cognitive Level: Application
Concept: Patient-Centered Care; Elimination

24. ANSWER: 2.

Rationales:

1. Tap water is hypotonic, which can cause water intoxication and fluid and electrolyte imbalance, not excessive interstitial fluid loss. In addition, this is medical terminology that may not be understood.

2. The large volume of instilled tap water distends the colon, which, in turn, stimulates peristalsis; it also softens feces. This terminology should be understood.

3. Soap is not added to a tap-water enema. Soapsuds enemas work by irritating the mucosa and distending the colon, which, in turn, stimulates peristalsis. In addition, this is medical terminology that may not be understood.

4. A tap-water enema is hypotonic, not hypertonic. In addition, this is medical terminology that may not be understood.

Content Area: Bowel Elimination
Integrated Processes: Communication/Documentation; Nursing Process: Implementation
Client Need: Physiological Integrity; Basic Care and Comfort
Cognitive Level: Application
Concept: Patient-Centered Care; Elimination

25. ANSWER: 3.

Rationale:

Solve the problem by using the formula for ratio and proportion.

$$\frac{\text{Desire 15 mg}}{\text{Have 5 mg}} \times \frac{x\ \text{tablet}}{1\ \text{tablet}}$$

$$5x = 15 \times 1$$
$$5x = 15$$
$$x = 15 \div 5$$
$$x = 3\ \text{tablets}$$

Content Area: Bowel Elimination
Integrated Processes: Nursing Process: Planning
Client Need: Physiological Integrity; Pharmacological and Parenteral Therapies
Cognitive Level: Application
Concept: Medication; Elimination

26. ANSWER: 2, 3.

Rationales:

1. Washing the anal area before collecting the specimen will wash away the pinworm eggs deposited on the skin around the anus.

2. Collecting the specimen upon awakening and before toileting and bathing ensures the greatest opportunity to collect eggs that were deposited during the night on the skin around the anus.

3. Using a piece of cellophane tape pressed against the anus and then applied to a slide, is the standard test for pinworm eggs deposited on the perianal skin surface during the night.

4. This is unsafe. Inserting a cotton-tipped swab into the anus and rectum places the child at risk for injury to the intestinal mucosa.

5. The eggs of pinworms, not the actual worms, are collected in the tape test for pinworms; the tape test for pinworms does not require sterile technique. The parent should wash the hands thoroughly before and after the procedure.

TEST-TAKING TIP: Identify the options that are opposites. Options 2 and 5 are opposites. Option 2 describes steps that are implemented immediately upon awakening, and option 5 describes actions that are implemented at night. More often than not, a correct answer is one of the opposites. Examine options 2 and 5 carefully. Identify the clang association. The word *specimen* in the stem and in option 2 is a clang association.

Content Area: Bowel Elimination
Integrated Processes: Teaching/Learning; Nursing Process: Implementation
Client Need: Physiological Integrity; Reduction of Risk Potential
Cognitive Level: Application
Concept: Patient-Centered Care; Elimination

27. ANSWER: 2, 3, 4, 5.

Rationales:

1. Cranberry juice is not associated with a blockage of the intestines after a colostomy. Cranberry juice is a beverage that may help control gas or odor.

2. Green beans are considered a "stringy" food that has the potential to cause an intestinal obstruction after a colostomy and therefore should be avoided. However, if the beans are cut into tiny pieces and chewed thoroughly, a client may tolerate green beans without experiencing an obstruction.

3. Fresh pears should be avoided because their tough skin is associated with blockage of the intestines after a colostomy. However, if the skin is removed, the inside of the pear is cut into tiny pieces, and the fruit is chewed thoroughly, a client may tolerate a pear without experiencing an obstruction.

4. Popcorn should be avoided because it produces a large amount of undigested fiber and could cause a blockage of the intestine after a colostomy.

5. Rice is stripped of its fiber when processed and is a starchy food associated with alleviating diarrhea. Because it is low in fiber, it prolongs transit time of

stool through the intestines, allowing more time for fluid absorption, resulting in a harder, dryer stool. Excessively hard, dry stool can cause an intestinal obstruction.

TEST-TAKING TIP: Identify the word in the stem that indicates negative polarity. The word *avoid* in the stem indicates negative polarity. The question is asking, "Which foods should *not be eaten* because they can cause an intestinal blockage?"

Content Area: Bowel Elimination
Integrated Processes: Teaching/Learning; Nursing Process: Implementation
Client Need: Physiological Integrity; Basic Care and Comfort
Cognitive Level: Application
Concept: Patient-Centered Care; Elimination

28. ANSWER: 2.
Rationales:
1. Although you want to teach the client to expect an increase in flatus after the procedure, it is not the priority.
2. These signs and symptoms may indicate bowel perforation, hemorrhage, or infection and should be reported immediately to the primary health-care provider.
3. High-fiber food should be avoided for 48 hours, not for a week, after the procedure if a polyp was excised or biopsy was taken during the procedure. High-fiber food has roughage which can injure the site of the polyp or biopsy, causing bleeding.
4. The client can lift light items but not heavy items for a week after the procedure if a polyp was excised or biopsy was taken during the procedure. This reduces the risk of bleeding at the site of the polyp or biopsy.

TEST-TAKING TIP: Identify the option with a specific determiner. Option 4 contains the word *anything* which is a specific determiner.

Content Area: Bowel Elimination
Integrated Processes: Teaching/Learning; Nursing Process: Implementation
Client Need: Physiological Integrity; Reduction of Risk Potential
Cognitive Level: Application
Concept: Patient-Centered Care; Elimination

29. ANSWER: 4.
Rationales:
1. Chyme is the matter produced by gastric digestion of food.
2. Melena is dark, tarry stool caused by digested blood.
3. Meconium is the term used to describe the initial stool passed by an infant. It is greenish black in color and generally occurs during the first 2 to 3 days after birth.
4. Steatorrhea is frothy, odorous stool with an excessive amount of fat; this is associated with malabsorption syndromes.

Content Area: Bowel Elimination
Integrated Processes: Communication/Documentation; Nursing Process: Implementation
Client Need: Physiological Integrity; Physiological Adaptation
Cognitive Level: Comprehension
Concept: Elimination

30. ANSWER: 1, 2.
Rationales:
1. A client's activity level is prescribed by a primary health-care provider. Providing for a client's activity, such as ambulating, sitting in a chair, or remaining in bed, is a dependent function of the nurse.
2. Administering a medication, such as docusate sodium (Colace), requires a prescription from a primary health-care provider and is a dependent function of the nurse.
3. Although providing a diet is based on a prescription by a primary health-care provider and therefore a dependent function of the nurse, suggesting which foods on the tray that are best for a client with constipation is associated with client teaching. Client teaching is an independent function of the nurse.
4. Implementing some measures to prevent complications of immobility, such as having a client turn from side to side, does not require a prescription from a primary health-care provider and therefore is an independent function of the nurse. Movement promotes intestinal peristalsis.
5. Assisting a client with toileting is an independent function of the nurse. Responding to the urge to defecate helps prevent constipation because the longer feces remain in the large intestine, the more water is reabsorbed, resulting in hard stools.

Content Area: Bowel Elimination
Integrated Processes: Nursing Process: Implementation
Client Need: Physiological Integrity; Basic Care and Comfort
Cognitive Level: Analysis
Concept: Elimination

31. ANSWER: 2.
Rationales:
1. Although this regimen may cause a deficient fluid volume, it is not as serious a consequence as another option presented. Fluids can be taken up to 8 hours before the test and intravenous fluids are administered during the test.
2. NuLYTELY (420 grams of polyethylene glycol (PEG) 3350, 5.72 grams sodium bicarbonate, 11.2 grams of sodium chloride, and 1.4 grams of potassium chloride) is an osmotic that draws water into the intestinal lumen. Bisacodyl (Dulcolax) is an intestinal stimulant that also expands intestinal fluid volume. These medications act together to pull fluid, which pulls electrolytes, into the intestinal lumen where they are excreted. Electrolyte imbalances can result in dysrhythmias that can be life threatening.
3. Although abdominal cramps may result from the cleansing regimen, cramping will not precipitate a life-threatening condition.
4. This bowel cleansing regimen will result in stools that will be frequent and liquid in consistency. This is the purpose of the regimen; an empty bowel allows for inspection of the intestinal mucosa without being impeded by feces.

TEST-TAKING TIP: Identify the obscure clang association. The words *sodium* in the stem and *hyponatremia* in option 2 is an obscure clang association.

Content Area: Bowel Elimination
Integrated Processes: Nursing Process: Evaluation
Client Need: Physiological Integrity; Pharmacological and Parenteral Therapies
Cognitive Level: Application
Concept: Fluid and Electrolyte Balance

32. **ANSWER: 1, 4, 5.**
    Rationales:
    1. Specimens are collected from three consecutive bowel movements.
    2. Specimens do not need to be collected in the morning. A client may not have a bowel movement every day.
    3. A thin layer of stool is all that is necessary to achieve an accurate result.
    4. Collecting the specimen in a dry, clean container inserted under the seat of the toilet helps to ensure that the specimen is not contaminated with toilet water. A specimen contaminated with water or urine may cause an inaccurate test result.
    5. Nonsteroidal anti-inflammatory medications and aspirin should be avoided before testing for occult blood because these medications can cause false-positive results.
    TEST-TAKING TIP: Identify the clang association. The word *test* in the stem and in options 1 and 5 are clang associations. Examine options 1 and 5 carefully.
    Content Area: Bowel Elimination
    Integrated Processes: Teaching/Learning; Nursing Process: Implementation
    Client Need: Physiological Integrity; Reduction of Risk Potential
    Cognitive Level: Application
    Concept: Patient-Centered Care; Elimination

33. **ANSWER: 4, 5, 3, 2, 1.**
    Rationales:
    4. Clarifying exactly when the client had the last bowel movement should be the first intervention to determine if the client is constipated. This is part of assessment. Some clients believe that they are constipated if they do not have a bowel movement every day or every other day.
    5. After constipation is confirmed, other issues related to constipation (e.g., amount of fiber and fluid in the diet and the amount of exercise) can be explored. This is part of assessment.
    3. After constipation has been confirmed and other data collected, the nurse can make recommendations to help resolve the problem. Constipation is a human response that nurses are legally permitted to treat. Adequate fluid intake promotes a soft stool.
    2. A laxative should not be prescribed until other less-invasive interventions are attempted.
    1. Obtaining a prescription for an enema should be the last intervention to be performed among the options presented. Less-invasive interventions should be attempted first.
    Content Area: Bowel Elimination
    Integrated Processes: Communication/Documentation; Nursing Process: Planning

Client Need: Physiological Integrity; Basic Care and Comfort
Cognitive Level: Analysis
Concept: Patient-Centered Care; Elimination

34. **ANSWER: 3.**
    Rationales:
    1. Prolonging the time between opiate administrations will decrease constipation but will reduce its pain control abilities. Pain must be treated effectively and interventions implemented to cope with the potential side effects.
    2. Although explaining why ingesting yogurt daily is important, it is not as important an intervention when compared to the information in another option. Yogurt may help constipation, but it is more effective in maintaining normal intestinal flora when receiving an antibiotic.
    3. An opioid will decrease peristalsis; therefore, a high-fiber diet is most effective in preventing constipation because it increases the bulk in the intestine, increasing peristalsis.
    4. This is unnecessary. The administration of oxygen will not prevent respiratory depression associated with the administration of morphine sulfate. If respiratory depression occurs, oxygen may be prescribed to increase oxygen to body cells.
    TEST-TAKING TIP: Identify the option that denies the client's feelings, concerns, or needs. Option 1 denies the client's need to have adequate medication to address pain caused by fractures of the extremities and orthopedic surgery.
    Content Area: Bowel Elimination
    Integrated Processes: Teaching/Learning; Nursing Process: Implementation
    Client Need: Physiological Integrity; Pharmacological and Parenteral Therapies
    Cognitive Level: Application
    Concept: Medication; Elimination

35. **ANSWER: 1.**
    Rationales:
    1. For a nasogastric tube to function effectively, the tubing must be connected appropriately, intact, and patent to allow drainage to flow to the collection container.
    2. Wall suction establishes negative pressure, which facilitates the flow of fluid from the client to the collection container; it does not rely on gravity.
    3. Wall suction works by establishing negative pressure. The position of the client is irrelevant.
    4. Humidification is associated with the administration of oxygen, not removal of fluid from the stomach via a nasogastric tube to intermittent wall suction.
    TEST-TAKING TIP: Identify the clang association. The word *tube* in the stem and *tubing* in option 1 is a clang association.
    Content Area: Bowel Elimination
    Integrated Processes: Nursing Process: Implementation
    Client Need: Physiological Integrity; Reduction of Risk Potential
    Cognitive Level: Application
    Concept: Safety

Chapter 24

Perioperative Care

NURSING CONCEPTS

Collaboration
Comfort
Communication
Elimination
Fluid and Electrolyte Balance
Hematologic Regulation
Infection
Inflammation
Legal

Mobility
Nutrition
Oxygenation
Patient-Centered Care
Perfusion
Safety
Sensory Perception
Tissue Integrity

KEY TERMS

Atelectasis—Collapsed or airless alveoli due to inadequate lung expansion

Conscious sedation—Administration of an intravenous agent to produce a depressed level of consciousness that allows a client to follow directions but to feel little or no pain

Dehiscence—Separation of one or more layers of a surgical wound before healing

Epidural anesthesia—Agent injected via a catheter into the epidural space to relieve pain while the client is awake and aware of surroundings

Evisceration—Spilling of abdominal contents from a surgical abdominal wound as a result of dehiscence

Hemorrhage—Uncontrolled internal or external bleeding

Hemovac drain—Drainage tube placed in the body near an operative site and attached to a round, collapsible reservoir with springs that, when compressed, establishes low negative pressure, which pulls drainage into the device

Hypervolemia—Excess fluid within the intravascular compartment.

Hypovolemia—Insufficient circulating blood volume

Hypovolemic shock—Severe insufficient circulating blood volume due to loss of 30%, or 1,500 mL, or more of circulating blood volume

Hypoxemia—Inadequate oxygen in the blood

Jackson-Pratt drain—Thin tube placed in the body near an operative site and connected to a self-suction bulb that is compressed to establish low negative pressure, which pulls drainage into the bulb

Laparoscopic surgery—Minimally invasive surgery using a thin lighted tube (laparoscope) and other instruments inserted through small incisions, allowing the surgical field to be visualized on a video monitor connected to the scope

Malignant hyperthermia—Rapid increase in heart and respiratory rates, progressing to hyperthermia, dysrhythmias, and respiratory and metabolic acidosis precipitated by anesthesia in clients with a rare autosomal dominant trait

Patient-controlled analgesia—Device that administers an intravenous analgesic at an hourly dose to manage pain at a consistent, tolerable level and allows the client to compress a trigger to deliver an extra dose as needed; however, a "lockout" prevents excessive doses when the trigger is pushed prematurely

Penrose drain—Soft, flat tube placed in the body near an operative site to drain blood, pus, tissue, and debris into a gauze dressing via gravity and capillary action

Continued

KEY TERMS—cont'd

Postoperative ileus (paralytic ileus, adynamic ileus)— Cessation of intestinal peristalsis characterized by lack of forward movement of intestinal contents

Pulmonary embolus—A thrombus that travels via venous circulation to the lung, obstructing a pulmonary artery

Robotic surgery—Surgery involving the use of mechanical arms to hold surgical instruments that are controlled by a surgeon sitting at a console

Spinal anesthesia—Agent injected via a lumbar puncture into the cerebrospinal fluid in the subarachnoid space to block movement and sensation below the level of the injection

Surgical safety check ("time-out")—Safety measure performed at various times during the perioperative period to verify the client's name, surgical procedure, and surgical site

Robotic telesurgery—Robotic surgery implemented remotely, in which the surgeon's console is located in one location and is connected to the surgical system at the client's location

Thrombophlebitis—Inflammation of a vein often with formation of a blood clot (thrombus)

Urinary retention—Inability to empty the bladder completely, resulting in excessive urine accumulation

I. Introduction

Perioperative nursing includes the care that is delivered by nurses to clients during the preoperative and postoperative phases of the surgical experience. Nurses must understand that surgery is an invasive procedure that has various purposes, degrees of urgency, and levels of risk and can be performed in a variety of settings. In addition, numerous personal risk factors can affect a client's surgical outcome. Nurses must identify the presence of these risk factors and implement appropriate nursing care during each of the phases of the surgical experience to meet the individual needs of clients.

A. Purposes of surgery
   1. *Ablative:* Surgical removal of a body part, pathway, or function (e.g., appendectomy, colectomy, amputation, and obliteration of ectopic foci in the heart).
   2. *Cosmetic:* Surgery to improve appearance (e.g., liposuction, facelift, and rhinoplasty).
   3. *Curative:* Surgical excision or repair of a diseased organ to reestablish function (e.g., complete removal of a cancerous tumor and repair of an aortic aneurysm).
   4. *Diagnostic and explorative:* Surgery to validate a diagnosis (e.g., cardiac catheterization, biopsy of a mass, and identification of a cause of gastrointestinal [GI] bleeding).
   5. *Palliative:* Surgery to reduce symptoms without curing (e.g., resection of a nerve root or partial removal of a mass) to provide for comfort.
   6. *Reconstructive and restorative:* Surgery to restore function or appearance (e.g., repair of a torn ligament, internal fixation of a fracture, or cleft lip repair).
   7. *Transplant:* Replacement of a diseased body part (e.g., kidney, heart, or lung transplant or joint replacement).

B. Degree of urgency
   1. Elective.
      a. When surgery is advised but the client's life is not imminently threatened.
      b. Allows for client preparation.
      c. Associated with low morbidity and mortality.
      d. Examples: Cataract extraction, knee replacement, and breast reduction.
   2. Urgent.
      a. When surgery is necessary within 24 hours of diagnosis.
      b. Allows for some client preparation.
      c. Reduces the risk of complications that can occur with a delay.
      d. Examples: Open reduction internal fixation of a fracture and removal of a cancerous tumor.
   3. Emergency.
      a. When immediate surgery is necessary to preserve life and/or function.
      b. Limits time for history taking and client preparation.
      c. Associated with increased morbidity and mortality due to concurrent conditions.
      d. Examples: Subdural hematoma, hemorrhaging, coronary artery bypass, and traumatic amputation.

C. Level of risk of surgery
   1. Major.
      a. Involves a high degree of risk.
      b. Associated with prolonged and/or complicated surgical procedures, blood loss, total or partial removal of a structure or organ, open abdominal or thoracic surgery, and potential postoperative complications.
      c. Examples: Cardiac surgery, removal of a kidney (nephrectomy), removal of a section of the large intestine (colectomy), and organ transplantation.

2. Minor.
   a. Involves a low degree of risk.
   b. Associated with few potential complications.
   c. Generally performed on an outpatient basis or in a surgical center.
   d. Examples: Hernia repair, arthroscopy, and cataract extraction.
D. Factors affecting surgical risk
   1. Age.
      a. Older adults.
         (1) Decreased physiological reserves, such as decreased cardiac output, cough reflex, immunity, vital capacity, subcutaneous tissue, blood oxygenation, glomerular filtration rate, and basal metabolic rate.
         (2) Increased comorbidities, such as heart disease, obstructive lung disease, diabetes, and peripheral vascular disease.
         (3) Increased calcium and cholesterol deposits within small arteries that increase the risk of hypertension, fluid and electrolyte imbalances, and shock when blood loss occurs.
      b. Infants and children.
         (1) Immature immune, renal, cardiovascular, and biliary systems.
         (2) Limited ability to regulate body temperature due to underdeveloped shivering reflex.
         (3) Limited response to anesthesia that causes vasodilation and heat loss.
         (4) Increased psychological and physiological stress because of an inability to understand what is happening and separation from parents.
         (5) Limited circulating blood volume, which increases the risk of hypovolemic shock and fluid and electrolyte imbalances, such as fluid volume deficit or excess.
   2. Medical history.
      a. Cardiovascular disease, such as hypertension, heart failure, and myocardial infarction, affects the ability to maintain cardiac efficiency.
      b. Kidney dysfunction, such as acute or chronic kidney disease, reduces the ability to excrete medications and regulate fluid and electrolyte balance.
      c. Lung diseases, such as asthma, emphysema, and bronchitis, decrease pulmonary function and increase the risk of postoperative pneumonia and atelectasis.
      d. Neurological disorders, such as spinal cord injury, are associated with vasomotor instability; people with seizure disorders commonly have an increased number of seizures during the perioperative period.
      e. Liver disease, such as cirrhosis, increases the risk of hemorrhage because of an inability to make prothrombin and increases the risk of toxic reactions to medications and anesthesia because of an inability to detoxify these agents.
      f. Coagulation disorders can contribute to hemorrhage due to delayed clotting mechanisms or risk of brain attack and intravascular clotting due to hypercoagulation.
      g. Diabetes mellitus increases the risk of infection and delayed wound healing because of a reduced ability to metabolize carbohydrates, proteins, and fat. Blood glucose levels are elevated in response to the stress of surgery.
      h. Current acute infections challenge physiological and energy reserves, increasing the potential for postoperative complications; upper respiratory infections increase the risk of pneumonia and atelectasis, particularly with general anesthesia.
      i. A decreased immune system, such as from cancer and its treatments (e.g., radiation, chemotherapy), bone marrow alterations, immunosuppressives to prevent organ transplant rejection, and steroids to reduce inflammatory disorders, places the client at risk for postoperative infection and delayed wound healing.
      j. Allergies and intolerances can cause uncomfortable—and life-threatening—integumentary and respiratory system reactions; some clients are allergic to prescription and nonprescription drugs, tape, latex, soaps, and ointments.
   3. Medications.
      a. Anticoagulants: Prolong blood coagulation time, causing bleeding.
      b. Antidepressants: Interact with anesthetics and may decrease blood pressure.
      c. Antidysrhythmics: Impair cardiac conduction during anesthesia.
      d. Antihypertensives: May interact with anesthetic agents, causing hypotension, bradycardia, and reduced circulation.
      e. Corticosteroids: Impair wound healing, suppress immunity, and increase the risk of excess fluid volume.
      f. Diuretics: May alter fluid and electrolyte balance, precipitating fluid volume deficit, hyponatremia, and hypokalemia.
      g. Anxiolytics and sedatives: May interact with anesthetic agents, causing respiratory depression.
   4. Herbal products.
      a. Ephedra (to lose weight): Increases the risk of dysrhythmias.
      b. Feverfew (to limit migraine headaches): Increases the risk of bleeding.

c. Ginkgo biloba (to increase memory): Affects platelet activity and increases the risk of postoperative bleeding.

d. Ginseng (to increase energy and immunity): Affects platelet activity and increases the risk of postoperative bleeding; may also increase hypoglycemia with insulin administration when a perioperative client has diabetes.

e. Kava (to promote relaxation): Intensifies the effects of sedatives.

f. Vitamin E (to increase immunity): In high doses, may increase the risk of bleeding.

5. Tobacco smoking.
   a. Increases respiratory complications because anesthesia is a respiratory irritant that stimulates the production of secretions.
   b. Nicotine constricts blood vessels.

6. Illegal drug use: May increase tolerance to anesthetics and analgesics, requiring higher doses to obtain a therapeutic effect.

7. Alcohol misuse.
   a. Alcohol potentiates the action of analgesics and anesthetic agents.
   b. Associated malnutrition delays wound healing.
   c. Associated liver disease and portal hypertension increase the risk of complications, such as hemorrhage.
   d. Withdrawal begins 24 hours after alcohol deprivation.

8. Nutritional status.
   a. Inadequate nutrition increases the risk of infection and delays wound healing.
   b. Increased protein, zinc, and vitamins C and A intake support wound healing.
   c. Daily requirement of 1,500 kcal is needed to maintain basic metabolic needs; because the metabolic rate increases during wound healing, this amount may have to be increased.

9. Obesity.
   a. Presence of comorbidities associated with obesity, such as sleep apnea, hypertension, coronary artery disease, and diabetes mellitus, may increase the risk of perioperative complications.
   b. Obesity decreases postoperative ventilation due to thoracic and abdominal weight impinging on the expansion of the thoracic cavity during inhalation, which may result in respiratory and cardiac postoperative complications.
   c. Fragility of adipose tissue and limited circulation in adipose tissue are associated with increased wound complications, such as delayed wound healing, separation of the wound edges (*dehiscence*), protrusion of the abdominal viscera through the incision (*evisceration*), and wound infection.

10. Fluid and electrolyte balance.
    a. Surgical trauma increases blood glucose and breaks down protein, resulting in a negative nitrogen balance, which impairs wound healing and increases the risk of infection.
    b. Adrenocortical stress response causes sodium and water retention and hypokalemia, which increases the risk of dysrhythmias.

11. Cognitive status: Impaired cognitive function, such as dementia, delirium, developmental delays, mental illness, confusion, and disorientation, may interfere with the ability to understand teaching or give consent.

12. Emotional health.
    a. Anxiety and a feeling of unease are common reactions.
    b. Clients may express emotions via angry, argumentative, demanding, or overly critical behaviors.

13. Extent of the incision: The larger the incision, the more trauma to body tissues.

DID YOU KNOW?

Historically, all surgery was performed through open incisions. Minimally invasive surgery was introduced with the advent of laparoscopic surgery. **Laparoscopic surgery** involves the insertion of a thin, lighted tube (laparoscope) and other instruments through small incisions, allowing the surgical field to be visualized by the surgeon on a video monitor connected to the scope. The laparoscopic approach causes less tissue trauma, thereby reducing the length of recovery. Laparoscopic surgery moved to a more complex level with the invention of robotic surgery. **Robotic surgery** involves a system that holds surgical instruments that, when moved by a surgeon sitting at a console, are more deliberate and precise than the human hand. Initially, these consoles were in close proximity to the client; however, in 1996, robotic telesurgery was introduced. **Robotic telesurgery** involves a computerized interface that transmits the surgical field over the Internet to a console at a great distance from the client. The continued growth in technology and miniaturization of instruments is predicted to result in robotic devices so small that they will be inserted into the body and directed to the surgical site, where they can be manipulated by the surgeon via computer commands. This technology is not so far-fetched when one notes that only several years elapsed between the first laparoscopic cholecystectomy in 1986 and laparoscopic surgery becoming the industry standard in the early 1990s for such surgeries as cholecystectomy, hysterectomy, and hernia and joint repair.

E. Surgical settings
1. Primary health-care provider's offices.
   a. Allow procedures to be performed at the time of an office visit.
   b. Are convenient for clients and primary health-care providers.
   c. Examples: Biopsy, minor plastic surgery, and dermal procedures.
2. Ambulatory surgery centers.
   a. Allow clients to be admitted for surgery in the morning and to be discharged later that day when stable.
   b. Used for surgeries that have minimal risk.
   c. Allow surgeries to be minimally disruptive to a client's usual routine.
   d. Allow the diagnostic surgical workup to be done on an outpatient basis.
   e. Typically have 23-hour admission, which allows monitoring for complications and pain control after surgery.
   f. Examples: Hernia repair, lumpectomy, laparoscopic cholecystectomy, angioplasty, tonsillectomy, and arthroscopy.
3. Hospital-based settings.
   a. Allow clients to be admitted to the hospital before surgery to perform diagnostic tests and/or correct problems (e.g., fluid and electrolyte imbalances) that may negatively impact the client's status during the perioperative period.
   b. Allow clients to remain in the hospital after major surgery that requires continued medical and nursing care.
   c. Allow clients admitted for same-day surgery (ambulatory surgery) to be admitted to the hospital after surgery if their status is unstable or a complication occurs.
   d. Examples: Joint replacement, gastric bypass, and emergency exploratory surgery.

F. Anesthesia
1. General.
   a. Loss of sensation and consciousness.
   b. Agent administered via IV or inhalation.
   c. Used for major surgery.
   d. Advantages.
      (1) Leaves client unconscious and motionless, with muscles relaxed.
      (2) Allows dose to be adjusted to age, physical condition, and length of procedure.
   e. Disadvantages.
      (1) Depresses the respiratory system, including cough and gag reflexes, increasing the risk of pneumonia and atelectasis.
      (2) Depresses the circulatory system, increasing the risk of thrombophlebitis.
      (3) Causes postoperative throat discomfort when an endotracheal tube is used.

      (4) Can lead to life-threatening complications, such as brain attack, malignant hyperthermia, and cardiac arrest.
   f. Stages.
      (1) Stage I: Beginning anesthesia, drowsiness, dizziness, and depressed pain sensation.
      (2) Stage II: Excitement, spasmodic muscles, irregular breathing, intact swallowing reflexes, and possible vomiting.
      (3) Stage III: Regular, rhythmic breathing; depressed reflexes and vital functions; relaxed skeletal muscles; constricted pupils; absent eyelid reflexes; and client readiness for surgery.
      (4) Stage IV: Complete respiratory depression; rapid, thready pulse.
2. Conscious sedation (moderate sedation).
   a. **Conscious sedation** produces a depressed level of consciousness (LOC) that allows the client to follow directions but causes the client little or no pain and usually prevents the client from remembering the proceedings of the procedure.
   b. Involves IV administration of sedatives and/or analgesic medications.
   c. Used for minor surgery and uncomfortable or painful diagnostic procedures.
   d. Advantages.
      (1) Allows for quick reversal of effects.
      (2) Allows the client to respond to commands and be aroused easily by touch or speech.
      (3) Allows the client to retain protective airway reflexes and spontaneous ventilation; vital signs usually remain stable.
   e. Disadvantages.
      (1) May cause discomfort in some clients, and some clients experience awareness of the procedure.
      (2) Requires client safety to be maintained during recovery (e.g., vital signs monitored every 15 minutes until fully awake and stable; client cannot drive after the procedure).
   f. Uses.
      (1) Endoscopies, such as colonoscopy and bronchoscopy.
      (2) Cosmetic surgery.
3. Regional anesthesia.
   a. Causes loss of sensation in a specific area while the client remains conscious.
   b. Given via a catheter.
   c. Types.
      (1) **Spinal anesthesia.**
         (a) Agent injected via a lumbar puncture into the cerebrospinal fluid in the subarachnoid space (Fig. 24.1).

Fig 24.1 Spinal and epidural anesthesia. (From Williams and Hopper [2015]. *Understanding medical surgical nursing,* 5th ed. Philadelphia: F. A. Davis Company, with permission.)

    (b) Blocks movement and sensation below the level of the injection.

    (c) Advantages: Usually does not cause respiratory depression; allows the client to be awake and aware of surroundings.

    (d) Disadvantages: May cause hypotension, urinary retention, nausea and vomiting, and/or headache from leakage of cerebrospinal fluid; agent may migrate upward in spinal cord, depressing respirations and heart rate.

    (e) Uses: Surgical procedures in the lower abdomen, pelvis, or extremities.

  (2) **Epidural anesthesia.**

    (a) Agent injected via a catheter into the epidural space (see Fig. 24.1); the catheter can be left in place and taped along the client's back and over the shoulder for easy access.

    (b) Advantages: Depth of anesthesia is less than general, and ability to move is maintained; client is awake and aware of surroundings; is safer than a spinal because it does not enter the subarachnoid space.

    (c) Disadvantages: Dose is higher than a spinal; if accidentally injected too deeply, hypotension and respiratory paralysis requiring mechanical ventilation may occur.

    (d) Uses: Pain, postoperative analgesia, and cesarean and vaginal births.

  (3) Local.

    (a) Agent injected into a specific area.

    (b) Advantages: Allows the client to be awake and aware of surroundings; has no systemic effects.

    (c) Disadvantages: May cause local skin reactions, such as itching and rash.

    (d) Uses: Minor procedures, such as suturing a laceration and biopsy.

  (4) Nerve block.

    (a) Injected into and around a nerve or group of nerves *(plexus).*

    (b) Advantages: Allows the client to be awake and aware of surroundings; usually has no systemic effects.

    (c) Disadvantages: Has the potential for systemic absorption.

    (d) Uses: Anesthetize the facial nerves, brachial plexus, and perineum for repair of an episiotomy.

  (5) Topical.

    (a) Agent is applied directly to the surface of the skin or mucous membranes.

    (b) Advantages: Allows agents to be promptly absorbed and act quickly.

    (c) Disadvantages: Requires an applicator or gloved hand to prevent exposure of the agent to the caregiver.

    (d) Uses: Reduce cutaneous neuropathic pain; limits pain of an injection.

G. Phases of perioperative nursing care

  1. Preoperative: Nursing care that is administered before the client has surgery.

  2. Intraoperative: Nursing care that is administered when the client is in the surgical suite.

  3. Postoperative: Nursing care that is administered after the client has surgery.

II. Preoperative Nursing Care

The preoperative period begins when the client and primary health-care provider agree that surgery is necessary or desired and ends when the client is transferred to the surgical suite. The reengineering of the health-care system, resulting in same-day surgery that negates the need for overnight hospital stays (e.g., outpatient surgery, ambulatory surgery), has dramatically changed the role of nurses during this phase. During the preoperative period, nurses are still responsible for collecting client information, helping with identification of health problems and risk factors that may impact surgery, preparing clients physically just prior to surgery, and participating in obtaining signatures for consents for surgery. However, the teaching role of the nurse has become most significant because the majority of clients are now responsible for their own care before and after a surgical experience. Pre-operative teaching decreases client concerns, prepares clients for the surgical experience, and limits the risk of postoperative complications.

A. Collect client information
1. Collect data from all sources, including the client, significant other, family members, medical record, and health team members.
2. Collect a health history.
3. Collect a spiritual and cultural history.
4. Perform a physical assessment.
5. Perform a mental and emotional assessment. Notify the primary health-care provider if a client expresses feelings of impending doom because this finding may herald the potential for an increase in mortality.
6. Identify factors that affect surgical risk, such as age-related issues and allergies (e.g., latex allergy) (Box 24.1).
7. Assess knowledge of surgery and perioperative care.
8. Assess past coping strategies and available support systems.

B. Informed consent for surgery and related nursing care (See "Informed Consent" in Chapter 3, Legal and Ethical Issues.)

C. Review common preoperative screening results
1. Complete blood count: Indicates the oxygen-carrying capacity of the blood and the status of immune function.
2. Urinalysis: Detects abnormal components, such as protein or glucose, or signs of infection, such as presence of casts or cloudy urine.
3. Chest x-ray: Assesses pulmonary status and the size of the heart.

4. Electrocardiogram: Identifies cardiac disease or dysrhythmias; usually for clients age 40 and older.
5. Blood urea nitrogen: Assesses kidney function.
6. Fasting blood glucose: Detects the possibility of diabetes mellitus.
7. Platelet count and partial thromboplastin time: Assess clotting ability and identify the risk of hemorrhage.
8. Type and cross-match blood: Prepare for possible blood transfusion.
9. Electrolyte panel: Provides data about fluid and electrolyte status.
10. Serum total protein and albumin: Assess nutritional status.
11. Pregnancy test: Detects pregnancy; implemented for all females of childbearing age.
12. Ensure that the test results are in the client's clinical record.
13. Report abnormal results to the primary health-care provider.

D. Implement bowel preparation
1. Teach the necessity of bowel preparation, which generally is done only for GI procedures to avoid the risk of contaminating the operative site.
2. Teach specific preparations, such as a low-residue diet for several days followed by medications, such as NuLYTELY and/or enemas, the day before and/or day of surgery.
3. Assess for clinical indicators of deficient fluid volume, hyponatremia, and hypokalemia.
4. Teach that bowel function may take 24 to 72 hours to return after GI surgery.

E. Administer or withhold medications
1. Administer routine medications as prescribed. *Note:* Many medications are withheld the day of surgery.

DID YOU KNOW?

Some medications that clients routinely take should be adjusted or discontinued before surgery. For example:
- Anticoagulants, such as clopidogrel (Plavix) and warfarin (Coumadin), increase bleeding and usually are discontinued 2 to 10 days before surgery.
- Aspirin and NSAIDs, such as ibuprofen (Advil, Motrin), increase bleeding time and usually are discontinued 5 to 10 days before surgery.
- Insulin doses must be adjusted according to the client's response to stress and the amount of glucose in intravenous solutions administered during and after surgery.

2. Administer medications when notified to do so by the health team in the surgical suite ("on call"), usually because the medication's onset and duration of action are synchronized with other drugs, anesthesia, and the surgical procedure.

Box 24.1 Latex Allergy and Related Nursing Care

- *Identify clients at risk, such as those with a history of multiple surgeries or medical procedures and health-care workers. Note: Latex allergy commonly is caused by excessive exposure to latex.*
- *Schedule latex-intolerant clients for the first surgery of the day so that the operating room has not been exposed to latex from a prior surgical procedure.*
- *Ensure a latex-free environment, such as by using percutaneous, mucosal, parenteral, and inhalation latex-free supplies.*
- *Identify latex allergy responses in an anesthetized client, such as flushing, urticaria, facial swelling, bronchospasm, hypotension, and anaphylaxis.*

3. Administer medications as prescribed.
   a. Antibiotics.
      (1) Limit microorganisms that can cause an infection.
         (a) May be given to prevent bacterial endocarditis in the presence of a history of rheumatic, congenital, or valvular disease.
         (b) Required with "dirty" wounds, such as traumatic injury, perforated thoracic or abdominal cavity, and devitalized tissue.
         (c) Recommended with surgery that requires entry into the genitourinary, GI, or biliary tract and with neck dissections and orthopedic surgery.
      (2) Usually administered 1 hour before surgery.
      (3) Examples are cefazolin (Ancef) and clindamycin (Cleocin).
   b. Anticholinergics.
      (1) Dry oral and respiratory secretions and help prevent laryngospasm, airway irritability, and risk of aspiration.
      (2) Usually administered just before the client is transferred to the surgical suite.
      (3) Examples are scopolamine and atropine.
   c. Antiemetics.
      (1) Reduce the risk of postoperative nausea and vomiting.
      (2) Usually administered just before the client is transferred to the surgical suite.
      (3) Examples are ondansetron (Zofran) and famotidine (Pepcid).
   d. Anxiolytics, sedatives, and hypnotics.
      (1) Ease anxiety, relax skeletal muscles, and facilitate anesthesia induction.
      (2) Usually administered just before the client is transferred to the surgical suite.
      (3) Examples are temazepam (Restoril), alprazolam (Xanax), and midazolam (Versed).
   e. Antisecretories.
      (1) Decrease gastric fluid volume and acidity.
      (2) Usually administered just before the client is transferred to the surgical suite.
      (3) Examples are cimetidine (Tagamet), ranitidine (Zantac), omeprazole (Prilosec), and pantoprazole (Protonics).
   f. Opioid analgesics.
      (1) Provide sedation and decrease the amount of anesthetic needed.
      (2) Usually administered just before the client is transferred to the surgical suite.
      (3) Examples are fentanyl (Sublimaze) and morphine sulfate.

   g. Anticoagulants.
      (1) Intravenously administered heparin must be withheld for 4 hours before surgery.
      (2) Subcutaneously administered heparin or low-molecular-weight heparin must be withheld for 12 hours before surgery.
      (3) Warfarin (Coumadin) must be withheld for a prescribed amount of time as indicated by the primary health-care provider; international normalized ratio (INR) must be stabilized before surgery.
4. Document medications administered and the client's response; notify the primary health-care provider if a drug has to be withheld (e.g., antihypertensive when a client's blood pressure is outside indicated parameters).

F. Maintain nothing-by-mouth (NPO) status
   1. Dietary restrictions may be necessary preoperatively because general anesthesia decreases GI motility and may cause vomiting.
   2. Teach about the length of time of NPO before surgery.
      a. Varies according to the type of surgery, client's status, and primary health-care provider's preference.
      b. Most primary health-care providers still prescribe NPO after midnight the day before surgery; however, the American Society of Anesthesiologists recommends a more liberal time frame (Box 24.2).

G. Detach removable items and indicate the presence of implanted devices
   1. Document the presence of a pacemaker, implanted defibrillator, implanted infusion ports, or any implanted metal, such as screws and plates.
   2. Remove any nail polish, makeup, false eyelashes, and hairpieces.
   3. Remove all prosthetic and metal items, such as artificial limbs, hearing aids, dentures, prosthetic eyes, contact lenses, eyeglasses, jewelry, body piercings, and hair pins and clips.

Box 24.2 Maintaining Nothing-By-Mouth (NPO) Status

Age	Solids	Clear Liquids
<6 months	4 hours	2 hours
6 to 36 months	6 hours	3 hours
>36 months including adults	6 hours	2 hours

In an Emergency: Nasogastric aspiration is performed to decrease risk of pulmonary aspiration

Adapted from: American Society of Anesthesiologist Task Force on Perioperative Fasting (1999).

H. Implement skin preparation
  1. Teach the client to wash, scrub, or shower the surgical area with antibacterial solution the night before and/or day of surgery as prescribed. *Note:* Final skin preparation occurs during the intraoperative phase.
  2. Remove hair as prescribed. *Note:* Hair removal is rarely performed because abrasions and nicks increase the risk of infection. Hair removal, if required, is done in the preoperative holding area with clippers, which are less likely to cause injury.

DID YOU KNOW?
Removal of hair (e.g., mustache, beard, and hair on head) before a procedure or surgery requires the client's written consent.

I. Implement urinary preparation
  1. Instruct the client to void just before being transported to the surgical suite.
  2. Insert an indwelling urinary catheter if prescribed to ensure an empty bladder, reduce the risk of injury during pelvic surgery, and allow for hourly monitoring of urinary output.
  3. Attach tubing to frame of bed or stretcher, not a side rail.

J. Implement safety protocols
  1. Raise the side rails on a client's bed immediately after administering preoperative medications that depress the central nervous system.
  2. Raise the side rails and secure client straps when a client is on a stretcher being transported to the surgical suite.
  3. Complete a preoperative checklist (Fig. 24.2).
  4. Complete a surgical safety check ("time-out") (Box 24.3).

K. Provide preoperative teaching regarding postoperative nursing care (See "Postoperative Nursing Care" in this chapter.)
L. Document all nursing assessments, interventions, and client responses

III. Intraoperative Nursing Care

The intraoperative period begins when the client is admitted to the surgical suite and ends when the client is transferred to the postanesthesia care unit (PACU). Nurses who work in a surgical suite engage in activities to maintain client safety and an aseptic environment as well as prevent postoperative complications and function as client advocates. With reengineering in health-care agencies, other certified personnel (e.g., surgical technologist) are more involved in direct client care. In addition, in today's health-care environment, recent-graduate registered nurses (RNs) rarely begin their practice in the surgical suite. For these reasons, the NCLEX-RN no longer asks questions in relation to the intraoperative period. However, the following information is included to provide a basic understanding of the intraoperative period.

A. Scrub nurse
  1. Can be an RN, a licensed practical nurse, or a certified surgical technologist.
  2. Prepares and maintains the sterility of the field and hands sterilized equipment to the surgical team members.
  3. Participates in the surgical safety checks ("time-outs").
  4. Uses vigilance and caution with sharps; counts all sharps, instruments, and sponges with circulating nurse before close of incision.

B. Circulating nurse (RN)
  1. Provides emotional support to the client.
  2. Ensures safety of environment (e.g., grounding of client and all electrical equipment).
  3. Ensures that the preoperative checklist is completed.
  4. Participates in the surgical safety checks ("time-outs").
  5. Assists with positioning of the client; provides supplies, equipment, and medications; manages specimens.
  6. Monitors I&O and blood loss.
  7. Counts all gauze sponges, sharps, and instruments with the scrub nurse before incision closure.

MAKING THE CONNECTION

Surgical Sponge Counts and Client Safety
A surgical sponge retained in the body after a surgical incision is closed can cause many problems. Not only can it lead to infection, but it also requires additional surgery for its removal and is considered professional malpractice. Historically, two nurses are responsible for counting the number of sponges before and after surgery to detect discrepancies that can help to identify retained sponges. Today, however, new technology provides other ways to double-check a sponge count by identifying whether a sponge is still in the wound and where it is located. For example, radiofrequency identification technology enables an operating room nurse to scan a client's surgical wound to identify the presence of a chip-embedded sponge. Activation of the scanner when it is held over the client's surgical wound alerts the nurse that a surgical sponge is still in the wound. In addition, some sponges have bar codes that are scanned before surgery and before the incision is closed to help account for the presence of all sponges.

PRE-OP SURGICAL CHECKLIST

Patient _____ Surgeon _____
    Last name   First name   Last name   First name

Patient Identification Number _____ Date of Surgery _____ Time of Surgery _____

- -

Date   **RN Initial**   **Patient Information**
____   _____   ID band on
____   _____   Allergy band on
____   _____   Allergies: _____
____   _____   Advanced directives completed (specify): _____

Medical Information
____   _____   History and physical completed
____   _____   Laboratory studies completed
                    RBC _____ HgB _____ HCT _____ WBC _____ Platelets _____
                    Potassium _____ Urinalysis _____
                    Pregnancy test: Serum _____ Urine _____
                    PT _____ PTT _____ Bleeding time _____
                    Type and screen _____ Crossmatch _____ - _____ units
____   _____   ECG completed: Yes _____ No _____
____   _____   Chest x-ray completed: Yes _____ No _____

Surgical Information
____   _____   Procedure to be performed: _____
____   _____   Site identified by surgeon with X and initials
____   _____   Consent signed
____   _____   Preoperative teaching performed (specify): _____
____   _____   OR prep completed (specify): _____

Day of Surgery
____   _____   Next of kin (specify): _____ Location of family (specify): _____
____   _____   NPO as ordered (specify): _____
____   _____   Hospital gown, head and foot coverings on
____   _____   Jewelry removed—disposition (specify): _____
____   _____   Dentures/bridges, prosthesis, contact lenses, eyeglasses, and hearing aids
                    removed—disposition (specify): _____
____   _____   Hair pins, makeup, nail polish, and one acrylic nail removed
____   _____   Antiembolism stockings on: Yes _____ No _____
____   _____   IV access in place: Yes _____ No _____

Prior to Transfer to Surgical Suite
____   _____   Preoperative medications given (specify): _____
____   _____   Side rails up
____   _____   Voided: Yes _____ No _____ Retention catheter in place: Yes _____ No _____
____   _____   Vital signs: T _____ P _____ R _____ BP _____

- -

Time-Out Safety Check
Patient identification (specify) _____
Procedure to be performed (specify) _____
Site of procedure (specify) _____
Comments:

Verified by: 1. Name (print) _____ Signature _____ Date/Time: _____
Verified by: 2. Name (print) _____ Signature _____ Date/Time: _____

Fig 24.2 Preoperative surgical checklist.

Box 24.3 Surgical Safety Check

- *Surgical safety checks (sometimes called "time-outs") are implemented to avoid wrong-person, wrong-procedure, and wrong-site surgical errors.*
- *Surgical safety checks are completed verbally, with the client If possible, and with participation of all health team professionals who are responsible for the client's care.*
- *Surgical safety checks are completed at specific times, such as before transfer to the surgical suite from the unit; on admission to the surgical holding area; before anesthesia induction; before the surgeon makes the surgical incision; and before the client leaves the surgical suite.*
- *Surgical safety checks involve three steps.*
  1. *Verify the name of the client: Ask the client his or her name and date of birth; check the arm band for the client's name, date of birth, and hospital number; use the arm-band bar code to verify this information if the client's arm band has a bar code.*
  2. *Verify the procedure: Have the client state the name of the surgery or procedure; this may be done by the surgeon if the client is not able to do so.*
  3. *Verify the surgical site: Have the client identify the surgical site if able. The surgical team should identify the location of the site; verify that the surgical site is clearly marked according to policy, such as with the word yes, and that the mark is visible after the client is draped for surgery. Also, verify that the mark includes the initials of the surgeon. The surgeon should mark the site before surgery, preferably the day before surgery, when the client is awake and aware.*

C. Anesthesiologist
  1. Transports the client to the PACU with assist from circulating nurse.
  2. States own name and gives report to the nurse receiving the client in the PACU.
     a. Client name, age, procedure, history, and current health problems.
     b. Intraoperative problems and how addressed; estimated blood loss; fluid and blood products administered.
     c. Location and condition of incision and dressing, location and status of tubes and drains, type of oxygen therapy; pain management interventions, and physical status (e.g., vital signs, O_2 saturation, respiratory status, and urine output).

D. Intraoperative complications
  1. Hypoxemia.
     a. **Hypoxemia** is deficient oxygen in the blood due to aspiration of secretions or vomitus.
     b. Caused by loss of cough reflex secondary to anesthesia and positioning that allows the pressure of abdominal organs to impinge on the diaphragm, limiting lung expansion.
  2. Hypothermia.
     a. Body temperature less than 98.6°F.
     b. Caused by exposure of body and internal organs to cool operating room temperature.
     c. Body heat lost by radiation, convection, evaporation, and conduction.
  3. Malignant hyperthermia.
     a. **Malignant hyperthermia** is the Rapid increase in heart and respiratory rates, progressing to hyperthermia, dysrhythmias, and respiratory and metabolic acidosis.
     b. Caused by anesthesia in clients with a rare autosomal dominant trait.
  4. Paresthesia.
     a. Numbness, prickly, stinging, or burning feeling indicating trauma to a nerve.
     b. Caused by prolonged placement in one position or inadequate use of protective devices, such as a mattress or foam/gel pads, that results in excessive pressure on peripheral nerves.
  5. Pressure ulcers.
     a. Damage to surface and underlying tissue integrity.
     b. Caused by prolonged placement in one position that compresses capillaries, interfering with oxygen to cells.
  6. Hemorrhage, hypovolemia, and hypovolemic shock.
     a. Uncontrolled internal or external bleeding (**hemorrhage**), insufficient circulating blood volume (**hypovolemia**), and severe blood and/or fluid loss that results in an inadequate cardiac output (**hypovolemic shock**).
     b. Precipitated by excessive blood loss, inadequate blood components, fluid loss, or inadequate fluid intake.

IV. Postoperative Nursing Care

The postoperative period begins when the client is admitted to the PACU and ends when the client has healed from surgery. Nurses caring for clients immediately after surgery focus on supporting clients during their recovery from anesthesia and maintaining airway, breathing, and circulation after the trauma of surgery. After clients are stable and are returned to a surgical unit or are being prepared for discharge home, the focus of nursing care shifts to meeting individual client needs. These needs include caring for tubes, drains, and wounds; managing pain; maintaining a balance among activity, rest, and sleep; maintaining fluid and nutritional intake; and promoting fecal and urinary elimination. These needs are met directly by nurses, or nurses reinforce the preoperative teaching so that clients can perform competent self-care in the home.

A. Receive report when client is admitted to the PACU or surgical unit
  1. General information: Identity of client using two indicators, age, procedure, name of primary health-care provider, and significant other.

2. Client history: Information such as allergies and acute and chronic health problems.
3. Intraoperative and PACU management: Type and duration of anesthesia, medications used, problems addressed, estimated blood loss, fluid and blood administration, urine output, and client responses.
4. Current physical, emotional, and mental status of the client.
   a. Use a scoring system, such as the Aldrete score, to objectively measure client status during the PACU stay; the Aldrete score assesses extent of activity, respirations, circulation, LOC, and O_2 saturation on a scale of 0 to 2 for each assessment.
   b. Determine when the clinical criteria for discharge from the PACU are met.
      (1) Stable vital signs.
      (2) Presence of spontaneous respiration and effective ventilatory functioning.
      (3) Easy arousal.
      (4) Absence of complications.
      (5) Aldrete score of 8 to 10; transfer the client to the intensive care unit if a score of 8 to 10 is not achieved within 4 hours postoperatively.
B. Maintain the client's respiratory function
   1. Assessments.
      a. Rate and rhythm of respirations; determine whether respirations are within or outside expected limits.
      b. Depth of respirations and use of accessory muscles.
      c. Breath sounds.
      d. Presence of artificial airway.
      e. Presence of gag and cough reflexes.
      f. Amount and characteristics of sputum; productive or nonproductive cough.
      g. Type and flow of oxygen delivery system.
      h. Pulse oximetry measurements.
      i. Clinical indicators of atelectasis, pneumonia, and pulmonary embolus.
   2. Nursing care.
      a. Maintain the client's airway and suction it if necessary. (See Table 19.7, "Types of Artificial Airways and Related Nursing Care," in Chapter 19, Oxygenation.)
      b. Administer oxygen as prescribed. (See Table 19.6, "Oxygen Delivery Systems," in Chapter 19, Oxygenation.)
      c. Position the client on the side unless contraindicated, and maintain functional alignment to allow secretions to exit the mouth and promote a patent airway.
      d. Remove the airway or endotracheal tube when the gag reflex returns to prevent vomiting; usually done in the PACU.

e. Promote lung expansion to prevent atelectasis and pneumonia.
   (1) Elevate the head of the bed.
   (2) Encourage coughing and deep breathing; teach the client to splint an abdominal incision with a pillow or the hands to limit pain and increase the depth of inhalations.
   (3) Encourage the use of an incentive spirometer 10 times every hour when awake (Fig. 24.3A and B).
   (4) Encourage in-bed activity or progressive ambulation if permitted.
f. Notify the rapid response team and primary health-care provider if the client's oxygen saturation is less than acceptable compared per agency policy or the surgeon's preset parameters (e.g., less than 92%) or if the client exhibits clinical indicators of atelectasis, pneumonia, or pulmonary embolus.

Fig 24.3 Incentive spirometry. (A) Voldyne volumetric deep-breathing exerciser. (B) Client using an incentive spirometer. (From [A] Williams and Hopper [2015]. *Understanding medical surgical nursing*, 5th ed. Philadelphia: F. A. Davis Company, with permission; [B] Wilkinson and Treas [2011]. *Fundamentals of nursing*, Vol. 1, 2nd ed. Philadelphia: F. A. Davis Company, with permission.)

3. Postoperative respiratory complications.
   a. **Atelectasis:** Collapsed or airless alveoli due to inadequate lung expansion.
      (1) Assessments.
         (a) Dyspnea, tachypnea, and pleural pain.
         (b) Reduced or absent breath sounds and crackles.
         (c) Tachycardia.
         (d) Decreased oxygen saturation.
         (e) Anxiety.
         (f) Diaphoresis.
      (2) Nursing care.
         (a) Raise head of bed to promote lung expansion.
         (b) Administer humidified oxygen as prescribed.
         (c) Monitor for clinical indicators of progression to pneumonia.
   b. Pneumonia: Inflammation of the lungs caused by a microorganism.
      (1) Assessments.
         (a) Dyspnea, tachypnea, and chest pain.
         (b) Decreased breath sounds, crackles, and wheezes.
         (c) Blood-tinged and/or purulent sputum; cough that usually is productive.
         (d) Increased temperature.
         (e) Decreased oxygen saturation.
         (f) Increased white blood cell count.
         (g) Infiltrates on chest x-ray examination.
         (h) Identification of causative microorganism on culture of sputum.
      (2) Nursing care.
         (a) Raise head of bed to promote lung expansion.
         (b) Suction the airway to maintain patency if necessary.
         🛑 (c) Maintain droplet transmission-based precautions if required.
         (d) Administer humidified oxygen as prescribed.
         (e) Balance rest and activity.
         (f) Teach pursed-lip breathing to facilitate exhalation.
         (g) Increase oral and/or IV fluid intake as prescribed to liquefy respiratory secretions.
         (h) Teach client to dispose of tissues contaminated with sputum into a bag impervious to fluid; provide frequent oral hygiene.
         (i) Administer prescribed medications, such as antibiotics, mucolytics, and bronchodilators.
         (j) Provide chest physiotherapy if prescribed.
   c. **Pulmonary embolus:** Obstruction of a pulmonary artery caused by a blood clot (thrombus) that originated in a lower extremity and traveled to the lung.
      (1) Assessments.
         (a) Sudden chest pain, frequently unilateral.
         (b) Shortness of breath *(dyspnea)*.
         (c) Absent breath sounds in affected area of lung.
         (d) Blood-tinged sputum *(hemoptysis)*.
         (e) Tachycardia; decreased blood pressure.
         (f) Cyanosis.
      (2) Nursing care.
         (a) Maintain bedrest.
         (b) Elevate the head of the bed.
         (c) Provide humidified oxygen.
         🛑 (d) Notify the rapid response team and the primary health-care provider immediately.
         (e) Administer prescribed fibrinolytic therapy if prescribed.
         (f) Administer analgesics and anticoagulants (e.g., heparin progressing to warfarin [Coumadin]) as prescribed.
         (g) Prepare the client for insertion of an inferior vena cava filter if scheduled.
         (h) Assess the client's lower extremities for clinical indicators of thrombophlebitis.
C. Maintain the client's circulatory function
   1. Assessments.
      a. Continuous cardiac monitoring while in the PACU; heart rate and rhythm and blood pressure routinely after discharge from the PACU based on the client's status or agency protocol.
      b. Skin color (e.g., pink, dusky, blotchy, cyanotic).
      c. I&O, including blood loss via incision, wound drains, and tubes.
      d. Hourly urine as prescribed if a urinary retention catheter is present; expect hourly output to be more than 30 mL.
      e. Neurovascular status of the extremities, such as pedal pulse, capillary refill, color, temperature, movement, and sensation.
      f. Clinical indicators of thrombophlebitis, hemorrhage, and hypovolemic shock.

2. Nursing care.
  a. Promote venous return to prevent venous stasis, thrombophlebitis, and pulmonary embolus.
    (1) Maintain the use of a venous compression device or antiembolism stockings if prescribed (Fig. 24.4A and B).
    (2) Teach the client to prevent popliteal pressure: Avoid crossing the legs, placing pillows behind the knees, and positioning the bed in the contour position ("gatching" the bed); avoid keeping the legs dependent to prevent venous stasis; avoid massaging the legs to prevent a thrombus from becoming an embolus.
    (3) Encourage the client to perform postoperative leg exercises (Box 24.4).
    (4) Administer prescribed prophylactic anticoagulants, such as low-molecular-weight heparin (e.g., dalteparin [Fragmin], enoxaparin [Lovenox]).
  b. Encourage oral fluid intake if permitted; administer IV fluids as prescribed.
  c. Notify the primary health-care provider if hourly urine output is less than 30 mL/hr.

Fig 24.4 Lower extremity compression devices. (A) Sequential compression device. (B) Antiembolism stockings. (From Wilkinson and Treas [2016]. *Fundamentals of nursing,* Vol. 1, 3rd ed. Philadelphia: F. A. Davis Company, with permission.)

Box 24.4 Postoperative Leg Exercises

Flex the knee while sliding the foot on the mattress toward the buttocks.

A

Extend the knee while sliding the foot on the mattress away from the buttocks; press the back of the knee against the bed with the leg extended and the foot dorsiflexed.

B

Raise and lower the leg while keeping the knee extended.

C

Keep the knee extended while flexing the foot toward the abdomen (dorsiflexion) and then away from the abdomen (plantar flexion).

D

Rotate the ankle while maintaining the foot in dorsiflexion.

E

  d. Notify the rapid response team and primary health-care provider if the client exhibits clinical indicators of thrombophlebitis, hemorrhage, or hypovolemic shock.

3. Postoperative circulatory complications.
  a. **Thrombophlebitis:** Inflammation of a vein often with formation of a blood clot (thrombus) due to injury to a vein, external pressure behind the knees, or venous pooling secondary to immobility.
    (1) Assessments.
      (a) Discomfort or pain, such as burning, achiness, or cramping in an extremity, usually the calf of a lower extremity.
      (b) Pain on dorsiflexion of a foot (Homan sign); this sign should never be elicited intentionally because doing so can dislodge a thrombus, causing a pulmonary embolus.

(c) Erythema, edema, and warmth in the affected area.

(d) Bilateral measurements of calf and thigh circumferences may identify an increase in the circumference of the affected extremity.

(2) Nursing care.

🛑 (a) Institute bedrest immediately.

(b) Elevate the affected extremity on a pillow.

(c) Notify the primary health-care provider.

(d) Encourage oral fluid intake and IV fluids as prescribed.

(e) Apply warm soaks to the affected area if prescribed.

(f) Administer anticoagulants as prescribed, usually IV heparin, progressing to warfarin (Coumadin).

(g) Prepare the client for insertion of an inferior vena cava filter if scheduled.

(h) Administer prescribed medications, such as antibiotics and analgesics.

b. Hemorrhage and hypovolemic shock: **Hemorrhage** is the loss of blood from the circulatory system that is difficult to control. **Hypovolemic shock** is the severe loss of blood and fluid (class III and class IV hemorrhage) that make the heart unable to pump enough blood to the body.

(1) Assessments.

(a) Internal or external bleeding; blood emanating from a wound, drain, or tube or into a body cavity; arterial blood—bright red blood characterized by spurts; venous blood—dark red blood characterized by a continuous flow.

(b) Class I hemorrhage (up to 15% blood loss; 750 mL): No change in vital signs, pale skin, and slight anxiety.

(c) Class II hemorrhage (15% to 30% blood loss; 750 to 1,500 mL): Tachycardia; tachypnea; increased diastolic blood pressure; narrowed pulse pressure; restlessness; anxiety; pale, cool, clammy skin; confusion; prolonged capillary refill; and urine output 20 to 30 mL/hr.

(d) Class III hemorrhage (30% to 40% blood loss; 1,500 to 2,000 mL): Systolic blood pressure 100 mm Hg or less; tachycardia more than 120 beats/min; tachypnea more than 30 breaths/min; cool, pale, clammy skin; confusion;

agitation; prolonged capillary refill; and urine output 20 mL or less per hour.

(e) Class IV hemorrhage (more than 40% blood loss; more than 2,000 mL): Systolic blood pressure less than 70 mm Hg; tachycardia more than 140 beats/min; pronounced tachypnea; extremely pale, sweaty, cool skin; absent capillary refill; negligible urine output; and state of dying (moribund).

(2) Nursing care.

(a) Apply direct pressure to the site of bleeding.

(b) Reinforce the dressing over the wound.

(c) Ensure that the venous access device is #18 gauge to allow for fluid and blood resuscitation.

🛑 (d) Notify the rapid response team and primary health-care provider.

(e) Administer IV fluids as prescribed; usually normal saline or lactated Ringer's solution given at a rate to maintain permissive hypotension so that clotting factors are not diluted.

(f) Administer blood and blood products as prescribed, usually whole blood or fresh frozen plasma.

(g) Maintain the airway if compromised; administer oxygen.

(h) Administer prescribed inotropic therapy (e.g., dopamine, noradrenaline).

(i) Prepare the client for surgery to repair the site of bleeding.

D. Maintain safety when the client's central nervous system is depressed

1. Assessments.

a. LOC.

b. Orientation to time, place, and person.

c. Ability to follow commands.

d. Movement of the extremities.

2. Nursing care.

a. Ensure that the client's airway remains patent.

b. Keeping side rails up, maintaining the integrity of all catheters and monitoring lines.

c. Call the client by name.

d. Reorient the client to time, place, and person.

E. Manage the client's pain and support comfort

1. Assessments.

a. Pain location, intensity, quality, onset, duration, nonverbal clues, and aggravating and relieving factors.

b. Use an objective pain scale to assess pain intensity, such as a numeric pain scale, the Wong-Baker FACES pain scale, or the FLACC pain scale. (See Figs. 15.2 and 15.3, in Chapter 15, Pain, Comfort, Rest, and Sleep).

c. Client responses to interventions, especially 20 minutes after receiving an analgesic; respiratory status after receiving a medication that depresses the central nervous system.

2. Nursing care.

a. Validate and accept the client's description of pain because pain is a subjective experience.

b. Give medication before pain becomes severe.

c. Progress from least invasive independent nursing interventions to dependent nursing interventions.

d. Institute independent nursing interventions to reduce pain and promote comfort.

(1) Place the client in a position of comfort if not contraindicated; support the body in functional alignment.

(2) Suggest distractions, such as music, television, and reading.

(3) Use relaxation techniques, such as warm blankets, back rub, imagery, and progressive muscle relaxation.

(4) Organize care so that the client has uninterrupted periods of rest and sleep.

(5) Maintain an environment conducive to rest and sleep, such as by limiting noise, lowering lights, and setting a comfortable environmental temperature.

e. Institute dependent nursing interventions to reduce pain and promote comfort.

(1) Implement thermal therapy (e.g., heat or cold) as prescribed.

(a) Heat dilates blood vessels and relaxes muscles.

(b) Cold anesthetizes nerve endings and constricts blood vessels, limiting edema.

(2) Administer prescribed analgesics to reduce pain and anxiolytics, sedatives, and hypnotics to reduce anxiety and promote rest and sleep. (See Table 15.4, "Nonopioid Analgesics"; Table 15.5, "Opioid (Narcotic) Analgesics"; and Table 15.8, "Anxiolytics, Sedatives, and Hypnotics" in Chapter 15 , Pain, Comfort, Rest and Sleep, for information about these medications and related nursing care.)

(a) Medications can be administered by a nurse via the oral, Sub-Q, IM, IV, or transdermal routes.

(b) Medications can be controlled by a client via the intravenous or epidural route (**patient controlled anesthesia** [PCA]). (See "Maintain Patient-Controlled Anesthesia" in Chapter 15, Pain, Comfort, Rest and Sleep.)

(3) Administer an antiemetic to limit nausea and vomiting. (See Table 20.8, "Antiemetics and Related Nursing Care," Chapter 20, Nutrition.)

F. Maintain the Client's Position and Promote Activity

1. Assessments.

a. Intolerance to positioning, such as reports of discomfort or pain.

b. Intolerance to activity, such as shortness of breath, respirations more than 24 breaths/min, or heart rate more than 95 beats/min after 3 minutes of rest.

c. Skin over bony prominences for clinical indicators of pressure.

d. Clinical indicators of orthostatic hypotension when moving to an upright position.

2. Nursing care.

a. Position according to the client's needs and/or primary health-care provider's prescription.

(1) Semiconscious or lethargic client: Place in a side-lying position with the head slightly elevated to allow secretions to drain from the mouth.

(2) After spinal anesthesia: Keep flat for 8 to 12 hours to avoid a headache associated with cerebrospinal fluid leakage.

(3) After surgery that causes edema in an extremity (e.g., mastectomy or internal fixation of a fracture): Elevate the extremity higher than the heart to promote venous drainage and reduce edema.

(4) After head and neck surgery (e.g., craniotomy, radical neck dissection, and rhinoplasty): Keep the head of the bed elevated to limit cerebral and tissue edema.

(5) After spinal surgery: Keep flat and roll the entire body as one unit (*logrolling*) when turning to maintain alignment of the spine.

(6) After open reduction and internal fixation (ORIF) of a hip fracture: Use an abduction pillow to avoid internal and external rotation of involved leg to prevent femoral head dislocation (Fig. 24.5).

(7) After total joint replacement (hip, knee or elbow): Use a continuous passive motion (CPM) machine if prescribed (Fig. 24.6 and Box 24.5).

Fig 24.5 Abduction pillow.

Fig 24.6 Continuous passive motion machine. (From Burton and Ludwig [2015]. *Fundamentals of nursing care: Concepts, connections & skills,* 2nd ed. Philadelphia: F. A. Davis Company, with permission.)

b. Change the client's position at least every 2 hours.
c. Assist with or provide range-of-motion exercises.
d. Encourage in-bed activities, such as turning from side to side, if permitted.
e. Assist with and encourage being out of bed and ambulating if prescribed.

G. Maintain the client's urinary elimination
1. Assessments.
    a. Amount and characteristics of urine, such as color, clarity, and odor.
    b. Urge to void, hesitancy, and frequency.
    c. Patency of urinary retention catheter if present.
    d. Clinical indicators of urinary retention.

> **Box 24.5 Continuous Passive Motion Machine and Related Nursing Care**
>
> • *Position sheepskin on the platform, especially at the gluteal fold, where there is a risk of pressure.*
> • *Position the client's extremity on the platform so that the knee/elbow is centered over the break in the platform.*
> • *Ensure that the extremity is in alignment with the client's hips/torso or shoulder.*
> • *Set the degree of flexion, speed, and time on and off the machine as prescribed; speed and degree of flexion increase as recovery progresses.*
> • *Position the controller within easy reach of the client so that the client can shut off the machine if unable to tolerate the procedure.*
> • *Assess the client's skin, and provide skin care when the client's extremity is removed from the device.*
> • *Evaluate and document the client's response to continuous passive motion.*

2. Nursing care.
    a. Document the time and amount of the first voiding.
    b. Promote urination. (See "Nursing Care to Assist Clients With Urinary Elimination" in Chapter 22, Urinary Elimination.)
    c. Provide care related to an indwelling urinary catheter. (See "Nursing Care for Clients With an Indwelling Urinary Catheter" in Chapter 22, Urinary Elimination.)
    d. **Follow predetermined protocol or notify the primary health-care provider if the client does not void within 8 hours after surgery because a straight catheter or urinary retention catheter will be necessary to empty the bladder.**
3. Postoperative urinary elimination complications
    a. Urinary retention: Inability to empty the bladder completely, resulting in excessive urine accumulation due to decreased bladder tone related to anesthetics, analgesics, manipulation during surgery, or pelvic inflammation. (See "Urinary Retention" in Chapter 22, Urinary Elimination.)
    b. Urinary tract infection: Invasion of the bladder by bacteria, viruses, or fungi. (See "Urinary Tract Infection" in Chapter 22, Urinary Elimination.)

H. Maintain the client's fluid and electrolyte balance
1. Assessments.
    a. I&O and daily weight.
    b. Clinical indicators of electrolyte imbalances. (See Table 21.1, "Electrolyte Imbalances and Specific Nursing Care," in Chapter 21, Fluid, Electrolyte, and Acid-Base Balance.)
    c. Clinical indicators of hypervolemia and hypovolemia. (See "Deficient Fluid Volume" and

"Excess Fluid Volume" in Chapter 21, Fluid, Electrolyte, and Acid-Base Balance.)

2. Nursing care.

 a. Administer IV fluids and electrolytes as prescribed.

 b. Notify the primary health-care provider if electrolyte imbalances, excess fluid volume, or deficient fluid volume occur.

3. Postoperative fluid and electrolyte complications.

 a. **Hypovolemia:** Deficient fluid in the intravascular compartment.

 (1) Assessments.

 (a) Decreased blood pressure; orthostatic hypotension.

 (b) Thirst; dry mucous membranes.

 (c) Loss of skin elasticity; flushed, dry skin.

 (d) Weight loss.

 (e) Decreased urine output.

 (f) Weak, thready pulse.

 (g) Atonic muscles; weakness; lethargy.

 (h) Mental confusion.

 (2) Nursing care.

 (a) Encourage oral fluid intake and administer IV fluids as prescribed.

 (b) Provide for safety, particularly in relation to orthostatic hypotension and mental confusion.

 (c) Provide frequent oral hygiene and skin care.

 b. **Hypervolemia:** Excess fluid within the intravascular compartment.

 (1) See "Excess Fluid Volume" in Chapter 21, Fluid, Electrolyte, and Acid-Base Balance.

 (2) See "Complications of Intravenous Solutions and Related Nursing Care" in Chapter 21, Fluid, Electrolyte, and Acid-Base Balance.

I. Maintain the client's nutritional status

1. Assessments.

 a. Verify dietary prescription.

 b. Presence of gag and swallowing reflexes.

 c. Presence and quality of bowel sounds; dietary intake usually resumes after intestinal peristalsis returns, which can be verified by bowel sounds and the passing of flatus.

 d. I&O.

 e. Amount of food ingested.

2. Nursing care.

 a. Maintain NPO status until a diet is prescribed.

 (1) Remove the water pitcher from the bedside.

 (2) Teach the client about the restrictions.

 b. Provide meticulous mouth care.

 c. Maintain an aesthetically pleasant environment, such as avoiding odors by uncovering the meal tray before entering the room to dissipate food odors, using an air freshener, and storing the bedpan and urinal.

 d. Initiate the prescribed diet, which varies depending on the type of surgery and the organs involved.

 (1) Begin usually with ice chips and then progress to clear liquids, to full liquids, to soft, to regular as tolerated.

 (2) Advance the diet to the next level if the client has no nausea, vomiting, or other signs of GI distress if progression is left to the nurse's judgment.

 🛑 e. Encourage intake of foods high in protein and vitamin C to promote wound healing, if permitted.

 f. Assist weak clients with meals; obtain a prescription for between meal supplements if a client's intake is inadequate.

3. Postoperative complications related to nutritional status.

 a. Nausea and vomiting: *Nausea* is an unpleasant wavelike sensation in the throat, epigastrium, or abdomen. *Vomiting* is the ejection of stomach contents from the mouth in response to pain, anxiety, decreased intestinal peristalsis, or administration of oral intake before return of peristalsis after receiving anesthesia.

 (1) Assessments.

 (a) Precipitating factors such as pain, anxiety, and hypoactive or absent bowel sounds.

 (b) Client reports feeling nauseated.

 (c) Frequent swallowing.

 (d) Retching or gagging.

 (e) Ejection of gastric contents.

 (2) Nursing care.

 (a) Reinstitute NPO status.

 (b) Notify the primary health-care provider because vomiting can precipitate fluid and electrolyte imbalances.

 (c) Administer prescribed antiemetics and antisecretories. (See Table 20.9 for "Antiemetics" and Table 20.10 for "Antisecretory Agents" in Chapter 20, Nutrition, for additional information about these medications and related nursing care.)

 (d) Administer prescribed IV fluids and electrolytes.

 (e) Maintain nasogastric (NG) decompression if a nasogastric tube is inserted (Fig. 24.7). A tube is inserted into a naris, down the esophagus, and into the stomach to remove gastric contents when attached to suction

Fig 24.7 Nasogastric tube for gastric decompression. (From Wilkinson and Treas [2016]. *Fundamentals of nursing,* Vol. 2, 3rd ed. Philadelphia: F. A. Davis Company, with permission.)

(gastric decompression) or remove toxic matter from the stomach through repeated irrigations *(lavage)*.

- Secure the tube to the nose; provide skin care to the nares and frequent mouth care.
- ⛔ • **Ensure correct placement of the tube; for example, aspirate gastric contents, auscultate sound of 15 to 30 mL of instilled air entering the stomach.**
- Maintain suction as prescribed: Low intermittent suction for a single-lumen tube; low continuous suction for a double-lumen tube with a blue "pigtail."
- Maintain patency of a single-lumen tube (e.g., Levin): Instill 30 mL of air into the tube; instill 30 mL of normal saline into the tube after verifying tube placement.
- Maintain patency of a double-lumen tube (e.g., Salem sump): Keep the blue pigtail higher than the drainage catheter; instill 30 mL of air into the blue pigtail to ensure patency of air vent tube.

- Have the client cough periodically to increase intra-abdominal and intra-thoracic pressure that moves tube contents toward the collection container.
- Instill solution as prescribed to dilute gastric contents, usually 30 to 50 mL of normal saline.

(f) Monitor for clinical indicators of fluid volume deficit and electrolyte imbalances, such as metabolic alkalosis, because hydrochloric acid is part of gastric secretions. (See "Metabolic Alkalosis" in Table 21.2 in Chapter 21, Fluid, Electrolyte, and Acid-Base Balance)

(g) Empty the collection container, and document the amount and characteristics.

b. Inadequate nutritional intake.

(1) See "Enteral Nutrition" in Chapter 20, Nutrition.

(2) See "Parenteral Nutrition" in Chapter 20, Nutrition.

J. Maintain the client's bowel elimination

1. Assessments.

a. Frequency, amount, and characteristics of stool.

b. Presence and extent of bowel sounds in all four quadrants of the abdomen.

c. Contour of the abdomen to identify abdominal distention.

d. Amount and characteristics of drainage from GI or biliary tubes.

2. Nursing care.

a. Document the time and characteristics of the first bowel movement.

b. Encourage fluids if permitted; administer IV fluids if prescribed.

c. Encourage dietary fiber if permitted.

d. Encourage bed exercises and progressive ambulation if permitted.

e. Promote defecation.

(1) Maintain the client's usual routine for defecation.

(2) Provide privacy and time to defecate.

(3) Encourage assumption of a sitting position for defecation if permitted; provide a commode at the bedside if the client is permitted out of bed but is unable to ambulate safely.

f. Administer a stool softener if prescribed.

g. Care for a tube placed in the common bile duct that exits the abdomen and drains bile into a collection bag via gravity (biliary tube, T-tube); generally anchored with a suture to prevent dislodgement.

(1) Assess the area around the insertion site for clinical indicators of inflammation or infection.

(2) Assess the amount and characteristics of drainage; expect 300 to 500 mL in first 24 hours; report output of more than 500 mL; after 4 days, output should be less than 200 mL daily; expect color to be green-brown.

(3) Clean the insertion site and cover the site with a sterile dressing as prescribed.

🛑 h. **Notify the primary health-care provider if the client develops abdominal distension, constipation, or postoperative ileus.**

3. Postoperative intestinal complications.
   a. Abdominal distention: Excessive flatulence within the intestine, resulting from reduced peristalsis due to manipulation of the intestines during surgery, anesthesia, opioids, and immobility.
      (1) Assessments.
         (a) Enlarged, taut abdomen.
         (b) Abdominal discomfort.
         (c) Hyperactive bowel sounds.
      (2) Nursing care.
         (a) Teach client to avoid carbonated beverages and foods that produce gas.
         (b) Teach client to avoid drinking through a straw to limit swallowing air.
         (c) Encourage the client to move from side to side and assume a knee chest position to facilitate passage of flatus.
         (d) Administer an antiflatulent as prescribed. (See Table 23.5, "Antiflatulent and Related Nursing Care" in Chapter 23, Bowel Elimination.)
         (e) Administer a return-flow enema (e.g., Harris flush, Harris drip) as prescribed to siphon flatus out of the intestines. See section "Return-flow enema (Harris flush, Harris drip)" in Table 23.2 in Chapter 23, Bowel Elimination.
         (f) Insert a rectal tube as prescribed to facilitate the expulsion of flatus.
            • Attach a collection container to the end of a 22 to 34 French rectal tube; usually a vented plastic bag or urine collection bag.
            • Insert the lubricated rectal tube past the external and internal sphincters of the rectum (4 to 5 inches) and tape in place.
            • Remove the tube after 15 to 20 minutes to avoid pressure necrosis of the rectal mucosa and loss of the

neuromuscular response; can be repeated every 2 to 3 hours if flatus persists.

   b. Constipation: No stool or decreased frequency of bowel movements due to reduced peristalsis as a result of manipulation of the intestines during surgery, anesthesia, opioids, and immobility.
      (1) Assessments.
         (a) No stool, less than 2 stools a week, or hard, dry stool.
         (b) Absent or decreased bowel sounds.
         (c) Rectal pressure.
      (2) Nursing care.
         (a) Encourage increased fluid intake if permitted.
         (b) Encourage increased intake of dietary fiber if permitted.
         (c) Encouraged increased ambulation if permitted.
         (d) Administer a laxative or cathartic as prescribed. (See Table 23.4, "Laxatives and Cathartics and Related Nursing Care," in Chapter 23, Bowel Elimination.)
         (e) Administer an enema as prescribed.

   c. **Postoperative ileus (paralytic ileus, adynamic ileus):** Cessation of intestinal peristalsis characterized by a lack of forward movement of intestinal contents; GI secretions continue accumulating in the GI tract; due to anesthesia, opioids, handling of the intestines during surgery, infection, or electrolyte imbalance.
      (1) Assessments.
         (a) Absent stool.
         (b) Absent bowel sounds.
         (c) Abdominal distension.
         (d) Abdominal cramps.
         (e) Fecal vomiting.
      (2) Nursing care.
         (a) Follow prescriptions concerning conservative interventions (e.g., administer small frequent oral fluids in an attempt to stimulate peristalsis; reinstitute NPO status if the client vomits; notify primary health-care provider if bowel sounds do not begin within 48 hours).
         (b) Assist with insertion and maintenance of a nasoenteric tube as prescribed. A long tube with a weighted tip (e.g., Cantor, Miller-Abbott) is inserted via a naris and advanced along the GI tract into the duodenum to remove secretions and gas from the small intestine. Also used for clients with small bowel obstructions; used

for 3 to 5 days and if unsuccessful surgery is performed.

- Position the client in a semi- to high-Fowler position while the tube is passed through a naris and advanced to the stomach.
- Turn the client on the right side to facilitate passage of the tube through the pyloric sphincter into the duodenum.
- Permit client to assume position of comfort after tube is in the duodenum.
- Monitor the markings on the tubing to determine placement.
- Allow the tube to advance via peristalsis or advance it a specified length (e.g., inch per hour) as prescribed.
- Verify placement of the tube via radiography or a scan as prescribed.
- Secure tube to the naris when the tube has reached the desired site.

(c) Provide meticulous and frequent oral hygiene and nares care when a GI tube is in place; pressure of tube can cause an alteration in tissue integrity. (See Fig. 20.8 in Chapter 20, Nutrition.)

(d) Administer IV fluids and electrolytes, such as potassium, as prescribed.

K. Manage the client's operative site
1. Assess the wound, cleanse the wound, apply a dressing: See "Commonalities of Nursing Care for Clients With All Types of Wounds," in Chapter 16, Inflammation, Infection, Immunity, and Wound Care.
2. Use the principles of surgical asepsis when caring for a client's wound: See Table 16.3, "Principles of Surgical Asepsis and Related Nursing Care," in Chapter 16, Inflammation, Infection, Immunity, and Wound Care.
3. Portable wound drainage system.
   a. A catheter inserted into the body near the operative site and connected to a collection container that is compressed to establish low negative pressure, which pulls drainage into the container (e.g., **Jackson Pratt drain** [Fig. 24.8]; **Hemovac drain** [Fig. 24.9]).
   b. Teach the client that the drain will remove fluid that causes swelling and pain and will limit the potential source of infection.
   c. Maintain and teach the client how to care for the drain.
      (1) Maintain the collection container below the insertion site to augment the negative pressure of the system.

Fig 24.8 Jackson-Pratt drain. (From Wilkinson and Treas [2016]. *Fundamentals of nursing*, Vol. 1, 3rd ed. Philadelphia: F. A. Davis Company, with permission.)

Fig 24.9 Hemovac drain. (Adapted from Wilkinson and Treas [2016]. *Fundamentals of nursing*, Vol. 1, 3rd ed. Philadelphia: F. A. Davis Company, adapted with permission.)

(2) Attach tubing to gown or clothing to prevent tension on the tubing.
(3) Empty the collection container when half full to prevent weight from pulling on the tubing and to maintain negative pressure; as drainage in the collection container increases, negative pressure decreases.
(4) Wear clean gloves when emptying the collection container.
(5) Empty the collection container by opening the port and draining the contents into a collection container without touching the inside of the port; avoid touching the collection container with the port to maintain sterility.
(6) Reestablish negative pressure by compressing the collection container, close the port, and release the hand compressing the container.
(7) Assess drainage for amount and characteristics.
(8) Discard drainage in a toilet and flush the toilet twice.

CASE STUDY: Putting It All Together   *cont'd*

- Vital signs are stable: Temperature, 98.8°F (tympanic route); pulse, 80 beats/min, regular rhythm; respirations, 16 breaths/min, shallow; oxygen saturation 98% with oxygen via nasal cannula at 2L; blood pressure, 110/68 mm Hg; no jugular vein distention or adventitious breath sounds noted; pedal pulses palpable; 1+ dependent edema of lower extremities; skin pink and dry; capillary refill 2 to 3 seconds.
- Client is able to move from side to side with help; alert when stimulated and capable of summoning help; deep breathing and coughing on request; cough nonproductive.
- Client in low-Fowler position; sequential venous compression device in place; dressing dry and intact.
- IVF: 0.9% sodium chloride 125 mL/hr; site in right median cubital vein dry and intact; no clinical indicators of infiltration or inflammation noted at IV site.
- IV morphine sulfate via a PCA pump: Basal rate 1.5 mg/hour; PCA dose 1 mg; lockout interval 12 minutes; maximum dose over 4 hours, 26 mg.
- Client states that incisional pain is constantly at a level 2, using a numerical scale of 0 to 10, and tolerable.

Postoperative Prescriptions

NG tube (Salem sump tube) to low continuous wall suction.

NPO except ice chips and sips of water with oral medications.

Strict I&O.

IVF: 0.9% sodium chloride 125 mL/hr.

CBC, basic metabolic panel daily.

Heparin 5,000 units Sub-Q, every 12 hours.

Blood glucose monitoring every 2 hours times 12 hours then every 6 hours, regular insulin coverage:

Serum glucose 150–200 mg/dL—2 units Sub-Q.
Serum glucose 201–300 mg/dL—4 units Sub-Q.
Serum glucose 301–350 mg/dL—8 units Sub-Q.
Serum glucose 351–400 mg/dL—10 units Sub-Q.
Call primary health-care provider if serum glucose is less than 90 mg/dL or more than 400 mg/dL.

Vital signs, BP, and pulse oximetry every 4 hours.

PCA morphine sulfate: Basal rate 1.5 mg/hr; PCA dose 1 mg; lockout interval 12 minutes; maximum dose over 4 hours, 26 mg.

Sequential compression device when in bed.

Early ambulation: Dangle client on side of bed this p.m.; day 1 postop: Ambulate with assist 25 feet at least 2 times and OOB in a chair for at least 20 minutes times 2; day 3 postop: Ensure client is OOB (walking frequently and in a chair) at least 6 hours daily; progressively increase walking distance as tolerated.

Urinary retention catheter to gravity; assess hourly output for 4 hours then every shift; notify primary health-care provider if less than 50 mL/hr.

Case Study Questions

A. What is the purpose of this client's surgery: ablative, curative, explorative, palliative, or restorative?

_____

B. What degree of surgical urgency is this client's medical condition: elective, urgent, or emergency?

_____

C. Is the risk of this client's surgery considered to be major or minor? Explain your answer.

_____

1. _____

2. _____

3. _____

4. _____

5. _____

CASE STUDY: Putting It All Together

cont'd

Case Study Questions

D. Identify the clinical criteria required for discharge from the PACU.

1. _____
2. _____
3. _____
4. _____
5. _____

E. Identify at least 10 nursing interventions associated with the client's Jackson-Pratt drains and explain why they are employed.

1. _____
2. _____
3. _____
4. _____
5. _____
6. _____
7. _____
8. _____
9. _____
10. _____

F. Which postoperative complication is a serious concern in relation to the drugs that the client was taking before the surgery?

_____

G. For what clinical indicators of stage II hemorrhage (blood loss of 750 to 1,500 mL) should the nurse assess the client?

1. _____
2. _____
3. _____
4. _____
5. _____
6. _____
7. _____
8. _____
9. _____
10. _____

continued.

CASE STUDY: Putting It All Together

cont'd

Case Study Questions

H. What are the four most common postoperative concerns that require preventive measures that are associated with this client's obesity and diabetes? Explain your answer.

1. _____
2. _____
3. _____
4. _____

I. Identify at least six nursing interventions that the nurse should employ to reduce the risk of a postoperative wound infection.

1. _____
2. _____
3. _____
4. _____
5. _____
6. _____

J. What nursing interventions should the nurse implement to prevent a postoperative pulmonary embolus? Explain your answer.

1. _____
2. _____
3. _____
4. _____
5. _____

K. A nurse assesses the client's blood glucose level and it is 285 mg/dL. What should the nurse do?

_____

REVIEW QUESTIONS

Be sure to read the Introduction for valuable test-taking tips.

1. A nurse is caring for a postoperative client who has a history of cigarette smoking. For what complication should the nurse initially monitor the client?
   1. Airway patency
   2. Dependent edema
   3. Respiratory infection
   4. Pulmonary hemorrhage

2. What should a nurse do when assessing for the presence of dehiscence after a client had abdominal surgery? **Select all that apply.**
   1. Monitor urine output.
   2. Assess for hypertension.
   3. Observe for broken sutures.
   4. Assess for tissue extruding from wound.
   5. Monitor volume of serosanguineous drainage.

3. Before abdominal surgery, the nurse teaches the client leg and ankle pumping exercises that are to be done during the postoperative period. Which postoperative complication does the nurse explain will be prevented by these exercises?
   1. Atelectasis
   2. Adynamic ileus
   3. Wound infection
   4. Thrombophlebitis

4. A nurse in the postanesthesia care unit receives a client transferred from the operating room. Which assessment should the nurse perform **first**?
   1. Vital signs
   2. Urinary output
   3. Airway patency
   4. Wound dressing

5. A client goes to the outpatient clinic to be prepared for extensive head and neck surgery for a cancerous tumor of the jaw. Which intervention is the priority?
   1. Initiate discharge planning with a home health agency.
   2. Teach postoperative deep breathing and coughing exercises.
   3. Ensure that the client understands the rationale for leg exercises.
   4. Review methods of communicating with the health team after the surgery.

6. A nurse is caring for a client who had an esophagogastroduodenoscopy 2 hours ago. The nurse has to attend a meeting and provides information to the nurse accepting responsibility for the client. What information is **most** important for the relieving nurse to know about this client?
   1. Vital signs are stable.
   2. Reports a sore throat.
   3. Gag reflex returned 5 minutes ago.
   4. Voided a sufficient quantity 1 hour ago.

7. A primary health-care provider prescribes the removal of a client's nasogastric (NG) tube. The nurse explains what is to be done, provides privacy, washes the hands, and dons clean gloves before implementing the procedure. Place the following steps in the order in which they should be implemented by the nurse.
   1. Instruct the client to take a deep breath.
   2. Remove adhesive tape from the client's nose.
   3. Place a disposable pad across the client's chest.
   4. Fold the tube on itself and quickly and carefully remove the tube.
   5. Shut off the suction and separate the tube from the suction device.
   Answer: _____

8. A nurse is providing preoperative teaching for a client who is scheduled for laparoscopic surgery for removal of the gallbladder (cholecystectomy). Which information is **most** important to teach the client preoperatively?
   1. Performing ankle pumping exercises
   2. Planning to be out of work for six weeks
   3. Avoiding taking drugs that may increase bleeding
   4. Self-administering a hypertonic enema the night before the procedure

9. A client is admitted to the postanesthesia care unit (PACU) after having a partial gastrectomy. Which nursing interventions should the nurse implement? **Select all that apply.**
   1. Monitor the pulse oximeter.
   2. Auscultate the client's breath sounds.
   3. Assess the depth and rate of respirations.
   4. Clamp the nasogastric tube intermittently.
   5. Maintain the client in the dorsal recumbent position.
   6. Push the trigger on the PCA pump when the client states the presence of pain.

10. A nurse in the postanesthesia care unit (PACU) is caring for a client whose skin becomes cold and clammy; pulse is 112 beats/min; respirations are 30 breaths/min; blood pressure is 84/50 mm Hg; and surgical dressing is saturated with blood. Place the following steps in the order in which they should be implemented.
    1. Retake the client's vital signs.
    2. Activate the rapid response team.
    3. Change the nasal cannula to a face mask.
    4. Place the bed in the Trendelenburg position.
    5. Increase the flow rate of the intravenous solution.
    Answer: _____

11. A client is transferred from the operating room to the postanesthesia care unit (PACU). What should the PACU nurse assess **first**?
    1. Cardiovascular status
    2. Level of consciousness
    3. Oxygen saturation level
    4. Adequacy of the airway

12. A client is transferred from the operating room to the postanesthesia care unit (PACU). What should the nurse assess **first** from among the options presented?
    1. Presence of pain
    2. Level of consciousness
    3. Indicators of fluid overload
    4. Patency of a urinary catheter

13. A nurse is caring for a client wearing the device illustrated in the photograph. What is the expected result that the nurse can anticipate when this client wears this device? **Select all that apply.**

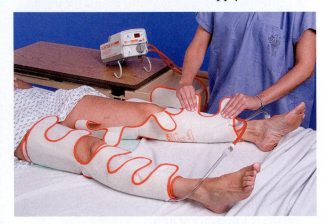

    1. Increased venous return
    2. Minimized muscle atrophy
    3. Reduced lower extremity edema
    4. Increased risk of thrombophlebitis
    5. Reduced lower extremity discomfort

14. A client is scheduled for a colon resection and is to receive general anesthesia. Which data collected during a nursing history and physical should cause the **most** concern?
    1. History of a latex allergy
    2. Blood pressure of 140/84 mm Hg
    3. Smokes 2 packs of cigarettes a day
    4. Presence of vesicular breath sounds

15. A nurse on a surgical unit is caring for a group of postoperative clients. Which nursing interventions included in the clients' plans of care help reduce the risk of both hypostatic pneumonia and deep vein thrombosis? **Select all that apply.**
    1. Increase fluid intake to 3,000 mL daily.
    2. Encourage coughing and deep breathing.
    3. Ambulate 100 feet in the hall four times daily.
    4. Encourage changing position from side to side when in bed.
    5. Teach how to don compression stockings before getting out of bed in the morning.

16. A nurse is caring for a client with a Hemovac. The collection chamber is half filled with drainage and requires emptying. Place the steps in the order in which they should be implemented.
    1. Don clean gloves.
    2. Open the port of the collection chamber.
    3. Press down firmly on the top of the chamber.
    4. Empty the contents into a container for measurement.
    5. Close the drainage port while maintaining compression of the collection chamber.
    Answer: _____

17. What is **most** important for the nurse to include in preoperative teaching?
    1. Plan for pain management
    2. Potential complications to be avoided
    3. Risk factors associated with the type of anesthesia
    4. Detailed information related to the type of surgery

18. A nurse is providing preoperative teaching for a client who is scheduled for surgery in the morning. Antiembolism stockings are prescribed as a component of postoperative care. The client asks, "Why do I need to wear these ugly stockings?" What information is important for the nurse to include in a response to the client's question? **Select all that apply.**
    1. Helps prevent muscle atrophy
    2. Reduces the risk of a deep vein thrombosis
    3. Supports venous blood return from the legs
    4. Minimizes joint contractures when ambulating
    5. Keeps the legs warm while in the postanesthesia care unit

19. Which nursing actions are associated with caring for a client with a portable wound drainage system like the one in the photograph? **Select all that apply.**

1. Discard drainage in a toilet.
2. Document the characteristics of the drainage.
3. Empty the collection container only when it becomes full.
4. Maintain medical asepsis when emptying the collection container.
5. Verify that the volume of drainage is consistent with expectations.

20. A nurse is caring for a client who is obese and is scheduled for abdominal surgery in the morning. Which information is **most** important to include in a preoperative teaching plan for this client?
1. How to cough and deep breathe effectively
2. What to do to prevent a wound infection
3. What to do to safely ambulate in the hall
4. How to exit the bed independently

21. A nurse in the postanesthesia care unit (PACU) is caring for a client who had debulking surgery for ovarian cancer. The client's apical pulse is 128 beats/min, respirations are 22 breaths/min, blood pressure is 88/60 mm Hg, and two portable wound drainage devices are both half full of sanguineous drainage. What should the nurse do **first**?
1. Call the surgeon immediately.
2. Empty the collection containers.
3. Palpate the abdomen for urinary distention.
4. Increase the flow rate of the intravenous solution.

22. A nurse is caring for a client with a Salem sump tube attached to continuous low suction following abdominal surgery. The client reports feeling nauseated and begins to vomit. The nurse identifies that the client's abdomen is distended. Which are acceptable actions associated with ensuring that this sump tube is patent? **Select all that apply.**
1. Ensure the tubing is free from kinks and is not being compressed.
2. Reposition the client and instruct the client to cough.
3. Administer the prescribed antiemetic to the client.
4. Instill the blue pigtail with thirty milliliters of air.
5. Change to intermittent suction until patent.

23. Eight hours after surgery, a nurse identifies that a client has not voided. Which actions by the nurse are appropriate? **Select all that apply.**
1. Catheterize the client.
2. Palpate the client's bladder for fullness.
3. Increase the rate of the intravenous fluids.
4. Encourage the client to drink more fluids.
5. Cover the suprapubic area with a warm towel while running water in the sink.

24. A nurse is caring for a client who just returned from the postanesthesia care unit after abdominal surgery. What should the nurse do **first** when the client begins to vomit red-colored emesis?
1. Assist the client to the lateral position.
2. Increase the flow rate of the intravenous fluid.
3. Document the volume of effluent, including its characteristics.
4. Call the blood bank to deliver a unit of packed red blood cells.

25. A nurse is developing a preoperative plan of care for a client scheduled for intestinal surgery. The nurse should ensure that the surgeon has prescribed a medication from which drug classification to be administered to the client preoperatively?
1. Opioid
2. Antibiotic
3. Antiemetic
4. Thrombolytic

26. A nurse is caring for a client who recently returned to the surgical unit from the postanesthesia care unit after intestinal surgery. The nurse identifies abdominal distention and the absence of bowel sounds. Which nursing intervention addresses the nurse's main concern?
1. Inspect proximity of wound edges.
2. Ensure patency of the nasogastric tube.
3. Encourage an increase in oral fluid intake.
4. Assess for clinical indicators of hypovolemia.

27. A nurse is caring for a semiconscious client in the postanesthesia care unit. The client begins to try to expel the oropharyngeal airway. What should the nurse do?
    1. Maintain the use of wrist restraints until the client is fully alert.
    2. Explain to the client that the airway needs to remain in place.
    3. Remove the airway from the client's mouth.
    4. Place the client in the lateral position.

28. In which position should the nurse maintain a client after spinal anesthesia?
    1. Sitting
    2. Supine
    3. Contour
    4. Orthopneic

29. A nurse is caring for a client 6 hours after surgery for repair of a deep 7-inch long laceration of an abdominal muscle as a result of a motorcycle accident. In addition, the client is currently engaged in chemotherapy for stage II lung cancer. Which is the important concern of the nurse after reviewing the client's clinical record and interviewing the client?
    1. Hemorrhage
    2. Risk for infection
    3. Respiratory distress
    4. Electrolyte imbalance

Client's Clinical Record

Progress Notes 0800

Moderate amount of serosanguineous drainage noted on abdominal dressing. Reinforced with one abdominal pad. IV running at 100 mL/hr via an infusion pump; IV insertion site clean, dry, and intact; no S&S of phlebitis or infiltration. Voided 450 mL of clear, straw-colored urine at 0730.

Vital Signs

Temperature: 100.4°F
Pulse: 90 beats/min
Respirations: 24 breaths/min and shallow
Blood pressure: 120/80 mm Hg
Oxygen saturation: 95%

Laboratory Results

Hb: 15.5 g/dL
RBC: 5.6 mm^3
Platelet count: 200,000 mm^3
WBC: 2.5 mm^3
Serum potassium: 4.5 mEq/L
Serum sodium: 140 mEq/L

30. A nurse is caring for a postoperative client who had abdominal surgery and who has an impaired immune system because of corticosteroid therapy. Which nursing intervention is essential when caring for this client?
    1. Maintaining medical asepsis when changing the dressing
    2. Suggesting ingesting foods high in protein
    3. Instituting neutropenic precautions
    4. Encouraging fluid intake

31. A nurse is caring for a postoperative client who is experiencing nausea and vomiting. What is **most** important for the nurse to do?
    1. Encourage deep breathing.
    2. Use room-deodorizing sprays.
    3. Provide frequent oral hygiene.
    4. Maintain prescribed NPO status.

32. A nurse working in the ambulatory surgical center is admitting a 65-year-old male client scheduled for elective bowel surgery in 2 hours. After reviewing the client's preoperative blood tests, interviewing the client, and taking the vital signs, what information is **most** important for the nurse to report to the primary health-care provider?
    1. Client's BP is elevated.
    2. Client took a sip of water today.
    3. Client ingested clopidogrel yesterday.
    4. Client's Hb is lower than the expected range.

Client's Clinical Record

Client Interview

Client stated that he completed the bowel prep, ingested a clear liquid diet for 2 days, and did not eat or drink anything since 12 midnight. He said that he stopped taking his last dose of clopidogrel yesterday morning but had his vitamins 2 hours ago with a little sip of water.

Vital Signs

Temperature: 99°F
Pulse: 88 beats/min, regular
Respirations: 22 breaths/min
Blood pressure: 140/88 mm Hg

Laboratory Test Results

Hb: 15 g/dL
RBC: 5.1 mm^3
Platelets: 280,000 mm^3
WBC: 6 mm^3

33. Versed 2.5 mg IV push is prescribed for preoperative sedation. It is available in 5 mg/mL. How many milliliters should the nurse prepare to administer to the client?

    Answer: _____ mL

34. A nurse receives a client in the postanesthesia care unit after 4 hours of abdominal surgery. An hour later the client regains consciousness, is trembling, and reports feeling cold. The monitor indicates that the client's heart rate and respirations are within expected limits. What should the nurse do first?

    1. Take the client's temperature.
    2. Notify the surgeon of the client's status.
    3. Cover the client with a heated bath blanket.
    4. Continue to monitor the status of the client.

35. A client has an open reduction and internal fixation of a fractured hip. The client arrives in the postanesthesia care unit with prescription for an abduction pillow. What should the nurse do until the pillow is received from central supply?

    1. Place trochanter rolls on both lateral sides of the body from the waist to the knees.
    2. Place 3 pillows between the client's thighs while the client is in the supine position.
    3. Put 2 pillows under both knees while the client is in the supine position.
    4. Position the client on the unoperated side.

REVIEW ANSWERS AND RATIONALES

1. ANSWER: 1.

Rationales:

1. Smoking increases mucus production and destroys the protective action of cilia; a smoker is at risk for ineffective airway clearance.

2. Dependent edema is related to heart and peripheral vascular diseases, not smoking.

3. Although the nurse should monitor the client for signs of respiratory infection, this is not the priority at this time. An infection will not occur until several days later.

4. Pulmonary hemorrhage is an unlikely occurrence; it can occur with tissue erosion associated with lung cancer.

TEST-TAKING TIP: Identify the word in the stem that sets a priority. The word *initially* in the stem sets a priority. Use the principle of the ABCs (Airway, Breathing, and Circulation) when setting a priority. Option 1 is clearly associated with Airway. Options 2 and 4 are associated with Circulation. Options 3 and 4 are associated more with Breathing because infection causes inflammation, which can reduce the surface area of the lung, affecting breathing.

Content Area: Perioperative
Integrated Processes: Nursing Process: Evaluation
Client Need: Physiological Integrity; Reduction of Risk Potential
Cognitive Level: Application
Concept: Oxygenation

2. ANSWER: 3, 5.

Rationales:

1. Urine output is unrelated to dehiscence.

2. Hypertension is unrelated to dehiscence.

3. Sutures that break no longer hold the wound edges together, allowing the wound to separate and indicating dehiscence. Dehiscence most frequently occurs 5 to 14 days postoperatively. It is precipitated by increased intra-abdominal pressure associated with coughing, vomiting, and distension; obesity is a risk factor.

4. Tissue extruding from an incision is known as evisceration, not dehiscence.

5. An increase in serosanguineous drainage from an incision is associated with dehiscence. Serous fluid and blood seep out of the incision when the wound edges are no longer approximated.

Content Area: Perioperative
Integrated Processes: Nursing Process: Evaluation
Client Need: Physiological Integrity; Reduction of Risk Potential
Cognitive Level: Application
Concept: Tissue Integrity

3. ANSWER: 4.

Rationales:

1. Leg and ankle pumping exercises will not prevent atelectasis. Deep breathing and coughing are the most effective actions to prevent collapse of alveoli (atelectasis).

2. Leg and ankle pumping exercises will not prevent an adynamic ileus. Early ambulation is the most effective intervention to reduce the likelihood of the absence of peristaltic motility lasting longer than 72 hours (adynamic ileus, postoperative ileus).

3. Leg and ankle pumping exercises will not prevent a wound infection. Maintaining medical and surgical asepsis will help prevent a wound infection.

4. Leg and ankle pumping exercises, early ambulation, and the use of antiembolism stockings increase venous return, thereby minimizing venous stasis and thrombophlebitis.

Content Area: Perioperative
Integrated Processes: Teaching/Learning; Nursing Process: Implementation
Client Need: Physiological Integrity; Reduction of Risk Potential
Cognitive Level: Application
Concept: Patient-Centered Care; Perfusion

4. ANSWER: 3.

Rationales:

1. Although vital signs are important and are associated with Breathing and Circulation, another option has priority.

2. Although assessing urinary output is important because it assesses glomerular filtration rate and the adequacy of Circulation, it is not associated with Airway or Breathing; another option has priority.

3. Airway patency always is the priority because adequate ventilation is essential for life.

4. Although assessing the dressing is important to assess for hemorrhage, which is associated with Circulation, it is not the priority.

TEST-TAKING TIP: Identify the word in the stem that sets a priority. The word *first* in the stem sets a priority. Use the principle of the ABCs (Airway, Breathing, and Circulation) when setting a priority. Option 3 is associated with Airway.

Content Area: Perioperative
Integrated Processes: Nursing Process: Evaluation
Client Need: Physiological Integrity; Reduction of Risk Potential
Cognitive Level: Application
Concept: Oxygenation

5. ANSWER: 4.

Rationales:

1. Discharge planning generally is initiated on admission to the hospital when a discharge planner is assigned responsibility for assessing the needs of the client in preparation for discharge.

2. With extensive head and neck surgery, the client will have either an endotracheal tube or tracheostomy to facilitate respirations as well as suctioning if necessary to clear the airway.

3. Although the client should be taught about performing leg exercises after surgery, this is not the priority associated with the type of surgery the client will experience.

4. Establishing a method of communication for use after head and neck surgery is the priority because the client will most likely have an endotracheal tube or tracheostomy tube in place. This intervention is important because it meets the emotional and safety needs of the client when the client knows how to make needs known to the health-care team.

TEST-TAKING TIP: Identify the word that sets a priority. The word *priority* indicates that the question is asking what should be done first.

Content Area: Perioperative
Integrated Processes: Teaching/Learning; Nursing Process:
Implementation
Client Need: Physiological Integrity; Reduction of Risk Potential
Cognitive Level: Application
Concept: Patient-Centered Care; Communication

6. **ANSWER: 3.**
Rationales:
1. Stable vital signs are expected; this indicates that the
client is responding safely after the procedure.
2. A sore throat is expected after this procedure because of
irritation of the mucous membranes from the tube inserted
into the esophagus.
3. **During an esophagogastroduodenoscopy, a local anes-**
thetic is sprayed into a client's posterior pharynx to lessen
the gag reflex. The client is kept on NPO status until the
gag reflex returns. When the gag reflex returns, liquids
are permitted; eventually the client is instructed to eat a
light diet during the first 12 to 24 hours.
4. Although assessing urinary output is important because
it assesses the glomerular filtration rate and adequacy of
Circulation, it is not associated with Airway or Breathing.
Voiding urine in a sufficient quantity after the procedure
is expected. Urinary retention is not associated with this
procedure because conscious sedation, not general
anesthesia, is used.
TEST-TAKING TIP: Identify the word in the stem that sets a
priority. The word *most* in the stem sets a priority. Use the
principle of the ABCs (Airway, Breathing, and Circulation)
when establishing a priority. Option 3 is associated with
Airway, which is the priority. Option 2 is associated with
Breathing. Options 3 and 4 are associated with circulation.
Option 4 indicates that the client's voiding pattern is of a
sufficient quantity. Assessing adequacy of urinary output is
associated with Circulation (cardiac output must be main-
tained to ensure an adequate glomerular flow rate).
Content Area: Perioperative
Integrated Processes: Communication and Documentation;
Nursing Process: Evaluation
Client Need: Safe and Effective Care Environment;
Management of Care
Cognitive Level: Application
Concept: Oxygenation

7. **ANSWER: 3, 5, 2, 1, 4.**
Rationales:
3. **A disposable pad protects the client from contact with**
gastric secretions.
5. **Shutting off the suction and separating the tube from**
the suction device prepares for removal of the tube. This
is done before removing the tape from the client's nose.
2. **Removal of adhesive tape from the client's nose allows**
for unrestricted removal of the tube.
1. **Instructing the client to take a deep breath helps mini-**
mize the risk of accidental aspiration of gastric secretions.
4. **Folding the tube on itself clamps the tube with the**
fingers, which helps prevent aspiration of gastric contents
exiting from the tube during its withdrawal. Quickly and
carefully removing the tube minimizes discomfort and
the risk of trauma.

Content Area: Perioperative
Integrated Processes: Nursing Process: Planning
Client Need: Physiological Integrity; Reduction of Risk Potential
Cognitive Level: Analysis
Concept: Oxygenation

8. **ANSWER: 3.**
Rationales:
1. Although exercises that increase venous return should be
encouraged to reduce the risk of a thrombus and pulmonary
emboli, it is not the priority.
2. Generally, clients are advised that they can return to their
usual activities within 7 to 10 days, not 6 weeks. People who
perform heavy manual labor may require 2 to 4 weeks to
recuperate.
3. **Medications that can cause bleeding, such as aspirin,**
clopidogrel (Plavix), and warfarin (Coumadin), increase
the risk of postoperative bleeding and should be avoided
before surgery. The primary health-care provider will
determine how many days before and after surgery the
client should avoid drugs that increase bleeding time.
4. Generally, an enema the night before this surgery is unnecessary because the bowel is not involved in this surgery.
TEST-TAKING TIP: Identify the word in the stem that sets a
priority. The word *most* in the stem sets a priority.
Content Area: Perioperative
Integrated Processes: Teaching/Learning; Nursing Process:
Implementation
Client Need: Physiological Integrity; Reduction of Risk
Potential
Cognitive Level: Application
Concept: Medication; Hematologic Regulation

9. **ANSWER: 1, 2, 3.**
Rationales:
1. **The pulse oximeter informs the nurse about the**
client's oxygen saturation. If it decreases below 92%,
the primary health-care provider should be informed.
Generally, clients in the postanesthesia care unit (PACU)
receive oxygen until they awaken from anesthesia and the
oxygen saturation level is stabilized within the expected
range (95% to 100%).
2. **Auscultating for breath sounds monitors lung func-**
tion. Absence of breath sounds indicates a pneumothorax
or atelectasis. Adventitious breath sounds, such as
rhonchi or crackles, indicate the accumulation of fluid
in the lung. Maintaining an airway and providing for
adequate oxygenation is a critical role of the nurse in
the PACU.
3. **A gastrectomy is surgery performed just below the**
diaphragm. Deep breaths can be painful postoperatively.
The depth and rate of respirations should be monitored.
4. Generally, an NG tube is used for decompression of the
stomach after gastric surgery. It should be attached to
intermittent suction if it is a single-lumen tube or continuous suction if it is a double-lumen tube. It should not be
clamped without a prescription. Several days after surgery,
an NG tube may be prescribed to be clamped periodically
to determine whether gastric emptying is occurring. The
NG tube will be removed once it is determined that gastric
emptying is occurring.

5. Postoperatively, the head of the bed should be elevated to the low Fowler position after a client has general anesthesia. Gravity moves the abdominal organs away from the diaphragm, which facilitates respirations and helps prevent aspiration.
6. Only the client should activate the trigger on a patient-controlled analgesia pump.
Content Area: Perioperative
Integrated Processes: Nursing Process: Implementation
Client Need: Physiological Integrity; Physiological Adaptation
Cognitive Level: Application
Concept: Oxygenation

10. ANSWER: 2, 5, 4, 3, 1.
Rationales:
2. The client's signs and symptoms indicate impending hypovolemic shock. The nurse should mobilize professionals from a variety of health-care disciplines to assist with this emergency.
5. Increasing the flow rate of the IV will immediately increase the circulating blood volume.
4. The Trendelenburg position uses the principle of gravity to increase blood return from the legs, which brings more blood to the brain and vital organs. This takes more time to accomplish than increasing the intravenous flow rate but less time than setting up an oxygen delivery system.
3. Exogenous oxygen will increase the partial pressure of oxygen within the circulatory system. A nasal cannula delivers 24% to 44% oxygen depending on the oxygen liter flow, whereas a simple face mask delivers 40% to 60% oxygen depending on the oxygen liter flow.
1. The vital signs should be obtained to determine the client's response to interventions.
Content Area: Perioperative
Integrated Processes: Communication and Documentation; Nursing Process: Planning
Client Need: Physiological Integrity; Physiological Adaptation
Cognitive Level: Analysis
Concept: Perfusion

11. ANSWER: 4.
Rationales:
1. The client's cardiovascular status should be assessed after two other assessments indicate that the client's oxygen needs are met.
2. The client's level of consciousness should be assessed after 3 other assessments are done first.
3. The client's oxygen saturation level may be monitored as part of an assessment of the client's respiratory status. This occurs after another critical assessment is completed first.
4. The nurse should follow the ABCs of assessing Airway, Breathing, and Circulation, in that order. Maintaining the airway is always the priority to ensure that oxygen can reach the lungs.
TEST-TAKING TIP: Identify the word in the stem that sets a priority. The word *first* in the stem sets a priority. A nurse should follow the ABCs (Airway, Breathing, and Circulation)

as a guide when establishing a priority. Option 4 is associated with airway, which is the priority.
Content Area: Perioperative
Integrated Processes: Nursing Process: Evaluation
Client Need: Physiological Integrity; Reduction of Risk Potential
Cognitive Level: Application
Concept: Oxygenation

12. ANSWER: 3.
Rationales:
1. Although it is important to assess the client's level of pain, it is not the most important assessment that should be performed among the options presented.
2. Although it is important to assess a client's level of consciousness, it is not the most important assessment that should be performed among the options presented.
3. Of the options presented, none refer to airway or breathing. However, assessing a client for signs of fluid volume excess is associated with circulation. Often, clients are administered a large volume of IV solutions during surgery to ensure that the client's circulating blood volume is adequate and that the glomerular filtration rate is sufficient to maintain kidney function. The nurse should assess clients for fluid excess or deficit when in the PACU.
4. Although assessing the patency of a urinary catheter is important, it is not the most important assessment that should be performed among the options presented.
TEST-TAKING TIP: Identify the word in the stem that sets a priority. The word first in the stem sets a priority. The nurse should use the ABCs (Airway, Breathing, and Circulation) as a guide when setting a priority. No option refers to Airway or Breathing. Option 3 relates to circulation. Examine option 3 carefully.
Content Area: Perioperative
Integrated Processes: Nursing Process: Evaluation
Client Need: Physiological Integrity; Reduction of Risk Potential
Cognitive Level: Application
Concept: Fluid and Electrolyte Balance

13. ANSWER: 1, 3, 5.
Rationales:
1. This is a sequential compression device used to prevent deep vein thrombosis by facilitating venous return. It will intermittently inflate chambers and then deflate chambers in the device in a sequential pattern from distal to proximal, thereby promoting venous return.
2. This is a sequential compression device; it will not minimize muscle atrophy.
3. This is a sequential compression device used to prevent deep vein thrombosis by facilitating venous return. When lower extremity venous return is promoted, it reduces lower extremity edema.
4. The risk of thrombophlebitis is reduced, not increased, with a sequential compression device. Venous stasis is a risk factor of thrombophlebitis.
5. Dependent edema can cause discomfort as fluid collects in the interstitial spaces and dermal tissue

becomes taut. This device will promote venous return
and limit peripheral edema.
Content Area: *Perioperative*
Integrated Processes: *Nursing Process: Evaluation*
Client Need: *Physiological Integrity; Reduction of Risk
Potential*
Cognitive Level: *Analysis*
Concept: *Perfusion*

14. **ANSWER: 3.**
    Rationales:
    1. The hospital and operating room can be modified and
    controlled to ensure a latex-free environment.
    2. Slight hypertension may be in response to anxiety
    associated with the impending surgery. Just before surgery,
    clients are given medications that reduce anxiety and
    induce relaxation, which will decrease the blood pressure.
    **3. Usually, general anesthesia is administered via a
    combination of inhalation and the intravenous route.
    A client with a history of smoking is at an increased risk
    for pulmonary complications with general anesthesia.
    The lungs may be impaired as a result of inhaled toxins
    associated with smoking. Also, inhaled anesthetic agents
    are eliminated via the lungs, which may be inefficient
    because of lung impairment.**
    4. Vesicular breath sounds are noiseless breath sounds that
    are normal and expected.
    TEST-TAKING TIP: Identify the word in the stem that sets a
    priority. The word *most* in the stem sets a priority.
    Content Area: *Perioperative*
    Integrated Processes: *Nursing Process: Analysis*
    Client Need: *Physiological Integrity; Reduction of Risk
    Potential*
    Cognitive Level: *Application*
    Concept: *Oxygenation*

15. **ANSWER: 1, 3, 4.**
    Rationales:
    **1. Increasing fluid intake will reduce the viscosity of
    circulating blood, helping to reduce the risk of a deep
    vein thrombosis. Also, it reduces the viscosity of
    respiratory secretions, facilitating expectoration of
    respiratory secretions; this minimizes pooling of secre-
    tions in the lungs, which provides a medium for bacte-
    rial growth.**
    2. Coughing and deep breathing will facilitate lung expan-
    sion and expectoration of secretions, reducing the risk of
    hypostatic pneumonia; it does not reduce the risk of deep
    vein thrombosis.
    **3. Ambulation requires contraction of muscles of the
    legs, which increases venous return. Also, it increases the
    depth of respirations as the body needs more oxygen to
    meet the needs of muscles. Deep respirations aerate the
    distal alveoli, preventing the accumulation of fluid.
    Accumulated fluid precipitates hypostatic pneumonia.
    4. Changing position from side to side requires the
    client to use leg muscles to turn, which increases venous
    return. It also allows fluid in the lung to move via gravity
    to dependent sections of the pulmonary system; this in
    turn facilitates aeration and expansion of alternate lung
    areas as the client changes position.**

5. Compression stockings provide external pressure
facilitating venous return, thereby reducing the risk of
deep vein thrombosis. Compression stockings will not
reduce the risk of hypostatic pneumonia.
Content Area: *Perioperative*
Integrated Processes: *Communication and Documentation;
Nursing Process: Planning*
Client Need: *Physiological Integrity; Reduction of Risk
Potential*
Cognitive Level: *Analysis*
Concept: *Perfusion*

16. **ANSWER: 1, 2, 4, 3, 5.**
    Rationales:
    **1. Donning clean gloves protects the nurse from
    potential contact with drainage from the collection
    chamber.
    2. The port to the collection chamber is opened so
    that the contents can be emptied into a container for
    measurement.
    4. The content is emptied into a container with marks in-
    dicating fluid volume to ensure an accurate measurement
    of the drainage.
    3. Once the collection chamber is empty, the chamber is
    compressed firmly. This is the first step in reestablishing
    negative pressure within the portable wound drainage
    system.
    5. The port is closed before compression of the chamber
    is released. This reestablishes negative pressure. Negative
    pressure establishes a vacuum and the resulting suction
    pulls drainage from the wound.**
    Content Area: *Perioperative*
    Integrated Processes: *Nursing Process: Planning*
    Client Need: *Physiological Integrity; Physiological
    Adaptation*
    Cognitive Level: *Analysis*
    Concept: *Tissue Integrity*

17. **ANSWER: 1.**
    Rationales:
    **1. Most clients anticipate some discomfort/pain
    after surgery, and this concern should be addressed
    to decrease anxiety.**
    2. Teaching should focus on the activities that prevent
    complications. Stressing potential complications may
    cause unnecessary anxiety.
    3. It is the surgeon's, not the nurse's, responsibility to
    review the risks and benefits of surgery.
    4. It is the surgeon's, not the nurse's, responsibility to
    discuss the type of surgery that is planned when securing
    the consent for surgery.
    TEST-TAKING TIP: Identify the word in the stem that sets a
    priority. The word *most* in the stem sets a priority. Identify
    equally plausible options. Options 2, 3, and 4 are all equally
    plausible; they all have the potential to raise anxiety.
    Identify the unique option. Option 1 is unique because it
    is the only option that will reduce anxiety that the client
    may have about postoperative pain.
    Content Area: *Perioperative*
    Integrated Processes: *Teaching/Learning; Nursing Process:
    Implementation*

*Client Need: Physiological Integrity; Reduction of Risk
Potential*
Cognitive Level: Application
Concept: Patient-Centered Care; Comfort

18. **ANSWER: 2, 3.**
Rationales:
1. Only active contraction of muscles will prevent muscle
atrophy.
**2. Antiembolism stockings are elastic and provide
counter pressure supporting muscles in the legs, facilitating venous return to the heart. Avoiding venous stasis
helps to minimize the risk of thrombophlebitis.**
**3. Antiembolism stockings are elastic and provide
counter pressure supporting muscles in the legs
facilitating venous return to the heart.**
4. Antiembolism stockings do not prevent contractures;
placing joints through their full range of motion several
times a day prevents contractures.
5. The purpose of antiembolism stockings is not to keep
the legs warm. Blankets may be used to provide warmth if
it is considered necessary.
Content Area: Perioperative
*Integrated Processes: Teaching/Learning; Nursing Process:
Implementation*
*Client Need: Physiological Integrity; Reduction of Risk
Potential*
Cognitive Level: Application
Concept: Patient-Centered Care; Perfusion

19. **ANSWER: 1, 2, 5.**
Rationales:
**1. Discarding drainage in a toilet is the correct way to
manage disposal of drainage from a portable wound
drainage system. It prevents exposure of others to the
client's body fluids.**
**2. Documenting the characteristics of drainage is
important information to include in the client's
clinical record.**
3. The drainage collection container should be emptied
when half full because a full container may place tension
on the insertion site. Also, the extent of negative pressure
within the device decreases as the container fills with
drainage, impeding its effectiveness.
4. Sterile technique, not medical asepsis, is required when
emptying the drainage collection container; this minimizes
the introduction of pathogens to the wound bed via the
container and tubing of the device.
**5. Verifying that the volume of drainage is consistent
with expectations is an important action when caring for
a client with a wound drainage system. The tubing may
be clogged or kinked if there is too little drainage. The
client may be hemorrhaging if there is too much
drainage. The nurse must respond to both events; the
nurse can milk the tubing to relieve a clogged tube or
straighten it manually if it is kinked; the nurse should
notify the surgeon if the drainage is a larger volume than
that which is expected.**
TEST-TAKING TIP: Identify the option with a specific
determiner. The word *only* in option 3 is a specific determiner. Rarely is an option with a specific determiner the

correct answer. Identify the clang associations. The word
drainage in the stem and in options 1, 2, and 5 are clang
associations. Examine options 1, 2, and 5 carefully.
Content Area: Perioperative
Integrated Processes: Nursing Process: Evaluation
*Client Need: Physiological Integrity; Physiological
Adaptation*
Cognitive Level: Analysis
Concept: Tissue Integrity

20. **ANSWER: 1.**
Rationales:
**1. Individuals who are obese have more adipose tissue in
the torso, which can limit the person's ability to take a
deep breath, increasing the risk of respiratory complications. Also, intrathoracic pressure increases as the lungs
expand on inspiration, causing an increase in intra-
abdominal pressure and resulting in abdominal pain.
To avoid this painful response, clients may take shallow
breaths, thereby increasing the risk of respiratory
complications. Clients should be taught to splint the
incisional area when coughing and deep breathing to
prevent dehiscence.**
2. Although it is important to teach a client how to prevent
a wound infection, it is not the priority at this time.
3. The nurse can teach the client how to safely ambulate in
the hall when assisting the client to ambulate postoperatively.
4. Although a nurse may teach a client preoperatively how
to exit the bed postoperatively, it is not as important as another option. The nurse has time during the postoperative
period to teach the client how to safely accomplish this activity of daily living.
TEST-TAKING TIP: Identify the word in the stem that sets a
priority. The word *most* in the stem sets a priority. Identify
equally plausible options. Options 3 and 4 are equally
plausible; both are associated with mobility and one
option is no better than the other. Identify the unique
option. Option 1 is unique because it identifies two
interventions, not one—cough and deep breathe.
Content Area: Perioperative
*Integrated Processes: Teaching/Learning; Nursing Process:
Planning*
*Client Need: Physiological Integrity; Reduction of Risk
Potential*
Cognitive Level: Application
Concept: Patient-Centered Care; Oxygenation

21. **ANSWER: 4.**
Rationales:
1. Although calling the surgeon is important and should be
done eventually, it is more important that the nurse have
more data and institute emergency standing protocols.
2. Emptying the collection containers is unsafe at this
time. Emptying the collection containers will take time,
delaying addressing the client's low blood pressure.
3. Palpating the abdomen for urinary distention will not
correct the low blood pressure. A client with this type of
surgery will have a urinary retention catheter in place and
should not experience urinary retention.
**4. Increasing the IV flow rate will increase the circulating
blood volume, which will help raise the blood pressure;**

once this is done, the nurse can assess the client to identify additional data before notifying the surgeon. Nurses
in a PACU have standing protocols that permit them to
increase an IV flow rate if a blood pressure is less than
expected during a potential emergency.

TEST-TAKING TIP: Identify the word in the stem that sets a
priority. The word *first* in the stem sets a priority.
Content Area: Perioperative
Integrated Processes: Nursing Process: Implementation
*Client Need: Physiological Integrity; Reduction of risk
Potential*
Cognitive Level: Application
Concept: Perfusion

22. **ANSWER: 1, 2, 4.**
    Rationales:
    **1. An NG tube must be unobstructed for negative
    pressure to reach the stomach. The fact that the client
    is vomiting and the abdomen is distended indicates that
    secretions are accumulating in the stomach. The first
    nursing measure is to ensure that the tube is free from
    factors that can cause obstruction of the tube, such as
    kinks in the tubing or compression of the tube.**
    **2. Repositioning the client and instructing the client
    to cough will alter the pressure in the tubing, often
    alleviating an obstruction.**
    3. Administering the prescribed antiemetic to the client
    will not address the problem of an obstructed NG tube.
    **4. Once the other interventions that are correct answers
    fail to reestablish the flow of secretions from the tube,
    30 mL of air can be added via the blue pigtail. This may
    clear secretions from the blue tube that are preventing
    air from entering the stomach, thereby reestablishing
    suction.**
    5. The primary health-care provider has prescribed contin-
    uous suction, not intermittent suction; in addition, a
    Salem sump tube is a double-lumen tube that must use
    continuous suction to function properly.

    TEST-TAKING TIP: Identify the clang association. The word
    tube in the stem and the word *tubing* in option 1 is a clang
    association. More often than not, an option with a clang
    association is a correct answer. Examine option 1 carefully.
    Content Area: Perioperative
    *Integrated Processes: Communication and Documentation;
    Nursing Process: Implementation*
    *Client Need: Physiological Integrity; Reduction of Risk
    Potential*
    Cognitive Level: Application
    Concept: Oxygenation

23. **ANSWERS: 2, 5.**
    Rationales:
    1. Catheterizing a client should never be done without
    a prescription from the client's primary health-care
    provider.
    **2. Palpating and percussing the client's bladder for
    fullness should be performed first to determine if the
    client has urinary retention. If the bladder is not full,
    the client may be experiencing kidney dysfunction.**
    3. The nurse should never increase the IV flow rate with-
    out a prescription from the client's primary health-care

provider. A standing prescription would not exist for this
situation.
4. Encouraging the client to drink more fluids should not
be done until the cause of the client's status is confirmed.
**5. Placing a warm towel over the client's lower abdomen
may relax the urinary sphincters and the sound of
running water in the clients' sink may psychologically
precipitate voiding.**
Content Area: Perioperative
Integrated Processes: Nursing Process: Implementation
*Client Need: Physiological Integrity; Physiological
Adaptation*
Cognitive Level: Application
Concept: Elimination

24. **ANSWER: 1.**
    Rationales:
    **1. The initial concern is that the client may aspirate the
    vomitus. Turning the client to the lateral position will
    facilitate movement of vomitus out of the mouth,
    thereby reducing the risk of aspiration.**
    2. Although increasing the flow rate of the intravenous
    fluid is something the nurse may do after it is determined
    that the client has a problem maintaining the blood
    pressure, it is not the first action that the nurse should
    implement. A standing protocol would have to exist for
    the nurse to implement this action without first notifying
    the primary health-care provider.
    3. Although documenting the amount and characteristics
    of the emesis is important, it is not the priority at this time.
    4. Although calling the blood bank to deliver a unit of
    packed red blood cells is an action that the nurse may
    implement if it is determined that the client is hemorrhag-
    ing, it is not the priority at this time. In addition, adminis-
    tering a blood product requires a prescription from the
    primary health-care provider.

    TEST-TAKING TIP: Identify the word in the stem that sets a
    priority. The word *first* in the stem sets a priority.
    Content Area: Perioperative
    Integrated Processes: Nursing Process: Implementation
    *Client Need: Physiological Integrity; Physiological
    Adaptation*
    Cognitive Level: Application
    Concept: Oxygenation

25. **ANSWER: 2.**
    Rationales:
    1. Opioids are prescribed postoperatively, not preopera-
    tively. An opioid is a central nervous system depressant
    used to manage pain.
    **2. An antibiotic generally is prescribed prophylactically
    preoperatively when a surgeon plans to enter the abdom-
    inal cavity, thoracic cavity, GI tract, or biliary tract;
    surgically repair a traumatic wound (dirty wound); or
    perform a neck dissection. There is an increased risk
    of infection associated with these areas of the body.**
    3. An antiemetic generally is not administered preopera-
    tively. An antiemetic is prescribed postoperatively to treat
    nausea and vomiting.
    4. An anticoagulant, not a thrombolytic, may be prescribed
    prophylactically to reduce the risk of thrombophlebitis or a

pulmonary embolus. Thrombolytics are prescribed to dissolve clots in blood vessels or venous/arterial catheters after they occur, not before they occur.

Content Area: Perioperative
Integrated Processes: Communication and Documentation; Nursing Process: Planning
Client Need: Physiological Integrity; Pharmacological and Parenteral Therapies
Cognitive Level: Application
Concept: Medication; Collaboration

26. **ANSWER: 2.**
    Rationales:
    1. Although the nurse may be concerned about an increased risk of dehiscence due to the presence of abdominal distension, another option directly addresses the potential cause of the abdominal distension. The risk of dehiscence will decrease after abdominal distension is reduced. Also, dehiscence is most common 5 to 14 days after surgery, not immediately after surgery.
    2. Identifying whether the nasogastric (NG) tube is patent is the most important intervention. The concern is that the NG tube is not maintaining decompression of the upper GI tract in the presence of a postoperative ileus. A postoperative ileus is a common response to the handling of the bowel during surgery and the effects of anesthesia. The tube may be occluded due to an obstruction within or kink in the tubing.
    3. After bowel surgery, a client generally is not permitted fluids by mouth until peristalsis returns. Peristalsis is indicated by the presence of bowel sounds.
    4. Absent bowel sounds and abdominal distension are not clinical indicators of hypovolemia. Clinical indicators of hypovolemia include decreased blood pressure and urinary output, tachycardia, tachypnea, restlessness, and anxiety.
    TEST-TAKING TIP: Identify the word in the stem that sets a priority. The word *main* in the stem sets a priority.
    Content Area: Perioperative
    Integrated Processes: Nursing Process: Evaluation
    Client Need: Physiological Integrity; Reduction of Risk Potential
    Cognitive Level: Analysis
    Concept: Oxygenation

27. **ANSWER: 3.**
    Rationales:
    1. Wrist restraints are inappropriate to manage this situation.
    2. The client is semiconscious and probably will not comprehend an explanation at this time. Leaving the airway in place is unsafe.
    3. An attempt to expel the airway indicates that the client is recovering from the anesthesia and is becoming more alert. As the effects of anesthesia decrease, the gag reflex returns. The use of an oropharyngeal airway in the presence of the gag reflex will cause choking and retching, which may precipitate vomiting. Vomiting should be avoided because it may result in aspiration.
    4. Placing the client in the lateral position does not address the issue of the client attempting to expel the airway.

Content Area: Perioperative
Integrated Processes: Nursing Process: Evaluation
Client Need: Physiological Integrity; Physiological Adaptation
Cognitive Level: Application
Concept: Oxygenation

28. **ANSWER: 2.**
    Rationales:
    1. The sitting position elevates the head of the bed, which can precipitate a postdural puncture headache after spinal anesthesia.
    2. A postdural puncture headache can occur as a result of leakage of cerebrospinal fluid when the needle hole in the dura does not close immediately after spinal anesthesia. Cerebrospinal fluid leakage reduces pressure on the spinal cord, resulting in a headache. Positioning a client in the supine position helps to reduce postdural puncture headaches.
    3. The contour position elevates the head of the bed, which can precipitate a postdural puncture headache after spinal anesthesia.
    4. The orthopneic position elevates the head of the bed, which can precipitate a postdural puncture headache after spinal anesthesia.
    TEST-TAKING TIP: Identify the unique option. Option 2 is unique. It is the only option that positions the client flat in bed. Options 1, 3, and 4 require the head of the bed to be elevated.
    Content Area: Perioperative
    Integrated Processes: Nursing Process: Implementation
    Client Need: Physiological Integrity; Physiological Adaptation
    Cognitive Level: Application
    Concept: Neurologic Regulation

29. **ANSWER: 2.**
    Rationales:
    1. The client is not hemorrhaging. Serosanguineous drainage is expected. A blood pressure of 120/80 mm Hg is within the expected range of 90 to 120 mm Hg for the systolic blood pressure and 60 to 80 mm Hg for the diastolic blood pressure. If the client were hemorrhaging, the blood pressure would be lower than the expected range. A hemoglobin level of 15.5 g/dL is within the expected range of 14 to 18 g/dL for an adult male. An RBC count of 5.6 mm^3 is within the expected range of 5.0 to 5.80 mm^3 for an adult male. If the client were hemorrhaging, the hemoglobin and RBC counts would be lower than the expected ranges. A platelet count of 200,000 mm^3 is within the expected range of 150,000 to 450,000 mm^3 for an adult. If the platelet count were lower than the expected range, the client would be at risk for hemorrhage. If the drainage changes to sanguineous (abundance of blood), the client may be hemorrhaging. If the serosanguineous drainage continues to be profuse, the primary health-care provider should be notified because this is an unexpected response that requires further assessment.

2. Infection is a concern because the client's WBC count is lower than the expected range of 4.5 to 11.0 mm³, which most likely is a complication of the chemotherapy for stage II lung cancer. Also, the client has a temperature of 100.4°F, which is higher than the expected range of approximately 97.5°F to 99.5°F. This may be a response to inflammation associated with trauma and surgery, but it could indicate the presence of infection.

3. The client is not experiencing respiratory distress. The slightly elevated respirations are most likely a response to the increased temperature. Shallow respirations may be a defensive response to avoid discomfort associated with the abdominal wall trauma when taking a deep breath. Taking a deep breath increases thoracic exertion, which in turn will increase intra-abdominal pressure causing discomfort at the injured site.

4. The client is not experiencing an electrolyte imbalance. A serum potassium level of 4.5 mEq/L is within the expected range of 3.5 to 5.0 mEq/L, and a serum sodium level of 140 mEq/L is within the expected range of 135 to 145 mEq/L.

TEST-TAKING TIP: Identify the unique option. Option 2 is unique because it is the only option that involves a "risk for" concern.

Content Area: *Perioperative*
Integrated Processes: *Communication and Documentation; Nursing Process: Analysis*
Client Need: *Physiological Integrity; Physiological Adaptation*
Cognitive Level: *Analysis*
Concept: *Hematologic Regulation*

30. ANSWER: 3.
Rationales:

1. Surgical, not medical, asepsis should be employed when changing a client's surgical dressings or when emptying drains.

2. Although suggesting that the client ingest high-protein foods facilitates wound healing, it is not as essential as another option.

3. **Neutropenic precautions protect the client from pathogens. When a client has impaired immunity, the white blood cell count is low, which decreases a person's ability to fight infection. The client is placed in a private room, caregivers and visitors must wear gowns and masks, and strategies, such as wet dusting and mopping; banning of dried, fresh, or potted flowers; a diet of well-cooked food; omission of fresh vegetables and fruit; frequent hand hygiene; meticulous and frequent oral care; and having the client wear an N95 respirator when being transported for essential reasons, are implemented to protect the client from pathogens.**

4. Although encouraging fluid intake is important to meet fluid requirements and to flush the urinary tract of microorganisms, it is not as essential as another option.

TEST-TAKING TIP: Identify the word in the stem that sets a priority. The word *essential* in the stem sets a priority.

Content Area: *Perioperative*
Integrated Processes: *Nursing Process: Implementation*

Client Need: *Safe and Effective Care Environment; Safety and Infection Control*
Cognitive Level: *Application*
Concept: *Medication; Safety*

31. ANSWER: 4.
Rationales:

1. Deep breathing and coughing generally are suggested to minimize the risk of hypostatic pneumonia after anesthesia and surgery.

2. Although room-deodorizing sprays may be used to cover up offensive odors, this intervention is not as important as another option.

3. Although frequent oral hygiene should be provided for the client who is experiencing nausea and vomiting, it is not as important as another option.

4. **The primary health-care provider prescribed that the client be NPO (nothing-by-mouth). This is the most important intervention of the options presented. Until the cause of the nausea and vomiting is identified, the client should be NPO. In addition, drinking and eating may exacerbate nausea and vomiting.**

TEST-TAKING TIP: Identify the word in the stem that sets a priority. The word *most* in the stem sets a priority. Identify the unique option. Option 4 is unique because it is the only option that involves an intervention prescribed by the primary health-care provider. The other actions are all independent nursing interventions. Also, option 4 is the only option with capital letters, making it unique.

Content Area: *Perioperative*
Integrated Processes: *Communication and Documentation; Nursing Process: Implementation*
Client Need: *Physiological Integrity; Physiological Adaptation*
Cognitive Level: *Application*
Concept: *Oxygenation*

32. ANSWER: 3.
Rationales:

1. Although the systolic blood pressure is 20 mm Hg above the expected range for a systolic blood pressure (<120 mm Hg), it is not unusual for a person 65 years of age. In addition, the slight elevation of the systolic pressure most likely is associated with the psychological and physical stress of preparing for bowel surgery.

2. A little sip of water is not critical 2 hours before general anesthesia. This fluid will pass through the stomach in 2 hours and not be a risk factor for aspiration.

3. **Clopidogrel (Plavix) is a platelet aggregation inhibitor. It is recommended that clopidogrel be discontinued 5 to 7 days before surgery because it can cause bleeding and hemorrhage. This is important information that must be reported to the primary health-care provider immediately. Surgery may need to be postponed.**

4. An Hb level of 15 g/dL is within the expected range of 14 to 18 g/dL for an adult male.

TEST-TAKING TIP: Identify the word in the stem that sets a priority. The word *most* in the stem sets a priority.

Content Area: *Perioperative*
Integrated Processes: *Communication and Documentation; Nursing Process: Analysis*

Client Need: Physiological Integrity; Pharmacological and Parenteral Therapies
Cognitive Level: Analysis
Concept: Medication; Communication

33. **ANSWER: 0.5.**
Rationale:
Solve the problem by using ratio and proportion.

$$\frac{\text{Desire 2.5 mg}}{\text{Have 5 mg}} = \frac{x \text{ mL}}{1 \text{ mL}}$$
$$5x = 2.5 \times 1$$
$$5x = 2.5$$
$$x = 2.5 \div 5$$
$$x = 0.5 \text{ mL}$$

Content Area: Perioperative
Integrated Processes: Nursing Process: Planning
Client Need: Physiological Integrity; Pharmacological and Parenteral Therapies
Cognitive Level: Application
Concept: Medication; Safety

34. **ANSWER: 3.**
Rationales:
1. Although this may eventually be done, it is not the priority. The client's heart rate and respirations are within expected limits, indicating that the client is not exhibiting malignant hyperthermia.
2. Notifying the surgeon is not necessary. The client's status is not unstable.
3. **Feeling cold postoperatively is a common response. Clients may feel cold because of exposure to the cool environmental temperature of the operating room. Also,** body heat can be lost via radiation, convection, evaporation, and conduction. One or more heated bath blankets should be placed over the client to promote comfort and help conserve body heat.
4. Although continuing to monitor the client will be done, it does not address the client's problem.
Content Area: Perioperative
Integrated Processes: Nursing Process: Evaluation
Client Need: Physiological Integrity; Basic Care and Comfort
Cognitive Level: Application
Concept: Comfort

35. **ANSWER: 2.**
Rationales:
1. Although trochanter rolls will prevent external rotation of the hips, they will not promote abduction or prevent adduction.
2. **The pillows between the thighs prevent internal rotation and adduction of the hips. The supine position prevents hip flexion. Both interventions prevent trauma to the operative site.**
3. Flexing the knees is unsafe because it will cause hip flexion, which will traumatize the operative site.
4. Positioning the client on the unoperated side without an abduction pillow is unsafe because it will promote adduction.
Content Area: Perioperative
Integrated Processes: Nursing Process: Implementation
Client Need: Physiological Integrity; Reduction of Risk Potential
Cognitive Level: Application
Concept: Mobility

Comprehensive Final Exam

REVIEW QUESTIONS

Be sure to read the Introduction for valuable test-taking tips.

1. Which actions are associated with a first-level need according to Maslow's hierarchy of needs? **Select all that apply.**
   1. Eating a sandwich for lunch
   2. Inviting friends over for a party
   3. Taking a nap after working out at a gym
   4. Getting a haircut before the holiday season
   5. Locking the car door when alone in the car
   6. Taking a bottle of water along when going for a walk

2. A nurse identifies a 1-cm superficial circular break in the skin over the right trochanter of a client during an admission assessment. What should the nurse do **first**?
   1. Initiate a turning schedule.
   2. Complete a skin assessment form.
   3. Inform the primary health-care provider of the client's status.
   4. Start wound care based on the agency's pressure ulcer protocol.

3. Which situations may lead to a legal action for assault? **Select all that apply.**
   1. A nurse threatens a client with inserting a tube to feed the client if the client does not eat all the food on a meal tray.
   2. A nurse administers a medication that the client has refused by telling the client that it is different from the refused medication.
   3. A nurse uses a restraint when a client attempts to leave the hospital before the primary health-care provider writes a discharge prescription.
   4. A nurse tells a client who has a prescription for bedrest that unless the client stays in bed the four side rails on the bed will have to be raised.
   5. A nurse is heard by a client's relative telling another nurse on an elevator that the client contracted hepatitis C from IV drug use when, in fact, the client contracted the disease via a blood transfusion.

4. A nurse is caring for a group of clients who each have an intestinal diversion for fecal matter. The nurse should be concerned about the client with which ostomy if the fecal matter has a loose consistency?
   1. Ileostomy
   2. Cecostomy
   3. Sigmoid colostomy
   4. Ascending colon colostomy

5. A nurse caring for a newly admitted client reviews the information in the client's admission history and performs a chart review. The nurse should assess the client for which additional human response based on the data collected?
   1. Peripheral edema
   2. Burning on urination
   3. Suprapubic distension
   4. Decreased blood pressure

Client's Clinical Record

Admission History

An 85-year-old male came to the emergency department reporting urinary frequency and urgency, increased nocturia, and weakness and tiredness. The client has not been eating well for the last few days but states that he is drinking lots of fluids. Client states, "Usually when I used to go to the bathroom to urinate, it took a long time to start the stream. Now I barely make it to the bathroom in time." The client's abdomen is soft and nontender.

Vital Signs Sheet

Temperature: 100.6°F, oral route.
Respirations: 24 breaths/minute, regular.
Pulse: 86 beats/minute, regular.

Urinalysis Results

White blood cell count increased.
Red blood cell count increased.
Glucose negative.
Ketones negative.
Protein negative.
Nitrites positive.

---

6. A nurse assesses four clients to determine their hygiene needs. The nurse should anticipate that the client with which problem will have the **greatest** difficulty having hygiene needs met by the nurse?
   1. Pain
   2. Dementia
   3. Impaired vision
   4. Limited mobility

7. A client with the diagnosis of stage 4 pancreatic cancer is consulting with a discharge planner regarding the most appropriate level of care required after palliative surgery. The client is able to provide self-care but will need pain management. Which setting is **most** appropriate for this client?
   1. Home hospice care
   2. Rehabilitation facility
   3. Skilled nursing facility
   4. Assistive living apartment

3/6

8. A client comes to the emergency department reporting a sore throat and earaches. The client has a history of diverticulitis and emphysema with shortness of breath. Which routes can the nurse use to obtain this client's temperature safely? **Select all that apply.**
   1. Oral
   2. Skin
   3. Rectal
   4. Axillary
   5. Temporal
   6. Tympanic

9. A nurse is teaching a group of clients about diabetes mellitus. Which participant should the nurse anticipate will have the **most** difficulty following a medical regimen associated with a chronic health problem?
   1. Adolescent
   2. Older adult
   3. Young adult
   4. Middle-aged adult

10. A nurse is caring for an older adult who is hearing impaired. What should the nurse do to facilitate communication? **Select all that apply.**
    1. Talk at a slow rate.
    2. Use shorter phrases.
    3. Speak in a low tone of voice.
    4. Overarticulate when speaking.
    5. Stand so that the nurse's face can be seen easily.

11. A client is frustrated about not being able to perform activities of daily living (ADLs) without help. What should the nurse do to reduce the client's frustration? **Select all that apply.**
    1. Disregard the client's behavior.
    2. Offer the client choices about care.
    3. Distract the client by discussing the news.
    4. Assist the client to recognize personal limitations.
    5. Have the client engage in activities that can be completed successfully.

12. A client comes to the emergency department and reports pain in the hip. Which client assessments reflect chronic pain rather than acute pain? **Select all that apply.**
    1. Variable breathing patterns
    2. Decreased blood pressure
    3. Slow monotonous speech
    4. Increased heart rate
    5. Pressured speech
    6. Dilated pupils

13. What action is unrelated to maintaining airborne precautions for a client with a diagnosis of suspected primary tuberculosis?
    1. Donning a gown when entering the room
    2. Wearing a respirator mask when in the room
    3. Maintaining negative air pressure within the room
    4. Having the client wear a surgical mask when transported outside the room

14. A nurse is to administer eardrops to an adult. The nurse verifies the original prescription, washes the hands, and collects the medication, following the three checks and ten rights associated with medication administration. The nurse then dons clean gloves. Place the following steps in the order in which they should be implemented.
    1. Pull the auricle of the ear up and back gently.
    2. Apply slight pressure several times to the tragus of the ear.
    3. Instruct the client to remain in a side-lying position for 5 to 10 minutes.
    4. Position the client in a side-lying position with the affected ear facing up.
    5. Hold the dropper a half inch above the ear canal and instill the drops so that they fall on the side of the ear canal.
    Answer: 4, 1, 5, 2, 3

15. At a nursing organization meeting, the vice president for nursing informs the nurse managers that each client care unit must engage in one nursing research project a year as part of attaining Magnet status. A nurse manager holds a unit meeting to inform the nursing staff of this new initiative. Which nurse manager statement provides the **best** introduction?
    1. "To improve the status of the hospital in the community, we must become involved in nursing research."
    2. "I know that it will require more effort, but you will find it very rewarding to engage in nursing research."
    3. "We have a great opportunity to expand our involvement within our profession by performing nursing research."
    4. "I have just received a new edict from nursing administration that we have to get involved in nursing research."

16. Before going to lunch, a nurse provides information to the nurse accepting responsibility for a client who returned 2 hours ago after a fiberoptic colonoscopy. Which information is **most** important for the covering nurse to know about this client?
    1. Gag reflex is present
    2. Reports mild abdominal pain
    3. Passing flatus for the last hour
    4. Dozing intermittently since the procedure

5/5

17. Which nursing assessments indicate a period of exacerbation? **Select all that apply.**
1. Client's symptoms have returned despite adhering to the medical regimen.
2. Client's status is unchanged following a course of chemotherapy.
3. Client reports long-standing joint pain from rheumatoid arthritis.
4. Client had an allergic response to a prescribed medication.
5. Client states that the back spasms are acting up again.

18. A client who misuses alcohol is admitted to the hospital for detoxification. The client is intoxicated and agitated. The client's agitation increases and the client becomes verbally abusive to the nurse. What should the nurse do **next**?
1. Obtain a prescription for a physical restraint for the client.
2. Offer emotional support while touching the client's shoulder.
3. Stand between the client and the exit to the room while talking with the client.
4. Approach the client's bedside and state that using bad language is unacceptable.

19. Which statement by the nurse **best** helps a client clarify values regarding a health-care decision that was not supported by the client's family or primary health-care provider?
1. "There were many possible options. What motivated you to make your decision?"
2. "Your decision was courageous. I give you credit for taking control of your future."
3. "Why did you choose your decision? It was not what your loved ones and doctor preferred."
4. "Your decision would not have been my choice. But everyone has a right to self-determination."

20. A nurse is obtaining a blood specimen for monitoring a blood glucose level by using a lancet. Which actions are appropriate when implementing this procedure? **Select all that apply.**
1. Use the first drop of blood that appears at the puncture site.
2. Select an index finger for performing the puncture to acquire a drop of blood.
3. Apply pressure with gauze to the puncture site for half a minute after the procedure.
4. Place the hand in a dependent position before inserting the lancet to obtain the blood specimen.
5. Milk the finger from the palm of the hand to the distal part of the finger to bring more blood to the area.

21. A client with moderate cognitive impairment who lives in an assisted living facility has been having more difficulty providing self-care over the past year. Which intervention is **most** significant to ensure that the client is receiving adequate nutrition?
1. Feed the client meals.
2. Weigh the client weekly.
3. Give the client a liquid supplement between meals.
4. Provide the client with opportunities to choose foods that are preferred.

22. A client is receiving an enteric-coated iron preparation. The client asks, "Why can't I just chew this pill so it is easier to take?" Which is the **best** response by the nurse?
1. "It has to dissolve slowly in your mouth for best absorption."
2. "If you can stand the taste, you are more than welcome to do that."
3. "If you break the tablet in your mouth, the medication can stain your teeth."
4. "If the tablet coating is damaged, the drug will be deactivated by gastric enzymes."

23. A nurse plans to provide foot care for an older adult. What actions should the nurse include in this procedure? **Select all that apply.**
1. Soak the feet for 30 minutes.
2. Push the cuticles back gently with a washcloth.
3. Dry each foot thoroughly, especially between the toes.
4. Clean under nails with an orangewood stick while a foot is in the water.
5. Soak the feet one at a time in water that has a temperature of 115° to 120°F.

24. A client who had a brain attack (cerebrovascular accident) is experiencing hemiparesis and fatigue. The nurse plans to progress from passive range-of-motion (ROM) exercises to active ROM exercises as prescribed. What should the nurse do to **best** facilitate teaching sessions with this client?
1. Plan teaching sessions for after lunch.
2. Have another nurse assist with teaching sessions.
3. Conduct client teaching sessions that are 15 minutes in length.
4. Medicate the client for pain 30 minutes before a teaching session.

25. A client is to receive a prescribed drug for the first time at 10 a.m. The laboratory report indicates a newly elevated creatinine level at 6 a.m. Which nursing action is **most** important when caring for this client?
    1. Assess the client for clinical manifestations of drug toxicity.
    2. Call the pharmacist to ensure that it is safe to administer the medication.
    3. Withhold the medication until repeat test results are within the normal range.
    4. Inform the primary health-care provider of the client's impaired kidney function.

26. With which clients should a nurse protect oneself from potential exposure to HIV when providing direct physical care? **Select all that apply.**
    1. Client who is crying
    2. Man who is diaphoretic
    3. Woman who is menstruating
    4. Client who is incontinent of feces
    5. Client who requires the insertion of an intravenous catheter

27. Which skill should the nurse implement **first** when assessing a client's abdomen?
    1. Palpation
    2. Inspection
    3. Percussion
    4. Auscultation

28. A client is admitted to a medical unit from the emergency department with the diagnosis of pneumonia. The client is in the high-Fowler position and is receiving oxygen 2 L via nasal cannula. The nurse obtains the client's vital signs, performs a focused assessment, and verifies the primary health-care provider's prescriptions. What should be the nurse's **next** intervention?
    1. Suction the client's airway.
    2. Administer the clarithromycin as prescribed.
    3. Obtain a sputum specimen for culture and sensitivity.
    4. Insert a circulatory access device and administer the prescribed intravenous fluids.

Client's Clinical Record

Vital Signs

Temperature: 101.4°F, orally.
Pulse: 98 beats/minute, regular rhythm, radial.
Respirations: 28 breaths/minute, shallow, regular rhythm.
Blood pressure: 138/84 mm Hg.

Primary Health-Care Provider's Prescriptions

Bedrest.
Regular diet.
Droplet precautions.
Culture and sensitivity of sputum.
Clarithromycin (Biaxin) 500 mg twice a day by mouth.
Guaifenesin (Mucinex) 200 mg every 6 hours by mouth.
Acetaminophen (Tylenol) 325 mg every 6 hours for a temperature more than 101°F.
IVF: 0.9% sodium chloride at 100 mL/hour.
Oxygen 2 L via nasal cannula.
Incentive spirometer.
Monitor vital signs and pulse oximetry every 4 hours.

Physical Assessment

Reports shortness of breath, a feeling of tightness in the chest on inhalation, and excessive coughing after a deep breath. Coughing is frequent and produces thick yellow sputum. Breaths are rapid and shallow. Crackles in lower lobes bilaterally and bronchial wheezes heard on auscultation. Dull percussion over lower lobes bilaterally.

29. Which actions are associated with the analysis step of the nursing process? **Select all that apply.**
    1. A nurse takes the vital signs when a client reports dizziness.
    2. A nurse groups collected information into related categories.
    3. A nurse determines that a client is at risk for a pressure ulcer because of immobility and edema.
    4. A nurse and client decide that within two days the client will learn how to transfer from a bed to a chair safely.
    5. A nurse concludes that further intervention is necessary when the client does not accurately prepare an insulin injection.

30. A nurse enters the room of a client who is scheduled to go for surgery within the hour. The nurse observes the client gazing out the window and that the client's eyes are filled with tears. The nurse asks, "Are you okay?" The client responds, "Don't worry. I'll be fine." What is the nurse's **most** appropriate response?
    1. "What are you thinking about?"
    2. "I'll be here if you need to talk."
    3. "Don't you think everything will be all right?"
    4. "When people cry, it usually means something is wrong."

7/2

31. Which statements by a client experiencing insomnia indicate that the nurse must provide further education? **Select all that apply.**
1. "I enjoy a walk after dinner."
2. "I always have a snack just before I go to bed."
3. "I drink a big glass of wine when watching television at night."
4. "I like to set my bedroom temperature at a cool setting at night."
5. "I take a nap when I get home from work each day for about an hour."

32. A nurse is providing morning care to a hospitalized client. Which statement by the nurse is **most** important before leaving the room after providing care?
1. "Push your call bell if you need anything after I leave."
2. "Would you like the door to your room closed?"
3. "Your lunch will be served at around noon."
4. "Is your room temperature comfortable?"

33. A primary health-care provider prescribes 1,000 mL of 0.9% NaCl to be administered every 8 hours and an antibiotic to be administered intravenously twice a day. The instructions accompanying the antibiotic indicate that it should be diluted in 100 mL of sterile water. The first dose was administered at 8 p.m. A nurse working the 7 a.m. to 7 p.m. shift the next day continues to implement the primary health-care provider's prescription. The antibiotic was administered via a circulatory access device at a different site than the primary infusion. How much intravenous fluid did the client receive during the 7 a.m. to 7 p.m. shift? **Record your answer using a whole number.**
Answer: _____ 1600 _____ mL

34. A person who fell down the basement stairs at home is brought to the hospital by the spouse. The client, who has a psychiatric history, is actively hallucinating and the spouse is upset. The primary health-care provider prescribes a computed tomography scan with contrast. What should the nurse do?
1. Ask the client about having an allergy to shellfish.
2. Determine if the client currently is taking any medications.
3. Obtain an informed consent for the procedure from the spouse.
4. Explain the procedure in detail to limit the anxiety that both are experiencing.

35. Which is **most** effective in helping a client who has an activity intolerance to shower safely at home?
1. Advise the use of a shower chair.
2. Suggest using a handheld faucet.
3. Encourage the installation of handrails.
4. Recommend placing a nonskid mat in the shower stall.

36. Omeprazole, a proton-pump inhibitor, is prescribed for a client with gastroesophageal reflux disease. The prescription states to take 20 mg by mouth once a day. Which instruction should the nurse give the client regarding this medication?
1. "Take the medication several hours before an antacid."
2. "Sprinkle the capsule contents in applesauce."
3. "Take the medication with food."
4. "Swallow the capsule whole."

37. A nurse is teaching a professional athlete with hypertension the reasons for taking all of the prescribed antihypertensive medications, including a diuretic once a day. The client states, "I take my other medications, but I have stopped taking the diuretic because there are no toilets near our outside training facilities. What is the nurse's **best** reply?
1. "It must be difficult to be taking all these drugs."
2. "It is important that you follow the prescriptions exactly."
3. "Let's explore a time when it is convenient to take the diuretic."
4. "The other drugs provide an insufficient response without the diuretic."

38. A nurse is caring for clients on a surgical unit. Which client should the nurse assess **first**?
1. A client experiencing nausea and vomiting for several hours
2. A client asking for pain medication for incisional pain on a level 3
3. A client reporting chest pain 3 days after admission for a fractured pelvis
4. A client requesting to see the surgeon before signing the consent form for morning surgery

39. A nurse is preparing a medication to be administered to a client. The nurse identifies that the name of the medication on the unit dose package is not the same as the name on the medication administration record. What should the nurse do?
1. Give it if the dose of the drug is the same as what is indicated on the prescription.
2. Call the primary health-care provider and ask if the drug provided is the drug prescribed.
3. Ask another nurse on the unit who is more familiar with drugs if it is equivalent to the prescription.
4. Check a drug information resource to determine if the name on the unit dose package is a generic form of the drug.

40. Which nursing interventions are important when assisting a client to eat? **Select all that apply.**

1. Offer to toilet the client before the meal.
2. Place the client in an upright position for the meal.
3. Engage the client in conversation when feeding the client.
4. Open containers, cut meat, and apply condiments to the client's food.
5. Ask the client's preference regarding the order of foods and fluids to ingest.
6. Ensure the client has swallowed the previous bite before assisting with another bite.

41. A nurse responds to a call light of a client who had a colon resection 2 days ago for the removal of a cancerous tumor. The client states, "It feels very wet and funny under my dressing." Which additional information collected by the nurse supports the conclusion that the client may be experiencing dehiscence? **Select all that apply.**

1. Client described throbbing pain at the site of the incision.
2. Client stated, "I just felt a popping sensation at my incision."
3. Client informed the nurse of voiding excessively during the night.
4. Client stated, "My stomach feels better when I keep my knees bent."
5. Client reported just having had an intense episode of coughing that brought up phlegm.

42. An 84-year-old man is admitted to a long-term care facility because his daughter can no longer care for him. The nurse reviews the client's family history and, when the client is brought to the unit, interviews the client and performs a physical assessment. Which nursing intervention addresses this client's **most** important need?

1. Use a product to thicken liquids before giving them to the client.
2. Maintain splints and braces on extremities at all times.
3. Apply an external urinary drainage device at night.
4. Encourage the client to explore feelings.

Client's Clinical Record

Family History

The client's wife died 10 years ago. Approximately 5 years ago, the client had a brain attack, resulting in right-sided hemiplegia and expressive aphasia. The client moved into his daughter's home after discharge from the hospital. The daughter provided almost constant care and supervision of her father. The daughter has two children in college and must go to work to earn money to add to her husband's income to pay for tuition.

Physical Assessment

The client has right hemiplegia and wears a hand and forearm splint on the right arm and a brace on the right leg to manage footdrop. The client needs assistance with all activities of daily living. The client usually is continent of urine and feces but occasionally experiences functional urinary incontinence. Transfer from bed to chair or wheelchair is accomplished with a mechanical lift. The ability to chew and swallow solid food safely is intact, but the client occasionally chokes when drinking liquids.

Client Interview

The client has expressive aphasia but was able to write short phrases and use a picture board and gestures to express his needs. The client was oriented to time, place, and person. He indicated that he understands where he is, but he does not want to be here. The client was crying and pulled himself to the side of the bed in an attempt to get out of bed. The client indicated that he is angry with his daughter and will do whatever his daughter wants if he can go back home. The client banged the bed with his left hand several times and wrote, "WANT TO GO HOME."

---

43. A nurse and a nursing assistant are working together caring for a group of clients in a district. Which activities are appropriate for the nurse to assign to the nursing assistant? **Select all that apply.**

1. Turning and repositioning a client who had spinal surgery
2. Giving a bath and oral care to a client receiving contact precautions
3. Providing range-of-motion exercises while administering a bed bath
4. Reassessing the signs and symptoms of a client with a wound infection
5. Assisting a client to the bathroom the first time after returning from surgery

44. A nurse is teaching the spouse of an immobile client how to position the client. Which observations indicate to the nurse that the client was correctly positioned when supine? **Select all that apply.**

1. The client's heels are placed on a pillow.
2. A pillow is placed between the client's legs.
3. A pillow is placed under the client's head and shoulders.
4. The client's hands are turned with the palms facing the ceiling.
5. A trochanter roll is positioned from the client's hip to the knee bilaterally.

45. A nurse accidentally administers an opioid to a client. What should the nurse do **first**?
1. Call the nursing supervisor.
2. Administer the antidote immediately.
3. Instruct the client to drink a glass of water.
4. Contact the client's primary health-care provider.

46. A nurse is caring for a client who has an elevated temperature and identifies that the client's skin is flushed and feels warm. The nurse should assess the client for which additional clinical manifestation that supports the conclusion that the client's fever is in the defervescence phase?
1. Pallor
2. Malaise
3. Sweating
4. Shivering

47. A primary nurse is observing a licensed practical nurse (LPN) change a dressing on a client's abdominal wound. Which action by the LPN requires the primary nurse to interrupt the procedure?
1. Using nonsterile gloves to remove the soiled dressing
2. Removing sterile gloves and applying tape to secure the dressing
3. Touching the sterile irrigating container with the neck of the bottle of normal saline
4. Failing to wash the hands between removing the soiled dressing and donning sterile gloves

48. A 12-year-old child is receiving intravenous patient-controlled analgesia postoperatively. The nurse teaches the child and parents about the trigger connected to the pump and how basal and bolus doses of the analgesic help relieve pain. Later when the child is sleeping, the nurse observes one of the parents pushing the trigger to deliver a bolus dose of medication. What should the nurse do **first**?
1. Review with the parents that the child is still receiving medication even if not pushing the trigger.
2. Tell the parents to stop pushing the trigger when the child is sleeping.
3. Notify the primary health-care provider of the parent's behavior.
4. Increase the dosage of the basal dose.

49. A client is diagnosed as having herpes simplex type 2, and acyclovir is prescribed during outbreaks of lesions. Which statement indicates that the client understands the nurse's instructions about this medication?
1. "I should discontinue the medication if I develop dizziness."
2. "I have to increase fiber in my diet because the medication may cause constipation."
3. "I must take my pulse before I take this medication because it can raise my heart rate."
4. "I need to take the medication as soon as I feel tingling in the area where I get the sores."

50. A nurse is caring for a client who is receiving an anticoagulant. When assisting the client with hygiene, the client expresses a desire to shave himself. Which is **most** important for the nurse to teach the client to do?
1. Use a safety razor when shaving.
2. Use an electric razor when shaving.
3. Apply some aftershave lotion on the skin after shaving.
4. Wrap the face with a hot towel for a few minutes before shaving.

51. A client is diagnosed with inflammation of the right lower lobe (RLL) of the lung (pleurisy). The nurse identifies the presence of a pleural friction rub. Where was the stethoscope placed on the client's chest when the pleural friction rub was heard?

1. A
2. B
3. C
4. D

5/5

52. A nurse is admitting a client to an acute care facility. The nurse should explain to the client that the **most** important member of the health-care team is which person?
1. Client
2. Primary nurse
3. Nurse manager
4. Nurse practitioner

53. A bladder-retraining program is prescribed for a client who is incontinent of urine after therapy for bladder cancer. Which nursing interventions when implemented effectively promote a successful bladder-retraining program? **Select all that apply.**
1. Teach relaxation techniques
2. Follow the scheduled program.
3. Place a commode at the bedside.
4. Wash the perineal area every shift.
5. Maintain a strict record of fluid balance.

54. A nurse is caring for two clients who just had surgery. One client has a Jackson-Pratt drain, and the other client has a Penrose drain. Which nursing interventions are common to both types of drains? **Select all that apply.**
1. Maintaining negative pressure in the collection device
2. Emptying the collection device when it is half full
3. Assessing tissue integrity around the drain site
4. Shortening the drain an inch daily
5. Assessing color of the drainage

55. A nurse is designing a teaching plan for a client who speaks a different language. What is a reliable way for the nurse to facilitate client understanding of the information?
1. Arrange a telephone translation service to be used during the teaching session.
2. Have a staff member who is from the same country act as an interpreter.
3. Provide a pamphlet with pictures to reinforce what is being taught.
4. Use a translation book that will aid in the conversion of words.

56. A nurse is caring for a client who tends to become confused. Which information communicated to the client is the **best** intervention to prevent falls in a hospital setting?
1. "I am going to care for you today and I will be here whenever you call me for help."
2. "When you finish in the bathroom, activate the call light and I will help you back to your bed."
3. "When you decide you want to walk around the unit, I would appreciate it if you would use the walker."
4. "I am going to transfer you to your wheelchair now and move you to an area near the nurses' station."

57. A nurse is assessing the physical status of several clients. Which client problem should be the nurse's **greatest** concern?
1. Tenting of skin
2. Difficulty breathing
3. Erythema over the greater trochanter
4. Body weight inadequate in relation to height

58. A nurse is caring for an obese client with an abdominal surgical incision that has a separation of wound edges with a large amount of exudate. The primary health-care provider prescribes a wet to moist dressing with sterile normal saline every 6 hours. What should the nurse do when implementing this procedure?
1. Secure the dressing using Montgomery straps.
2. Cleanse the wound with half-normal saline and peroxide.
3. Ensure the gauze packing is saturated and dripping with saline.
4. Dry the wound by patting with gauze from the skin toward the wound.

59. Which actions should a nurse implement when administering eyedrops to a client with an eye infection? **Select all that apply.**
1. Put on sterile gloves.
2. Pull the upper lid toward the forehead.
3. Draw the skin under the eye downward.
4. Administer drops into the conjunctival sac.
5. Wipe from the outer toward the inner canthus.

60. Which data that the nurse documents in the client's clinical record is objective information? **Select all that apply.**
1. Client statements of always feeling hungry as the reason for excessive eating
2. Observation of the client avoiding eye contact when talking with the nurse
3. Assessment of the presence of bladder spasms after the client urinates
4. Presence of a pleural friction rub at the height of inspiration
5. Reports of epigastric discomfort after meals

61. A nurse observes a client sitting in bed crying. The nurse enters the room, sits in a chair next to the bed, and states, "You seem upset." The client says, "I will be fine," but continues to cry. What is the **best** intervention by the nurse?
1. State, "I will be at the nurses' station if you decide you want to talk."
2. Say, "It is important that you talk about what is bothering you."
3. Remain seated in the chair for several minutes
4. Leave the room so that the client has privacy

7/1

62. A nurse is purchasing toys for children in the child life center. Identify the toys that the nurse purchased that are appropriate for the ages of children progressing from infants to adolescents.
1. Chess set
2. Plastic rattles
3. Decks of cards
4. Pounding board
5. Construction set
Answer: ___2, 4, 5, 3, 1___

63. A nurse is assessing a postoperative client's incision. Which clinical manifestations support the conclusion that the client has a wound infection versus an expected local response to the stress of surgery? **Select all that apply.**
1. Redness
2. Swelling
3. Warm to touch
4. Purulent drainage
5. Elevated temperature

64. A nurse is performing range-of-motion exercises for a client who had a brain attack (cerebrovascular accident) to prevent contractures. How should the nurse move the client's hip when performing internal rotation?
1. Position the leg behind the body.
2. Move the leg laterally across the midline of the body.
3. Turn the leg and foot pointing away from the other leg.
4. Rotate the leg and foot pointing inward toward the other leg.

65. A resident in a nursing home wanders during the night and scares other residents by going into their rooms. What is the **most** effective intervention that the nurse should implement to address this situation?
1. Explain to others that the resident means no harm.
2. Position a bed alarm on the wandering resident's bed.
3. Close the doors of the other residents' rooms during the night.
4. Place bolsters against four side rails of the wandering resident's bed.

66. A nurse manager allows the staff to self-arrange days off on a monthly calendar. One nurse tells the nurse manager that no one wants to complain but that one of the nurses attempts to take all the holidays and most of the weekends off. What is the nurse manager's **best** response?
1. "Why didn't you meet with the nurse and attempt to work it out?"
2. "Will the other nurses be willing to confront the nurse if you all approach the nurse together?"
3. "I guess I will have to change the system of selecting days off because this system is not working."
4. "I will arrange a meeting so that we can meet together to fix the process so that it is fair to everyone."

67. A nurse teaches a client who is lactose intolerant about foods to avoid. Which foods eliminated from the diet by the client indicate an understanding about foods that contain lactose? **Select all that apply.**
1. Soy milk
2. Fruit cocktail
3. Creamed soup
4. Cottage cheese
5. Vegetable juice

68. A nurse must administer a medication through a nasogastric tube that is being used for gastric decompression. What is the **most** important intervention by the nurse?
1. Instill an ounce of water before instilling the medication.
2. Use high pressure via a piston syringe to instill the medication.
3. Shut off the negative pressure after the medication is administered.
4. Determine accurate placement of the nasogastric tube before the medication is administered.

69. A nurse is caring for a group of clients on a surgical unit. Which clinical finding warrants immediate nursing action?
1. Mildly active bowel sounds 3 days after a colon resection
2. Dark pink urine immediately after a transurethral resection of the prostate
3. Reduced breath sounds on the left side 1 day after a wedge resection of the right lung
4. Greenish drainage from a nasogastric tube immediately after an abdominal cholecystectomy

70. A nurse is developing a teaching plan for adults who are overweight. What teaching method is **most** effective to promote behavioral changes?
   1. Online course
   2. Series of lectures
   3. Group instruction
   4. Colorful pamphlets

71. A client has bilateral wrist restraints because of repeated attempts to pull out tubes. How frequently should the nurse release the restraints, exercise the client's hands and wrists, and document this activity?
   1. Every hour
   2. Every shift
   3. Every 4 hours
   4. Every 2 hours

72. A nurse is assessing a client's pain. What question obtains information about whether the client is experiencing radiating pain?
   1. "What is the extent of your pain on a zero to ten numerical scale?"
   2. "Was the onset of pain gradual over a period of time?"
   3. "Did the pain start in one area and extend to another?"
   4. "Does the pain tend to come and go?"

73. A hospitalized client reports an inability to urinate. What should the nurse do to obtain more information about this problem? **Select all that apply.**
   1. Perform a straight catheterization.
   2. Initiate intake and output monitoring.
   3. Assess the client's lower abdomen for bladder distension.
   4. Implement a bladder ultrasound scan according to protocol.
   5. Ask the client about the time and amount of the last voiding.
   6. Obtain the client's weight to compare to the weight on admission to the hospital.

74. A female client on bedrest asks the nurse what she can do to prevent her hair from becoming tangled and matted. What should the nurse encourage the client to avoid?
   1. Conditioning the hair after shampooing
   2. Washing the hair with soap
   3. Placing the hair in braids
   4. Brushing the hair daily

75. A client is taking furosemide daily because of hypertension. Which foods should the nurse teach the client to consume on a regular basis? **Select all that apply.**
   1. Ten grapes
   2. Five dried figs
   3. One baked potato
   4. Half of a grapefruit
   5. One cup of cooked spinach

76. A person calls the nursing unit of a hospital stating, "I am a lawyer and must speak with a client on the unit because there is a family emergency." What is the nurse's **most** appropriate intervention?
   1. Bring the client to the telephone to talk with the lawyer.
   2. Refuse to discuss anything regarding the client with the lawyer.
   3. Inform the lawyer that the presence of a client cannot be confirmed or denied.
   4. Take the lawyer's phone number and give it to the client without revealing that the client is on the unit.

77. A nurse is caring for a client who was admitted to the hospital because of a fecal impaction. The nurse identified that inadequate fiber, fluid, and activity contributed to this client's problem. In addition, which medication that the client is taking may have contributed to the fecal impaction?
   1. Warfarin
   2. Metronidazole
   3. Ferrous sulfate
   4. Magnesium/aluminum hydroxide

78. A nurse is caring for an older adult who had a brain attack (cerebrovascular accident) and has a residual problem with chewing and swallowing. What is the **greatest** risk considering the client's physical status?
   1. Aspiration
   2. Constipation
   3. Fluid volume deficit
   4. Inadequate nutrition

79. A nurse is assessing a client with the medical diagnosis of dehydration. Which assessments should the nurse document on the client's record to support this diagnosis? **Select all that apply.**
   1. Low urine specific gravity
   2. Bounding radial pulse
   3. Straw-colored urine
   4. Sunken eyeballs
   5. Flat neck veins
   6. Tenting of skin

80. A client who is a Christian Scientist is admitted to the hospital for medical management and dialysis for renal failure. Which intervention is important for the nurse to implement when caring for this client?
   1. Ensure that pork and pork products are eliminated from the client's diet.
   2. Position the client's bed so that the feet are facing toward the entrance to the room.
   3. Encourage expression of feelings regarding the medical management of the client's problem.
   4. Support the client's desire to wear an amulet around the neck to chase away evil spirits and support health.

6/4

Comprehensive Final Exam   **837**

81. A nurse is completing the assessment phase of the nursing process for a group of clients with four different human responses. For which human responses did the nurse use the physical examination method of auscultation? **Select all that apply.**
1. Bruit
2. Lesion
3. Ascites
4. Distention
5. Borborygmi

82. A nurse is caring for a client who is dying. Which assessments identified by the nurse indicate that the client is soon approaching the active phase of dying? **Select all that apply.**
1. Increased periods of sleep
2. Marked decrease in urine output
3. Decreased intake of food and liquid
4. Mottling of the skin of the extremities
5. Reports seeing persons who have died

83. Total parenteral nutrition is prescribed for a client. What should the nurse do when administrating total parenteral nutrition to this client? **Select all that apply.**
1. Remove the solution from the refrigerator 15 minutes before the infusion.
2. Change the intravenous tubing set every 24 hours.
3. Assess for placement of the tube in the stomach.
4. Use intravenous tubing that has an inline filter.
5. Warm the solution in a microwave oven.
6. Monitor blood glucose levels routinely.

84. Penicillin V potassium 250 mg by mouth every 6 hours is prescribed for a client with a staphylococcal infection. The pharmacy provides penicillin V potassium 125 mg per 5 mL. How much solution should the nurse administer? **Record your answer using a whole number.**
Answer: _____10_____ mL

85. A nurse is writing progress notes for a variety of clients. Which documentation meets the criteria for a legal record?
1. Client tolerated being out of bed in a chair for 1 hour.
2. Client urinated 350 mL of clear amber urine at 8 a.m.
3. Client received the prn antiemetic at 2 p.m.
4. Client reported pain at a level of 5.

86. While assisting a client to eat, the other client in the room begins to choke on food and is unable to speak. According to the American Heart Association, what should the nurse do **first?**
1. Initiate the abdominal thrust maneuver.
2. Instruct the client to swallow forcefully.
3. Clap between the client's scapulae several times.
4. Wait to see if the client can cough up the obstruction.

87. A urinalysis is prescribed for a client with an indwelling urinary catheter. Which actions are implemented when collecting a urine specimen from the port of a urinary retention catheter? **Select all that apply.**
1. Wear sterile gloves to collect the specimen.
2. Clean the specimen port with an alcohol swab.
3. Release the clamp after collecting a urine specimen.
4. Separate the catheter from the tubing to collect the specimen.
5. Transfer urine to a sterile container designed for a urine specimen.
6. Clamp the drainage tubing just below the level of the specimen port for about 15–30 minutes.

88. A nurse is assessing a 78-year-old adult. What cognitive changes should the nurse anticipate that the client will report?
1. "My short-term memory is better than my long-term memory."
2. "It takes longer for me to learn something new."
3. "My level of intelligence has been decreasing."
4. "I get easily confused."

89. Which nursing interventions should be implemented regardless of the oxygen delivery system being used? **Select all that apply.**
1. Obtain routine pulse oximetry measurements.
2. Ensure the oxygen mask is securely placed over the nose and mouth.
3. Flood the reservoir with oxygen before attaching the mask to the client.
4. Set the oxygen flow rate at a minimum of between two and four liters per minute.
5. Assess the client's skin on the face and ears for trauma to determine if the oxygen device is too tight.

90. A nurse is transferring a client from a bed to a chair. Which principles of the mechanics of movement are important for the nurse to employ? **Select all that apply.**
1. Avoid twisting the upper body toward the direction of the move.
2. Have the client wear a gait belt during the transfer.
3. Ensure that the bed is higher than the chair.
4. Keep arms in a locked position.
5. Place the feet wide apart.
6. Bend at the waist.

91. Which nursing actions demonstrate the evaluation step of the nursing process? **Select all that apply.**
    1. Having a client provide a return demonstration of administration of an injection
    2. Identifying a skin lesion during a client's admission physical examination
    3. Determining activity intolerance after ambulating a client
    4. Connecting a contributing factor to a problem statement
    5. Formulating an intervention to address a risk factor

92. A nurse enters a client's room and observes smoke coming out of an air-conditioning duct. The nurse transfers the client into a wheelchair, moves the client into the corridor, and closes the door to the client's room while exiting the room. What should the nurse do **next**?
    1. Report the fire.
    2. Attempt to put out the fire.
    3. Close the doors on the unit.
    4. Evacuate all the clients to another unit.

93. A nurse is assessing a client for signs and symptoms of electrolyte imbalances. What clinical manifestation helps to differentiate hypernatremia from hyponatremia?
    1. Vomiting
    2. Confusion
    3. Increased thirst
    4. Muscle weakness

94. A client self-administers a bowel prep consisting of NuLYTELY and bisacodyl the night before a colonoscopy. For what most serious adverse effect should the nurse assess for when the client arrives in the morning for the colonoscopy?
    1. Deficient fluid volume
    2. Intestinal cramping
    3. Hypernatremia
    4. Diarrhea

95. When talking to the school nurse about his decision to drop out of high school and marry his girlfriend who is pregnant, a student says, "I need to do this. It is the right thing to do." What defense mechanism should the nurse determine is being used?
    1. Projection
    2. Suppression
    3. Introspection
    4. Intellectualization

96. A nurse identifies that a client has inadequate circulation to the right foot as evidenced by prolonged capillary refill, yellow brittle toenails, and an absent pedal pulse. What pulse should the nurse assess **next**?

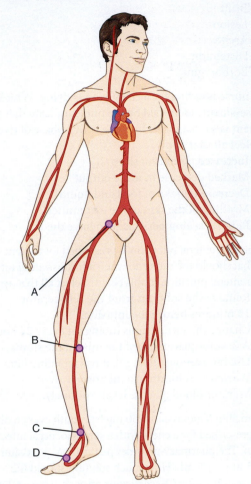

1. A
2. B
3. C
4. D

97. A nurse is assessing a client's urinary status. Which question is appropriate when collecting data about reflex incontinence?
    1. "Have you ever had an involuntary loss of urine without sensing the need to void?"
    2. "Have you ever lost control of urine after a strong sense of the need to void?"
    3. "Do you ever experience urinary dribbling when you sneeze or cough?"
    4. "Do you ever experience a weak urinary stream when you pass urine?"

3/0

98. A nurse is determining if a prescribed opioid dose is appropriate for a 3-year-old child. What **most** essential information should the nurse gather to assist with this determination?
1. Obtain the child's weight.
2. Take the child's vital signs.
3. Assess the child's level of pain.
4. Explore the child's reaction to previous analgesics.

99. A client with esophageal reflux has been experiencing heartburn, regurgitation, and a hoarse voice. What should the nurse encourage the client to do to minimize these signs and symptoms? **Select all that apply.**
1. Eat within one hour before going to bed.
2. Drink a glass of warm water at bedtime.
3. Elevate the head of the bed on blocks.
4. Recline for half an hour after meals.
5. Avoid foods high in fat.

61/100

100. The number of client falls on a medical-surgical unit increased by 20% in the last 3 months, and the nurse manager forms a committee to address this issue. First the committee members analyzed the factors precipitating the falls. What should the committee members do **next**?
1. Implement a plan of action.
2. Choose a solution to address the issue.
3. Explore possible strategies to prevent future falls.
4. Arrange for an in-service program for the nurses involved with the falls.

REVIEW ANSWERS AND RATIONALES

1. ANSWER: 1, 3, 6.
Rationales:
1. Food is a basic requirement of life. Eating food meets a physiological (first-level) need according to Maslow's hierarchy of needs.
2. Inviting friends over for a party is an example of a third-level need, the need for love and belonging.
3. To function properly the body requires a balance between rest and activity. Taking a nap after exercise meets a physiological (first-level) need according to Maslow's hierarchy of needs.
4. Getting a haircut before the holiday season is an example of a fourth-level need, the need for self-esteem.
5. Locking car doors when alone in the car is an example of a second-level need, the need for safety and security.
6. Taking a bottle of water along when going for a walk is an example of meeting a physiological (first-level) need according to Maslow's hierarchy of needs.
Content Area: Evidenced-Based Practice
Integrated Processes: Nursing Process: Implementation
Client Need: Health Promotion and Maintenance
Cognitive Level: Analysis
Concept: Evidenced-Based Practice

2. ANSWER: 2.
Rationales:
1. This is premature at this time; it should be done eventually.
2. Assessment is the first step of the nursing process. Risk factors for skin breakdown should be identified first before the nurse can formulate a plan of care.
3. This is not a life-threatening situation and is not the first action. Notification of the primary health-care provider about the client's status should be done eventually.
4. This is an intervention, part of the implementation phase of the nursing process. Other steps of the nursing process must be completed first.
TEST-TAKING TIP: Identify the word in the stem that sets a priority. The word *first* in the stem sets a priority. Identify the option that is unique. Option 2 is unique because it is an action that is an assessment and the other options are interventions other than assessment. Identify the clang associations. The words *skin* and *assessment* in the stem and in option 2 are clang associations.
Content Area: Tissue Integrity and Hygiene
Integrated Processes: Nursing Process: Assessment
Client Need: Physiological Integrity; Reduction of Risk Potential
Cognitive Level: Application
Concept: Tissue Integrity

3. ANSWER: 1, 4.
Rationales:
1. In this scenario, the nurse could be sued for assault. An unjustifiable threat to touch another person is assault.
2. In this scenario, the nurse could be sued for battery. Clients have a right to refuse treatment. Touching another person without consent, such as administering a medication against the wishes of a client, is battery.

3. In this scenario, the nurse could be sued for false imprisonment and battery. The nurse unjustifiably touched and detained the client without consent.
4. In this scenario the nurse is threatening the client in an unjustifiable, offensive manner. Also, raising all the side rails of a bed is considered a restraint that requires a prescription. The nurse should provide teaching regarding the client's physiological need to maintain bedrest.
5. In this scenario, the nurse could be sued for slander. Spoken words that are untrue and can cause defamation of character are considered slander.
Content Area: Legal and Ethical Issues
Integrated Processes: Nursing Process: Evaluation
Client Need: Safe and Effective Care Environment; Management of Care
Cognitive Level: Analysis
Concept: Legal

4. ANSWER: 3.
Rationales:
1. Liquid fecal effluent from an ileostomy is expected because fluid is absorbed in the transverse and descending colon. An ileostomy is a surgically created opening (stoma) in the small intestine (ileum).
2. Liquid fecal effluent from a cecostomy is expected because fluid is absorbed in the transverse and descending colon. A cecostomy is a surgically created opening (stoma) in the proximal part of the large intestine.
3. Stool from a sigmoid colostomy is soft to formed stool. Loose stool should be reported because it indicates diarrhea, which may be due to a gastrointestinal problem that requires medical intervention.
4. Liquid fecal effluent from an ascending colon colostomy is expected because fluid is absorbed in the transverse and descending colon.
TEST-TAKING TIP: Identify the key words in the stem that indicate negative polarity. The words *be concerned* are the key words that indicate negative polarity. The question is asking, "Which ostomy *should not produce* loose fecal matter?"
Content Area: Bowel Elimination
Integrated Processes: Nursing Process: Evaluation
Client Need: Physiological Integrity; Physiological Adaptation
Cognitive Level: Analysis
Concept: Elimination

5. ANSWER: 2.
Rationales:
1. There is less concern about assessing for the presence of peripheral edema than another concern. The absence of protein in the urine generally rules out upper urinary system impairment, which could cause fluid volume excess. Also, the client is not reporting a decrease in urine output.
2. The clinical indicators of increased vital signs, elevated white and red blood cells, nitrites in the urine, and urinary frequency and urgency support the conclusion that the client most likely has a urinary tract infection. The slow urinary stream indicates that the client may have an enlarged prostate gland associated with aging, contributing to urinary stasis. Urinary stasis is a risk factor for a

urinary tract infection. **A burning sensation on urination is associated with bacteria in the urine that irritates the mucous membranes of the urinary system.**

3. Suprapubic distension is associated with urinary retention. There are no data that indicate the presence of urinary retention, such as anuria, eliminating small amounts of urine frequently (overflow incontinence), or a feeling of fullness in the suprapubic area. Also, assessment revealed that the client's abdomen was soft and nontender.

4. The blood pressure increases, not decreases, in response to the increased metabolic rate associated with a fever.

TEST-TAKING TIP: Identify the clang association. The word *urination* in option 2 and the repetitious use of words associated with the urinary system within the data, such as *urinary frequency, nocturia* (urinating at night), and *to urinate,* are clang associations. Examine option 2 carefully.
Content Area: Urinary Elimination
Integrated Processes: Communication and Documentation; Nursing Process: Assessment
Client Need: Physiological Integrity; Physiological Adaptation
Cognitive Level: Analysis
Concept: Patient-Centered Care; Elimination

6. ANSWER: 2.
Rationales:

1. A nurse can address a client's pain control needs before providing care so that interventions can be performed within a tolerable pain level.

2. A client with dementia may have difficulty interpreting environmental stimuli and perceive hygiene care as a threat. This may cause the client to become frightened or anxious and resist hygiene interventions.

3. A client with impaired vision generally can understand directions regarding the setup of the overbed table with hygiene equipment placed according to the numbers of a clock. Assistance by the nurse may be provided to complete the care.

4. A client with impaired mobility generally can participate in hygiene care, even if it is just the ability to make choices regarding preferences. Clients with impaired mobility should be encouraged to participate to their best ability, with the balance of care provided by the nurse.

TEST-TAKING TIP: Identify the word in the stem that sets a priority. The word *greatest* in the stem sets a priority.
Content Area: Tissue Integrity and Hygiene
Integrated Processes: Nursing Process: Analysis
Client Need: Physiological integrity; Basic Care and Comfort
Cognitive Level: Analysis
Concept: Cognition

7. ANSWER: 1.
Rationales:

1. Most people prefer to return home if appropriate supportive care is available. Hospice programs are designed to meet the needs of individuals with less than 6 months to live. Hospice programs approach a client's needs comprehensively, with an increase in services as a client's condition requires more constant and varied interventions.

2. No data indicate the need for rehabilitation services.

3. The client does not need constant services of a skilled nurse.

4. This requires a major environmental change. This alternative is not capable of meeting this client's physical and emotional needs when the disease progresses.

TEST-TAKING TIP: Identify the word in the stem that sets a priority. The word *most* in the stem sets a priority. Identify the word that is a clang association. The word *care* is used twice in the stem. The word *care* in option 1 is a clang association. Examine option 1 carefully. More often than not, the option with a clang association is the correct answer.
Content Area: Health-Care System
Integrated Processes: Nursing Process: Planning
Client Need: Safe and Effective Care Environment, Management of Care
Cognitive Level: Analysis
Concept: Health-Care System

8. ANSWER: 2, 4, 5.
Rationales:

1. The oral route is contraindicated in a client with shortness of breath. The client may become short of breath while the lips are sealed around the probe long enough to obtain a reading.

2. Skin strips designed to assess body temperature can be placed against a client's skin, usually the forehead. This route is safe for the client in this scenario.

3. The rectal route is contraindicated in a client with anal or large intestine problems. A rectal probe may traumatize the intestinal mucosa and perforate the intestine.

4. The axillary route, under the client's arm, is a safe route to obtain this client's temperature. It will take longer to obtain a measurement at this site and the result will not be as accurate as other routes because an axillary temperature lags behind core temperatures during rapid temperature changes.

5. The temporal route will reflect the core body temperature without jeopardizing the client's physical status.

6. The tympanic route is contraindicated in a client with an ear infection because it may traumatize the ear as well as produce an inaccurate measurement due to the presence of inflammation in the ears.
Content Area: Physical Assessment
Integrated Processes: Nursing Process: Planning
Client Need: Physiological Integrity; Reduction of Risk Potential
Cognitive Level: Analysis
Concept: Thermo-regulation

9. ANSWER: 1.
Rationales:

1. Adolescents have few rigid routines, have busy schedules, and are influenced by peer pressure, which are factors that influence a person's ability to follow a medical regimen. Also, adolescents feel omnipotent, operate most often in the present, and have less ability to appreciate the long-term consequences of inadequate self-care than an older person.

2. More often than not, an older adult is capable of recognizing the importance of appropriate self-care when faced with a chronic health condition.

3. Although a young adult may have some difficulty adjusting to a life-long health problem, a young adult is better able to recognize that appropriate self-care is important than a client in another option.

4. More often than not, a middle-aged adult is capable of recognizing the importance of appropriate self-care when faced with a chronic health condition.

TEST-TAKING TIP: Identify the word in the stem that sets a priority. The word *most* in the stem sets a priority. Identify the option that is unique. Option 1 is unique because it is the only option that contains one word and it is the only option that does not contain the word *adult.*

Content Area: Development Across the Life Span
Integrated Processes: Teaching/Learning; Nursing Process: Analysis
Client Need: Health Promotion and Maintenance
Cognitive Level: Analysis
Concept: Growth and Development

10. **ANSWER: 3, 5.**
    Rationales:
    1. People should talk at a moderate, not slow, rate when communicating with a person who is hearing impaired. When talking slowly, people tend to overarticulate, which makes it more difficult to interpret what is being said.
    2. Longer, not shorter, phrases facilitate understanding. Additional words support a clearer message.
    3. Older adults have more difficulty hearing high-pitched, rather than low-pitched, tones. Using a lower tone of voice may increase what the client can hear.
    4. Overarticulation should be avoided because it is harder for a deaf person to understand than when the person speaking articulates normally.
    5. Standing so that the nurse's face can be seen easily facilitates lip reading. The nurse should gently touch the person and ensure that the person's attention is secured before initiating conversation.
    Content Area: Communication, Collaboration, and Documentation
    Integrated Processes: Communication and Documentation; Nursing Process: Implementation
    Client Need: Psychosocial Integrity
    Cognitive Level: Application
    Concept: Communication

11. **ANSWER: 2, 5.**
    Rationales:
    1. All behavior has meaning and requires recognition.
    2. Offering choices empowers a client to make decisions. This places a client in control and supports feelings of independence.
    3. Using distraction denies the client's concerns. Client concerns should be addressed.
    4. Pointing out limitations may intensify the client's feelings of dependence.
    5. Focusing on those activities that can be performed successfully emphasizes what the client can do and is motivating.
    TEST-TAKING TIP: Identify the options that deny that client's feelings. Options 1 and 3 deny the client's feelings.

Identify the clang association. The word *activities* in the stem and in option 5 is a clang association.
Content Area: Psychosocial Health
Integrated Processes: Caring, Communication and Documentation; Nursing Process: Implementation
Client Need: Psychosocial Integrity
Cognitive Level: Application
Concept: Self

12. **ANSWER: 1, 2, 3.**
    Rationales:
    1. Variable breathing patterns are associated with chronic pain because of its relationship to the parasympathetic nervous system. An increased respiratory rate is associated with acute pain because of its relationship to the sympathetic nervous system.
    2. The blood pressure is decreased with chronic pain because of its relationship to the parasympathetic nervous system. The blood pressure is increased with acute pain because of its relationship to the sympathetic nervous system.
    3. Slow, monotonous speech is associated with chronic pain because of its relationship to the parasympathetic nervous system. Pressured speech is associated with acute pain; it is a sympathetic nervous system response.
    4. An increased heart rate is associated with acute pain because of its relationship to the sympathetic nervous system. The heart rate will be decreased with chronic pain because of its relationship to the parasympathetic nervous system.
    5. Loud, rapid speech (pressured speech) is associated with acute pain because of its relationship to the sympathetic nervous system.
    6. Dilated pupils are associated with acute pain because of its relationship to the sympathetic nervous system. Constricted pupils are related to chronic pain because of the relationship to the parasympathetic nervous system.
    TEST-TAKING TIP: Identify the options that are opposites. Options 3 and 5 are opposites. Examine them carefully because one of them is among the correct options.
    Content Area: Pain, Comfort, Rest, and Sleep
    Integrated Processes: Nursing Process: Assessment
    Client Need: Physiological Integrity; Pharmacological and Parenteral Therapies
    Cognitive Level: Analysis
    Concept: Comfort

13. **ANSWER: 1.**
    Rationales:
    1. Wearing a gown is not necessary to maintain airborne precautions for a client with a diagnosis of primary tuberculosis. The pathogenic organism is transmitted to others via airborne respiratory secretions. However, a gown is necessary whenever the caregiver has a likelihood of coming into contact with blood, body fluids, excretions, secretions, contaminated items, or nonintact skin.
    2. A respiratory device (N95 respirator) is necessary to protect a caregiver from the *M. tuberculosis* emanating from the client's respiratory tract.
    3. A room with negative air pressure, air change of 6 to 12 air changes per hour, and either discharge of air to the

outside or a filtration system for the air in the room is essential to maintain airborne precautions for a client with a diagnosis of suspected or known tuberculosis.

4. Placing a surgical mask on the client when being transported for a procedure outside the room is essential to maintaining airborne precautions. This protects others and the environment from contamination from pathogens emanating from the client's respiratory tract.

TEST-TAKING TIP: Identify the word in the stem that indicates negative polarity. The word *unrelated* indicates negative polarity. The test-taker must identify the intervention that is *not necessary* to maintaining airborne precautions.

Content Area: Inflammation, Infection, Immunity, and Wound Care
Integrated Processes: Nursing Process: Implementation
Client Need: Safe and Effective Care Environment; Safety and Infection Control
Cognitive Level: Analysis
Concept: Infection

14. **ANSWER: 4, 1, 5, 2, 3.**
    Rationales:
    4. The side-lying position enables medication to flow by gravity into the ear canal.
    1. Pulling the auricle of the ear up and backward straightens the ear canal, facilitating distribution of the medication.
    5. Holding the dropper a half inch above the ear canal avoids contamination of the dropper. Directing the flow of medication to the side of the ear canal prevents injury to the tympanic membrane as the drop enters the ear canal.
    2. Applying gentle pressure to the tragus of the ear facilitates complete distribution of the medication to all surfaces of the ear canal, which promotes its absorption.
    3. Remaining in a side-lying position for 5 to 10 minutes allows for more contact of the medication with the ear canal and tympanic membrane and prevents the medication from exiting the ear.
    Content Area: Medication
    Integrated Processes: Nursing Process: Planning
    Client Need: Physiological Integrity; Pharmacological and Parenteral Therapies
    Cognitive Level: Analysis
    Concept: Medication; Safety

15. **ANSWER: 3.**
    Rationales:
    1. Although this is a true statement, its tone is autocratic. It is not a visionary, charismatic approach.
    2. This statement begins with a negative tone; in addition, it may be false reassurance for some staff members. The nurse manager should accentuate the positive.
    3. This statement is inspiring and motivating; it creates excitement and relates a new initiative to the role of the nurse.
    4. An edict is a proclamation, directive, or an order to do something. This approach is autocratic.
    TEST-TAKING TIP: Identify the word in the stem that sets a priority. The word *best* in the stem sets a priority.

Content Area: Leadership and Management
Integrated Processes: Communication and Documentation; Nursing Process: Implementation
Client Need: Safe and Effective Care Environment; Management of Care
Cognitive Level: Analysis
Concept: Leadership and Management

16. **ANSWER: 2.**
    Rationales:
    1. Generally, conscious sedation, not general anesthesia, is used to sedate a client for a colonoscopy. Conscious sedation does not cause the loss of the gag reflex.
    2. A serious concern after a fiberoptic colonoscopy is bowel perforation. A symptom of bowel perforation is abdominal pain. Although the client's pain is mild, it should be assessed frequently to ensure that it does not intensify. In addition, the nurse should assess for rectal bleeding, abdominal distention, fever, and malaise, which are all associated with bowel perforation after a colonoscopy.
    3. Passing flatus is an expected response after a colonoscopy because air is introduced into the intestine to distend the lumen for improved visibility.
    4. Dozing intermittently is expected because of the effects of the conscious sedation used during the procedure.
    TEST-TAKING TIP: Identify the word in the stem that sets a priority. The word *most* in the stem sets a priority. All the options reflect information that should be communicated, but one is *most* essential.
    Content Area: Bowel Elimination
    Integrated Processes: Communication and Documentation; Nursing Process: Evaluation
    Client Need: Safe and Effective Care Environment; Management of Care
    Cognitive Level: Application
    Concept: Elimination

17. **ANSWER: 1, 5.**
    Rationales:
    1. This statement indicates the concept of exacerbation, a return of signs and symptoms or an increase in the severity of signs and symptoms of a disease.
    2. This statement reflects a course of therapy that is ineffective. The client's status remained the same.
    3. This statement reflects the concept of chronicity. Chronicity refers to a disease of long duration or progressive deterioration over a long period of time.
    4. This statement does not relate to an exacerbation. This statement refers to an immune response to an antigen, the prescribed medication.
    5. This statement refers to the concept of exacerbation, a return or intensification of signs and symptoms of a disease process.
    Content Area: Physical Assessment
    Integrated Processes: Nursing Process: Analysis
    Client Need: Physiological Integrity; Physiological Adaptation
    Cognitive Level: Analysis
    Concept: Cellular Regulation

18. ANSWER: 3.

Rationales:

1. Obtaining a prescription for a restraint is premature. Verbal interactions, one to one observation, or a prescribed sedative are less-restrictive measures than a physical restraint.

2. Touching the client's shoulder may be viewed as aggressive by the client and elicit a hostile physical response. A nurse should never touch an agitated, intoxicated client without the client's permission.

3. Increasing agitation and verbal abuse may be precursors to physical abuse. The nurse should stand in an area that will provide an escape if the client attempts physical aggression.

4. This may be viewed as aggressive by the client and precipitate an altercation. A minimum of 3 feet should be maintained between the nurse and client.

TEST-TAKING TIP: Identify the word in the stem that sets a priority. The word *next* in the stem sets a priority. Identify options that are opposites. Options 3 and 4 are opposites. Option 3 positions the nurse at a distance from the client, while option 4 has the nurse in close proximity to the client. Consider these options carefully.

Content Area: *Safety*
Integrated Processes: *Communication and Documentation; Nursing Process: Implementation*
Client Need: *Safe and Effective Care Environment; Safety and Infection Control*
Cognitive Level: *Application*
Concept: *Violence*

19. ANSWER: 1.

Rationales:

1. The response in option 1 is open-ended and non-committal about the client's decision. It provides an opportunity for the client to explore the reasons for the decision.

2. This statement does not provide the client the opportunity to explore the reasons for the decision. Also, the nurse should not voice personal opinions that could make it difficult for the client to change the decision in the future.

3. This statement is a challenging statement that puts the client on the defensive.

4. This statement is judgmental. The second sentence does not invite the client to explore the reasons for the decision.

TEST-TAKING TIP: Identify the word in the stem that sets a priority. The word *best* in the stem sets a priority. Identify the options that are not client centered. Options 3 and 4 are judgmental and focus on other people's opinions. These options are not client centered and can be eliminated.

Content Area: *Psychosocial Health*
Integrated Processes: *Caring, Communication and Documentation; Nursing Process: Implementation*
Client Need: *Psychosocial Integrity*
Cognitive Level: *Analysis*
Concept: *Communication*

20. ANSWER: 3, 4.

Rationales:

1. The first drop of blood should not be used because it may contain a large volume of serous fluid, which may produce an inaccurate result.

2. The index finger should be avoided because it is reported to be a more painful site than other fingers.

3. Applying 30 seconds of pressure generally is sufficient to stop bleeding from a lancet wound.

4. Placing the hand in the dependent position will increase blood flow to the distal portion of the finger.

5. Squeezing the puncture site should be avoided because it will increase serum and dilute the blood specimen resulting in a false low blood glucose level.

TEST-TAKING TIP: Identify the clang association. The word *lancet* in the stem and in option 4 is a clang association. Identify the unique option. Option 3 is unique. It is the only option that does not contain the word *blood*. Examine unique options carefully. Often they are one of the correct answers in a multiple-response question.

Content Area: *Nutrition*
Integrated Processes: *Nursing Process: Implementation*
Client Need: *Physiological Integrity; Reduction of Risk Potential*
Cognitive Level: *Application*
Concept: *Metabolism*

21. ANSWER: 2.

Rationales:

1. Feeding the client will not evaluate the adequacy of the diet; also, the client should be encouraged to be as independent as possible.

2. Weighing the client weekly will reflect if the client is maintaining or losing weight. Maintenance of weight indicates that the client is receiving adequate nutrition.

3. Although giving a liquid supplement between meals is an appropriate action, it does not evaluate the adequacy of the client's diet. In addition, adding a supplement between meals requires a prescription from the primary health-care provider.

4. Encouraging the client to choose foods that are preferred may be beyond the cognitive ability of the client, which may increase frustration, anxiety, and agitation. Also, it does not reflect the client's nutritional status.

TEST-TAKING TIP: Identify the word in the stem that sets a priority. The word *most* in the stem sets a priority.

Content Area: *Nutrition*
Integrated Processes: *Nursing Process: Evaluation*
Client Need: *Physiological Integrity; Reduction of Risk Potential*
Cognitive Level: *Application*
Concept: *Nutrition*

22. ANSWER: 4.

Rationales:

1. A lozenge or troche, not an enteric-coated medication, is designed to dissolve slowly in the pocket between the gum and cheek (buccal cavity).

2. The enteric coating is not to protect the mouth from the taste of the medication.

3. The potential to stain the teeth is not the reason why an enteric-coated medication should not be chewed before swallowing.

4. An enteric-coated medication is designed to dissolve in the intestines. This is either because the drug is caustic to the stomach mucosa or because the drug is deactivated by gastric enzymes.

TEST-TAKING TIP: Identify the word in the stem that sets a priority. The word *best* in the stem sets a priority.

Content Area: Medication
Integrated Processes: Communication and Documentation, Teaching/Learning; Nursing Process: Implementation
Client Need: Physiological Integrity; Pharmacological and Parenteral Therapies
Cognitive Level: Application
Concept: Medication; Safety

23. **ANSWER: 2, 3, 4.**
    Rationales:
    1. Five to 10 minutes generally is the length of time the nurse should soak a client's feet. It is enough time to precipitate relaxation and soften debris without excessively removing natural oils that can lead to cracks in the skin.
    2. Cuticles should be pushed back gently with a wash cloth; a wash cloth is rough enough to push back the cuticles without causing trauma.
    3. Drying the feet thoroughly, especially between the toes, helps prevent maceration of the skin and reduces the risk of a fungal infection.
    4. Using the flat side of an orangewood stick to clean under nails while the foot is in the water facilitates removing debris caught under the nail.
    5. Although the nurse should soak each foot separately and change water and towels between the feet, the water should be 105°F to 115°F to avoid burning the skin.

    TEST-TAKING TIP: Identify the clang associations. The word *foot* in the stem and in options 3 and 4 are clang associations.

    Content Area: Tissue Integrity and Hygiene
    Integrated Processes: Nursing Process: Planning
    Client Need: Physiological Integrity; Basic Care and Comfort
    Cognitive Level: Application
    Concept: Tissue Integrity

24. **ANSWER: 3.**
    Rationales:
    1. Teaching sessions should be conducted early in the morning before the client becomes fatigued. Fatigue will interfere with learning.
    2. Two nurses are unnecessary; one nurse is capable of teaching this client active range-of-motion exercises.
    3. The client is experiencing fatigue. Teaching sessions should be kept short so that learning can occur before the client becomes fatigued.
    4. There are no data that indicate that the client is in pain.

    TEST-TAKING TIP: Identify the word in the stem that sets a priority. The word *best* in the stem sets a priority.

Content Area: Teaching and Learning
Integrated Processes: Teaching/Learning; Nursing Process: Planning
Client Need: Health Promotion and Maintenance
Cognitive Level: Application
Concept: Patient-Centered Care

25. **ANSWER: 4.**
    Rationales:
    1. The client has not yet received the medication.
    2. Although the nurse may call the pharmacist for an opinion, it is the nurse's responsibility to intervene in this situation.
    3. The laboratory results may never return to the expected (normal) range. Also, this is not within the scope of nursing practice, except for with a few medications where exact parameters are identified by the primary health-care provider.
    4. The primary health-care provider should be informed of the client's impaired kidney function because the dose of the medication may need to be reduced or the drug canceled to avoid drug toxicity. Impaired kidney function may interfere with the ability to excrete the drug.

    TEST-TAKING TIP: Identify the word in the stem that sets a priority. The word *most* in the stem sets a priority.

    Content Area: Medication
    Integrated Processes: Communication and Documentation; Nursing Process: Implementation
    Client Need: Safe and Effective Care Environment; Management of Care
    Cognitive Level: Application
    Concept: Medication; Communication

26. **ANSWER: 3, 5.**
    Rationales:
    1. HIV is not transmitted via tears.
    2. HIV is not transmitted via sweat.
    3. HIV is transmitted via blood and body fluids, such as semen, vaginal secretions, and breast milk. The nurse must use measures associated with standard precautions for protection from exposure to blood and body fluid.
    4. HIV is not transmitted via feces.
    5. HIV is transmitted via blood and body fluids, such as semen, vaginal secretions, and breast milk. An intravenous catheter is inserted directly into a vein, which may expose the nurse to the client's blood. The nurse must use measures associated with standard precautions to prevent exposure to the client's blood.

    Content Area: Safety
    Integrated Processes: Nursing Process: Planning
    Client Need: Safe and Effective Care Environment; Safety and Infection Control
    Cognitive Level: Application
    Concept: Safety

27. **ANSWER: 2.**
    Rationales:
    1. Palpating the abdomen first may alter the findings of inspection, auscultation, and percussion.
    2. Inspection should occur before touching the client. Inspection involves assessing for visual clues of pathology.

Options 1, 3, and 4 are all skills that require the nurse to touch the client's abdomen in some way. The least intrusive assessment method of inspection should be performed first, followed progressively by auscultation, percussion, and palpation.

3. Percussion should be done after inspection and auscultation.

4. Auscultation should be done after inspection and before any other hands-on assessments are implemented.

TEST-TAKING TIP: Identify the word in the stem that sets a priority. The word *first* in the stem sets a priority. Identify the unique option. Option 2 is unique; it is the only option that does not require the nurse to touch the client. Consider this option carefully.

Content Area: Physical Assessment
Integrated Processes: Nursing Process: Implementation
Client Need: Health Promotion and Maintenance
Cognitive Level: Application
Concept: Patient-Centered Care

28. **ANSWER: 3.**
Rationales:

1. Although the client has excessive respiratory secretions, the client is capable of clearing the airway as evidenced by the productive cough. Suctioning can be traumatic to the mucous membranes when it is unnecessary.

2. Although administering the clarithromycin should be done eventually, administering the clarithromycin first is inappropriate.

3. **A sputum specimen must be obtained before antibiotic therapy is instituted. The results of the culture and sensitivity may be inaccurate if an antibiotic is administered before the sputum specimen is obtained.**

4. Although inserting a circulatory access device and administering the prescribed intravenous fluids should be done, they are not the priority. This intervention will take time that will delay another intervention that is more important.

TEST-TAKING TIP: Identify the word in the stem that sets a priority. The word *next* in the stem sets a priority.

Content Area: Oxygenation
Integrated Processes: Communication and Documentation; Nursing Process: Implementation
Client Need: Physiological Integrity; Reduction of Risk Potential
Cognitive Level: Analysis
Concept: Patient-Centered Care; Infection

29. **ANSWER: 2, 3.**
Rationales:

1. Taking a client's vital signs in response to a client's report of dizziness is an example of assessment.

2. **Clustering collected data into related categories allows the nurse to organize and manage information so that interpretations about the information can be made.**

3. **Determining that a client is at risk for impaired skin integrity because of reduced mobility and edema is associated with the analysis step of the nursing process. Making connections among human responses, contributing factors to illness, disease or injury, and**

potential negative future developments is part of the analysis step of the nursing process.

4. Identifying a desired outcome is part of the planning step of the nursing process.

5. Revising a plan of care in response to a client not achieving a desired outcome (the ability to accurately prepare an insulin injection) is part of the evaluation step of the nursing process.

Content Area: Critical Thinking and the Nursing Process
Integrated Processes: Nursing Process: Analysis
Client Need: Safe and Effective Care Environment; Management of Care
Cognitive Level: Application
Concept: Patient-Centered Care

30. **ANSWER: 1.**
Rationales:

1. **This is a question that offers the client an opportunity to discuss thoughts, feelings, or concerns with the nurse.**

2. Although this is a supportive statement, it is not the most inviting response.

3. This is a biased question and may not elicit a true response by the client.

4. This is a gross generalization. Nurses should not make assumptions.

TEST-TAKING TIP: Identify the word in the stem that sets a priority. The word *most* in the stem sets a priority.

Content Area: Communication, Collaboration, and Documentation
Integrated Processes: Caring, Communication and Documentation; Nursing Process: Implementation
Client Need: Psychosocial Integrity
Cognitive Level: Application
Concept: Communication

31. **ANSWER: 3, 5.**
Rationales:

1. Activity performed 2 hours before bedtime will not interfere with sleep and is appropriate. Activity during the day or early evening stimulates physical functioning and increases mental activity.

2. A snack is appropriate because it prevents hunger and promotes sleep if it contains the amino acid L-tryptophan.

3. **Alcohol shortens sleep onset, but its rapid metabolism causes rebound arousal, resulting in shortened REM sleep. Also, it may cause early morning awakening secondary to a full bladder because alcohol acts as a mild diuretic.**

4. Although excessively cold environmental temperatures will cause frequent awakenings, a cool environmental temperature usually is comfortable for sleeping.

5. **Daytime naps, particularly later in the afternoon, can interfere with sleep at night. Awakening from a nap that is an hour long usually occurs during stage 4 NREM sleep. This is the stage of deepest sleep and the individual may awaken groggy and confused. Daytime naps should not exceed 20 minutes; naps this long may be refreshing and not interfere with nighttime sleeping.**

TEST-TAKING TIP: Identify the word in the stem that indicates negative priority. The word *further* in the stem indicates negative polarity. The question is asking, "What should the client with insomnia *not do?*" Identify the option that contains a specific determiner. The word *always* in option 2 is a specific determiner. More often than not, options with specific determiners are distractors and can be eliminated.

Content Area: Pain, Comfort, Rest, and Sleep
Integrated Processes: Teaching/Learning; Nursing Process: Evaluation
Client Need: Physiological Integrity; Basic Care and Comfort
Cognitive Level: Application
Concept: Sleep and Rest

32. ANSWER: 1.
Rationales:
1. This is the most important statement because it addresses maintaining the client's safety and security. This statement tells the client how to alert the nurse in an emergency or call for any reason that the client desires assistance.
2. Although offering choices supports independence, which is important, another statement is more important because it addresses maintaining the client's safety and security.
3. Although clients generally want to know when meals are served, another statement is more important because it addresses maintaining the client's safety and security.
4. Although the nurse should ensure that the room temperature is comfortable, another statement is more important because it addresses maintaining the client's safety and security.

TEST-TAKING TIP: Identify the word in the stem that sets a priority. The word *most* in the stem sets a priority. Identify the clang association. The word *leaving* in the stem and the word *leave* in option 1 is a clang association. Identify equally plausible options. Options 2 and 4 are equally plausible. They both have to do with comfort of the environment. Option 2 is no better than option 4. Eliminate both options from further consideration.

Content Area: Safety
Integrated Processes: Communication and Documentation; Nursing Process: Implementation
Client Need: Safe and Effective Care Environment; Safety and Infection Control
Cognitive Level: Application
Concept: Safety

33. ANSWER: 1,600.
Rationale:
To determine the hourly volume of intravenous fluid to be administered, divide 1,000 mL by 8 hours (1,000 ÷ 8 = 125). To identify the total volume of intravenous fluid for a 12-hour period, multiply the hourly rate by 12 hours (125 × 12 = 1,500). During the 7 a.m. to 7 p.m. shift, the antibiotic was administered once at 8 a.m. The total volume of fluid administered intravenously was 1,500 + 100 = 1,600 mL.

Content Area: Fluid, Electrolyte, and Acid-Base Balance
Integrated Processes: Nursing Process: Evaluation
Client Need: Physiological Integrity; Pharmacological and Parenteral Therapies

Cognitive Level: Application
Concept: Medication; Fluid and Electrolyte Balance

34. ANSWER: 3.
Rationales:
1. The client is actively hallucinating and is not a reliable source of information. In addition, research has demonstrated that an allergy to seafood and shellfish does not place a person at an increased risk of having a reaction to contrast dyes. Seafood and shellfish allergies are due to the protein content of these foods, not the iodine content.
2. Although the nurse should collect information about medications that the client is taking, it is not the priority in this scenario.
3. The client has a psychiatric diagnosis and is actively hallucinating. The client is incompetent and cannot sign a valid consent. The client's significant other should be asked to sign the consent.
4. An involved, detailed explanation may increase anxiety. Significant information should be provided in language that can be understood by the spouse and client, even if the client is physiologically or psychologically impaired.

TEST-TAKING TIP: Identify the option with a clang association. The word *spouse* in the stem and in option 3 is a clang association.

Content Area: Legal and Ethical Issues
Integrated Processes: Communication and Documentation; Nursing Process: Implementation
Client Need: Safe and Effective Care Environment; Management of Care
Cognitive Level: Application
Concept: Legal

35. ANSWER: 1.
Rationales:
1. A shower chair permits the client to sit during the procedure. This negates the need to stand on a wet, slippery surface and use excess energy to stand while bathing.
2. A handheld faucet will increase the risk of a fall because one hand is occupied holding the shower faucet while the other hand is used for washing; this leaves no hand to hold onto a handrail.
3. Although handrails in a shower stall will contribute to better balance and reduce the risk of a fall, it does not address the client's activity intolerance.
4. Although a nonskid mat should be used in a shower stall to help prevent a fall, it does not address the client's activity intolerance.

TEST-TAKING TIP: Identify the word in the stem that sets a priority. The word *most* in the stem sets a priority. Identify the clang associations. The word *shower* in the stem and in options 1 and 4 are clang associations. Examine options with clang associations carefully.

Content Area: Safety
Integrated Processes: Teaching/Learning; Nursing Process: Implementation
Client Need: Safe and Effective Care Environment; Safety and Infection Control
Cognitive Level: Application
Concept: Safety

36. ANSWER: 4.

Rationales:

1. Omeprazole (Prilosec) can be taken concurrently with an antacid; no drug-drug interaction occurs that interferes with absorption of the medication.

2. A capsule of omeprazole (Prilosec) should not be opened, crushed, or chewed. The pellets in the capsule are designed for delayed absorption.

3. Omeprazole (Prilosec) should be given before food is eaten, preferably breakfast.

4. A capsule of omeprazole (Prilosec) should be swallowed whole and should not be opened, crushed, or chewed. The pellets in the capsule are designed for delayed absorption.

TEST-TAKING TIP: Identify the options that are opposites. Options 2 and 4 are opposites. Examine these options carefully because one of the opposite options is commonly the correct answer.

Content Area: Medication

Integrated Processes: Communication and Documentation, Teaching/Learning; Nursing Process: Implementation

Client Need: Physiological Integrity; Pharmacological and Parenteral Therapies

Cognitive Level: Application

Concept: Medication; Safety

37. ANSWER: 3.

Rationales:

1. Although this statement focuses on feelings, it is not the most appropriate nursing statement because the client is not in denial; the client is following the rest of the medication regimen.

2. This is a rigid response that denies the client's concern.

3. The client is taking the other medications and probably would take the diuretic if there were accessible bathroom facilities. An alternate time of day to take the diuretic should be explored to address the client's concern and to ensure that all the prescribed medications are taken.

4. Although this may be a true statement, it does not address the client's concern.

TEST-TAKING TIP: Identify the word in the stem that sets a priority. The word *best* in the stem sets a priority. Identify the option that has a specific determiner. Option 1 contains the word *all,* which is a specific determiner. Most options with a specific determiner are distractors and can be eliminated. Identify the option that denies the client's concern. Option 2 denies the client's concern. Identify the options with a clang association. The stem and options 3 and 4 contain the word *diuretic.* Examine options 3 and 4 carefully.

Content Area: Fluid, Electrolyte, and Acid-Base Balance

Integrated Processes: Communication and Documentation; Nursing Process: Implementation

Client Need: Health Promotion and Maintenance

Cognitive Level: Application

Concept: Medication; Health Promotion

38. ANSWER: 3.

Rationales:

1. The client has been experiencing nausea and vomiting for several hours. This is not a new event. However, the nurse should be monitoring this client on a regular basis for electrolyte imbalances and administering an antiemetic if prescribed.

2. Pain on a level of 3 generally is considered tolerable. The client's pain level should be periodically reassessed.

3. Any client reporting chest pain should be assessed immediately. The client may have a pulmonary emboli or myocardial infarction. Both of these events require emergency interventions and the primary health-care provider to be notified immediately.

4. Although this is important for the nurse to explore and resolve, this client's need is not the priority in this situation.

TEST-TAKING TIP: Identify the word in the stem that sets a priority. The word *first* in the stem sets a priority.

Content Area: Perioperative

Integrated Processes: Nursing Process: Assessment

Client Need: Safe and Effective Care Environment; Management of Care

Cognitive Level: Analysis

Concept: Patient-Centered Care

39. ANSWER: 4.

Rationales:

1. This action is unsafe. Many drugs have similar doses.

2. It is not necessary to call the primary health-care provider. There are other resources that can be accessed to safely manage this concern.

3. This action is unsafe. The other nurse may not provide the nurse administering the drug with accurate information.

4. This is the most appropriate way to verify if the name of the medication on the unit dose package is equivalent to the name of the medication on the medication administration record. A drug usually has only one generic name, but a drug may have many trade names.

TEST-TAKING TIP: Identify the options that contain a clang association. The word *dose* in the stem and in option 1 is a clang association; the words *unit dose package* in the stem and in option 4 is a clang association. Examine options 1 and 4 carefully.

Content Area: Medication

Integrated Processes: Nursing Process: Implementation

Client Need: Physiological Integrity; Pharmacological and Parenteral Therapies

Cognitive Level: Application

Concept: Medication; Safety

40. ANSWER: 1, 2, 5, 6.

Rationales:

1. Toileting the client before the meal prevents the need to interrupt the meal if the client has to attend to elimination needs.

2. An upright position uses gravity to facilitate movement of food from the mouth to the stomach; this is a safety precaution. Eating in a recumbent position promotes aspiration of food.

3. This is unsafe. Attempting to speak while chewing or swallowing may result in aspiration.

4. The nurse should not cut meat or apply condiments to the client's food without direction from the client.

5. Asking about preferences is a client-centered response; it supports the client as an individual who is the center of the health team.

6. Ensuring that the client has swallowed the previous bite is a safety precaution. It prevents overloading the mouth with food, interfering with the ability to chew and swallow safely.

Content Area: Nutrition
Integrated Processes: Nursing Process: Implementation
Client Need: Physiological Integrity; Basic Care and Comfort
Cognitive Level: Application
Concept: Nutrition

41. ANSWER: 2, 5.

Rationales:

1. Throbbing pain at the incision site most likely is associated with the trauma of surgery and the inflammatory process, not dehiscence.

2. Clients with dehiscence often state that they feel a popping sensation at the site of the incision; it is the release of tension due to the separation of wound edges.

3. This is unrelated to dehiscence. Diuresis is expected because the levels of glucocorticoids and mineralocorticoids increased in response to the stress of surgery return to expected levels after surgery.

4. Keeping the knees bent minimizes abdominal discomfort because it reduces tension on the incisional site. In addition, when dehiscence is identified the client should be placed in the low-Fowler position with the knees bent.

5. An activity that uses the Valsalva maneuver (e.g., coughing, bearing down with a bowel movement, and moving from a lying down to a sitting position) increases intra-abdominal pressure that will put tension on the suture line.

Content Area: Perioperative Care
Integrated Processes: Communication and Documentation; Nursing Process: Assessment
Client Need: Physiological Integrity; Physiological Adaptation
Cognitive Level: Application
Concept: Tissue Integrity

42. ANSWER: 4.

Rationales:

1. Occasional difficulty with swallowing liquids should be managed by giving small amounts of liquid while the client is in the Fowler position. Direct supervision is essential. Clients should enjoy meals in their usual form until difficulty progresses to a point where it may be unsafe; then a thickening product may be used.

2. Although this is important, it is not the priority. In addition, splints and braces must be removed for hygiene, skin care, and range-of-motion exercises.

3. Although this may be done, it is not the priority. Initially, the nurse should design a bladder-retraining program that includes interventions, such as toileting the

client before going to bed at night and the first thing in the morning, every 2 hours when awake, or 30 minutes before a documented pattern of incontinence. An external urinary drainage device should be used as a last resort.

4. The client is experiencing a major change in living arrangements and may be coping with a sense of rejection or punishment. The nurse should stay with the client and encourage the expression of feelings.

TEST-TAKING TIP: Identify the word in the stem that sets a priority. The word *most* in the stem sets a priority. Identify the option with a specific determiner. Option 2 contains the word *all*, which is a specific determiner. Identify the unique option. Option 4 is unique because it is the only one that addresses the emotional domain. Options 1, 2, and 3 all refer to physiological issues.

Content Area: Psychosocial Health
Integrated Processes: Caring, Communication and Documentation; Nursing Process: Planning
Client Need: Health Promotion and Maintenance
Cognitive Level: Analysis
Concept: Patient-Centered Care; Stress

43. ANSWER: 2, 3.

Rationales:

1. A client with spinal surgery should have assistance with turning and positioning by a licensed professional. Nursing knowledge and skill are necessary to maintain alignment of the vertebral column of clients who have had spinal surgery.

2. These activities are within the legal role of unlicensed assistive personnel; the activities are routine ADLs.

3. Range-of-motion (ROM) exercises and a bed bath are routine activities that unlicensed assistive personnel are taught to administer. Nursing assistants are instructed to interrupt ROM and inform a licensed nurse if excessive resistance or pain occurs.

4. Assessment is within the legal role of a licensed nurse, not unlicensed assistive personnel.

5. A nurse should assist a postoperative client to the bathroom the first time after surgery. This provides an opportunity for the nurse to assess the client's strength and physical ability. In addition, postoperative clients may have IVs, indwelling catheters, etc. that require the nurse's expertise when transferring and ambulating.

Content Area: Leadership and Management
Integrated Processes: Nursing Process: Planning
Client Need: Safe and Effective Care Environment; Management of care
Cognitive Level: Analysis
Concept: Leadership and Management

44. ANSWER: 3, 5.

Rationales:

1. A pillow should be positioned under the client's calves, not heels, so that the heels are slightly elevated off the surface of the mattress. This reduces pressure on the heels that can cause pressure ulcers.

2. A pillow between the legs is used for the side-lying, not supine, position.

3. A pillow placed under the client's head and shoulders keeps the head and neck in functional alignment and prevents hyperextension of the head.

4. This is an awkward position because it places strain on the structures of the arms. Functional alignment of the arms is best achieved with the arms and hands resting on the bed with the palms of the hands facing the side of the body or facing the mattress.

5. A trochanter roll helps to maintain functional alignment by preventing external rotation of the hip.

Content Area: Mobility
Integrated Processes: Teaching/Learning; Nursing Process: Evaluation
Client Need: Physiological Integrity; Basic Care and Comfort
Cognitive Level: Application
Concept: Patient-Centered Care; Mobility

45. ANSWER: 4.

Rationales:

1. Informing the nursing supervisor should be done after another more important intervention.
2. This is not within the legal practice of nursing. This is a dependent function of the nurse.
3. This will not safely meet the client's need at this time.
4. When a medication error is made, the nurse must immediately contact the client's primary health-care provider, particularly when the medication error may harm or kill the client.

TEST-TAKING TIP: Identify the word in the stem that sets a priority. The word *first* in the stem sets a priority.

Content Area: Medication
Integrated Processes: Communication and Documentation; Nursing Process: Implementation
Client Need: Safe and Effective Care Environment; Management of Care
Cognitive Level: Application
Concept: Medication; Safety

46. ANSWER: 3.

Rationales:

1. Pallor occurs in response to vasoconstriction related to the onset, not defervescence, stage of a fever.
2. Malaise, a vague feeling of discomfort, is associated with the course (plateau) phase of a fever. This response occurs because of irritation of cellular function related to the increase in temperature and by-products of pyrogenic activity.
3. Sweating (diaphoresis) occurs in the defervescence (fever abatement/flush phase) phase of a fever when the cause of the temperature subsides and the set point of the hypothalamic thermostat is reduced. The usual heat loss responses include diaphoresis; warm, flushed skin; and decreased shivering as vasodilation occurs during the defervescence stage of a fever.
4. Shivering is a heat production response that occurs during the onset stage of a fever before the new set point of the hypothalamic thermostat adjusts to a higher level.

Content Area: Physical Assessment
Integrated Processes: Nursing Process: Analysis
Client Need: Physiological integrity; Reduction in Risk Potential
Cognitive Level: Analysis
Concept: Thermo-regulation

47. ANSWER: 3.

Rationales:

1. Sterile gloves are not necessary to remove a soiled dressing. A nurse wears clean gloves for protection from the client's body fluids.
2. The outside of the client's dressing is not considered sterile. A nurse can apply tape to secure the dressing with ungloved hands.
3. A sterile container should not be touched with a bottle of normal saline that is contaminated on the outside. Only sterile objects can touch a sterile field or sterile item for sterility to be maintained. If a sterile object or field is touched by a nonsterile object, it is contaminated and is no longer sterile.
4. This is acceptable practice. To wash the hands at this time requires the nurse to leave the bedside with the wound exposed. If the sterile field was already established, the nurse would have to leave it unattended, which is a violation of a principle of surgical asepsis. If a sterile field is unattended, it is considered contaminated because its sterility cannot be validated when outside the nurse's visual field.

TEST-TAKING TIP: Identify the word in the stem that indicates negative polarity. The word *interrupt* in the stem indicates negative polarity. What action by the LPN is unacceptable? Identify the unique option. Option 3 is the only option that does not contain the word *dressing*, making this option unique. Option 3 is the only option that relates to something other than a dressing. Also, it is the only option that does not contain the word *dressing*.

Content Area: Inflammation, Infection, Immunity, and Wound Care
Integrated Processes: Nursing Process: Evaluation
Client Need: Safe and Effective Care Environment; Management of Care
Cognitive Level: Analysis
Concept: Infection

48. ANSWER: 1.

Rationales:

1. The nurse should provide further teaching in an attempt to change the parent's behavior. The parents may stop pushing the trigger if they understand that the child is still receiving an analgesic even when not pushing the trigger.
2. This is an authoritative intervention. A less aggressive approach should be used to change the parent's behavior.
3. This is unnecessary. The nurse should notify the primary health-care provider if the basal and bolus doses are inadequate to control the child's pain.
4. This intervention requires a prescription. This action is a dependent function of the nurse.

TEST-TAKING TIP: Identify the word in the stem that sets a priority. The word *first* in the stem sets a priority. Using the test-taking tip, "Identify the clang associations," will not help in answering this question because each option has a clang association with a word or words in the stem.

Content Area: Pain, Comfort, Rest, and Sleep
Integrated Processes: Teaching/Learning; Nursing Process: Implementation

Client Need: Physiological Integrity; Pharmacological and
Parenteral Therapies
Cognitive Level: Application
Concept: Comfort

49. ANSWER: 4.
Rationales:
1. A medication should not be discontinued without
collaboration with the primary health-care provider. Safety
precautions should be taken if the client develops dizziness
or fatigue.
2. Acyclovir (Zovirax) will not precipitate constipation; it
may cause anorexia, nausea, vomiting, and diarrhea.
3. Taking the pulse before the administration of
acyclovir (Zovirax) is unnecessary; it does not
influence the heart rate.
**4. Acyclovir (Zovirax) should be taken at the first
indication of an outbreak, such as itching (pruritus),
tingling, or pain at the site where lesions develop
(usually the perineal area).**
TEST-TAKING TIP: Identify the unique option. Option 4
is unique. It relates to what should be done before the
medication is taken. Options 1, 2, and 3 all relate to adverse
effects of the medication.
Content Area: Inflammation, Infection, Immunity, and
Wound Care
Integrated Processes: Communication and Documentation,
Teaching/Learning; Nursing Process: Evaluation
Client Need: Physiological Integrity; Pharmacological and
Parenteral therapy
Cognitive Level: Application
Concept: Medication; Infection

50. ANSWER: 2.
Rationales:
1. The use of a safety razor is contraindicated when
receiving an anticoagulant. Although a safety razor is
safer than a straight edge razor, it still has a sharp blade
that can cut the skin.
**2. An electric razor is designed to trim facial hair with
sharp blades safely confined within the shaving surface
of the razor. This type razor minimizes the risk of
incurring a break in the skin, which may bleed
excessively when a person is receiving an anticoagulant.**
3. Although aftershave lotion may provide comfort, it does
not provide for client safety.
4. Wrapping the face with a warm, not hot, towel often is
done before shaving to soften hair. However, it should be
avoided when receiving anticoagulants because this action
causes vasodilation. If a break in the skin should occur
when shaving, bleeding may be excessive.
TEST-TAKING TIP: Identify equally plausible options.
Options 3 and 4 are equally plausible; both are actions
that are associated with skin care. One is no better than
the other. Identify options that are opposites. Options 1
and 2 are opposites. A safety razor has exposed blades and
does not use electricity. An electric razor has unexposed
blades and uses electricity.
Content Area: Tissue Integrity and Hygiene
Integrated Processes: Teaching/Learning; Nursing Process:
Implementation

Client Need: Physiological Integrity; Pharmacological and
Parenteral Therapy
Cognitive Level: Application
Concept: Medication; Safety

51. ANSWER: 2.
Rationales:
1. Soft, low-pitched, breezy sounds heard in the periphery
of the lungs are called vesicular breath sounds; they reflect
expected sounds in the tiny airways of the lungs.
**2. A low-pitched, grating sound usually heard during
the height of inspiration reflects the sound of inflamed
pleura rubbing together. A pleural friction rub is heard
at the lateral anterior base of the lung, indicated as RLL
in the figure.**

3. Loud, high-pitched, hollow, blowing sounds heard over
the trachea anteriorly are called bronchial breath sounds;
these sounds are expected breath sounds and do not
indicate the presence of pleurisy.
4. Medium-pitched, medium-intensity, blowing sounds
heard on inspiration and expiration when the stethoscope
is over the major bronchi are called bronchovesicular
breath sounds; they are expected breath sounds and are
not indicative of pleurisy.
Content Area: Oxygenation
Integrated Processes: Nursing Process: Implementation
Client Need: Physiological Integrity; Physiological
Adaptation
Cognitive Level: Analysis
Concept: Oxygenation

52. ANSWER: 1.
Rationales:
**1. The client is the most important member of the
health-care team. All activities of the members of the
team focus on the needs of the client.**
2. Although the primary nurse is an important member
of the health-care team, the nurse assumes a lesser role
compared to a person in another option.

3. Although the nurse manager is an important member of the health-care team, the nurse manager assumes a lesser role compared to a person in another option.

4. Although the nurse practitioner is an important member of the health-care team, the nurse practitioner assumes a lesser role compared to a person in another option.

TEST-TAKING TIP: Identify the word in the stem that sets a priority. The word *most* in the stem sets a priority. Identify the unique option. Option 1 is unique because it is the only option that does not include the word *nurse* and it only has one word and options 2, 3, and 4 all have two words.

Content Area: Health-Care System
Integrated Processes: Communication and Documentation; Nursing Process: Implementation
Client Need: Safe and Effective Care Environment; Management of Care
Cognitive Level: Comprehension
Concept: Health Care System

53. **ANSWER: 1, 2.**
Rationales:

1. **Using relaxation techniques when the urge to void is felt may postpone voiding, thereby increasing bladder capacity.**

2. **Toileting times are purposely scheduled in response to times of fluid intake and the client's usual elimination pattern; the schedule must be followed exactly to increase success.**

3. Placing a commode at the bedside is unnecessary. The client should use the bathroom to maintain privacy.

4. Washing the perineal area does not contribute to a client's ability to regain continence.

5. The pattern of voiding, not fluid balance relative to fluid intake, is significant.

TEST-TAKING TIP: Identify the option with a clang association. The word *program* in the stem and option 2 is a clang association.

Content Area: Urinary Elimination
Integrated Processes: Nursing Process: Planning
Client Need: Physiological Integrity; Physiological Adaptation
Cognitive Level: Application
Concept: Elimination

54. **ANSWER: 3, 5.**
Rationales:

1. Penrose drains function on the principle of gravity and drainage flows directly into a gauze dressing, not a collection device. With a Jackson-Pratt drain, negative pressure is established when the opened collection device is compressed and then closed. The negative pressure establishes gentle suction that pulls drainage from the wound into the collection device. It should be emptied of drainage when half full and negative pressure reestablished to ensure adequacy of the negative pressure.

2. Penrose drains drain directly into a gauze dressing. They do not have a collection chamber.

3. **Both drains pierce the skin and therefore interrupt the first line of defense against infection. The site of entry of the drains should be assessed for signs of inflammation and infection.**

4. Penrose drains are shortened regularly as healing takes place. Jackson-Pratt drains are not shortened; generally they are removed once drainage decreases to less than 10 mL daily.

5. **The color of the drainage of both tubes should be assessed and the results documented.**

TEST-TAKING TIP: Identify the clang associations. The word *drain* in the stem and in options 3 and 4 and the word *drainage* in option 5 are clang associations. Examine these options carefully.

Content Area: Perioperative Care
Integrated Processes: Nursing Process: Implementation
Client Need: Physiological Integrity; Physiological Adaptation
Cognitive Level: Analysis
Concept: Tissue Integrity

55. **ANSWER: 1.**
Rationales:

1. **A telephone translation service employing competent, certified translators ensures that translations will be accurate.**

2. Using a staff member to translate a conversation may not ensure accuracy in the translation because the staff member may not be fully competent in the required language. Also, people in different regions of a country may speak a different dialect.

3. Pictures can reinforce learning, but teaching should use the spoken word.

4. A translation book will assist in communicating but cannot guarantee comprehension because the client may have a different interpretation of words.

TEST-TAKING TIP: Identify the option with a clang association. The word *teaching* in the stem and in option 1 is a clang association. Give option 1 careful consideration.

Content Area: Communication, Collaboration, and Documentation
Integrated Processes: Communication and Documentation; Nursing Process: Planning
Client Need: Safe and Effective Care Environment; Management of Care
Cognitive Level: Application
Concept: Communication

56. **ANSWER: 4.**
Rationales:

1. Although this is something the nurse should instruct the client to do, this client is confused at times and cannot be relied upon to call for help when it is needed.

2. A confused client should not be left unattended in the bathroom; also, the client may not understand how to use a call light device.

3. A confused client who needs a walker should not be permitted to walk unattended.

4. **This is the best intervention of the options presented to help keep a client safe from falls. By positioning the client's wheelchair next to the nurses' station, staff members can continuously supervise a confused client.**

TEST-TAKING TIP: Identify the word in the stem that sets a priority. The word *best* in the stem sets a priority. Identify

equally plausible options. Options 1 and 2 are equally plausible. Both options instruct the client to call for help. Option 1 is no better than option 2.
Content Area: *Safety*
Integrated Processes: *Communication and Documentation; Nursing Process: Implementation*
Client Need: *Safe and Effective Care Environment; Safety and Infection Control*
Cognitive Level: *Application*
Concept: *Safety*

57. **ANSWER: 2.**
Rationales:
1. Although this reflects dehydration and is an important assessment, it is not the priority among the options presented.
2. Ensuring adequate gas exchange is the priority; inadequate gas exchange is life threatening.
3. Although this reflects a stage I pressure ulcer and is an important assessment, it is not the priority among the options presented.
4. Although this may reflect inadequate nutrition and is an important assessment, it is not the priority among the options presented.
TEST-TAKING TIP: Identify the word in the stem that sets a priority. The word *greatest* in the stem sets a priority. Use the ABCs (Airway, Breathing, and Circulation) to identify the priority.
Content Area: *Physical Assessment*
Integrated Processes: *Nursing Process: Analysis*
Client Need: *Safe and Effective Care Environment; Management of Care*
Cognitive Level: *Analysis*
Concept: *Patient-Centered Care; Oxygenation*

58. **ANSWER: 1.**
Rationales:
1. Montgomery straps are paired adhesive straps applied several inches on either side of a wound with central sections that can be folded back, allowing access to the primary dressing. On the leading edge of each of the central sections are perforations that allow for a method of securing one side to the other. It is used to secure a primary dressing without having to replace the tape every time the dressing is changed.
2. Wound care is a dependent function of the nurse; half-normal saline solution and peroxide were not prescribed. Normal saline solution was prescribed because it is isotonic. Research demonstrates that peroxide is caustic to new granulating tissue and counterproductive to the healing process.
3. The gauze packing should not be dripping wet. It should be moist enough to promote granulation of tissue without causing maceration of tissue.
4. Gently wiping away, not toward, the wound avoids contaminating the wound with skin flora. Patting violates surgical asepsis. One 4×4 gauze pad should be used for each swipe from the edge of the wound outward away from the center of the wound.
Content Area: *Inflammation, Infection, Immunity, and Wound Care*

Integrated Processes: *Nursing Process: Implementation*
Client Need: *Physiological Integrity; Physiological Adaptation*
Cognitive Level: *Application*
Concept: *Tissue Integrity*

59. **ANSWER: 3, 4.**
Rationales:
1. Clean, not sterile, gloves should be worn to protect the nurse from the client's body fluids. The client has an infection, and a discharge may be present.
2. Pulling the upper lid toward the forehead is unrelated to the administration of eyedrops.
3. The lower lid should be moved by placing a finger just below the lower eyelashes and exerting gentle pressure downward toward the bony prominence of the cheek. This exposes the conjunctival sac.
4. Drops should be placed in the conjunctival sac to prevent trauma to the eyeball. The fluid disperses when the eye is closed gently after the insertion of the drops.
5. A new cotton ball for each stroke should be moved from the inner to the outer canthus to prevent debris from entering the lacrimal duct. The eye should be cleansed before the procedure to remove debris and wiped gently after the procedure to remove excess fluid that may have leaked onto the cheek.
TEST-TAKING TIP: Identify the options that are opposites. Options 2 and 3 are opposites. They are moving opposite eyelids in opposite directions. More often than not one of the opposites is among the right answers. Identify the clang association. The word *eye* in the stem and in option 3 is a clang association.
Content Area: *Medication*
Integrated Processes: *Nursing Process: Implementation*
Client Need: *Physiological Integrity; Pharmacological and Parenteral Therapies*
Cognitive Level: *Application*
Concept: *Medication; Safety*

60. **ANSWER: 2, 4.**
Rationales:
1. Feeling hungry is subjective, not objective, information. Subjective data involve feelings, sensations, and concerns reported by the client. Subjective data are not observable and can be described only by the client.
2. Objective data are observable and measurable and can be confirmed by another person though the use of the senses. In this situation, the client is observed avoiding eye contact when talking with the nurse.
3. Bladder spasms are subjective, not objective, data. They can be reported only by the client. The client generally will report feeling abdominal cramping and pain in the lower abdomen when bladder spasms occur.
4. A pleural friction rub can be heard by auscultation when a stethoscope is placed over the base of the lung at the height of inhalation when a client has pleurisy. It is a rubbing or grating sound as one layer of the pleural membrane slides over the other during breathing.

5. Reports of epigastric discomfort are subjective, not objective, information. Discomfort can be reported only by the client.

TEST-TAKING TIP: The word *always* in option 1 is not a true specific determiner. The word is used in a sentence by the client when explaining the reason for excessive eating. Coincidentally, option 1 is a distractor because reporting *always feeling hungry* is subjective data.

Content Area: Critical Thinking and the Nursing Process
Integrated Processes: Nursing Process: Assessment
Client Need: Safe and Effective Care Environment; Management of Care
Cognitive Level: Analysis
Concept: Patient-Centered Care

61. **ANSWER: 3.**
Rationales:
1. Leaving the client's room while the client is in distress without providing an opportunity for the client to express feelings, needs, or concerns is inappropriate.
2. Forcing a client to talk about concerns is inappropriate; nurses must proceed at the client's pace.
3. Remaining seated in the room with the client for several minutes allows the client to gather personal thoughts and not feel abandoned by the nurse.
4. Leaving the room while the client is upset without giving the client a chance to express concerns may be viewed by the client as abandonment.

TEST-TAKING TIP: Identify the word in the stem that sets a priority. The word *best* in the stem sets a priority. Identify opposite options. Options 3 and 4 are opposites. More often than not one of the options that is an opposite is the correct answer. Examine options 3 and 4 carefully. Identify the equally plausible options. Options 1 and 4 are equally plausible. They both leave the client when the client is upset. Eliminate options 1 and 4. Identify the option that denies the client's feelings. Option 4 denies the client's feelings.

Content Area: Communication, Collaboration, and Documentation
Integrated Processes: Caring, Communication and Documentation; Nursing Process: Implementation
Client Need: Psychosocial Integrity
Cognitive Level: Application
Concept: Communication

62. **ANSWER: 2, 4, 5, 3, 1.**
Rationales:
2. Infants are developing sensorimotor skills and enjoy the sounds associated with rattles. They become interactive with toys and demonstrate preferences by 3 to 6 months of age.
4. Toddlers are mastering gross and fine motor skills; they enjoy the autonomy of playing with a pounding toy.
5. Preschoolers are developing mastery of fine motor skills. Construction toys allow them to engage in endeavors with purpose and that require skill.
3. School-aged children enjoy associate play and games with increasing complexity.
1. Adolescents develop formal operational thought and are capable of following the rules of complex games.

Content Area: Development Across the Life Span
Integrated Processes: Nursing Process: Implementation
Client Need: Health Promotion and Maintenance
Cognitive Level: Analysis
Concept: Growth and Development

63. **ANSWER: 4, 5.**
Rationales:
1. Redness (erythema) indicates the presence of the inflammatory response; the wound may or may not be infected.
2. Swelling (edema) indicates the presence of the inflammatory response; the wound may or may not be infected.
3. A wound that is warm to the touch is a result of an increase in circulation to the area that is indicative of the inflammatory response; the wound may or may not be infected.
4. Thick fluid that appears yellow, green, tan, or brown exiting from a wound is purulent drainage. The drainage is debris consisting of fluid, cells, or cellular material escaped from blood vessels as a result of an infection.
5. An elevated temperature indicates the presence of infection. An elevated temperature is the body's effort to establish a hostile environment that impedes the replication of a pathogenic microorganism.

Content Area: Inflammation, Infection, Immunity, and Wound Care
Integrated Processes: Nursing Process: Evaluation
Client Need: Physiological Integrity; Physiological Adaptation
Cognitive Level: Application
Concept: Infection

64. **ANSWER: 4.**
Rationales:
1. This movement achieves hyperextension.
2. This movement achieves adduction.
3. This movement achieves external rotation.
4. This movement achieves internal rotation.

TEST-TAKING TIP: Identify the options that are opposites. Options 3 and 4 are opposites. Examine options 3 and 4 carefully.

Content Area: Mobility
Integrated Processes: Nursing Process: Implementation
Client Need: Physiological Integrity; Basic Care and Comfort
Cognitive Level: Application
Concept: Mobility

65. **ANSWER: 2.**
Rationales:
1. This explanation does not protect the other residents from becoming scared when the wandering resident enters their rooms.
2. The alarm will ring when the resident exits the bed. When the alarm rings, the nurse can immediately intervene to walk with the resident or engage the resident in a distracting activity. This is the only action among the options offered that effectively protects the other residents.

3. Some residents may feel isolated if the door is closed. Closing the doors of all residents' rooms at night violates the right of residents to have their doors remain open. Also, a closed door may not stop a wandering resident from entering another resident's room.

4. The wandering resident may climb over a bolster and rail causing a safety concern for the resident. A bolster generally is used to remind a resident to call for assistance when wanting to get of bed, not to keep a resident from climbing out of bed. Four raised side rails are considered a restraint and requires a prescription from the primary health-care provider.

TEST-TAKING TIP: Identify the word in the stem that sets a priority. The word *most* in the stem sets a priority. Identify the central persons in the question. The other residents are the central persons in the question. The question is asking, "Which intervention is most effective in protecting the other residents from the resident who is wandering at night?" Identify the options that deny residents' feelings, concerns, and rights. Option 1 denies the other residents' feelings and concerns. Delete option 1 from further consideration. Option 3 denies the other residents' rights to have their doors left open at night. Delete option 4 from further consideration. Identify the clang association. The word *wanders* in the stem and the word *wandering* in option 2 is a clang association.

Content Area: Safety
Integrated Processes: Caring; Nursing Process: Implementation
Client Need: Safe and Effective Care Environment; Safety and Infection Control
Cognitive Level: Application
Concept: Safety

66. ANSWER: 4.
Rationales:
1. This is an inappropriate, confrontational response.
2. This action is too confrontational and divisive. Also, the nurse manager is abdicating an important role of a manager.
3. This response is too autocratic.
4. **The whole team should discuss the issue and negotiate an equitable process so that it is fair to everyone.**

TEST-TAKING TIP: Identify the word in the stem that sets a priority. The word *best* in the stem sets a priority. Identify the option that denies the nurse's concerns. Option 1 denies the nurse's concerns. Identify the clang associations. The word *nurse* in the stem and in options 1 and 2 are clang associations. However, in this question, this tip will not help you focus in on a correct answer because in this question options 1 and 2 are distractors. More often than not, *but not always*, an option with a clang association is the correct answer.

Content Area: Leadership and Management
Integrated Processes: Caring, Communication and Documentation; Nursing Process: Implementation
Client Need: Safe and Effective Care Environment; Management of Care
Cognitive Level: Analysis
Concept: Leadership and Management

67. ANSWER: 3, 4.
Rationales:
1. Soy milk is lactose free and does not have to be avoided when on a lactose-free diet.
2. Fruit cocktail is lactose free and does not have to be avoided when on a lactose-free diet.
3. **Creamed soup has milk, which contains lactose, and should be avoided by a client following a lactose-free diet.**
4. **Cottage cheese is a dairy product. It contains curds that are produced by coagulating milk in a process called curdling. Milk and dairy products should not be consumed by people who are lactose intolerant.**
5. Vegetable juice is lactose free and does not have to be avoided when on a lactose-free diet.

TEST-TAKING TIP: Identify the words in the stem that indicate negative polarity. The words *avoid* and *eliminated* in the stem indicate negative polarity.

Content Area: Nutrition
Integrated Processes: Teaching/Learning; Nursing Process: Evaluation
Client Need: Physiological Integrity; Basic Care and Comfort
Cognitive Level: Application
Concept: Nutrition

68. ANSWER: 4.
Rationales:
1. Although this should be done before and after administration of a medication to help keep the tube patent, it is not the priority.
2. A piston syringe can be used, but the medication should be instilled slowly; gravity flow is preferred. This intervention is not the priority.
3. The negative pressure should be shut off immediately before instillation of the medication, otherwise the medication will be withdrawn by the negative pressure before it can be absorbed. The negative pressure should be kept off for 30 minutes after medication administration as well to promote absorption.
4. **It is important to identify that the tube is in the stomach. If it inadvertently moved into the esophagus or the trachea, instillation of liquid may be aspirated or flood the respiratory tract, respectively.**

TEST-TAKING TIP: Identify the word in the stem that sets a priority. The word *most* in the stem sets a priority. Identify the words that are a clang association. The words *nasogastric tube* in the stem and option 4 is clang association. Consider option 4 carefully.

Content Area: Medication
Integrated Processes: Nursing Process: Implementation
Client Need: Physiological integrity; Pharmacological and Parenteral Therapies
Cognitive Level: Analysis
Concept: Medication; Safety

69. ANSWER: 3.
Rationales:
1. Mildly active bowel sounds 3 days after a colon resection reflects a return of peristalsis, which is expected.

2. Dark pink urine immediately after a transurethral resection of the prostate is expected. If it becomes red or does not become lighter in color several hours after surgery, it may indicate excessive bleeding, which should be reported to the primary health-care provider.

3. The client has an already reduced surface area for the exchange of oxygen and carbon dioxide as a result of the wedge resection of the right lung. Reduced breath sounds on the nonoperative lung indicate a problem that will further compromise respiratory function. This should be reported to the primary health-care provider immediately.

4. Greenish drainage from a nasogastric tube after an abdominal cholecystectomy is the expected color of gastric secretions.

TEST-TAKING TIP: Identify the word in the stem that sets a priority. The word *immediate* in the stem sets a priority. Use the ABCs (Airway, Breathing, and Circulation) when examining options to establish the priority. No option presents a concern with airway. Option 3 is associated with breathing.

Content Area: Perioperative Care
Integrated Processes: Nursing Process: Evaluation
Client Need: Safe and Effective Care Environment; Management of Care
Cognitive Level: Analysis
Concept: Patient-Centered Care; Oxygenation

70. ANSWER: 3.
Rationales:

1. An online course is most effective when cognitive learning is required.

2. Lectures are effective for large groups, but interaction among members of the group is not promoted.

3. Overeating has an emotional component. Clients interacting with each other within a group have the opportunity for affective learning that involves changes in feelings, values, attitudes, and beliefs. Also, group members can provide support when designing and maintaining new behaviors.

4. Written materials are effective when cognitive learning is required.

TEST-TAKING TIP: Identify the word in the stem that sets a priority. The word *most* in the stem sets a priority.

Content Area: Teaching and Learning
Integrated Processes: Teaching/Learning; Nursing Process: Planning
Client Need: Health Promotion and Maintenance
Cognitive Level: Application
Concept: Patient-Centered Care

71. ANSWER: 4.
Rationales:

1. Range-of-motion (ROM) exercises every hour are unnecessary unless the client has an extenuating circumstance, such as a neuromusculoskeletal or peripheral circulation problem.

2. ROM exercises once a shift is too long between releasing restraints and performing ROM and may result in contractures.

3. ROM exercises every 4 hours is too long between releasing restraints and performing ROM and may result in contractures.

4. Every 2 hours is often enough to perform ROM exercises to prevent contractures unless there are extenuating circumstances, such as when a client has a neuromusculoskeletal or peripheral circulation problem.

Content Area: Safety
Integrated Processes: Communication and Documentation; Nursing Process: Planning
Client Need: Safe and Effective Care Environment; Safety and Infection Control
Cognitive Level: Application
Concept: Safety

72. ANSWER: 3.
Rationales:

1. Rating the intensity of pain on an objective scale assesses the severity of pain.

2. Information about the onset of pain assists in distinguishing the difference between acute and chronic pain, not radiating pain.

3. Pain that extends via direct extension from a point of origin to another close-lying area is known as radiating pain.

4. Pain that comes and goes is known as intermittent pain; it is associated with exacerbations and remissions of an illness.

Content Area: Pain, Comfort, Rest, and Sleep
Integrated Processes: Communication and Documentation; Nursing Process: Assessment
Client Need: Physiological Integrity; Reduction of Risk Potential
Cognitive Level: Application
Concept: Comfort

73. ANSWER: 3, 4, 5.
Rationales:

1. A nurse cannot catheterize a client without a prescription.

2. Intake and output monitoring will take a minimum of hours, which could place the client in physical jeopardy.

3. The client has identified a potential urinary problem that may be urinary retention. Assessing the suprapubic area is part of a focused assessment.

4. A bladder ultrasound scan will provide data about the volume of urine in the bladder.

5. The client has identified a potential urinary problem that may be urinary retention. Determining the time and amount of the client's last voiding is part of a focused assessment.

6. Body weights are inappropriate and ineffective when assessing for urinary retention. Daily weights are used for assessing for fluid retention associated with heart failure, edema, and ascites. One liter of fluid is equal to 2.2 pounds.

TEST-TAKING TIP: Identify the obscure clang association. The word *urinate* in the stem and *voiding* in option 5 is an obscure clang association. Examine option 5 carefully.

Content Area: Urinary Elimination
Integrated Processes: Nursing Process: Assessment
Client Need: Physiological Integrity; Reduction of Risk Potential
Cognitive Level: Application
Concept: Elimination

74. **ANSWER: 2.**
   Rationales:
   1. Conditioners moisturize the hair, which makes the strands supple, preventing tangles.
   2. Soap is drying because it removes natural secretions that keep the hair supple. When shampooing is necessary, a gentle moisturizing shampoo should be used.
   3. Braids organize the strands of hair, which limits movement of hair into mats and tangles because of friction and pressure.
   4. Brushing distributes oils along hair shafts, keeping them supple, preventing tangles and matting.
   TEST-TAKING TIP: Identify the word in the stem that indicates negative polarity. The word *avoid* in the stem indicates negative polarity. The question is asking, "What action will promote tangles and matting of hair?"
   Content Area: Tissue Integrity and Hygiene
   Integrated Processes: Teaching/Learning; Nursing Process: Implementation
   Client Need: Physiological Integrity; Basic Care and Comfort
   Cognitive Level: Application
   Concept: Tissue Integrity

75. **ANSWER: 2, 3, 5.**
   Rationales:
   1. Ten grapes contain only 116 mg of potassium.
   2. Five dried figs contain 712 mg of potassium. Furosemide (Lasix) is not a potassium-sparing diuretic, and a client may develop hypokalemia unless foods high in potassium are consumed.
   3. One baked potato contains 610 mg to 1081 mg of potassium, depending on its size.
   4. Half of a grapefruit contains only 165 mg of potassium.
   5. One cup of cooked spinach contains 839 mg of potassium.
   Content Area: Fluid, Electrolyte, and Acid-Base Balance
   Integrated Processes: Teaching/Learning; Nursing Process: Implementation
   Client Need: Physiological Integrity; Basic Care and Comfort
   Cognitive Level: Application
   Concept: Medication; Fluid and Electrolyte Balance

76. **ANSWER: 4.**
   Rationales:
   1. Bringing the client to talk with the lawyer without written consent from the client is a breach of Health Insurance Portability and Accountability Act (HIPAA) regulations.
   2. Refusing to discuss anything regarding the client indirectly implies that the client is on the unit. Also, it does not provide the client with potentially important information.
   3. Although this is correct, it is not the best choice in this scenario because the client is not given potentially important information.

4. **It is against HIPAA regulations to reveal that a client is on the unit without written consent from the client. The nurse should take the lawyer's phone number and pass it on to the client without revealing to the caller that the client is on the unit. It is important to relay crucial information to the client without violating HIPAA regulations.**
   TEST-TAKING TIP: Identify the word in the stem that sets a priority. The word *most* in the stem sets a priority.
   Content Area: Legal and Ethical Issues
   Integrated Processes: Communication and Documentation; Nursing Process: Implementation
   Client Need: Safe and Effective Care Environment; Management of Care
   Cognitive Level: Application
   Concept: Legal

77. **ANSWER: 3.**
   Rationales:
   1. Side effects of warfarin (Coumadin), an anticoagulant, are bruising, melena, hematuria, epistaxis, bleeding gums, anemia, and thrombocytopenia, not constipation.
   2. Metronidazole (Flagyl) is an anti-infective; generally, diarrhea, not constipation, is a side effect. It depletes the natural flora in the colon and permits other organisms that do not belong in the colon to grow, causing diarrhea. For example, *Clostridium difficile* causes pseudomembranous colitis, a profuse infectious diarrhea.
   3. Constipation is a common side effect of ferrous sulfate (Feosol); iron interferes with myoglobin, which helps provide oxygen to muscles, including those associated with the bowel, resulting in decreased bowel motility.
   4. Magnesium salts in magnesium/aluminum hydroxide (Maalox) may increase peristalsis, causing diarrhea, not constipation.
   Content Area: Bowel Elimination
   Integrated Processes: Nursing Process: Analysis
   Client Need: Physiological Integrity; Pharmacological and Parenteral Therapies
   Cognitive Level: Analysis
   Concept: Medication; Elimination

78. **ANSWER: 1.**
   Rationales:
   1. Difficulty chewing results in food particles that are dangerously large at the time of swallowing, and difficulty swallowing may result in secretions, fluids, or solids entering the tracheobronchial tree rather than the esophagus. The client is at risk for aspiration.
   2. Although constipation may occur because the client may avoid eating foods high in fiber due to the fact that they are difficult to chew, this is not the priority. High-fiber drinks and stool softeners may be prescribed to prevent constipation.
   3. Fluid volume deficit can be prevented with adequate supervision (e.g., high-Fowler position when drinking small amounts of fluid at a time) and the use of products that thicken the fluid into a gelatin-like consistency.

4. Inadequate nutrition can be prevented by ordering food with an altered consistency (e.g., soft, chopped, pureed) along with supplemental nutritional drinks.

TEST-TAKING TIP: Identify the word in the stem that sets a priority. The word *greatest* in the stem sets a priority.
Content Area: Safety
Integrated Processes: Nursing Process: Analysis
Client Need: Safe and Effective Care Environment; Reduction of Risk Potential
Cognitive Level: Application
Concept: Safety

79. **ANSWER: 4, 5, 6.**
Rationales:
1. A low urine specific gravity reflects diluted urine, which indicates that the client may have an excess, not deficient, fluid volume.
2. A bounding pulse indicates an increase in circulating blood volume and is a sign of an excess fluid volume, not dehydration.
3. Straw-colored urine indicates that the client probably is in fluid balance.
4. Seventy percent of body fluids are in the intracellular compartment. When cells lose fluid due to dehydration, they become smaller, including the cells in and around the eyes.
5. When a person is dehydrated there is less fluid in the intravascular compartment. As a result the neck veins, which tend to be prominent, appear flat.
6. Skin turgor refers to expected skin fullness or the ability of the skin and underlying tissue to return to their regular position after being pinched and lifted. When there is decreased skin turgor because of dehydration, the skin remains pinched or "tented" for a longer time after it is released than well-hydrated skin.
Content Area: Fluid, Electrolyte, and Acid-Base Balance
Integrated Processes: Communication and Documentation; Nursing Process: Assessment
Client Need: Physiological Integrity; Physiological Adaptation
Cognitive Level: Analysis
Concept: Fluid and Electrolyte Balance

80. **ANSWER: 3.**
Rationales:
1. Eating pork and pork products is not prohibited by the Christian Science religion; this is prohibited by people who practice Judaism or Hinduism.
2. This is not a belief of the Christian Science religion. Observant Jewish people believe that the feet should not face toward the exit of a room unless one has died.
3. The client may feel guilty about seeking traditional medical care. Traditional medicine and drugs to treat illness are not accepted by the Christian Science religion. It is believed that illness is caused by ignorance, fear, or sin and that the client will return to health with prayers and Christian Science treatment.
4. Amulets to ward off evil spirits are associated with Native American cultures, not the Christian Science religion.

TEST-TAKING TIP: Identify the option that is unique. Option 3 is unique because it is the only option associated with requiring a response from the client. Identify the option with a clang association. The words *medical management* in the stem and in option 3 is a clang association. Examine option 3 carefully.
Content Area: Diversity and Spirituality/Religion
Integrated Processes: Caring; Communication and Documentation; Nursing Process: Implementation
Client Need: Psychosocial Integrity
Cognitive Level: Application
Concept: Spirituality

81. **ANSWER: 1, 5.**
Rationales:
1. A bruit is the sound produced by the turbulence of blood flow within a vessel. A stethoscope can auscultate the abnormality of a bruit in the venous/arterial system.
2. A lesion is observed via inspection, not by auscultation.
3. Ascites is assessed by inspection and palpation, not auscultation.
4. Distention of the abdomen is assessed by inspection and palpation, not auscultation.
5. Borborygmi are the gurgling sounds that occur as gas flows through liquid in the intestine. They can be heard when auscultating the abdomen for bowel sounds.
Content Area: Physical Assessment
Integrated Processes: Nursing Process: Assessment
Client Need: Health Promotion and Maintenance
Cognitive Level: Analysis
Concept: Patient-Centered Care

82. **ANSWER: 1, 3, 5.**
Rationales:
1. Increased periods of sleep occur before the active phase of dying as the person attempts to conserve energy.
2. A marked decrease in urine output occurs during the active phase of dying as the kidneys fail to produce urine.
3. Reduced intake of food and fluid occurs before the active phase of dying because it requires too much energy to eat and drink the volume of food and fluid normally ingested. During the active phase of dying a person generally does not eat or drink at all.
4. Mottling, cyanosis or bluish or purple coloring, of the skin of the extremities occurs during the active phase of dying as the person's blood pressure falls as the body is no longer able to circulate adequate oxygen to the extremities.
5. The phenomenon of "seeing people who have died" is commonly associated with the time before a person is actively dying. It is unexplained.

TEST-TAKING TIP: Identify the clang association. The word *dying* in the stem and the word *died* in option 5 is a clang association.
Content Area: Grief and Loss
Integrated Processes: Nursing Process: Assessment
Client Need: Psychosocial Integrity
Cognitive Level: Application
Concept: Grief and Loss

83. ANSWER: 2, 4, 6.
    Rationales:
    1. The solution should be removed from the refrigerator 1 hour before administration so that it warms to room temperature to prevent pain, venous spasms, and hypothermia.
    2. Total parenteral nutrition intravenous tubing should be changed every 24 hours to minimize the risk of infection.
    3. This is unnecessary. Total parenteral nutrition is administered via a vein into the circulatory system, not the stomach. Viability of the intravenous catheter insertion site should be assessed.
    4. Intravenous infusion sets with an inline filter should be used for the administration of total parenteral nutrition. It decreases the infusion of particles that increase the incidence of phlebitis and bacterial infection.
    5. Total parenteral nutrition solutions should never be warmed in a microwave oven or by submerging the bag in warm water. Accelerating warming can cause the solution to precipitate, resulting in catheter occlusion or an embolus when administered.
    6. Total parenteral nutrition solutions are high in glucose (usually dextrose). Blood glucose levels should be monitored routinely, usually a minimum of every 6 hours.
    Content Area: Nutrition
    Integrated Processes: Nursing Process: Implementation
    Client Need: Physiological Integrity; Pharmacological and Parenteral Therapies
    Cognitive Level: Application
    Concept: Nutrition

84. ANSWER: 10.
    Rationale:
    Use ratio and proportion to answer the question.

$$\frac{\text{Desire } 250 \text{ mg}}{\text{Have } 125 \text{ mg}} = \frac{x \text{ mL}}{5 \text{ mL}}$$
$$125x = 250 \times 5$$
$$125x = 1{,}250$$
$$x = 1{,}250 \div 125$$
$$x = 10 \text{ mL}$$

    Content Area: Medication
    Integrated Processes: Nursing Process: Planning
    Client Need: Physiological integrity; Pharmacological and Parenteral Therapies
    Cognitive Level: Application
    Concept: Medication; Safety

85. ANSWER: 2.
    Rationales:
    1. The word *tolerated* is too general. The nurse should use specific, descriptive terminology to communicate the client's status after being in the chair.
    2. This documentation is specific, descriptive, and has a time frame.
    3. The situation indicating the need for a prn medication must be included in the documentation. In addition, the specific drug, dose, route, and client response should be included.

4. Pain assessment should include location, severity, and characteristics of the pain. The specific pain scale should be referenced (e.g., 5 on a scale of 0 to 10).
Content Area: Communication, Collaboration, and Documentation
Integrated Processes: Communication and Documentation; Nursing Process: Evaluation
Client Need: Safe and Effective Care Environment; Management of Care
Cognitive Level: Application
Concept: Communication

86. ANSWER: 1.
    Rationales:
    1. The inability to speak indicates a total obstruction. The abdominal thrust maneuver pushes trapped air out of the lungs, forcing out the food causing the obstruction.
    2. Attempting to swallow may cause the food to move further down the respiratory passages.
    3. Clapping between the scapulae several times may cause aspirated food to lodge deeper in the respiratory passages and is contraindicated.
    4. Waiting is unsafe. Letting the client cough is appropriate if there is a partial obstruction.
    TEST-TAKING TIP: Identify the opposite options. Options 1 and 4 are opposites. Identify the unique option. Option 1 is the only option without the word *client*.
    Content Area: Oxygenation
    Integrated Processes: Nursing Process: Implementation
    Client Need: Physiological Integrity; Physiological Adaptation
    Cognitive Level: Application
    Concept: Oxygenation

87. ANSWER: 2, 3, 6.
    Rationales:
    1. Sterile gloves are not necessary to maintain sterile technique when collecting a urine specimen from a closed urinary catheter and collection set. A sterile syringe protects the client from the introduction of microorganisms into the urinary catheter, and clean gloves protect the nurse from the client's body fluids.
    2. Collecting a urine specimen from a urinary drainage tube requires piercing of a port with a sterile needle attached to a sterile syringe for the purpose of withdrawing urine. Sterile technique must be maintained, which includes removing microorganisms on the port of the drainage tubing with an alcohol swab. This is necessary because the urinary retention catheter that is part of the closed urinary drainage system enters the bladder, a sterile body cavity.
    3. A clamp is used to occlude the tubing of a urinary catheter so that fresh urine can collect in the tubing proximal to the clamp. After the specimen is collected from a port proximal to the clamp, the clamp should be released immediately to allow urine to flow out of the bladder via the unobstructed tubing.
    4. Generally, urinary retention catheters are closed systems whereby the catheter, tubing, and collection bag are permanently connected to prevent separation. A closed

system reduces the risk of entry of microorganisms, which in turn reduces the risk of a urinary tract infection.

5. A sterile specimen cup is not necessary for a urinalysis. However, the use of a sterile specimen cup and maintenance of sterile technique are essential when collecting a sterile urine specimen for a culture and sensitivity examination.

6. Clamping the drainage tubing just below the level of the specimen port for 15 to 30 minutes allows fresh urine to collect above the specimen port.

TEST-TAKING TIP: Identify the clang associations. The word *urine* in the stem and in options 3 and 5 are clang associations. The word *port* in the stem and in options 2 and 6 are clang associations. Identify the unique option. Option 6 is unique because it is the only option with numbers. Examine options 2, 3, 5, and 6 carefully. Options 2, 3, and 6 are correct answers.

Content Area: Urinary Elimination
Integrated Processes: Nursing Process: Implementation
Client Need: Physiological Integrity; Reduction of Risk Potential
Cognitive Level: Application
Concept: Elimination

88. **ANSWER: 2.**
    Rationales:
    1. The opposite is true in older adults; long-term memory is better than short-term memory.
    2. Mental acuity slows in older adults, and it may take longer to learn something new. Teaching sessions should be short and frequent to allow for repetition and reinforcement.
    3. A person's IQ does not change as one ages.
    4. People who get easily confused usually have a cognitive disorder (e.g., learning disability, dementia).
    Content Area: Development Across the Life Span
    Integrated Processes: Communication and Documentation; Nursing Process: Assessment
    Client Need: Health Promotion and Maintenance
    Cognitive Level: Application
    Concept: Growth and Development

89. **ANSWER: 1, 5.**
    Rationales:
    1. Pulse oximetry measures the percentage of arterial oxygen saturation by assessing the percentage of hemoglobin molecules carrying oxygen. This measurement monitors the client's status and the effectiveness of oxygen therapy.
    2. Not all oxygen delivery systems cover both the nose and mouth. Nasal prongs and a face tent do not cover the nose and mouth.
    3. This is not an intervention that is appropriate for all oxygen delivery systems. This is done just with partial-rebreather and nonrebreather masks.
    4. Liter flow rates depend on the oxygen flow rate required by the device and the primary health-care provider's prescription. A simple facemask is set between 5 and 10 L/min. Nasal prongs are set between 1 and 6 L/min. Partial-rebreather and nonrebreather masks are set between 6 and 15 L/min. The liter flow rate for a Venturi

mask is set between 4 and 15 L/min, depending on the size of valve used. A face tent is set between 8 and 12 L/min.

5. All oxygen delivery systems anchor the device around the head with an elastic band or tubing; this can cause pressure, resulting in ischemia and skin breakdown.

TEST-TAKING TIP: Identify the unique option. Option 1 is the only option that contains the word *oximetry* rather than *oxygen*.

Content Area: Oxygenation
Integrated Processes: Nursing Process: Evaluation
Client Need: Physiological Integrity; Physiological Adaptation
Cognitive Level: Analysis
Concept: Oxygenation

90. **ANSWER: 1, 2, 3, 5.**
    Rationales:
    1. The nurse's body should remain in functional alignment when moving in the direction of the planned move. When the upper body is twisted (torqued), undue stress and strain are placed on muscles, joints, tendons, ligaments, and bones. Twisting the upper body should be avoided to prevent self-injury.
    2. A gait belt (transfer belt) is an assistive device that provides a secure mechanism to hold a client when performing a transfer or ambulating. It helps to ensure the safety of the client and health team member.
    3. Gravity facilitates the transfer when the bed is higher than the chair. The client is moving downward rather than upward, which requires more energy.
    4. The arms should be flexed so that the elbows can act as fulcrums while the arms act as levers.
    5. A wide base of support keeps the greatest mass of the body (torso) in the center of gravity, which provides stability.
    6. The nurse should bend the knees, not the waist. Bending the knees uses the large muscles of the legs rather than the weaker muscles of the back to assist with a transfer.
    TEST-TAKING TIP: Identify the clang association. The word *movement* in the stem and the word *move* in option 1 is a clang association.
    Content Area: Mobility
    Integrated Processes: Nursing Process: Implementation
    Client Need: Safe and Effective Care Environment; Safety and Infection Control
    Cognitive Level: Application
    Concept: Mobility

91. **ANSWER: 1, 3.**
    Rationales:
    1. A return demonstration of a skill by a client allows the nurse to evaluate if the client can perform the skill. A return demonstration is an effective way to evaluate teaching that was conducted in the psychomotor (doing) domain.
    2. Identifying a skin lesion during an admission physical is associated with the assessment, not evaluation, step of the nursing process.
    3. Determining whether a client has activity intolerance after ambulation is part of the evaluation step of the

nursing process. Evaluation is the process whereby the nurse reassesses the client after nursing care is provided to identify the client's response (actual outcome), which is then compared with the goal/expected outcome identified in the plan of care.

4. Connecting a contributing factor to a problem statement is part of the analysis/diagnosis, not evaluation, step of the nursing process.

5. Formulating an intervention to address a risk factor is part of the planning step of the nursing process as a nurse designs a plan of care to meet client needs.

Content Area: Critical Thinking and the Nursing Process
Integrated Processes: Nursing Process: Evaluation
Client Need: Safe and Effective Care Environment; Management of Care
Cognitive Level: Analysis
Concept: Patient-Centered Care

92. **ANSWER: 1.**
Rationales:
1. **The nurse should report the fire as soon as the safety of the client in immediate danger is ensured. This guarantees that additional staff members and the fire department are notified to assist in this emergency. Remember the mnemonic RACE: Rescue, Alarm, Confine, and Extinguish.**
2. Attempting to put out the fire is premature and unsafe at this time.
3. Closing all the doors on the unit is premature and unsafe at this time.
4. The evacuation of all clients is premature at this time.
TEST-TAKING TIP: Identify the word in the stem that sets a priority. The word *next* in the stem sets a priority. Identify the option with a specific determiner. Option 4 contains the word *all*, which is a specific determiner. More often than not, an option with a specific determiner is a distractor. Although the word *door* in the stem may be interpreted as a clang association with the word *doors* in option 3, the words are different in that the *door to the client's room* is different from the *doors on the unit*. Although a clang association usually helps you to focus on the correct answer, unfortunately in this question it does not.
Content Area: Safety
Integrated Processes: Nursing Process: Implementation
Client Need: Safe and Effective Care Environment, Safety and Infection Control
Cognitive Level: Analysis
Concept: Safety

93. **ANSWER: 3.**
Rationales:
1. Nausea and vomiting occur with both hypernatremia and hyponatremia because the resting membrane potential of cells is altered with sodium imbalances.
2. Confusion occurs with both hypernatremia and hyponatremia because altered serum sodium levels interfere with cerebral functioning.
3. **Dry, sticky mucous membranes and increased thirst are associated with hypernatremia; hypernatremia often is associated with fluid volume deficit. The compensatory**

mechanism of thirst should increase the intake of fluid to return the elevated serum sodium level to its expected level of 135 to 145 mEq.
4. Sodium is a component of the sodium-potassium pump that is involved with muscle contraction. An increase or decrease in serum sodium will result in muscle weakness and fatigue.
Content Area: Fluid, Electrolyte, and Acid-Base Balance
Integrated Processes: Nursing Process: Assessment
Client Need: Physiological Integrity, Physiological Adaptation
Cognitive Level: Analysis
Concept: Fluid and Electrolyte Balance

94. **ANSWER: 3.**
Rationales:
1. Although this regimen may cause a fluid volume deficit, it is not as serious a consequence as another option presented. Fluids can be taken up to 8 hours before the test and intravenous fluids are administered during the test.
2. Although abdominal cramps may result from the cleansing regimen, it will not precipitate a life-threatening condition.
3. **NuLYTELY is an osmotic bowel prep that draws water into the intestinal lumen. Bisacodyl (Dulcolax) is an intestinal stimulant that expands intestinal fluid volume. These products both pull sodium into the intestinal lumen where it is excreted, resulting in a decreased serum sodium level (hyponatremia). Sodium is essential in the functioning of the sodium-potassium pump that is essential for muscle contraction. Hyponatremia can interfere with the contraction of the heart, resulting in dysrhythmias that can be life threatening.**
4. This bowel-cleansing regimen will result in stools that will be liquid in consistency. This is the purpose of the regimen; an empty bowel allows for inspection of the intestinal mucosa without being impeded by the presence of feces.
TEST-TAKING TIP: Identify the word in the stem that sets a priority. The word *most* in the stem sets a priority.
Content Area: Bowel Elimination
Integrated Processes: Nursing Process: Evaluation
Client Need: Physiological Integrity; Pharmacological and Parenteral Therapies
Cognitive Level: Application
Concept: Fluid and Electrolyte Balance

95. **ANSWER: 4.**
Rationales:
1. No data demonstrate that the student is blaming others (projection).
2. No data demonstrate the intentional dismissing of the event from the mind and opinions.
3. No data demonstrate that the student is concentrating thoughts and emotions on his inner self (introspection).
4. **The student is using intellectual reasoning (intellectualization) to avoid confronting the unconscious conflict and the stress of having to cope with his girlfriend's pregnancy.**

Content Area: Psychosocial Health
Integrated Processes: Communication and Documentation;
Nursing Process: Analysis
Client Need: Psychosocial Integrity
Cognitive Level: Analysis
Concept: Stress

96. ANSWER: 3.
Rationales:
1. This site is appropriate for assessing the femoral pulse. This site should be assessed next if palpation of the popliteal pulse reveals an absent pulse or a pulse volume of 1+.
2. This site is appropriate for assessing the popliteal pulse. This site should be assessed next if palpation of the dorsalis pedis pulse reveals an absent pulse or a pulse volume of 1+.
3. The next proximal pulse should be assessed in an extremity when a distal peripheral pulse is absent or its pulse volume is 1+. The next site is the posterior tibial pulse. The extent of adequacy or inadequacy of circulation to the extremity must be determined.

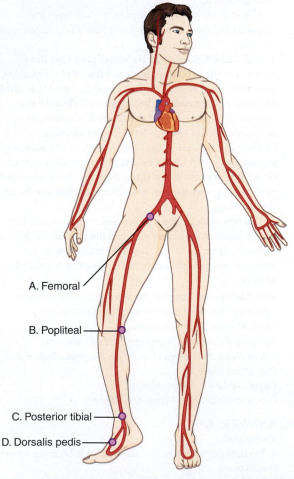

A. Femoral

B. Popliteal

C. Posterior tibial

D. Dorsalis pedis

4. This site is appropriate for assessing the dorsalis pedis pulse. The dorsalis pedis pulse is another name for the pedal pulse. The nurse has already identified that the pedal pulse is absent.
Content Area: Physical Assessment
Integrated Processes: Nursing Process: Assessment
Client Need: Physiological Integrity; Physiological Adaptation

Cognitive Level: Analysis
Concept: Perfusion

97. ANSWER: 1.
Rationales:
1. An involuntary loss of urine without the sensation of the need to void describes reflex incontinence. A relevant factor is spinal cord dysfunction (e.g., loss of cerebral awareness, impairment of the reflex arc).
2. Urinary incontinence after a strong sense of insistence to void describes urge incontinence, not reflex incontinence. Urge incontinence usually is associated with bladder spasms or contractions; also known as an overactive bladder.
3. Experiencing urinary dribbling with increased intra-abdominal pressure (e.g., sneezing, coughing, or lifting with a full bladder) describes stress incontinence, not reflex incontinence. Stress incontinence usually occurs in women who have had numerous pregnancies, a large fetus, or multiple births (e.g., twins, triplets). This also can occur with urinary retention with overflow (overflow incontinence).
4. A weak urinary stream is not associated with reflex incontinence. A weak urinary stream is associated with hyperplasia of the prostate gland or any condition that narrows the diameter of the urethra.
TEST-TAKING TIP: Identify the options that are opposites. Option 1 and option 2 are opposites. More often than not, the correct answer is one of the options that are opposites.
Content Area: Urinary Elimination
Integrated Processes: Communication and Documentation;
Nursing Process: Assessment
Client Need: Safe and Effective Care Environment;
Reduction of Risk Potential
Cognitive Level: Application
Concept: Elimination

98. ANSWER: 1.
Rationales:
1. The weight, age, and body surface area of a child must be obtained to individualize a safe, effective analgesic dose specific to the child. The processes of drug absorption, distribution, biotransformation, and excretion, all influenced by age, weight, and body surface area, can alter the safety and effectiveness of a drug.
2. Although vital signs should be assessed before and after administering an analgesic, this information is not as significant as body weight in determining the appropriate dose of a medication for a child.
3. Although the child's level of pain should be assessed before administering an analgesic, this information does not influence the safe dose for a child.
4. Although this information may influence future doses of analgesics, it is not as essential as another factor.
TEST-TAKING TIP: Identify the word in the stem that sets a priority. The word *most* in the stem sets a priority.
Content Area: Medication
Integrated Processes: Nursing Process: Assessment
Client Need: Physiological Integrity; Pharmacological and Parenteral Therapies
Cognitive Level: Application
Concept: Medication; Safety

99. ANSWER: 3, 5.

Rationales:

1. Food should be avoided 3 hours before bedtime to minimize the risk of regurgitation and aspiration.
2. This is contraindicated for clients with esophageal reflux. Fluids should be avoided 3 hours before bedtime to minimize the risk of regurgitation and aspiration.
3. Elevating the head of the bed on blocks uses gravity to keep food in the stomach, thereby reducing the risk of regurgitation and aspiration.
4. The client should remain in an upright position for 1 to 2 hours after meals; gravity helps to keep food in the stomach and allows time for food to progress into the jejunum.
5. Foods high in fat relax the lower esophageal sphincter and take longer to exit the stomach, both of which promote reflux of gastric contents. Foods high in fat should be avoided.

TEST-TAKING TIP: Identify the unique options. Option 3 is unique because all the other options relate to something that should be done in relation to food or fluid, while option 3 does not. Option 5 is unique because all the other options relate to something the nurse should teach the client to do, while option 5 is something the client should avoid. Examine options 3 and 5 carefully.

Content Area: Nutrition
Integrated Processes: Teaching/Learning; Nursing Process: Implementation
Client Need: Physiological Integrity; Physiological Adaptation
Cognitive Level: Application
Concept: Nutrition

100. ANSWER: 3.

Rationales:

1. Implementing a plan of action is premature without further information. More data must be collected and examined to make an informed decision.
2. Choosing an initial solution without further information may not be the best intervention to address the cause of the falls.
3. All possible strategies should be explored. One or more strategies may be selected to address the issue of the falls.
4. This is a punitive approach; quality improvement initiatives should focus on arriving at a positive outcome. All members of the unit should be involved in an in-service program if this strategy is part of the plan of action.

TEST-TAKING TIP: Identify the word in the stem that sets a priority. The word *next* in the stem sets a priority. Identify options with clang associations. The word *falls* in the stem and in options 3 and 4 are clang associations. An option with a clang association is often the correct answer; examine these options carefully. Identify equally plausible options. Options 1 and 2 are equally plausible, and therefore both can be eliminated from consideration.

Content Area: Leadership and Management
Integrated Processes: Nursing Process: Assessment
Client Need: Safe and Effective Care Environment; Management of Care
Cognitive Level: Application
Concept: Quality Improvement

Case Study Answers

Chapter 1—Safety

A. 1. Impaired mobility associated with left-sided hemiplegia that required a sling on the left arm and a below-the-knee leg brace to prevent footdrop and facilitate walking increased the client's risk of a fall.

2. The client is 72 years old. With age, flexibility, muscle strength, voluntary and autonomic reflexes, cognitive awareness and ability to manage multiple incoming stimuli decline.

3. Furosemide (Lasix) might have caused postural hypotension when the client suddenly stood at the side of the bed, resulting in syncope and a fall.

4. Scatter rugs are unstable objects that can precipitate a fall.

B. The priority concern is the client's safety. The client is confused; she is not aware of the time of day or that she is in a hospital. She is receiving an opioid for pain, which can cause lethargy and reduce cognition and perception. In addition, she is trying to get out of the bed immediately after orthopedic surgery while attached to intravenous tubing and a urinary retention catheter. The scenario provides no evidence that the client is experiencing hemorrhage. The dressing is dry and intact and vital signs are within expected limits, indicating hemodynamic stability and absence of blood loss. The client is receiving IV fluids and is voiding a sufficient quantity of urine hourly; therefore, fluid balance is not the priority. The client rates her pain as a level 3 on a 0-to-10 pain scale, which is considered tolerable; therefore, pain control is not an issue at this time.

C. 1. Ensure that the client is wearing an identity wrist band.

2. Check on the client frequently.

3. Orient the client to the environment frequently.

4. Keep the call bell and personal items within reach.

5. Keep the bed in the lowest position with two side rails raised.

6. Keep wheels on movable objects locked.

7. Inspect all equipment before use.

8. Maintain adequate lighting in the environment for day, evening, and night.

9. Answer the call bell immediately.

D. 1. Apply a wristband that indicates that the client is at risk for falls.

2. Employ other acceptable indicators to notify nursing staff members that the client is at risk for falls (e.g., red socks, flower or butterfly insignia on door).

3. Address the client's risk of falls in the nursing plan of care.

4. Employ nonrestrictive safety measures, such as a bed alarm, position-sensitive ankle alarm, bed bolsters, and wedges for positioning.

5. Document the outcomes of the use of nonrestrictive safety equipment. Only when nonrestrictive measures are ineffective can a nurse seek a prescription for a restraint.

E. 1. Explain the reason for the restraint to the client.

2. Ensure that the V opening of the vest is in the front and that the closure is at the back of the restraint.

3. Ensure that there are two fingerbreadths between the client's body and the vest to ensure that the client is able to breathe easily.

4. Secure the ties of the vest to the frame of the bed, not the side rails, using a quick-release knot.

5. Check on the client every 30 minutes to ensure that the client can breathe easily and that the vest is not too tight.

6. Remove the vest restraint every 2 hours to assess skin integrity; provide for activity, such as range-of-motion; and massage skin surfaces, such as the client's back and along the lower edge of the vest. Encourage coughing and deep breathing during this time. Reapply the vest, and reposition the client.

7. Meet hydration, nutrition, elimination, and emotional needs while the client is restrained.

8. Delegate application and restraint release to unlicensed assistive personnel if necessary, but remember that evaluation of the client's status and response to the restraint must be implemented by the nurse.

9. Ensure that the primary health-care provider assesses the client's need for the restraint and renews the prescription every 24 hours.

10. Discontinue use of the restraint as soon as possible.

Chapter 2—Communication, Collaboration, and Documentation

A. 1. The nurse pulled a curtain around the client's stretcher. *This action provides some privacy and communicates respect.*
   2. The nurse made eye contact with the client. *This action communicates that the nurse's attention is focused on the client.*
   3. The nurse introduced himself and explained what he was going to do. *This action supports the client's right to know who is providing care and what is going to be done.*
   4. The nurse faced the client at the head of the bed. *Facing a client enables the client to see the nurse's face, particularly the lips, which facilitates the reception of verbal messages. In addition, it projects the nurse's voice toward the client, not away from the client.*
   5. The nurse asked the client's preference regarding the daughter and grandson staying or leaving the area during the interview. *This action supports the client's right to make personal decisions regarding confidentiality and demonstrates respect for the client. Also, the daughter's presence may contribute to the client's emotional comfort.*

B. 1. The emergency department was filled with noise and commotion. *These can be distracting and interfere with reception of messages.*
   2. The stretcher was placed in the alcove of a hallway. *This action does not provide for complete privacy and makes it difficult to communicate owing to a noisy, distracting environment.*
   3. The grandson was pulling on the bed linen at the foot of the client's bed. *The grandson's behavior can be distracting.*
   4. The nurse was unable to sit at the bedside when conducting the interview because of the hazard of the chair blocking the hallway. *Standing may convey that the nurse is in a rush and not focused on the client.*
   5. The daughter and grandson were at the client's bedside. *The presence of the daughter and grandson may prevent the client from being open to discuss information that the client does not want them to know.*

C. 1. The nurse observed the client's nonverbal behavior. The nurse identified that the client was grimacing and rubbing her right hip; breathing in short, shallow breaths; shaking her head from side to side; and closing her eyes before speaking. These behaviors indicate that the client may be having pain. The nurse should ask appropriate questions in relation to the observations that indicate that the client may be having pain. *This*

ensures that the nonverbal behavior is congruent with what the client verbalizes before concluding that the client is in pain.
   2. The nurse made a reflective statement: "It must be frustrating to know that you did everything right and still had something like this happen." *Reflection encourages further discussion by focusing on emotional themes and feelings. In addition, it indicates active listening.*
   3. The nurse asked direct questions, such as, "What is the intensity of your pain on a scale of 0 to 10?" and "Tell me the location of the pain and what it feels like." *A direct question is used to collect objective information rapidly. In an emergency situation, the nurse wants to quickly obtain information about the location, intensity, and characteristic of the client's pain.*
   4. The nurse asked a clarifying question: "Can you explain in more detail what you mean by 'crazy'?" The client's message was unclear. *The nurse's response encouraged the client to elaborate and explain more fully what was meant by the word "crazy."*
   5. The nurse touched the client's arm when the client began to cry. *Touch communicates caring, concern, and encouragement.*
   6. The nurse used the technique of validation by stating, "It's okay to cry. You had a lot happen to you today." *The first sentence demonstrated acceptance of the client's crying. The second sentence corroborated that the client experienced a difficult event.*

D. 1. The nurse used medical jargon when using the word ORIF (which stands for "open-reduction internal fixation"). *Using medical jargon communicates a lack of interest in the client's understanding of the situation. It also communicates a demeanor of superiority and even arrogance.*
   2. The nurse provided false reassurance by saying, "Everything is going to be fine." *False reassurance minimizes the client's concerns and violates trust.*
   3. The nurse demonstrated nonacceptance of the client's feelings by saying, "Try to be strong and a good role model for your grandson." *This statement could be interpreted as the nurse saying, "Stop your crying. You're being a big baby."*

Chapter 3—Legal and Ethical Issues

A. Informed consent should be obtained from the infant's mother after the primary health-care provider has given the mother adequate information about the care to be provided. When a client is an infant, a parent, even if younger than 18 years of age, has the authority to give consent. Because the infant's mother appears dazed and is accompanied by her parent, the nurse must determine whether the mother understands the information surrounding the care to be provided, is giving consent voluntarily, and is alert and has intact cognition. When a person is incapable of participating in the decision-making process (e.g., is an infant or child or has impaired cognition), a surrogate decision maker must be identified. Most states specify the order of priority, such as parents of minors, durable power of attorney for health care, court-appointed guardian, spouse, or partner.

B. 1. This question is inappropriate. It is a probing question that violates the person's rights to privacy. The only purpose this question serves is to satisfy the nurse's curiosity.

2. This question is appropriate. Alcohol crosses the placenta and can negatively impact a fetus, resulting in health problems in the infant during the neonatal period.

3. This question is inappropriate because it is prying into personal information that has no bearing on the present situation. It is a probing question that violates the person's rights to privacy. The mother is the infant's legal guardian. Legally, the father does not have to be involved in the infant's care.

4. This question is appropriate. Many drugs can cross the placenta and negatively impact a fetus, resulting in health problems in the infant during the neonatal period.

5. This question is appropriate. Health problems in a pregnant woman, whether they are related or unrelated to the pregnancy, may negatively impact a fetus, resulting in health problems in the infant during the neonatal period.

6. This question is inappropriate at this time. The mother of the infant appeared dazed, did not make eye contact, and rarely answered the nurse's questions during the initial assessment. The infant's and mother's physical and emotional conditions must be assessed and addressed before future plans can be explored.

C. The nurse intentionally touched the mother in an angry manner when the nurse grabbed the mother's arm and pulled her back to the unit, saying firmly, "Where do you think you are going? Stay here. Your baby needs you!" The nurse's behavior constitutes battery, which occurs when someone touches a person's body or clothing or anything held by or attached to the person in an angry, willful, negligent, or violent manner without consent.

D. The triage nurse made the following statement, "The baby's mother is on drugs. She had no business getting pregnant in the first place." This statement was made without any verifiable data and was made loud enough for other health team members to hear. The nurse could be liable for slander, a form of defamation. Defamation, a quasi-intentional tort, occurs when false, derogatory information is communicated to others that harms a person's reputation, holds the person up to ridicule or contempt, or causes the person to be avoided.

Chapter 4—Health-Care System

A. Immunizations are a form of primary health care. Primary health care focuses on maintaining an optimum level of wellness and implementing interventions to decrease the risk of disease or disability.

B. Complete physical examinations, bone density testing, and mammograms are forms of secondary health care. Secondary health care focuses on early detection and intervention to cure disease and minimize further impairment. Treatment includes acute medical care and surgery.

C. Receiving physical therapy and modifying a home to support a person's independence and safety are associated with tertiary health care. Tertiary health care focuses on rehabilitation, health restoration, and palliative care. It maximizes the ability to accomplish activities of daily living, which supports independence in light of a chronic or irreversible condition.

D. Hospice care focuses on maintaining comfort and quality of life for dying clients and provides emotional support for grieving family members. The location of hospice care varies depending on the client's condition and the ability of family members to provide care at home. This family has indicated the desire to care for their loved one at home, so services (e.g., direct physical care, management of pain, emotional support, and advocacy within the health-care system) should be made available to assist them with this goal.

Chapter 5—Leadership and Management

A. 1. The director of nursing seems to prefer the transformational leadership style. The director has a vision that nurses should be expanding their roles within the profession of nursing and implementing evidence-based practice. The statement made to the nurse managers incorporated the director of nursing's vision concerning these topics; was optimistic and energetic; and attempted to inspire others to be committed to the initiative.

2. The nurse manager of the medical unit seems to prefer the autocratic leadership style. The nurse manager was controlling, did not involve staff members in designing the project, and made decisions for the unit. This autocratic style stifles creativity and ultimately may limit commitment of others to the initiative.

B. 1. The director of nursing seems to prefer theory Y of human relations–oriented management, as evidenced by the director's involvement of the nurse managers in identifying a goal (conducting a research project) and inspiring them to achieve it. The director also gave the nurse managers and staff nurses the autonomy to achieve the goal and ensured that a consultant would be hired to support and assist them in attaining the goal. Approaches that encourage participation and creativity and provide support and appreciation are typical of a person who believes in theory Y management.

   2. The nurse manager of the medical unit seems to prefer theory X of human relations–oriented management. An authoritarian approach with strict rules and threats of consequences ("I expect you all to participate in this project, and if you don't, I will have to include that information in your next evaluation.") are typical of a person who believes in theory X management.

C. Examples of resistance.

   1. The nurse manager's statements: "I can't believe we are now going to have to do research projects. Don't you think we do enough already?" and "We are going to be conducting a research project on our unit. I am not thrilled about having to do this, but we have no choice." Both of these statements were attempts to influence others to reach a negative attitude regarding the initiative.

   2. The nurse manager's statement: "Let's talk with the other nurse managers and see if we can reverse this decision." This statement reflects an attempt to organize resistance.

   3. Two nurse mangers did not attend the meeting, stating that they were too busy, and one nurse manager took a day off to avoid the meeting. These avoidance behaviors are forms of passive resistance.

D. 1. Power of authority: Both the director of nursing and nurse managers have power by virtue of their positions within the organization.

   2. Power of coercion: The nurse manager of the medical unit used the power of coercion when threatening staff members with a negative evaluation if they did not participate in the initiative.

   3. Power of expertise: The director of nursing assured the nurse managers that the budget had enough money to hire a nurse researcher to assist the nurses with their projects.

Chapter 6—Critical Thinking and the Nursing Process

A. 1. Skin pale and intact.
   2. Nailbeds pale.
   3. Respirations 23 breaths/minute.
   4. Temperature 97.8°F with temporal scanner thermometer.
   5. Clean and well-groomed appearance.
   6. Apical pulse rate 95 beats/minute.
   7. Blood pressure 160/86 mm Hg.
   8. Vesicular breath sounds.
   9. Slight expiratory wheeze.
   10. Hyperactive bowel sounds.
   11. Tympany when the abdomen was percussed.
   12. Skin dry, warm, and tenting.
   13. Delayed capillary refill.
   14. Slight abdominal distention over suprapubic area.
   15. No lower extremity edema.

B. 1. Client has felt bloated and uncomfortable in the abdominal area for the past several months.
   2. Client does not feel that he empties the bladder fully after voiding.
   3. Client is afraid that he might become impotent and experience urinary incontinence after the surgery.
   4. Client trusts the urologist.
   5. Client verbalizes that he recognizes that the surgery is necessary.
   6. Client stated, "Having cancer puts a big monkey wrench into my retirement plans. I hope I'll live long enough to do a little traveling."
   7. Wife stated, "I don't care if we can't travel. I don't want my husband to die."

C. 1. The client is the only primary source of data. The client is the most valuable source of data because the data collected are most recent, unique, and specific to the client. Only the client can exhibit clinical indicators and share sensations, feelings, and concerns.

   2. The wife is a secondary source of data. A spouse or other family member can provide supplemental information about a client, such as communicating the client's likes and dislikes, functioning before and after the occurrence of the health problem, and similarities and differences in the client's behavior.

   3. The primary health-care provider is a secondary source of data. A primary health-care provider provides supplemental information about the client within the client's frame of reference.

   4. The nurse is a secondary source of data. A nurse provides supplemental information about the client within the client's frame of reference. The nurse obtained a drug handbook and reviewed the side effects of terazosin (Hytrin). Tertiary sources of data include textbooks, policy and procedure manuals, and commonalities among clients with comparable health problems.

Chapter 7—Evidenced-Based Practice

A. 1. Effective breathing promotes the exchange of oxygen and carbon dioxide, which is essential to maintaining life. Air, water, elimination, sleep, activity, sex, and maintenance of body temperature are some of the basic physiological needs necessary for survival. Physiological needs are first-level needs according to Maslow's hierarchy of needs.

2. Although fall prevention is important, it is not the client's priority need. The prevention of falls is related to maintaining client safety. Safety and security needs are second-level needs according to Maslow's hierarchy of needs.

3. Although the needs to be accepted and loved by another are important, they are not the client's priority needs. Giving and receiving affection and maintaining positive relationships with significant others and members of the community are related to love and belonging needs, which are third-level needs according to Maslow's hierarchy of needs.

4. Although the client may have a decreased self-regard, it is not the client's priority need. Feelings of confidence and self-respect are related to self-esteem needs. Self-esteem needs are fourth-level needs according to Maslow's hierarchy of needs.

B. 1. **The physiological-physical mode** relates to basic physiological issues such as oxygenation. The client has increasing shortness of breath and fatigue. The client has so much phlegm that she coughs all the time, can hardly breathe, and is exhausted all the time.

2. **The self-concept mode** relates to threats to the physical or personal self. It includes anxiety and guilt as it relates to physical stressors. The client states that she should have given up smoking when she was diagnosed with emphysema and if she had to do it over again she would do things differently.

3. **The role function mode** relates to the inability to maintain personal life roles. The client states that she has gotten so sick she is on sick-leave from work and she cannot do her usual chores around the house.

4. **The interdependence mode** relates to issues that interrupt a client's ability to maintain significant relationships. There is stress between the client and her significant other. The client was reluctant to come to the clinic but her partner insisted. Her partner hates that she always smells like smoke.

C. The client's statement, "The smoking finally got the best of me. I guess I should have stopped smoking when I was diagnosed with emphysema. If I had to do it over, I would do a lot of things differently," indicates that the client is struggling with Erikson's developmental task of integrity versus despair and tasks related to later maturity in Havighurst's developmental theory. According to Erikson, people 65 years and older are reviewing their life and determining whether their experiences and decisions have been positive or negative. Eventually, they may come to the conclusion that their life accomplishments are acceptable and they develop feelings of self-worth and integrity. On the other hand, if they regret previous actions or decisions, they may develop negative feelings of self-regard and despair. According to Havighurst, tasks that individuals in later maturity are coping with include adjusting to physiological changes of aging and alterations in health. The physiological changes related to aging and emphysema and their impact on quality of life create challenges for the client.

D. The health belief model proposes that a relationship exists between a person's beliefs and behaviors. The theory stipulates that the likelihood of implementing a healthy action is dependent on several factors.

1. The individual's perceived susceptibility to a disease: The client in the scenario already has emphysema; it was diagnosed 10 years ago.

2. The individual's perceived severity of the disease: The client now understands the severity of the disease, as evidenced by the statement: "I have so much phlegm; I cough all the time. I can hardly breathe, and I'm exhausted all the time."

3. The individual's perceived benefits of and perceived barriers to adopting a specific action, as evidenced by the statements, "The smoking finally got the best of me. I guess I should have stopped smoking when I was diagnosed with emphysema. If I had to do it over, I would do a lot of things differently" (benefit) and "I've been smoking since I was 15 years old, but I can't stop" (barrier).

   The client probably did not stop smoking (a major precipitating cause of emphysema) previously because the clinical manifestations of emphysema were tolerable, the pleasures of smoking were more intense than the perceived benefit of stopping smoking, and the client did not have adequate support systems to make the behavioral change. The client now is making statements that indicate a readiness for change. However, if the actions are to be implemented and maintained, the client will require intrapersonal strength, support from significant others, and health-care resources.

Chapter 8—Teaching and Learning

A. The nurse addressed all three learning domains.

1. **Cognitive domain:** During the client's initial hospitalization, the nurse discussed information about diabetes, made a referral to a nutritionist to

provide dietary teaching, and reinforced this teaching at mealtimes. During the counseling center visit, the nurse gave the client written materials and a CD about diabetes and related self-care activities.

2. **Affective domain:** During hospitalization, the nurse initially gave the client the opportunity to discuss his shock and disbelief that he had diabetes, and then the nurse met with the client daily to explore the client's feelings about having diabetes. During the counseling center visit, the nurse continued to explore the client's feelings and concerns to identify the etiology of the client's nonadherence to the medical regimen. The nurse recommended that the client attend a support group for clients with diabetes.

3. **Psychomotor domain:** Before hospital discharge, the nurse taught the client how to perform self-blood glucose monitoring (SBGM) and self-administer a subcutaneous injection. During the counseling center visit, the nurse reviewed SBGM and self-administration of a subcutaneous injection and had the client perform return demonstrations.

B. 1. **The client is a kinesthetic learner.** A kinesthetic learner learns best when processing information by doing. The client stated, "I learn new things better if I can actually do what I am supposed to do."

2. **The client has an external locus of control.** A person who has an external locus of control generally is motivated by pressure or rewards outside of the self, not from within. The client stated, "My wife would kill me if I didn't come this time" and "My wife is on my tail all the time. She doesn't let me out of the house without me taking the insulin."

C. 1. The client is in denial. The client stated, "I can't believe I have to take insulin. No one in my family who has diabetes has to take insulin," and he failed to adhere to the medical regimen. The wife stated, "He's had type 2 diabetes for several years, but he didn't take his pills consistently then and he doesn't take his insulin consistently now, never does the fingerstick test, and eats anything he wants."

2. The client did not attend the first scheduled follow-up visit at the diabetes counseling center. The client came to the next visit because of coercion by his wife. The client stated, "My wife would kill me if I didn't come this time."

3. The client stipulates, "I am not going to give myself insulin at work where everyone can see."

D. 1. **Learning takes place within the learner:** The nurse collected information about what the client already knew about diabetes so that teaching could move from what was familiar to the unknown. The nurse matched teaching strategies to the client's learning style (kinesthetic learner) and learning needs (SBGM and self-administration of a subcutaneous injection) when using the teaching strategy of demonstration and return demonstration of self-care skills.

2. **Learning occurs best in an environment that is physically and emotionally conducive to learning:** The nurse addressed the client's fears and concerns on several occasions before beginning teaching SBGM and self-administration of a subcutaneous injection.

3. **Motivation facilitates learning:** The nurse identified client behaviors that indicated the client's lack of readiness to learn (e.g., client statements indicating denial, failure to attend a counseling appointment, nonadherence to the medical regimen) and explored the client's feelings and concerns to determine the cause of nonadherence to the medical regimen. The nurse accepted the client nonjudgmentally and delayed teaching psychomotor skills.

4. **Literacy, language, and communication are essential components of the teaching and learning process:** The nurse in the hospital used repetition of information in the teaching plan to reinforce learning. The nurse met with the client daily to discuss information about diabetes, explored the client's feelings about having diabetes, and reviewed the principles of a diabetic diet at mealtimes. During the follow-up counseling visit the nurse again explored the client's feelings and concerns and reinforced previous teaching. During the visit the nurse demonstrated the procedures for SBGM and self-administration of a subcutaneous injection and had the client perform return demonstrations. The nurse also gave the client booklets with illustrations and a CD about these procedures.

E. 1. **One-to-one discussion:** In the hospital, the nurse met with the client daily and discussed information about diabetes, explored the client's feelings about having diabetes, and reviewed the diabetic diet at mealtimes. At the subsequent counseling center visit, the nurse primarily provided care in the affective domain by exploring the client's feelings and concerns and referring the client to a support group. This client was attempting to cope emotionally with a chronic health problem with multiple lifestyle changes. One-to-one discussion promotes the nurse-client relationship, allows the nurse to individualize instruction so that it is client centered, and provides an opportunity to address identified concerns

2. **Demonstration:** In the hospital and the subsequent counseling center visit, the nurse demonstrated how to perform SBGM and self-administer

a subcutaneous injection. The nurse also had the client perform a return demonstration of these skills. This client was a kinesthetic learner who learns best when processing information by doing. Demonstration involves hands-on manipulation of equipment with time to practice a skill. During a return demonstration, the nurse can evaluate the client's performance and intervene immediately if further teaching is required. This approach is especially useful when learning a psychomotor skill.

3. **Support group:** The client was referred to a support group for individuals with diabetes. The client initially was having difficulty accepting the diagnosis and adjusting to the medical regimen. A group provides an opportunity for two or more individuals to interact, thereby enhancing learning with the exchange of information. It is particularly effective when addressing issues related to feelings and concerns (affective domain).

F. 1. **Printed materials:** The nurse gave the client printed materials about diabetes while the client was in the hospital and provided additional printed materials (e.g., booklets and written instructions with illustrations about self-care procedures) when the client attended the follow-up counseling session. Written materials support the comprehension of complex concepts and relationships, can be read at the learner's own pace, provide reinforcement of verbal instruction and psychomotor skills, and can be in the client's first language.

2. **Audiovisual aids:** The nurse gave the client a CD that included a demonstration of SBGM and self-administration of a subcutaneous injection. Audiovisual aids present information that stimulates both the eyes and ears. A CD can be used to provide new information or reinforce previous learning.

3. **Equipment and models:** The nurse taught SBGM and administration of a subcutaneous injection in the hospital and during the follow-up counseling session. Blood glucose monitoring equipment, a syringe, a vial, and a model of a client's abdomen were used to learn the skills necessary for self-care. These items stimulate learning because the client has the opportunity to touch and manipulate actual equipment that will be used in the home. The use of equipment and models is extremely effective when teaching psychomotor skills.

Chapter 9—Medication

A. 1. Older adults have a decreased rate of medication metabolism and excretion, which increases the risk of drug toxicity.

2. This client stated that he is forgetful and does not always take his medication every day and also stated that he avoids taking furosemide (Lasix) sometimes because stopping to urinate is inconvenient. Omission of doses does not provide adequate treatment of the client's medical conditions. Also, a forgetful person may accidentally take a double dose of medication, not remembering that the medication was already taken, leading to drug toxicity.

3. The client's limited income may prevent the client from filling his medication prescriptions.

B. 1. Construct a calendar of days and times medications are to be taken.

2. Instruct the client to place medications or signs regarding the medications in a prominent place in the home.

3. Teach the client how to use a divided pill container to minimize the risk of missed doses. If the client is unsure of having taken daily medications, the client only has to refer to the divided-dose container to see if the medications are there or have already been ingested.

C. 1. The furosemide (Lasix) 40 mg IVPB prescription does not contain the frequency at which this medication is to be given.

2. The famotidine (Pepcid) 20 mg bid prescription does not contain the route through which this medication is to be given.

3. The docusate sodium (Colace) 1 tab PO bid prescription does not contain the milligrams contained in 1 tab.

D. 1. Repeat the prescription back to the primary health-care provider for confirmation.

2. Have another nurse listen in to the conversation on the telephone and countersign the prescription.

3. Ensure that the primary health-care provider countersigns the prescription within 24 hours.

Chapter 10—Development Across the Life Span

A. **Assessments that meet developmental norms.**

1. Turns from abdomen to back and from back to abdomen. *This task is usually achieved by age 6 months.*

2. Holds on to the mother and refuses to go to the nurse. *Fear of strangers is common by age 6 to 8 months.*

3. Reacts to simple commands. *This task occurs by age 9 months.*

4. Enjoys peek-a-boo. *This task occurs by age 7 months.*

Assessments that indicate a developmental delay.

1. Is not sitting. *This task is expected by age 7 months.*

2. Is not crawling or pulling self up. *This task is expected by age 9 months.*

3. Is not using a pincer grasp. *This task is expected by age 9 months.*

B. Data typically associated with toddlers:
1. Sucks thumb while holding a security blanket. *These actions are common toddler behaviors that provide self-comfort.*
2. Is fearful of loud noises. *Fear is a common response of toddlers to loud noises because they may perceive it as a threat.*
3. Is always saying "mine" and "no." *Saying "mine" is associated with an increased concept of ownership and the egocentric nature of toddlers. Saying "no" is related to the need to be independent and is common during toddlerhood.*

Data that raise a cause for concern include:
1. Has 14 teeth. *This finding reflects a developmental delay because a toddler should have 20 teeth.*
2. Has made no progress with daytime bladder and bowel control. *Daytime bowel and bladder control should be achieved by age 3 years.*

C. 1. **Cluster:** Climbs stairs using right foot first for each step; hops on two feet. *Most children are able to climb stairs while alternating their feet by age 3 years. Most children are able to hop on one foot by age 4 years.*
Nursing intervention: Consult with the primary health-care provider to ensure that the child is evaluated by a physical therapist and receives physical therapy. Teach the mother to praise the child's accomplishments and to provide supervision, especially when climbing stairs, to maintain safety.
2. **Cluster:** Needs help with dressing and undressing; is unable to tie shoes. *By age 5 years, children should have the coordination to dress and undress themselves and tie their shoes.*
Nursing intervention: Consult with the primary health-care provider to ensure that the child is evaluated by an occupational therapist and receives occupational therapy. Teach the mother to praise the child's accomplishments, encourage self-care activities of daily living, encourage choices, and provide toys that require fine motor skills (e.g., threading beads, age-appropriate crafts, and age-appropriate construction sets).
3. **Cluster:** Does not print letters; has a limited vocabulary. *Children who are 5 years old should be able to print a few letters. By age 3 years, children should know 900 words; by age 4 years, children should know 1,500 words; and by age 5 years, children should know 2,100 words.*
Nursing intervention: Arrange for the child's school district to provide an educational evaluation and receive educational support. Teach the mother to praise the child's progress, work with the child using appropriate activity books that support success, and read to the child.
4. **Cluster:** Is difficult to understand when speaking; has a limited vocabulary. *Children should have totally intelligible speech by age 5 years and should know 2,100 words.*
Nursing intervention: Consult with the primary health-care provider to ensure that the child is evaluated by a speech therapist and receives speech therapy. Teach mother to follow-through with speech exercises daily.

D. 1. Demonstrate some simple chair exercises that the grandmother can accomplish several times a day. *These exercises will increase muscle tone and strength.*
2. Teach safety precautions, such as principles associated with using a walker, the need to keep feet wide apart for a wide base of support, and the need to rise slowly. Also suggest removing any scatter rugs from the environment. *These actions will reduce the risk of a fall.*
3. Assess the grandmother for the risk of suicide. *Risk of suicide increases secondary to multiple losses, such as loss of husband and loss of home and friends due to moving into the daughter's home.*
4. Spend some time encouraging the grandmother to reminisce. *Reminiscence is a component of the task of integrity versus despair associated with older adulthood.*
5. Suggest that the daughter give her mother simple chores to do, such as folding laundry or reading to the toddler and 5-year-old. *These activities contribute to a feeling of task accomplishment and contribution to family life, which should support self-esteem.*
6. Assess the client's perineal area. *This assessment provides information necessary to establish a skin care program to maintain tissue integrity.*

Chapter 11—Diversity and Spirituality/Religion

A. "People who are dying go through various stages. Toward the end of life it is common to see a decreased interest in activities and people as the person prepares to let go of the present life."
B. 1. Assign a female caregiver to provide care to the client.
2. Position the bed so that the client's head is facing toward Mecca.
3. Allow the client to wear her small leather bag around her neck that contains her religious articles.
4. Ensure that the hospital gown and sheets cover the client's body adequately to meet the cultural need to keep covered.

5. Meet any spiritual needs such as a request for a family member or representative to provide a ritual bath after death.

C. 1. Explain the stages of death and dying to family members so that they understand their loved one's behavior and that dying clients may interact minimally with family members.

2. Involve family members in direct care if it is their and the client's wish.

3. Support the comfort of family members. Encourage them to take care of their own needs such as food and rest.

4. Keep family members informed about signs of active dying (e.g., falling BP, diaphoresis, mottled and cold skin.)

5. Explain that moaning and groaning are common when death is near and may not mean that the client is in pain.

6. Encourage that they occasionally talk to their family member even if the client is unconscious.

7. Allow adequate time for family members to remain with the body until they are ready to move on.

8. Accept family member's behavior after the death of a loved one.

Chapter 12—Psychosocial Health

A. 1. **Situational.**
   a. Single parent after abandonment by wife.
   b. Hospitalization and rehabilitation that will require prolonged treatment.
   c. Children living with neighbors.
   d. On medical leave from his job.

2. **Psychosocial.**
   a. Inability to provide for the daily care of his children.
   b. High cost of hospitalization and rehabilitation.
   c. Altered body image as a result of the initial injury and healing ("I look like a monster").
   d. Fears about how his appearance will affect his relationship with his children and coworkers.
   e. Potential for altered family dynamics associated with separation from his children.
   f. Financial concerns related to an inability to work, high cost of hospitalization and rehabilitation, and possible inadequate health insurance.

3. **Developmental.**
   a. Stress of raising three children with little help.
   b. Potential inability to be a wage earner and provide for his children.

4. **Microbiological.**
   a. Risk for microbiological stress as a result of multiple open wounds due to the burn injury.

   b. Potential for decreased immune status due to multiplicity of stresses.

5. **Physiological.**
   a. Pain associated with the burn injury and its treatment.
   b. Potential for fluid and electrolyte imbalances related to the consequences of the burn injury.

B. 1. **Stressors:** See answers to question number 1.

2. **Appearance:** Partial-thickness burns (erythema and blanching with pressure) on the neck, hands, and lower arms, involving more than 12% of the body, and patches of deep partial-thickness burns (erythema, moist blebs, and blisters) on the face, chest, and anterior upper arms, involving 5% of the body. Singed hair on the forehead and sides of the head, absence of eyebrows and eyelashes, singed nostril hair, and sooty sputum noted.

3. **General attitude:** Openly and willingly shared concerns and feelings. Maintained eye contact most of the time.

4. **Activity and behavior:** Increase in muscle tension, voice tremors when talking, and restlessness, as evidenced by nervously moving about in bed and shaking a lower leg; gestures congruent with expressed feelings, evidenced by shaking his head, shrugging his shoulders, and drawing his hand across his throat as if he were cutting his throat.

5. **Sensory and cognitive status:** Alert and oriented to time, place, and person. Able to recall events surrounding the fire. Appropriately receiving and responding to verbal messages.

6. **Thought processes:** Thought processes were well organized, but talked in a rapid manner (pressured speech) when discussing the fire. Content of verbalizations indicated suicide ideation: "Maybe it would be better for the kids if I just killed myself."

7. **Judgment and insight:** Stated, "I have been able to deal with what life has tossed at me because I always want to do right by my kids, but this is more than I can handle. Maybe it would be better for the kids if I just killed myself."

8. **Mood:** Client's data indicate depression as evidenced by a sad facial expression and tone of voice, the comment "Maybe it would be better if I just killed myself," slumped posture, and avoidance of eye contact at times. Client data such as increased muscle tension, pressured speech when discussing the event, voice tremors when talking, and restless behavior (e.g., nervously moving about in bed, shaking a lower leg) indicate anxiety.

9. **Affect:** Varied emotional expression based on content of verbalization. Affect was congruent with mood.

10. **Speech:** Pressured speech when discussing the event, exhibited voice tremors when talking, and at times was hesitant when he became emotional.

11. **Self-concept and self-esteem:** Said he was able to deal with what life had tossed his way in the past but that this event was more than he could handle; believes that he looks like a monster; afraid that his face may scare his children and that he may have to get a new job that enables him to stay in the house so that he does not scare others.

12. **Perception:** No altered perception identified.

13. **Impulse control:** No evidence of a lack of impulse control.

14. **Potential for violence:** Risk for suicide as evidenced by the statement, "Maybe it would be better for the kids if I just killed myself."

15. **Family and social systems:** No evidence of family other than children. One neighbor is caring for his three children until other arrangements can be made.

16. **Spiritual status:** No evidence of spiritual status at this time.

17. **Signs and symptoms of anxiety:** Demonstrating an increase in muscle tension, pressured speech when discussing the event, voice tremors when talking, and restless behavior (e.g., nervously moving about in bed, shaking a lower leg). Several comments indicate that he was worried about finances, anticipation of his children's and coworkers' responses to his appearance, and the need for a change in job in the future.

18. **Use of defense mechanisms:** Used projection when he told his children to "be strong." Used suppression when he said, "This is really going to set me back, but I am not going to worry about that now."

C. The client's statement, "Maybe it would be better for the kids if I just killed myself," is the most important information. Suicide ideation can progress to actual suicide.

D. 1. Provide constant observation and a safe environment.
2. Identify if the client's behavior involves giving away possessions or putting affairs in order as precursors to a suicide attempt.
3. Ask the client whether he has a plan and means to carry out suicide.
4. Focus on strengths rather than weaknesses.
5. Address factors that precipitated the suicide crisis.
6. Encourage exploration of consequences of suicide, such as impact on others if successful, feelings about death, and reasons for living.
7. Assist with problem-solving; help the client to prioritize problems and focus on one at a time.

8. Help the client write a list of sources of support, community resources, and ways to ask for help.
9. Accept feelings of worthlessness, helplessness, and powerlessness as real to the client.
10. Minimize isolation; involve the client in activities.
11. Assist the client to identify and replace self-deprecating thoughts with positive thoughts through cognitive restructuring.
12. Avoid false reassurance and overly cheerfulness.
13. Implement measures to support self-esteem.
14. Monitor risk of suicide as depression lifts and energy increases.

Chapter 13—Grief and Loss

A. The client is experiencing complicated grieving. Complicated (dysfunctional) grieving occurs over an extended length of time (more than 2 years) or involves excessive intensity of emotion or maladaptive responses. It has been 3 years since the client's wife died. The client said that he goes to the cemetery every day and has left the house just as it was the day she passed away. He said, "I just can't go through her clothes or change anything in the house."

B. The client is in the stage of depression. The client recognizes the full impact of his losses. He stated he cannot take care of himself, will have to move into an assisted living facility, and is not well enough to walk his daughter down the aisle. While crying he said, "I am so lonely and sad."

C. 1. Death of his wife 3 years ago.
2. Loss of the ability to walk.
3. Loss of independence.
4. Loss of dignity.
5. Inability to walk his daughter down the aisle on her wedding day.
6. Loss of his home necessitated by the need to move into an assisted living facility.
7. Loss of most of his wife's belongings when he moves into an assisted living facility.

Chapter 14—Physical Assessment

A. 1. Thermometer to obtain the client's body temperature.
2. Sphygmomanometer and stethoscope to obtain the client's blood pressure.
3. Pulse oximetry machine to obtain the client's oxygen saturation level.
4. Stethoscope to listen to the client's apical pulse, breath sounds, and bowel sounds.
5. Ophthalmoscope to assess the client's red eye reflex.
6. Otoscope to assess the client's external auditory canal.

B. 1. **Inspection:** The nurse observed the movement of the client's chest or abdomen to determine the rate and depth of respirations and the intercostal, supra-clavicular, and trapezius muscles to determine the degree of effort necessary for breathing. The nurse inspected the external auditory canal to determine the presence of cerumen. The nurse inspected the eyes to identify that they were glazed and had a limited red eye reflex. The nurse also observed the abdomen to determine if it appeared distended.

2. **Auscultation:** The nurse used auscultation to obtain the client's blood pressure, to listen to the lungs to determine the presence of adventitious breath sounds (e.g., crackles), and to listen to the abdomen to identify the extent of bowel sounds.

3. **Percussion:** The nurse used percussion to identify musical sounds associated with air in the stomach or intestines (tympany).

4. **Palpation:** The nurse used palpation to obtain the radial pulse.

C. 1. **Presence and volume of peripheral pulses:** The nurse should assess the peripheral pulses, beginning with the most distal in the extremity and progressing to the most proximal. Begin with the dorsalis pedis (top of foot slightly above the space between the big and second toe), then the posterior tibial (medial surface of the ankle behind the medial malleolus), and finally the popliteal (behind the knee). They should be assessed for presence, strong volume (obliterated only with moderate pressure), and symmetry. Absent or weak pulses and asymmetry of pulses indicate impaired arterial circulation.

2. **Length of capillary refill:** Compression of the nailbed or tip of the toe should occlude circulation in the capillary bed, causing the area to appear blanched. Release of compression should result in return of circulation and the color that was present before the compression. This assessment should take less than 3 seconds (may take 4 to 5 seconds in older adults) if cardiac output and circulation to the distal extremity are adequate. If capillary refill takes longer than 3 seconds (4 or 5 in older adults), then further assessment of the cardiovascular system is required.

3. **Color and texture of nails:** The color under nails should be a variation of pink, and the nails should be translucent. If the toenails are thick, yellow, and brittle, the client might have inadequate circulation to the distal extremity or a fungal infection under the nail.

4. **Color, texture, and temperature of skin:** Inspection should reveal that the skin is similar in color to the rest of the client's body and its texture is smooth and supple. The skin should be warm to the touch. If the skin is pale, mottled, or red in color, the texture is rough and dry, and the surface temperature is cool to the touch, distal arterial circulation is impaired.

5. **Sensation:** The client should be able to tell what toes are being touched and distinguish between dull and sharp stimuli (e.g., cotton ball versus end of a paper clip). Impaired sensation indicates peripheral nervous system impairment.

6. **Mobility:** The client should be able to curl toes downward (flexion), straighten toes (extension), spread toes apart (abduction), and bring toes together (adduction). If the client is unable to perform range of motion of the toes, motor function may be impaired.

D. A systematic approach must be used when auscultating for sounds produced by the heart, lungs, and intestines to ensure that all areas of significance are assessed. In addition, an appropriate amount of time should be spent at each location, particularly when sounds are complex, difficult to hear, or infrequent.

Chapter 15—Pain, Comfort, Rest, and Sleep

A. 1. Malignant tumor physiologically causing visceral pain.
2. Seven-month duration of the pain experience.
3. Emotions, such as feeling helpless and feeling like a burden.
4. Emotions, such as feeling angry and afraid.
5. Wife killed by a drunk driver 4 months ago.
6. Unfamiliar environment.
7. Noisy and busy environment interfering with rest; constant fatigue.
8. Pain and suffering perceived as penance for wrongdoings during the war.
9. Multiplicity of stressors impacting ability to adapt.

B. 1. "Is there a pattern to the pain?"
2. "What initiates or increases the pain?"
3. "How long does the pain last when it starts?"
4. "What helps to diminish or eliminate the pain?"
5. "Is the pain deep or superficial, and does it radiate to other areas of the body?"
6. "Is this pain different from the pain that you have been experiencing all along?"

C. 1. Assess the client's pain on an ongoing basis.
2. Accept the client's perception of pain.
3. Be nonjudgmental.
4. Validate the client's pain.
5. Treat the client with respect and provide for privacy.
6. Provide opportunities for making choices and being involved in planning care to support independence.

7. Encourage family members to be involved and to provide direct care if desired by the client and family members.

8. Maintain an attitude of caring that precipitates nursing behaviors, such as responding to needs immediately, ensuring continuity of care, and providing information and teaching that are client centered.

9. Provide emotional support and answer questions the client has to relieve anxiety and fears; use interviewing techniques to encourage the client to express feelings and concerns.

10. Use distraction techniques, such as soft music, television, and conversation.

11. Alter irritating stimuli, such as by limiting noise in the environment, closing curtains or doors, dimming environmental lights, and adjusting room temperature to the client's preference.

12. Teach relaxation techniques, such as diaphragmatic breathing, guided imagery, and progressive muscle relaxation.

13. Provide physical comfort measures, such as supporting positioning; providing backrubs; providing for hygiene, oxygen, nutrition, and elimination needs.

14. Pace care to minimize fatigue and the risk of activity intolerance.

15. Accommodate the client's desired spiritual needs, especially related to his perception that the suffering he is experiencing is penance for past wrongdoings.

16. Teach the client the need to inform the nurse immediately if the pain level increases, so that appropriate interventions can be implemented before the pain becomes severe.

17. Correct misconceptions regarding drug tolerance as well as physical and psychological dependence.

18. Evaluate the client's response to nursing intervention, such as the extent of pain relief; decrease in vital signs, particularly respirations; and presence of constipation.

19. Notify the primary health-care provider when an analgesic is ineffective.

20. Document nursing care delivered and the client's response in the client's clinical record.

D. 1. Administer morphine sulfate 6 mg Sub-Q every 4 hours prn for severe pain.

2. Administer oxycodone 2.5 mg + acetaminophen 325 mg (Percocet), 1 tablet PO every 6 hours prn for mild pain and 2 tablets PO every 6 hours prn for moderate pain.

3. Administer acetaminophen (Tylenol) 500 mg, 1 capsule PO every 4 hours prn for temp over 101°F.

4. Administer docusate sodium (Colace) 100 mg PO every 12 hours.

5. Administer sennosides (Senokot) 2 tablets PO h.s. prn for constipation.

Chapter 16—Inflammation, Infection, Immunity, and Wound Care

A. The nurse should collect the wound specimen for C&S first, before the first dose of antibiotic is administered. This is done so that the antibiotic does not influence the results of the culture and sensitivity test.

B. 1. Place the client in a private room or place the client with another client who has the same microorganism *(cohort)* after the client's organism is identified and after consultation with infection control personnel.

2. Implement hand hygiene before entering and when leaving the client's room.

3. Don gloves and a gown after hand hygiene before entering the client's room.

4. When leaving the room, but while still inside the room, untie the ties at the waist, remove gloves, untie ties of the mask and dispose of the mask in an appropriate trash container, and remove the gown by touching only the inside of the gown and place it in an appropriate trash container.

5. Wear other PPE (e.g., mask and face shield) if splashing of body fluids is anticipated.

6. Dedicate client-care equipment so that microorganisms are not transmitted to others via multiple use.

7. Limit the client's movement outside of the isolation room to medically necessary purposes. Infected or colonized areas of the body must be contained and covered when the client is transported outside the room for essential medical purposes. Two people should transport the client. One person is responsible for touching unclean surfaces, such as elevator buttons, and one person is gowned and gloved ready to care for the client if necessary.

C. 1. Importance of leaving belongings in the anteroom outside the client's isolation room.

2. Importance of and proper methods for implementing hand hygiene (i.e., use soap and water meticulously for 15 seconds) before entering the room and putting on an isolation gown and gloves.

3. Proper removal of contaminated gloves and gown without contaminating self or the environment.

4. Proper disposal of contaminated gloves and gown without contaminating the environment.

5. Importance of and proper method for implementing hand hygiene after disposing of contaminated gloves and gown and before leaving the client's room.

D. Yes. Alcohol-based and non–alcohol-based hand sanitizers can be used to reduce the risk of transmission of MRSA when soap and water are not available. However, hand hygiene with soap and water is most effective in preventing the spread of bacterial pathogens.

Chapter 17–Mobility

A. 1. **Ineffective airway clearance:** Maintaining a patent airway is always a priority. A patent airway is necessary to permit exchange of oxygen and carbon dioxide. This client has a diagnosis of pneumonia and is experiencing thick, yellow secretions and a nonproductive cough. Thick secretions can obstruct the airway, causing a life-threatening situation.

2. **Risk for injury:** The client is experiencing multiple problems that place him at risk for injury, such as altered mobility due to Parkinson disease, fatigue related to activity, orthostatic hypotension when changing position, and a history of falls.

3. **Impaired walking:** Walking is the least of the client's problems at this time. Although impaired walking is a problem evidenced by small, shuffling steps with involuntary accelerations due to the effects of Parkinson disease, the client at this time will most likely have a prescription for bedrest. Bedrest is prescribed to minimize exertion. Exertion taxes the respiratory system, which is already compromised by the inflammatory process and thick secretions associated with pneumonia.

B. Propulsive gait and cogwheel gait are terms used to describe the small, shuffling steps with involuntary accelerations associated with Parkinson disease.

C. Stage II pressure ulcer.

D. 1. **Increased cardiac workload:** Decreased gravity pressure redistributes blood from the legs to other parts of the body, resulting in an increase in heart rate, stroke volume, and cardiac output. The heart must work harder when a client is in the supine position than in an erect position.

2. **Thrombus formation:** Venous stasis results from lack of muscle contraction in the legs that promote venous return. In addition, pressure on blood vessels from bedbound or sitting positions causes intima damage that begins the cascade of clot formation. A pulmonary embolus results if a thrombus moves from its place of origin to the lungs.

E. 1. Encourage in-bed exercises to promote muscle contraction and venous return.

2. Encourage the client to change position every 1 to 2 hours to avoid constant pressure on body parts, helping to prevent damage to venous intima or tissue hypoxia.

3. Encourage fluid intake if not restricted to prevent dehydration and hypercoagulability.

4. Apply prescribed venous compression devices to the legs to promote venous return.

5. Teach the client to avoid the Valsalva maneuver, which causes a surge of blood flow when the held breath is released that can dislodge a thrombus if present.

6. Teach the client not to massage the legs, which can dislodge a thrombus if present.

F. 1. Assess the client's status, such as presence of joint stiffness, swelling, or pain; physical ability to perform or assist with exercise; level of motivation; and cognitive ability to follow instructions.

2. Begin each movement with the extremity in functional alignment.

3. Put each joint through the fullest range while moving to the point of resistance.

4. Support each joint distal and proximal to the joint being ranged.

5. Implement range-of-motion exercises slowly, smoothly, and rhythmically; repeat each movement three to five times.

6. Monitor the client's physical, verbal, and nonverbal responses to interventions.

7. Document interventions, extent of mobility of joints, and the client's responses.

G. 1. Seek the assistance of another caregiver to move the client up in bed. *This action shares the stress and strain between two caregivers, decreasing the risk of injury to nursing team members.*

2. Raise the client's bed to waist level. *This places the bed at a working height, which avoids unnecessary stress and strain on the nurse's joints, ligaments, tendons, muscles, and bones.*

3. Lower the head of the client's bed when moving the client up in bed. *This position uses gravity to facilitate moving the client up toward the head of the bed.*

4. Position a pull sheet under the client. *Doing so reduces the risk of shearing forces and also causes less strain and stress on the client than moving the client up by holding on to the client's upper body and extremities. Also, it shares the workload between two caregivers.*

5. Position your body so that you are facing the head of the bed before moving the client. *This position limits stress and strain on the nurse's anatomical structures.*

6. Keep your neck, back, pelvis, and feet in alignment. *Doing so avoids twisting, which stresses anatomical structures.*

7. Spread your feet apart with one foot in front of the other. *Doing so increases stability because the wider the base of support, the more centered is the body mass.*

8. Contract gluteal, abdominal, leg, and arm muscles before the actual move. *This prepares the muscles for action.*

9. Use leg muscles and flex the knees, hips, and ankles when moving the client up in bed. *Doing so permits the larger muscles of the body to provide the power and decreases strain on back muscles.*

10. Move the client toward the head of the bed on the count of three. *Doing so coordinates the action of the two caregivers and the client.*

Chapter 18—Tissue Integrity and Hygiene

A. The nurse must determine whether the client prefers to have only female caregivers. A woman who follows the Islamic faith cannot be touched by a man other than her husband.

B. 1. Identify the size and shape of the lesion in millimeters.
2. Identify the depth of the lesion.
3. Identify the color of the lesion.
4. Identify the presence of exudate and its color and odor if present.

C. 1. The client's wound may be infected.
2. The client may be reluctant to seek assistance with hygiene, grooming, and urine incontinence because privacy and modesty are a hallmark of the Islamic faith.
3. The client may limit activity because it may precipitate pain.
4. The client may be dehydrated. Often, clients who are incontinent of urine do not drink adequate fluid to avoid the frequency of incontinent episodes.
5. The client's skin may be dry and fragile due to the aging process.
6. The client's perineal area may be excoriated because of constant exposure to urea on the surface of the skin.

D. 1. Assign a female caregiver to provide client care if this is the client's preference.
2. Provide a complete bath less frequently according to a client's preference to avoid drying the skin.
3. Keep the client's perineal area clean and dry. Check the client frequently for incontinence of urine and provide perineal care and dry linens and clothing as necessary.
4. Use mild cleansing products to maintain pH balance of the skin and prevent removal of natural moisturizers and lipids that protect the skin.
5. Use a soft cloth and pat skin surfaces dry to avoid damage by abrasion.
6. Apply a moisturizer or emollient after bathing and at least twice a day to make the skin supple and less dry.

E. 1. **Eye:** Each stroke should begin at the inner canthus and progress toward the outer canthus. *This action minimizes secretions from entering the lacrimal duct that is located at the inner canthus.*
2. **Extremities:** Each stroke should begin at the distal portion of the extremity (e.g., fingers and toes) and progress toward the proximal portion of the extremity (e.g., axilla and genital area). *This action promotes venous return.*
3. **Female genitalia:** Each stroke should begin at the top of the labia majora and labia minora and progress toward the anus. *This action follows the principle of "clean to dirty" and prevents fecal material from contaminating the vagina and urinary meatus.*
4. **Male genitalia:** Each stroke should begin at the penile head and using a circular motion progress down the shaft of the penis toward the suprapubic area. This action follows the principle of "clean to dirty" by cleaning the area around the urinary meatus first and then moving toward more soiled perineal areas. *This action prevents dirty matter from entering the urinary meatus. If the client is uncircumcised, then the foreskin must be retracted before cleaning the penis and returned to its natural position after cleaning the penis to prevent constriction of blood flow (phimosis) that can precipitate edema, pain, and even necrosis of the glans penis.*

Chapter 19—Oxygenation

A. **Stridor** is a sign of a potential medical emergency that requires immediate medical intervention. It is a harsh, high-pitched breath sound generally heard on inspiration and is associated with a narrowed or obstructed airway, which can be life threatening. A severe allergic reaction to an allergen, such as smoke from a fire, can cause irritation and inflammation of the respiratory tract mucosa, laryngeal spasm, swelling of the tongue, and irritation and edema of the vocal cords. The client should be assessed frequently for the reoccurrence of stridor because an airway obstruction can be life threatening.

B. 1. **Use of accessory muscles of respiration:** Contraction of the intercostal, abdominal, and trapezius muscles and lifting of the shoulders on inhalation help expand the chest cavity.
2. **Nasal flaring:** Widening of the nares during inhalation decreases airway resistance.
3. **Grunting immediately before exhalation:** A closed glottis at the height of inspiration keeps the alveoli open to enhance gas exchange; the grunt occurs when air is expelled through the larynx.
4. **Pursed-lip breathing:** Exhalation through the mouth with lips positioned to create a small opening prolongs exhalation, keeping alveoli open

longer for gas exchange and more efficient expulsion of trapped air.

5. **Barrel chest:** An increased anteroposterior-to-lateral ratio is associated with chronic retention of carbon dioxide. An expected anteroposterior-to-lateral ratio should be 1:2.

6. **Clubbing of the fingers:** Bulbous swelling of the soft tissue of the end of the phalanx of the fingers causes the nail plates to be equal to or greater than 180°.

7. **Presence of sputum and its characteristics:** Sputum color other than clear may indicate a respiratory problem; for example, yellow-green sputum may indicate infection.

8. **Productive or nonproductive cough:** A productive cough indicates the presence of respiratory secretions. A nonproductive cough indicates an inability to raise secretions if secretions are present, which places the client at risk for impaired gas exchange.

9. **Decreased oxygen saturation level:** A decreased oxygen saturation level indicates the presence of hypoxemia.

C. 1. **Two-pack-a-day smoker with a 20-year history of smoking who experienced secondhand smoke exposure as a child.**
   a. Tobacco smoke contains tars, toxins, and nicotine, which are known to precipitate damage to lung tissue.
   b. Tobacco smoke contains nicotine, which constricts bronchioles.
   c. Tobacco smoke causes mucous membrane inflammation, increases respiratory secretions, breaks down elastin, and decreases the numbers and efficiency of cilia.
   d. Prolonged tobacco use results in chronic bronchitis, smaller diameter of the airways, and loss of alveolar elasticity, leading to emphysema.

2. **Older age.**
   a. As people age, lung compliance and lung elasticity decrease and airway resistance increases, leading to impaired ventilation.
   b. Drier mucus, fewer cilia, a reduced cough efficiency, air trapping in the alveoli, and a decline in immunity in older adults increase the risk of respiratory tract infections.
   c. Other problems, such as gastroesophageal reflux disease (GERD), may result in aspiration, which can precipitate a respiratory infection.

3. **Obesity.**
   a. Excess abdominal adipose tissue limits chest expansion and gas exchange in the alveoli.
   b. Obesity increases the risk of sleep apnea due to an increase in neck girth and fat deposits in the upper airway that obstruct the pharynx.

4. **Smoke from the neighborhood fire.**
   a. Smoke is a pulmonary allergen that can precipitate a respiratory hypersensitivity response.

5. **History of asthma.**
   a. Airborne allergens, such as secondhand smoke, can contribute to asthma and other lung diseases, causing a person to experience chronic airway inflammation and sensitivity to various triggers, instigating an allergic reaction.
   b. Smoke from burning wood and tobacco is a common trigger for an allergic reaction for many individuals who have asthma.

D. 1. Factors to assess.
   a. Vital signs, especially for quality, rate, pattern, and depth of respirations; breathing effort; adventitious breath sounds; oxygen saturation; and signs of hypoxemia (tachycardia, restlessness, headache, lethargy, and confusion).
   b. Clinical indicators of atelectasis (e.g., diminished chest excursion, tachycardia, dyspnea, chest pain, reduced breath sounds, crackles, low oxygen saturation).
   c. Skin color for pallor or cyanosis.
   d. Ability to cough effectively.

2. Support the client in the orthopneic or high-Fowler position.

3. Maintain body alignment for optimal respiratory excursion.

4. Encourage the client to change position every 2 hours.

5. Encourage the intake of 2 to 3 L of fluid by mouth daily if permitted.

6. Encourage coughing and deep breathing every few hours and use of an incentive spirometer, if prescribed.

7. Teach abdominal and pursed-lip breathing techniques.

8. Encourage rest and limit physical activities.

9. Increase activities as tolerated (e.g., progress from passive ROM exercises to active ROM exercises as tolerated).

10. Pace care and schedule rest periods to avoid activity intolerance.

11. Provide for the client's hygiene and grooming needs and increase the client's participation in activities of daily living as tolerated.

12. Anticipate needs.

13. Provide emotional support.

14. Teach about prescribed medications and the use of a medication delivery device, such as metered-dose inhaler and home nebulizer, as indicated.

15. Refer the client to a home health agency if oxygen therapy is required at home.

Chapter 20—Nutrition

A. Nurse's response: Breastfeeding is recommended during the first year of life because it provides the most appropriate nutrients for an infant. It reduces food allergies and intolerances versus cow's milk and is easier to digest. It is convenient, it is the right temperature, and it is economical. Cow's milk is too concentrated for an infant's kidneys to manage, is a poor source of iron and vitamin C and E, and may cause gastrointestinal bleeding.

B.
1. Teach the mother to provide her toddler with opportunities to explore foods with different textures and tastes.
2. Teach the mother to avoid using food, such as ice cream, to motivate, bribe, or punish because this may cause inappropriate food attitudes.
3. Teach the mother to avoid serving hot dogs and peanut butter because they are associated with an increased risk for choking. In addition, French fries are high in calories, "bad fat" (trans fat, unsaturated fat), and salt and are known to increase cholesterol levels contributing to cardiovascular disease.

C.
1. Spending an excessive amount of time in the bathroom. The adolescent may be engaging in activities such as self-induced vomiting or excessive use of diuretics and laxatives.
2. Gorging followed by self-induced vomiting. Binging and purging are associated with the eating disorder bulimia nervosa.
3. Spending an excessive amount of time exercising. Exercising is an attempt to lose weight.
4. Complaining of a sore throat. A sore throat may indicate mucosal contact with gastric acid during vomiting.
5. Excessive dental caries, enamel erosion, and staining of teeth. These signs may be due to contact with gastric acid during vomiting.
6. Diarrhea. This can result from excessive laxative use.
7. Dehydration. This can result from the excessive use of diuretics and laxatives.
8. Excessive weight loss and muscle wasting. These are signs of malnutrition.
9. Arrested sexual development; amenorrhea. Adequate nutrition and body weight are essential for functioning of the endocrine and reproductive systems.

D.
1. Encourage the grandmother to make an appointment with a dentist for dental care.
2. Encourage the grandmother to chop or puree her food until dental care is implemented.
3. Encourage the intake of foods high in nutritive value to ensure adequate nutritional intake.
4. Encourage between meal snacks that are high in nutritive value to meet caloric needs.
5. Encourage the avoidance of salt when cooking and suggest the use of alternate spices.
6. Provide the grandmother with information about local senior citizens organizations to increase her social life with peers.

E.
1. Teach the mother how to maintain a balanced daily diet to meet nutritional needs of herself and her infant.
2. Encourage the avoidance of alcohol, caffeine, and medications not specifically prescribed by her primary health-care provider because these are transferred via breast milk.
3. Teach the mother to avoid tobacco use because it decreases milk production and is an unhealthy habit.

F.
1. Encourage consultation with a primary health-care provider and a nutritionist to determine a weight reduction regimen that is appropriate for a lactating mother.
2. Encourage the mother to use a food diary to help develop insight into eating habits.
3. Help the mother to identify realistic objectives and to review them weekly.
4. Help the mother to understand that healthy eating needs to be an enduring lifestyle change.
5. Explain how to read a nutrition facts label to identify foods that are high in calories, fat, and carbohydrates that should be reduced when on a weight reduction diet.
6. Teach the mother to avoid food shopping when hungry to reduce the temptation to buy inappropriate comfort foods.
7. Encourage the intake of fresh fruits and vegetables.
8. Encourage incorporation of nutritious morning and afternoon snacks into the meal plan to minimize the desire to graze throughout the day.
9. Encourage the mother to serve food on small plates, take small bites, chew food well, eat slowly and put the fork or spoon down between bites.
10. Encourage participation in an exercise program to increase the resting metabolic rate.
11. Encourage adequate sleep because sleep deprivation negatively affects the hormones leptin and ghrelin that regulate appetite. This may be a challenge with an infant or young child in the household.
12. Encourage participation in a support group, such as Weight Watchers or Overeaters Anonymous, where a person is weighed weekly to evaluate progress and where emotional support is provided.

Chapter 21—Fluid, Electrolyte, and Acid-Base Balance

A. 1. Client states, "I can't seem to keep anything down."
2. Client reports feeling weak and dizzy.
3. Client reports experiencing nausea, vomiting, and diarrhea for 3 days.
4. Client reports currently taking hydrochlorothiazide (HCTZ).

B. 1. Vital signs that indicate hypovolemia.
2. Tenting over sternum.
3. Sticky, dry oral mucosa, cracked lips.
4. Oliguria and dark amber urine.
5. Weight loss of 5 pounds.
6. Unsteadiness when transferring from chair to bed.

C. Dehydration.

D. 1. **Temperature of 99°F:** An older adult may have an inefficient thermoregulatory mechanism resulting in a decrease in perspiration. The temperature increases because a dehydrated older adult is less able to cool the body via vaporization due to the decrease in perspiration.
2. **Weak, thready pulse of 126 beats/minute with a regular rhythm:** As blood volume decreases, the heart contracts more quickly but less powerfully, causing a rapid, weak, thready pulse.
3. **Blood pressure of 98/64 mm Hg; orthostatic hypotension when moving from sitting to standing position:** Orthostatic hypotension is caused by hypovolemia associated with dehydration. When a client moves from a lying down to a sitting position or from a sitting to a standing position, fluid pools in the lower extremities until the baroreceptors react to the change in position and precipitate vasoconstriction.
4. **Respirations of 26 breaths/minute with a regular rhythm:** Respirations increase in an attempt to increase the amount of oxygen reaching body cells; the need for oxygen increases when the body's metabolic rate increases.
5. **Cracked lips, sticky and dry oral mucosa, and tenting (decreased turgor):** Fluid moves from within cells (intracellular compartment) to between cells (interstitial compartment) and then into blood vessels (intravascular compartment) in an attempt to maintain the circulating blood volume.
6. **Fatigue and weakness:** Fatigue and weakness are caused by electrolyte imbalances, such as a low potassium level (hypokalemia) and a high sodium level (hypernatremia).
7. **Oliguria and concentrated urine:** Oliguria and concentrated urine occur as the body attempts to conserve water; the urine that is excreted is more concentrated (less diluted) due to a higher percentage of waste product to water than when water is not being conserved by the kidneys.
8. **Five-pound weight loss in less than 1 week:** One liter of fluid weighs 2.2 pounds. The client lost over 3.6 L of fluid in less than 1 week. A quick weight loss is related to fluid loss, not a loss of tissue mass.

E. 1. **Elevated serum Na$^+$:** An increased serum sodium level indicates dehydration because the number of sodium ions increases in relation to the amount of the remaining circulating volume (hemoconcentration). Normal serum sodium is 135 to 145 mEq/L.
2. **Elevated blood urea nitrogen:** Elevated blood urea nitrogen levels occur due to hemoconcentration related to dehydration. Normal levels are 8 to 21 mg/dL.
3. **Elevated urine specific gravity:** Increased urine specific gravity levels occur due to concentration of urine as the body attempts to conserve water. Normal range is 1.001 to 1.029.
4. **Elevated serum creatinine:** An increased serum creatinine level is associated with dehydration due to hemoconcentration. Normal range is 0.5 to 1.2 mg/dL.
5. **Elevated hemoglobin:** With dehydration, the total blood volume decreases, but the volume of RBCs remains the same, resulting in hemoconcentration. The normal range is 14 to 18 g/dL in a male; critical levels are 20 g/dL or more.
6. **Elevated hematocrit:** Hematocrit reflects the proportion of red blood cells (RBC) to blood plasma. Total blood volume is decreased with dehydration, but the number of RBCs remains the same, resulting in hemoconcentration. Normal hematocrit levels are 40% to 50%; critical levels are more than 60%.
7. **Decreased serum K$^+$:** A decreased serum potassium level results from gastrointestinal losses due to vomiting and diarrhea as well as losses via the kidneys in response to diuretic therapy. Normal serum potassium levels are 3.5 to 5 mEq/L; critical levels are less than 2.5 mEq/L.

F. 1. **Vital signs.**
a. Assess vital signs every 4 hours and when necessary.
2. **Diagnostic tests.**
a. Obtain a stool specimen for culture and sensitivity (C&S).
b. Obtain a urine specimen for C&S and urinalysis.
c. Obtain blood specimens for complete blood count (CBC) and basic metabolic panel (BMP).
3. **Nutrition.**
a. Maintain NPO status.
4. **Activity.**
a. Transfer the client to a chair for 1 hour two times daily.

5. **Hydration.**
   a. Monitor I&O and weight daily.
   b. Assess for nausea and vomiting.
   c. Administer IVF 1,000 mL 0.45% NaCl, 20 mEq KCl, at 125 mL/hour.
6. **Hygiene.**
   a. Provide frequent mouth care.
   b. Apply a water-soluble lubricant to the lips.
   c. Keep skin and linens clean and dry.
   d. Provide perianal hygiene immediately after an episode of diarrhea.
   e. Apply skin barrier ointment to the perianal area per protocol.
   f. Provide privacy and use room deodorizers.
7. **Prescribed medications.**
   a. Discontinue hydrochlorothiazide and explain to the client the rationale for it being discontinued.
   b. Ondansetron (Zofran ODT) 8 mg sublingual every 8 hours prn for nausea.
   c. Acetaminophen (Tylenol) 325 mg every 4 hours prn for temperature more than 101°F.
   d. Ensure that KCl 20 mEq is added to IVF 1,000 mL 0.45% NaCl.
8. **Health teaching.**
   a. Teach about foods high in potassium to include in the diet if a non–potassium-sparing diuretic is prescribed.
   b. Teach the importance of and proper technique for taking blood pressure and weight daily when at home.

G. 1. **Vital signs:** Assess the client's vital signs to determine whether temperature, pulse, and respirations are decreasing and blood pressure is increasing, indicating a movement toward fluid balance and an appropriate circulating blood volume.
   2. **Laboratory results:** Monitor the laboratory results of a CBC and BMP to determine the client's fluid volume and electrolyte status in response to the therapeutic regimen. Specific laboratory results should be moving toward the normal range.
   3. **Intake and output (I&O):** Monitor I&O to identify a greater intake versus output until dehydration is resolved and then ensure that intake and output remain balanced.
   4. **Complications of fluid overload:** Assess for clinical indicators of the complication of fluid overload in response to excessive rehydration therapy, such as bounding pulse; increased blood pressure; increased respirations and pulse; distended neck veins; decreased HCT, Hb level, and BUN levels; and signs of pulmonary edema with severe fluid overload, such as presence of crackles, dyspnea, and shortness of breath.

Chapter 22–Urinary Elimination

A. 1. **Age:** Older adults experience a decline in urinary system functioning. They are less able to filter waste and maintain acid-base and fluid and electrolyte balance. They also experience a loss of bladder tone, contributing to urgency, frequency, and incomplete emptying of the bladder. Most importantly, this client is experiencing an enlarged prostate, which is associated with aging.
   2. **Alcohol intake:** Excessive alcohol intake reduces the release of antidiuretic hormone, increasing urine production.
   3. **Caffeine intake:** Caffeine increases urine production.
   4. **Sodium intake:** Potato chips contain a large amount of sodium, which produces water retention, causing a decrease in urine production.
   5. **Smoking history:** Nicotine irritates the detrusor muscle, causing bladder contractions and urinary urgency.
   6. **Sedentary lifestyle:** Lack of exercise leads to decreased bladder tone, which can cause incomplete emptying of the bladder when voiding. Stasis of urine in the bladder can contribute to urinary tract infections.
   7. **Enlargement of the prostate:** Prostate enlargement can cause a narrowing of the urethra, resulting in incomplete emptying of the bladder and eventual obstruction, causing urinary retention.
   8. **Comorbidity of heart disease:** Heart disease can diminish blood flow through the kidneys, reducing the glomerular filtration rate (GFR).
   9. **Sharing a bathroom with others:** Sharing a bathroom may cause a delay in responding to the need to empty the bladder, which can decrease bladder tone and contribute to urinary stasis.
   10. **History of urinary tract infections:** An enlarged prostate (an obstructive problem) increases the risk of urinary retention, which leads to the potential for urinary tract infection.
   11. **Medications:** Many classifications of drugs can be nephrotoxic or cause urinary retention. The client is receiving a diuretic, an antihistamine, and an antidepressant, which can cause side effects associated with the urinary system.

B. 1. Presence of small, frequent incontinence episodes.
   2. Presence of urinary dribbling.
   3. Presence of urgency.
   4. Presence of blood in the urine.
   5. Decreased daily urine output.
   6. Sudden weight gain.
   7. Dependent edema.

C. 1. **Hydrochlorothiazide 50 mg PO daily in a.m.:** Diuretics interfere with water reabsorption, causing an increase in urine output.

2. **Loratadine (Claritin) 10 mg PO daily:** Antihistamines have an anticholinergic effect that inhibits involuntary contractions of the bladder, which increases the capacity of the bladder and delays the urge to void; urinary retention is a side effect.

3. **Sertraline (Zoloft) 50 mg PO hour of sleep:** This selective serotonin reuptake inhibitor (SSRI) may cause urinary side effects, such as frequency or urinary retention.

D. **Common principles associated with caring for clients with any type of urinary catheter.**

1. Place the collection bag and tubing below the level of the bladder.
2. Curl excess tubing on the bed.
3. Secure the catheter to the client's anterior thigh or abdomen for a male client.
4. Ensure that the client is not lying on the tubing and that the tubing is under, not passed through, the side rails.
5. Assess the catheter frequently to ensure tube patency.
6. Ask the client about the presence or absence of bladder spasms.
7. Administer pain medication as prescribed and needed.
8. Assess the amount and characteristics of urine; assess hourly volumes as prescribed to assess GFR, and notify the primary health-care provider if output is equal to or less than 30 mL/hour.
9. Maintain safety when ambulating a client with a urinary catheter; hold the catheter tubing so that the client does not step on it and to ensure that it does not drag along the floor.
10. Teach the client about self-care management of the urinary catheter.
11. Document the client's status, care provided, and client responses in the client's clinical record.

Specific principles when caring for a client with a triple-lumen urinary catheter for continuous bladder irrigation.

1. Maintain the irrigating solution flow rate as prescribed, usually a prescribed amount of flow or to "keep output pink."
2. Increase the irrigating solution flow rate to keep the output free from blood clots.
3. Deduct the volume of irrigating solution from the urinary output to accurately document urine output.

Chapter 23—Bowel Elimination

A. 1. Fecal urgency.
2. Hyperactive bowel sounds.
3. Flatus.
4. Anorexia.

5. Nausea and vomiting.
6. Blood in the stool (frank or occult).

B. 1. Decreased tissue turgor.
2. Furrows of the tongue.
3. Flushed, dry skin and mucous membranes.
4. Sunken eyeballs.
5. Hypotension and orthostatic hypotension.
6. Atonic muscles.
7. Mental confusion.
8. Decreased urine output.

C. After having surgery for a total knee replacement, the client experienced a wound infection requiring antibiotic therapy. Antibiotics can suppress the normal GI flora, permitting opportunistic infections to flourish in the bowel. Stool that is malodorous and greenish in color is indicative of *Clostridium difficile* infection. *C. difficile* is a bacterium that causes diarrhea and can extend to a life-threatening inflammation of the colon (pseudomembranous colitis).

D. Stool specimens for C&S, ova and parasites, and *C. difficile* should be collected first. If an antibiotic is implemented before collecting stool specimens, the test results may be inconclusive. Microorganisms might not grow after exposure to an antibiotic or their volume in the specimen may decrease, causing uncertain test results.

E. 1. Factors to assess.
   a. Vital signs and BP every 4 hours.
   b. Daily weight.
   c. Stool for frequency, amount, consistency, color, odor, and other characteristics.
   d. Clinical indicators of fluid volume deficit and electrolyte imbalances.
   e. Perianal area for excoriation.
   f. Bowel sounds.
2. Maintain contact precautions.
3. Monitor I&O.
4. Assist with elimination, provide for privacy, and use air fresheners discretely.
5. Provide perineal care, such as providing for hygiene and using a protective skin barrier or emollient, per protocol.
6. Maintain NPO status and progress the client's diet as prescribed.
7. Increase oral fluid intake gradually once permitted because large amounts can precipitate peristalsis.
8. Administer prescribed metronidazole (Flagyl).
9. Administer D_5 in 0.45% NaCl at 125 mL/hour.
10. Provide health teaching once client is advanced to a regular diet.
   a. Discourage intake of spicy and fatty foods, caffeine, and high-fiber foods until after the acute infection is resolved.
   b. Discourage the intake of hot and cold fluids because they stimulate peristalsis.

c. Encourage intake of foods high in sodium, such as tomatoes and bouillon, and foods high in potassium, such as bananas, oranges, apricots, and potatoes, as the diet is advanced.

d. Teach the client to perform perianal skin care after each bowel movement.

11. Evaluate the client's responses to nursing interventions.

12. Document assessments, interventions, and client responses in the client's clinical record.

Chapter 24—Perioperative Care

A. Curative. Removal of the uterus, fallopian tubes, and ovaries is curative in its purpose. Excision or repair of a diseased organ via surgery is a therapeutic intervention to achieve a cure.

B. Elective. Because this client is diagnosed with a benign fibroid of the uterus, the client's surgery is considered to be elective. Elective surgery includes surgical interventions that are advised but are for reasons that do not imminently threaten the client's life.

C. Major. This surgery is considered major surgery because the incision enters the abdominal cavity and requires the removal of organs and structures. Also, the client is at risk for postoperative complications because of the client's age, obesity, and preexisting conditions of diabetes and hypertension.

1. Older adults experience a decrease in physiological reserves, such as decreased cardiac output, cough reflex, immunity, vital capacity, subcutaneous tissue, blood oxygenation, glomerular filtration rate, and basal metabolic rate.

2. Older adults experience increased calcium and cholesterol deposits within small arteries that increase the risk of hypertension, fluid and electrolyte imbalances, and shock when blood loss occurs.

3. Obesity can decrease postoperative ventilation and cardiac function.

4. Obesity is associated with increased wound complications, such as delayed wound healing, dehiscence (separation of the wound edges), evisceration (protrusion of the abdominal viscera through the incision), and wound infection because adipose tissue contains a limited blood supply.

5. Diabetes mellitus increases the risk of infection and delayed wound healing because of a reduced ability to metabolize carbohydrates, proteins, and fat.

D. 1. Stable vital signs.

2. Presence of spontaneous respirations or effective mechanical ventilator function.

3. Easy arousal.

4. Absence of complications.

5. Aldrete score of 8 to 10.

E. 1. Assign each drainage device a number to ensure that each site is assessed independently. Generally, when drainage volume from a device decreases to less than 10 mL in 24 hours, it is discontinued.

2. Assess the area around the drain insertion sites for clinical indicators of inflammation or infection; this supports early treatment if these problems occur.

3. Cover the sites with sterile dressings to protect the exit wounds from environmental pathogens.

4. Maintain the collection bulbs below the insertion sites because this uses gravity to move drainage toward the bulbs. This is in addition to the negative pressure within the portable wound drainage system.

5. Secure collection bulbs in place and attach them to the client's gown to prevent tension on the tubing.

6. Empty a collection bulb when half full to prevent the weight of a bulb from pulling on the tubing; a less than half-full bulb maintains effective negative pressure. As the volume of drainage in a bulb increases, the extent of negative pressure decreases.

7. Maintain sterility when opening and closing a drainage port to prevent contamination of the port and drain.

8. Wear gloves when emptying the bulb to protect self from the client's body fluids. To empty the bulb open the port and drain the contents into a measuring container without touching the inside of the port; do not touch the measuring container with the port to maintain port sterility and reduce the risk of infection.

9. Compress the collection bulb, close the port, and release the hand compressing the bulb to reestablish negative pressure.

10. Measure the volume and characteristics of drainage to assess the status of the drainage. Expect drainage to progress from sanguinous to serosanguineous to serous. Notify the primary health-care provider if the volume of drainage is greater than the amount expected.

11. Discard drainage in the toilet and flush twice, remove and dispose gloves, and wash your hands to limit the spread of microorganisms.

12. Document the volume and characteristics of drainage; if more than one device is present, document findings according to the assigned number of the device to ensure the accuracy of the status of each device.

F. Postoperative hemorrhage is a concern because the client was taking clopidogrel (Plavix), which has antiplatelet activity. In addition, the client was taking ginseng, which also has antiplatelet activity. Having taken clopidogrel and ginseng recently increases the risk of postoperative bleeding.

G. 1. Tachycardia.
2. Tachypnea.
3. Increased diastolic blood pressure.
4. Narrowed pulse pressure.
5. Pale, cool, clammy skin.
6. Prolonged capillary refill.
7. Urine output less than 20 to 30 mL/hour.
8. Restlessness.
9. Anxiety.
10. Confusion.

H. 1. **Pneumonia** is a concern because obesity interferes with a client's ability to deep breathe, thereby leading to stagnation of respiratory secretions.
2. **Wound infection** is a concern because of the size and depth of the wound required to accomplish the surgery. In addition, the client's comorbidity of diabetes increases the risk of wound infection because elevated levels of serum glucose support growth of pathogens and because a reduced ability to metabolize carbohydrates, proteins, and fat delays wound healing.
3. **Thromboembolism** is a concern because of venous relaxation that occurs during anesthesia and atherosclerosis associated with diabetes.
4. **Wound dehiscence and evisceration** are a concern with obesity because excessive weight places added stress and strain on the incision and adipose tissue contains a limited blood supply, delaying wound healing. The client's comorbidity of diabetes additionally contributes to delayed wound healing because of a reduced ability to metabolize carbohydrates, proteins, and fat.

I. 1. Engage in meticulous hand hygiene practices.
2. Change wound dressing as prescribed, keeping the wound clean and dry.
3. Maintain sterile technique when changing dressings or when opening and closing drains.
4. Encourage foods high in protein and vitamin C to promote wound healing.
5. Encourage fluid intake as prescribed.
6. Administer antibiotics prophylactically as prescribed.
7. Ensure that roommates are free from infection.
8. Ensure that the client's environment is meticulously cleaned.

9. Ensure that family members and visitors understand that they should not visit the client if they have an infection.

J. 1. Encourage exercises, such as performing flexion and extension of the ankles (ankle pumping) and knees and raising the legs off of the bed, to facilitate venous return. Doing so minimizes venous stasis, thereby reducing the risk of thrombophlebitis. Matter associated with thrombophlebitis can become an embolus that gets carried via the vasculature and lodges in a pulmonary vessel, which is a life-threatening condition.
2. Teach the client to avoid using pillows behind the knees and raising the lower portion of the bed into the contour position (gatching the bed); this minimizes popliteal pressure and increases venous blood flow, preventing venous stasis.
3. Apply prescribed antiembolism stockings or sequential compression devices to facilitate venous return, which minimizes venous stasis, thereby reducing the risk of thrombophlebitis.
4. Provide progressive ambulation as prescribed to facilitate venous return, which minimizes venous stasis, thereby reducing the risk of thrombophlebitis. Activity, such as ambulation, increases the depth and rate of respirations as the body attempts to bring more oxygen to muscles. When respirations increase in depth, the lower areas of lungs are aerated, thereby minimizing the risk of stasis of pulmonary secretions.
5. Administer prescribed prophylactic heparin 5,000 units Sub-Q every 12 hours; this interferes with normal coagulation to decrease the risk of thrombus formation.

K. The nurse should verify the prescription for regular insulin coverage and administer the dose based on the client's blood glucose result. The prescription indicates that a serum glucose level of 201 to 300 mg/dL requires administration of 4 units of regular insulin via the subcutaneous route. Therefore, the nurse should administer 4 units of regular insulin via the subcutaneous route.

Bibliography

Chapter 1—Safety

Akron Children's Hospital. (n.d.). *Gun safety.* Retrieved July 19, 2016, from https://www.akronchildrens.org/cms/kidshealth/efef5a40d0022cdc/index.html.

American Academy of Pediatrics. (n.d.). *Forward-facing car seats for toddlers & preschoolers.* Retrieved July 19, 2016, from https://www.healthychildren.org/English/safety-prevention/on-the-go/Pages/Forward-Facing-Car-Seats-for-Toddlers-Preschoolers.aspx.

American Academy of Pediatrics. (2016). *Rear-facing car seats for infants & toddlers.* Retrieved July 19, 2016, from https://www.healthychildren.org/English/safety-prevention/on-the-go/Pages/Rear-Facing-Car-Seats-for-Infants-Toddlers.aspx.

Booth, J., & Edwards, A. R. (2011). *Four-point restraint.* Retrieved July 19, 2016, from http://emedicine.medscape.com/article/1941454-overview#a1.

Centers for Disease Control and Prevention. (2002). Guideline for hand hygiene in health-care settings: Recommendations of the Healthcare Infection Control Practices Advisory Committee and the HICPAC/SHEA/APIC/IDSA Hand Hygiene Task Force. *MMWR Recommendations and Reports, 51*(RR-16), 1–44. Retrieved July 16, 2016, from http://www.cdc.gov/mmwr/PDF/rr/rr5116.pdf.

Centers for Disease Control and Prevention. (2012). *10 Leading causes of death by age group, United States—2012.* Retrieved July 19, 2016, from http://www.cdc.gov/injury/wisqars/pdf/leading_causes_of_death_by_age_group_2012-a.pdf.

Centers for Disease Control and Prevention. (2013). *Hand hygiene saves lives.* Retrieved July 18, 2016, from http://www.cdc.gov/cdctv/healthyliving/hygiene/hand-hygiene-saves-lives.html.

Centers for Disease Control and Prevention. (2015). *Important facts about falls.* Retrieved July 19, 2016, from http://www.cdc.gov/homeandrecreationalsafety/falls/adultfalls.html.

Centers for Disease Control and Prevention. (2015). *Leading causes of death.* Retrieved July 19, 2016, from http://www.cdc.gov/nchs/fastats/leading-causes-of-death.htm.

Centers for Disease Control and Prevention. (2016). *2014 Nonfatal data, injury prevention & control: Data & statistics (WISQARTS™).* Retrieved July 19, 2016, from http://www.cdc.gov/injury/wisqars/index.html.

Centers for Disease Control and Prevention. (2016). *Home & recreational safety: Unintentional drowning: Get the facts.* Retrieved July 19, 2016, from http://www.cdc.gov/HomeandRecreationalSafety/Water-Safety/waterinjuries-factsheet.html.

Giardino, A., DeLago, C., Kersten, H., Matz, P., McGregor, R., Smals, L., & Spector, N. (2007). *Child safety: A pediatric guide for parents, teachers, nurses and caregivers.* St. Louis, MO: STM Learning.

Halm, M. (2009). Hourly rounds: What does the evidence indicate? *American Journal of Critical Care, 18*(6), 581–584. Retrieved May 29, 2012, from http://ajcc.aacnjournals.org/content/18/6/581.full.

Institute for Healthcare Improvement. (n.d.). *Patient safety.* Retrieved July 19, 2016, from http://www.ihi.org/Topics/PatientSafety/Pages/default.aspx.

Maslow, A. H. (1970). *Motivation and personality* (2nd ed.). New York: Harper & Row.

Morse, J. (2009). *Preventing patient falls: Establishing a fall intervention program* (2nd ed.). New York: Springer.

National Highway Traffic Safety Administration. Seat belt use in 2015–overall results. *Traffic safety facts.* Retrieved July 19, 2015, from https://crashstats.nhtsa.dot.gov/Api/Public/ViewPublication/812243.

National Patient Safety Foundation. (n.d.). *NPSF at a glance.* Retrieved July 20, 2016, from http://www.npsf.org/?page=npsfataglance.

National Safety Council. (n.d.). *Hot cars, improper safety seats, teen driver error all put children at risk.* Retrieved July 19, 2016, from http://www.nsc.org/learn/safety-knowledge/Pages/Child-Passenger-Safety.aspx.

Nelson, A. (Ed.). (2009). *The illustrated guide to safe patient handling and movement.* New York: Springer.

O'Donnell, J. (2014). New regulations sought for child car seats. *USA Today,* January 23.

Privitera, M. (Ed.). (2011). *Workplace violence in mental and general health settings.* Sudbury, MA: Jones & Bartlett.

Sherwood, G., & Barnsteiner, J. (Eds.). (2012). *Quality and safety in nursing: A competency approach to improving outcomes.* Hoboken, NJ: Wiley-Blackwell.

The Joint Commission. (2016). 2016 *National patient safety goals.* Retrieved July 19, 2016, from https://www.jointcommission.org/standards_information/npsgs.aspx.

The Leapfrog Group. (n.d.). *Safe practices.* Retrieved July 19, 2016, from http://www.leapfroggroup.org/ratings-reports/safe-practices.

Tideiksaar, R. (2010). *Falls in older people: Prevention and management* (4th ed.). Baltimore, MD: Health Professions Press.

University of Michigan Health System. (2010). *Gun safety for kids and youth.* Retrieved July 20, 2016, from www.med.umich.edu/yourchild/topics/guns.htm.

U.S. Department of Labor & Occupational Safety and Health Administration. (n.d.). *OSHA law & regulations.* Retrieved July 20, 2016, from https://www.osha.gov/law-regs.html.

Wall, J., Churan, B., Campbell, S., & Davis, J. (2000). The timed get-up-and-go test revisited: Measurement of the component tasks. *Journal of Rehabilitation Research & Development, 37*(1), 109–114.

World Health Organization. (2012). *Falls.* Retrieved July 20, 2016, from http://www.who.int/mediacentre/factsheets/fs344/en/.

Chapter 2—Communication, Collaboration, and Documentation

Antai-Otong, D. (2006). *Nurse-client communication: A life span approach.* Burlington, MA: Jones & Bartlett Learning.

Arnold, E., & Boggs, K. (2015). *Interpersonal relationships: Professional communication skills for nurses* (7th ed.). St. Louis, MO: Elsevier Health Sciences.

Diefenbeck, C., Paulanka, B., & Phillips, K. (2011). *Interpersonal skills for healthcare professionals—Student version.* Philadelphia: F. A. Davis.

Haig, K., Sutton, S., & Whittington, J. (2006). SBAR: A shared mental model for improving communication between clinicians. *Joint Commission Journal on Quality and Patient Safety, 32*(3). Retrieved July 17, 2016, from http://www.1000livesplus.wales.nhs.uk/sitesplus/documents/1011/Whittington_SBAR_JtCommJ_Mar06.pdf.

Institute for Healthcare Improvement. (2016). *SBAR technique for communication: A situational briefing model.* Kaiser Permanente of Colorado. Retrieved July 16, 2016, from http://www.ihi.org/resources/Pages/Tools/SBARTechniqueforCommunicationASituationalBriefingModel.aspx.

Institute for Safe Medication Practices (ISMP). (2012). *ISMP's list of error-prone abbreviations, symbols, and dose designations.* Retrieved July 15, 2016, from http://www.ismp.org/Tools/errorproneabbreviations.pdf.

Munoz, C., & Luckman, J. (2005). *Transcultural communication in nursing* (2nd ed.). Clifton Park, NY: Cengage Learning.

Riley, J. (2017). *Communication in nursing* (8th ed.). St. Louis, MO: Elsevier Health Sciences.

Schuster, P. (2010). *Communication for nurses: How to prevent harmful events and promote patient safety.* Philadelphia: F. A. Davis.

Sheldon, L. (2013). *Communication for nurses: Talking with patients* (3rd ed.). Sudbury, MA: Jones & Bartlett.

The Joint Commission. (2016). *Facts about the official "Do Not Use" list.* Retrieved July 16, 2016, from https://www.jointcommission.org/facts_about_do_not_use_list/.

Webb, L. (Ed.). (2011). *Nursing: Communication skills in practice.* New York: Oxford University Press.

Chapter 3—Legal and Ethical Issues

American Hospital Association. (2003). *The patient care partnership: Understanding expectations, rights and responsibilities.* Retrieved July 15, 2016, from www.aha.org/content/00-10/pcp_english_030730.pdf.

American Nurses Association. (2013). *Position statement: Euthanasia, assisted suicide, and aid in dying.* Retrieved November 16, 2016, from http://www.nursingworld.org/MainMenuCategories/EthicsStandards/Ethics-Position-Statements/Euthanasia-Assisted-Suicide-and-Aid-in-Dying.pdf.

American Nurses Association (ANA). (2015). *Code of Ethics for Nurses.* Retrieved November 16, 2016 from http://www.nursingworld.org/MainMenuCategories/EthicsStandards/CodeofEthicsforNurses.aspx.

American Nurses Association. (2016). *Nurses' bill of rights.* Retrieved July 15, 2016, from http://nursingworld.org/NursesBillofRights.

Burkhardt, M. A., & Nathaniel, A. (2014). *Ethics & issues in contemporary nursing* (4th ed.). Stamford, CT: Cengage Learning.

Guido, G. W. (2013). *Legal and ethical issues in nursing* (6th ed.). Saddle River, NJ: Pearson.

International Council of Nurses (ICN). (2012). *Code of Ethics for Nurses.* Retrieved November16, 2016, from http://www.icn.ch/who-we-are/code-of-ethics-for-nurses/.

Pozgar, G. D. (2016). *Legal and ethical issues for health professionals.* Burlington, MA: Jones & Bartlett Learning.

Chapter 4—Health-Care System

Centers for Disease Control and Prevention. (2015). *About CDC's office of minority health & health equity (OMHHE).* Retrieved July 16, 2016, from http://www.cdc.gov/minorityhealth/OMHHE.html.

Institute of Medicine of the National Academies. (2011). *Leading health indicators for healthy people 2020: Letter report.* Retrieved February 22, 2017, from http://www.nationalacademies.org/hmd/~/media/Files/Report%20Files/2011/Leading-Health-Indicators-for-Healthy-People-2020/Leading%20Health%20Indicators%202011%20Report%20Brief.pdf

International Council of Nurses. (2016). *Definition of nursing.* Retrieved July 15, 2016, from www.icn.ch/who-we-are/icn-definition-of-nursing/.

International Council of Nurses. (2016). *Who we are.* Retrieved July 15, 2016, from http://www.icn.ch/who-we-are/icn-definition-of-nursing/.

National League for Nursing. (2011). *National league for nursing mission, goals and objectives.* Retrieved July 15, 2016, from http://dlsii.com/blog/uncategorized/nationalleaguefornursingmissiongoalsandobjectives/.

National Student Nurses Association. (n.d.). *About us.* Retrieved July 15, 2016, from http://nsna.org/AboutUs.aspx.

Nies, M., & McEwen, M. (2014). *Community/public health nursing: Promoting the health of populations* (6th ed.). St. Louis, MO: Elsevier Health Sciences.

Selekman, J. (Ed.). (2012). *School nursing: A comprehensive text* (2nd ed.). Philadelphia: F. A. Davis.

Sigma Theta Tau International (STTI). (2016). *STTI organizational fact sheet.* Retrieved July 16, 2016, from http://www.nursingsociety.org/connect-engage/about-stti/sigma-theta-tau-international-organizational-fact-sheet.

Stanhope, M., & Lancaster, J. (2013). *Foundations of nursing in the community: Community-oriented practice* (4th ed.). St. Louis, MO: Elsevier Health Sciences.

Stanhope, M., & Lancaster, J. (2016). *Public health nursing: Population-centered health care in the community* (9th ed). Maryland Heights, MO: Elsevier Health Sciences.

U.S. Department of Health and Human Services. (2010). *Healthy people 2020.* Washington, DC.

U.S. Department of Health and Human Services. (2012). *About healthy people: Introducing healthy people 2020.* Retrieved July 16, 2016, from https://www.healthypeople.gov/2020/About-Healthy-People.

U.S. Department of Health and Human Services. (2017). *Healthy people 2020 leading health indicators: Progress update.* Retrieved February 22, 2017, from https://www.healthypeople.gov/2020/leading-health-indicators/Healthy-People-2020-Leading-Health-Indicators%3A-Progress-Update.

Watkins, D., & Cousins, J. (Eds.). (2010). *Public health and community nursing: Frameworks for practice* (3rd ed.). Philadelphia: Elsevier Health Sciences UK.

Chapter 5—Leadership and Management

American Nurses Association. (2013). *ANA principles for delegation.* Available from www.nursingworld.org.

American Nurses Association & National Council of State Boards of Nursing. (2005). *Joint statement on delegation.* Retrieved July 15, 2016, from www.ncsbn.org/Delegation_joint_statement_NCSBN-ANA.pdf.

American Nurses Credentialing Center. (2016). *Magnet recognition program overview.* Retrieved July 15, 2016, from http://www.nursecredentialing.org/Magnet/ProgramOverview.

Bennis, W., Spreitzer, G. M., & Cummings, T. G. (Eds.). (2001). *The future of leadership: Today's top leadership thinkers speak to tomorrow's leaders.* San Francisco: Jossey-Bass.

Finkelman, A. (2016). *Leadership and management for nurses: Core competencies for quality care* (3rd ed.). Upper Saddle River, NJ: Pearson Education.

Hargrove-Huttel, R. A., & Colgrove, K. (2009). *Client management and leadership success: A course review applying critical thinking to test taking.* Philadelphia: F. A. Davis.

Huston, C. J., & Marquis, B. L. (2014). *Leadership roles and management functions in nursing: Theory and application* (8th ed.). Philadelphia: Lippincott Williams & Wilkins & Wolters Kluwer.

Jones, R. P. (Ed.). (2007). *Nursing leadership and management: Theories, processes, and practice.* Philadelphia: F. A. Davis.

Lee, J. A. (1981). *The gold and the garbage in management theories and prescriptions.* Athens, OH: Ohio University Press.

Lewin, K. (1964). *Field theory in social science.* Portland, ME: Harper Torchbook: The Academy Library, originally published in 1951 by New York: Harper & Row.

Locke, E. A. (1982). The ideas of Frederick Taylor: An evaluation. *Academy of Management Review, 7*(1), 14–24.

McGregor, D. (2006). *The human side of enterprise: Annotated edition.* New York: McGraw-Hill.

National Council of State Boards of Nursing. (2005). *Working with others: A position paper.* Retrieved July 15, 2016, from www.ncsbn.org/Working_with_Others.pdf.

New York State Nurses Association. (2004). *Position Statement: Registered Professional Nursing's Utilization of Unlicensed Assistive Personnel.* Retrieved October 25, 2012, from www.nysna.org/practice/positions/position1_04.htm.

Porter-O'Grady, T., & Malloch, K. (2014). *Quantum leadership: A textbook of new leadership* (4th ed.). Boston: Jones & Bartlett.

Trofino, J. (1995). Transformational leadership in health care. *Nursing Management, 26*(8), 42–47.

Venes, D. (Ed.). (2013). *Taber's cyclopedic medical dictionary* (2nd ed.). Philadelphia: F. A. Davis.

Weiss, S. A., & Tappen, R. M. (2015). *Essentials of nursing leadership and management* (6th ed.). Philadelphia: F. A. Davis Company.

White, R. K., & Lippitt, R. (1972). *Autocracy and democracy: An experimental inquiry.* London: Greenwood Press.

Chapter 6—Critical Thinking and the Nursing Process

Ackley, B., & Ladwig, G. (2014). *Nursing diagnosis handbook: An evidence-based guide to planning care* (10th ed.). St. Louis, MO: Elsevier Health Sciences.

Alfaro-LeFevre, R. (2014). *Applying nursing process: The foundation for clinical reasoning* (8th ed.). Philadelphia: Lippincott Williams & Wilkins.

Bulechek, G. M., Butcher, H. K., Dochterman, J. M., & Wagner, C. (2013). *Nursing interventions classification (NIC)* (6th ed.). St. Louis, MO: Elsevier.

Carpenito-Moyet, L. J. (2005). *Understanding the nursing process: Concept mapping and care planning for students.* Philadelphia: Lippincott Williams & Wilkins.

Doenges, M., & Moorhouse, M. (2013). *Application of nursing process and nursing diagnosis: An interactive text for diagnostic reasoning* (6th ed.). Philadelphia: F. A. Davis.

Gulanick, M., & Myers, J. (2013). *Nursing care plans: Diagnoses, interventions, and outcomes* (8th ed.). St. Louis, MO: Elsevier Health Sciences.

Henderson, V. (1964). The nature of nursing. *American Journal of Nursing, 64*(8), 62–68.

Maslow, A. H. (1970). *Motivation and personality* (2nd ed.). New York: Harper & Row.

Moorhead, S., Johnson, M., Maas, M. L., & Swanson, E. (2014). *Nursing outcomes classification (NOC)* (5th ed.). St. Louis, MO: Elsevier.

Murray, M., & Atkinson, L. (2000). *Understanding the nursing process in a changing care environment* (6th ed.). Columbus, OH: McGraw-Hill.

NANDA International. (2011). *Nursing diagnoses 2015–17: Definitions and classifications.* Hoboken, NJ: Wiley-Blackwell.

University of Iowa, College of Nursing. (n.d.). *Center for nursing classification and clinical effectiveness (CNC).* Retrieved July 18, 2016, from http://www.nursing.uiowa.edu/center-for-nursing-classification-and-clinical-effectiveness.

Wilkinson, J. (2011). *Nursing process and critical thinking* (5th ed.). Upper Saddle River, NJ: Pearson Education.

Chapter 7—Evidenced-Based Practice

Accrediting Commission for Education in Nursing. *Mission/purpose/goals.* Retrieved November 19, 2016, http://www.acenursing.org/mission-purpose-goals/.

Ackley, B. J., Ladwig, G. B., Swan, B. A., & Tucker, S. J. (2008). *Evidence-based nursing care guidelines: Medical-surgical interventions.* St. Louis, MO: Elsevier Health Sciences.

American Nurses Association (ANA). *About ANA.* Retrieved November 19, 2016, from http://nursing-world.org/aboutana.

American Nurses Association. (2015). *Nursing: Scope and standards of practice* (3rd ed.). Silver Springs, MD: Nursesbooks.org: The Publishing Program of ANA.

American Nurses Association. (2016). *What is nursing?* Retrieved July 15, 2016, from http://www.nursing-world.org/EspeciallyForYou/What-is-Nursing.

Anspaugh, D., Hamrick, M., & Rosato, R. (2011). *Wellness: Concepts and applications* (8th ed.). Columbus, OH: McGraw-Hill.

Becker, M. H., & Maiman, L. A. (1975). Sociobehavioral determinants of compliance with health and medical care recommendations. *Medical Care, 13*(1), 10–24.

Carpenito, L. J. (2016). *Handbook of nursing diagnosis* (15th ed.). Philadelphia: Wolters Kluwer.

Catalano, J. (2015). *Nursing now: Today's issues, tomorrow's trends* (7th ed.). Philadelphia: F. A. Davis.

Dearholt, S. L., & Dang, D. (2012). *Johns Hopkins nursing evidenced based practice model and guidelines* (2nd ed.). Indianapolis, IN: Sigma Theta Tau International.

Doenges, M., Moorhouse, M., & Murr, A. (2016). *Nursing diagnosis manual: Planning, individualizing, and documenting client care* (5th ed.). Philadelphia: F. A. Davis Company.

Dunn, H. L. (1959). High-level wellness for man and society. *American Journal of Public Health and the Nation's Health, 49*(6), 786–792.

Erikson, E. H. (1963). *Childhood and society* (2nd ed.). New York: Norton.

Fowler, J. W. (1981). *Stages of faith: The psychology of human development and the quest for meaning.* New York: Harper& Row.

Gordon, M. (1994). *Nursing diagnosis: Process and application* (3rd ed.). St. Louis, MO: Mosby.

Havighurst, R. J. (1971). *Developmental tasks and education* (3rd ed.). New York: Longman.

Hopp, L., & Rittenmyer, L. (2012). *Introduction to evidenced-based practice: A practical guide for nursing.* Philadelphia: F. A. Davis.

Huston, C. J. (2017). *Professional issues in nursing: Challenges and opportunities*. Philadelphia: Lippincott Williams & Wilkins & Wolters Kluwer.

International Council of Nurses. *Our mission, strategic intent, core values and priorities*. Retrieved November 19, 2016 from http://www.icn.ch/who-we-are/our-mission-strategic-intent-core-values-and-priorities/.

International Council of Nurses. (2002). *The definition of nursing*. Retrieved November 19, 2016, from http://www.icn.ch/who-we-are/icn-definition-of-nursing/.

Kohlberg, L. (1968). Moral development. In D. L. Sills (Ed.), *International encyclopedia of social science* (Vol. 18). New York: Macmillan.

Kübler-Ross, E. (1969). *On death and dying*. New York: Macmillan.

Leininger, M. M. (2002). *Transcultural nursing: Concepts, theories, and practices* (3rd ed.). New York: McGraw-Hill.

Maslow, A. H. (1954). *Motivation and personality*. New York: Harper & Row, Publishers.

Maslow, A. H. (1970). *Motivation and personality* (2nd ed.). New York: Harper & Row.

Melnyk, B., & Fineout-Overholt, E. (2015). *Evidenced-based practice in nursing & healthcare: A guide to best practice* (3rd ed.). Philadelphia: Lippincott Williams & Wilkins & Wolters Kluwer.

Myers, J., Sweeney, T., & Witmer, J. (2000). The wheel of wellness counselling for wellness: A holistic model for treatment planning. *Journal of Counselling & Development, 78*(3), 251–267.

NANDA International. *Nursing diagnoses 2015–2017: Definitions and classifications* (10th ed.). Hoboken, NJ: Wiley-Blackwell.

National League for Nursing (NLN). *Mission and goals*. Retrieved, November 19, 2016, from http://www.nln.org/search?query=mission.

National Student Nurses Association (NSNA). *About us*. Retrieved, November 19, 2016, from http://www.nsna.org/AboutUs.aspx.

Orem, D. (2001). *Nursing: Concepts of practice* (6th ed., p. 126). St. Louis, MO: Mosby.

Piaget, J. (1952). *The origins of intelligence in children*. New York: International University Press.

Rogers, M. E. (1990). Nursing: Science of unitary, irreducible human beings. In E. A. M. Barrett (Ed.), *Visions of Rogers' science-based nursing* (Pub. No. 15-2285). New York: National League for Nursing Press.

Rosenstock, I. M. (1974). Historical origins of the health belief model. In M. H. Becker (Ed.), *The health belief model and personal health behavior*. Thorofare, NJ: Slack.

Roy, C. (2003). *The Roy adaptation model*. Retrieved July 15, 2016, from www.bc.edu/schools/son/faculty/featured/theorist/Roy_Adaptation_Model.html.

Sadock, B., & Sadock, V. (2014). *Kaplan & Sadock's synopsis of psychiatry* (11th ed.). Philadelphia: Lippincott Williams & Wilkins.

Sigma Theta Tau International. *STTI Organizational fact sheet*. Retrieved, November 19, 2016, from http://www.nursingsociety.org/connect-engage/about-stti/sigma-theta-tau-international-organizational-fact-sheet.

U.S. Department of Health and Human Services & Health Resources and Services Administration. (2010). *The registered nurse population: Initial findings from the 2008 National Sample Survey of Registered Nurses*. Retrieved July 18, 2016, from http://bhpr.hrsa.gov/healthworkforce/rnsurveys/rnsurveyfinal.pdf.

Watson, J. (1988). *Nursing: Human science and human care. A theory of nursing* (Pub. No. 15-2236). New York: National League for Nursing Press.

World Health Organization (WHO). (1948). *Preamble to the constitution of the World Health Organization as adopted by the International Health Conference*. New York, 19–22 June 1946; signed on 22 July 1946 by the representatives of 61 states (Official Records of the WHO, no. 2, p. 100) and entered into force on 7 April 1948.

Chapter 8—Teaching and Learning

Anderson, A., & Klemm, P. (2008). The Internet: Friend or foe when providing patient education? *Clinical Journal of Oncology Nursing, 12*(1), 55–63.

Bastable, S. (2013). *Nurse as educator: Principles of teaching and learning for nursing practice* (4th ed.). Sudbury, MA: Jones & Bartlett.

Bastable, S. (2017). *Essentials of patient education* (2nd ed.). Sudbury, MA: Jones & Bartlett.

Bietz, J., & Snarponis, J. A. (2006). Strategies for online teaching and learning: Lessons learned. *Nurse Educator, 31*(1), 20–25.

Bradshaw, M., & Lowenstein, A. (Eds.). (2016). *Innovative teaching strategies in nursing and related health professions* (7th ed.). Sudbury, MA: Jones & Bartlett.

Canobbio, M. (2005). *Mosby's handbook of patient teaching* (3rd ed.). St. Louis, MO: Elsevier Health Sciences.

Doak, C., Doak, L., & Root, J. (1995). *Teaching patients with low literacy skills* (2nd ed.). Philadelphia: Lippincott Williams & Wilkins.

Dreeben, O. (2010). *Patient education in rehabilitation*. Sudbury, MA: Jones & Bartlett.

Falvo, D. (2011). *Effective patient education: A guide to increased adherence* (4th ed.). Sudbury, MA: Jones & Bartlett.

Lowenstein, A., Foord-May, L., & Romano, J. (2009). *Teaching strategies for health education and health promotion: Working with patients, families, and communities.* Sudbury, MA: Jones & Bartlett.

Miller, M., & Stoeckel, P. (2016). *Client education: Theory and practice* (2nd ed.). Sudbury, MA: Jones & Bartlett.

Piaget, J. (1952). *The origins of intelligence in children.* New York: International University Press.

Redman, B. (2007). *The practice of patient education: A case study approach* (10th ed.). St. Louis, MO: Elsevier Health Sciences.

Roberts, D. (2004). Advocacy through patient teaching. *MedSurg Nursing, 13*(6), 363, 382.

U.S. Department of Health and Human Services, Office of Disease Prevention and Health Promotion. (n.d.). *Health literacy basics.* Retrieved July 18, 2016, from http://health.gov/communication/literacy/quickguide/factsbasic.htm.

Chapter 9—Medication

Adams, M., & Urban, C. (2015). *Pharmacology: Connections to nursing practice* (3rd ed.). Upper Saddle River, NJ: Prentice Hall.

Adams, M., et al. (2013). *Pharmacology for nurses: A pathophysiologic approach* (4th ed.). Upper Saddle River, NJ: Prentice Hall.

Broyles, B., et al. (2013). *Pharmacological aspects of nursing care* (8th ed.). Clifton Park, NY: Cengage Learning.

Edmunds, M. (2015). *Introduction to clinical pharmacology* (8th ed.). St. Louis, MO: Elsevier Health Sciences.

Giangrasso, A., & Shrimpton, D. (2012). *Dosage calculations: A multi-method approach.* Upper Saddle River, NJ: Prentice Hall.

Hargrove-Huttel, R., & Colgrove, K. (2014). *Pharmacology success* (2nd ed.). Philadelphia: F. A. Davis.

Horntvedt, T. (2015). *Calculating dosages safely: A dimensional analysis approach* (Rev. Reprint). Philadelphia: F. A. Davis.

Kee, J., & Marshall, S. (2016). *Clinical calculations* (8th ed.). St. Louis, MO: Elsevier Health Sciences.

Lesmeister, M. (2013). *Math basics for the health care professional* (4th ed.). Upper Saddle River, NJ: Pearson.

Lilley, L., et al. (2014). *Pharmacology and the nursing process* (8th ed.). St. Louis, MO: Elsevier Health Sciences.

Macklin, D., Chernecky, C., & Infortuna, M. H. (2011). *Math for clinical practice* (2nd ed.). Maryland Heights, MO: Elsevier Health Sciences.

Morris, D. (2014). *Calculate with confidence* (6th ed.). St. Louis, MO: Elsevier Health Sciences.

National Coordinating Council for Medication Error Reporting and Prevention. (2015). *Recommendations to reduce medication errors associated with verbal medication orders and prescriptions.* Retrieved July 20, 2016, from http://www.nccmerp.org/recommendations-reduce-medication-errors-associated-verbal-medication-orders-and-prescriptions.

Ogden, S., & Fluharty, L. (2016). *Calculation of drug dosages: A work text* (10th ed.). St. Louis, MO: Elsevier Health Sciences.

Phillips, L. (2014). *Manual of I.V. therapeutics: Evidence-based practice for infusion therapy* (6th ed.). Philadelphia: F. A. Davis.

Raines, V. (2010). *Davis's basic math review for nurses: With step-by-step solutions.* Philadelphia: F. A. Davis.

Right Diagnosis. (n.d.). *Chronic illness.* Retrieved July 20, 2016, from http://www.rightdiagnosis.com/c/chronic/intro.htm#whatis.

Tomlinson, G., & Ennis, D. (2011). *Pocket I.V. drugs.* Philadelphia: F. A. Davis.

Ulbricht, C. (2011). *Davis's pocket guide to herbs and supplements.* Philadelphia: F. A. Davis.

U.S. Food and Drug Administration. (2015). *How to dispose of unused medicines.* Retrieved July 20, 2016, from http://www.fda.gov/ForConsumers/ConsumerUpdates/ucm101653.htm#1.

U.S. Food and Drug Administration. (2015). *Strategies to reduce medication errors: Working to improve medication safety.* Retrieved July 15, 2016, from http://www.fda.gov/Drugs/ResourcesForYou/Consumers/ucm143553.htm.

U.S. Food and Drug Administration. (2016). *Orange book: Approved drug products with therapeutic equivalence evaluations.* Retrieved July 20, 2016, from http://www.accessdata.fda.gov/scripts/cder/ob/default.cfm.

U.S. Pharmacopeial Convention. (n.d.). *About us.* Retrieved July 20, 2016, from http://www.usp.org./about-usp.

Vallerand, A., Sanoski, C., & Deglin, J. (2015). *Davis's drug guide for nurses* (15th ed.). Philadelphia: F. A. Davis.

Workman M., et al. (2016). *Understanding pharmacology: Essentials for medication safety* (2nd ed.). St. Louis, MO: Elsevier Health Sciences.

Chapter 10—Development Across the Life Span

Anderson, M. (2016). *Caring for older adults holistically* (6th ed.). Philadelphia: F. A. Davis.

Carlson, D., & Pfadt, E. (2009). *Clinical coach for effective nursing care for older adults.* Philadelphia: F. A. Davis.

Centers for Disease Control and Prevention. (2015). *Childhood obesity facts.* Retrieved July 16, 2016, from http://www.cdc.gov/obesity/data/childhood.html.

Centers for Disease Control and Prevention. (2015). *Obesity prevalence maps.* Retrieved July 15, 2016, from http://www.cdc.gov/obesity/data/prevalence-maps.html.

Centers for Disease Control and Prevention. (2016). *Sexual risk behaviors: HIV, STD, & Teen Pregnancy Prevention*. Retrieved November 23, 2016, from http://cdc.gov/Healthy Youth/sexualbehaviors/.

Centers for Disease Control and Prevention & National Center for Health Statistics (NCHS). (2009). *Delayed childbearing: More women are having their first child later in life* (NCHS Data Brief No. 21). Retrieved July 16, 2016, from http://www.cdc.gov/nchs/data/databriefs/db21.htm.

Chapman, L., & Durham, R. (2013). *Maternal-newborn nursing: The clinical components of nursing care* (2nd ed.). Philadelphia: F. A. Davis.

Colyar, M. (2011). *Assessment of the school-age child and adolescent*. Philadelphia: F. A. Davis.

Doenges, M., Moorhouse, M. F., & Murr, A. C. (2014). *Nursing care plans: Guidelines for individualizing client care across the life span* (9th ed.). Philadelphia: F. A. Davis Company.

Edelman, C. L., Kudzma, E. C., & Mandle, C. L. (2014). *Health promotion throughout the life span* (8th ed.). St. Louis, MO: Elsevier Health Sciences.

Holloway, B. W., Moredich, C., & Aduddell, K. (2011). *OB/GYN & peds notes: Nurse's clinical pocket guide* (2nd ed.). Philadelphia: F. A. Davis.

Jenny, C. (2011). *Child abuse and neglect: Diagnosis, treatment and evidence*. St. Louis, MO: Elsevier Health Sciences.

Lange, J. (2012). *The nurse's role in promoting optimal health of older adults: Thriving in the wisdom years*. Philadelphia: F. A. Davis.

Leifer, G., & Hartston, H. (2012). *Growth and development across the lifespan: A health promotion focus* (2nd ed.). St. Louis, MO: Elsevier Health Sciences.

Linnard-Palmer, L. (2010). *Peds notes: A nurse's clinical pocket guide*. Philadelphia: F. A. Davis.

Livingston, G., & Cohn, D. (2010). *The new demography of American motherhood*. Retrieved July 15, 2016, from www.pewresearch.org/pubs/1586/changing-demographic-characteristics-american-mothers.

Meiner, S. (2014). *Gerontologic nursing* (5th ed.). St. Louis, MO: Elsevier Health Sciences.

Nagtalon-Ramos, K. (2014). *Maternity-newborn nursing care: Best evidence-based practices*. Philadelphia: F. A. Davis.

Polan, E., & Taylor, D. (2015). *Journey across the life span: Human development and health promotion* (5th ed.). Philadelphia: F. A. Davis.

Renz, M., & Kyburz, M. (2016). *Hope and grace: Spiritual experience in severe distress, illness and dying*. London: Jessica Kingsley Publisher.

Richardson, V. (2014). *Pediatric success: A course review applying critical thinking skills to test-taking* (2nd ed.). Philadelphia: F. A. Davis.

Stanley, M., Blair, K., & Beare, P. (2005). *Gerontological nursing: Promoting successful aging with older adults* (3rd ed.). Philadelphia: F. A. Davis.

Touhy, T., & Jett, K. (2014). *Ebersole and Hess' gerontological nursing & healthy aging* (4th ed.). St. Louis, MO: Elsevier Health Sciences.

U.S. Department of Health and Human Services & Administration on Aging. (2011). *A profile of older Americans: 2014*. Retrieved July 15, 2016, from http://www.aoa.acl.gov/aging_statistics/profile/2014/docs/2014-profile.pdf.

Chapter 11–Diversity and Spirituality/Religion

Centers for Disease Control and Prevention. (2011). *Fact sheet: Tuberculosis in minorities*. Retrieved July 11, 2012, from www.cdc.gov/tb/publications/factsheets/specpop/resources_TB_Minorities.htm.

Centers for Disease Control and Prevention. (2015). *Health disparities in TB*. Retrieved July 18, 2016, from http://www.cdc.gov/tb/topic/populations/HealthDisparities/default.htm.

Doka, K. (2011). *Living with grief: Spirituality and end of life care*. Washington, DC: Hospice Foundation in America.

Leininger, M. M., & McFarland, M. R. (2015). *Culture care diversity & universality: A worldwide nursing theory* (3rd ed.). Boston: Jones & Bartlett.

National Institutes of Health. (2013). *Fact sheet: Health disparities*. Retrieved July 18, 2016, from https://report.nih.gov/nihfactsheets/Pdfs/HealthDisparities (NIMHD).pdf.

Pew Research Center. (2012). *91.7%—Minorities account for nearly all U.S. population growth*. Retrieved July 18, 2016, from http://www.pewresearch.org/daily-number/minorities-account-for-nearly-all-u-s-population-growth/.

Purnell, L., & Paulanka, B. (2013). *Transcultural health care: A culturally competent approach* (4th ed.). Philadelphia: F. A. Davis.

Ray, M. (2016). *Transcultural caring dynamics in nursing and health care* (2nd ed.). Philadelphia: F. A. Davis.

Stuart, B., Cherry, C., & Stuart, J. (2011). *Pocket guide to culturally sensitive health care*. Philadelphia: F. A. Davis.

U.S. Census Bureau. (2015). *2014 National population projections*. Retrieved July 17, 2016, from http://www.census.gov/population/projections.

Chapter 12–Psychosocial Health

American Psychiatric Association. (2013). *Diagnostic and statistical manual of mental disorders* (5th ed.). Arlington, VA: American Psychiatric Publishing.

Coopersmith, S. (1968). *The antecedents of self-esteem.* San Francisco: Freeman Press.

Drench, M. E. (2011). *Psychosocial aspects of healthcare* (3rd ed.). Upper Saddle River, NJ: Pearson Education.

Erikson, E. H. (1963). *Childhood and society* (2nd ed.). New York: Norton.

Falco, D. (2014). *Medical and psychosocial aspects of chronic illness and disability* (5th ed). Sudberry, MA: Jones & Bartlett Learning.

Kaakinen, J., Gedaly-Duff, V., Coehlo, D., & Hanson, S. (2015). *Family health care nursing: Theory, practice, and research* (5th ed.). Philadelphia: F. A. Davis.

Katz, A. (2015). *Meeting the needs for psychosocial care in young adults with cancer.* Pittsburgh, PA: Oncology Nursing Society.

Thompson, R. (2009). *The handbook of child life: A guide for pediatric psychosocial care.* Springfield, IL: Charles C. Thomas Publisher Ltd.

Tracey, M. (2012). The top 10 reasons against the use of no-suicide contracts. *Genesee Health System: Hope and Health in the Community,* January 11. Retrieved July 17, 2016, from http://gencmh.org/News/Quality Matters/tabid/315/Article/129/the-top-10-reasons-against-the-use-of-no-suicide-contracts.aspx.

Varcarolis, E. M. (2013). *Essentials of psychiatric mental health nursing* (2nd ed., Rev. Reprint). St. Louis, MO: Elsevier Health Services.

Chapter 13—Grief and Loss

Ad Hoc Committee of the Harvard Medical School. (1968). A definition of irreversible coma: Report of the ad hoc committee of the Harvard medical school to examine the definition of brain death. *Journal of the American Medical Association, 205*(6), 337–340.

Chabad.org. *From life to life: Death, mourning and hope in Jewish tradition & practice.* Retrieved July 18, 2016, from http://www.chabad.org/generic_cdo/aid/266275/jewish/Death-Mourning.htm.

Cox, G. R., & Stevenson, R. G. (Eds.). (2013). *Final acts: The end of life, hospice and palliative care.* Amityville, NY: Baywood Publishing Company.

Doka, K. (1996). *Living with grief: After sudden loss suicide, homicide, accident, heart attack, stroke.* Washington, DC: Hospice Foundation in America.

Doka, K. (2000). *Living with grief: Children, adolescents and loss.* Washington, DC: Hospice Foundation in America.

Doka, K. (2003). *Living with grief: Loss in later life.* Washington, DC: Hospice Foundation in America.

Doka, K. (2005). *Living with grief: Alzheimer's disease.* Washington, DC: Hospice Foundation in America.

Doka, K. (2007). *Living with grief: Before and after the death.* Washington, DC: Hospice Foundation in America.

Doka, K. (2011). *Living with grief: Spirituality and end of life care.* Washington, DC: Hospice Foundation in America.

Doka, K. J., & Davidson, J. (1997). *Living with grief when illness is prolonged.* Washington, DC: Hospice Foundation in America.

Doka, K. J., & Jennings, B. (2005). *Living with grief: Ethical dilemmas at the end of life.* Washington, DC: Hospice Foundation of America.

Engel, G. (1964). Grief and grieving. *American Journal of Nursing, 64*(9), 93–98.

Hogan, M. (2012). *Anticipatory grief.* Ashland, OR: Sacred Vigil Press.

Kübler-Ross, E. (1969). *On death and dying.* New York: Macmillan.

Marques, S. M. (2015). *Now and at the hour of our death.* Los Angeles: High Wycombe.

Niethammer, D., et al. (2012). *Speaking honestly with sick and dying children and adolescents: Unlocking the silence.* Baltimore, MD: The Johns Hopkins University Press.

Pantilat, S. Z., et al. (2015). *Hospital-based palliative medicine: A practical, evidenced-based approach.* Hoboken, NJ: John Wiley & Sons.

President's Commission for the Study of Ethical Problems in Medicine and Biomedical and Behavioral Research. (1981). *Defining death: A report on the medical, legal, and ethical issues in the determination of death.* Washington, DC: U.S. Government Printing Office.

Smith, F., & Himmel, S. (2013). *Changing the way we die: Compassionate end of life care and the hospice movement.* Berkeley, CA: Viva Editions/Cleis Press Inc.

Spiro, H., & Wandel, L. P. (Eds.). (1996). *Facing death: Where culture, religion and medicine meet.* New Haven, CT: Yale University Press.

Wilkinson, J., & Treas, L. (2015). *Fundamentals of nursing* (3rd ed.). Philadelphia: F. A. Davis.

Wright, L. (2005). *Spirituality, suffering, and illness: Ideas for healing.* Philadelphia: F. A. Davis.

Yoder, G., & Wolfelt, A. D. (2012). *Companioning the dying: A soulful guide for caregivers.* Fort Collins, CO: Companion Press.

Zerwekh, J. (2006). *Nursing care at the end of life: Palliative care for patients and families.* Philadelphia: F. A. Davis.

Chapter 14—Physical Assessment

Centers for Disease Control and Prevention. (2012). *High blood pressure facts.* Retrieved July 18, 2016, from http://www.cdc.gov/bloodpressure/facts.htm.

Centers for Disease Control and Prevention. (2013). Racial/ethnic disparities in the awareness, treatment, and control of hypertension–United States, 2003–2010. *Morbidity and Mortality Weekly Report (MMWR), 62*(18), 351–355. Retrieved July 18, 2016, from http://www.cdc.gov/mmwr/preview/mmwrhtml/mm6218a2.htm.

Dillon, P. (2015). *Nursing health assessment: The foundation of clinical practice* (3rd ed.). Philadelphia: F. A. Davis.

Hurst, J. (2011). *Anatomy & physiology in a flash! Book & flash cards: An interactive, flash-card approach.* Philadelphia: F. A. Davis.

Jones, S. (2012). *Pocket anatomy and physiology* (2nd ed.). Philadelphia: F. A. Davis.

Lee, A. H. (2005). Why is carcinoma of the breast more frequent in the upper outer quadrant? A case series based on needle core biopsy diagnoses. *Breast, 14*(2), 151–152. Retrieved July 18, 2016, from www.ncbi.nlm.nih.gov/pubmed/15767185.

Mayo Clinic. What to expect during a clinical breast exam. *Healthy lifestyle women's health.* Retrieved July 18, 2016, from http://www.mayoclinic.org/healthy-lifestyle/womens-health/in-depth/breast-lump/art-20044839?pg=2.

National Comprehensive Cancer Network. *Your best resource in the fight against cancer.* (n.d.). Retrieved July 18, 2016, from https://www.nccn.org/.

Perloff, D., Grim, C., Flack, J., Frohlich, E. D., Hill, M., McDonald, M., et al. (1993). Human blood pressure determination by sphygmomanometry. *Circulation, 88*(5 Pt 1), 2460–2470.

Saslow, D., Hannan, J., Osuch, J., Alciati, M. H., Baines, C., Barton, M., et al. (2004). Clinical breast examination: Practical recommendations for optimizing performance and reporting. *CA: A Cancer Journal for Clinicians, 54*(6), 327–344.

Scanlon, V., & Sanders, T. (2014). *Essentials of anatomy and physiology* (7th ed.). Philadelphia: F. A. Davis.

Selye, H. A. (1936). Syndrome produced by diverse nocuous agents. *Nature, 138*(3479), 32.

Shimek, J. M., Emmanuel, J., Orris, P., & Chartier, Y. (Eds.). (2011). *Replacement of mercury thermometers and sphygmomanometers in health care: Technical guidance.* Retrieved July 16, 2016, from http://apps.who.int/iris/bitstream/10665/44592/1/9789241548182_eng.pdf.

Terndrup, T., Allegra, J. A., & Kealey, J. A. (1989). A comparison of oral, rectal, and tympanic membrane-derived temperature changes after ingestion of liquids and smoking. *American Journal of Emergency Medicine, 7*(2), 150–154.

The World Medical Association, Inc. (2008). *WMA statement on reducing the global burden of mercury.* Retrieved July 18, 2016, from http://www.wma.net/en/30publications/10policies/m36/index.html.

U.S. Environmental Protection Agency. (2002). *Eliminating mercury in hospitals: Environmental best practices for health care facilities.* Retrieved July 18, 2016, from https://www3.epa.gov/region9/waste/p2/projects/hospital/mercury.pdf.

Weber, J., & Kelley, J. (2014). *Health assessment in nursing* (5th ed.). Philadelphia: Lippincott Williams & Wilkins.

Wijkicks, E. F., Bamlet, W. R., Maramattom, B. V., Manno, E. M., & McClelland, R. L. (2005). Validation of a new coma scale: The FOUR score. *Annals of Neurology, 58*(4), 585–593.

Wilson, S., & Giddens, J. (2013). *Health assessment for nursing practice* (5th ed.). St. Louis, MO: Elsevier Health Sciences.

Chapter 15–Pain, Comfort, Rest, and Sleep

Brody, L. T., & Hall, C. M. (2011). *Therapeutic exercise: Moving toward function* (3rd ed.). Philadelphia: Lippincott Williams & Wilkins & Wolters Kluwer.

Colten, H., & Altevogt, B. (Eds.). (2006). *Sleep disorders and sleep deprivation: An unmet public health problem.* Washington, DC: National Academies Press.

Cranwell-Bruce, L. (2009). PCA delivery systems. *Medsurg Nursing, 18*(2), 127–129, 133.

Gloth, F. M., III (Ed.). (2011). *Handbook of pain relief in older adults: An evidence-based approach* (2nd ed.). New York: Humana Press/Springer Science+Business Media.

Griensven, H. V., Strong, J., & Unruh, A. M. (Eds.). (2014). *Pain: A textbook for health professionals* (2nd ed.). St. Louis, MO: Elsevier Health Sciences.

Hockenberry, M., & Wilson, D. (2015). *Wong's nursing care of infants and children* (10th ed.). St. Louis, MO: Elsevier Health Sciences.

Johnston, N., & Scholler-Jaquish, A. (Eds.). (2007). *Meaning of suffering: Caring practices in the health professions.* Madison, WI: University of Wisconsin Press.

Kolcaba, K. (1994). A theory of holistic comfort for nursing. *Journal of Advanced Nursing, 19*(6), 1178–1184.

Kolcaba, K. (2003). *Comfort theory and practice.* New York: Springer.

Kolcaba, K., & DiMarco, M. (2005). Comfort theory and its application to pediatric nursing. *Pediatric Nursing, 31*(3), 187–194.

Kuebler, K., Heidrich, D., & Esper, P. (2007). *Palliative and end-of-life care: Clinical practice guidelines* (2nd ed.). St. Louis, MO: Elsevier Health Sciences.

Macintyre, P., & Schug, S. (2015). *Acute pain management: A practical guide* (4th ed.). St. Louis, MO: Elsevier Health Sciences.

Mann, E., & Carr, E. (2006). *Essential clinical skills for nurses: Pain management.* Malden, MA: Blackwell.

Melzack, R., & Wall, P. (1965). Pain mechanisms: A new theory. *Science, 150*(3699), 971–979.

Merkel, S. I., Voepel-Lewis, T., & Malviya, S. (1997). *FLACC Behavioral Pain Assessment Scale.* Retrieved October 18, 2012, from http://wps.prenhall.com/wps/media/objects/3103/3178396/tools/flacc.pdf.

Morgan, K., & Closs, S. J. (1999). *Sleep management in nursing practice: An evidence-based guide.* Philadelphia: Elsevier Health Sciences.

Oakes, L. (2011). *Compact clinical guide to infant and child pain management: An evidence-based approach for nurses.* New York: Springer.

Pantley, E. (2005). *The no-cry sleep solution for toddlers and preschoolers: Gentle ways to stop bedtime battles and improve your child's sleep.* New York: McGraw-Hill.

Pasero, C., & McCaffery, M. (2011). *Pain assessment and pharmacologic management.* St. Louis, MO: Elsevier Health Sciences.

Quinlan-Colwell, A., & D'Arcy, Y. (2012). *Compact clinical guide to geriatric pain management: An evidence-based approach for nurses.* New York: Springer.

Redeker, N., & McEnany, G. (2011). *Sleep disorders and sleep promotion in nursing practice.* New York: Springer.

Sackheim, K. A. (Ed.). (2015). *Pain management and palliative care: A comprehensive guide.* New York: Springer.

U.S. Department of Health and Human Services. (2012). *Key sleep disorders.* Retrieved July 20, 2016, from http://www.cdc.gov/sleep/about_sleep/key_disorders.html.

Wright, S. (2014). *Pain management in nursing practice.* Thousand Oaks, CA: Sage Publications.

Chapter 16–Inflammation, Infection, Immunity, and Wound Care

American Nurses Association. (1980). *Nursing: A social policy statement.* Kansas City, MO: American Nurses Association.

Centers for Disease Control and Prevention. (1989). Guidelines for prevention of transmission of human immunodeficiency virus and hepatitis B virus to health-care and public-safety workers: A response to P.L. 100-607, The Health Omnibus Programs Extension Act of 1988. *MMWR Supplements, 38*(S-6), 3–37. Retrieved July 16, 2016, from http://www.cdc.gov/mmwr/preview/mmwrhtml/00001450.htm.

Centers for Disease Control and Prevention. (2002). Guideline for hand hygiene in health-care settings: Recommendations of the Healthcare Infection Control Practices Advisory Committee and the HICPAC/SHEA/APIC/IDSA Hand Hygiene Task Force. *MMWR Recommendations and Reports, 51*(RR-16), 1–44. Retrieved July 16, 2016, from http://www.cdc.gov/mmwr/PDF/rr/rr5116.pdf.

Centers for Disease Control and Prevention. (2012). *Top CDC recommendations to prevent healthcare-associated infections.* Retrieved July 18, 2016, from http://www.cdc.gov/HAI/pdfs/hai/top-cdc-recs-factsheet.pdf.

Centers for Disease Control and Prevention. (2013). *Hand hygiene saves lives.* Retrieved July 18, 2016, from http://www.cdc.gov/cdctv/healthyliving/hygiene/hand-hygiene-saves-lives.html.

Centers for Disease Control and Prevention. (2015). *Get smart: Know when antibiotics work.* Retrieved May 24, 2012, from http://www.cdc.gov/getsmart/community/index.html.

Centers for Disease Control and Prevention. (2016). *Recommended adult immunization schedule—United States, 2016.* Retrieved July 18, 2016, from http://www.cdc.gov/vaccines/schedules/downloads/adult/adult-combined-schedule.pdf.

Centers for Disease Control and Prevention. (2016). *Recommended immunization schedule for persons aged 0 through 18 years—United States, 2016.* Retrieved July 18, 2016, from http://www.cdc.gov/vaccines/schedules/downloads/child/0-18yrs-schedule.pdf.

Centers for Disease Control and Prevention. (2016). *Healthcare-associated infections (HAI) topics.* Retrieved July 16, 2016, from http://www.cdc.gov/hai/.

Clancy, C. (2008). *Simple steps can reduce health care-associated infections.* Agency for Healthcare Research and Quality, Rockville, MD. Retrieved July 18, 2016, from http://archive.ahrq.gov/news/columns/navigating-the-health-care-system/070108.html.

Collier, K. S., Protus, B., & Bohn, C. L. (2013). *Wound care at end of life: A guide for hospice professionals.* Montgomery, AL: HospiScript Services, a Catamaran Company.

Daniels, S. (2007). Protecting patients from harm: Improving hospital care for surgical patients. *Nursing, 37*(8), 36–41.

Hess, C. T. (2013). *Clinical guide to skin and wound care* (7th ed.). Philadelphia: Lippincott Williams & Wilkins & Wolters Kluwer.

Holcomb, S. (2008). MRSA infections. *Nursing, 38*(6), 33.

Jernigan, J., & Kallen, A. (2010). Methicillin-resistant *staphylococcus aureus* (MRSA) infections, *Division of Healthcare Quality Promotion*, Centers for Disease Control and Prevention. Retrieved July 18, 2016, from http://www.cdc.gov/HAI/pdfs/toolkits/MRSA_toolkit_white_020910_v2.pdf.

Kennamer, M. (2007). *Basic infection control for health care providers* (2nd ed.). Clifton Park, NY: Cengage Learning.

Liu, C., Bayer, A., Cosgrove, S. E., Daum, R. S., Fridkin, S. K., Gorwitz, R. J., et al. (2011). *Clinical practice guidelines by the Infectious Diseases Society of America for the treatment of methicillin-resistant* Staphylococcus aureus *infections in adults and children.* Retrieved May 30, 2012, from http://www.idsociety.org/uploadedFiles/IDSA/Guidelines-Patient_Care/PDF_Library/MRSA.pdf.

Mazurek Melnyk, B., & Fineout-Overholt, E. (2015). *Evidence-based practice in nursing and healthcare: A guide to best practice* (3rd ed.). Philadelphia: Wolters Kluwer Health/Lippincott Williams & Wilkins.

Motacki, K., O'Mara, N. B., & Kapoian, T. (Eds.). (2011). *An illustrated guide to infection control.* New York: Springer.

Perry, C. (2007). *Infection prevention and control.* Hoboken, NJ: Wiley-Blackwell.

Safe Care Campaign. Urinary tract infections. *Preventing Healthcare and Community Associated Infections.* Retrieved July 16, 2016, from http://www.safecarecampaign.org/uti.html.

Siegel, J. D. (2006). *Management of multidrug-resistant organisms in healthcare settings.* Retrieved July 18, 2016, from http://www.cdc.gov/hicpac/pdf/MDRO/MDROGuideline2006.pdf.

Siegel, J. D., Rhinehart, E., Jackson, M., Chiarello, L., & the Healthcare Infection Control Practices Advisory Committee. (2007). *Guideline for isolation precautions: Preventing transmission of infectious agents in healthcare settings.* Retrieved December 2, 2016, from http://www.cdc.gov/ncidod/dhqp/pdf/isolation2007.pdf

Sussman, C., & Bates-Jensen, B. (2012). *Wound care: A collaborative practice manual for health professionals* (4th ed.). Philadelphia: Lippincott Williams & Wilkins & Wolters Kluwer.

U.S. Department of Labor & Occupational Safety and Health Administration. (n.d.). *Bloodborne pathogens and needlestick prevention.* Retrieved July 19, 2016, from https://www.osha.gov/SLTC/bloodbornepathogens/index.html.

World Health Organization (WHO). (n.d.). *Prevention of hospital-acquired infections: A practical guide* (2nd ed.). Retrieved July 19, 2016, from http://www.who.int/csr/resources/publications/drugresist/en/whocdscsreph200212.pdf?ua=1.

World Health Organization (WHO). (2015). *Antibiotic resistance: Fact sheet.* Retrieved July 19, 2016, from http://www.who.int/mediacentre/factsheets/antibiotic-resistance/en/.

Yamamoto, L., & Marten, M. (2007). Listen up, MRSA: The bug stops here. *Nursing, 37*(12 Pt 1), 51–55.

Chapter 17—Mobility

Berman, A., & Snyder, S. (2016). *Kozier and Erb's fundamentals of nursing: Concepts, process, and practice* (10th ed.). Upper Saddle River, NJ: Prentice Hall.

Burton, M., & Ludwig, L. (2014). *Fundamentals of nursing care: Concepts, connections and skills* (2nd ed.). Philadelphia: F. A. Davis.

Calais-Germain, B. (2007). *Anatomy of movement* (rev. ed.). Vista, CA: Eastland Press.

Dziedzic, M. E. (2014). *Fast facts about pressure ulcer care for nurses: How to prevent, detect, and resolve them in a nutshell.* New York: Springer.

Olson, E., Johnson, B., & Thompson, L. (1990). The hazards of immobility. 1967. *American Journal of Nursing, 90*(3), 43–48.

Thomas, D. R., & Compton, G. A. (Eds.). *Pressure ulcers in the aging population.* New York: Springer.

Wilkinson, J., & Treas, L. (2015). *Fundamentals of nursing* (3rd ed.). Philadelphia: F. A. Davis.

Chapter 18—Tissue Integrity and Hygiene

Baranoski, S., & Ayello, E. (2016). *Wound care essentials: Practice principles* (4th ed.). Philadelphia: Lippincott Williams & Wilkins.

Burton, M., & Ludwig, L. (2014). *Fundamentals of nursing care: Concepts, connections and skills* (2nd ed.). Philadelphia: F. A. Davis.

Cowdell, F. (2010). Promoting skin health in older people. *Nursing Older People, 22*(10), 21–26.

Cowdell, F. (2011). Older people, personal hygiene, and skin care. *Medsurg Nursing, 20*(5), 235–240.

Dillon, P. (2015). *Nursing health assessment: The foundation of clinical practice* (3rd ed.). Philadelphia: F. A. Davis.

Wilkinson, J., & Treas, L. (2015). *Fundamentals of nursing* (3rd ed.). Philadelphia: F. A. Davis.

Williams, L., & Hopper, P. (2014). *Understanding medical surgical nursing* (5th ed.). Philadelphia: F. A. Davis.

Chapter 19—Oxygenation

Berman, A., Snyder, S., & McKinney, D. (2011). *Nursing basics for clinical practice.* Upper Saddle River, NJ: Prentice Hall.

Burton, M., & Ludwig, L. (2014). *Fundamentals of nursing care: Concepts, connections and skills* (2nd ed.). Philadelphia: F. A. Davis.

Coviello, J. (2013). *Auscultation skills: Breath and heart sounds* (5th ed.). Philadelphia: Lippincott Williams & Wilkins.

Dillon, P. (2015). *Nursing health assessment: The foundation of clinical practice* (3rd ed.). Philadelphia: F. A. Davis.

Potter, P. A., Perry, A. G., Stockert, P., & Hall, A. (2017). *Fundamentals of nursing* (9th ed.). St. Louis, MO: Elsevier Health Sciences.

Sheldon, L. (2008). *Quick look nursing: Oxygenation* (2nd ed.). Sudbury, MA: Jones & Bartlett.

Venes, D. (Ed.). (2013). *Taber's cyclopedic medical dictionary* (22nd ed.). Philadelphia: F. A. Davis.

Wilkinson, J., & Treas, L. (2015). *Fundamentals of nursing* (3rd ed.). Philadelphia: F. A. Davis.

Williams, L., & Hopper, P. (2014). *Understanding medical surgical nursing* (5th ed.). Philadelphia: F. A. Davis.

Chapter 20—Nutrition

American Diabetes Association. (2015). *Checking your blood glucose level.* Retrieved July 20, 2016, from http://www.diabetes.org/living-with-diabetes/treatment-and-care/blood-glucose-control/checking-your-blood-glucose.html.

Centers for Disease Control and Prevention & National Center for Health Statistics. (2014). *Fast stats: Obesity and overweight.* Retrieved July 20, 2016, from http://www.cdc.gov/nchs/fastats/obesity-overweight.htm.

Dudek, S. (2014). *Nutrition essentials for nursing practice* (7th ed.). Philadelphia: Lippincott Williams & Wilkins.

Eating Disorder HOPE. (2010). *Eating disorder statistics & research.* Retrieved July 15, 2016, from http://www.eatingdisorderhope.com/information/statistics-studies.

Garcia, J., & Chambers, E. (2010). Managing dysphagia through diet modifications. *American Journal of Nursing, 110*(11), 26–33.

Gedney, L. (2013). *Healthy eating: What is calorie-dense vs. nutrient-dense food?* New York: Demand Media, retrieved July 7, 2013, from http://healthyeating.sfgate.com/caloriedense-vs-nutrientdense-food-5391.html.

Geissler, C., & Powers, H. (2009). *Fundamentals of human nutrition: For students and practitioners in the health sciences.* New York: Elsevier Health Sciences UK.

Grodner, M., Roth, S., & Walkingshaw, B. (2016). *Nutritional foundations and clinical applications: A nursing approach* (6th ed.). St. Louis, MO: Elsevier Health Sciences.

Lopez-Jimenez, F. (2015). *Rhabdomyolysis from statins: What's the risk?* Retrieved December 8, 2016 from http://www.mayoclinic.org/diseases-conditions/high-blood-cholesterol/expert-answers/rhabdomyolysis/FAQ-20057817

Lutz, C., & Przytulski, K. (2004). *Nutri-notes: Nutrition & diet therapy pocket guide.* Philadelphia: F. A. Davis.

Lutz, C., & Przytulski, K. (2015). *Nutrition and diet therapy* (6th ed.). Philadelphia: F. A. Davis.

Metheny, N., Eisenberg, P., & McSweeney, M. (1988). Effect of feeding tube properties and three irrigants in clogging rates. *Nursing Research, 37*(3), 165–169.

Moore, M. (2009). *Mosby's pocket guide to nutritional assessment and care* (6th ed.). St. Louis, MO: Elsevier Health Sciences.

National Osteoporosis Foundation. (n.d.). *What is osteoporosis and what causes it?* Retrieved July 15, 2016, from https://www.nof.org/patients/what-is-osteoporosis/.

Nix, S. (2017). *Williams' basic nutrition & diet therapy* (15th ed.). St. Louis, MO: Elsevier Health Sciences.

O'Keefe, S. J. D. (2015). *The principles and practice of nutritional support.* New York: Springer.

Rivero, E. (2009). Elderly women with Dowager's hump may be at higher risk of earlier death. *UCLA Newsroom,* May 26, 2009.

Schlenker, E., & Roth, S. (2015). *Williams' essentials of nutrition and diet therapy* (11th ed.). St. Louis, MO: Elsevier Health Sciences.

Smith, R., & Meyers, S. (2005). 2 devices that unclog feeding tubes. *Modern Medicine.* Retrieved July 20, 2016, from www.modernmedicine.com/modernmedicine/article/articleDetail.jsp?id=142656.

Sorte, J., Daeschel, I., & Amador, C. (2013). *Nutrition, health, and safety for young children: Promoting wellness* (2nd ed.). Upper Saddle River, NJ: Pearson.

Stanfield, P., & Hui, Y. (2010). *Nutrition and diet therapy* (5th ed.). Sudbury, MA: Jones & Bartlett.

Talbott, S., & Hughes, K. (2007). *Health professional's guide to dietary supplements.* Philadelphia: Lippincott Williams & Wilkins.

U.S. Food and Drug Administration. (2004). *Changes to the nutrition facts label.* Retrieved July 20, 2016, from http://www.fda.gov/Food/GuidanceRegulation/GuidanceDocumentsRegulatoryInformation/LabelingNutrition/ucm385663.htm#images.

U.S. Food and Drug Administration & Center for Nutrition Policy and Promotion. (2011). *10 tips to a great plate.* Retrieved July 20, 2016, from http://www.choosemyplate.gov/sites/default/files/tentips/DGTipsheet1ChooseMyPlate.pdf.

U.S. Food and Drug Administration & ChooseMyPlate.Gov. (n.d.). *Dietary guidelines for Americans 2015–2020.* Retrieved July 20, 2016, from http://www.choosemyplate.gov/dietary-guidelines.

Chapter 21—Fluid, Electrolyte, and Acid-Base Balance

Chernecky, C., Macklin, D., & Murphy-Ende, K. (2006). *Saunder's nursing survival guide: Fluids and electrolytes* (2nd ed.). Philadelphia: Elsevier Health Sciences.

Hale, A., & Hovey, M. (2012). *Fluid and electrolyte notes: Nurse's clinical pocket guide.* Philadelphia: F. A. Davis.

Hale, A., & Hovey, M. (2014). *Fluid, electrolytes and acid-base imbalances: Content review PLUS practice questions.* Philadelphia: F. A. Davis.

Kee, J., Paulanka, B., & Polek, C. (2010). *Fluids and electrolytes with clinical applications* (8th ed.). Clifton Park, NY: Cengage Learning.

Kee, J., Paulanka, B., & Polek, C. (2010). *Handbook of fluid, electrolyte and acid-base imbalances* (3rd ed.). Clifton Park, NY: Cengage Learning.

Metheny, N. (2012). *Fluid & electrolyte balance: Nursing considerations* (5th ed.). Sudbury, MA: Jones & Bartlett Learning.

Phillips, L. (2005). *IV therapy notes: Nurse's clinical pocket guide.* Philadelphia: F. A. Davis.

Phillips, L. (2014). *Manual of I.V. therapeutics: Evidence-based practice for infusion therapy* (6th ed.). Philadelphia: F. A. Davis.

Van Leeuwen, A., Poelhuis-Leth, D., & Bladh, M. (2015). *Davis's comprehensive handbook of laboratory and diagnostic tests with nursing implications* (6th ed.). Philadelphia: F. A. Davis.

Westgard, E. (2011). *Clinical coach for fluid & electrolyte balance.* Philadelphia: F. A. Davis.

Chapter 22—Urinary Elimination

Boltz, M., Capezuti, E., Fulmer, T., & Zwicker, D. (Eds.). (2012). *Evidence-based geriatric nursing protocols for best practice* (4th ed.). New York: Springer.

Downey, P. (Ed.). (2005). *Introduction to urological nursing.* Philadelphia: Whurr.

Gray, M., & Moore, K. (2009). *Urologic disorders: Adult and pediatric care.* St. Louis, MO: Elsevier Health Sciences.

National Kidney Foundation. (n.d.). *How your kidneys work.* Retrieved July 20, 2016, from https://www.kidney.org/search-results?solr-keywords=how+your+kidneys+work.

Newman, D., & Wein, A. (2009). *Managing and treating urinary incontinence* (2nd ed.). Baltimore: Health Professions Press.

Thiedke, C. C. (2003). Nocturnal enuresis. *American Family Physician, 67*(7), 1499–1506. Retrieved October 18, 2012, from http://www.aafp.org/afp/2003/0401/p1499.html.

Wilkinson, J., & Treas, L. (2015). *Fundamentals of nursing* (3rd ed.). Philadelphia: F. A. Davis.

Chapter 23—Bowel Elimination

Breckman, B. (2006). *Stoma care and rehabilitation.* St. Louis, MO: Elsevier Health Sciences.

Burch, J. (Ed.). (2008). *Stoma care.* Hoboken, NJ: Wiley-Blackwell.

Colwell, J., Goldberg, M., & Carmel, J. (2004). *Fecal & urinary diversions: Management principles.* St. Louis, MO: Elsevier Health Sciences.

Doughty, D. (2006). *Urinary & fecal incontinence: Current management concepts* (3rd ed.). St. Louis, MO: Elsevier Health Sciences.

Meiner, S. (Ed.). (2004). *Care of gastrointestinal problems in the older adult.* New York: Springer.

Ogilvie, J., Hicks, L., & Kalloo, A. (2008). *Johns Hopkins manual of gastrointestinal endoscopic procedures* (2nd ed.). Thorofare, NJ: Slack.

Porrett, T., & McGrath, A. (2005). *Stoma care: Essential clinical skills for nurses.* Malden, MA: Blackwell.

Scanlon, V., & Sanders, T. (2017). *Essentials of anatomy and physiology* (7th ed.). Philadelphia: F. A. Davis.

Chapter 24—Perioperative Care

Aldrete, J. A. (1995). Post-anesthesia recovery score revisited. *Journal of Clinical Anesthesia, 7*(1), 89–91.

Aldrete, J. A., & Kroulik, D. (1970). A postanesthetic recovery score. *Anesthesia and analgesia, 49*(6), 924–934.

American Society of Anesthesiologists Task Force on Preoperative Fasting. (1999). Practice guidelines for preoperative fasting and the use of pharmacologic agents to reduce the risk of pulmonary aspiration: Application to healthy patients undergoing elective procedures. *Anesthesiology, 90*(3), 896–905. Retrieved December 12, 2016 from https://www.ncbi.nlm.nih.gov/pubmed/10078693.

Browne, N., Flanigan, L., McComiskey, C., & Pieper, P. (2013). *Nursing care of the pediatric surgical patient* (3rd ed.). Burlington, MA: Jones & Bartlett Learning.

Cabanas, J., Manning, J., & Cairns, C. (2016). Fluid and blood resuscitation. In J. Tintinalli, J. S. Stapczynski, D. Cline, O. J. Ma, R. Cydulka, & G. Meckler (Eds.), *Tintinalli's emergency medicine: A comprehensive study guide* (8th ed., pp. 172–176). New York: McGraw-Hill.

Girard-Powell, V. (Ed.). (2010). *Pain, analgesia and anesthesia, an issue of perioperative nursing clinics.* St. Louis, MO: Elsevier Health Sciences.

Goldman, M. (2008). *Pocket guide to the operating room* (3rd ed.). Philadelphia: F. A. Davis.

Hopper, P., & Williams, L. (Eds.). (2014). *Understanding medical surgical nursing* (4th ed.). Philadelphia: F. A. Davis.

Litwack, K. (2009). *Clinical coach for effective perioperative nursing care.* Philadelphia: F. A. Davis.

Mishra, R. (2011). *History of minimal access surgery.* Retrieved July 15, 2016, from https://www.laparoscopy hospital.com/history_of_laparoscopy.htm.

Pudner, R. (Ed.). (2010). *Nursing the surgical patient* (3rd ed.). Philadelphia: Elsevier Health Sciences UK.

Shippee-Rice, R., Fetzer, S., & Long, J. (2012). *Gerioperative nursing care: Principles and practices in surgical care of the older adult.* New York: Springer.

Smeltzer, S., Bare, B., Hinkle, J., & Cheever, K. (2014). *Brunner and Suddarth's textbook of medical surgical nursing* (13th ed.). Philadelphia: Lippincott Williams & Wilkins & Wolters Kluwer.

Timmins, F., & McCabe, C. (2009). *Day surgery: Contemporary approaches to nursing care.* Hoboken, NJ: Wiley-Blackwell.

Watson, D. (2011). *Perioperative safety.* St. Louis, MO: Elsevier Health Sciences.

Wicker, P., & O'Neill, J. (2010). *Essential clinical skills: Caring for the perioperative patient* (2nd ed.). Hoboken, NJ: Wiley-Blackwell.

Williams, L., & Hopper, P. (2015). *Understanding medical surgical nursing* (5th ed.). Philadelphia: F. A. Davis.

Woodhead, K., & Fudge, L. (2012). *Manual of perioperative care: An essential guide.* Hoboken, NJ: Wiley-Blackwell.

Index

Note: Page numbers followed by *b* indicate boxes, *f* indicate figures, and *t* indicate tables.